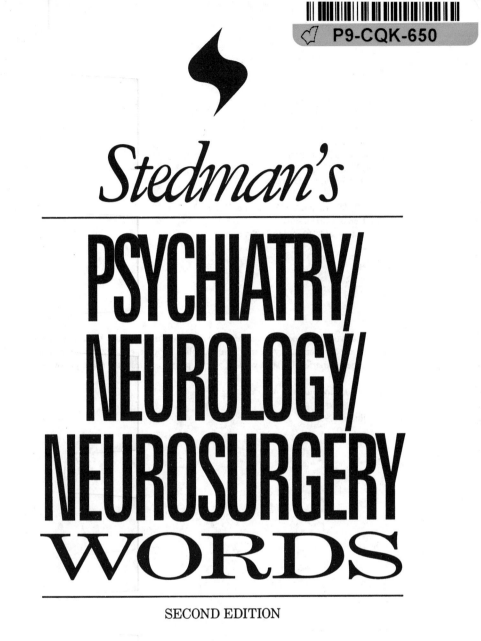

Stedman's
PSYCHIATRY/ NEUROLOGY/ NEUROSURGERY WORDS

SECOND EDITION

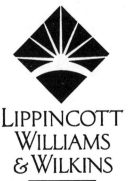

LIPPINCOTT
WILLIAMS
& WILKINS

Series Editor: Maureen Barlow Pugh
Managing Editor: Beverly J. Wolpert
Database Content Editor: Jennifer Schmidt
Art Direction: Jonathan Dimes
Production Manager: Patricia Smith
Typesetter: Peirce Graphic Services, Inc.
Printer & Binder: Victor Graphics

Printed in the United States of America

Second Edition, 1999

00

4 5 6 7 8 9 10

Stedman's Word Book Series:

Stedman's Abbreviations, Acronyms & Symbols, 2 ed.—
#0-683-40459-8

Stedman's Cardiology & Pulmonary Words, 2 ed.—#0-683-40081-9

Stedman's Dermatology & Immunology Words—#0-683-40080-0

Stedman's GI & GU Words, 2 ed.—#0-683-18145-9

Stedman's Medical Speller, 2 ed.—#0-683-40023-1

Stedman's Medical & Surgical Equipment Words, 2 ed.—
#0-683-18144-0

Stedman's OB-GYN Words, 2 ed.—#0-683-07967-0

Stedman's Ophthalmology Words—#0-683-07952-2

Stedman's Orthopaedic & Rehab Words, 3 ed.—#0-683-30778-9

Stedman's Pathology & Lab Medicine Words, 2 ed.—#0-683-40191-2

Stedman's Plastic Surgery/ENT/Dentistry Words—#0-683-40460-1

Stedman's Psychiatry/Neurology/Neurosurgery Words, 2 ed.—
#0-683-30775-4

Stedman's Radiology & Oncology Words, 2 ed.—#0-683-07966-2

Stedman's Surgery Words—#0-683-40190-4

Other References from Stedman's

Stedman's Medical Eponyms—#0-683-07965-4

Stedman's WordWatcher 1995–1997—#0-683-40313-3

Available directly from the publisher
Call TOLLFREE 1.800.527.5597

Your Medical Word Resource Publisher

We strive to provide you with the most up-to-date and accurate word references available. Your use of this word book will prompt new editions, which we will publish as often as updates and revisions justify. We welcome your suggestions for improvements, changes, corrections, and additions—whatever will make this Stedman's product more useful to you. Please use the postpaid card at the back of this book, and send your recommendations care of "Stedman's" at Lippincott Williams & Wilkins.

292.84	-Induced Mood Disorder	296.25	In Partial Remission	307.47	Nightmare Disorder
	-Induced Psychotic	296 21	Mild	V71.09	No Diagnosis on Axis II
	Disorder	296.22	Moderate	V71.09	No Diagnosis or Condition on
292.11	With Delusions	296.23	Severe Without Psychotic		Axis I
292.12	With Hallucinations		Features	V15.81	Noncompliance With
292.89	Intoxication	296.24	Severe With Psychotic		Treatment
292.81	Intoxication Delirium		Features	300.3	Obsessive-Compulsive
292.89	Persisting Perception	296.20	Unspecified		Disorder
	Disorder	608.89	Male Dyspareunia Due to . . .	301.4	Obsessive-Compulsive
292.9	-Related Disorder NOS		[Indicate the General		Personality Disorder
301.50	Histrionic Personality Disorder		Medical Condition]	V62.2	Occupational Problem
307.44	Hypersomnia related to . . .	302.72	Male Erectile Disorder		Opioid
	[Indicate the Axis I or Axis II	607.84	Male Erectile Disorder Due to	305.50	Abuse
	Disorder]		. . . [Indicate the General	304.00	Dependence
302.71	Hypoactive Sexual Desire		Medical Condition]	292.84	-Induced Mood Disorder
	Disorder	608.89	Male Hypoactive Sexual		-Induced Psychotic Disorder
300.7	Hypochondriasis		Desire Disorder Due to . . .	292.11	With Delusions
313.82	Identity Problem		[Indicate the General	292.12	With Hallucinations
312.30	Impulse-Control Disorder		Medical Condition]	292.89	-Induced Sexual
	NOS	302.74	Male Orgasmic Disorder		Dysfunction
	Inhalant	V65.2	Malingering	292.89	-Induced Sleep Disorder
305.90	Abuse	315.1	Mathematics Disorder	292.89	Intoxication
304.60	Dependence		Medication-Induced	292.81	Intoxication Delirium
292.89	-Induced Anxiety Disorder	333.90	Movement Disorder NOS	292.9	-Related Disorder NOS
292.84	-Induced Mood Disorder	333.1	Postural Tremor	292.0	Withdrawal
292.82	-Induced Persisting	293.9	Mental Disorder NOS Due to	313.81	Oppositional Defiant Disorder
	Dementia		. . . [Indicate the General	625.8	Other Female Sexual
	-Induced Psychotic		Medical Condition]		Dysfunction Due to . . .
	Disorder	319	Mental Retardation, Severity		[Indicate the General
292.11	With Delusions		Unspecified		Medical Condition]
292.12	With Hallucinations	317	Mild Mental Retardation	608.89	Other Male Sexual
292.89	Intoxication	315.32	Mixed Receptive-Expressive		Dysfunction Due to . . .
292.81	Intoxication Delirium		Language Disorder		[Indicate the General
292.9	-Related Disorder NOS	318.0	Moderate Mental Retardation		Medical Condition]
307.42	Insomnia Related to . . .	293.83	Mood Disorder Due to . . .		Other (or Unknown)
	[Indicate the Axis I or Axis II		[Indicate the General		Substance
	Disorder]		Medical Condition]	305.90	Abuse
312.34	Intermittent Explosive	296.90	Mood Disorder NOS	304.90	Dependence
	Disorder	301.81	Narcissistic Personality	292.89	-Induced Anxiety Disorder
312.32	Kleptomania		Disorder	292.81	-Induced Delirium
315.9	Learning Disorder NOS	347	Narcolepsy	292.84	-Induced Mood Disorder
	Major Depressive Disorder,	V61.21	Neglect of Child	292.83	-Induced Persisting
	Recurrent	995.52	Neglect of Child (if focus of		Amnestic Disorder
296.36	In Full Remission		attention is on victim)	292.82	-Induced Persisting
296.35	In Partial Remission		Neuroleptic-Induced		Dementia
296.31	Mild	333.99	Acute Akathisia		-Induced Psychotic
296.32	Moderate	333.7	Acute Dystonia		Disorder
296.33	Severe Without Psychotic	332.1	Parkinsonism	292.11	With Delusions
	Features	333.82	Tardive Dyskinesia	292.12	With Hallucinations
296.34	Severe With Psychotic	333.92	Neuroleptic Malignant	292.89	-Induced Sexual
	Features		Syndrome		Dysfunction
296.30	Unspecified		Nicotine	292.89	-Induced Sleep Disorder
	Major Depressive Disorder,	305.10	Dependence	292.89	Intoxication
	Single Episode	292.9	-Related Disorder NOS	292.9	-Related Disorder NOS
296.26	In Full Remission	292.0	Withdrawal	292.0	Withdrawal

Contents

Acknowledgments

An important part of our editorial process is the involvement of medical transcriptionists—as advisors, reviewers and/or editors.

We extend special thanks to Martha Richards, RRA, for reviewing, proofreading, and researching questions related to *Stedman's Neurology Words* and to Jeanne Bock, CSR, RPR, MT, for completing the same challenging steps with *Stedman's Psychiatry Words*.

We also extend special thanks to Ellen Atwood; Renée Hentz, CMT; and again, to Jeanne Bock for editing the new terms added to *Stedman's Psychiatry/Neurology/Neurosurgery Words, Second Edition,* helping to resolve many difficult content questions, and contributing much of the material for the appendices.

Thanks as well to our MT Editorial Advisory Board for *Stedman's Psychiatry/Neurology/Neurosurgery Words, Second Edition,* including Amelia M. Duquette, CMT; Robin A. Koza; Seamond Roberts, CMT; Wendy Ryan, ART; Jane Saville; and Karen Thomas-Bates, CMT. These medical transcriptionists served as important contributors, editors, and advisors.

Other important contributors to this edition include Susan Couper, CMT; Diane Edgar; Sheila L. Hatch, MT; Darcy Johnson; Kathryn Mason, CMT; Averill Ring, CMT; and Jenifer Walker, MA.

Barb Ferretti played an integral role in the process by reviewing the content files for format, updating the database, and providing a final quality check.

As with all our *Stedman's* word references, this resource incorporates the suggestions and expertise of our many contacts in the medical transcriptionist community. Thanks to all of our advisory board participants, reviewers, and editors; AAMT meeting attendees; and others who have written us with requests and comments—keep talking, and we'll keep listening.

Editor's Preface

When is a word a word? What is the difference between a "neologism," which indicates a psychiatric disturbance, and a new word? (*See below for the answer.) How about knowing for an absolute certainty that a particular sequence of letters can't possibly be a real word, only to look it up and find out that it is? When is it useful? When is it applicable or pertinent? When, oh when, is it spelled right?

These are but a few of the myriad challenges in using medical language in general, and the specific editorial processes involved in revising and updating Stedman's specialty word books.

Creating new and revised word books involves many steps, which incorporate looking at thousands of possible inclusions, and then winnowing until only the specialty-specific or pertinent words are left. The end result is a timely, reliable, useful, and quick reference. Working medical transcriptionists do not have the time to discourse etymology and diphthongs while under turnaround or production pressure, but the references they use must be built upon accuracy while reflecting usage.

Of continuing and increasing concern in these days of automation, optical character recognition, voice technologies, and more sophisticated "spillchuckers" is the fact that there may be no such thing as an insignificant error or harmless "typo" in a medical record. Medical transcriptionists have a direct effect on healthcare, as there can be far-reaching medical, legal, social, and even health-endangering repercussions from even a single erroneous term included in a medical record. To bring this point solidly home, get a copy of your own medical records and proofread!

Stedman's Psychiatry/Neurology/Neurosurgery Words, Second Edition, is a reflection of not only the growth and updates in terminology for psy-

---

*New terms are constantly being added to the medical vocabulary for the express purpose of conveying precise information, unlike neologisms which have meaning only to their creator.

chiatric, medical neurology, and neurosurgical specialties, but also incorporates the rapidly evolving recognition of the mind/body continuum, exemplified by efforts to discontinue rigid classification of various conditions as solely of the mind or distinctly originating from and affecting only the body.

Of special consideration for this edition was how to incorporate the extensive and growing lists of "street language." This richly expressive jargon includes a seemingly endless variety of names for drugs of abuse and for criminal or subculture activities, words that will be encountered by MTs in many psychiatric and neurologic reports. This informal language is not subject to the regular rules of spelling and grammar most likely by virtue of its being spoken rather than written. We've attempted to include at least one acceptable spelling; there may be many more.

Ellen Atwood

Publisher's Preface

Stedman's Psychiatry/Neurology/Neurosurgery Words, Second Edition offers an authoritative assurance of quality and exactness to the wordsmiths of the healthcare professions—medical transcriptionists, medical editors and copy editors, health information management personnel, court reporters, and the many other users and producers of medical documentation.

For years we have received requests for a single word book covering the overlapping specialities of psychiatry, neurology, and neurosurgery so that terms in each area would be easier to find, rather than requiring access to several references. Recently, we have also received requests for updates to *Stedman's Neurosurgery Words* and *Stedman's Psychiatry Words*. As the requests continued, we realized that medical language professionals needed a comprehensive, current reference for psychiatry, neurology, and neurosurgery terminology.

Users will find thousands of words encompassing the function and structure of the brain, spinal cord, and peripheral nerves (neuroanatomy), along with disorders of the nervous system (neurology) and the mind (psychiatry). This collection includes terminology used in psychiatric and neuroradiologic diagnosis and testing, including MRI, CAT, SPECT, and PET, as well as in treatments, such as electric stimulation, drugs, and herbs. Users will also find words for surgical instruments, implantable stimulators, and spinal instrumentation, in addition to terminology associated with acute and chronic pain, aging, stroke, mood and personality disorders, substance abuse counseling, mind/body connections, and genetic, degenerative, and traumatic disorders and diseases.

This compilation of 110,000 entries, fully cross-indexed for quick access, was built from a base vocabulary of more than 65,000 medical words, phrases, abbreviations and acronyms. The extensive A-Z list was developed from the database of *Stedman's Medical Dictionary* and supplemented by terminology found in current medical literature (please see list of References on page xvi).

We at Lippincott Williams & Wilkins strive to provide you with the most up-to-date and accurate word references available. Your use of this word book will prompt new editions, which we will publish as often as updates and revisions justify. We welcome your suggestions for improvements, changes, corrections, and additions—whatever will make this *Stedman's* product more useful to you. Please complete the postpaid card at the back of this book, and send your recommendations care of "Stedman's" at Lippincott Williams & Wilkins.

Explanatory Notes

Medical transcription is an art as well as a science. Both are needed to correctly interpret the dictation of a physician, whose language is a product of education, training, and experience. This variety in medical language means that there are several acceptable ways to express certain terms, including jargon. *Stedman's Psychiatry/Neurology/Neurosurgery Words, Second Edition* provides variant spellings and phrasings for many terms. These elements, in addition to complete cross-indexing, make *Stedman's Psychiatry/Neurology/Neurosurgery Words, Second Edition* a valuable resource for determining the validity of terms as they are encountered.

Alphabetical Organization

Alphabetization of main entries is letter by letter as spelled, ignoring punctuation, spaces, prefixed numbers, Greek letters, or other characters. For example:

adrenaline
adrenergic
β-adrenergic
adrenocortical

In subentry alphabetization, the abbreviated singular form or the spelled-out plural form of the noun main entry word is ignored.

Format and Style

All main entries are in **boldface** to expedite locating a sought-after term, to enhance distinction between main entries and subentries, and to relieve the textual density of the pages.

Irregular plurals and variant spellings are shown on the same line as the singular or preferred form of the word. For example:

claustrum, pl. **claustra**

arachnoidea, arachnoides

Hyphenation

As a rule of style, multiple eponyms (e.g., Mears-Rubash approach) are hyphenated. Also, hyphens have been added between a manufacturer and one or more eponyms (e.g., Vital-Metzenbaum dissecting scissors). Please note that hyphenation is a question of style, not of accuracy, and thus is a matter of choice.

Possessives

Possessive forms have been dropped in this reference for the sake of consistency and conformance with the guidelines of the American Association for Medical Transcription (AAMT) and other groups. Please note, however, that retaining the possessive is a question of style, not of accuracy, and thus is a matter of choice. To form the possessive of a word, simply add the apostrophe or apostrophe "s" to the end of the word.

Cross-indexing

The word list is an index-like main entry-subentry format that contains two combined alphabetical listings:

(1) A *noun* main entry-subentry organization, which is typical of the A-Z section of medical dictionaries like **Stedman's:**

clip
    Adson scalp c.
    aneurysm c.

defense
    character d.
    ego d.

(2) An *adjective* main entry-subentry organization, which lists words and phrases as you hear them. The main entries are the adjectives or modifiers in a multi-word term. The subentries are the nouns around which the terms are constructed and to which the adjectives or modifiers pertain:

target
    t. acquisition
    t. localization

venous
    v. aneurysm
    v. angioma

This format provides the user with more than one way to locate and identify a multi-word term. For example:

nerve
medial planter n

medial
m. planter nerve

axis
neural a.

neural
n. axis

It also allows the user to see together all terms that contain a particular descriptor, as well as all types, kinds, or variations of a noun entity. For example:

frequency
f. curve
f. distribution
dominant f.
gene f.

polioencephalitis
p. infectiva
inferior p.
superior hemorrhagic p.

Wherever possible, abbreviations are separately defined and cross-referenced. For example:

BEAM
brain electrical activity mapping

brain
b. electrical activity mapping (BEAM)

mapping
brain electrical activity mapping (BEAM)

References

In addition to the manufacturers' literature we gather at various medical meetings, scientific reports from hospitals, and the lists of our MT Editorial Advisory Board members (from their daily transcription work), we used the following sources for new words for *Stedman's Psychiatry/Neurology/Neurosurgery, Second Edition:*

Books

Agur AMR, Lee MJ. Grant's atlas of anatomy, 9th ed. Williams & Wilkins, 1991.

American Psychiatric Association. Diagnostic and statistical manual of mental disorders, 4th ed. Washington DC: American Psychiatric Association, 1994.

Dorland's illustrated medical dictionary, 28th ed. Philadelphia: WB Saunders Company, 1994.

Forbis P. The psychiatry word book with street talk terms. Philadelphia: F. A. Davis, 1993.

Goldman MA. Pocket guide to the operating room. Philadelphia: F. A. Davis, 1996.

Kaplan HI, Sadock BJ. Kaplan and Sadock's synopsis of psychiatry. 8th ed. Baltimore: Williams & Wilkins, 1997.

Lance LL. Quick look drug book. Baltimore: Lippincott Williams & Wilkins, 1999.

Orthopedic/neurology words and phrases. Modesto: Health Professions Institute, 1994.

Pyle V. Current medical terminology, 5th ed. Modesto: Health Professions Institute, 1994.

Rowland LP. Merritt's textbook of neurology. Baltimore: Williams & Wilkins, 1997.

Sloane SB. The medical word book, 3rd ed. Philadelphia: WB Saunders Company, 1991.

Stedman's medical dictionary, 26th ed. Baltimore: Williams & Wilkins, 1995.

Stedman's neurosurgery words. Baltimore: Williams & Wilkins, 1993.

Stedman's psychiatry words. Baltimore: Williams & Wilkins, 1992.

Stedman's WordWatcher 1995–1997. Baltimore: Williams & Wilkins, 1998.

Journals

American Academy of Child and Adolescent Psychiatry. Baltimore: Williams & Wilkins, 1995–1998.

American Journal of Psychiatry. Washington DC: American Psychiatric Press, 1997–1999.

Clinical Psychiatry News. Rockville, MD: International Medical News Group, 1998–1999.

Journal of Developmental and Behavioral Pediatrics. Baltimore: Williams & Wilkins, 1995.

Journal of Neurology. Charlottesville, VA: American Association of Neurological Surgeons, 1995–1996.

Journal of the American Association for Medical Transcription. Modesto: American Association for Medical Transcription, 1995–1999.

MT Monthly. Gladstone, MO: Computer Systems Management, 1994–1999.

Neurology. Philadelphia: Lippincott Williams & Wilkins, 1994–1999.

Neurology Reviews. Clifton, NJ: Partners in Medical Communication, 1998.

Neurosurgery. Baltimore: Lippincott Williams & Wilkins, 1996–1998.

Perspectives on the Medical Transcription Profession. Modesto: Health Professions Institute, 1993–1998.

Psychiatric Annals. Thorofare, NJ: Slack Inc., 1998–1999.

Stedman's WordWatcher. Baltimore: Williams & Wilkins, 1995–1997.

The Latest Word. Philadelphia: WB Saunders Company, 1994–1999.

The Neuroscientist. Baltimore: Lippincott Williams & Wilkins, 1995–1998.

Websites

http://www.medscape.com/Medscape/psychiatry/journal/1998/v03.n02/mh3208.mcdo/ca-mh3208.mcdo.html

http://www.medscape.com/Medscape/psychiatry/journal/1997/v02.n05/mh3118.frances/mh3118.frances.html

http://www.medscape.com/govmt/NIMH/SchizophreniaBulletin/1998/v24.n01/sb2401..02.lehm/sb2401.02.lehm.01.html

http://www.medscape.com/SCP/IIM/1998/v15.n08/m3128.bale/m3128.bale-01.html

http://www.medscape.com/moffitt/CancerControl/1998/v05.n02/cc0502.06.mikk/cc 0502.06.mikk.01.html

http://www.medscape.com/govmt/NIMH/SchizophreniaBulletin/1997/v23.n03/sb2303..07.boge/sb2303.07.boge.html

http://www.medscape.com/SCP/IIM/1998/v15.n07/m4724.harr/m4724.harr-01.html

http://www.medscape.com/govmt/NIMH/SchizophreniaBulletin/1998/v24.n02/sb2402..10.weic/sb2402.10.weic-01.html

http://www.medscape.com/govmt/NIMH/SchizophreniaBulletin/1998/v24.n02/sb2402..08.donn/sb2402.08.donn-01.html

http://www.mwsearch.com

http://www.rxlist.com

http://www.virtualdrugstore.com

α (*var. of* alpha)

A
- A deux
- A fiber
- A reflex
- A Sales Potential Inventory for Real Estate (ASPIRE)
- A scale

A2
- Criterion A.

1a
- interferon-β 1a (IFN-B1a)

A9 neuron

AA
- Academic Alertness
- achievement age
- Alcoholics Anonymous
- amino acid
- anaplastic astrocytoma
- anticipatory avoidance

AAA
- acute anxiety attack

AAF
- altered auditory feedback

AAI
- Adolescent Alienation Index

AAMI
- age-associated memory impairment

a-amino-3-hydroxy-5-methylisoxazole-4-propionic acid (AMPA)

AAO
- awake, alert, and oriented

Aarskog syndrome

AAT
- Academic Aptitude Test
- Auditory Apperception Test

AB, ab
- abortion

ABA
- applied behavioral analysis
- Apraxia Battery for Adults

abactio

abactus venter

A/B/A design

Abadie sign of tabes dorsalis

abalienate

abalienatio mentis

abandoned child

abandonment
- a. concern
- emotional a.
- fear of a.
- imagined a.
- perceived emotional a.
- real a.

abarognosis

abasia
- atactic a., ataxic a.
- a. atactica
- choreic a.
- frontal a.
- hysterical a.

- paralytic a.
- paroxysmal trepidant a.
- spastic a.
- trembling a.
- a. trepidans

abasia-astasia

abasic, abatic

abatement

abaxial, abaxile

abaxonal

abbau

Abbokinase

Abbott fluorescence polarization immunoassay technique

Abboxapam

Abbreviated
- A. Conners Teacher Questionnaire
- A. Conners Teacher Rating Scale (ACTRS)
- A. Injury Score (AIS)

ABC
- Aberrant Behavior Checklist
- Assessment of Basic Competencies
- ABC Inventory - Extended

ABCD
- Arizona Battery for Communication Disorders of Dementia

Abderhalden-Fauser reaction

abdominal
- a. brain
- a. discomfort
- a. epilepsy
- a. migraine
- a. neuralgia
- a. pain
- a. reflex
- a. trauma

abdominal-diaphragmatic respiration

abducens
- a. nerve
- a. nerve palsy
- a. nerve paralysis
- a. nerve paresis
- nervus a.
- a. nucleus
- a. pathway

abducent

abducentis
- nucleus a.

abduction
- a. nystagmus
- a. weakness

abductor pollicis brevis

Abercrombie neuronal cell count formula

aberrant
- a. artery
- a. autocrine control
- a. behavior
- A. Behavior Checklist (ABC)
- a. bundle
- a. cycle

aberrant *(continued)*
    a. ganglion
    a. gene
    a. motivational syndrome
    a. pattern
    a. regeneration
aberration
    autosomal a.
    chromosomal a.
    intersegmental a.
    mental a.
    a. of perception
    semantic a.
    sexual a.
aberrometer
ABES
    Adaptive Behavior Evaluation Scale
abeyance
ABI
    ankle-brachial index
ABIC
    Adaptive Behavior Inventory for
    Children
ability
    a. to abstract and calculate
    abstracting a.
    abstractive a.
    ACER Test of Reasoning A.
    attentional a.
    attention shift a.
    auditory a.
    bathing and dressing a.
    a. battery
    cognitive a.
    communication a.
    conceptual a.
    concrete abstractive a.
    constructional a.
    coping a.
    crystallized a.
    disturbance in perceptual motor a.
    drawing a.
    eidetic a.
    fluid a.
    focal a.
    Full Scale Broad Cognitive A.
    general learning a.
    Group Tests of Musical A.
    Illinois Test of Psycholinguistic A.
    (ITPA)
    impaired concentration a.
    impaired thinking a.
    intellectual a.
    language a.
    learning a.
    MacQuarrie Test for Mechanical A.
    mathematical a.
    McCarthy Scales of Children's A.
    (MCSA, MSCA)
    Measures of Musical A.
    memory a.
    mental a.
    motor a.
    occupational a.

    oral sensory a.
    perceptual motor a.
    Porch Index of Communicative A.
    (PICA)
    positive a.
    premorbid a.
    primary a.
    Primary Mental A.
    psychic a.
    psycholinguistic a.
    RBH Test of Learning A.
    reality testing a.
    reasoning a.
    reduced attention a.
    response generalization general
    learning a.
    sequencing a.
    shift a.
    spatial a.
    special a.
    synthesizing a.
    a. to take criticism
    Test of Syntactic A. (TSA)
    The Henmon-Nelson Tests of
    Mental A.
    thinking a.
    thoroughness, reliability, efficiency,
    analytic a. (TREA)
    verbal conceptualization a.
    verbal and oral language a.
    visuomotor a.
    word-finding a.
    writing a.
Ability-to-Benefit Admissions Test
ab initio
abiotic
abiotrophy
ABLA test
ablation
    Amytal a.
    choroid plexus a.
    stereotactic surgical a.
    total pituitary a.
ablative central neurosurgical procedure
ABLB
    alternate binaural loudness balance
ABLE
    Adult Basic Learning Examination
ablienation
ablutomania
abnegation
abneural
abnormal
    a. asymmetry
    a. behavior during sleep
    a. brain structure
    a. dermatoglyphic
    a. development
    a. EEG
    a. EEG tracing
    a. epileptic neuron
    a. gait
    a. involuntary movement
    a. involuntary movement disorder
    (AIMD)

A. Involuntary Movements Scale (AIMS)
a. mood
a. muscle response (AMR)
a. pathologic condition
a. perception
a. physiological event during sleep
a. position of distal limbs
a. psychology
a. responsiveness
a. sleep-wake schedule
a. stoppage of sound
a. ventilation
abnormalities in sleep-wake timing mechanism
abnormality
a. of affect
autosomal a.
bony a.
brain a.
bulbar a.
chromosomal a.
CNS a.
convergence a.
cranial nerve a.
cytoarchitectonic a.
cytoskeletal a.
electrolyte a.
endogenous a.
eye movement a.
food intake a.
frontal plane growth a.
gain-of-function a.
gait a.
G protein a.
hallucal a.
inherited a.
insulin a.
interictal epileptiform a.
laboratory a.
lateralizing a.
metabolic a.
migration a.
movement a.
nonspecific a.
oculomotor a.
perceptual a.
performance a.
polysomnographic a.
pupillary a.
pursuit a.
saccadic a.
sleep a.
sleep-wake a.
soft tissue a.
spinal cord injury without radiological a. (SCIWORA)
startle a.
structural brain a.
torsional a.
transient signal a.
vocal pitch a.
X-linked a.
ABO antigen compatibility
aboiement

abolic syndrome
aboriginal therapy
abort
abortifacient
abortion (AB, ab)
criminal a.
elective a.
induced a.
missed a.
spontaneous a.
therapeutic a. (TAB)
abortive neurofibromatosis
abortus
Brucella a.
aboulia (*var. of* abulia)
about face
above-average
a.-a. intelligence
a.-a. student
ABR
auditory brainstem response
ABR audiometry
abract set
Abraham view of depressive disorder
Abramson catheter
abreaction
hypnotic a.
motor a.
abreactive drug
abrin
Abrodil
abrosia
abrupt
a. onset
a. topic shift
ABS
acute brain syndrome
Adaptive Behavior Scale
aloin, belladonna, strychnine
abscess
actinomycotic brain a.
arthrifluent a.
Aspergillus cerebral a.
brain a.
cerebral a.
cranial epidural a.
daughter a.
encapsulated brain a.
epidural a.
extradural a.
frontal a.
intracranial epidural a.
intradural a.
otic a.
parasitic brain a.
periapical a.
pituitary a.
Pott a.
psoas a.
retropharyngeal a.
spinal epidural a. (SEA)
sterile a.
subdural a.
subgaleal a.

abscess *(continued)*
    thecal a.
    tuberculous a.
abscise
abscissa
abscission
absence
    atonic a.
    a. attack
    atypical a.
    automatic a.
    complex a.
    a. of depressed mood
    a. of elevated mood
    enuretic a.
    a. epilepsy
    epileptic a.
    a. episode
    fantasy a.
    a. of feeling
    hypertonic a.
    a. of insight
    leave of a. (LOA)
    myoclonic a.
    pure a.
    retrocursive a.
    a. seizure
    simple a.
    a. status
    sternutatory a.
    subclinical a.
    a. syndrome
    tussive a.
    typical a.
    vasomotor a.
absent
    a. ataxia
    a. drive
    a. pupil
    a. reflex
    a. sexual desire
    a. spinous process
    a. state
    a. without leave (AWOL)
absenteeism
absentia
    a. epileptica
    epileptica a.
    in a.
Absidia **infection**
absinthe, absinth
    a. addiction
    a. addiction or dependence
absinthism
absolute
    a. agraphia
    a. alcohol
    a. band amplitude
    a. construction of phases
    a. diet
    a. EP amplitude
    a. field
    a. impression
    a. inversion

    a. measurement
    a. neutrophil count (ANC)
    a. pitch
    a. quantity
    a. rating scale
    a. refractory period
    a. scotoma
    a. sensitivity
    a. terminal innervation ratio
    a. threshold
    a. unconsciousness
absolutism
    cultural a.
    phenomenal a.
absorbable gelatin sponge
absorbed mania
absorptiometry
    dual-energy x-ray a. (DEXA)
absorption
    a. of inhalant
    transdermal a.
abstinence
    alcohol a.
    alimentary a.
    caffeine a.
    a. delirium
    drug a.
    nicotine a.
    opiate a.
    a. phenomenon
    rule of a.
    sexual a.
    a. symptom
    a. syndrome
    a. syndrome alcoholic psychosis
abstract
    a. attitude
    a. behavior
    a. concept
    a. conceptualization
    a. expression
    a. idea
    a. intelligence
    a. interpretation
    a. logical thought
    a. modeling
    a. perception
    Personal Values A. (PVA)
    a. reasoning
    a. theory
    a. thinking
    a. versus representational
    a. wit
abstracting
    a. ability
    a. disability
abstraction ladder
abstractive ability
absurdities test
absurdity
abulia, aboulia
    cyclic a.
    social a.
abulic mental change
abulomania

A

abundancy motive
abuse
    adolescent a.
    adult a.
    aerosol spray a.
    a. of the aged
    alcohol a.
    amphetamine a.
    amyl nitrate a.
    animal a.
    antidepressant-type a.
    anxiolytic a.
    barbiturate a.
    benzodiazepine a.
    caffeine a.
    cannabis a.
    a. case (AC)
    cathartic a.
    chemical a.
    child a.
    chronic alcohol a.
    cocaine a.
    Committee on Family Violence and
      Sexual A.
    a. counseling
    a. criterion
    drug a.
    elder a.
    emotional a.
    ethanol a.
    geriatric a.
    hallucinogen a.
    hypnotic a.
    Index of Spouse A.
    inhalant a.
    IV drug a.
    laxative a.
    liability a.
    long-term course of a.
    LSD a.
    maladaptive pattern of substance a.
    marijuana a.
    medication a.
    mental a.
    methamphetamine a.
    morphine a.
    narcotic a.
    National Institute on Drug A.
      (NIDA)
    nicotine a.
    nondependent adult a.
    a. of nonprescribed drug
    nonprescription drug a.
    opioid a.
    parent a.
    patent medicinal a.
    a. of patent medicinals
    PCP a.
    perpetuator of a.
    phencyclidine a.
    physical a.
    polydrug a.
    polysubstance a.
    prescription drug a.
    problems related to a.
    psychoactive drug a.
    psychoactive substance a.
    psychological a.
    ritual a.
    sadistic a.
    sedative a.
    sexual a.
    spouse a.
    stimulant a.
    substance a.
    survivor of child a.
    sympathomimetic a.
    tobacco a.
    tranquilizer a.
    twelve-step program for
      substance a.
    verbal a.
    victim a.
    vocal a.
abused
    a. child
    a. drug
    a. patient
abused-child
    a.-c. hotline
    a.-c. syndrome
abused-wife hotline
abuse/neglect
    suspected child a. (SCAN)
abuser
    Alliance for Mentally Ill
      Chemical A.'s
    anxious substance a.
    child a.
    drug a.
    spouse a.
    substance a.
abusive vocal behavior
AC
    abuse case
    alcoholic cirrhosis
    alternating current
    anterior commissure
a.c.
    before meals
ACA
    anterior cerebral artery
    anterior choroidal artery
academic
    A. Alertness (AA)
    A. Alertness Test
    A. Aptitude Test (AAT)
    a. difficulty
    a. inhibition
    A. Instruction Measurement System
    a. inventory
    a. orientation (AO)
    A. Orientation scale
    a. preparation
    a. psychiatry
    A. Readiness Scale (ARS)
    a. skills disorder
    a. underachievement disorder
academically understimulating
  environment

acalculia
aphasic a.
visual-spatial a.
acanthamebiasis
Acanthamoeba
Acanthamoeba infection
Acanthamoeba meningitis
acanthesthesia
acapnia
acarbose
acarinatum syndrome
acarophobia
ACAS
asymptomatic carotid artery stenosis
asymptomatic carotid atherosclerosis
study
ACASH
Automated Child/Adolescent Social
History
acatalepsia
acatamathesia
acataphasia (*var. of* akataphasia)
acatastasia
acatastatic
acathexia, acathectic
acathexis
acathisia (*var. of* akathisia)
ACB
asymptomatic carotid bruit
Acc
accommodation
accelerans
accelerant
accelerated
a. heart rate
a. interaction
a. reaction
a. speech
acceleration
educational a.
a. extension injury
positive a.
accelerator
Bevatron a.
a. fiber
isocentric linear a.
linear a. (LINAC)
a. nerves
Philips linear a.
stereotactic linear a.
accelerometer
accent
word a.
accented vowel
acceptable behavior
acceptance
A. of Disability Scale
group a.
Access
A. Management Survey (AMS)
access
arterial a.
a. to health care services
lexical a.
Survey of Employee A. (SEA)

accessing cue
accessorius
nervus a.
a. willisii
accessory
a. chromosome
a. cramp
a. cuneate nucleus
a. flocculus
Isola spinal implant system a.
a. middle cerebral artery
a. nerve
a. nerve paresis
a. oculomotor nucleus
a. olivary nuclei
a. sign
a. symptom
ACCI
Adult Career Concerns Inventory
accident
alcohol-related risk for a.
all-terrain vehicle a.
ATV a.
cerebrovascular a. (CVA)
compensable a.
fatal a.
horseback riding a.
motorcycle a. (MCA)
a. neurosis
a. prevention
a. reduction
a. repeater
a. risk
skateboarding a.
vascular a.
vehicular a.
accidental
a. affair
a. crisis
a. death
a. error
a. experience
a. hanging
a. homosexuality
a. hypothermia
a. image
a. overdose
a. pregnancy
a. psychosis
a. stimuli
a. suicide
accident-prone behavior
accidents as major childhood stressor
accommodation (Acc)
auditory a.
a. curve
a. disorder
interpersonal a.
a. of nerve
passive a.
a. reflex
reflex a.
visual a.
accompli
fait a.

accomplished suicide
accomplishment quotient (AQ)
accoucheur's hand
accountability
    Foundation for A. (FaAct)
accountable for action
Accounting Program Admission Test (APAT)
ACCSCI
    acute central cervical spinal cord injury
Accu-Flo
    A.-F. CSF reservoir
    A.-F. dura film
    A.-F. polyethylene bur hole cover
    A.-F. silicone rubber bur hole cover
    A.-F. ventricular catheter
acculturation
    a. problem
    a. problem with expression of customs
    a. problem with expression of habits
    a. problem with expression of political value
    a. problem with expression of religious value
    psychological a.
accumbens neuron
accuracy test
Accura shunt
accurate empathy (AE)
Accuray Neurotron 1000 machine
accusation
    false a.
accusatory hallucination
Accusway balance measurement system
ACD
    Assessment of Career Development
ACDM
    Assessment of Career Decision Making
Ace
    A. halo-cast assembly
    A. halo pelvic girdle
    A. Hershey halo jig
    A. low profile MR halo
    A. Mark III halo
    A. Trippi-Wells tong cervical traction
    A. universal tong cervical traction
acenesthesia
acephalgic migraine
acephalous
Acephen
ACER
    A. Advanced Test B90
    A. Applied Reading Test
    A. Test of Basic Skills - Blue Series
    A. Test of Basic Skills - Green Series
    A. Test of Reasoning Ability
acerbophobia
acerophobia
acervuline

acervulus
Aceta
acetaldehyde
acetaminobenzoate
    deanol a.
acetaminophen
    a., aspirin, and caffeine
    butalbital and a.
    chlorzoxazone and a.
    a. and codeine
    a. and dextromethorphan
    a. and diphenhydramine
    hydrocodone and a.
    a., isometheptene, and dichloralphenazone
    oxycodone and a.
    a. and phenyltoloxamine
    a. poisoning
    propoxyphene and a.
    propoxyphene napsylate and a.
acetanilid
acetate
    amyl a.
    butyl a.
    cortisone a.
    Cortone a.
    cyproterone a. (CPA)
    desmopressin a.
    desoxycorticosterone a.
    glatiramer a.
    Hydrocortone A.
    levomethadyl a.
    medroxyprogesterone a.
    mepazine a.
    methylprednisolone a.
    paramethasone a.
    potassium a.
    sodium a.
acetazolamide
ACE Test
acetohexamide
acetone
acetonide
    triamcinolone a.
acetophenazine
acetophenetidin
acetous
acetrizoate
acetrizoic acid
acetum
N-acetylaspartate (NAA)
acetylcarbromal
acetylcholine (ACH, ACh)
    a. as neurotransmitter
    a. cholinergic receptor
    a. esterase
    a. receptor (AChR)
acetylcholinesterase (ACHE)
acetylcysteine
    10% a. 0.05% isoproterenol hydrochloride solution
acetyl-L-carnitine
acetylphosphate
acetylsalicylic acid

acetyltransferase
    choline a.
acetylureas
ACF
    anterior cervical fusion
ACG
    Assessment of Core Goals
ACH, ACh
    acetylcholine
        ACH receptor
achalasia
    cricopharyngeal a.
    esophageal a.
ACHE
    acetylcholinesterase
ache
    brain a.
acheiria, achiria
Achenbach
    A. Child Behavior Checklist
    A. Child Behavior Test
Aches-N-Pain
achievement
    a. age (AA)
    assessment of academic a.
    a. battery
    a. behavior
    A. Checklist (ACL)
    a. drive
    educational a.
    a. ethics
    exaggerated a.
    expected level of a.
    Kaufman Test of Educational A.
      (K-TEA)
    math a.
    a. motivation
    a. motive
    motive a.
    a. need (n-Ach)
    a. quotient (AQ)
    a. ratio (AR)
    reading a.
    school a.
    a. test (AT)
    a. through counseling and treatment
      (ACT)
    vocational a.
Achilles
    A. heel
    A. jerk
    A. tendon reflex
achiria (*var. of* acheiria)
achlorhydria
achluophobia
achondroplasia
achondroplastic dwarfism
AChR
    acetylcholine receptor
achromatic
    a. color
    a. color response
achromatic-chromatic scale
achromatism

achromatopsia
    central a.
achromians
    incontinentia pigmenti a.
acid
    a-amino-3-hydroxy-5-methylisoxazole-
      4-propionic a. (AMPA)
    acetrizoic a.
    acetylsalicylic a.
    adenylic a.
    amidotrizoic a.
    amino a. (AA)
    aminocaproic a.
    aminohydroxybutyric a.
    amoxicillin-clavulanic a.
    arachidonic a.
    ascorbic a.
    aspartic a.
    barbituric a.
    battery a.
    benzoic a.
    carbonic a.
    carboxylic a.
    cis-parinaric a.
    clavulanic a.
    clorazepic a.
    cyclic deoxyribonucleic a. (cDNA)
    deoxyribonucleic a. (DNA)
    diatrizoic a.
    diethylenetriamine penta-acetic a.
      (DTPA)
    differential display of messenger
      ribonucleic a.
    docosahexanoic a.
    eicosapentaenoic a.
    epsilon-aminocaproic a.
    essential amino a.
    ethacrynic a.
    ethylenediaminetetraacetic a.
      (EDTA)
    excitatory amino a. (EAA)
    a. flashback
    folic a.
    gadolinium diethylenetriamine penta-
      acetic a. (Gd-DTPA)
    gamma aminobutyric a. (GABA)
    gamma linolenic a.
    ganglioside monosialic a.
    glutamic a.
    glutaric a.
    homocysteine a.
    homovanillic a. (HVA)
    5-hydroxyindoleacetic a. (5-HIAA)
    inhibitory amino a. (IAA)
    iobenzamic a.
    iobutoic a.
    iocarmic a.
    iodamic a.
    iodoalphionic a.
    iodoxamic a.
    ioglicic a.
    ioglycamic a.
    iopanoic a.
    iophenoxic a.
    ioprocemic a.

iopronic a.
iosefamic a.
ioseric a.
iosumetic a.
ioteric a.
iothalamic a.
iotroxic a.
ioxaglic a.
ioxithalamic a.
iozomic a.
ipodate a.
kynurenic a.
a. lipase
long-chain fatty a.
lysergic a.
a. maltase deficiency (AMD)
mefenamic a.
messenger ribonucleic a. (mRNA)
metrizoic a.
myristic a.
neuroactive amino a.
nitric a. (NO)
okadaic a.
Owsley's a.
oxolinic a.
palmitic a.
phenylpyruvic a.
a. phosphatase
polyanhydroglucuronic a.
potassium citrate and citric a.
ribonucleic a. (RNA)
serum folic a.
sialic a.
super a.
a. test
tolfenamic a.
tranexamic a.
triiodobenzoic a.
tyropanoic a.
uric a.
valproic a.
vanilla mandelic a.
y-aminobutyric a.

acid-base
a.-b. balance
a.-b. disturbance
a.-b. imbalance

acidemia
methylmalonic a.
organic a.
proprionic a.

acidification treatment
acidogenic
acidophil adenoma
acidophilic pituitary tumor
acidosis
extracellular a.
hypokalemic metabolic a.
lactic a.
metabolic a.
respiratory a.

acid-Schiff
periodic a.-S. (PAS)

aciduria
alpha-methylacetoacetic a.

argininosuccine a.
glutaric a. type I
methylmalonic a.
organic a.
pipoglutamic a.

Acinetobacter
Ackerman-Schoendorf Scales for Parent Evaluation of Custody (ASPECT)
ACL
Achievement Checklist
Adjective Checklist

Acland clip
ACLC
Assessment of Children's Language Comprehension

ACM
acute confusional migraine

acme
acmesthesia
ACN
acute conditioned neurosis

acne
acnes
Propionibacterium a.

ACO
alert, cooperative, and oriented
Assessment of Conceptual Organization

ACOA
adult child of alcoholic

ACoA
anterior communicating artery

acoasm, akoasm
ACO: Improving Writing, Thinking and Reading Skills
acolasia
AComA
anterior communicating artery

aconuresis
acoria
acorn
a. bit
a. drill

acosmia
Acosta
A. disease
A. syndrome

acouasm (*var. of* acousma)
acouesthesia
acoupedic rehabilitation
acoupedics
acousma, acouasm
acousmatagnosis
acousmatamnesia
acoustic
a. agnosia
a. agraphia
a. analysis
a. aphasia
a. area
a. bone window
a. center
a. crest
a. energy
a. evoked potential
a. feedback

acoustic *(continued)*
   a. immittance measurement test
   a. input
   a. interface
   a. irritability
   a. lemniscus
   a. meatus
   a. nerve
   a. nerve complex
   a. nerve sheath tumor
   a. neurasthenia
   a. neurilemoma
   a. neurinoma
   a. neuroma
   A. Neuroma Registry
   a. noise
   a. papilla
   a. phonetics
   a. pressure
   a. radiation
   a. reflex
   a. reflex threshold
   a. resonance
   a. schwannoma
   a. signal
   a. spectrum
   a. startle
   a. stria
   a. trauma
   a. trauma deafness
   a. tubercle
acoustical shadowing
acoustic-amnestic aphasia
acousticofacial
   a. crest
   a. ganglion
acousticomotor epilepsy
acousticooptics
acousticopalpebral reflex
acousticophobia
acoustics
AC-PC
   anterior commissure-posterior
   commissure
   AC-PC line
ACQ Behavior Checklist
acquiesce
acquiescence
   response a.
   social a. (SA, sa)
acquiescent-response set
acquired
   a. agraphia
   a. character
   a. dementia
   a. demyelinative neuropathy
   a. drive
   a. dyslexia
   a. epilepsy
   a. epileptic aphasia
   a. fluent aphasia
   a. folie morale
   a. hepatocerebral degeneration
   a. hepatocerebral syndrome

   a. hydrocephalus
   a. immunodeficiency syndrome
   (AIDS)
   a. immunodeficiency syndrome
   dementia complex
   a. knowledge
   a. nystagmus
   a. paranoia
   a. reflex
   a. sexual dysfunction
   a. spinal stenosis
   a. toxoplasmosis
acquired-type
   a.-t. disorder
   a.-t. dyspareunia
acquisita
   myotonia a.
acquisition
   psychosocial skill a.
   reading skills a.
   target a.
   a. time
acquisitive
   a. instinct
   a. spirit
Acra-clip system
Acra-Cut
   A.-C. blade
   A.-C. cranial perforator
   A.-C. cranioblade
   A.-C. wire pass drill
Acra-gun system
acral
acrasia
Acremonium alabamensis
acrescentism
   emotional a.
acroagnosis
acroanesthesia
acroataxia
acrobrachycephaly
acrocentric chromosome
acrocephalosyndactyly
acrocephaly
acrocinesis
acrocinetic
acrocyanosis
acrodermatis chronica atrophicans
acrodynia
acrodysesthesia
acroedema
acroesthesia
acrognosis
acrohypothermia
acrolect
acrolein
acromania
acromegalia *(var. of* acromegaly*)*
acromegalic neuropathy
acromegaloid-hypertelorism-pectus
acromegaloid personality
acromegaly, acromegalia
   hypothalamic a.
acromelalgia

acromial
    a. dimple
    a. reflex
acromicria
acronarcotic
acroneurosis
acroparesthesia syndrome
acropathy
    mutilating a.
acrophase
acrophobia
acrosclerosis
across identity state
acrotrophodynia
acrotrophoneurosis
acrylaldehyde
acrylamide
    a. monomer
    a. peripheral neuropathy
acrylic
    a. cranioplasty
    a. glue
    a. prosthesis
ACS
    acute confusional state
ACT
    achievement through counseling and
      treatment
    adaptive control of thought
    American College of Testing
    anxiety control training
    atropine coma therapy
      ACT Evaluation/Survey Service
act
    Age Discrimination in
      Employment A.
    Americans with Disabilities A.
      (ADA)
    assaultive a.
    biologic a.
    Community Mental Health
      Centers A.
    compulsive a.
    consummatory a.
    Controlled Substances A. (CSA)
    criminal a.
    Drug Induced Rape Prevention and
      Punishment A.
    Employee Retirement Income
      Security A. (ERISA)
    a. ending
    frequency of violent a.
    Gann A.
    a. of God
    habitual a.
    Harrison Antinarcotic A.
    imperious a.
    impulsive a.
    Individuals with Disabilities
      Education A. (IDEA)
    instrumental avoidance a.
    mental a.
    psychology a.
    rape a.
    reflex a.

    sadistic rape a.
    sensorimotor a.
    serious assaultive a.
    speech a.
    suicide a.
    symptomatic a.
    Terazoff A.
    Uniform Determination of
      Death A.
    a. utilitarianism
    violent a.
    a. and volition
ACTeRS
    ADD-H: Comprehensive Teacher's
      Rating Scale, Second Edition
ACTH
    adrenocorticotropic hormone
act-habit
Acthar
ACTH-producing adenoma
Actidose-Aqua
Actidose With Sorbitol
actin
acting
    a. in
    a. out
    a. out behavior
    a. out defense mechanism
    a. out potential
    a. out tendency
actinic keratosis
Actinomadura madurae
actinomycin D
actinomycosis
    a. lymphocytic meningitis
actinomycotic brain abscess
actinoneuritis
action
    accountable for a.
    affirmative a.
    amphetamine-like a.
    anatonistic a.
    antigonadal a.
    a. of arrest
    automatic a.
    calorigenic a.
    chance a.
    chemical a.
    compulsive a.
    consensual a.
    consequences of a.
    cumulative drug a.
    a. current
    duration of drug a.
    a. dystonia
    effective a.
    a. group
    a. guide
    independent a.
    a. instrument
    intensified a.
    a. interpretation
    irrational a.
    a. level
    a. location

action (*continued*)
    missing in a. (MIA)
    morphine-like a.
    a. organization
    a. painting
    a. pattern
    a. potential
    raptus a.
    a. recipient
    a. research
    scotomata of a.
    seriously wounded in a. (SWA)
    a. system
    tendency of a.
    thermogenic a.
    toxic a.
    a. tremor
    uncontrollable a.
    viscoelastic a.
    wounded in a.
action-group process
activa
    oneirodynia a.
    A. tremor control system
    A. Tremor Control System implant
    A. tremor control therapy
activated
    a. epilepsy
    a. sleep
    a. state
activation
    a. defect
    EEG a.
    enzyme a.
    nociceptor a.
    parahippocampal a.
    a. pattern
    peripheral nociceptor a.
    phasic a.
    prefrontal a.
    semantic a.
    a. technique
    a. theory of emotion
    transient channel a.
activator
    plasminogen a. (PA)
    recombinant tissue plasminogen a.
    a. table
    tissue plasminogen a. (t-PA)
active
    a. algolagnia
    a. analysis
    a. analytical psychotherapy
    a. bilingualism
    a. castration complex
    a. concretization
    a. daydream technique
    a. delirium
    a. desire
    a. displacement of emotive energy
    a. euthanasia
    a. fantasizing
    a. filter
    a. friendliness

    a. hostility index (AHI)
    a. immunity
    a. incontinence
    a. integral range of motion (AIROM)
    a. intervention
    a. mode of consciousness
    a. modification
    a. movement
    a. negativism
    a. nymphomania
    a. passivity
    a. phase
    a. phase of schizophrenia
    a. placebo
    a. psychoanalysis
    a. psychotic symptom
    a. recreation
    a. sleep
    a. surface electrode
    a. therapist
    a. therapy
    a. transport
    a. treatment
    a. trigger
    a. vocabulary
    a. voice
actively aggressive reaction type
active-passive model
active-phase
    a.-p. symptom
    a.-p. symptoms of schizophrenia
activities
    a. of daily living (ADL)
    a. of daily living skills
    a. therapist
Activities Therapist, Registered (ATR)
activity
    adolescent sexual a.
    aimless motor a.
    alpha a.
    antisocial a.
    asymmetrical generalized epileptiform a.
    a. and attention disturbance
    autonomic a.
    background a.
    barbiturate-induced spindle-like a.
    a. and behavior
    beta a.
    bilateral a.
    blocking a.
    brain opioid a.
    brain wave a.
    burst of delta a.
    a. catharsis
    cerebral antioxidant a.
    C fiber a.
    constricted a.
    cortical-subcortical network a.
    criminal a.
    delta a.
    a. deprivation
    desynchronization a.
    diffuse distribution of a.

diminished pleasure in
  everyday a.'s
discontinuous a.
a. displacement
dopaminergic a.
a. drive
dynamic physical a.
efferent sympathetic a.
electrocerebral a.
electrographic seizure a.
electrooculographic a.
emotional a.
epileptiform a.
excessive diffuse low and medium
  wave beta a.
excessive motor a.
extracellular calcium a.
extracerebral a.
fast a.
fine motor a.
focal delta slow wave a.
focal epileptiform a.
frontal intermittent rhythmic
  delta a. (FIRDA)
functional a.
goal-directed a.
graded a.
gross motor a. (GMA)
group a.
a. group psychotherapy
a. group therapy (AGT)
hedonistic a.
high-frequency a.
high-risk a.
high voltage slow and sharp a.
ictal epileptiform a.
impulsive a.
interictal epileptiform a.
intermittent rhythmic delta a.
  (IRDA)
lambdoid a.
lateralized a.
leisure a.
level of a.
a. level
limited a.
locomotor a.
a. log
A. Loss Assessment (ALA)
low-amplitude a.
low-frequency a.
low-voltage a.
lysosomal enzymatic a.
major life a.
masochistic sexual a.
masturbatory a.
mental a.
MFD a.
monomorphic a.
monorhythmic frontal delta a.
monorhythmic sinusoidal delta a.
motor a.
neuronal a.
neuronal spike a.
nighttime a.

noncerebral a.
nonepileptiform a.
nonproductive a.
occipital dominant intermittent
  rhythmic delta a.
occipital intermittent rhythmic
  delta a. (OIRDA)
occupational a.
organized a.
orogenital a.
oxygen-depriving a.'s
paroxysmal a.
paroxysmal alpha a.
pathologic spontaneous a. (PSA)
A. Pattern Indicator (API)
peak level of drug a.
peripheral electromyographic a.
persistent motor a.
a. playing
a. pleasure
polymorphic delta a. (PDA)
polyphasic a.
polyrhythmic a.
posterior dominant a.
posttraumatic epileptiform a.
propagation of a.
pseudoepileptiform a.
psychomotor a.
purposeless motor a.
a. quotient
random a.
rapid change in a.
a. record
reflex neurologic a.
religious a.
REM a.
repetitious a.
repetitive motor a.
restricted a.
a. restriction
rhythmic spindle-shaped a.
risk a.
runs of a.
scattered dysrhythmic slow a.
seizure a.
self-care a.
sentinel a.
serotonergic a.
sexual a.
sigma a.
sleep a.
slow-frequency EEG a.
slow wave a.
social a.
solitary a.
spectral peak frequency of a.
spiking a.
spontaneous a.
stereotyped a.
stream of mental a.
a. system
thalamocortical a.
a. theory of aging
theta a.
triphasic slow wave a.

activity *(continued)*
    unilateral epileptiform a.
    unilateral focus of a.
    vacuum a.
    voyeuristic a.
    a. wheel
    widespread distribution of a.
activity-interview group psychotherapy (A-IGP)
activity-reactivity
    autonomic a.-r.
actograph
actometer
Actonel
Actron
ACTRS
    Abbreviated Conners Teacher Rating Scale
actual
    a. derailment
    a. mortality
    a. neurosis
    a. self
actus reus
actylate
ACU
    acute care unit
ACU-dyne antiseptic
acuesthesia
acuity
    auditory a.
    central vision a.
    A. of Psychiatric Illness scale
    sensory a.
    visual a.
aculalia
acumen
acuology
acupressure
acupuncture
acupuncturist
acusticus
    nervus a.
    nucleus a.
    porus a.
acute
    a. acquired hemiplegia
    Adjustment Disorder, A.
    a. affective reflex
    a. African sleeping sickness
    a. alcoholic delirium
    a. alcoholic mania
    a. alcoholic myopathy
    a. alcohol intoxication
    a. alcoholism
    a. amnesia
    a. amphetamine poisoning
    a. angular kyphosis
    a. anoxia
    a. anterior poliomyelitis
    a. anxiety
    a. anxiety attack (AAA)
    a. anxiety depression
    a. aphonia

    a. atrophic paralysis
    a. brachial radiculitis
    a. brain syndrome (ABS)
    a. bulbar poliomyelitis
    a. burst injury
    a. care unit (ACU)
    a. central cervical spinal cord injury (ACCSCI)
    a. cerebellar ataxia
    a. cerebellar hemispheric lesion
    a. cerebral tremor
    a. chorea
    a. conditioned neurosis (ACN)
    a. confusional insanity
    a. confusional migraine (ACM)
    a. confusional migraine headache
    a. confusional state (ACS)
    a. confusional state arteriosclerotic dementia
    a. dangerousness
    a. dementia
    a. disseminated encephalomyelitis (ADE, ADEM)
    a. drug toxicity
    a. drunkenness
    a. epidemic leukoencephalitis
    a. exacerbation
    a. fracture
    a. genomic response
    a. hallucinatory mania
    a. hallucinatory paranoia
    a. hallucinosis
    a. head trauma
    a. hemorrhagic encephalitis
    a. hemorrhagic leukoencephalitis
    a. homosexual panic
    a. hydrocephalus
    a. idiopathic polyneuritis
    a. inflammatory demyelinating polyradiculoneuropathy (AIDP)
    a. inflammatory demyelinating polyradiculopathy (AIDP)
    a. inflammatory polyneuropathy (AIP)
    a. intensive treatment (AIT)
    a. intermittent porphyria
    a. intoxication
    a. ischemic brachial neuropathy
    a. lead poisoning
    a. lung injury (ALI)
    a. maladjustment situational
    a. melancholia
    a. necrotizing encephalitis
    a. necrotizing hemorrhagic leukoencephalitis
    a. neuronal toxicity
    pain disorder, a.
    a. painful polyneuropathy
    A. Panic Inventory
    a. paranoid reaction nonorganic
    a. paranoid schizophrenic reaction (APSR)
    a. partial myelopathy
    a. phase
    A. Physiology Score

a. posterior multifocal placoid pigment
a. primary dementia
a. primary hemorrhagic meningoencephalitis
a. psychosis
a. psychotic break
a. purulent meningitis
a. schizophrenia
a. schizophrenic attack
a. schizophrenic episode
a. seizure
a. severe hypotension
a. situational depression
a. situational disturbance
sleeplessness associated with a.
a. steroid quadriplegic myopathy
a. stress disorder (ASD)
a. stress situational reaction
a. stroke
a. subdural hematoma
a. therapy
a. tolerance
a. toxic encephalopathy
a. transverse myelitis
a. transverse myelopathy (ATM)
a. trypanosomiasis
a. tubular necrosis
a. undifferentiated schizophrenic reaction (AU/SR)
a. whiplash

acutely acquired hemiplegia
acute-onset paraparesis
Acutrim
acyanotic
acyclic
acyclovir
AD
addict
adherent
admitting diagnosis
Alzheimer disease
AD Scale
ad
a. hominem
a. lib
a. nauseam
Ad7C cerebrospinal fluid test
ADA
Americans with Disabilities Act
ADA diet
ADAD
Adolescent Drug and Alcohol Diagnostic Assessment
adamantinoma
pituitary a.
ADAMHA
Alcohol, Drug Abuse, and Mental Health Administration
Adamkiewicz
artery of A.
Adams-Stokes
A.-S. disease
A.-S. syndrome
Adapin Oral

adaptability
cultural a.
a. profile
a. to stress
adaptation
air pollution a. (APA)
alloplastic a.
a. approach
autoplastic a.
Balthazar Scales for Adaptive Behavior II: Scales of Social A.
brightness a.
cross a.
dark a.
disease a.
a. disease
failure in social a.
fascicular a.
a. level theory
a. mechanism
migration a.
a. period
positive a.
a. reaction
reality a.
a. skill
social a.
a. syndrome
a. syndrome of Selye
a. time
adaptational
a. approach
a. dynamics
a. psychodynamic
adaptation-promoting therapy
Adapted Sequenced Inventory of Communication Development (A-SICD)
adapter, adaptor
Brown-Roberts-Wells ring a.
halo-ring a.
Telestill photo a.
adaptive
a. approach
a. behavior
A. Behavior Composite percentile
A. Behavior Evaluation Scale (ABES)
a. behavior inventory
A. Behavior Inventory for Children (ABIC)
A. Behavior Scale (ABS)
a. capacity
a. control of thought (ACT)
a. defense mechanism
a. delinquency
a. equipment
a. hypothesis
a. process
a. response
a. skill
a. skill domain
a. style
a. technique
a. testing

ADAS
    Alzheimer Disease Assessment Scale
    ADAS noncognitive subscale
adatanserin
ADC
    affective disorders clinic
    Aid to Dependent Children
    AIDS dementia complex
ADD
    attention deficit disorder
ADDBRS
    Attention Deficit Disorder Behavior
    Rating Scale
Adderall II
ADDES
    Attention Deficit Disorders Evaluation
    Scale
ADD-HA
    attention deficit disorder with
    hyperactivity
ADD-H: Comprehensive Teacher's
Rating Scale, Second Edition
(ACTeRS)
addict (AD)
    drug a.
    fellow drug a.
    food a.
    gambling a.
    narcotic a.
    object a.
    sex a.
addicting drug
addiction
    absinthe a.
    alcohol a.
    barbiturate a.
    biologic roots of a.
    a. center
    chemical a.
    cocaine a.
    cross a.
    drug a.
    enema a.
    ethyl alcohol a.
    heroin a.
    iatrogenic a.
    Internet a.
    laxative a.
    methadone a.
    methamphetamine a.
    methyl alcohol a.
    methylated spirit a.
    morphine a.
    narcotic a.
    nicotine a.
    object a.
    opiate a.
    opium a.
    a. organic psychosis
    polydrug a.
    polysubstance a.
    polysurgical a.
    proneness to a.
    a. psychiatry
    psychological a.

    relationship a.
    a. relationship
    A. Research Center Inventory
    a. root
    sedative a.
    A. Severity Index (ASI)
    sexual a.
    substance a.
    surgical a.
    sympathomimetic a.
    a. syndrome
    tobacco a.
    true a.
    work a.
addiction-prone personality (APP)
addiction-type organic psychosis
addictive
    a. behavior
    a. disease unit (ADU)
    a. disorder
    a. drug
    a. personality
    a. potential of drug
    a. risk
addictologist, addictology
Addison-Biermer anemia
Addison disease
addisonia
addisonian anemia
addition articulation
additive
    food a.
    a. W
addressability
    content a.
adduction weakness
adductor
    a. reflex
    a. spasmodic dysphonia
ADE, ADEM
    acute disseminated encephalomyelitis
A-delta fiber
ademonia
adendric, adendritic
adenine
    a. arabinoside
    a. molecule
adenocarcinoma
    mucin-secreting a.
adenohypophyseal, adenohypophysial
    a. cell
    a. compromise
    a. neoplasia
adenohypophysectomy
adenohypophysis
    agranular chromophobe cells in a.
adenohypophysitis
    allergic a.
    lymphocytic a.
adenoid
    a. cystic carcinoma
    a. type
adenoid-type adenoma
adenoma
    acidophil a.

ACTH-producing a.
adenoid-type a.
basophilic a.
choroid plexus a.
chromophil a.
chromophobic a.
cutaneous a.
endocrine-inactive pituitary a.
eosinophil a.
fetal a.
follicle-stimulating/luteinizing
  hormone a.
glycoprotein-secreting a.
gonadotropin-producing a.
growth hormone-producing a.
growth hormone-secreting a.
hypersecretory a.
intraspinal a.
invasive pituitary a.
islet cell a.
mixed growth hormone-prolactin
  cell a.
null-cell a.
pituitary a.
prolactin-producing a.
sebaceous a.
suprasellar a.
thyrotropin-producing a.
undifferentiated cell a.
adenomatoid
adenomectomy
  transsphenoidal selective a.
adenoneural
adenopathy
adenosine
  a. monophosphate
  a. triphosphatase
  a. triphosphate (ATP)
adenovirus
adenylate cyclase
adenylic acid
adequacy
  nutritional a.
adequate
  a. diet
  a. stimulus
  a. treatment
ADH
  alcohol dehydrogenase
  antidiuretic hormone
ADHD
  attention deficit hyperactivity disorder
  ADHD rituals
ADHD-PI
  attention deficit hyperactivity disorder-
  predominantly inattentive
adherent (AD)
adhesio, pl. adhesiones
  a. interthalamica
  a. interthalamica tumor
adhesion
  arachnoid a.
  interthalamic a.
  neuronal a.

adhesive
  a. arachnoiditis
  a. otitis media
ADI
  Adolescent Diagnostic Interview
  Adolescent Drinking Index
adiabatic fast passage
adiadochokinesis, adiadochocinesia,
  adiadochocinesis
adiaphoria
Adie
  A. tonic pupil
  A. tonic pupil syndrome
Adie-Holmes pupil
adience
adient behavior
adinazolam
Adipex-P
adipiodone
adipocele
adipocellular
adipocyte
adipogenesis
adipoid
adipolysis
adipometer
adiposalgia
adipose graft
adiposis cerebralis
adiposity
adiposogenital
  a. degeneration
  a. dystrophia
  a. dystrophy
  a. syndrome
adiposogenitalis
  dystrophia a.
adipsia, adipsy
aditus, pl. aditus
  a. ad aqueductum cerebri
  a. ad infundibulum
adjective
  A. Checklist (ACL)
  A. Rating Form (ARF)
adjoining pedicle
adjunctive
  a. individual session
  a. screw fixation
  a. therapy
  a. treatment
adjust
  a. repetitive behavior
adjustability
  3D positional a.
adjustable pedicle connector
adjustment
  attitude a.
  cultural a.
  A. Disorder, Acute
  A. Disorder, Chronic
  a. disorder with anxiety
  a. disorder with depressed mood
  a. disorder with disturbance of
    conduct

adjustment *(continued)*
a. disorder with mixed anxiety and depressed mood
a. disorder with mixed disturbance of emotions
emotional a.
a. following migration
a. interface disorder
a. inventory
inventory a.
life-cycle a.
marital a.
a. measure
a. mechanism
a. method
occupational a.
partial a.
personal a.
premorbid a.
a. process
psychological a.
a. reaction
a. reaction of adolescence
a. reaction of childhood
a. reaction conduct disorder
a. reaction disturbance
a. reaction of infancy
a. reaction of later life
a. reaction of menopause
a. reaction of middle age
a. reaction physical symptom
school a.
sexual a.
a. therapy
A. and Value
vocational a.
Vocational Evaluation and Work A. (VEWA)
Walker-McConnell Scale of Social Competence and School A.
withdrawal a.
adjuvant
Freund a.
a. whole-brain radiation therapy
Adkins spinal fusion
ADL
activities of daily living
adrenoleukodystrophy
extended ADL
ADL index
instrumental ADL
Northwick Park Index of Independence in ADL
ADL scale
ADL test
adlerian
a. psychoanalysis
a. psychology
a. psychotherapy
a. theory
Adler theory
Adlone Injection
ADLR
advanced design LINAC radiosurgery

ADmark Assay
administration
Alcohol, Drug Abuse, and Mental Health A. (ADAMHA)
anal a.
avenues of a.
Drug Enforcement A. (DEA)
enema drug a.
Food and Drug A. (FDA)
method of a.
parenteral drug a.
Social Security A. (SSA)
Veterans A. (VA)
administrative
a. psychiatry
a. segregation
a. therapy
admiration
excessive a.
need for a.
admissible
a. admission
a. evidence
admission
admissible a.
elective a.
first a.
informal a.
involuntary a.
prior to a. (PTA)
temporary a.
voluntary a.
admitting diagnosis (AD)
adnata
alopecia a.
adnerval, adneural
adolescence
adjustment reaction of a.
anxiety disorder of a.
avoidant disorder of a.
crushes in a.
a. developmental stage
disorder of infancy, childhood, or a.
early a.
emancipation disorder of a.
emotional disturbance of a.
fearfulness disorder of a.
gender identity disorder in a.
GID of a.
identity disorder of a.
introverted disorder of a.
late a.
middle a.
oppositional disorder of a.
overanxious disorder of a.
reaction of a.
sensitivity reaction of a.
withdrawal reaction of a.
adolescent
a. abuse
A. Alienation Index (AAI)
a. anxiety
autistic-presymbiotic a.
a. behavior

communication with a.
a. counseling
a. crisis
a. culture
delinquent a.
a. depression
Diagnostic Achievement Test
for A.'s
A. Diagnostic Interview (ADI)
Diagnostic Interview for Children
and A.'s
Diagnostic Interview for Children
and A.'s-Revised (DICA-R)
A. Drinking Index (ADI)
A. Drug and Alcohol Diagnostic
Assessment (ADAD)
a. drug use
evaluation of a.
Fullerton Language Test for A.'s
a. group therapy
a. guardedness
a. homosexuality
a. insanity
a. inventory
a. language quotient
A. Language Screening Test
"Let's Talk" Inventory for A.'s
A. Life Change Event
Questionnaire (ALCEQ)
Life Event Scale A.'s
limit-setting for a.
a. mania
Methodology for Epidemiology in
Children and A.'s (MECA)
Minnesota Multiphasic Personality
Inventory, A. (MMPI-A)
A. Multiphasic Personality
Inventory
a. negativism
a. neurotic delinquency
Offer Self-Image Questionnaire
for A.'s
a. onset
opinions toward a.'s (OTA)
a. pedophilia
a. personal identity
Personal Problems Checklist
for A.'s (PPC)
a. population
a. pregnancy
A. Problem Severity Index (ASPI)
a. psychiatry
a. psychology
a. psychotherapy
Responsibility and Independence
Scale for A.'s (RISA)
A. Self-Report Trauma
Questionnaire
A. Separation Anxiety Test
a. sexual activity
a. sexual change
a. sexual ideation
a. sexual identity
South Oaks Gambling Screen
for A.'s

a. suicide
a. support group
a. thinking
a. turmoil
a. turmoil reaction
a. voice
**Adolescent-Coping Orientation for
Problem Experiences**
**Adolescent-Family Inventory of Life
Events and Changes**
adolescent-onset
a.-o. conduct disorder
a.-o. epilepsy
adolescent-parent interview
adopt
adopted child
adoptee
a. family method
putative a.
adoption study
adoptive
a. care
a. caregiver
a. family
a. immunotherapy
ADP-ribosylation
pertussis-toxin-catalyzed
A.-r.
Adprin-B
Extra Strength A.-B.
ADR
adverse drug reaction
adrenal
a. axis
a. cortex
a. cortical hyperfunction
a. cortical insufficiency
a. crisis
a. disorder
a. gland
a. hyperplasia
a. medulla
a. medulla graft
a. medulla transplantation
adrenalectomy
adrenalin
adrenalin-mecholyl test
adrenarche
adrenergic
a. block
a. blockade
a. blocking agent
a. fiber
a. hyperstimulation
a. innervation
a. neurotransmission
a. receptor
a. synapse
a. system
adrenergic-response state
adrenochrome
adrenocortical
a. coma
a. insufficiency

adrenocorticotropic
- a. compromise
- a. hormone (ACTH)

adrenocorticotropin
adrenogenital syndrome
adrenoleukodystrophy (ADL, ALD)
adrenoleukodystrophy-adrenomyeloneuropathy (ALD-AMN)
adrenoleukomyeloneuropathy
adrenomedullary
adrenomyeloneuropathy (AMN)
adrenopathy
adrenopause
adriamycin
adroit
adromia
ADRS
Alzheimer Disease Rating Scale
Adson
- A. bipolar forceps
- A. brain-exploring cannula
- A. brain-extracting cannula
- A. brain suction tip
- A. brain suction tube
- A. clip-introducing forceps
- A. conductor
- A. cranial rongeur
- A. cup forceps
- A. dissecting hook
- A. dressing forceps
- A. dural hook
- A. dural knife
- A. dural needle holder
- A. dural protector
- A. dural protector guide
- A. elevator
- A. enlarging bur
- A. ganglion scissors
- A. hemilaminectomy retractor
- A. hemostatic forceps
- A. hypophyseal forceps
- A. knot tier
- A. laminectomy chisel
- A. modified maneuver
- A. needle
- A. nerve hook
- A. perforating bur
- A. right-angle knife
- A. scalp clip
- A. test
- A. tissue forceps
- A. wire saw

Adson-Anderson cerebellar retractor
Adson-Brown forceps
Adson-Mixter neurosurgical forceps
Adson-Rogers cranial bur
ADT
Auditory Discrimination Test
AdTech
- A. electrode guide
- A. electrode strip

Adtech Spencer platinum depth electrode
adterminal

ADU
addictive disease unit
adult
- a. abuse
- a. acid maltase deficiency
- Anxiety Scales for Children and A.'s (ASCA)
- Apraxia Battery for A.'s (ABA)
- A. Basic Learning Examination (ABLE)
- A. Career Concerns Inventory (ACCI)
- a. child of alcoholic (ACOA)
- consenting a.
- Culture-Free Self-Esteem Inventories for Children and A.'s
- A. Diagnostic and Treatment Center
- a. ego state
- Elizur Test of Psycho-Organicity: Children and A.'s
- a. foster home
- gender identity disorder in a.'s
- General Ability Measure for A.'s (GAMA)
- a. group therapy
- a. home
- a. motivation
- A. Neuropsychological Questionnaire (ANQ)
- nonconsenting a.
- North American Depression Inventories for Children and A.'s
- A. Performance Level Survey (APLS)
- A. Personal Adjustment and Role Skills
- A. Personal Data Inventory (APDI)
- A. Personality Inventory (API)
- physical abuse of a.
- A. Protective Services (APS)
- a. pseudohypertrophic muscular dystrophy
- Reitan-Indiana Neuropsychological Test Battery for A.'s
- a. respiratory distress syndrome (ARDS)
- a. Reye syndrome
- Scholastic Abilities Test for A.'s (SATA)
- a. scoliosis
- a. scoliosis patient
- a. scoliosis surgery
- A. Self-Expression Scale (ASES)
- sexual abuse of a.
- a. situational stress reaction (ASSR)
- a. social dysfunction
- stress effect on a.
- subclinical rhythmic epileptiform discharge of a. (SREDA)
- A. Suicidal Ideation Questionnaire (ASIQ)
- a. survivor of neglect

adulterate drug

adulteration of cocaine
adulterous
adultery
adulthood
    a. developmental stage
    early a.
    gender identity disorder of a.
    GID of a.
    late a.
    middle a.
    a. psychiatry
    young a.
adultomorphic
    a. behavior
    a. behavior role
    a. stance
adultomorphism
adult-onset
    a.-o. dystonia
    a.-o. epilepsy
    a.-o. obesity
advance
    phase a.
advanced
    a. cortical disease
    a. dementia
    a. design LINAC radiosurgery
      (ADLR)
    A. Placement Examination (APE)
    A. Placement Program (APP)
    A. Progressive Matrices
    a. sleep-phase pattern
    a. sleep-phase syndrome
advancement
    frontoorbital a.
    monobloc a.
    transcranial frontofacial a.
AdVans three dimensional digitizer
advantage
    economic a.
    a. by illness
    law of a.
    take a.
adventitial neuritis
adventitious
    a. motor flow
    a. movement
    a. reinforcement
adversary model
adverse
    a. drug reaction (ADR)
    a. effects of medication
    a. selection
    a. side effect
adversive attack
advertising psychology
advice
    against medical a. (AMA)
    discharged against medical a.
      (DAMA)
    medical a.
    signed out against medical a.
      (SOAMA)

Advil
    Children's A.
    A. Cold & Sinus Caplets
advocacy research
ADW
    assault with a deadly weapon
adynamia episodica hereditaria
adynamic ileus
AE
    accurate empathy
    anoxic encephalopathy
AED
    antiepileptic drug
Aedes aegypti
aego-dystonic
aegypti
    Aedes a.
aelurophobia (*var. of* ailurophobia)
AEP
    auditory evoked potential
AEq
    age equivalent
AER
    apical ectodermal ridge
    average evoked response
AERA
    average evoked response audiometry
aerasthenia, aeroasthenia
aeroacrophobia
aerodromophobia
aerodynamic speech analysis
aeroneurosis
aerophagia, aerophagy
aerophilus
    Haemophilus a.
aerophobia
aerosialophagy
Aerosol
    Fluro-Ethyl A.
aerosol
    a. inhalant
    a. spray abuse
    a. spray dependence
aeruginosa
    Pseudomonas a.
aerumna
Aesculap
    A. ABC cervical plating system
    A. bipolar cautery
    A. skull perforator
AESP
    applied extrasensory projection
aesthetic, esthetic
    environmentally a.
    a. pleasure
    a. value
AF
    alleged father
    anterior frontal
    arcuate fasciculus
    atrial fibrillation
AFDC
    Aid to Families with Dependent Children
affair
    accidental a.

affair *(continued)*
    extramarital a.
    instrumental a.
    withdrawal from social a.
affect
    abnormality of a.
    ambivalent a.
    angry a.
    apathetic a.
    appropriate a.
    assessment of a.
    A. Balance Scale
    bland a.
    a. block
    blunted a.
    broad a.
    charge of a.
    congruent a.
    constricted a.
    constriction of a.
    cooling of a.
    depressed a.
    depressive a.
    diminution of a.
    disorder of a.
    a. displacement
    displacement of a.
    a. display
    drama a.
    dramatic a.
    dull a.
    dysphoric a.
    elated a.
    emptiness of a.
    a. energy
    energy a.
    euphoric a.
    facial a.
    a. fantasy
    a.-fantasy
    a. fixation
    fixation of a.
    flat a.
    flattened a.
    fluctuating a.
    garrulous a.
    a. hunger
    impaired a.
    inappropriate a.
    incongruous a.
    infantile a.
    intense a.
    A. Intensity Measure
    a. intensity problem
    a. inversion
    isolation of a.
    labile range of a.
    a. memory
    modulated a.
    a. modulation
    a.-modulation
    mood and/or a. (M/A)
    negative a.
    normal a.

    painful a.
    predominant a.
    preservation of a.
    range of a.
    removed a.
    a. response
    restricted range of a.
    reversal of a.
    schizophrenic a.
    shallow a.
    shallowness of a.
    short-lived schizophrenic a.
    silly a.
    solemn a.
    a. spasm
    a. state
    strangulated a.
    superficial a.
    transformation of a.
    transposition of a.
    unstable a.
    vacuous a.
    a. within normal range
affectation
affected
    a. by feeling
    germinally a.
    a. pain
    proportion of survivors a. (PSA)
affection
    masked a.
affectional
    a. attachment
    a. bond
    a. drive
    a. life change
affectionate transference
affectionless character
affective
    a. ambivalence
    a. amnesia
    a. arousal
    a. bipolar disorder
    a. blunting
    a. cathexis
    a. change
    a. constriction
    a. depressive reaction
    a. determined disorder
    a. discharge
    a. disease
    a. disharmony
    a. disorders clinic (ADC)
    a. disorder syndrome
    a. disturbance
    a. dyscontrol
    a. dysregulation
    a. eudemonia
    a. experience
    a. expression
    a. feeblemindedness
    a. flattening
    a. function
    a. hallucination
    a. imagery

a. incontinence
a. insanity
a. instability
a. interaction
a. lability
a. melancholia
a. monomania
a. need
a. neurotic personality disorder
a. paranoid organic psychosis
a. and paranoid state
permissive hypothesis of a.
a. personality
a. prodrome of epilepsy
a. prodrome of migraine
a. psychosis
a. ratio
a. reaction type
a. reactivity
a. responsiveness
a. rigidity
a. separation
a. slumber
a. spectrum disorder
a. stupor
A. Style Index
a. suggestion
a. symptom of seizure
a. tone
affective-arousal theory
affectivity
flattened a.
a. ratio
affect-laden
a.-l. delusion
a.-l. paranoia
affectless
affectomotor pattern
affectosymbolic
afferent
a. digital lesion
a. digital nerve
a. feedback
a. fiber
a. motor aphasia
a. motor unit
a. nerve lesion
a. neuron
a. pupillary defect
a. stimulus interaction
affiliation
religious a.
affiliative
a. bonding
a. drive
a. need
affinin
affinity
affirmation
affirmative action
affirming the consequent
affix afflict
afflict
affix a.
affricate

AFI
amaurotic familial idiocy
afibrinogenemia
AFQT
Armed Forces Qualification Test
A-frame electrode
African
A. American vernacular English
East A.
A. sleeping sickness
A. trypanosomiasis
West A.
A. woodbine
after
a. glide
a. meals (p.c.)
afteraction
aftercare
a. group
a. worker
afterdischarge threshold
aftereffect
a. of drinking
figural a.
afterhyperpolarization
afterimage
memory a.
positive a.
Purkinje a.
afterloading catheter
aftermath of trauma
after-nystagmus
cycles of a.-n.
afterperception
afterpotential
aftersensation
aftershock
psychic a.
aftersound
aftertaste
aftertest
afterthought
aftertouch
aftervision
AG
angular gyrus
against medical advice (AMA)
agaric
fly a.
agarose
a. gel electrophoresis
low-melt temperature a.
agastroneuria
AGCT
Army General Classification Test
age
achievement a. (AA)
adjustment reaction of middle a.
anatomical a.
a. at onset
basal mental a.
Binet a.
biologic a.
bone a. (BA)
calendar a.

age *(continued)*
    ceiling a.
    characteristic a.
    chronologic a.
    Composite Psycholinguistic A.
    a. of consent
    a. correction
    a. correction procedure
    critical a.
    a. critique
    de retour a.
    developmental a.
    a. discrimination
    A. Discrimination in Employment
      Act
    educational a. (EA)
    a. effect
    emotional a.
    a. equivalent (AEq)
    a. equivalent scale
    functional a.
    a. group
    individual's a.
    legal a.
    mental a. (MA)
    middle a.
    new a.
    a. norm
    old a.
    a. peer
    physiological a.
    A. Projection Test (APT)
    a. ratio
    a. of reasoning
    a. regression
    relation to a.
    a. scale
    a. score
    social a. (SA, sa)
    stated a.
    stress effect in old a.
    test a. (TA)
    a. transition
    typical a.
age-appropriate
    a.-a. behavior
    a.-a. societal norm
**age-associated memory impairment
  (AAMI)**
aged
    abuse of the a.
Agee
    3M A. carpal tunnel release
      system
    A. technique
age-grade scaling
ageism
age-level behavior
age-matched individual
agency
    Federal Emergency Management A.
      (FEMA)
    health systems a. (HSA)

    home-service a.
    social service a.
agency-centered consultation
agenesis
    callosal a.
    corpus callosum a.
    a. of corpus callosum
    gonadal a.
    Pang type a.
    partial a.
    sacral a.
    sacrococcygeal a.
    total a.
agent
    adrenergic blocking a.
    alkylating a.
    alpha adrenergic blocking a.
    alpha receptor blocking a.
    anabolic a.
    antianxiety a.
    antibradycardiac a.
    antidepressant a.
    antidipsotropic a.
    antifibrinolytic a.
    antihypertensive a.
    antipanic a.
    antiparkinsonism a.
    antipsychotic a.
    anxiolytic a.
    azaspirodecanedione a.
    beta adrenergic blocking a.
    blocking a.
    butyrophenone a.
    calcium channel blocking a.
    catalytic a.
    causative a.
    cerebral vasodilating a.
    change a.
    a. of change
    chelating a.
    chemical a.
    chemotherapeutic a.
    contrast a.
    dibenzoxozepine a.
    etiological a.
    excitatory a.
    fibrinolytic a.
    ganglionic blocking a.
    heterocyclic a.
    hyperosmotic a.
    lacing a.
    MAOI-serotonergic a.
    monoamine oxidase inhibitor a.
    monoamine oxidase inhibitor-
      serotonergic a.
    monoamine oxidase inhibitor-
      tricyclic a.
    mood-stabilizing a.
    narcotic a.
    neuroleptic a.
    neuromuscular blocking a.
    offending a.
    a. orange
    phenothiazine a.
    possessing a.

a. provocateur
psychedelic a.
psychotomimetic a.
sedative-hypnotic a.
susceptibility a.
tantalum powder contrast a.
therapeutic a.
transforming a.
transmissible a.
in utero teratologic a.

agent-action
agent, action, and object
agent-object
agerasia
age-related
a.-r. cognitive decline
a.-r. deterioration
a.-r. feature
a.-r. hearing loss
a.-r. pharmacodynamics

age-specific feature
ageusia, ageustia
ageusic aphasia
agglutination
image a.

aggravated assault
aggregate
epileptic neuronal a.
gaze coordinating a.
neuronal a.

aggregated
technetium 99m albumin a.

aggregation
familial a.
a. problem

aggression
a. to animals
antipredatory a.
antisocial a.
authoritarian a.
destructive a.
domestic a.
healthy a.
hostile a.
husband-to-wife a.
identifying with a.
indirect a.
instrumental a.
inward a.
passive a.
a. to people and animals
physical a.
territorial a.
unassertive a.
verbal a.
wife-to-husband a.
a. without provocation

aggressive
a. behavior
a. behavior syndrome
a. behavior theory
a. disorder
a. drive
a. fantasy
a. impulse

a. instinct
a. invasion
a. obsession
oral a.
a. outburst
a. papillary middle ear tumor
(APMET)
passive a. (PA)
a. personality
a. predatory type
a. reaction
a. scale

aggressiveness
hostile a.

aggressor
identification with the a.

aging
activity theory of a.
biologic changes associated with a.
brain a.
cybernetic theory of a.
eversion theory of a.
neuroanatomy of a.
precocious a.
a. theory

agitans
paralysis a.
spasmus a.

agitata
amentia a.
cephalea a.
melancholia a.

agitated
a. behavior
a. depression
a. melancholia
a. patient
a. state

agitatio
animi a.

agitation
a. catatonic schizophrenia
emotional a.
extreme a.
mental a.
nighttime a.
onset of a.
physical a.
psychomotor a.
purposeless a.
unpredictable a.
unrelieved a.
untriggered a.
violent a.

agitative feature
agitographia
agitolalia
agitophasia
aglossia
agnathia
agnathous
agnea
agnesis
Kaplan a.
Toriello-Carey a.

agnesis *(continued)*
    Vici a.
    Wilson a.
AgNOR
    argyrophil organizer region protein
agnosia
    acoustic a.
    apperceptive visual a.
    associative visual a.
    auditory sound a.
    autotopagnosia a.
    body-image a.
    color a.
    corporal a.
    facial a.
    finger a.
    generalized auditory a.
    ideational a.
    localization a.
    object a.
    optic a.
    position a.
    selective auditory a.
    somatagnosia a.
    spatial a.
    tactile a.
    time a.
    topographical a.
    verbal auditory a.
    verbal visual a.
    visual a.
    visual-spatial a.
agnostic
    a. alexia
    a. behavior
agonadal
agonadism
agonist
    dopamine a.
    D_2-selective dopamine a.
    inverse a.
    M1 a.
    a. medication
    partial a.
    a. therapy
    vasopressin receptor a.
agonist/antagonist medication
agoramania
agoraphobia
    Mobility Inventory for A.
    panic disorder with a.
    panic disorder without a.
    a. without history of panic
      disorder
agoraphobic
    A. Cognitions Questionnaire
    panic a.
    panic a.
agrammatica
agrammatic speech
agrammatism agraphia
agrammatologia

agranular
    a. chromophobe cells in
      adenohypophysis
    a. cortex
agranulocytosis
    clozapine-induced a.
agraphia
    absolute a.
    acoustic a.
    acquired a.
    agrammatism a.
    a. alexia
    alexia with a.
    alexia without a.
    amnemonic a.
    a. amnemonica
    aphasic a.
    apraxic a.
    atactic a.
    a. atactica
    cerebral a.
    developmental a.
    jargon a.
    lexical a.
    literal a.
    mental a.
    motor a.
    musical a.
    optic a.
    phonological a.
    pure a.
    spatial a.
    verbal a.
agraphic
agreed-on
    a.-o. pattern
    a.-o. routine
agreement
    reciprocal a.
    separation a.
    subject-verb a.
agriothymia hydrophobica
agromania
agrypnia
agrypnocoma
agrypnodal coma
agrypnotic
AGS Early Screening Profile
AGT
    activity group therapy
agyiomania
agyiophobia
agyria
AH
    alcoholic hepatitis
    ataxic hemiparesis
AH4 Group Intelligence Test
**AH5 Group Test of High Grade
Intelligence**
**AH6 Group Test of High Level
Intelligence**
AHC
    alternating hemiplegia of childhood

AHI
active hostility index
anterior horn index
ahylognosia
ahypnia, ahypnosia
AI
allergy index
anxiety index
artificial intelligence
autoimmune
AICA
anterior inferior cerebellar artery
anterior inferior cerebral artery
anterior inferior communicating artery
Aicardi syndrome
aichmophobia
aid
Compoz Nighttime Sleep A.
A. to Dependent Children (ADC)
Electric Kool A.
electronic a.
external memory a.
A. to Families with Dependent
Children (AFDC)
first a.
functional a.
sexual a.
visual a.
walking a.
aide
child-care a.
home-health a.
aidoiomania
AIDP
acute inflammatory demyelinating
polyradiculoneuropathy
acute inflammatory demyelinating
polyradiculopathy
AIDS
acquired immunodeficiency syndrome
AIDS dementia complex (ADC)
AIDS encephalopathy
AIDS neuropathy
person with AIDS
aids
daily-living a.
eating a.
AIDS-related
A.-r. complex (ARC)
A.-r. myelopathy
A.-r. toxoplasmosis
A-IGP
activity-interview group psychotherapy
AIH
anterior interhemispheric approach
ailment
functional a.
ailurophilia
ailurophobia, aelurophobia
AIM
Artificial Intelligence in Medicine
aim
a. inhibition
instinctual a.

partial a.
a. transference
AIMD
abnormal involuntary movement disorder
aiming test
aimless
a. behavior
a. motor activity
a. wandering
AIMS
Abnormal Involuntary Movements Scale
AIN
American Institute of Nutrition
Ainsworth Strange Situation Test
AIP
acute inflammatory polyneuropathy
air
a. blade
a. blast
complemental a.
a. conduction
a. conduction deafness
a. conduction test
a. conduction testing
a. contrast study
cork the a.
a. drill
a. drinking
a. embolism
a. embolus
a. encephalopathy
a. hunger
a. plasma spray (APS)
a. plethysmography
a. pollution adaptation (APA)
a. pollution index
a. pollution syndrome (APS)
a. pressure effect
recycled a.
a. swallowing
tidal a.
a. tube
a. ventriculography
a. wastage
air-blade sound
air-bone gap
air-brain interface
Airlife MediSpacer
AIROM
active integral range of motion
airplane glue dependence
air-powered drill
AIRS
Amphetamine Interview Rating Scale
airstream mechanism
airway
artificial a.
a. control
a. edema
esophageal a.
a. protection
AIS
Abbreviated Injury Score
AIT
acute intensive treatment

AKA
   alcoholic ketoacidosis
   also known as
akari
      Rochalimaea a.
akataphasia, acataphasia
akathisia, acathisia
      neuroleptic dose-dependent a.
      neuroleptic-induced a.
Akerfeldt Test
akinesia
   a. algera
   a. amnestica
      neuroleptic-induced a.
   reflex a.
akinesthesia
akinetic
   a. apraxia
   a. autism
   a. depression
   a. drop attack
   a. drop spell
   a. epilepsy
   a. mania
   a. mutism
   a. psychosis
   a. seizure
   a. spell
   a. stupor
akinetic-abulic syndrome
Akineton
akoasm (*var. of* acoasm)
Akros
      A. extended care mattress
      A. pressure mattress
AK-Taine
aktamathesia
aktanoesis
Akureyri disease
AL
   annoyance level
ALA
   Activity Loss Assessment
ala, gen. and pl. **alae**
   a. cerebelli
   a. cinerea
   alae lingulae cerebelli
   a. lobuli centralis
   nasal a.
alabamensis
      Acremonium a.
alacrity
alae (*gen. and pl. of* ala)
alalia
   a. cophica
   a. organica
   a. physiologica
   a. prolongata
alanine
   a. aminotransferase (ALT)
   a. transaminase (ALT)
   a. tRNA
Al-Anon
alanyl
alanyl-tRNA synthetase

alar
   a. flutter
   a. lamina of neural tube
   a. ligament
   a. plate
   a. plate of neural tube
   a. screw
alarm
   a. clock headache
   a. reaction (AR)
   a. reaction stage
   ventilator a.
alarmist
alaryngeal speech
Alateen
alba
Albany Panic and Phobia Questionnaire
albedo
Albee
      A. lumbar spinal fusion
      A. olive-shaped bur
      A. shelf procedure
Albee-Delbert operation
albendazole therapy
Albenza
Albert Grass Heritage PSG
albicans
      Cryptococcus a.
albinism
albino
albocinereous
Albright disease
albumin
      technetium 99m macroaggregated a.
   a. transfusion
albuminocytologic dissociation
albuminurophobia
albuterol
ALC
   Alternative Lifestyle Checklist
   approximate lethal concentration
Alcadd Test
Alcaine
Alcar
ALCEQ
   Adolescent Life Change Event
      Questionnaire
alchemy
Alcock test
alcohol
      absolute a.
   a. abstinence
   a. abuse
   a. abuse scale
   a. acquired (non-wilsonian) chronic
      hepatocerebral degeneration
   a. acute intoxication
   a. addiction
   a. amnestic disorder
      amyl a.
   a. as cause of seizure
   A. Assessment and Treatment
      Profile
   a. binge
      blood a. (BA)

cannabis and a.
a. cerebellar degeneration
a. consumption
a. counseling
a. dehydrogenase (ADH)
a. delirium
a. dependence
a. derivative
a. detoxification
a. drinking
ethyl a.
a. habit
a. idiosyncratic intoxication
a. intolerance
a. intoxication-related disorder
isopropyl a.
methyl a.
a. on breath (AOB)
a. pathological intoxication
pathologic reaction to a.
a. poisoning
polyvinyl a. (PVA)
a. problem
a. related (AR)
toxic effects of a.
A. Usage Questionnaire (AUQ)
a. use disorder
A. Use Inventory (AUI)
a. withdrawal hallucinosis
a. withdrawal seizure
a. withdrawal syndrome
a. withdrawal tremulousness
alcohol-Antabuse reaction
alcohol-associated dementia
Alcohol, Drug Abuse, and Mental Health Administration (ADAMHA)
alcoholic
adult child of a. (ACOA)
a. amblyopia
amblyopia a.
a. amentia
a. amnesia
A.'s Anonymous (AA)
a. ataxia
a. binge
a. blackout
a. brain syndrome
a. cardiomyopathy
child of a. (COA)
a. cirrhosis (AC)
closet a.
a. coma
a. confusional state
a. delirium tremens
a. delirium withdrawal
a. dementia
a. deterioration
detoxified a.
a. drunkenness
a. epilepsy
a. family
a. gastritis
a. hallucination
a. hepatitis (AH)
inactive a. (IA)

a. insanity
a. intoxication
a. jealousy
a. ketoacidosis (AKA)
a. Korsakoff psychosis
a. liver disease (ALD)
a. liver disease-type organic psychosis
a. malabsorption syndrome
a. mania
a. myocardiopathy
a. myopathy
newly abstinent a.
a. organic mental disorder
a. pancreatitis
a. paralysis
a. paranoia
a. paranoid state
a. paraplegia
a. paresis
a. pellagra encephalopathy
a. peripheral neuropathy
a. polyneuropathy
a. possible pancreatic encephalopathy
a. pseudoparesis
a. rehabilitation
a. stupor
a. symptom
a. twilight state
type I a.
type II a.
alcoholicum
delirium a.
alcohol-induced
a.-i. anxiety
a.-i. nighttime sleep
a.-i. organic mental syndrome
a.-i. paranoid state
a.-i. peripheral neuropathy
a.-i. persisting dementia
a.-i. psychotic disorder with delusions
a.-i. psychotic disorder with hallucinations
a.-i. sexual dysfunction
alcoholism
acute a.
alpha a.
antisocial a.
a. associated with dementia
beta a.
chronic a.
delirium a.
delta a.
dementia associated with a.
developmentally cumulative a.
developmentally limited a.
Diagnostic Questions for Early or Advanced A.
epsilon a.
essential a.
Feighner criteria for a.
gamma a.
McAndrews A.

alcoholism *(continued)*
    mental disorder due to a.
    negative-affect a.
    a. organic psychosis
    reactive a.
    regressive a.
    Semi-Structured Assessment for the
      Genetics of A.
alcohol-methadone interaction
alcoholomania
alcoholophilia
alcoholophobia
alcohol-positive history (APH)
alcohol-precipitated epilepsy
alcohol-related
    a.-r. birth defect (ARBD)
    a.-r. insomnia
    a.-r. risk for accident
    a.-r. risk for suicide
    a.-r. risk for violence
    a.-r. seizure
    a.-r. use disorder, not otherwise
      specified
ALD
    adrenoleukodystrophy
    alcoholic liver disease
    Appraisal of Language Disturbances
Aldactazide
Aldactone
ALD-AMN
    adrenoleukodystrophy-
      adrenomyeloneuropathy
    ALD-AMN complex
aldehyde dehydrogenase
Aldoclor
aldolase
Aldomet
Aldoril
aldose reductase
aldosterone deficiency
alector
alektorophobia
alemmal
alendronate
alert
    a. awake state
    a. inactivity
    a. and oriented
alert, cooperative, and oriented (ACO)
alerting
    a. effect
    a. maneuver on
      electroencephalogram
    a. mechanism
    a. stimulus
    a. stimulus on electroencephalogram
alertness
    Academic A. (AA)
    level of a.
    a. level
    state of a.
    visual a.
alethia
Aleve

Alexander
    A. deafness
    A. disease
    A. technique
alexia
    agnostic a.
    agraphia a.
    a. anterior
    anterior a.
    auditory a.
    central a.
    cortical a.
    incomplete a.
    literal a.
    motor a.
    musical a.
    optical a.
    posterior a.
    pure a.
    sensory a.
    subcortical a.
    tactile a.
    verbal a.
    visual a.
    a. with agraphia
    a. without agraphia
alexithymia
alexithymic
    a. behavior
    a. personality
Alfenta Injection
alfentanil
algedonic
algera
    akinesia a.
    analgesia a.
    aphagia a.
    dyskinesia a.
algesia
algesichronometer
algesiogenic
algesiometer, algesimeter
    Aly a.
    Björnström a.
algesthesia
algetic
algica
    synesthesia a.
alglucerase
algodystrophy
algogenesia
algogenic psychosyndrome
algolagnia
    active a.
    passive a.
algolagniac
algolagnist
algologist
algology
algometer
algoneurodystrophy
algophilia, algophily
algophobia
algopsychalia

algorithm
    bone a.
    diagnostic a.
    Fourier transform a.
    hydrophobicity a.
    interpolation a.
algospasm
ALI
    acute lung injury
alias
    use of a.
aliasing
    frequency a.
    a. on electroencephalogram
alibi
alibiing
Alice in Wonderland syndrome
aliele
alielism
alielomorph
alien
    ego a.
    a. hand sign
    a. limb phenomenon
    a. obsession
    a. thought
alienate
alienatio mentis
alienation
    a. coefficient
    social a.
alignment
    pen a.
    sagittal anatomic a.
aliment
alimentary
    a. abstinence
    a. edema
    a. obesity
    a. orgasm
    a. seizure
alimentation
    enteral a.
    forced a.
    parenteral a.
alimentotherapy
aliphatic
    a. chain
    a. phenothiazine
aliquorrhea
aliquot
alkali
alkaline phosphatase
alkaloid
    belladonna a.
    ergot a.
    a. neuropathy
    opium a.
    rauwolfia a.
    vinca a.
alkalosis
    metabolic a.
    respiratory a.
    tetany of a.
Alka-Mints

alkaptonuria
Alksne iron suspension
alkyl
    amino-keto a.
alkylating agent
allachesthesia
Allah
all-American drug
alleged father (AF)
allele
    wild-type a.
allelic
    a. heterogeneity
    a. loss
allelomorph
allemand
    vice a.
Allen
    A. picture
    A. test
allenian
    a. theory
    a. therapy
allergen
allergenic
allergic
    a. adenohypophysitis
    a. angiitis
    a. encephalomyelitis
    a. encephalopathy
    a. jaundice
    a. psychogenic disorder
    a. reaction
    a. salute
allergy index (AI)
AllerMax Oral
allesthesia, alloesthesia
    visual a.
alleviating
    a. aggressive behavior
    a. violence
    a. violence in aggressive behavior
Allevyn dressing
alliance
    therapeutic a.
    working a.
Alliance for Mentally Ill Chemical Abusers
allied
    A. Health Professions Admission Test
    a. reflex
alligator
    a. cup forceps
    a. MacCarty scissors
all-median nerve hand
allobarbital
allocentric
allochiria, allocheiria
allocinesia (*var. of* allokinesis)
allocortex
allocortical cortex
allodynia
alloerotic
alloerotism, alloeroticism

alloesthesia (*var. of* allesthesia)
allogamy
allograft
 a. bone grafting
 fibular a.
 a. iliac bone
 a. strut
 Tutoplast a.
allogrooming
allokinesis, allocinesia
allolalia
allomeric function
allomorph
allonomous
allopathic species
allopathy
allophasis
allophone tabulation
alloplastic
 a. adaptation
 a. cranioplasty
 a. material
alloplasty
allopsychic delusion
allopsychosis
allopurinol
all-or-none reaction
allotoxin
allotriogeustia, allotriogeusia
allotriophagia, allotriophagy
allotriorhexia
allotriosmia
allotropic personality
allowance
 recommended daily a. (RDA)
Allport
 A. A-S Reaction Study
 A. group relations theory
 A. personality trait theory
Allport-Vernon-Linzey Study of Values
all-terrain
 a.-t. vehicle (ATV)
 a.-t. vehicle accident
all-trans retinoic acid receptor
allude
all-ulnar nerve hand
allusion in wit
allusive thinking
alma
 perdida del a.
almond nucleus
Alnico Magneprobe magnet
alogia
alogical thinking
aloin, belladonna, strychnine (ABS)
along
 getting a.
aloof
alopecia
 a. adnata
 androgenic a.
 a. areata
 a. capitis totalis
 a. celsi
 Celsus a.

cicatricial a.
a. cicatrisata
a. circumscripta
a. congenitalis
congenital sutural a.
a. disseminate
a. dynamica
a. follicularis
a. hereditaria
Johnston a.
a. leprotica
a. liminaris frontalis
lipedematous a.
male pattern a.
a. marginalis
a. medicamentosa
moth-eaten a.
a. mucinosa
a. neurotic
a. parviculata
patterned a.
a. pityrodes
postoperative pressure a.
postpartum a.
premature a.
a. presenilis
psychogenic a.
self-induced a.
a. senilis
stress-induced a.
a. symptomatica
syphilitic a.
a. syphilitica
a. totalis
a. toxica
traction a.
traumatic a.
a. triangularis congenitalis
trichotillomania-induced a.
a. universalis
Alor 5/500
Alpers disease
alpha, α
 a. activity
 a. adrenergic blocking agent
 a. adrenergic blocking drug
 a. adrenergic receptor
 a. adrenergic stimulating drug
 a. alcoholism
 a. apparent
 a. arc
 a. block
 a. blocking
 a. cell
 a. error
 a. ET
 a. ethyltryptamine
 a. examination
 a. factor
 a. feedback
 a. fetoprotein
 a. fiber
 a. frequency
 a. frequency band
 a. frequency coma

a. frequency range
a. index
a. interferon
a. level
a. mannosidosis
a. methyldopa
a. motor neuron
a. movement
a. pattern
a. receptor blocking agent
a. rhythm
a. spindle
a. state
a. tocopherol
a. verbal test
a. wave
a. wave strain
a. wave training
alpha-2 antagonist
alphabet
Initial Teaching A.
dl-**alpha-difluoromethylornithine (DFMO)**
alphalytic
alpha-methylacetoacetic aciduria
alpha-methyldopa-induced mood disorder
alphamimetic
alphaprodine hydrochloride
Alphavirus
alphoid
alpidem
alpinism
alprazolam
alprenolol
ALPS
Aphasia Language Performance Scale
ALS
amyotrophic lateral sclerosis
antilymphocyte serum
ALSD
Alzheimer-like senile dementia
alseroxylon
ALS-like syndrome
also known as (AKA)
ALS-PD
amyotrophic lateral sclerosis-Parkinson dementia
ALS-PD complex
Alström-Haligren syndrome
Alstrom syndrome
ALT
alanine aminotransferase
alanine transaminase
alteration
genomic a.
a. in identity
NMDA receptor a.
a. in rate of speech
reactive ego a.
receptor a.
a. in time perception
altered
a. auditory feedback (AAF)
a. level of consciousness
a. life circumstance
a. mental status

a. mentation
a. mind-body perception
a. sensation
a. sensory perception
a. state
a. state of consciousness (ASC)
a. vision
a. voice
alterego
alter ego
alternans
hemiplegia a.
alternate
a. binaural loudness balance (ABLB)
a. binaural loudness balance test
a. forms reliability coefficient
a. hemianesthesia
a. identity
a. monaural loudness balance (AMLB)
a. motion rate (AMR)
a. response test
a. uses test
alternating
a. behavior
a. bipolar disorder
a. current (AC)
a. hemiplegia of childhood (AHC)
a. hypoglossal hemiplegia
a. insanity
a. mydriasis
a. nystagmus
a. personality
a. perspective
a. psychosis
a. pulse
a. role
a. skew deviation
a. tremor
alternation
triple a.
alternative
a. behavior
a. criterion B for dysthymic disorder
a. diagnosis
a. dimensional descriptors for schizophrenia
graft material a.
least restrictive a.
a. lifestyle
A. Lifestyle Checklist (ALC)
a. occipital artery middle cerebral artery (AOA-MCA)
a. perspective
pharmaceutical a.
a. psychosis
a. school
a. treatment
viable a.
althesin
altitude
a. anoxia

altitude *(continued)*
    a. disease
    a. sickness
altitudinal hemianopia
altophobia
altricial
altricious
altrigendrism
Altropane
altruistic
    a. behavior
    a. personality
    a. role
    a. suicide
aluminum
    a. contouring template set
    a. cranioplasty
    a. glycinate
    a. hydroxide
    a. hydroxide with magnesium
      hydroxide and simethicone
    a. intoxication
    a. master rod
Alupent
Alurate
alvei (*pl. of* alveus)
alveolar hypoventilation syndrome
alveolus, pl. **alveoli**
alveus, pl. **alvei**
Aly algesiometer
alymphoplasia
    thymic a.
Alzheimer
    A. atrophic dementia
    A. basket
    A. disease (AD)
    A. Disease Assessment Scale
      (ADAS)
    A. disease noncognitive subscale
    A. Disease Rating Scale (ADRS)
    A. neurofibrillary degeneration
    A. sclerosis
    A. syndrome
    A. tangles
Alzheimer-like senile dementia (ALSD)
AM
    amplitude modulation
AMA
    against medical advice
amacrine cell
amalgam
    emotional a.
    emotional-object a.
Amanita
    A. *muscaria*
    A. *phalloides*
amanitin
amanitoxin
amantadine hydrochloride
Amaphen
amasesis
amathophobia
amative
amatory

amaurosis
    central a.
    a. centralis
    cerebral a.
    epileptoid a.
    a. fugax
    hysteric a.
    Leber congenital a.
    a. partialis fugax
    partialis fugax a.
    reflex a.
    toxic a.
    uremic a.
amaurotic
    a. axonal idiocy
    a. familial idiocy (AFI)
amaxomania
amaxophobia, hamaxophobia
amazonian
ambageusia
ambenonium
ambidexterity
ambidextrism
ambidextrous
Ambien
ambient
    a. air pressure
    a. behavior
    a. cistern
    a. noise
    a. temperature
ambiguity
    lexical a.
    role a.
    structural a.
    a. tolerance
ambiguous
    a. figure
    a. genitalia
    a. nucleus
ambiguus
    nucleus a.
ambilaterality
ambilevosity
ambilevous
ambiopia
ambisexual
ambisinister
ambisinistrous
ambisyllabic
ambitendency
ambivalence
    affective a.
    dual a.
    a. of the intellect
    a. of the will
ambivalent
    a. affect
    a. feeling
    a. quotient
ambiversion
ambivert
amblyaphia
amblygeustia

amblyopia
    alcoholic a.
    a. alcoholic
    arsenic a.
    color a.
    a. ex anopsia
    hysteric a.
    nutritional a.
    tobacco a.
    tobacco-alcohol a.
    toxic a.
    traumatic a.
ambon
ambulans
    paroniria a.
ambulation
    brace-free a.
    a. index
    a. skills
ambulatory
    a. automatism
    a. care
    a. EEG recording
    a. schizophrenia
    a. status
AMD
    acid maltase deficiency
AME
    A. microcurrent TENS unit
    A. PinSite shield
amebiasis
    cerebral a.
    Entamoeba histolytica cerebral a.
    Iodamoeba buetschlii cerebral a.
amebic
    a. aneurysm
    a. meningoencephalitis
ameboid
    a. astrocyte
    a. cell
ameboidism
ameliorate
amelioration
    tendency toward a.
amendment
    Drug Abuse Control A.'s (DACA)
amenia
amenomania
amenorrhea
    dietary a.
    dysponderal a.
    emotional a.
    nutritional a.
    pathologic a.
    physiological a.
    premenopausal a.
    primary a.
    secondary a.
    stress-related a.
amenorrheic
amentia
    a. agitata
    alcoholic a.
    a. attonita
    eclamptic a.

    isolation a.
    nevoid a.
    a. occulta
    a. paranoides
    a. phenylpyruvic
    phenylpyruvic a.
    primary a.
    Stearns alcoholic a.
AmerAsian
Amerge
americamania
American
    A. Academy of Otolaryngology
    A. Academy of Pediatrics
    A. Academy of Psychiatry and Law
    A. Academy of Stress Disorders
    A. College of Testing (ACT)
    A. dream
    A. Drug and Alcohol Survey
    A. Institute of Nutrition (AIN)
    A. Law Institute Formulation
    A. Law Institute formulation of insanity
    A. Law Institute rule
    A. Law Institute Test
    A. Musculoskeletal Tumor Society rating scale
    A. Optical (AO)
    A. Optical Hardy-Rand-Rittler color plate
    A. Psychiatric Association Index
    A. Psychiatry Association/Center for Mental Health Services
    A. silk suture
    A. Society for Testing and Materials
    A. Spinal Cord Injury Association classification
    A. Sterilizer operating table
    A. Veterans of World War II (AMVET)
    A.'s with Disabilities Act (ADA)
americanize
Ames demonstration
ametamorphosis
A-methaPred Injection
a-methylparatyrosine
AMI
    Athletic Motivation Inventory
Amicar
Amidate
amide
    lysergic acid a.
amidone
amidotrizoic acid
amikacin sulfate
Amikin
amiloride and hydrochlorothiazide
amimia
    amnesic a.
    ataxic a.
    expressive a.
amine
    biogenic a.

amine *(continued)*
    secondary a.
    tricyclic secondary a.
    tricyclic tertiary a.
amineptine
amino
    a. acid (AA)
    a. acid neurotransmitter
    a. acid transporter
aminoaciduria
    arginase deficiency a.
    argininosuccinic a.
    Baló a.
    carnosinemia a.
    cystathioninuria a.
    a. deficiency
    Devic a.
    histidinemia a.
    hydroxyisovaleric a.
    hyper-β-alaninemia a.
    hyperlysinemia a.
    hyperprolinemia a.
    isovaleric acidemia a.
    Marchiafava-Bignami a.
    methylmalonic a.
    neonatal tyrosinemia a.
    primary a.
    Schilder a.
    sulfite oxidase deficiency a.
    tyrosinemia a.
aminobenzoate
    butyl a.
    sodium a.
aminocaproic acid
aminoglutethimide
aminoglycoside
aminohydroxybutyric acid
amino-keto alkyl
aminopenicillin
aminophylline
4-aminopyridine
21-aminosteroid U74006F
aminotransferase
    alanine a. (ALT)
    aspartate a. (AST)
Amipaque
amisulpride
Amitone
Amitril
amitriptyline
    a. and chlordiazepoxide
    a. hydrochloride
    a. hydrochloride and
      chlordiazepoxide
    a. and perphenazine
amitriptyline-induced mood disorder
amixia
AML
    Automated Multitest Laboratory
AMLB
    alternate monaural loudness balance
Ammon
    A. horn
    A. horn sclerosis

ammonia intoxication
ammonium
    a. bromide
    a. chloride
    a. chloride delirium
    a. salicylate
    a. valerate
Ammons quick test
AMN
    adrenomyeloneuropathy
amnalgesia
amnemonic
    a. agraphia
    a. aphasia
amnemonica
    agraphia a.
amnesia
    acute a.
    affective a.
    a. after trance
    alcoholic a.
    amnesic a.
    antegrade a.
    anterograde a.
    asymmetrical a.
    audioverbal a.
    auditory a.
    autohypnotic a.
    axial a.
    Broca a.
    catathymic a.
    childbirth a.
    a. in children
    chronic a.
    circumscribed a.
    complete a.
    concussion a.
    continuous a.
    cortical a.
    degree of a.
    dissociative a.
    emotional a.
    episodic a.
    epochal a.
    evidence of a.
    a. evidence
    executive (or frontal) deficit
      transient global a.
    generalized a.
    global a.
    hippocampal a.
    hypnotic a.
    hysterical a.
    ictal a.
    infantile a.
    Korsakoff a.
    korsakoffian a.
    lacunar a.
    localized a.
    a. loss of memory
    neurological a.
    nonpathological a.
    olfactory a.
    organic a.
    partial a.

patchy retrograde a.
polyglot a.
postconcussive a.
postelectroconvulsive a.
posthypnotic a.
posttraumatic a. (PTA)
pretraumatic a.
profound a.
psychogenic a.
residual a.
retroactive a.
retroanterograde a.
retrograde a.
reversible a.
selective a.
shrinking retrograde a.
a. for sleep and dreaming
a. for sleep-terror event
subsequent a.
systematized a.
tactile a.
toxin-provoked a.
transient global a. (TGA)
traumatic a.
a. traumatica
true a.
verbal a.
visual a.
amnesiac
amnesic
a. amimia
a. amnesia
a. aphasia
a. apraxia
a. color blindness
a. state
amnesic-confabulatory syndrome
amnestic
a. aphasia
a. apraxia
a. confabulatory alcoholic psychosis
a. disorder
a. disorder due to a general
medical condition
a. dysnomia
a. episode
a. state
a. syndrome alcoholic psychosis
a. syndrome drug psychosis
amnestica
akinesia a.
amnestic-confabulatory syndrome
amniography
amobarbital
a. elixir
a. interview
a. and secobarbital
a. sodium
amodiaquine
amoeba
amok syndrome
amoral
a. behavior
a. psychopathic personality
a. trends psychopathic personality

amorophony
amorous paranoia
amorphagnosia
amorphism
amorphosynthesis
Amostat
amotivated behavior
amotivation
denial of a.
amotivational syndrome
amoxapine
amoxicillin
amoxicillin-clavulanic acid
AMPA
a-amino-3-hydroxy-5-methylisoxazole-4-
propionic acid
ampakine CX-516
Ampalex
ampere
amperozide
ampheclexis
Amphedroxyn
amphetamine (AMT)
a. abuse
a. aspartate
a. challenge test
a. delirium
a. delusional disorder
a. dependence
dextroamphetamine and a.
gamma hydroxybutyrate and a.'s
a. hydrochloride
a. inhaler
A. Interview Rating Scale (AIRS)
a. intoxication
a. intoxication, with perceptual
disturbance
a. look-alike
a. overdose
a. phosphate
a. poisoning
a. psychosis
racemic a.
smokable a.
substituted a.
a. sulfate
a. use disorder
a. withdrawal
amphetamine-induced
a.-i. anxiety
a.-i. psychotic disorder with
delusions
a.-i. psychotic disorder with
hallucinations
a.-i. sexual dysfunction
amphetamine-like
a.-l. action
a.-l. substance
amphetamine/methamphetamine
analog of a.
phencyclidine and a.
amphetamine-related disorder
amphicrania
amphierotism
amphigenesis

amphigenic inversion
amphigonadism
amphimixis
amphithymia
amphitypia
amphoric
amphoriloquy
amphorophony
amphotericin B
amphotonia, amphotony
ampicillin sodium
ampicillin-sulbactam
amp joint
amplification
    memory a.
    a. reaction
amplifier
    Botox injection a.
    compression a.
    gradient a.
    power a.
Ampligen
amplitude
    absolute band a.
    absolute EP a.
    asymmetry a.
    CMAP a.
    compound muscle action
     potential a.
    local reduction in a.
    a. modulation (AM)
    peak-to-peak a.
    reduction of a.
    relative band a.
    sensory nerve action potential a.
    SNAP a.
    very low a.
    waveform a.
ampullaris
    neuroepithelium cristae a.
ampullary
    a. crest
    a. limbs of semicircular ducts
amputation
    a. doll
    a. neuroma
amputee
AMR
    abnormal muscle response
    alternate motion rate
AMS
    Access Management Survey
    auditory memory span
Amsler grid testing
Amsterdam-type retardation
Amsustain
AMT
    amphetamine
    Anxiety Management Training
AMTR
    anteromedial temporal lobe resection
amuck
amulet
amurakh

amusia
    expressive a.
    motor a.
    sensory a.
    vocal a.
amusing aspect
AMVET
    American Veterans of World War II
amychophobia
amyelencephalia
amyelia
amyelinated
amyelinic
amyeloic, amyelonic
amyelous
amygdala, gen. and pl. amygdalae
    a. cerebelli
    nucleus amygdalae
amygdalar epilepsy
amygdaline
amygdalofugal
    a. fiber
    a. pathway
amygdalohippocampectomy
amygdaloid
    a. complex
    a. nucleus
    a. stimulation
    a. tubercle
amygdaloidectomy
amygdalotomy
amyl
    a. acetate
    a. alcohol
    a. chloride
    a. nitrate abuse
    a. nitrate inhalant
    a. nitrite
    a. salicylate
    a. valerate
amylase
    serum a.
amylobarbitone
amyloid
    a. angiopathy
    a. angiopathy cerebral
    beta a.
    congophilic a.
    a. deposition
    a. neuropathy
    a. precursor protein
    a. precursor protein gene
amyloidoma
amyloidosis
    cerebrovascular a.
    familial a.
    metabolic a.
    a. peripheral neuropathy
    skeletal a.
amyloidosis-Dutch type
amylophagia
amyoesthesia, amyoesthesis
amyoplasia congenita
amyostasia
amyosthenia

amyotaxy, amyotaxia
amyotonia congenita
amyotrophia
amyotrophic
    a. lateral sclerosis (ALS)
    a. lateral sclerosis-Parkinson
      dementia (ALS-PD)
    a. lateral sclerosis-Parkinson
      dementia complex
    a. type of spongiform
      encephalopathy
amyotrophy
    Aran-Duchenne a.
    asthmatic a.
    benign focal a.
    brachial a.
    diabetic a.
    dystonic a.
    hemiplegic a.
    juvenile a.
    monomelic a.
    neuralgic a.
    a. parkinsonism
    primary progressive a.
    progressive nuclear a.
    progressive spinal a.
    syphilitic a.
amyotrophy-parkinsonism
AMY plaque
amytal
    A. ablation
    A. interview
    A. Sodium
    sodium a.
AN
    anorexia nervosa
anabolic
    a. agent
    a. androgenic
    a. steroid
anabolism
anacamptometer
anacatesthesia
anachronism
    EEG a.
anachronobiology
Anacin
Anacin-3
anaclasis
anaclitic
    a. depression
    a. psychotherapy
    a. relationship
    a. therapy
anacoluthon
anacusis
ANAD
    anorexia nervosa and associated disorders
Anadenanthera
Anadrol
Anafranil
anaglyphoscope
anagoge, anagogy
anagogic
    a. interpretation

    a. symbolism
    a. tendency
anakatesthesia
anal
    a. administration
    a. canal
    a. character
    a. erotism
    a. fissure
    a. humor
    a. impotence
    a. intercourse
    a. masturbation
    a. personality
    a. phase
    a. rape
    a. rape fantasy
    a. reflex
    a. retention
    a. sadism
    a. sex
    a. sphincter
    a. sphincter manometry
    a. stage
    a. stage psychosexual development
    a. verge
anal-aggressive character
analeptic
anal-expulsive stage
analgesia
    a. algera
    a. dolorosa
    intrathecal morphine a.
    patient-controlled a. (PCA)
    pentazocine a.
analgesic
    controlled a.
    a. cuirass
    migraine-neuralgia a.
    nonnarcotic a.
analgesimeter
analgetic
analingus
analis
    coitus a.
anality
analog, analogue
    a. of amphetamine/methamphetamine
    a. to digital converter
    a. domain
    a. experiment
    a. filter
    libido a.
    a. marking
    a. of meperidine (PEPAP)
    a. of phencyclidine
    a. of phencyclidine thiophene
    a. study
    Vitamin D A.
analogic change
analogous
analogue (*var. of* analog)
analogy
analphabetic
anal-retentive personality

anal-sadistic love
analysand
analysis, pl. analyses
  acoustic a.
  active a.
  aerodynamic speech a.
  applied behavioral a. (ABA)
  auditory a.
  autoregressive model for signal a.
  behavioral a.
  best-fit a.
  biomechanical a.
  blind a.
  cephalometric a.
  cerebrospinal fluid a.
  chain a.
  character a.
  child a.
  classical a.
  clinical a.
  cluster a.
  compressed spectral a.
  computer-assisted EEG signal a.
  computerized EEG signal a.
  content a.
  contrastive a.
  control a.
  a. of coping style
  cost-benefit a.
  cost-reward a.
  a. of covariance (ANCOVA)
  critical a.
  Dasein a.
  deformity a.
  densitometric a.
  a. in depth
  Developmental Sentence A.
  didactic a.
  digital signal a.
  discriminant a.
  distal distinctive feature a.
  distinctive feature a.
  distributive a.
  DNA a.
  3D relationship a.
  ego a.
  electrooculographic a.
  error a.
  existential a.
  expectant a.
  factor a.
  fate a.
  feature a.
  feelings a.
  focused a.
  Fourier a.
  fractional a.
  furthest-neighbor a.
  gait a.
  grammatical a.
  handwriting a.
  haplotype a.
  harmonic a.
  hierarchical regression a.
  holistic a.

  a. of homonomy
  immunoblot a.
  impact a.
  individual a.
  interaction-process a.
  item a.
  job a.
  Kaplan-Meier survival a.
  kinesthetic a.
  kinetic a.
  latent class a.
  lay a.
  Leader Behavior A. II (LBAII)
  linear regression a.
  linkage a.
  Marriage Skills A. (MSA)
  methods a.
  minor a.
  mitochondrial deoxyribonucleic
    acid a.
  morphometric a.
  motivation a.
  multiple a.
  multivariate a.
  Natural Process A.
  neurometric a.
  occupational a.
  passive a.
  pattern a.
  perceptual a.
  personal document a.
  phenomenological a.
  philosophical a.
  phonemic a.
  phonetic a.
  phonological a.
  Picha-Seron Career A.
  policy a.
  power spectral a. (PSA)
  quantitative EEG a.
  quantitative motor unit potential a.
  A. of Readiness Skills
  regression a.
  a. of the resistance
  Sassouni a.
  Schicksal a.
  script a.
  segmental a.
  sequential multiple a. (SMA)
  short EEG epoch FFT a.
  signal a.
  situs a.
  solution a.
  sound a.
  Southern blot a.
  SPECT a.
  spectral a.
  substitution a.
  suprasegmental a.
  a. by synthesis
  a. and synthesis
  task a.
  task performance and a.
  Taylor-Johnson Temperament A.
    (T-JTA, TJTA)

therapeutic group a.
three-dimensional a.
total body neutron activation a.
  (TBNAA)
toxicological a.
traditional phonetic a.
training a.
Transactional A. (TA)
a. of transference
trial a.
a. of variance (ANOVA)
volumetric a.

analyst anchor test
analytic
a. boundary
a. couch
a. exegesis
a. frame
a. group psychotherapy
a. insight
a. interpretation
A. Learning Disability Assessment
a. method
a. neurosis
a. object
a. patient
a. psychiatry
a. rule
a. stalemate
a. treatment

analytical
a. breakdown
a. philosophy
a. play therapy
a. process
a. psychology
A. Reading Inventory

analyzer, analyzor
Axon sentinel-4 a.
breath a.
fast Fourier transformation
  spectrum a.
immunoturbidimetry a.
IVEC-10 neurotransmitter a.
noise a.
octave band a.
Time Use A.
wave a.

analyzing new information disturbance
Anametrin
anamnesis
associative a.
anamnestic response
ananabasia
ananastasia
anancasm
anancastia
anancastic
a. depression
a. neurosis
a. personality
anandamide
anandria
anapeiratic
anaphia, anhaphia

anaphor
anaphoric pronoun
anaphrodisia
anaphrodite
anaphylactic
a. shock
a. shock prophylaxis
anaphylactogenesis
anaphylactoid reaction
anaphylaxis
psychiatric a.
psychic a.
anaplasia
anaplastic
a. astrocytoma (AA)
a. ependymoma
a. focus
a. glioma
Anaprox
anaptic
anaptyxis
anarchic behavior
anarchis
anarchism
anarithmia literalis
anaritide
anarthria literalis
anastomosing fiber
anastomosis, pl. anastomoses
carotid-basilar a.
carotid-vertebral a.
cross-facial nerve graft a.
end-to-end a.
extradural a.
faciofacial nerve a.
faciohypoglossal a.
Galen a.
grafting a.
hypoglossal-facial nerve a.
intradural a.
intraterritorial anastomoses
leptomeningeal a.
Martin-Gruber a.
microneurovascular a.
microvascular a.
primary end-to-end a.
spinal accessory nerve-facial
  nerve a.
STA-MCA a.
temporal-cerebral arterial a.
anastomotic fiber
anatomic
a. hook
a. impotence
anatomical
a. age
a. midline
a. site of pain
a. snuffbox
a. variant
anatomy
biochemical a.
cervicothoracic pedicle a.
pedicle a.
surgical a.

anatonistic action
anatopism
anatripsis
anatriptic
anatrofin
anaudia
Anavar
anaxon, anaxone
ANB cephalometric measurement
ANC
    absolute neutrophil count
ancestor worship
ancestral spirit
anchone
anchor
    collapsing a.
    firing an a.
    Isola spinal implant system a.
    a. signs of withdrawal
    stacking a.
    stealing an a.
    a. symptom
    a. test
    traction a.
anchorage-dependent signal
anchoring
    perceptual a.
    a. point
anchors/responses
    integrating a.
ancillary care
ANCOVA
    analysis of covariance
ancraophobia
Ancylostoma ceylanicum
ancyroid, ankyroid
Andersch ganglion
Anderson-Adson scalp retractor
Andes disease
André anatomical hook
Andresen Six-Basic-Factors-Model
  Questionnaire (A-SBFM)
Andrews frame
Androcur
androgen
    a. insensitivity syndrome
    a. level
androgenesis
androgenic
    a. alopecia
    anabolic a.
androgynization
androgynoid
androgynous individual
androgyny
android
andromania
andromimetic
andromorphous
androphilia
androphobia
androsterone
anecdotal method
anecdote
anechoic chamber

anejaculatory orgasm
anelectrotonic zone
anelectrotonus
Anel method
anemia
    Addison-Biermer a.
    addisonian a.
    aplastic a.
    cerebral a.
    chlorotic a.
    Cooley a.
    drug-induced a.
    familial splenic a.
    Fanconi a.
    hemolytic a.
    iron deficiency a.
    macrocytic megaloblastic a.
    megaloblastic a.
    nutritional a.
    pernicious a.
    postoperative a.
    sickle cell a.
anemic
    a. anoxia
    a. hypoxia
anemometer
    warm-wire a.
anemophobia
anencephalia
anencephalous
anencephaly
anepia
anepithymia
anerethisia
Anergan
anergasia
anergastic
    a. organic psychosis
    a. reaction
anergia
    physical a.
anergic
    a. depression
    a. schizophrenic
    a. stupor
anergy
    denial of a.
    denial of anhedonia, amotivation
    or a.
Anestacon
anesthekinesia, anesthecinesia
anesthesia
    barbiturate burst-suppression a.
    block a.
    bulbar a.
    central a.
    closed a.
    combined a.
    compression a.
    conduction a.
    continuous intravenous regional a.
    (CIVRA)
    conversion a.
    corneal a.
    crash induction of a.

crossed a.
cutaneous a.
diagnostic a.
dissociated a.
dissociative a.
doll's head a.
a. dolorosa
electric a.
emotional a.
first stage of a.
frost a.
gauntlet a.
general endotracheal a.
general orotracheal a.
girdle a.
glove a.
gustatory a.
Gwathmey a.
halogenated inhalational a.
halothane a.
hypnotic a.
hysterical a.
infiltration a.
inhaled a.
insufflation a.
insulation a.
intravenous regional a. (IVRA)
isoflurane a.
laryngeal a.
local a.
Mayo block a.
mental a.
muscular a.
neuroleptic a.
olfactory a.
painful a.
perineural a.
peripheral a.
pharyngeal a.
pressure a.
primary a.
ring block a.
SAB a.
saddle-shaped a.
segmental a.
sensory a.
sexual a.
spinal a.
splanchnic a.
stocking a.
stocking-glove a.
tactile a.
thalamic hyperesthetic a.
thermal a.
thermic a.
traumatic a.
unilateral a.
visceral a.
anesthesimeter
anesthetic
a. conversion reaction
eutectic mixture of local a.'s
(EMLA)
a. leprosy
a. monitoring

anethopath
anethopathy, anetopathy
aneuploidy
aneuroid chest bellows
aneurolemmic
aneurysm
amebic a.
anterior circulation intracranial a.
anterior communicating artery a.
arteriosclerotic intracranial a.
arteriovenous a.
aspergillotic a.
atherosclerotic a.
bacterial a.
basilar apex a.
basilar artery trunk a.
basilar bifurcation a.
basilar tip a.
berry a.
bilobed a.
blister-like a.
carotid a.
carotid cave a.
carotid-ophthalmic artery a.
cavernous-carotid a.
cavernous sinus a.
cerebral a.
Charcot-Bouchard intracerebral a.
circle of Willis a.
cirsoid a.
clinoidal a.
a. clip
a. clip applicator
clip ligation of a.
a. clipping
coating of a.
congenital a.
cranial a.
de novo a.
dissecting a.
distal anterior cerebral artery a.
dolichoectatic a.
dome of a.
extracerebral a.
extracranial a.
feeding artery of a.
fundus of a.
fusiform a.
giant cervical carotid artery a.
great cerebral vein of Galen a.
hunterian ligation of a.
Hunt-Kosnik classification of a.
hypophysial a.
incidental a.
infectious a.
infraclinoid a.
internal carotid artery a.
intracavernous carotid a.
intracerebral a.
intracranial a.
intranidal a.
lower basilar a.
luetic a.
miliary a.
M1 segment a.

aneurysm *(continued)*
    multiple intracranial a.'s (MIA)
    mycotic a.
    mycotic intracranial a.
    neck of a.
    a. neck dissector
    a. needle
    neoplastic a.
    a. occlusion
    ophthalmic artery a.
    ophthalmic segment a.
    paraclinoid internal carotid artery a.
    a. of persistent trigeminal artery
      (APTA)
    PICA a.
    posterior communicating artery a.
    posterior fossa a.
    posterior inferior communicating
      artery a.
    precursor sign to rupture of a.
    prerupture of a.
    rebleeding of a.
    rerupture of a.
    ruptured a.
    saccular a.
    sellar a.
    serpentine a.
    spirochetal a.
    supraclinoid a.
    thrombosed a.
    a. trapping
    trapping of a.
    traumatic intracranial a. (TICA)
    unruptured a.
    unspecified a.
    vein of Galen a.
    venous a.
    vertebrobasilar a.
    wide-necked a.
    wrapping of a.
aneurysmal
    a. bleeding
    a. bone cyst
    a. bruit
    a. bulging
    a. clipping operation
    a. dilation
    a. dome
    a. hemorrhage
    a. rebleed
    a. rest
    a. rupture
    a. subarachnoid hemorrhage
      (ASAH)
aneurysmectomy
aneurysmoplasty
aneurysmorrhaphy
aneurysmotomy
Anexsia
Angell James dissector
Angelman syndrome
Angelucci syndrome
anger
    a. attack

    constant a.
    difficulty controlling a.
    a. dysregulation
    fit of a.
    ineffective a.
    intense a.
    irrational a.
    a. mallet
    marked a.
    outburst of a.
    a. reaction
    a. and violence psychiatric
      syndrome
angiitis
    allergic a.
    granulomatous a.
    isolated a.
    necrotizing a.
angina
    a. pectoris sine dolore
    Prinzmetal a.
anginophobia
angioarchitecture
angioblastic meningioma
angioblastoma
angiocentric immunoproliferative lesion
Angioconray
angiodysgenetic myelomalacia
angioedema
angioendothelioma
    malignant endovascular papillary a.
angioendotheliomatosis
    neoplastic a.
angiofibroma
    juvenile a.
    nasopharyngeal a.
angiogenesis
angiogenic
    a. inducer
    a. response
angioglioma
angiogliomatosis
angiogliosis
angioglomoid tumor
Angiografin
angiogram
    blush of dye on a.
    carotid a.
    cerebral digital a.
    digital subtraction a.
    four-vessel cerebral a.
    innominate a.
    intercostal artery a.
    internal carotid a.
    intraarterial digital subtraction a.
      (IADSA)
    magnetic resonance a.
    MR a.
    postembolization a.
    postoperative a.
    preoperative a.
    Seldinger a.
    small angle double incidence a.
      (SADIA)
    vertebral a.

angiogram-negative SAH
angiographic
- a. catheter
- a. finding
- a. recanalization
- a. reference system (ARS)
- a. road-mapping technique
- a. targeting
- a. targetry
- a. vasospasm

angiographically
- a. confirmed
- a. occult intracranial vascular malformation (AOIVM)
- a. occult vascular malformation (AOVM)
- a. visualized vascular malformation (AVVM)

angiography
- baseline a.
- cerebral a.
- closed a.
- contrast a.
- cut-film a.
- 2DFT time-of-flight MR a.
- digital a.
- digital intravenous a.
- digital subtraction a. (DSA)
- digital subtraction venous a.
- helical CT a.
- intracranial MR a.
- intraoperative a.
- magnetic resonance a. (MRA)
- open a.
- orthogonal a.
- preoperative a.
- spinal a.
- stereomagnification a.
- stereotactic a.
- superselective a.
- vertebral a.

angioid streak
angio image
AngioJet rapid thrombectomy system
angiokeratoma corporis diffusum
angiokinetic
angiolipoma
- epidural a.
- spinal epidural a.

angiolithic sarcoma
angioma
- arteriovenous interhemispheric a.
- capillary a.
- cavernous a.
- cerebral cavernous a.
- cutaneous a.
- encephalic a.
- extracerebral cavernous a.
- intracranial cavernous a.
- intradermal a.
- retinal a.
- supratentorial cavernous a.
- venous a.

angiomatosis
- cephalotrigeminal a.

cerebral a.
cerebroretinal a.
congenital dysplastic a.
corticomeningeal a.
cutaneomeningospinal a.
Divry-van Bogaert familial corticomeningeal a.
encephalotrigeminal a.
leptomeningeal a.
meningeal a.
mesencephalooculofacial a.
neurocutaneous a.
neuroretinal a.
oculoencephalic a.
Rendu-Osler a.
retinocerebral a.
telangiectatic a.

angionecrosis
angioneurectomy
angioneuredema
angioneurosis
angioneurotic edema
angioneurotomy
angioparalytic neurasthenia
angiopathic neurasthenia
angiopathy
- amyloid a.
- cerebral amyloid a.
- congenital dysplastic a.
- congophilic a.
- radiation a.

angiophacomatosis, angiophakomatosis
angioplastic meningioma
angioplasty
- balloon a.
- computed tomographic a. (CTA)
- percutaneous transluminal coronary a. (PTCA)
- transluminal a.

angioreticuloma
angiosarcoma
angiostrongyliasis
Angiostrongylus costaricensis
angiotensin II
angiotomomyelography
angiotropic lymphoma
angle
- cephalic a.
- cephalomedullary a.
- cephalometric a.
- cerebellopontine a.
- cervicothoracic pedicle a.
- Citelli a.
- craniofacial a.
- flip a.
- a. meningioma
- pedicle axis a.
- phase a.
- pontine a.
- a. position potentiometer
- pulse flip a.
- Rolando a.
- sagittal pedicle a.
- Schmidt-Fischer a.
- sinodural a.

angle (*continued*)
    sylvian a.
    tentorial a.
    transverse pedicle a.
    venous a.
angle-closure glaucoma
angled
    a. aneurysm clip
    a. awl
    a. needle
    a. nerve root retractor
anglomania
anglophilia
anglophobia
Angola
angophrasia
angor
    a. animi
    a. ocularis
    a. pectoris
angry
    a. affect
    a. behavior
    a. outburst
    a. reaction
    a. reaction to minor stimuli
    a. woman syndrome
    a. word exchange
angst
anguish
    existential a.
    post-binge a.
angular
    a. convolution
    a. frequency
    a. gyrus (AG)
    a. knife
    a. momentum
    a. position
angulation
    radii of a.
    radius of a.
    screw a.
anhalonine
anhaphia (*var. of* anaphia)
anhedonia
    orgasmic a.
    pervasive a.
anhedonia-asociality
anhedonism
anhydrase
    carbonic a.
anhydration
anhydrous
anhypnia
ani
    pruritus a.
aniconia
anicteric
anile
aniled sense of self
anileridine
anilides
anilinction

anilinctus
anilingus
anility
anima
animal
    a. abuse
    a. magnetism
    A. and Opposite Drawing Technique (AODT)
    a. phobia
    a. psychology
    a. tranquilizer
animal/insect phobia
animals
    aggression to a.
    aggression to people and a.
animal-type specific phobia
animate
animation
    suspended a.
animato
animi
    a. agitatio
    angor a.
    demissio a.
animistic thinking
animus
anisocoria
anisomastia
anisonucleosis
anisotrophy
    chemical shift a.
anisotropic 3DFT
anisotropy of white matter
ankle
    a. clonus
    a. jerk
    a. reflex
ankle-brachial index (ABI)
ankyloglossia
ankylosing spondylitis
ankylosis
    cricoarytenoid a.
ankylostoma
ankyroid (*var. of* ancyroid)
anlage, pl. **anlagen**
Annamese
Ann Arbor Learning Inventory and Remediation Program
annectent gyrus
Annett hand preference scale
annihilation anxiety
annihilator
annihilatory
anniversary
    a. date
    a. excitement
    a. hypothesis
    a. reaction
annoyance level (AL)
annular radial rupture
annulment
annulospiral
    a. ending

a. fiber
a. organ
annulus
a. fibrosus
a. fibrous disci intervertebralis
fissure of a.
a. tendineus
a. of Vieussens
a. of Zinn
annuracetam
ano
coitus in a.
anochlesia
anociassociation
anocithesia
anodal block
anode
anodyne
anoesis
anoetic
anoexigenic
anogenital
anoia
anomalotrophy
anomalous
a. branching
a. movement
a. nonrecurrent right inferior
laryngeal nerve
a. origin
a. sexual behavior
a. sexual urge
anomaly
Aristotle a.
autosomal a.
congenital a.
cranial a.
craniofacial a.
duplication a.
ear a.
laryngeal a.
megadolichobasilar a.
megadolichovertebrobasilar a.
metabolic a.
multiple congenital a. (MCA)
sexual a.
anomia
color a.
finger a.
tactile a.
anomic
a. aphasia
a. error
a. suicide
anomie
anonacein
anonymity
anonymous
Alcoholics A. (AA)
Cocaine A.
Codependents A. (CODA)
Dropouts A.
Gamblers A. (GA)
Narcotics A. (NA)
Overeaters A. (OA)

Parents A.
Schizophrenics A.
Workaholics A.
anophthalmia
X-linked a.
anopsia
amblyopia ex a.
Anoquan
anorectal
a. atresia
a. physiological dysfunction
a. spasm
anorectic, anoretic
A. Attitude Questionnaire
Anorex
anorexia
elective a.
a. nervosa (AN)
a. nervosa and associated disorders
(ANAD)
social a.
anorexiant
anorexic
A. Behavior Scale
a. fast
anorexigenic
anorgasmic
anorgasmy, anorgasmia
anorthography
anorthosis
anosmia
essential a.
functional a.
mechanical a.
reflex a.
respiratory a.
true a.
anosmic
anosodiaphoria
anosognosia
anosognosic
a. epilepsy
a. seizure
anosphrasia
anospinal center
anosteoplasia
anostosis
ANOVA
analysis of variance
anoxemia
anoxia
acute a.
altitude a.
anemic a.
birth a.
cerebral a.
corneal a.
fulminating a.
hypokinetic a.
metabolic a.
perinatal a.
perioperative a.
terminal a.
anoxic
a. damage

anoxic *(continued)*
    a. encephalopathy (AE)
    a. hypoxia
    a. ischemia
ANP
    atrial natriuretic peptide
ANQ
    Adult Neuropsychological Questionnaire
ANS
    autonomic nervous system
ansa, gen. and pl. **ansae**
    Haller a.
    lenticular a.
    ansae nervorum spinalium
    peduncular a.
    Reil a.
    Vieussens a.
Ansaid Oral
ANSER System
ansiform lobule
ansotomy
Anspach
    A. craniotome
    A. drill
    A. 65K drill
    A. 65K instrument system
    A. 65K neuro system
Anstie rule
answer
    bizarre a.
    irrelevant a.
    syndrome of approximate
      relevant a.'s
    syndrome of deviously relevant a.'s
Antabuse
antagonism
    pharmacological a.
    physiological a.
antagonist
    alpha-2 a.
    benzodiazepine a.
    beta-adrenergic a.
    excitotoxic neurotransmitter a.
    5HT1A a.
    a. medication
    narcotic a.
    opiate a.
    opioid a.
antagonistic
    a. behavior
    a. muscle strength
    a. reflex
antalgic
    a. gait
    a. limp
antaphrodisiac
antapoplectic
antasthenic
antebrachial cutaneous nerve
antebrachium
antecedent
    a. event
    a. variable
antecedent-consequence variable

antegrade amnesia
antepartum
antephialtic
antergia
anterior
    alexia a.
    a. alexia
    a. basal encephalocele
    a. bulb syndrome
    a. callosotomy
    a. cavernous sinus space
    a. C1-C2 screw approach
    a. C1-C2 screw fixation
    a. central convolution
    a. central gyrus
    a. cerebral artery (ACA)
    a. cervical approach to
      cervicothoracic junction
    a. cervical cord syndrome
    a. cervical discectomy and fusion
    a. cervical fusion (ACF)
    a. cervical spine surgery
    a. cervical surgery vocal cord
      damage
    a. cervicothoracic junction surgery
    a. choroidal artery (ACA)
    a. cingulate
    a. cingulate cortex
    a. cingulate gyrus
    a. cingulate gyrus tumor
    a. cingulate pathway
    a. cingulate prefrontal syndrome
    a. circulation intracranial aneurysm
    a. circulation stroke
    a. clinoid
    a. clinoid process
    a. colliculus
    a. column disruption
    a. column of medulla oblongata
    a. column osteosynthesis
    a. commissure (AC)
    a. commissure-posterior commissure
      line
    a. commissure-posterior commissure
      reference point
    a. communicating artery (ACoA,
      AComA)
    a. communicating artery aneurysm
    a. communicating artery distribution
      infarction
    a. construct
    a. cord impingement
    a. corpectomy
    a. correction
    a. cortex penetration
    a. cranial base
    a. cranial fossa surgery
    a. decompression
    a. digastric muscle
    a. discectomy
    a. distraction instrumentation
    a. extradural clinoidectomy
    a. extremity of caudate nucleus
    a. feature English phoneme
    a. frontal (AF)

a. funiculus
a. ground bundle
a. horn
a. horn cell disease
a. horn cell motor impairment
a. horn index (AHI)
a. inferior cerebellar artery (AICA)
a. inferior cerebral artery (AICA)
a. inferior communicating artery (AICA)
a. interbody fusion
a. interhemispheric approach (AIH)
a. intermediate groove
a. internal fixation device
a. internal stabilization
a. interosseous nerve
a. ischemic optic neuropathy
a. ischemic otic neuropathy
a. Kostuik-Harrington distraction system
a. limbic association area
a. limb of internal capsule
a. lobectomy
a. lobe of hypophysis
a. longitudinal ligament
a. lower cervical spine surgery
a. lumbar spine interbody fusion
a. lunate lobule
a. median fissure of medulla oblongata
a. median fissure of spinal cord
a. medullary velum
a. meningeal artery
a. metallic fixation
a. neutralization
a. notch of cerebellum
a. nuclei of thalamus
nucleus ventralis a.
a. parietal lesion
a. parolfactory sulcus
a. partial laryngectomy
a. part of pons
a. perforated substance
a. pillar of fornix
a. piriform gyrus
a. pituitary insufficiency
a. plate fixation
a. plexus
a. polar-amygdalar epilepsy
a. pyramid
a. rhizotomy
a. root
a. scalene muscle
a. screw fixation
a. serratus muscle
a. short-segment stabilization
a. speech zone
a. spinal artery
a. spinal artery syndrome
a. spinal fixation
a. spinal plating
a. stabilization procedure
a. surgical exposure
a. temporal artery (ATA)
a. temporal lobectomy (ATL)

a. triangle approach
a. tubercle of thalamus
a. vein of septum pellucidum
ventralis oralis a. (Voa)
a. vertical canal
a. white commissure
anteriorly retracted
anterior-posterior fusion with SSI
anterochiasmatic lesion
anterodorsalis
nucleus a.
anterodorsal thalamic nucleus
anterograde
a. amnesia
a. fast component neuropathy
a. loss of memory
a. memory
a. memory interference
anterolateral
a. cordotomy
a. groove
a. sulcus
a. tractotomy
anteromedial
a. approach
a. incision
a. retropharyngeal approach
a. temporal lobe resection (AMTR)
a. thalamic nucleus
anteromedialis
nucleus a.
anteromedian groove
anteromesial temporal lobectomy
anteroposterior
a. projection
a. talocalcaneal (APTC)
anterotic
anteroventralis
nucleus a.
anteroventral thalamic nucleus
anthelix
anthomania
anthophilous
anthophobia
anthracycline
lipophilic morpholino a.
anthrax
cerebral a.
anthrophobia
anthropocentric
anthropocentrism
anthropocracy
anthropogenic
anthropography
anthropoid
anthropological linguistics
anthropology
applied a.
criminal a.
cultural a.
medical a.
physical a.
anthropometric identification
anthropometrics
anthropometry

anthropomorphic face
anthropomorphism
anthropomorphize
anthroponomy
anthropopathism
anthropopathy
anthropophagus
anthropophilic
anthropophobia
anthroposcopy
anthypnotic (*var. of* antihypnotic)
anthysteric (*var. of* antihysteric)
antiacetylcholine
anti-AChE
    anticholinesterase
antiadrenergic effect
antiadrenogenic
antialias filtering
antianalytic
antiandrogen therapy
antianxiety
    a. agent
    a. medication
antiarrhythmic
antibiotic
    intrathecal a.
    a. penetration
    a. powder
antibradycardiac agent
antibrain
anticatalyst
anticataplectic
anticathexis
anticephalalgic
Anticept
anticholinergic
    a. delirium
    a. drug
    a. property
    a. side effect
    a. syndrome
anticholinesterase (anti-AChE)
anticipation
    a. of role
    a. of trigger
anticipatory
    a. anxiety
    a. autocastration
    a. avoidance (AA)
    a. coarticulation
    a. error
    a. grief
    a. guidance
    a. response
    a. and struggle behavior
anticipatory-maturation principle
anticoagulant
    lupus a. (LA)
anticoagulation
    A. Service
    a. therapy
anticonformity
anticonvulsant
    a. drug
    a. intoxication

    a. medication-induced postural
      tremor
    a. prophylaxis
    a. therapy
anticonvulsive
anticus
    scalenus a.
    tetanus a.
antidepressant
    a. agent
    atypical a.
    heterocyclic a. (HCA)
    a. medication
    a. medication-induced postural
      tremor
    monocyclic a.
    tetracyclic a.
    a. treatment
    a. treatment-induced manic episode
    triazolopyridine a.
    tricyclic a. (TCA)
antidepressant-resistant
antidepressant-type abuse
antidipsotropic agent
antidiuretic hormone (ADH)
antidopaminergic
antidote
    British anti-Lewisite a.
    a. drug
antidromic
    a. conduction studies
    a. response
antiemetic
antiepileptic
    a. drug (AED)
    a. drug-induced bone disease
    a. medication
antierotica
antiestrogenic
antiexpectancy speech
antiferromagnetism
antifetishism
antifibrinolytic
    a. agent
    a. therapy
antifreeze poisoning
antiganglioside
antigen-antibody
    a.-a. complex
    a.-a. reaction
antiglial fibrillary acidic protein
antigonadal action
antihallucinatory
antihelix
    double a.
antihemophilic
    a. factor A
    a. factor C
antihistamine
anti-human transferrin
antihypertensive
    a. agent
    a. medication
antihypnotic, anthypnotic
antihysteric, anthysteric

anti-immune
anti-inflammatory drug
anti-instinctual force
anti-intoxicant
anti-intraception
antiklisis
antilethargic
antilibidinal ego
antilymphocyte serum (ALS)
antimaniacal
antimanic
antimicrobial prophylaxis
antimigraine therapy
antimongolism
antimongoloid slant
antimotivational syndrome
antimuscarinic drug
antimyasthenic
antinarcotic
antineuralgic
antineuritic
antineurofilament
antinodal behavior
antinoise
antinomian
antinomy
antiobesity
antiobsessive
antioncogene
antipanic agent
antiparkinsonian
    a. medication
    a. response
antiparkinsonism agent
antipathy
antiphobic
antiphospholipid
    a. antibodies in stroke study
      (APASS)
    a. syndrome (APS)
antiplatelet therapy
antipoplectic
antiposia
antipredatory aggression
antiproliferative
antipsychiatry
antipsychomotor
antipsychotic
    a. agent
    atypical a.
    a. medication
    thioxanthene a.
    tricyclic a. (TCA)
antipyretic
antiresonance
antiresorptive
antireward system
antiruminant
antiseizure drug
anti-Semitism
antisense
    a. oligonucleotide
    a. strategy
antiseptic
    ACU-dyne a.

antiserotonergic effect
antisiphon device (ASD)
antisocial (AS)
    a. activity
    a. aggression
    a. alcoholism
    a. behavior
    a. compulsion
    a. neurotic personality
    a. personality (ASP)
    a. personality disorder (ASPD)
    a. psychopathic personality
    a. reaction
    a. scale
    a. tendency
    a. trends psychopathic
    a. trends psychopathic personality
antispasmodic
antispasticity
antistrophe
antisyphilitic
antitetanic
antithrombin
    a. III
    a. III deficiency
antitonic
antitoxin
    botulinum a.
antitragus
antitrismus
antitussive
antivenin
    a. (*Crotalidae*) polyvalent
    a. (*Micrur fulvius*)
Antivert
antiviral
    chemotherapy a.
Antizol
antlophobia
Anton
    A. Brenner Developmental Gestalt
      Test of School Readiness
    A. syndrome
Antoni
    A. A cell
    A. B cell
    A. pattern (type A & B)
    A. type A neurilemoma
    A. type B neurilemoma
Antoni-A neurinoma classification
antra (*pl. of* antrum)
Antrizine
antrophose
antrostomy
antrum, pl. antra
    mastoid a.
    maxillary a.
Anturane
Antyllus method
anum
    per a.
anuptophobia
anuria
anus, pl. anus

anus (*continued*)
    Bartholin a.
    a. cerebri
anvil
    Hurteau skull plate a.
Anxanil
anxietas presenilis
anxiety
    acute a.
    a. adjustment disorder
    adjustment disorder with a.
    adolescent a.
    alcohol-induced a.
    amphetamine-induced a.
    annihilation a.
    anticipatory a.
    anxiolytic-induced a.
    a. attack
    authority a.
    basic a.
    caffeine-induced a.
    cannabis-induced a.
    a. castration
    castration a.
    catastrophic a.
    childhood a.
    chronic a.
    clinically significant a.
    cocaine-induced a.
    a. control training (ACT)
    covert a.
    death a.
    debilitating a.
    dental a.
    a. depression
    desertion a.
    diffuse a.
    a. discharge
    a. disorder of adolescence
    a. disorder of childhood
    a. disorder due to a general
      medical condition
    A. Disorders Interview Schedule
    a. disturbance
    a. dream
    a. due to potential evaluation by
      others
    ego a.
    eighth-month a.
    elementary a.
    environmentally induced a.
    erotized a.
    examination a.
    excessive social a.
    existential a.
    extreme a.
    feelings of a.
    a. fixation
    focus of a.
    free-floating a.
    frequency of a.
    gender differences in a.
    generalized a.
    Hamilton Rating Scale for A.

    heterosexual a.
    a. hierarchy
    high a. (HA)
    high impulsiveness high a. (HIHA)
    high impulsiveness low a. (HILA)
    hypnotic-induced a.
    hyposomnia associated with a.
    a. hysteria
    id a.
    immediate a.
    a. index (AI)
    insomnia associated with a.
    instinctual a.
    intense a.
    intercourse a.
    intercurrent a.
    a. inventory
    a. level
    level of a.
    low a. (LA)
    A. Management Training (AMT)
    manifest a.
    marked a.
    masked a.
    moral a.
    morbid a.
    a. neurosis
    neutralized a.
    noetic a.
    nonpathological a.
    nonpsychotic a.
    normal a.
    a. object
    objective a.
    oral a.
    organic a.
    pain-type a.
    panic attack neurotic a.
    panic-type a.
    paradoxical a.
    peer a.
    performance a.
    persecutory a.
    pervasive a.
    phobic a.
    physical concomitant of a.
    a. preparedness
    a. prevention
    primal a.
    primary a.
    a. profile
    prominent a.
    provoked a.
    psychogenic a.
    a. psychoneurosis
    a. rating scale
    a. reaction
    a. reaction, mild (ARM)
    reactive depression and a.
    real a.
    reality a.
    reduction of a.
    a. reduction
    relaxation-induced a. (RIA)
    a. relief response

a. resolution
a. scale
A. Scale for the Blind (ASB)
A. Scale Questionnaire (ASQ)
A. Scales for Children and Adults
  (ASCA)
sedative-induced a.
a. sensitivity (AS)
A. Sensitivity Index (ASI)
a. sensitivity theory
separation a.
a. separation
severe a.
sexual a.
signal a.
situation a.
sleeplessness associated with a.
social a.
a. state (AS)
a. state neurotic disorder
A. States Inventory
a. status index (ASI)
a. status inventory (ASI)
stranger a.
substance-induced a.
superego a.
a. symptom
a. tension state (ATS)
test a.
theory of a.
a. tolerance
total phobic a. (TPA)
trait a.
transformation theory of a.
traumatic a.
true a.
a. typology
undue social a.
urethral a.
virginal a.

anxiety-avoiding personality disorder
anxiety-blissfulness psychosis
anxiety-induced impaired social
  functioning
anxiety-related
  a.-r. mental disorder
  a.-r. psychiatric syndrome
anxiogenic stimuli
anxiolytic
  a. abuse
  a. agent
  a. amnestic disorder
  a. delirium
  a. dependence
  a. drug
  a. effect
  a. intoxication
  a. medication
  a. response
  serotonergic a.
  a. substance
  a. use disorder
  a. withdrawal
anxiolytic-induced
  a.-i. anxiety

a.-i. persisting dementia
a.-i. psychotic disorder with
  delusions
a.-i. psychotic disorder with
  hallucinations
a.-i. sexual dysfunction
anxious
  a. arousal
  a. delirium
  a. depression
  a. expectation
  a. intropunitiveness
  a. mood
  a. mood adjustment reaction
  a. rumination
  a. substance abuser
anxious-fearful cluster
anxiousness
  S-R Inventory of A.
anxious-neurotic personality trait
anylcyclohexylamine intoxication
AO
  academic orientation
  American Optical
  avoidance of others
    AO dynamic compression plate
    AO dynamic compression plate
      construct
    AO fixateur interne
    AO fixateur interne instrumentation
    AO gouge
    AO group
    AO guidepin
    AO internal fixator
    AO notched instrumentation
    AO reconstruction plate
    AO stopped-drill guide
AOA-MCA
  alternative occipital artery middle
    cerebral artery
    AOA-MCA bypass
AO/ASIF fixateur interne
AOB
  alcohol on breath
AODT
  Animal and Opposite Drawing Technique
AOIVM
  angiographically occult intracranial
    vascular malformation
aortic
  a. arch syndrome
  a. body
  a. body tumor
  a. coarctation
  a. insufficiency
  a. nerve
aorticorenal ganglia
aortobifemoral bypass graft
aortocranial disease
AOVM
  angiographically occult vascular
    malformation
APA
  air pollution adaptation
  APA Index

Apacet
APACHE II measure of disease severity
apallesthesia
apallic
a. state
a. syndrome
apandria
apanthropia, apanthropy
aparalytic
apareunia
APASS
antiphospholipid antibodies in stroke study
apastia
APAT
Accounting Program Admission Test
apathetic
a. affect
a. akinetic mutism
a. hyperthyroidism
a. thyrotoxicosis
a. withdrawal
apathetic-type personality disorder
apathic
apathism
apathy
avolition a.
euphoric a.
a. syndrome
APC
aspirin, phenacetin, caffeine
APDI
Adult Personal Data Inventory
APE
Advanced Placement Examination
ape
a. fissure
a. hand
a. hand of syringomyelia
apeirophobia
APELL
Assessment Program of Early Learning Levels
aperient
aperiodic
a. complex
a. reinforcement
a. wave
aperitif
aperitive
aperta
rhinolalia a.
spina bifida a.
Apert syndrome
apertura, pl. aperturae
a. lateralis ventriculi quarti
a. mediana ventriculi quarti
apertural hypothesis
aperture
lateral a. of the fourth ventricle
median a. of the fourth ventricle
apex, gen. apicis, pl. apices
petrous a.
a. of tongue

Apfelbaum retractor
Apgar score
APH
alcohol-positive history
aphagia
a. algera
psychogenic a.
aphagopraxia
aphanisis
aphasia
acoustic a.
acoustic-amnestic a.
acquired epileptic a.
acquired fluent a.
afferent motor a.
ageusic a.
amnemonic a.
amnesic a.
amnestic a.
anomic a.
associative a.
atactic a.
ataxic a.
auditory a.
Bastian a.
Bedside Evaluation and Screening Test of A.
Benson-Geschwind classification of a.
Boston Assessment of Severe A. (BASA)
Broca a.
callosal disconnection syndrome a.
central a.
childhood a.
A. Clinical Battery
combined transcortical a.
commissural a.
complete a.
conduction a.
contiguity a.
contiguity disorder a.
cortical a.
developmental a.
a. disorder
dynamic a.
efferent motor a.
executive a.
expressive a.
expressive-receptive a.
fluent a.
frontocortical a.
frontolenticular a.
functional a.
gibberish a.
global a.
graphic a.
graphomotor a.
Grashey a.
hypophonic a.
ideomotor a.
impressive a.
infantile a.
intellectual a.
International Test for A.

A

isolation a.
jargon a.
Kussmaul a.
Language Modalities Test for A.
   (LMTA)
A. Language Performance Scale
   (ALPS)
lenticular a.
lethica a.
a. lethica
Lichtheim a.
major motor a.
Minnesota Differential Diagnosis
   of A. (MDDA)
Minnesota Test for the Differential
   Diagnosis of A. (MTDDA)
mixed a.
motor a.
nominal a.
nonfluent a.
optic a.
parietooccipital a.
partial nominal a.
pathematic a.
pictorial a.
pragmatic a.
psychogenic a.
psychosensory a.
pure a.
a. quotient (AQ)
Reading Comprehension Battery
   for A.
receptive a.
A. Screening Test (AST)
semantic a.
sensory a.
similarity disorder of a.
simple a.
speech reading a.
subcortical motor a.
subcortical sensory a.
syndrome a.
syntactic a.
syntactical a.
tactile a.
temporoparietal a.
thalamic a.
Token Test for A.
Token Test for Receptive
   Disturbances in A.
total a.
transcortical a.
traumatic a.
true a.
verbal a.
visual a.
Wernicke a.
aphasic, aphasiac
   a. acalculia
   a. agraphia
   a. disturbance
   a. error
   a. impairment
   a. migraine

a. migraine headache
a. patient
a. phonological impairment
a. seizure
aphasiologist
aphasiology
aphemesthesia
aphemia
   pure a.
aphephobia
aphilopony
aphonia
   acute a.
   conversion a.
   functional a.
   hysterical a.
   intermittent a.
   a. paralytica
   paralytica a.
   a. paranoica
   spastic a.
   tactile a.
aphonic episode
aphonogelia
aphonous
aphoria
aphorism
   Hippocratic a.
aphose
aphrasia paranoica
aphremia
aphrodisiac
aphrodisia phrenitica
aphrodisiomania
aphthongia
aphthous stomatitis
aphylactic
aphylaxis
API
   Activity Pattern Indicator
   Adult Personality Inventory
apical
   a. dendrite
   a. distraction
   a. ectodermal ridge (AER)
   a. process
   a. turn of the cochlea
apicalization
apices (*pl. of* apex)
apicis (*gen. of* apex)
apicoectomy
apiculate waveform
apimania
apiospermum
   Scedosporium a.
apiphobia
apituitarism
aplasia
   cerebral a.
   cochlear a.
   a. cutis congenita
   labyrinthine a.
   vertebral a.
aplastic anemia

APLD
    automated percutaneous lumbar
      discectomy
aplestia
APLS
    Adult Performance Level Survey
Aplysia californica
APMET
    aggressive papillary middle ear tumor
apnea
    central a.
    central sleep a.
    episodic a.
    mixed sleep a.
    obstructive a.
    obstructive sleep a.
    peripheral a.
    sleep a.
    sleep-induced a.
    true a.
apneic
    a. pause
    a. period
    a. seizure
apneusis
apneustic
    a. breathing
    a. period
apocalypse
apocalypticism
apocamnosis (*var. of* apokamnosis)
apocarteresis
apocleisis
apocope
apocrine
    a. cystadenoma
    a. gland
apocryphal
apodemialgia
apodictic
APOE
    apolipoprotein E
apoenzyme
apoferritin
apogee
apogeotropic nystagmus
apokamnosis, apocamnosis
apokemnophilia
apolar cell
apolegamic
apolipoprotein E (APOE)
apomorphine hydrochloride
aponeurectomy
aponeurorrhaphy
aponeurotica
    galea a.
aponeurotic reflex
aponia
apopathetic behavior
apophysary point
apophysial, apophyseal
    a. joint
    a. point
apoplectic
    a. coma

    a. cyst
    a. dementia
    a. hemorrhage
    a. type
apoplectica
    dementia a.
apoplecticus
    habitus a.
apoplectiform
    a. convulsion
    a. seizure
apoplectoid
apoplexy
    bulbar a.
    delayed a.
    embolic a.
    functional a.
    ingravescent a.
    neonatal a.
    pituitary a.
    pontile a.
    posttraumatic a.
    Raymond a.
    serous a.
    spasmodic a.
    spinal a.
    thrombotic a.
apopnixis
apoptosis
    thymocyte a.
aporia
aporioneurosis
aposematic
aposia
aposiopesis
apostasis
apostasy
apostatize
apotentiality
    cerebral a.
apothanasia
apotheosis
apotreptic therapy
apotropaic
APP
    addiction-prone personality
    Advanced Placement Program
apparatus, pl. **apparatus**
    autonomic a.
    C-arm fluoroscopic a.
    halo a.
    Horsley-Clarke stereotaxic a.
    Kandel stereotactic a.
    Mayfield-Kees skull fixation a.
    mental a.
    mitotic spindle a. (MSA)
    psychic a.
    Spiegel-Wycis human a.
    Wells stereotaxic a.
apparent
    alpha a.
    a. competence
    a. death
    a. origin

appeal
    fear a.
    sex a.
    snob a.
appearance
    asthenic a.
    beaten-metal a.
    body a.
    de novo a.
    a. deterioration
    disheveled a.
    haggard a.
    meningothelial a.
    pearl-chain a.
    physical a.
    ping-pong a.
    posterior beaten copper a.
    sloppy a.
    thumbprinting a.
    unkempt a.
appeaser
Appedrine
appendicular
    a. ataxia
    a. ataxis
apperception
    feeling a.
    tendentious a.
    a. test
apperceptive
    a. disorder
    a. distortion
    a. mass
    a. visual agnosia
appersonation, appersonification
appestat
appestatqualitative approach
appetence
appetite
    a. control
    a. disturbance
    insatiable a.
    loss of a.
    a. loss
    perverted a.
    a. psychogenic disorder
    a. suppressant
    voracious a.
appetition
appetitive
    a. behavior
    a. center
    a. drive
    a. phase
applicable
    not a.
application
    biofeedback a.
    clip a.
    force a.
    Harrington rod instrumentation
      force a.
    Isola spinal implant system a.
    paraspinal rod a.
    ritualized makeup a.

    transverse fixator a.
    vertebral plate a.
applicator
    aneurysm clip a.
    NeuroAvitene a.
    scalp clip a.
applied
    a. anthropology
    a. behavioral analysis (ABA)
    a. extrasensory projection (AESP)
    a. psychoanalysis
    a. psychology
    a. research
applier
    bayonet clip a.
    clip a.
    Crockard transoral clip a.
    Ligaclip a.
    Mayfield miniature clip a.
    Mayfield temporary aneurysm
      clip a.
    mini a.
    Olivecrona clip a.
    Raney scalp clip a.
    Sano clip a.
    Vari-Angle clip a.
appraisal
    Conflict Management A. (CMA)
    inflated a.
    A. of Language Disturbances
      (ALD)
    Manager Style A.
    vocational a.
    Watson-Glaser Critical Thinking A.
      (WGCTA)
apprehension
    a. expectation
    intense a.
    irresistible a.
    sensation-focused a.
    sense of a.
    a. span
    a. state
    a. test
apprehensiveness
    social a.
apprenticeship
apprise, apprize
approach
    adaptation a.
    adaptational a.
    adaptive a.
    anterior C1-C2 screw a.
    anterior interhemispheric a. (AIH)
    anterior triangle a.
    anteromedial a.
    anteromedial retropharyngeal a.
    appestatqualitative a.
    assertive-community treatment a.
    Bailey-Badgley anterior cervical a.
    basal interhemispheric a. (BIH)
    basal reader a.
    basal subfrontal a.
    behavioral a.
    buccopharyngeal a.

approach *(continued)*
  categorical a.
  cerebellopontine angle a.
  checklist a.
  Cloward cervical disk a.
  cluster a.
  combined anterior and posterior a.
  combined low cervical and
    transthoracic a.
  combined presigmoid-
    transtransversarium intradural a.
  combined transsylvian and middle
    fossa a.
  computer-assisted volumetric
    stereotactic a.
  condylar a.
  constructive a.
  contralateral transcallosal a.
  costotransversectomy a.
  cross-culture a.
  descriptive a.
  dimensional a.
  disease-oriented/medical model a.
  economic a.
  environmental a.
  ethical a.
  ethnographic a.
  extended subfrontal a.
  extreme lateral inferior
    transcondylar a.
  extreme lateral transcondylar a.
  far lateral inferior suboccipital a.
  foraminal a.
  freudian a.
  frontotemporal a.
  fundamental a.
  a. gradient
  Hardy a.
  Harmon cervical a.
  here-and-now a.
  high-risk a.
  idiographic a.
  inferior extradural a.
  inferior-lateral endonasal
    transsphenoidal a.
  inferior transvermian a.
  infratentorial lateral supracellular a.
  interdisciplinary a.
  interfascial a.
  interforniceal a.
  interhemispheric a.
  intradural a.
  intraforaminal a.
  intratentorial supracerebellar a.
  ipsilateral a.
  Kanavel a.
  labioglossomandibular a.
  labiomandibular a.
  language experience a. (LEA)
  lateral extracavitary a.
  lateral intradural a.
  linguistic a.
  low cervical a.
  mechanistic a.

  medial extradural a.
  middle cranial fossa a.
  middle fossa craniotomy a.
  middle fossa transtentorial
    translabyrinthine a.
  midline spinal a.
  mixture a.
  moisture fear-molar a.
  molar a.
  molecular a.
  Mutt and Jeff a.
  nomothetic a.
  nondirective a.
  oblique transcorporeal a.
  occipital interhemispheric a.
  operative a.
  orbital venous a.
  orbitozygomatic temporopolar a.
  organic a.
  petrosal a.
  posterior occipitocervical a.
  posterolateral a.
  presigmoid a.
  psychodynamic a.
  pterional a.
  qualitative a.
  quantitative a.
  regressive-reconstructive a.
  resection of pituitary tumor,
    transfacial a.
  retrolabyrinthine-presigmoid a.
  retrolabyrinthine-transsigmoid a.
  retromastoid a.
  retroperitoneal a.
  retropharyngeal a.
  retrosigmoid a.
  rhinoseptal a.
  sacral foraminal a.
  screw plate a.
  stabilization a.
  standard retroperitoneal flank a.
  stereotactic microsurgical a.
  sternum-splitting a.
  subchoroidal a.
  subfrontal transbasal a.
  sublabial midline rhinoseptal a.
  sublabial transseptal
    transsphenoidal a.
  suboccipital posterior fossa a.
  suboccipital transmeatal a.
  subtemporal infratemporal a.
  subtemporal keyhole a.
  superior intradural a.
  superior ophthalmic vein a.
  supracerebellar a.
  supraclavicular a.
  supraorbital pterional a.
  supratentorial a.
  sylvian a.
  task-oriented a.
  there-and-then a.
  thoracoabdominal a.
  thoracolumbar retroperitoneal a.
  transantral ethmoidal a.
  transcallosal transforaminal a.

transcavernous transpetrous apex a.
transcerebellar hemispheric a.
transchoroidal a.
transcochlear a.
transcortical transventricular a.
transcranial frontotemporoorbital a.
transcubital a.
transfacial transclival a.
transfrontal a.
transfrontonasoorbital a.
translabyrinthine and suboccipital a.
translabyrinthine transotic a.
transmandibular glossopharyngeal a.
transmaxillosphenoidal a.
transnasal a.
transnasoorbital a.
transoral a.
transpalatal a.
transpedicular a.
transperitoneal a.
transsinus a.
transsphenoidal a.
transsylvian a.
transtemporal a.
transtentorial a.
transthoracic a.
transtorcular a.
transuncodiscal a.
transvenous a.
transventricular a.
transzygomatic a.
ultrasound-guided transfrontal
  transventricular a.
Wiltberger anterior cervical a.
Wiltse paraspinal a.
yawn-sign a.

approach-approach conflict
approach-avoidance
a.-a. conflict
a.-a. stance
appropriate
a. affect
a. behavior
a. in gender
a. relationship
a. response
a. treatment
appropriateness of emotional response
approval loss
approximate
a. answers syndrome
a. lethal concentration (ALC)
approximating closure
approximation
a. conditioning
a. method
method of successive a.
successive a.
vocal fold a.
word a.
approximator
Neuromeet nerve a.
APR
auropalpebral reflex
apractagnosia

apractic (*var. of* apraxic)
apragmatism
apraxia
akinetic a.
amnesic a.
amnestic a.
A. Battery for Adults (ABA)
Bruns gait a.
buccofacial a.
callosal a.
cerebral mapping of a.
classic a.
congenital ocular motor a.
constructional a.
cortical a.
developmental articulatory a.
diagnostic a.
disconnection a.
dressing a.
facial a.
gait a.
ideational a.
ideatory a.
ideokinetic a.
ideomotor a.
innervation a.
innervatory a.
kinesthetic a.
left-sided a.
Liepmann a.
limb-kinetic a.
magnetic a.
motor a.
ocular a.
oculomotor a.
oral a.
pure limb a.
sensory a.
speech a.
transcortical a.
verbal a.
apraxic, apractic
a. agraphia
a. behavior
a. disorder
a. dysarthria
Apresazide
Apresoline
aprobarbital elixir
aprophoria
aprosexia
aprosody
a. of speech
speech a.
aprotinin
APS
Adult Protective Services
air plasma spray
air pollution syndrome
antiphospholipid syndrome
APS hydroxyapatite
apselaphesia
apsithyria
APSR
acute paranoid schizophrenic reaction

apsychia
apsychognosia
apsychosis
APT
Age Projection Test
APTA
aneurysm of persistent trigeminal artery
APTC
anteroposterior talocalcaneal
aptiganel hydrochloride
aptitude
a. battery
Detroit Test of Learning A.
(DTLA)
Detroit Test of Learning A.-Adult
(DTLA-A)
Detroit Test of Learning A. -
Primary, Second Edition (DTLA-
P:2)
Detroit Test of Learning A.,
Third A. (DTLA-3)
Hiskey-Nebraska Test of
Learning A. (HNTLA)
A. Interest Measurement
a. inventory
learning a.
mechanical a.
numerical a. (N)
A. Research Project (ARP)
A. Research Project Test
Science Research Associates
Mechanical A.
Short Form Test of Academic A.
(SFTAA)
spatial a.
A. Survey and Interest Schedule-
Interest Survey
A. Tests for School Beginners
(ASB, ATSB)
Aptitude-Intelligence Test Series
apyretic tetanus
AQ
accomplishment quotient
achievement quotient
aphasia quotient
Aquachloral Supprettes
AquaMEPHYTON Injection
aquaphobia
AquaSens
Aquatensen
aquatic rehabilitation
aqueduct
cerebral a.
a. cerebrum
cochlear a.
Cotunnius a.
forking of sylvian a.
gliosis of a.
mesencephalon a.
Monro a.
sylvian a.
a. of Sylvius
a. veil
ventricular a.

aqueductal
a. intubation
a. occlusion
a. plasty
a. stenosis
aqueductoplasty
aqueductus, pl. **aqueductus**
a. cerebri
a. cochlea
a. cotunnii
a. sylvii
aqueous
a. humor deficiency
a. povidone-iodine
AR
achievement ratio
alarm reaction
alcohol related
ara-a
arabinoside
adenine a.
arachibutyrophobia
arachidonic
a. acid
a. acid cascade
a. acid metabolism
arachnephobia, arachnophobia
arachnodactyly
congenital a.
contracture a.
arachnoid
a. adhesion
a. canal
a. cell
a. cyst
a. fibrosis
a. foramen
a. granulation
a. knife
a. layer
a. mater
a. membrane
a. nerve root sheath dilation
a. plane
a. sheath
a. sleeve
a. space
a. tissue
a. of uncus
a. villus
arachnoidal
a. gliomatosis
a. hyperplasia
a. root sleeve
arachnoidea, arachnoides
a. spinalis
arachnoiditis
adhesive a.
basilar a.
chiasmal a.
cysticerotic a.
fibrosing a.
neoplastic a.
obliterative a.
a. of opticochiasmatic cistern

ossifying a.
spinal cord a.
arachnoid-shape Beaver blade
arachnophobia (*var. of* arachnephobia)
Aramine
Arana-Iniquez
    A.-I. intracranial cyst removal
    A.-I. intracranial cyst removal
      technique
Aran-Duchenne
    A.-D. amyotrophy
    A.-D. disease
arankan
Arantius ventricle
araphia
ARAS
    ascending reticular activating system
ARBD
    alcohol-related birth defect
arbor, pl. **arbores**
arborescent
arborization
arbovirus, arborvirus
    a. meningoencephalitis
ARC
    AIDS-related complex
arc
    alpha a.
    beta a.
    a. de cercle
    Leksell a.
    monosynaptic reflex a.
    a. radius system
    reflex a.
    Sceratti a.
    sensorimotor a.
    spinal reflex a.
    stereotactic a.
    Y-shaped reference a.
arcade of Frohse
arc-centered guidance system
archaeopsychic
archaic
    a. brain
    a. inheritance
    a. residue
    a. thought
archaic-paralogical thinking
archaism
archenemy
archeokinetic
archetype
archfiend
archicerebellum
archicortex
archipallium
architectonics
architectural barrier
architecture
    a. of the brain
    sleep a.
Arclite 20,000 light source
arc-quadrant stereotactic system
Arctic hysteria

arcuate
    a. eminence
    a. fasciculus (AF)
    a. fiber
    a. movement
    a. nucleus
    a. visual field defect
arcuati
    nuclei a.
arcuatus
    nucleus a.
ardanesthesia
ardor
    veneris a.
ARDS
    adult respiratory distress syndrome
area
    acoustic a.
    anterior limbic association a.
    association a.
    auditory association a.
    auditory projection a.
    basic skill a.
    body surface a.
    Broca parolfactory a.
    Brodmann 41 a.
    Brodmann a. 44
    Brodmann cortical a.
    callosal a.
    catchment a.
    a. centralis
    conflict-free a.
    cross-sectional a. (CSA)
    cultural a.
    diencephalic transition a.
    drug-buying a.
    entorhinal a.
    excitable a.
    Flechsig a.
    formed response of colored a.
      (FC)
    frontal a.
    frontoorbital a.
    gasserian ganglion a.
    high density a.
    inferior vestibular a.
    insular a.
    language a.
    low-density a. (LDA)
    mesencephalic transition a.
    motor a.
    noneloquent a.
    olfactory a.
    oval a. of Flechsig
    parabrachial a.
    paracentral gray a.
    paraolfactory cortical a.
    parastriate a.
    parietal association a.
    parietotemporal a.
    a. parolfactoria Brocae
    parolfactory a.
    peristriate a.
    piriform a.
    Pitres a.

area *(continued)*
    postcentral a.
    a. postrema
    precentral a.
    precommissural septal a.
    prefrontal a.
    premotor a.
    preoptic a.
    prestriate a.
    pretectal a.
    primary visual a.
    Rolando a.
    a. sampling
    sclerotic a.
    sclerotome a.
    secondary visual a.
    sensorial a.
    sensorimotor a.
    sensory a.
    septal a.
    shading response to black a.'s (Fc)
    shading response to gray a.'s (Fc)
    silent a.
    skill a.
    somesthetic a.
    striate a.
    subcallosal a.
    superior vestibular a.
    supplementary motor a. (SMA)
    trigger a.
    vagus a.
    ventral regimental a.
    ventral tegmental a. (VTA)
    vestibular a.
    a. vestibularis inferior
    a. vestibularis superior
    visual a.
    watershed a.
    Wernicke 22 a.
    Wernicke 39 a.
    Wernicke 40 a.
areata
    alopecia a.
arecoline
Aredia
areflexia
    detrusor a.
    upper limb a.
arena
    association a.
arenacea
    corpora a.
    corpus a.
arenavirus infection
Arenberg-Denver inner-ear valve
  implant
ARF
    Adjective Rating Form
Argentinian hemorrhage fever
argentophilic plaque
Argesic-SA
arginase
    a. deficiency
    a. deficiency aminoaciduria

arginine
    a. vasopressin
    a. vasotocin (AVT)
argininemia
argininosuccine aciduria
argininosuccinicaciduria
argininosuccinic aminoaciduria
argon
    a. ion
    a. laser
argot
argument
    semantic a.
    sylleptic a.
Argyll
    A. ftrocar catheter
    A. Robertson pupil
argyrophil
    a. organizer region protein
      (AgNOR)
    a. plaque
argyrophilic plaque
arhinencephaly *(var. of* arrhinencephaly)
Aricept
Ariculin
Ariel computerized exercise system
Aries
Arigelucci syndrome
Aristocort Forte
aristogenics
aristotelian method
Aristotle anomaly
arithmetic
    Diagnostic Tests and Self-Helps
      in A.
    a. disorder
    a. grade equivalent
    A. Grade Rating
    a. mean
    a. problem
    a. sign
    a. subtest
arithmetica
    epilepsia a.
arithmetical
    a. developmental delay disorder
    a. learning retardation
    a. reasoning
    a. skills learning retardation
arithmomania
Arizona
    A. Battery for Communication
      Disorders of Dementia (ABCD)
    A. Sexual Experience Scale
Arlin Test of Formal Reasoning
ARM
    anxiety reaction, mild
arm
    a. dystonia
    mechanical articulated a.
    phantom a.
    a. phenomenon
    shot in the a.
    a. weakness
    Yasargil Leyla retractor a.

armamentarium
Armed
    A. Forces Qualification Test
    (AFQT)
    A. Services Vocational Aptitude
    Battery (ASVAB)
armistice
armor
    character a.
Army General Classification Test
    (AGCT)
Army-Navy retractor
Arnold
    A. bundle
    A. ganglion
    A. tract
Arnold-Chiari
    A.-C. deformity
    A.-C. malformation
    A.-C. syndrome
arobrea
    Datura a.
aromatherapy
Aromatic Ammonia Aspirols
aromatic hydrocarbons
around-the-clock observation
arousability factor
arousal
    affective a.
    anxious a.
    autonomic a.
    a. boost
    a. boost mechanism
    a. component of consciousness
    conditional a.
    confusional a.
    a. defect
    a. detection
    a. disorder
    a. dysfunction
    erotic a.
    a. from sleep
    a. function
    hyperactive sexual a.
    hypoactive sexual a.
    impaired a.
    increased a.
    inhibited sexual a.
    intense autonomic a.
    a. jag
    oxygen-deprived sexual a.
    penile a.
    a. reaction
    a. reduction mechanism
    a. reduction technique
    sense of a.
    sexual a.
    sleep a.
    a. state
    a. theory
aroused motive
ARP
    Aptitude Research Project
arrangement
    contractual a.

    Kahn Test of Symbol A. (KTSA)
    picture a.
    Task Force on Local A.'s
arranging
    ordering and a.
array
    compressed spectral a.
    percutaneous electrode a.
    a. processor
    rostrocaudal contact a.
    rostrocaudal epidural a.
    surface coil a.
    transverse tripolar epidural a.
arrest
    action of a.
    cardiac a.
    cardiopulmonary a.
    deep hypothermic circulatory a.
    a. of development
    false a.
    house a.
    locomotor a.
    a. reaction
    a. of schizophrenia
    speech a.
    a. of speech
arrested development
arrhigosis
arrhinencephaly, arhinencephaly,
    arrhinencephalia
arrhythmia
    cardiac a.
    ventricular a.
arrhythmokinesis
arrival
    dead on a. (DOA)
arrogantasemasia
arrogant behavior
ARS
    Academic Readiness Scale
    angiographic reference system
    ARS art test
arseniasis
arsenic
    a. amblyopia
    a. peripheral neuropathy
    a. poisoning
arsenical tremor
arsenicophagy
arsine
arson
    communicative a.
arsphenamine
art
    black a.
    a. test
    a. therapy
Artane
Artemisia vulgaris
arteria, gen. and pl. **arteriae**
    a. basilaris
    a. calcarina
    a. cerebelli inferior anterior
    a. cerebelli inferior posterior
    a. cerebelli superior

arteria *(continued)*
    a. cerebri anterior
    a. cerebri media
    a. cerebri posterior
    a. choroidea anterior
    a. choroidea posterior
arterial
    a. access
    a. bruit
    a. circle of cerebrum
    a. hemorrhage
    a. occlusive disease
    a. oxygen saturation
    a. photothrombosis
    a. vasospasm
arterialization
arterial-occlusive retinopathy
arteriography
    cerebral a.
    spinal a.
arteriolopathy
    retinocochleocerebral a.
arteriolosclerosis
arteriopalmus
arteriopathy
    autosomal-dominant a.
arteriosclerosis
    cerebral a.
    eccentric a.
    hyaline a.
arteriosclerotic
    a. brain disease
    a. brain disease-type organic
      psychosis
    a. brain disorder
    a. cardiovascular disease (ASCVD)
    a. dementia
    a. dementia confusional state
    a. depression
    a. intracranial aneurysm
    a. organic psychosis
    a. paranoid state
    paranoid-type a.
    a. psychosis confusional state
    subcortical a.
    uncomplicated a.
arteriovenous
    a. aneurysm
    a. fistula
    a. interhemispheric angioma
    a. malformation (AVM)
arteritica
    polymyalgia a.
arteritis, pl. **arteritides**
    cranial a.
    giant cell a.
    granulomatous a.
    Horton giant cell a.
    obliterative a.
    rheumatoid a.
    spinal a.
    spinal cord a.
    Takayasu a.

    temporal a.
    viral intracerebral a.
artery
    aberrant a.
    accessory middle cerebral a.
    a. of Adamkiewicz
    alternative occipital artery middle
      cerebral a. (AOA-MCA)
    aneurysm of persistent trigeminal a.
      (APTA)
    anterior cerebral a. (ACA)
    anterior choroidal a. (ACA)
    anterior communicating a. (ACoA,
      AComA)
    anterior inferior cerebellar a.
      (AICA)
    anterior inferior cerebral a. (AICA)
    anterior inferior communicating a.
      (AICA)
    anterior meningeal a.
    anterior spinal a.
    anterior temporal a. (ATA)
    ascending frontoparietal a.
    ASFP a.
    auditory a.
    axillary a.
    basal cerebral a.
    basilar a. (BA)
    Bernasconi-Cassinari a.
    calcarine a.
    callosomarginal a.
    caroticotympanic a.
    cerebellar a.
    cerebral a.
    a. of cerebral hemorrhage
    Charcot a.
    choroidal pericallosal a.
    cingulothalamic a.
    collicular a.
    common carotid a. (CCA)
    costocervical a.
    dolichoectatic a.
    dolicoectatic internal carotid a.
    dynamic entrapment of vertebral a.
    en passage feeder a.
    external carotid a. (ECA)
    extradural vertebral a.
    facial a.
    friable a.
    frontal a.
    frontopolar a. (FPA)
    giant tortuous basilar a.
    great anterior medullary a.
    a. of Heubner
    inferior cerebellar a.
    inferolateral pontine a.
    innominate a.
    internal carotid a. (ICA)
    ipsilateral middle cerebral a.
    left common carotid a.
    lenticulostriate a.'s
    LPCh a.
    maxillary a.
    maxillomandibular a.
    medial striate a.

medullary a.
meningeal a.
MHT a.
middle cerebral a. (MCA)
MPCh a.
nodular induration of temporal a.
a. occlusion
ophthalmic a.
paramedian thalamopeduncular a.
parent a.
pericallosal azygos a.
petrous carotid a.
pial a.
plexus of choroid a.
polar a.
pontine a.
popliteal a.
posterior cerebellar a.
posterior cerebral a. (PCA)
posterior choroidal a.
posterior communicating a.
   (PComA)
posterior inferior cerebellar a.
   (PICA)
posterior inferior communicating a.
   (PICA)
posterior spinal a.
posteroinferior cerebellar a. (PICA)
posterolateral spinal a. (PLSA)
primitive otic a.
primitive trigeminal a.
primordial inferior hypophyseal a.
radial a.
radiculospinal a.
recurrent perforating a.
spinal cord a.
splenial a.
stapedial a.
a. stenosis
subclavian a.
sulcocommissural a.
superficial temporal a. (STA)
superficial temporal artery-middle
   cerebral a. (STA-MCA)
superficial temporal artery-posterior
   cerebral a. (STA-PCA)
superficial temporal artery-superior
   cerebellar a. (STA-SCA)
superior cerebellar a.
superior hypophyseal a.
   (SupHypArt)
superior laryngeal a.
superior thyroid a.
supraclinoid carotid a.
supraclinoid internal carotid a.
supreme intercostal a.
telencephalic ventriculofugal a.
temporal a.
temporopolar a. (TPA)
thalamocaudate a.
thalamogeniculate a.
thalamoperforating a.
thyrocervical trunk of subclavian a.
trifurcation of middle cerebral a.
trigeminocerebellar a.

ventriculofugal a.
vermian a.
vertebral a. (VA)
vertebrobasilar a.
zygomaticoorbital a.
artery-to-artery embolism
artery-to-vein shunt
Artha-G
arthralgia
   migratory a.
   subtalar a.
   temporomandibular joint a.
arthresthesia
arthrifluent abscess
arthritic general pseudoparalysis
arthritidis
   Mycoplasma a.
arthritis, pl. arthritides
   cervical spine a.
   degenerative a.
   enteropathic a.
   A. Foundation Pain Reliever
   gouty a.
   hypertrophic a.
   juvenile rheumatoid a.
   neuropathic a.
   A. Pain Formula
   psoriatic a.
   rheumatoid a.
arthrodesis
   atlantoaxial a.
   Brooks atlantoaxial a.
   C1-C2 posterior a.
   cervical a.
   Cloward cervical a.
   De Andrade-McNab occipito-
      cervical a.
   extension injury posterior
      atlantoaxial a.
   flexion injury posterior
      atlantoaxial a.
   occipitocervical a.
   posterior a.
   posterior atlantoaxial a.
arthrogryposis congenita multiplex
Arthropan
arthropathy
   Charcot a.
   diabetic a.
   neuropathic a.
   sensory neurogenic a.
   tabetic a.
Arthur Point Scale of Performance
   Test
arthyreosis
articular
   a. corpuscle
   a. cortex
   a. leprosy
   a. mass separation
   a. mass separation fracture
   a. sensibility
articulation
   addition a.

articulation *(continued)*
 Assessment Link Between
  Phonology and A.
 atlantoaxial a.
 a. developmental delay disorder
 Goldman-Fristoe Test of A.
 a. index
 infantile a.
 Predictive Screening Test of A.
 a. of speech
 a. test
 Vermont spinal fixator a.
articulator
articulatory
 a. loop component
 a. tic
artifact
 asymmetric a.
 asymmetric a.
 ballistocardiographic a.
 beam hardening a.
 blink a.
 cardiac a.
 cardiac pacemaker a.
 chemical shift a.
 electrode-popping a.
 eye blink a.
 eye movement a.
 ferromagnetic a.
 Gibbs a.
 glossokinetic a.
 impedance a.
 lateralized a.
 line a.
 machine a.
 magnetic susceptibility a.
 motion a.
 movement a.
 nonbiological a.
 nonphysiologic a.
 oculographic a.
 a. on x-ray
 paper stop a.
 perspiration a.
 physiological a.
 pulsation a.
 pulse wave a.
 rhythmic a.
 spike-like a.
 stimulus a.
 susceptibility a.
 tissue magnetic susceptibility a.
 truncation a.
artificial
 a. airway
 a. assist
 a. disorder
 a. dream
 a. fecundation
 a. intelligence (AI)
 A. Intelligence in Medicine (AIM)
 a. language
 a. neural network
 a. neurosis

 a. penis
 a. vertebral body
artuum
 tremor a.
aryepiglottic fold neurofibroma
arylcyclohexylamine compound
AS
 antisocial
 anxiety sensitivity
 anxiety state
as
 also known a. (AKA)
 a. necessary (PRN)
ASA
 Darvon with ASA
 Lortab ASA
 ASA score
ASAH
 aneurysmal subarachnoid hemorrhage
asaphia
asapholalia
ASB
 Anxiety Scale for the Blind
 Aptitude Tests for School Beginners
A-SBFM
 Andresen Six-Basic-Factors-Model
  Questionnaire
ASC
 altered state of consciousness
ASCA
 Anxiety Scales for Children and Adults
ascendance-submission
ascending
 a. degeneration
 a. frontal convolution
 a. frontal gyrus
 a. frontoparietal (ASFP)
 a. frontoparietal artery
 a. myelitis
 a. neuritis
 a. paralysis
 a. parietal convolution
 a. parietal gyrus
 a. pitch break
 a. reticular activating system
  (ARAS)
 a. reticular arousal system
 a. technique
ascertainment
 method of a.
asceticism
Aschner treatment
Asch situation
ascorbate
 quinine a.
 sodium a.
ascorbic acid
Ascriptin
ascriptive responsibility
ASCVD
 arteriosclerotic cardiovascular disease
ASD
 acute stress disorder
 antisiphon device

asemasia, asemia
    a. graphica
    a. mimica
    a. verbalis
Asendin
asepsis
aseptic
    a. meningeal reaction
    a. necrosis
    a. uremic meningitis
ASES
    Adult Self-Expression Scale
asexual
ASFP
    ascending frontoparietal
    ASFP artery
ashen
    a. tuber
    a. tubercle
    a. wing
Asher physical build assessment technique
Ashworth
    A. scale
    A. score of muscle spasticity
ASI
    Addiction Severity Index
    Anxiety Sensitivity Index
    anxiety status index
    anxiety status inventory
A-SICD
    Adapted Sequenced Inventory of Communication Development
ASIF
    A. broad dynamic compression bone plate
    A. T plate
as-if
    a.-i. hypothesis
    a.-i. performance
    a.-i. personality
    pseudo a.-i.
ASIQ
    Adult Suicidal Ideation Questionnaire
asitia
Aslan endoscopic scissors
asocial
    a. acting out
    a. personality
asociality
    premorbid a.
    schizophrenia with premorbid a. (SPA)
asonia
asoticamania
ASP
    antisocial personality
aspartame
aspartame-restricted diet
aspartate
    a. aminotransferase (AST)
    amphetamine a.
aspartic
    a. acid
    a. proteinase

aspartylglycosaminuria
ASPD
    antisocial personality disorder
ASPECT
    Ackerman-Schoendorf Scales for Parent Evaluation of Custody
aspect
    amusing a.
    executive a.
    integrative a.
    ironic a.
    laminar cortex posterior a.
    marche a petits plantar a.
    prominent a.
    speech a.
Aspen
    A. electrocautery
    A. laparoscopy electrode
    A. ultrasound system
Asperger
    A. disorder
    A. syndrome
aspergilloma
aspergillosis
aspergillotic aneurysm
Aspergillus
    A. cerebral abscess
    A. *fumigatus*
    A. *niger*
Aspergum
aspermia
    psychogenic a. (PA)
asphalgesia
asphyctic syndrome
asphyxia
    autoerotic a.
    neonate a.
    traumatic a.
asphyxiant
asphyxiation
ASPI
    Adolescent Problem Severity Index
aspiny neuron
aspiration
    a. level
    level of a.
    needle a.
    negative a.
    stereotactic a.
    ultrasonic a.
aspirational group
aspirator
    Cavitron ultrasonic surgical a. (CUSA)
    Selector ultrasonic a.
    Sharplan Ultra ultrasonic a.
    Sonocut ultrasonic a.
    ultrasonic a.
    ultrasonic surgical a.
Aspir-code
ASPIRE
    A Sales Potential Inventory for Real Estate
aspirin
    Bayer A.

aspirin *(continued)*
    Bayer Buffered A.
    butalbital compound and a.
    carisoprodol and a.
    carotid artery stenosis with
      asymptomatic narrowing: operation
      versus a. (CASANOVA)
    a. and codeine
    a. combination
    a. effect
    Extra Strength Bayer Enteric
      500 A.
    A. Free Anacin Maximum Strength
    hydrocodone and a.
    a. and meprobamate
    methocarbamol and a.
    oxycodone and a.
    a. poisoning
    propoxyphene and a.
    Regular Strength Bayer Enteric
      500 A.
    Saint Joseph Adult Chewable A.
    a. with butalbital, phenacetin, and
      caffeine
aspirin, phenacetin, caffeine (APC)
aspirin, phenacetin, and caffeine tablets
Aspirols
    Aromatic Ammonia A.
Asprimox
ASQ
    Anxiety Scale Questionnaire
    Attitude to School Questionnaire
assassination
    character a.
assault
    aggravated a.
    a. and battery
    indecent a.
    personal a.
    sexual a.
    violent personal a.
    a. with a deadly weapon (ADW)
assaulter
    serial a.
assaultive
    a. act
    a. behavior
assay
    ADmark A.
    B_2-TFn a.
    CH50 a.
    chloride channel flux a.
    clonogenic cell a.
    cocaethylene a.
    drug a.
    enzyme-linked immunosorbent a.
      (ELISA)
    5-HT receptor a.
    5-hydroxytryptamine receptor a.
    immunosorbent a.
    involuntary repetitive movement
      disorder antineuronal antibody a.
    MAO spectrophotometric a.

    Minnesota-Hartford Personality A.
      (MHPA)
    plaque reduction a.
    radioimmunometric a.
    serotonin receptor a.
    tissue-based monoamine oxidase a.
A-S scale
assembly
    Ace halo-cast a.
    Brown-Roberts-Wells arc-ring a.
    cell a.
    cryocooler a.
    multiple hook a.
    object a. (OA)
    picture a.
assertion structured therapy
assertive
    a. behavior
    a. conditioning
    a. outreach
    a. training
assertive-community treatment approach
assertiveness
    a. skill
    a. training
assess
    Reitan (and Selz) rules to a.
assessing
    A. Specific Competencies
    A. Specific Employment Skill
      Competencies
assessment
    a. of academic achievement
    Activity Loss A. (ALA)
    Adolescent Drug and Alcohol
      Diagnostic A. (ADAD)
    a. of affect
    Analytic Learning Disability A.
    automated a.
    A. of Basic Competencies (ABC)
    a. battery
    behavior a.
    behavior-oriented a.
    A. of Career Decision Making
      (ACDM)
    A. of Career Development (ACD)
    CFQ-for-others a.
    A. of Chemical Health Inventory
    A. of Children's Language
      Comprehension (ACLC)
    closed-chain functional a.
    Cognitive Skills A. (CSA)
    Committee on Psychiatric Diagnosis
      and A.
    communication skills a.
    community a.
    A. of Conceptual Organization
      (ACO)
    A. of Core Goals (ACG)
    cultural a.
    Diagnostic and Therapeutic
      Technology A. (DATTA)
    Differential Aptitude Test for
      Personnel and Career A.
    disorganized speech a.

A

Early School A. (ESA)
Ego Function A.
environmental a.
Erhardt Developmental
  Prehension A. (EDPA)
Erhardt Developmental Vision A.
  (EDVA)
family a.
fantasy a.
Frenchay Dysarthria A.
functional a.
Functional Needs A. (FNA)
general personality a.
Graduate and Managerial A.
home a.
a. instrument
A. of Intelligibility of Dysarthric
  Speech
Interpersonal Language Skills
  and A. (ILSA)
a. inventory
Job Seeking Skills A.
language a.
Life History of Aggression A.
Limon Self-Image A.
A. Link Between Phonology and
  Articulation
luteal phase a.
A. in Mathematics
Moire topographic scoliosis a.
neurolinguistic a.
neurophysiological a.
neuropsychologic a.
performance a.
personality a.
A. of Positive Symptom
Practical Math A.
A. Program of Early Learning
  Levels (APELL)
projective personality a.
psychosocial a. (PA)
quality of life rehabilitation a.
quantified cognitive a.
a. questionnaire
rehabilitation a.
Rivermead Motor A.
Ross Information Processing A.
a. scale
Social and Occupational
  Functioning A. (SOFAS)
specialized language a.
Speech-Language Pathology
  Evaluation A.
Stone and Neale Daily Coping A.
A. of Suicide Potential
System of Multicultural
  Pluralistic A. (SOMPA)
task-oriented a.
videotape a.
in vivo stereological a.
Vocational Interest, Experience, and
  Skill A. (VIESA)
Vocational Interest and
  Sophistication A. (VISA)

Vulpe A.
Written Language A.
assets-liabilities technique
ASSI coagulator
assigned
  a. responsibility
  a. sex
Assigning Structure Stages Test
assignment
  random a.
  a. therapy
  writing a.
assimilated nasality
assimilating
  a. information
  a. information disturbance
assimilation
  cultural a.
  double a.
  a. effect
  information a.
  a. law
  law of a.
  progressive a.
  reciprocal a.
  regressive a.
  reproductive a.
  a. rule
  velar a.
  vowel a.
assist
  artificial a.
assistant
  physician's a. (PA)
  psychiatric a.
assisted
  a. suicide
  a. ventilation
assistive technology device (ATD)
associated
  a. descriptive feature
  a. disability
  a. disorder
  a. idea
  a. intervention
  a. laboratory finding
  a. movement
  a. physical examination finding
associate learning
associates
  paired a.
  Science Research A. (SRA)
association
  A. Adjustment Inventory
  a. area
  a. arena
  backward a.
  Benton Controlled Oral Word A.
  causal a.
  a. center
  a. characteristic
  characteristic a.
  clang a.
  a. coefficient
  consequence a.

association *(continued)*
    controlled a.
    co-occurring a.
    a. cortex
    a. deficit pathology
    direct a.
    a. disease
    dominant a.
    dream a.
    etiological a.
    false a.
    a. fiber
    a. fluency
    free a.
    frequency encountered a.
    freudian-free a.
    idea a.
    a. of ideas
    indirect a.
    induced a.
    law of a.
    a. learning
    loose a.
    loosening of a.'s (LOA)
    a. mechanism
    a. neurosis
    phoneme-grapheme a.
    preceding a.
    psychosis of a.
    a. reaction time
    schizophrenia with premorbid a.
    (SPA)
    a. sensation ratio
    a. of sounds and symbols
    sound-symbol a.
    subordinate a.
    a. system
    tangential a.
    temporal a.
    a. test
    a. tract
    word a.
associationism
associative
    a. anamnesis
    a. aphasia
    a. facilitation
    a. fluency
    a. inhibition
    a. learning
    a. linkage
    a. memory
    a. play
    a. reaction
    a. response to a white space on a
    card (Ds)
    a. shifting
    a. strength
    a. thinking
    a. visual agnosia
assonance
assortive mating
ASSR
    adult situational stress reaction

assuasive
assumed
    a. mean
    a. similarity
assumption
    Hodgkin-Huxley a.
    a. of new identity
    reality a.
    theoretical a.
assumptive
assurance
    quality a. (QA)
AST
    Aphasia Screening Test
    aspartate aminotransferase
astasia
astasia-abasia
    hysterical a.-a.
astatic
astemizole
astereocognosy
astereognosia
astereognosis
asteric seizure
asterion
asterixis
asteroides
    Nocardia a.
asthenia
    heat-induced a.
    mental a.
    neurocirculatory a.
    psychogenic a.
asthenic
    a. appearance
    a. constitutional type
    a. delirium
    a. diathesis
    a. neurosis
    a. personality
    a. personality disorder
    a. reaction
asthenology
asthenophobia
asthenopia
asthenospermia
asthma
    bronchial a.
    extrinsic a.
    intrinsic a.
    nervous a.
    sleep-related a.
asthmatic amyotrophy
astigmatism
astomia
Astoria
astragalectomy
astral projection
Astramorph PF Injection
astraphobia, astrapophobia,
  astropophobia
astroblastoma
astrocyte
    ameboid a.
    fibrillary a.

fibrous a.
gemistocytic a.
peripapullar a.
plasmatofibrous a.
protoplasmic a.
reactive a.
stellate a.
suspended embryonic a.
wedge-shaped a.
astrocytic
a. gliosis
a. reaction
a. signal
a. tumor
astrocytoma
anaplastic a. (AA)
brainstem a.
cerebellar a.
cerebral anaplastic a.
chiasmatic-hypothalamic pilocytic a.
diencephalic a.
fibrillary a.
gemistocytic a.
giant cell a.
grade I a.
grade II a.
grade III a.
grade IV a.
hypothalamic a.
intracranial a.
juvenile cerebellar a.
juvenile pilocytic a.
low-degree a.
low-grade a.
malignant a.
optic nerve a.
pilocytic juvenile a.
piloid a.
protoplasmic a.
pseudopalisading a.
subcortical protoplasmic a.
subependymal giant cell a.
subependymal glomerate a.
supratentorial a.
thalamic a.
astrocytosis cerebri
astroependymoma
astroglia cell
astrogliosis
astrology
astrophobia
astropophobia (*var. of* astraphobia)
astrotraveling
astyphia
ASVAB
Armed Services Vocational Aptitude
Battery
asyllabia
asylum psychiatry
asymbolia
asymmetric
a. artifact
a. hyperreflexia
a. motor neuropathy
a. nystagmus

asymmetrical
a. amnesia
a. generalized epileptiform activity
asymmetry
abnormal a.
a. amplitude
cerebral a.
cytoarchitectural a.
facial a.
functional a.
interhemispheric a.
left-right a.
leftward a.
mental a.
metabolic a.
a. and order effect
planum temporale a.
reflex a.
skull a.
asymptomatic
a. carotid artery stenosis (ACAS)
a. carotid atherosclerosis study
(ACAS)
a. carotid bruit (ACB)
a. hydrocephalus
a. neck bruit
a. neurosyphilis
a. seizure
asymptotic wish fulfillment
asynchronously
asynchrony
impulse a.
asyndesis
asyndetic thinking
asynergia
asynergy
asynesia
asynodia
AT
achievement test
ATA
anterior temporal artery
atactic
a. abasia
a. agraphia
a. aphasia
a. ataxia
a. paramyotonia
a. paraplegia
atactica
abasia a.
agraphia a.
atactilia
ataque de nervios
ataractic drug
ataralgesia
Atarax 100
ataraxia
ataraxy
atavism
atavistic regression
ataxia
absent a.
acute cerebellar a.
alcoholic a.

ataxia *(continued)*
    appendicular a.
    atactic a.
    autonomic a.
    autosomal dominant a.
    Biemond a.
    Briquet a.
    Broca a.
    Bruns a.
    cerebellar a.
    choreic a.
    a. conversion
    conversion a.
    crural a.
    early-onset a.
    echovirus infection a.
    episodic a. type 2 (EA-2)
    equilibratory a.
    familial paroxysmal kinesigenic a.
    familial spastic a.
    Friedreich a.
    Greenfield classification of
      spinocerebellar a.
    hand a.
    hereditary posterior column a.
    hereditary spinal a.
    hysterical a.
    infantile X-linked a.
    inherited a.
    intrapsychic a.
    ipsilateral cerebellar a.
    kinesigenic a.
    kinetic a.
    late-onset a.
    Leyden a.
    locomotor a.
    Marie a.
    mental a.
    mild a.
    moderate a.
    moral a.
    motor a.
    a. muscularis
    noothymopsychic a.
    ocular motor a.
    optic a.
    psychogenic a.
    sensory a.
    severe a.
    spinal a.
    spinocerebellar a.
    sporadic a.
    static a.
    a. telangiectasia
    truncal a.
    vasomotor a.
    vestibulocerebellar a.
ataxiadynamia
ataxiagram
ataxiagraph
ataxiameter
ataxiamnesic
ataxiaphasia

ataxic
    a. abasia
    a. amimia
    a. aphasia
    a. breathing
    a. cerebral palsy
    a. diplegia
    a. dysarthria
    a. feeling
    a. gait
    a. hemiparesis (AH)
    a. paramyotonia
    a. paraplegia
    a. respiration
    a. speech
    a. writing
ataxiophemia, ataxophemia
ataxiophobia, ataxophobia
ataxis
    appendicular a.
ataxophemia *(var. of* ataxiophemia)
ataxy
ATD
    assistive technology device
ATDP
    Attitudes Toward Disabled Persons
atelectasis
Ateles
    cerebral cortex of A.
atelesis
atelia
ateliosis
atelophobia
atenolol
    a. and chlorthalidone
atephobia
atheist
atheoretical
atherectomy
    directional coronary a. (DCA)
atheroembolism
    diffuse disseminated a.
atheroma
atheromata
atheromatosis
atheromatous disease
atherosclerosis
    carotid a.
    cerebral a.
atherosclerotic
    a. aneurysm
    a. disease
    a. heart disease
    a. infarction
    a. plaque
athetoid
    a. cerebral palsy
    a. dysarthria
    a. movement
athetosic, athetotic
    a. dysarthria
    a. dystonia
    a. idiocy

A

athetosis
    double congenital a.
    posthemiplegic a.
athletic
    a. constitutional type
    A. Motivation Inventory (AMI)
athrepsia, athrepsy
athymia
athymism
Ativan
ATL
    anterior temporal lobectomy
    ATL real-time Neurosector scanner
atlantal fracture
atlantoaxial
    a. arthrodesis
    a. articulation
    a. dislocation
    a. fixation
    a. fusion
    a. instability
    a. interval
    a. joint
    a. separation
    a. stabilization
    a. subluxation
atlantodental
atlantoepistrophic ligament
atlantomastoid
atlantooccipital
    a. joint
    a. separation
    a. stabilization
atlas
    a. burst fracture
    Schaltenbrand-Wahren stereotactic a.
    stereotactic a.
atlas-axis combination fracture
ATM
    acute transverse myelopathy
atmosphere
    a. effect
    emotional a.
    optimistic a.
    situationally appropriate a.
    situationally optimistic a.
    therapeutic a.
atmospheric
    a. condition
    a. perspective
ATMS
    Attitudes Toward Mainstreaming Scale
atocia
atolide
atomistic psychology
atonia, atony
atonic
    a. absence
    a. absence seizure
    a. bladder
    a. cerebral palsy
    a. epilepsy
    a. impotence
atonicity
atony (*var. of* atonia)

atopognosia, atopognosis
Atozine
ATP
    adenosine triphosphate
ATR
    Activities Therapist, Registered
atrabiliary
atrabilious
atracurium besylate
atraumatic
atremble
atremia
atresia
    anorectal a.
    aural a.
    laryngeal a.
    oral a.
atretic
atrial
    a. fibrillation (AF)
    a. myxoma
    a. natriuretic peptide (ANP)
atrioventricular block
at risk
atrium
atrocious
atrophedema
atrophia
atrophic
    a. dementia
    a. lesion
    a. neuroarthropathy
atrophica
    myotonia a.
atrophicans
    acrodermatis chronica a.
atrophoderma neuriticum
atrophy
    Behr complicated optic a.
    brain a.
    cerebellar vermian a.
    cerebral a.
    circumscribed cerebral a.
    cortical a.
    dentatorubral a.
    dentatorubropallidoluysian a.
    dorsum sellae a.
    Duchenne-Aran spinal muscular a.
    Erb a.
    facioscapulohumeral a.
    familial spinal muscular a.
    focal muscular a.
    frontotemporal brain a.
    Gudden a.
    hippocampal formation a.
    Hoffmann muscular a.
    Hunt a.
    idiopathic muscular a.
    infantile muscular a.
    infantile progressive spinal
      muscular a.
    ischemic muscular a.
    juvenile muscular a.
    Kugelberg-Welander juvenile spinal
      muscle a.

atrophy *(continued)*
  Leber hereditary optic a.
  Leber optic a.
  lobar a.
  Marie-Foix-Alajouanine cerebellar a.
  Menzel olivopontocerebellar a.
  monomelic muscular a.
  multiple system a.
  muscular a.
  myopathic a.
  neuritic a.
  neurogenic a.
  neurotrophic a.
  nutritional type cerebellar a.
  olivopontocerebellar a.
  optic a.
  parenchymatous a.
  perifascicular a.
  peroneal muscular a.
  Pick a.
  postneuritic a.
  primary optic a.
  progressive neuropathic muscle a.
  progressive postpolio muscle a.
    (PPPMA)
  pseudohypertrophic muscular a.
  scapulohumeral a.
  scapuloperoneal muscular a.
  spinal muscular a. (SMA)
  structural a.
  subcortical a.
  Sudeck a.
  sulcal a.
  temporal horn a.
  testicular a.
  transneuronal a.
  trophoneurotic a.
  vermian a.
  Vulpian a.
  Vulpian-Bernhardt spinal
    muscular a.
  Welander distal muscular a.
  Werdnig-Hoffmann spinal
    muscular a.
  X-linked recessive spinobulbar
    muscular a.
atropine coma therapy (ACT)
atropinics
ATS
  anxiety tension state
ATSB
  Aptitude Tests for School Beginners
attached
  a. cranial section
  a. craniotomy
attachment
  affectional a.
  avoidant a.
  a. behavior
  a. bond
  Bowlby theory of a.
  cerebellar a.
  clear-cut a.
  collodion a.

  continuity of a.
  a. disorder
  a. disorder of infancy
  dural a.
  a. figure
  Hardy a.
  Hudson cerebellar a.
  a. in infancy
  a. learning
  liquidation of a.
  locality a.
  maternal a.
  Mayfield-Kees table a.
  mother-child a.
  mother-infant a.
  object a.
  oscillations of a.
  resistant a.
  secure a.
  selective a.
  sense of a.
  social a.
  suffocating a.
  symbiotic a.
  a. theory
  unstable a.
  a. versatility
attachment/commitment
  emotional a.
attachment-in-the-making
attachment-separation disorder
attack
  absence a.
  acute anxiety a. (AAA)
  acute schizophrenic a.
  adversive a.
  akinetic drop a.
  anger a.
  anxiety a.
  biting a.
  bound panic a.
  cataleptic a.
  cephalgic a.
  character a.
  clawing a.
  crescendo transient ischemic a.
  cryptogenic drop a.
  cued a.
  cued panic a.
  dream anxiety a.
  drop a.
  epileptic drop a.
  factitious a.
  falling a.
  full-blown panic a.
  glottal a.
  jackknife a.
  kinesigenic a.
  limited-symptom a.
  masticatory a.
  motor jacksonian a.
  nocturnal panic a.
  obsessive a.
  oxygen radical a.
  panic a.

predisposed panic a.
psychomotor a.
psychotic a.
quiet biting a.
rage a.
recurrent panic a.
refreshing sleep a.
rock a.
salaam a.
schizophrenic a.
schizophreniform a.
sensory jacksonian a.
situationally bound panic a.
situationally predisposed panic a.
sleep a.
Stokes-Adams a.
transient hemisphere a. (THA)
transient ischemic a. (TIA)
twilight a.
uncinate a.
uncontrollable sleep a.
uncued panic a.
unexpected panic a.
vagal a.
vasospastic a.
vasovagal a.
vocal a.
word a.

attacker role

attainment

emotional a.
goal a.

ATTC

automated test target calibration

attempt

a. at a.
failed suicide a.
history of suicide a.
reconciliation a.
risk of suicide a.
suicide a. (SA)

attending

a. behavior
a. to language stage
a. physician

attention

a. alertness test
center of a.
a. and concentration
concentration and a.
controlled a.
covert visuospatial a.
a. deficit
a. deficit disorder (ADD)
A. Deficit Disorder Behavior
Rating Scale (ADDBRS)
a. Deficit Disorder Comprehensive
Teacher Rating Scale
A. Deficit Disorders Evaluation
Scale (ADDES)
a. deficit disorder with
hyperactivity (ADD-HA)
a. deficit hyperactivity disorder
(ADHD)

a. deficit hyperactivity disorder-
predominantly inattentive (ADHD-
PI)
disturbance of a.
fix and focus a.
Flowers Auditory Test of
Selective A. (FATSA)
a. fluctuation
a. focus
focus of clinical a.
focus-execute component of a.
free-floating a.
heightened a.
need for constant a.
Other Conditions That May Be a
Focus of Clinical A.
a. overload
a. problems syndrome
raptus of a.
a. reflex
selective a.
a. shift ability
a. to sound
a. span
span of a.
state of heightened a.
a. testing
Test of Variables of A. (TOVA)
vigility of ·a.
visuospatial a.
wandering a.

attentional

a. ability
a. bias
a. control
a. disturbance
a. impairment
a. processing
a. skills

attentional/executive system dysfunction

Attention-Deficit/Activity

A.-D. Disorder, Combined Type
A.-D. Disorder, Predominantly
Hyperactive-Impulsive Type
A.-D. Disorder, Predominantly
Inattentive Type

attention-deficit/hyperactivity

a.-d. disorder
a.-d. disorder, combined type

attention-deficit symptom

attention-focusing procedure

attention-seeking behavior

attenuation

a. of alpha rhythm on EEG
a. coefficient on MRI scan
intraaural a.
a. value on MRI scan

attitude

abstract a.
a. of active friendliness
a. adjustment
catatonoid a.
categorical a.
complacent a.
concrete a.

attitude *(continued)*
    concretizing a.
    counterphobic a.
    crucifixion a.
    cultural a.
    a. to death
    defeatist a.
    defense a.
    a. defense
    devil-may-care a.
    dionysian a.
    dog-eat-dog a.
    do-not-care a.
    emotional a.
    exposition a.
    fatalistic a.
    feminine a.
    forced a.
    gender-based a.
    holier-than-thou a.
    hyperdefensive a.
    illogical a.
    inappropriate a.
    inflexible a.
    a. inventory
    listening a.
    masculine a.
    maternal a.
    mummy a.
    negative a.
    neutral a.
    object a.
    objectifying a.
    oppositional a.
    overdependent a.
    passional a.
    passionate a.
    a. passionelle
    paternal a.
    phobic a.
    positive mental a.
    preadaptive a.
    primary oppositional a.
    a. reassessment
    referential a.
    a. restructuring
    rigid a.
    A. to School Questionnaire (ASQ)
    self-centered a.
    sexual a.
    stereotyped a.
    stilted a.
    a. survey
    A. Survey Program for Business and Industry
    Survey of School A.'s
    Survey of Study Habits and A.'s (SSHA)
    a. theory
    a. therapy
    a. tic
    A.'s Toward Disabled Persons (ATDP)
    A.'s Toward Mainstreaming Scale (ATMS)
    a. type

attitudinal
    a. group
    a. pathosis
    a. reflex
    a. type

attonita
    amentia a.
    cephalea a.
    melancholia a.

attonity

attraction
    gain-loss theory of a.
    magnetic a.

ATT/RhT
    atypical teratoid/rhabdoid tumor

attributable risk

attribute
    positive a.

attribute-entity

attribution
    dispositional a.
    environmental a.
    a. error
    error a.
    false a.
    personal a.
    situational a.
    a. theory

Attributional Style Questionnaire

ATV
    all-terrain vehicle
    ATV accident

atypia

atypical
    a. absence
    a. absence seizure
    a. antidepressant
    a. antipsychotic
    a. antipsychotic drug
    a. behavior
    a. bipolar disease
    a. child
    a. cleft
    a. course
    a. delusional experience
    a. depression
    a. development
    a. factitious disorder with physical symptoms
    a. feature
    a. giant cell tumor
    a. lymphocytosis
    a. mania
    a. or mixed organic brain syndrome
    a. mixed or other personality
    a. neuralgia
    a. neuroleptic
    a. neurotic anxiety state
    a. pain
    a. paraphilia
    a. presentation

a. psychosexual dysfunction
a. psychosis
a. puberty
a. schizophrenia
a. teratoid/rhabdoid tumor
  (ATT/RhT)
a. teratoma
a. tic
atypism
Aubert-Forster phenomenon
Aubert phenomenon
audible
a. blocking in speech
a. speech blockade
a. thought
audile
auding
audiobrain stimulation
audiofrequency eddy current
audiogenic
a. epilepsy
a. seizure
audiogram
pure tone a.
audiologic
audiologist
audiometric hearing
audiometry
ABR a.
automatic a.
average evoked response a.
  (AERA)
behavioral observation a. (BOA)
brainstem electrical response a.
impedance a.
pure-tone a.
audiophile
audioverbal amnesia
audiovisual
a. electroencephalogram (AVEEG)
a. training
audit
Management Transactions A.
  (MTA)
medical a.
patient-care a.
personal a.
Stress A.
audition
chromatic a.
gustatory a.
mental a.
auditive
auditognosis
auditory
a. ability
a. accommodation
a. acuity
a. alexia
a. amnesia
a. analysis
a. aphasia
A. Apperception Test (AAT)
a. artery
a. association area

a. aura
a. blending
a. brainstem response (ABR)
a. bulb
a. canal
a. closure
a. compound actional potential
a. comprehension
a. cortex
a. discrimination
A. Discrimination Test (ADT)
a. disorder
a. disorientation
a. distance cue
a. distortion
electric a.
a. evoked potential (AEP)
a. evoked response
a. fatigability
a. fatigue
a. feedback
a. ganglion
a. hallucination
a. hyperalgesia
a. hyperesthesia
a. imagery
a. koniocortex
a. learner
a. lemniscus
a. localization
a. memory
a. memory span (AMS)
a. nerve
a. nucleus
a. oculogyric reflex
a. pathway
a. processing
a. projection area
a. radiation
a. receptor cell
a. seizure
a. sequencing
a. skills
a. sound agnosia
a. space perception
a. stimulus
a. striae
a. symptom
a. synesthesia
a. system
a. threshold
a. tract
a. training
a. transfer deficit
a. vocabulary
auditory-verbal dysgnosia
Auerbach
A. ganglia
A. plexus
augment
augmentation
breast a.
thyroid a.
augmentative communication
augmented reality procedure

augmentor
  a. fiber
  a. nerve
augury
AUI
  Alcohol Use Inventory
AUQ
  Alcohol Usage Questionnaire
aura, pl. **aurae**
  auditory a.
  cephalic a.
  déjà vu a.
  electric a.
  epigastric a.
  epileptic a.
  gustatory a.
  a. hysterica
  hysterical a.
  a. hysterics
  intellectual a.
  a. intelligence
  a. interpretation
  jamais vu a.
  kinesthetic a.
  migraine with a. (MA)
  migraine without a. (MwoA)
  migrainous a.
  motor a.
  olfactory a.
  a. procursiva
  reminiscent a.
  sensory a.
  shimmering light with a.
  status a.
  tactile pricklings with a.
  tingling with a.
  uncinate a.
  visual shimmering with a.
  visual shining with a.
  visual sparkling with a.
  wavering light with a.
aural
  a. atresia
  a. pathology
aureus
  Staphylococcus a.
auricular
  a. ganglion
  a. lesion
auriculopalpebral reflex
auriculotemporal nerve syndrome
auropalpebral reflex (APR)
aurophobia
auroraphobia
auscultation
AU/SR
  acute undifferentiated schizophrenic
  reaction
Aussage test
austericity
Australian
  A. X disease
  A. X encephalitis
autarky, autarchy
autemesia

autesthetic
authoritarian
  a. aggression
  a. character
  a. conscience
  a. leader
  a. leadership pattern
  a. parent
  a. personality
  a. rejecting-neglecting parent
  a. submission
authority
  a. anxiety
  a. complex
  a. confusion
  a. figure
  a. figure fixation
  a. principle
authorization
  away without a. (AWA)
authorized leave
autia
autism
  akinetic a.
  Behavioral Observation Scale
    for A.
  childhood a.
  A. Diagnostic Interview
  early infantile a.
  infantile a.
  primary a.
  Ritvo-Freeman Real Life Rating
    Scale for A.
  A. Screening Instrument for
    Educational Planning
  secondary a.
  semantics of a.
autismus infantum
autistic
  A. Behavior Composite Checklist
    and Profile
  a. child
  a. disorder
  a. fantasy
  a. isolation
  a. phase
  a. proband
  a. psychopathy
  a. psychosis
  a. thinking
autistic-presymbiotic adolescent
Autley-Bixler syndrome
autoactivation
autoaggression
autoaggressive
  a. behavior
  a. behavior reflex
autoanalysis
autoanamnesis
autoantibody assay testing
autobiographical
  a. information
  a. life chart
  a. memory
autobiography

autocastration
  anticipatory a.
autocatharsis
autocerebral cooling
autochthonous
  a. delusion
  a. gestalt
  a. graft
  a. idea
  a. variable
autoclavable
  steam a.
autoclave
autoclitic operant
autocorrelation
autodysosmophobia
autoecholalia
autoechopraxis
autoerogenous
autoerotic asphyxia
autoerotism, autoeroticism
  secondary a.
autoerythrocyte sensitization syndrome
autofluorescence
autogenic training
autogenital stimulation
autogenous
  a. bone graft
  a. cable graft interposition VII-VII
    neuroanastomosis
  a. depression
  a. iliac bone
autognosis
autognostic
autograft bone grafting
autohemotherapy
autohypnosis
autohypnotic amnesia
autohypnotism
autoimmune (AI)
  a. deficiency
  a. disease
  a. obsessive-compulsive tic disorder
  a. thyroiditis
autoimmunity
  pituitary a.
autoinduction
  enzyme a.
autointoxication
autokinesia, autokinesis
autokinetic effect
autologous
  a. adrenal medullary tissue
  a. blood transfusion
  a. fat graft
  a. fibrin sealant glue
autolysis
automania
automanipulation
automate computed axial tomography
automated
  a. assessment
  A. Child/Adolescent Social History
    (ACASH)
  a. clinical record

A. Multitest Laboratory (AML)
a. percutaneous lumbar discectomy
  (APLD)
a. test target calibration (ATTC)
automatic
  a. absence
  a. action
  a. audiometry
  a. behavior
  a. chorea
  a. drawing
  a. epilepsy
  a. gain control
  a. judgment
  a. language
  a. memory
  a. movement
  a. obedience
  a. phrase level
  a. psychological process
  a. reactivity
  a. seizure
  a. speech
  a. thought
  a. volume control
  a. writing
automaticity of performance
automation
automatism
  ambulatory a.
  chewing a.
  command a.
  epileptic a.
  facial expression a.
  gestural a.
  ictal a.
  immediate posttraumatic a.
  lip smacking a.
  mumbling a.
  patting a.
  primary ictal a.
  scratching a.
  swallowing a.
  verbal a.
automatograph
automaton conformity
automization
automnesia
automorphic perception
automysophobia
autonarcosis
autonomasia
autonomic
  a. activity
  a. activity-reactivity
  a. apparatus
  a. arousal
  a. ataxia
  a. balance
  a. conditioning
  a. conversion reaction
  a. denervation
  a. disorder
  a. disorganization
  a. dysfunction

autonomic (*continued*)
  a. dysnomia
  a. dysreactivity
  a. dysregulation
  a. epilepsy
  a. ganglion
  a. hyperactivity
  a. hyperactivity sign
  a. hyperarousal
  a. hyperreflexia
  a. hyperventilation
  a. imbalance
  a. motor neuron
  a. motor pool
  a. nerve
  a. nervous system (ANS)
  a. neurogenic bladder
  a. neuropathy
  a. part
  a. reactivity
  a. response
  a. seizure
  a. side effect
  a. sympathomimetic drug
autonomic-affective law
autonomotropic
autonomous
  a. depression
  a. ego function
  a. psychotherapy
  a. stage
  a. superego
autonomy
  functional a.
  loss of a.
  a. loss
  a. of motives
  perseverative functional a.
  a. scale
  a. vs. shame and doubt
autonomy-heteronomy
autopagnosia
autopathography
autopathy
autophagia
autophagic
autophilia
autophobia
autophonia
autophonomania
autoplastic
  a. adaptation
  a. change
  a. symptom
autoplasty
autopsy
  brain a.
autopsychic
  a. delusion
  a. disorientation
  a. orientation
autopsychorhythmia
autopsychosis
autopsychotherapy

autopsy-negative death
autopunition
autoradiographic
  a. image
  a. localization
autoradiography
  quantitative receptor a.
autoregressive model for signal analysis
autoregulation
  cerebral pressure a.
  pressure a.
autoscope
autoscopic
  a. phenomenon
  a. psychosis
  a. syndrome
autoscopy
autosensitize
autosexing
autosexualism
autosexuality
autosmia
autosomal
  a. aberration
  a. abnormality
  a. anomaly
  a. dominant
  a. dominant ataxia
  a. dominant gene
  a. dominant inheritance
  a. dominant migraine
  a. dominant pattern
  a. recessive
  a. recessive inheritance
  a. trisomy
autosomal-dominant arteriopathy
autosomatognosis
autosomatognostic
autosome
autosuggestibility
autosymbolism
autosympathectomy secondary to neuropathy
autosynnoia
Autotechnicon
autotelic
autotherapy
autotomia
autotopagnosia agnosia
autotoxic
autotransfusion
autotrophic nutrition
autozygous
auxiliary
  a. ego
  a. organ
  a. solution
  a. therapist
  a. verb
auxoaction
auxotherapy
auxotox
avalanche
  law of a.
avascular necrosis

AVDO$_2$
cerebral arteriovenous oxygen content difference
AVEEG
audiovisual electroencephalogram
Avellis syndrome
Aventyl Hydrochloride
avenues of administration
average
a. conditioning
a. evoked response (AER)
a. evoked response audiometry (AERA)
a. evoked response technique
pure tone a. (PTA)
a. velocity
aversion
a. conditioning
a. depression
occasional sexual a.
a. reaction
a. response
school a.
sexual a.
a. therapy
aversion-covert conditioning
aversive
a. behavior
a. conditioning
a. control
a. drive
a. incentive
a. racism
a. stimulus
a. therapy
a. training
aviation medicine
aviator's
a. disease
a. effort syndrome
a. neurasthenia
avidin-biotin
a.-b. peroxidase complex
a.-b. stain technique
avidin-biotin-complex-peroxidase method
aviophobia
avis
nidus a.
avitaminosis B$_{12}$ peripheral neuropathy
Avitene
A. microfibrillator collagen hemostat
A. packing
A. solution
AVM
arteriovenous malformation
AVM nidus definition
avocation
avoidance
anticipatory a. (AA)
cognitive a.
a. conditioning
conflict a.
conscious a.
a. and escape learning

a. gradient
harm a.
incubation of a.
a. measure
a. of others (AO)
pain a.
passive a.
a. pattern
phobic a.
a. response
a. speaking
a. of speech dysfluency
a. symptom
a. syndrome
a. therapy
avoidance-avoidance conflict
avoidant
a. attachment
a. behavior
a. disorder of adolescence
a. disorder of childhood
a. neurotic personality disorder
a. personality
a. scale
avoidant-attached behavior
avoisomatognosis
avolition apathy
Avonex
AVT
arginine vasotocin
avulsion
brachial plexus a.
bypass coaptation for cervical nerve root a.
cauda equina a.
conus medullaris root a.
a. injury
nerve root a.
sacral plexus a.
third nerve a.
AVVM
angiographically visualized vascular malformation
AWA
away without authorization
awake, alert, and oriented (AAO)
awake state
award
potential external a.
awareness
body a.
closed a.
conscious a.
contingency a.
a. defect
a. deficit
emotional a.
environmental a.
heightened a.
interoceptive a.
lack of interoceptive a.
lapse of a.
leisure a.
mutual pretense a.
open a.

awareness *(continued)*
    phonemic a.
    postural a.
    reality a.
    sensory a. (SA)
    state of heightened a.
    subconscious a.
    suspected a.
    a. threshold
    a. training model
    visuospatial a.
away without authorization (AWA)
awl
    angled a.
    pointed a.
    reaming a.
    rectangular a.
    Swanson scaphoid a.
    T-handle bone a.
AWOL
    absent without leave
    AWOL ideation
axes (*pl. of* axis)
axial
    a. amnesia
    a. compression
    a. gradient
    a. gradiometer
    a. gripping strength
    a. hyperkinesis
    a. load
    a. loading
    a. loading fracture
    a. manual traction test
    a. musculature
    a. myopia
    a. neuritis
    a. pattern scalp flap
    a. plane angular deformity
      biomechanics
    a. projection
    a. spinal system
    a. spin-echo image
    a. stiffness
    a. traction
axial-occipital ligament
axifugal
axile corpuscle
axilla
    coitus in a.
axillary
    a. artery
    a. nerve
axiodrama
axiology
axiom
axiomatic
axion
axioplasm
axiramificate
axis, pl. axes
    A. I
    A. I disorder
    A. II

    A. II disorder
    A. III
    A. IV
    A. V
    adrenal a.
    basicranial a.
    cerebrospinal a.
    a. corpuscle
    a. cylinder
    defensive functioning a.
    encephalomyelonic a.
    endocrine axes
    hypothalamic hypophyseal
      gonadal a.
    hypothalamic-pituitary a.
    hypothalamic-pituitary-adrenal a.
    neural a.
    no diagnosis or condition on a.
    time a.
    visual a.
axis-atlas combination fracture
axoaxonic synapse
Axocet
axodendritic
    a. synapse
    a. tree
axofugal
axoid
Axokine
axolemma
axolysis
axon
    corticospinal a.
    a. flare
    a. guidance
    a. hillock
    myelination of a.
    a. reflex
    a. regeneration
    a. regrowth
    a. response
    A. sentinel-4 analyzer
    a. terminal
axonal
    a. degeneration
    a. idiocy
    a. injury
    a. loss
    a. neuropathy
    a. process
    a. regeneration
    a. terminal bouton
axonapraxia
axonapraxis
axonography
axonometer
**axonopathic neurogenic thoracic outlet
  syndrome**
axonopathy
axonotmesis
axonotmetic injury
axopetal
axoplasm degeneration
axoplasmic
    a. flow

a. flow and papilledema
a. transport
axosomatic synapse
Axostim nerve stimulator
Axotal
axotomy
delayed a.
instantaneous a.
peripheral nerve a.
primary a.
secondary a.
Axsain
Ayala disease
Ayers needle holder
azacyclonol
azaperone
azaspirodecanedione   agent
azathioprine
Azdone

azepindole
azidothymidine (AZT)
Azima battery
aziridinylbenzoquinone (AZQ)
azithromycin
azlocillin
azoospermia
Azorean disease
Azorean-Joseph-Machado disease
AZQ
aziridinylbenzoquinone
AZT
azidothymidine
Aztec idiocy
aztreonam
azumolene
azurophilic granule
azygous vein

β (*var. of* beta)
B
 B fiber
 B vitamin deficiency neuropathy
B1
 vitamin B1
B6
 vitamin B6
B12
 serum vitamin B12
 vitamin B12
1b
 interferon-β 1b (IFN-B1b)
BA
 basilar artery
 blood alcohol
 bone age
baah-ji
babbling
 non-reduplicated b.
 reduplicated b.
 social b.
Babcock forceps
Babinski
 B. percussion hammer
 B. phenomenon
 B. reflex
 B. sign
 B. syndrome
Babinski-Nageotte syndrome
baby
 battered b.
 b. habit
 war b.
BAC
 blood alcohol concentration content
bacampicillin
Bachelor of Social Work (BSW)
bacillary layer
bacilliformis
 Bartonella b.
bacillophobia
bacitracin solution
back
 b. of foot reflex
 b. pain
 b. phoneme
 b. vowel
backache
 psychogenic b.
back-formation word
background
 b. activity
 cultural b.
 b. disorganization
 ethnic b.
 b. interference
 b. masking
 b. noise
 regional b.
 b. rhythm
 sociocultural b.

backing to velars
Backlund
 B. biopsy needle
 B. stereotactic instrument
backout
 screw b.
backpack
 b. palsy
 b. paralysis
back-to-back
backward
 b. association
 b. coarticulation
 b. conditioning
 b. making technique
 b. visual masking
backwardness
 reading b.
baclofen
Bacon cranial rongeur
bacterial
 b. aneurysm
 b. endocarditis
 b. infection
 b. meningitis
 b. meningoencephalitis
 b. peripheral neuropathy
 b. toxin
bacteriophobia
bad
 b. blood
 b. conduct discharge (BCD)
 b. dream
 b. object
 b. PCP experience
 b. self
Badgley
 B. iliac wing resection
 B. laminectomy retractor
bad-me
bad-mouth
bad-people fear
Bad Wildungen Metz (BWM)
BAEP
 brainstem auditory evoked potential
BAER
 brainstem auditory evoked response
baffle
bag
 nuclear b.
bagger
bahnung
bah tschi
bail
 skip b.
Bailey
 B. conductor
 B. rib spreader
Bailey-Badgley
 B.-B. anterior cervical approach
 B.-B. cervical spine fusion

Baillarger
B. band
exterior band of B.
interior band of B.
B. line
Bailliart ophthalmodynamometer
bailout behavior
baked brain phenomenon
BAL
blood alcohol level
BAL in Oil
balance
acid-base b.
alternate binaural loudness b.
(ABLB)
alternate monaural loudness b.
(AMLB)
autonomic b.
b. control
core body b.
b. disorder
dopaminergic-cholinergic b.
dynamic ambulatory b.
dynamic standing b.
electrolyte b.
energy b.
family structural b.
fluid b.
genic b.
homeostatic b.
impaired b.
inhibition-action b.
b. mechanism
off b.
b. scale
sitting b.
spatial b.
standing b.
static and dynamic sitting b.
static and dynamic standing b.
static standing b.
structural b.
b. theory
water b.
balanced
b. diet
b. placebo
balancing subdural hematoma
balanus
balderdash
Balint syndrome
ball
b. of fire
B. operation
b. tip nerve hook
ball-and-field test
Ballantine hemilaminectomy retractor
baller
Baller-Gerold syndrome
ballet
B. disease
b. technique
b. therapy
ball-in-cone valve
balling

ballism
ballismus
ballistic
b. material
b. movement
ballistocardiographic artifact
ballistomania
ballistophobia
balloon
b. angioplasty
b. catheter
detachable b.
electrodetachable b.
latex b.
metrizamide-filled b.
nondetachable endovascular b.
nondetachable occlusive b.
occlusion balloon catheter with
silicone b.
b. occlusion test
silicone b.
Spiegelberg epidural b.
b. test occlusion
ballooned floor of ventricle
ballooning
b. of the sella
b. of vertebral interspace
balneology
balneotherapeutic
balneotherapy
Baló
B. aminoaciduria
B. concentric sclerosis
B. disease
B. sclerosis
Balthazar
B. Scales of Adaptive Behavior
(BSAB)
B. Scales for Adaptive Behavior
II: Scales of Social Adaptation
B. Scales for Adaptive Behavior I:
Scales of Functional Independence
Baltic
B. myoclonus epilepsy
B. syndrome
Bambalacha
Bamberger
B. disease
B. sign
bamboo spine
Bancaud
B. phenomenon on EEG
B. phenomenon on
electroencephalogram
band
alpha frequency b.
Baillarger b.
Bechterew b.
Broca diagonal b.
Büngner b.
Essick cell b.
b. frequency
Gennari b.
b. of Giacomini
b. heterotopia

B

b. of Kaes-Bechterew
b. keratopathy
oligoclonal b.
Osborn b.
peritumoral b.
Reil b.
b. spectrum
vocal b.
bandage
Comperm tubular elastic b.
Dressinet netting b.
hammock b.
band-like headache
band-pass filter
bandwidth
data acquisition b.
receiver b.
banging
head b.
sleep-related head b.
bangungut
banisterine
bank
blood b.
Traumatic Coma Data B. (TCDB)
bankruptcy
Bankson
B. Language Screening Test
(BLST)
B. Language Test-2 (BLT-2)
Bankson-Bernthal Test of Phonology
(BBTOP)
Bannayan syndrome
Bannister disease
Bannwarth syndrome
Banophen Oral
Banthine
Banting diet
BAP
Behavior Activity Profile
Behavioral Assessment of Pain
baptism by (with) fire
bar
dating b.
distraction b.
Dynamic mesh pre-angled
connecting b.
b. graph
Greenberg-type b.
Leyla self-retaining tractor b.
longitudinal spinal b.
b. reflex
screw alignment b.
baragnosis, barognosis
Bárány test
barb
Day B.
barbaralalia
barbed-wire
b.-w. disease
b.-w. psychosis
Barber Scales of Self-Regard for
Preschool Children
Barbita

barbital
sodium b.
barbitalism
barbitone
barbituism
barbiturate
b. abuse
b. addiction
b. burst-suppression anesthesia
b. dependence
b. intoxication
long-acting b.
b. overdose
b. peripheral neuropathy
b. poisoning
b. tolerance
ultrashort-acting b.
b. withdrawal
barbiturate-facilitated interview
barbiturate-induced
b.-i. coma
b.-i. death
b.-i. spindle-like activity
barbituric acid
Barbour technique
Barclay
B. Classroom Climate Inventory
(BCCI)
B. Learning Needs Assessment
Inventory (BLNAI)
Bardeen disk
Bardet-Biedl syndrome
baresthesia
baresthesiometer
bariatrics
barium
b. ferrite
b. sulfate
Barkman reflex
Barlow syndrome
Barnes
B. Akathisia Scale
B. dystrophy
Barnum effect
BARNY
Body Awareness Resource Network
baroceptor
barognosis (var. of baragnosis)
barophobia
baroreceptor
b. nerve
baroreflex
barostat
barotrauma
barotropism
Barouk microstaple
barracoon
Barranquilla Rapid Survey Intelligence
Test (BARSIT)
Barr chromatin body
barreflex
barrel
b. bur
b. field
b. staved graft

Barré-Lieou syndrome
barrenness
    inner b.
Barré sign
barrier
    architectural b.
    blood-brain b. (BBB)
    blood-brain-tumor b. (BBTB)
    blood-cerebrospinal fluid b., blood-
      CSF b.
    blood-thymus b.
    communication b.
    incest b.
    b. to intervention
    intra-blood-brain b. (IBBB)
    language b.
    protective b.
    b. response
    social b.
barrier-free environment
Barron-Welsh Art Scale (BWAS)
Barry Five Slate System
BARSIT
    Barranquilla Rapid Survey Intelligence
      Test
bart
    black b.
Bartel criteria
Barthel
    B. Activities of Daily Living
      Index
    B. ADL Index
Bartholin
    B. anus
    B. gland
bartholinitis
Bartonella bacilliformis
Bartschi-Rochaix syndrome
Bartter syndrome
Baruch law
baryesthesia
baryglossia
barylalia
baryphonia, baryphony
barythymia
BAS
    behavioral activation system
    British Ability Scale
BASA
    Boston Assessment of Severe Aphasia
basal
    b. cell nevus
    b. cell nevus syndrome
    b. cerebral artery
    b. diet
    b. endothelium-derived relaxing
      factor
    b. fluency
    b. ganglia
    b. ganglia calcification
    b. ganglia-cingulate gyrus-frontal
      lobe loop
    b. ganglia syndrome
    b. ganglia-thalamocortical motor
      circuit

    b. ganglionic lesion
    b. interhemispheric approach (BIH)
    b. joint reflex
    b. lamina
    b. lamina of neural tube
    b. line
    b. meningoencephalocele
    b. mental age
    b. metabolic rate (BMR)
    b. metabolism
    b. narcosis
    b. pitch
    b. plate of neural tube
    b. reader approach
    b. resistance level
    b. skull fracture
    b. subfrontal approach
    b. temperature
    b. vein of Rosenthal (BVR)
BASE
    Brief Aphasia Screening Examination
base
    anterior cranial b.
    b. of brain
    Brown-Roberts-Wells phantom b.
      (BRW-PB)
    b. component
    data b.
    ether b.
    b. head
    b. impulse
    phantom b.
    b. rate
    b. rule
    skull b.
    space b.
    b. structure
    b. word
basedowian insanity
Basedow pseudoparaplegia
baseline (BL)
    b. angiography
    behavioral b.
    b. monitoring
    Reid b.
    b. symptom
basement membrane (BM)
basiarachnitis
basiarachnoiditis
basic
    B. Achievement Skills Individual
      Screener
    b. anxiety
    B. Concept Inventory
    b. conflict
    b. diet
    B. Educational Skills Test
    b. fibroblast growth factor (bFGF)
    B. Inventory of Natural Language
    B. Language Concepts Test
    b. mistake
    b. mistrust
    B. Occupational Literacy Test
      (BOLT)
    b. personality

B. Personality Inventory (BPI)
b. personality type
B. Reading Inventory (BRI)
b. rest-activity cycle (BRAC)
b. rule
B. School Skills Inventory (BSSI)
B. School Skills Inventory battery
test
B. School Skills Inventory -
Diagnostic
B. School Skills Inventory-Screen
b. skill area
B. Skills Assessment Program
b. trust
basicranial
b. axis
b. flexure
basigenous
basilar
b. apex aneurysm
b. arachnoiditis
b. artery (BA)
b. artery migraine
b. artery migraine headache
b. artery thrombosis syndrome
b. artery trunk aneurysm
b. bifurcation
b. bifurcation aneurysm
b. crest of cochlear duct
b. ectasia
b. impression
b. insufficiency
b. invagination
b. lamina
b. leptomeningitis
b. membrane
b. meningitis
b. part of pons
b. skull fracture
b. sulcus
b. tip aneurysm
basilaris
membrana b.
basilar-vertebral artery disease
basilect
basilic
basing
missile b.
basiocciput tumor
basiphobia, basophobia
basis
biologic b.
b. cerebri
b. pedunculi
physiological b.
b. pontis
psychological b.
basistasiphobia, basistasophobia
basket
Alzheimer b.
b. cell
Moss-Harms b.
basolateral

basophilia
Cushing b.
pituitary b.
basophilic
b. adenoma
b. pituitary tumor
basophilism
basophil substance
basophobia (*var. of* basiphobia)
Bassen-Kornzweig
B.-K. disease
B.-K. peripheral neuropathy
B.-K. syndrome
Basser syndrome
Bassett electrical stimulation device
bastard
Bastian aphasia
Batelle Developmental Inventory
bathing and dressing ability
bathmophobia
bathmotropic
negatively b.
positively b.
bathophobia
bathos
bathroom privileges
bathyanesthesia
bathyesthesia
bathyhyperesthesia
bathyhypesthesia
bathypnea
batophobia
batrachophobia
Batson plexus
batt
battacca
battalion
battarism
battarismus
Battelle Developmental Inventory
Batten disease
Batten-Mayou disease
battered
b. baby
b. child
b. child syndrome (BCS)
b. infant syndrome
b. parent
b. spouse
b. spouse syndrome
b. wife
b. woman syndrome (BWS)
battery
ability b.
achievement b.
b. acid
Aphasia Clinical B.
aptitude b.
Armed Services Vocational
Aptitude B. (ASVAB)
assault and b.
assessment b.
Azima b.
Behavior Assessment B., 2nd
edition

battery *(continued)*
    Cambridge Test B.
    CERAD Assessment B.
    chemistry screening b. I (CSB I)
    chemistry screening b. II (CSB II)
    Children's Language B.
    Claybury Selection B.
    Clinical Support System B.
    Cognitive Control B.
    Cognitive Diagnostic B.
    Cognitive Skills Assessment B.
    Colorado Educational Interest B.
    Comprehensive Ability B. (CAB)
    Computer Operator Aptitude B.
      (COAB)
    Computer Programmer Aptitude B.
      (CPAB)
    diagnostic b.
    Diagnostic Achievement B., Second
      Edition (DAB-2)
    Diagnostic Skills B.
    educational achievement b.
    Effective School B. (ESB)
    electrophysiological b.
    Environmental Pre-Language B.
    Florida Kindergarten Screening B.
    Frostig Movement Skills Test B.
      (FMSTB)
    General Aptitude Test B. (GATB)
    G-F-W B.
    Goldman-Fristoe-Woodcock Auditory
      Skills Test B.
    Halstead-Reitan B. (HRB)
    Halstead-Reitan Neuropsychological
      Test B. (HRNTB)
    Hay Aptitude Test B.
    B. of Health Improvement (BHI)
    International Primary Factors
      test b.
    IPF test b.
    Jevs Work Sample B.
    Leisure Diagnostic B.
    Luria-Nebraska
      Neuropsychological B. (LNNB)
    Mental Deterioration B. (MDB)
    Michigan English Language
      Assessment B.
    Minnesota Clerical Assessment B.
      (MCAB)
    Motor Steadiness B.
    Multidimensional Aptitude B.
    Non-Reading Aptitude Test B.
      (NATB)
    Objective Analytic B.
    Pimsleur Language Aptitude B.
    quantitative electrophysiological b.
    Rand Functional Limitations B.
    Rand Physical Capacities B.
    Rand Social Health B.
    Rivermead Perceptual
      Assessment B. (RPAB)
    Schubert General Ability B.
    Social and Prevocational
      Information B. (SPIB)
    Special Aptitude Test B. (SATB)
    Specific Aptitude Test B.
    test b.
    b. test
    Trites Neuropsychological Test B.
    Valpar Work Sample B.
    Western Aphasia B. (WAB)
    Woodcock-Johnson
      Psychoeducational Test B.
      (WJPTB)
    Woodcock Language Proficiency B.
    Word Processor Assessment B.
    Work Sample B.

battle
    b. fatigability
    b. fatigue
    b. neurosis
    b. psychoneurosis
battledore incision
Battle sign
Battley sedative
Baxter disease
Bay Area Functional Performance Evaluation, Second Edition
Bayer
    B. Aspirin
    B. Buffered Aspirin
    B. Low Adult Strength
    B. Select Chest Cold Caplets
    B. Select Pain Relief Formula
Bayle disease
Bayley
    B. Behavior Record
    B. Infant Neurodevelopmental
      Screener (BINS)
    B. Scales of Infant Development
      (BSID)
Baylorfast diet
bayonet
    b. aneurysm clip
    b. clip applier
    b. forceps
    b. handle
BBB
    blood-brain barrier
BBRS
    Burks Behavior Rating Scale
BBT
    Bingham Button Test
BBTB
    blood-brain-tumor barrier
BBTOP
    Bankson-Bernthal Test of Phonology
BC
    behavior control
    birth control
BCCI
    Barclay Classroom Climate Inventory
BCD
    bad conduct discharge
BchE
    butylcholinesterase
BCP
    birth control pill
B-C powder

BCR
behavior control room
BCRS
Brief Cognitive Rating Scale
BCS
battered child syndrome
BDAC
Bureau of Drug Abuse Control
BDAE
Boston Diagnostic Aphasia Examination
BDD
body dysmorphic disorder
bdelygmia
BDI
Beck Depression Inventory
BDID
bystander dominates initial dominant
BDIS
Behavior Disorders Identification Scale
BDL
below detectable levels
BDNF
brain-derived neurotrophic factor
brain-derived neurotropic factor
BDRS
Blessed Dementia Rating Scale
beads
worry b.
BEAM
brain electrical activity mapping
beam
b. hardening artifact
high energy X-ray b.
laser b.
particle b.
proton b.
radiation b.
bearable
Beard disease
bearing
grudge b.
beast fetishism
beaten
b. copper cranium
b. copper pattern
beaten-metal appearance
beatific vision
beat vial
beau monde
Beaver
B. discission blade
B. keratome blade
Bechterew, Bechtereff
B. band
B. disease
B. nucleus
B. sign
Bechterew-Mendel reflex
Beck
B. Depression Inventory (BDI)
B. depression inventory score
B. Depression Scale
B. Hopelessness Scale (BHS)
B. Questionnaire
B. Suicide Intent Scale

B. Suicide Lethality Scale
B. view of depressive disorder
Becker
B. muscular dystrophy
B. variant
B. variant of Duchenne dystrophy
Becker-Kiener dystrophy
Becker-type tardive muscular dystrophy
Beckman-Adson laminectomy blade
Beckman-Eaton
B.-E. laminectomy
B.-E. laminectomy blade
B.-E. laminectomy retractor
Beckman retractor
Beckman-Weitlaner
B.-W. laminectomy
B.-W. laminectomy retractor
Beckwith-Wiedemann syndrome
beclouded dementia
bed
BioDyne b.
Burke Bariatric b.
Cardiopulmonary Paragon 8500 b.
Clinitron air b.
b. crisis
dynamic b.
Flexicair b.
high-air-loss b.
high muscular resistance b.
Keane Mobility b.
KinAir b.
Lapidus b.
low-air-loss b.
Magnum 800 b.
Medicus b.
Mega-Air b.
Mega Tilt and Turn b.
out of b. (OOB)
b. partner
Pulmonair 40 b.
Restcue b.
Skytron b.
SMI 3000 b.
SMI 5000 b.
Stryker b.
Thera Pulse b.
Tilt and Turn Paragon b.
tumor b.
Bedford Life Events and Difficulties Scale
bediamism
bedside
B. Evaluation and Screening Test of Aphasia
b. manner
b. multimodality monitoring
bedtime
Beery
B. Picture Vocabulary Screening (PVS)
B. Picture Vocabulary Screening Series
B. Picture Vocabulary Test and Beery Picture Vocabulary Screening Series

Beery (*continued*)
B. Test of Visual Motor Integration
B. Visual Motor Test
Beery-Buktinica
B.-B. Developmental Test
B.-B. Developmental Test of Visual Motor Integration
bees' nest
Beevor sign
before meals (a.c.)
Begbie disease
beggar
emotional b.
beginner
Aptitude Tests for School B.'s (ASB, ATSB)
BEHAVE-AD
Behavioral Pathology in Alzheimer Disease
BEHAVE-AD Rating Scale
behavior
aberrant b.
abstract b.
abusive vocal b.
acceptable b.
accident-prone b.
achievement b.
acting out b.
activity and b.
B. Activity Profile (BAP)
adaptive b.
addictive b.
adient b.
adjust repetitive b.
adolescent b.
adultomorphic b.
age-appropriate b.
age-level b.
aggressive b.
agitated b.
agnostic b.
aimless b.
alexithymic b.
alleviating aggressive b.
alleviating violence in aggressive b.
alternating b.
alternative b.
altruistic b.
ambient b.
amoral b.
amotivated b.
anarchic b.
angry b.
anomalous sexual b.
antagonistic b.
anticipatory and struggle b.
antinodal b.
antisocial b.
apopathetic b.
appetitive b.
appropriate b.
apraxic b.
arrogant b.

assaultive b.
assertive b.
b. assessment
B. Assessment Battery, 2nd edition
attachment b.
attending b.
attention-seeking b.
atypical b.
autoaggressive b.
automatic b.
aversive b.
avoidant b.
avoidant-attached b.
bailout b.
binge-eating b.
binge-eating/purging b.
bisexual b.
bizarre b.
borderline b.
catastrophic b.
catatonic motor b.
ceremonial b.
chain b.
b. chain
characteristic b.
chewing b.
child b.
child or adolescent antisocial b.
childhood cross-gender b.
choice b.
clinging b.
clinical b.
coercive b.
cognitive b.
collateral b.
collective b.
compelled b.
compensatory b.
competitive b.
complex motor b.
Comprehensive Test of Adaptive B.
compulsive drug-taking b.
compulsive sexual b.
consumer b.
contact b.
b. contract
contractual b.
b. control (BC)
b. control room (BCR)
cooperative b.
coping b.
copulatory b.
countertransference b.
courtship b.
covert b.
criminal b.
criterion b.
cross-dressing b.
cross-gender b.
crowd b.
cuddling b.
culturally appropriate avoidant b.
culturally sanctioned b.

cultural-related standards of sexual b.
cunning and hiding b.
cyclothymic-depressive b.
de-escalating aggressive b.
defensive b.
defiant b.
delinquent b.
delusional b.
demanding b.
dementia-related b.
dependent b.
destructive b.
b. determinant
developmentally appropriate avoidant b.
developmentally appropriate shy b.
deviant political b.
deviant religious b.
differential reinforcement of other b. (DRO)
diminution of goal-directed b.
direct self-destructive b. (DSDB)
discordant b.
discriminatory b.
disinhibited b.
disobedient b.
b. disorders of childhood
B. Disorders Identification Scale (BDIS)
disorganized b.
b. disruption
disruptive b.
disturbed eating b.
dominant-subordinate b.
drinking b.
driven motor b.
driving b.
drug-seeking b.
dysarthric b.
dysrhythmic aggressive b.
dyssocial b.
eating b.
eccentric b.
ecstatic b.
ego-dystonic b.
egosyntonic b.
elicited b.
embracing b.
emitted b.
empathic b.
entry b.
envious b.
erotic b.
eroticized b.
erratic b.
escape b.
estrous b.
ethical b.
ethnic relational b. (ERB)
B. Evaluation Scale-2 (BES-2)
evasive b.
excitable b.
exhibitionistic b.
experimental analysis of b.

explicit b.
exploitative-manipulative b.
exploratory b.
explosive aggressive b.
externalizing b.
extraindividual b.
extramarital b.
face-saving b.
failure to sustain consistent work b.
feeding b.
felony b.
fidgeting b.
b. field
finger-biting b.
fire-setting b.
flirtatious b.
following b.
freezing b.
gambling b.
gang b.
b. genetics
goal-directed b.
grossly disorganized b.
group b.
hair-pulling b.
hallucinatory b.
haughty b.
head-banging b.
health b.
helping b.
help-seeking b.
heterosexual b.
hiding b.
high-risk b.
homicidal b.
homosexual b.
hostile b.
hunting b.
hyperactive b.
hyperactive-impulsive combined b.
idiosyncratic b.
illness b.
imitative b.
immediacy b.
implicit b.
impulsive b.
inappropriate b.
inattentive b.
incoherent b.
incompatible b.
indirect self-destructive b. (ISDB)
infantile b.
ingratiating b.
initiation of goal-directed b.
innate b.
instinctive b.
intense sexual b.
intentional involuntary b.
interictal b.
intermittent explosive b.
interpersonal b.
intimidating b.
intrinsic b.
invariable b.

behavior *(continued)*
b. inventory
involuntary b.
irrational b.
irresponsible work b.
isolative b.
kinesic b.
kissing b.
knowledge, attitude, b. (KAB)
language b.
b. language
lawful b.
leadership b.
learned dysfunctional b.
life-threatening b. (LTB)
limit-testing b.
locality-specific pattern of
  aberrant b.
localization of b.
maladaptive b.
malevolent b.
management of assaultive b.
  (MAB)
manipulative b.
masochistic sexual b.
mass b.
maternal b.
mating b.
maze b.
mercurial b.
b. method
mischievous b.
mobbing b.
modeled b.
b. modification (B-mod)
b. modification program
molar b.
molecular b.
moral b.
motor b.
multidetermined b.
murderous predation b.
negative b.
negativistic b.
nodal b.
nonfunctional and repetitive
  motor b.
nonparaphilic compulsive sexual b.
nonproductive b.
nonverbal b.
nonviolent b.
normative b.
obedient b.
obsessive b.
odd b.
oddities of b.
oedipal b.
on-task b.
operant b.
operative b.
oral b.
out-of-control b.
overt b.
pacing b.

pain b.
paranoid b.
paraphiliac b.
parasuicidal b.
parental b.
Parent Rating of Student B.
passive b.
passive-aggressive b.
paternal b.
pathologic b.
b. pattern
pattern of antisocial b.
peculiar b.
pedophilic b.
petting b.
phobic b.
pressured b.
primary b.
B. Problem Checklist (BPC)
promiscuous sexual b.
provocative b.
psychomotor b.
psychotic b.
Pupil Record of Education B.
  (PREB)
purposeful b.
b. rating
B. Rating Instrument for Autistic
  and Other Atypical Children
B. Rating Profile, Second Edition
  (BRP-2)
b. rating scale
b. reaction
reckless b.
b. record
b. reflex
regressive b.
rehabilitation b.
b. rehearsal
relational b.
REM sleep b.
repetitious b.
repetitive checking b.
repetitive pattern of b.
repressive b.
respondent b.
restless b.
restricted b.
restricting b.
restrictive b.
b. reversal
risk-taking b.
risky b.
ritual b.
ritualistic b.
b. role
sadistic b.
b. sampling
Scale of Independent B.
seductive b.
self-damaging b.
self-defeating b.
self-destructive b.
self-dramatizing b.
self-injurious b. (SIB)

self-mutilating b.
self-punishing b.
self-stimulatory b.
semipurposeful b.
sensory/motor b.
b. setting
sex-role b.
sexual b.
sexually arousing b.
sexual predation b.
b. shaping
sissyish b.
sleepwalking b.
social b.
socially acceptable b.
socially unacceptable b.
social phobic-like b.
social stereotypical b.
sociopathic b.
spatial b.
speech b.
speech and language b.
splitting b.
stalking b.
standard b.
B. Status Inventory (BSI)
stereotyped pattern of b.
stereotypical b.
stimulation-bound b. (SBB)
structural analysis of social b.
struggle b.
B. Style Questionnaire (BSQ)
subliminal b.
submissive b.
substance-seeking b.
substituting b.
sucking b.
suicidal b.
superstitious b.
suspicious b.
target b.
Teacher Assessment of Social B.
  (TASB)
terminal achievement b.
terrorism b.
threatening b.
tic-like b.
tomboy b.
tool-using b.
trancelike b.
transference b.
b. type
type A b.
type B b.
typical b.
tyrannical b.
unacceptable b.
uncued b.
undersocialized conduct b.
unemployable unethical b.
unethical b.
unexpected b.
uninhibited b.
unlawful b.
unpurposeful b.

unusual b.
unvoluntary b.
usual b.
variable b.
verbal b.
violent b.
visuomotor b.
voluntary b.
voyeuristic b.
voyeuristic sexual b.
water-seeking b.
wild b.
behavioral
B. Academic Self-Esteem
b. activation system (BAS)
b. analysis
b. approach
B. Assessment of Pain (BAP)
B. Assessment of Pain
  Questionnaire (P-BAP)
B. Assessment Test
b. avoidance test for OCD
b. baseline
b. change
B. Checklist
b. consistency
b. contingency
b. contract
b. couples group therapy
b. criterion
b. development
B. Deviancy Profile
b. disorder
b. disorganization in schizophrenia
b. disturbance
b. dynamics
b. dyscontrol
b. dysfunction
b. dysfunction symptom
b. endocrinology
b. facilitation
b. flexibility
b. genetics
B. Health Systems (BHS)
b. immunogen
B. Inattention Test (BIT)
b. inhibition system (BIS)
b. management
b. manifestation
b. mapping
b. marital therapy (BMT)
b. medicine
b. memory
b. metamorphosis
b. model
b. modeling
b. monitoring
b. neuroanatomy
b. neurobiology
b. neurochemistry
b. neurology
b. objective
b. observation audiometry (BOA)
B. Observation Scale for Autism
b. oscillation

B

behavioral *(continued)*
    b. outburst
    b. pathogen
    B. Pathology in Alzheimer Disease
      (BEHAVE-AD)
    B. Pathology in Alzheimer Disease
      Rating Scale
    B. Performance Situation
    B. Problems Scale
    b. prosthesis
    b. psychiatry
    b. psychology
    b. psychotherapy
    b. rating scale
    b. reaction brain syndrome
    b. rehearsal
    b. repertoire
    b. research
    b. research orientation
    B. Scale for Developmentally
      Deviant Preschoolers
    b. science
    b. semantics
    b. sensitization
    b. set of disturbances
    b. technique
    b. theory
    b. theory of rumination
    b. toxicity
    b. transgression
    b. treatment
    b. undercontrol
    b. variability
behavior-altering substance
behavior-constraint theory
behaviorism
    eclectic b.
    operant b.
    radical b.
    Tolman purposive b.
behaviorist
behavioristic psychology
behavior-orientation
    Judgment of Occupational B.-o.
behavior-oriented assessment
behavior/personality
    type A b.
    type B b.
behavior-specimen recording
Behçet
    B. disease
    B. syndrome
behind the scale
Behn-Rorschach Test
Behr
    B. complicated optic atrophy
    B. syndrome
beigelii
    Trichosporon b.
Beimer-Clip aneurysm clip
being
    b. cognition
    b. motivation

    supreme b.
    b. value
Bekesy Functionality Detection Test
  (BFDT)
Bekhterev *(var. of* Bechtereff)
belief
    Christian b.
    cultural b.
    culture-bound b.
    delusional b.
    deviant b.
    dominant delusional b.
    endorsement of deviant thoughts
      and b.'s
    erroneous b.
    exaggerated b.
    false b.
    firmly held b.
    fixed b.
    fully organized b.
    internal world of b.
    loss of b.
    odd b.
    shared delusional b.
    sustained b.
    b. system of self-help
    traditional b.
    true b.
    unreasonable b.
    unshakable b.
believable
believe
    make b.
    This I B. (TIB)
Belix Oral
bell
    B. disease
    B. law
    B. mania
    B. Object Relations-Reality Testing
      Inventory
    b. and pad technique
    B. palsy
    B. paralysis
    B. phenomenon
    B. spasm
    B. Visible Speech
belladonna
    b. alkaloid
    b. and opium (B&O)
belladonna, phenobarbital, and
  ergotamine tartrate
Bellatal
belle
Bellergal-S
Bellevue Index of Depression
belligerent
Bell-Magendie law
bellows
    aneuroid chest b.
bell-shaped curve
belly dancer dyskinesia
Belmont collar
belonephobia

below-average student
below detectable levels (BDL)
Bel-Phen-Ergot S
Belyando spruce
bemar
    jinjinia b.
bemegride
bemidone
bemoan
Bem Sex-Role Inventory
bemuse
benactyzine hydrochloride
Benadryl
    B. Injection
    B. Oral
Ben-Allergin-50 Injection
benazepril and hydrochlorothiazide
Bence Jones protein
benchmark
bench warrant
bender
    French rod b.
    B. Gestalt (BG)
    B. Visual Gestalt drawing
    B. Visual-Motor Gestalt Test
    (BVMGT)
    B. Visual Retention Test
Bender-Gestalt
    B.-G. hexagon
    B.-G. Test (BGT)
    B.-G. Visual Motor Test
bending
    rod b.
    rule b.
    b. strength
bendroflumethiazide
beneceptor
Benedek reflex
Benedikt
    B. ipsilateral oculomotor paralysis
    B. syndrome
Benemid
benign
    b. brain neoplasm
    b. capillary hemangioblastoma
    b. cranial nerve tumors
    b. epileptiform transient of sleep
    (BETS)
    b. essential tremor
    b. exertional headache
    b. familial myoclonic epilepsy
    b. familial neonatal convulsion
    b. fasciculation with cramp
    b. focal amyotrophy
    b. focal of childhood epilepsy
    b. functional vertigo
    b. habit
    b. intracranial hypertension (BIH)
    b. lymphocytic choriomeningitis
    b. lymphocytic meningitis
    b. lymphoepithelial parotid tumor
    b. myalgic encephalitis
    b. myalgic encephalomyelitis
    b. neonatal familial seizure
    b. paralogia

    b. paroxysmal torticollis
    b. paroxysmal vertigo
    b. partial epilepsy of childhood
    b. positional paroxysmal vertigo
    b. psychopathy
    b. rolandic epilepsy
    b. senescent forgetfulness
    b. stupor
    b. tetanus
    b. X-linked recessive muscular
    dystrophy
Bennett Mechanical Comprehension Test
benoxaprofen
benperidol
benserazide
Benson-Geschwind classification of
  aphasia
bentazepam
Benton
    B. Controlled Oral Word
    Association
    B. Face Recognition Test
    B. Line Orientation Test
    B. Revised Visual Retention Test
    B. Visual Retention Test (BVRT)
bent-over neck
bent posture
Bentyl
benumb
benzamide
    substituted b.
benzathine penicillin
Benzedrine
benzenepropanamine
benzilate
    quinuclidinyl b.
benzisoxazole
benznidazole
benzoate
    caffeine and sodium b.
benzocaine
benzoctamine
benzodiazepine
    b. abuse
    b. antagonist
    b. dependence
    b. overdose
    b. receptor binding
    b. tolerance
    b. withdrawal
benzodiazepine-GABA-receptor complex
benzoic acid
benzoin
benzothiadiazide
benzothiazine
    dibenzepin b.
benzoylecgonine
benzphetamine hydrochloride
benztropine mesylate
BEP
    brain evoked potential
bereavement
    b. in children
    conjugal b.
    b. disorder

B

bereavement *(continued)*
    feigned b.
    b. stage
    traumatic b.
    uncomplicated b.
    unresolved b.
bereavement-related depression
Berenstein guiding catheter
Berger
    B. paresthesia
    B. rhythm
Bergeron
    B. chorea
    B. disease
Bergmann
    B. cord
    B. fiber
Bergstrom cannula
beriberi
    cerebral b.
    dry b.
    wet b.
Berliner percussion hammer
Bernard-Horner syndrome
Bernard puncture
Bernard-Soulier disease
Bernasconi-Cassinari artery
Bernhardt disease
Bernhardt-Roth syndrome
Bernoulli law
Bernreuter Personality Inventory
Bero Test
berry aneurysm
Bertillon cephalometer
BES-2
    Behavior Evaluation Scale-2
Bessman-Baldwin syndrome
best-fit
    b.-f. analysis
    b.-f. curve
bestialis
    mixoscopia b.
bestiality
best registration error
besylate
    atracurium b.
    mesoridazine b.
beta, β
    b. activity
    b. adrenergic blocking agent
    b. adrenergic medication
    b. adrenergic receptor
    b. alcoholism
    b. amyloid
    b. amyloid peptide
    b. arc
    b. blocker
    b. carboline
    b. cell
    b. endorphin
    b. error
    b. fiber
    b. glucuronidase

    b. hemolytic streptococcus meningitis
    b. histine
    b. hydroxybutyrate
    b. hypothesis
    b. index
    b. level
    b. mannosidosis
    b. movement
    b. pattern on EEG
    b. rhythm
    b. rhythm on EEG
    b. stimulant
    b. subunit
    b. test
    transforming growth factor b.
    b. wave
    b. wave on EEG
    b. weight
beta-adrenergic
    b.-a. antagonist
    b.-a. blocker
    b.-a. blocking drug
    b.-a. medication-induced postural tremor
beta-amyloid protein
Betachron E-R capsule
betacism
Betadine Helafoam solution
beta-emitting radiation
beta-hemolytic streptococcus
beta-human chorionic gonadotropin
beta-hydroxylase
    plasma dopamine b.-h. (DBH)
betamethasone
beta$_2$ microglobulin
Betaseron needle-free delivery system
Beta-Val
betel nut
bethanechol
BETS
    benign epileptiform transient of sleep
betterment
between
    betwixt and b.
between-group variance
betwixt and between
Betz cell
Beuren syndrome
Bevan-Lewis cell
Bevatron accelerator
bevel
Bexley-Maudsley Automated Psychological Screening
Bexophene
Beyer laminectomy rongeur
Bezold-Brucke phenomenon
Bezold ganglion
Bezold-Jarisch reflex
BFDT
    Bekesy Functionality Detection Test
bFGF
    basic fibroblast growth factor
BFQ
    Big Five Questionnaire

B

BG
    Bender Gestalt
BGT
    Bender-Gestalt Test
Bhakti yoga
BHI
    Battery of Health Improvement
BHS
    Beck Hopelessness Scale
    Behavioral Health Systems
Bianchi syndrome
bias
    attentional b.
    emotional b.
    evaluator b.
    exotic b.
    experimental b.
    experimenter b.
    free recall b.
    memory b.
    selection b.
    societal b.
    volunteer b.
BIB
    brought in by
biblicism
bibliokleptomania
bibliolater
bibliomania
bibliophile
bibliophobia
bibliotherapeutic strategy
bibliotherapy
bibrachial paresis
Bibring view of depressive disorder
bibulous
BICAP
    bipolar cautery probe
    BICAP cautery
    BICAP unit
bicarbonate
    potassium b.
    serum b.
    sodium b.
bicaudate ratio
biceps femoris reflex
bicerebral infarction
Bichat
    B. canal
    B. fissure
    B. foramen
Bicillin
bicircadian rhythm
bicisate
    technetium 99m b.
Bickerstaff
    B. encephalitis
    B. migraine
    B. migraine headache
BiCNU
    carmustine
biconditional
BICROS
    bilateral contralateral routing of signals
bicultural

bidialectalism
bidirectional selection study
biduous
Bidwell ghost
Biedl-Moon-Laurence syndrome
Bielschowsky
    B. disease
    B. head tilt test
    B. idiocy
    B. maneuver
Bielschowsky-Jansky disease
Biemond
    B. ataxia
    B. disease
    B. syndrome
Bier
    B. block
    B. lumbar puncture needle
    B. saw
Biernacki sign
bifid
    b. cranium
    b. hook
    b. tongue
    b. uvula
bifida
    cranial b.
    spina b.
bifidum
    cranium b.
bifrontal
    b. craniotomy
    b. headache
    b. incision
    b. malignant meningioma
bifunctional
bifurcated
bifurcation
    basilar b.
    carotid b.
    cervical carotid b.
bigamist
bigamy
Bigelow calvarium clamp
bigeminal body
Big Five Questionnaire (BFQ)
bigotry
BIH
    basal interhemispheric approach
    benign intracranial hypertension
bihemispheral insult
bilabial
bilateral
    b. abductor paralysis
    b. acoustic neuroma syndrome
    b. activity
    b. adductor paralysis
    b. arachnoid cyst
    b. centrocecal scotoma
    b. choroid plexus cyst
    b. contralateral routing of signals
       (BICROS)
    b. craniectomy
    b. ECT
    b. gaze palsy

bilateral *(continued)*
    b. hemisphere dysfunction
    b. hermaphroditism
    b. homonymous hemianopia
    b. hydrocephalus
    b. hyperreflexia
    b. independent periodic lateralizing epileptiform discharge (BIPLED)
    b. ligamentectomy
    b. myoclonic seizure
    b. occipital infarcts
    b. speech
    b. synchrony
    b. temporary tarsorrhaphy
    b. transfer
    b. upper brain stem infarction
    b. variable screw placement system
    b. ventral rhizotomy
bilayer
    lipid b.
bilharziasis
biliary dyskinesia
Biligrafin
Biligram
bilineal family
bilingual
bilingualism
    active b.
Bilingual Syntax Measure II Test (BSM)
Biliodyl
bilious headache
bilirachia
bilirubin encephalopathy
bilis
Bilivistan
bill
    b. of goods
    b. of particulars
    b. of rights
billet-doux
billingsgate
biloba
    Ginkgo b.
bilobed aneurysm
Bilopaque
Biloptin
biloquialism
bimanual coordination deficit
bimastoid line
bimedial
    b. frontal leukotomy
    b. leukotomy
bimodal distribution
binary principle
binaural shift
bind
    b. analysis date
    double b.
    b. over
binders
    breast b.
binding
    benzodiazepine receptor b.

    H-imipramine b.
    libido b.
    in vivo benzodiazepine receptor b.
Binet
    B. age
    B. scale
    B. test
Binet-Simon
    B.-S. scale
    B.-S. test
binge
    alcohol b.
    alcoholic b.
    b. buyer
    cocaine b.
    b. drinker
    b. drinking
    drug b.
    eating b.
    b. eating
    b. eating pattern
    b. gambling
    b. and purge
binge-eating
    b.-e. behavior
    b.-e. disorder
binge-eating/purging
    b.-e. behavior
bingeing *(var. of* binging)
Bingham Button Test (BBT)
Bing-Horton syndrome
binging, bingeing
Bing-Neel syndrome
Bing reflex
binocular
    b. acuity change
    b. perception
    b. vision
binomial
    b. distribution
    b. test
BINS
    Bayley Infant Neurodevelopmental Screener
Binswanger
    B. dementia
    B. disease
    B. encephalitis
    B. encephalopathy
bioactive
bioanalysis
bioassay
bioavailability
    neuroleptic b.
biobehavioral shift
Biobond
biocatalyst
bioccipital headache
bioceramic
    calcium phosphate b.
biochemical
    b. anatomy
    b. genetics
    b. imbalance

b. pathway
b. tumor marker
biochemorphology
biocidal
biocide
bioclimatology
biocompatible
biocybernetics
biocyclebiome
biodata
biodynamics
BioDyne bed
bioelectric potential
bioelement
bioenergetic
    b. deficiency
    b. therapy
bioenergetics
bioengineering
bioequivalence
bioequivalent
bioethics bionics
biofeedback
    b. application
    b. computer
    EEG b.
    electrodermal response b. (EDR)
    electromyography b.
    EMG b.
    galvanic skin response b.
    b. meter
    b. method
    temperature b.
    b. theory
    b. tones
    b. training
Biogel Sensor surgical glove
biogenesis
biogenetic mental law
biogenic
    b. amine
    b. amine hypothesis
    b. amine neurotransmitter
    b. psychosis
biogram
biographical
    b. data
    B. Inventory Form U
    b. memory
    b. method
biography
    reactions b.
biohazard
Biojector 2000 needle-free injection management system
biokinetics
biolinguistic
    b. language theory
    b. theory
biologic, biological
    b. act
    b. age
    b. basis
    b. causation
    b. changes associated with aging

chemical, radiological, and b.
    b. child
    b. clock
    b. consideration
    b. control
    b. data
    b. determinism
    b. diathesis
    b. drive
    b. dysfunction
    b. dysfunction symptom
    b. factor
    b. intelligence
    b. marker
    b. maturity
    b. measure
    b. predisposition
    b. process
    b. psychiatry
    b. research orientation
    b. response modifier
    b. rhythm
    b. roots of addiction
    b. sex
    b. sign depression
    b. status
    b. stress
    b. taxonomy
    b. theory
    b. therapy
    b. time
    b. viewpoint
    b. warfare
    b. weapon
biologism
biologos
biology
    b. of affective disease
    communications in behavioral b. (CBB)
    b. of deceit
bioluminescence
biolytic
biomagnetometer (BTi)
    37-channel b.
biomarker
biomathematics
biomechanical
    b. analysis
    b. factor
    b. testing
biomechanics
    axial plane angular deformity b.
    distraction instrumentation b.
    Dwyer instrumentation b.
    posterior fixation system b.
    Roy-Camille posterior screw plate fixation b.
biomedical
    b. engineering
    b. therapy
biomedicine
biometal
biometry
bion

bionergy
bionic
bionics
　　bioethics b.
bionomics
bionomy
biopercular syndrome
biophilia
biophysical
　　b. life change
　　b. system
biophysics
biophysiology
bioplastic
biopotential
biopsy
　　brain b.
　　CT-guided b.
　　endoscopic sphenoidal b.
　　image-guided stereotactic brain b.
　　leptomeningeal/wedge cortical b.
　　lumbar spine b.
　　meningeal b.
　　muscle b.
　　PET-guided stereotactic b.
　　stereotactic b.
　　sural nerve b.
　　targeted brain b.
　　thoracic spine b.
　　transnasal b.
　　Tru-Cut needle b. (TCNB)
biopsychic
biopsychology
biopsychosocial
　　b. history
　　b. model
　　b. paradigm
　　b. variable
biopterin
bioreversible
biorhythm
bioscience
bioscopy
biosis
biosocial
　　b. determinism
　　b. theory
Biosol
biosphere
biostatic
biostatistics
biosynthesis
　　heme b.
biosystematics
Biot
　　B. breathing
　　B. respiration
biotaxis
biotechnology
biotelemetry
biotic potential
biotin
biotoxication
biotoxicology
biotoxin

BioTrainer exercise meter
biotransformation
biotrepy
biotype
biotypology
biovular twin
BIOWARE software for Biodex
　　isokinetic exercise system
biparental
biparietal lesion
bipedal walking
biperiden
biphasic
　　b. action potential
　　b. symptom
Biphetamine
biplane roentgenogram
BIPLED
　　bilateral independent periodic lateralizing
　　epileptiform discharge
　　BIPLED on EEG
bipolar
　　b. affective disorder
　　b. affective psychosis
　　b. bayonet forceps
　　b. cautery
　　b. cautery probe (BICAP)
　　b. cautery scissors
　　b. cell
　　b. coagulating forceps
　　b. coagulation
　　b. coagulator
　　b. depression
　　b. depression disorder
　　b. diathermy forceps tip
　　b. electrocautery
　　b. electrocautery forceps
　　b. gradient
　　b. I disorder
　　b. I disorder, most recent episode
　　hypomanic
　　b. I disorder, most recent episode
　　mixed
　　b. I disorder, most recent episode
　　unspecified
　　b. I disorder, single manic episode
　　b. II
　　b. II disorder
　　b. illness (BPI)
　　b. long-shaft forceps
　　b. montage
　　b. neuron
　　B. Psychological Inventory (BPI)
　　b. type schizoaffective disorder
　　b. vertebral traction
bipole
　　narrow b.
　　wide b.
biportal technique
bipotentiality
biracial
Birbeck granule
birdcage resonator
birdlike facies
bird of passage

B

birth
>   b. anoxia
>   b. brain trauma organic psychosis
>   b. canal
>   b. certificate
>   complete b.
>   b. control (BC)
>   b. control pill (BCP)
>   b. control regimen
>   cross b.
>   b. cry
>   date of b.
>   b. date
>   b. defect
>   b. injury
>   live b.
>   multiple b.
>   b. order
>   b. palsy
>   premature b.
>   b. rate
>   season of b.
>   B. to Three Assessment and
>   Intervention System
>   B. to Three Developmental Scale
>   b. trauma
>   year of b. (YOB)

BIS
>   behavioral inhibition system

Bischof myelotomy

bisection
>   vertical line b.

bisensory method

bisexual
>   b. behavior
>   b. confusion
>   b. libido
>   b. orientation
>   b. pedophilia

bisexuality
>   theory of constitutional b.

bis-**guanylhydrazone**
>   methylglyoxal *bis*-g. (MGBG)

Bishop putty

bismuth

bisphosphonate

bisulfate
>   clopidogrel b.

BIT
>   Behavioral Inattention Test

bit
>   acorn b.
>   cannulated drill b.
>   drill guide with drill b.
>   Howmedica Microfixation System
>   drill b.
>   Leibinger Micro System drill b.
>   Luhr Microfixation System drill b.
>   Storz Microsystems drill b.
>   Synthes Microsystem drill b.

bitartrate
>   dihydrocodeine b.
>   dihydrocodeinone b.
>   hydrocodone b.
>   metaraminol b.

BITCH
>   Black Intelligence Test of Culture
>   Homogeneity

bite
>   rattlesnake b.
>   snake b.
>   spider b.

bitemporal
>   b. hemianopia
>   b. hemianopsia

biting
>   b. attack
>   lip b.
>   b. mania
>   nail b.
>   b. stage

biundulant
>   b. meningoencephalitis
>   b. viral encephalitis

bivalved speculum

bivariate

biventral lobule

bizarre
>   b. answer
>   b. behavior
>   b. behavior/formal thought disorder
>   b. delusion
>   b. gesture
>   b. idea
>   b. posture
>   b. thought process

Björnström algesiometer

BKV
>   BK virus

BK virus (BKV)

BL
>   baseline

black
>   b. art
>   b. bart
>   b. and blue
>   b. death
>   B. English
>   b. eyeblind
>   b. hand
>   B. Intelligence Test of Culture
>   Homogeneity (BITCH)
>   b. magic
>   b. patch psychosis
>   b. patch syndrome
>   b. tar heroin

black-and-white thinking

blacking out

blacklist

blackmail
>   emotional b.

black-market medication

blackout
>   alcoholic b.
>   b. threshold

Blacky picture

bladder
>   atonic b.
>   autonomic neurogenic b.
>   b. control

bladder *(continued)*
  cord b.
  nervous b.
  neurogenic b.
  pseudoneurogenic b.
  b. reflex
  reflex neurogenic b.
  stammering of the b.
  b. training
  uninhibited neurogenic b.
blade
  Acra-Cut b.
  air b.
  arachnoid-shape Beaver b.
  Beaver discission b.
  Beaver keratome b.
  Beckman-Adson laminectomy b.
  Beckman-Eaton laminectomy b.
  double-vector b.
  Meyerding laminectomy b.
  Meyerding-Scoville b.
  Micro-Aire b.
  retractor b.
  ribbon b.
  Scoville b.
  tapered b.
  b. of tongue
BLADES
  Bristol Language Development Scale
Blair-Ivy loop
Blake pouch
blame
  externalize b.
  b. psychology
blame-placing communication pattern
bland
  b. affect
  b. diet
blank
  Correctional Officers' Interest B.
  Crowley Occupational Interests B.
    (COIB)
  Dole Vocational Sentence
    Completion B.
  b. hallucination
  interest b.
  Leisure Activities B. (LAB)
  Personnel Reaction B.
  Rothwell-Miller Interest B.
  Rotter Incomplete Sentences B.
    (RISB)
  b. stare
  Strong Vocational Interest B.
    (SVIB)
  Vocational Interest B. (VIB)
blanket
  security b.
  thermal b.
blaspheme
blasphemous thought
blasphemy
blast
  air b.

  b. effect
  stoma b.
Blastomyces dermatitidis
blastomycosis
  nasopharyngeal b.
  spinal b.
blastomyocotic meningitis
blatherskite
bleeding
  aneurysmal b.
  b. disorder
  b. time
  b. of undetermined origin (BUO)
blend
  consonant b.
blended family
blending
  auditory b.
  sound b.
blennophobia
blennorrhagic swelling
blennorrhagicum
  keratoderma b.
Blenoxane
bleomycin sulfate
blepharedema
blepharism
blepharitis
blepharoconjunctivitis
blepharophimosis
blepharoplegia
blepharospasm, blepharospasmus
  essential b.
blepsopathia
blessed
  B. Behavior Scale
  B. Dementia Rating Scale (BDRS)
  B. IMC Test
  B. Information and Concentration
    Test
  B. Information-Memory-
    Concentration Test
Blessed-Roth Dementia Scale (BRDS)
Bleuler diagnostic system
BLHI
  Brief Life History Inventory
blind
  b. analysis
  Anxiety Scale for the B. (ASB)
  color b.
  double b.
  b. drunk
  b. faith
  b. headache
  B. Learning Aptitude Test
  b. matching technique
  b. spot
  b. study
  b. trust
blindness
  amnesic color b.
  cerebral b.
  b. cerebral
  concussion b.
  conversion b.

cortical psychic b.
developmental word b.
functional b.
hysterical b.
ipsilateral monocular b.
legal b.
letter b.
mind b.
b. monocular
monocular b.
music b.
note b.
object b.
psychic b.
sign b.
smell b.
soul b.
syllabic b.
taste b.
text b.
total monocular b. (TMB)
transient b.
word b.

blink
b. artifact
b. reflex
b. reflex latency
b. response

blinking
eye b.

blister-like aneurysm
blithely ignored need
BLNAI
Barclay Learning Needs Assessment
Inventory

bloc
en b.

Blocadren Oral
Bloch equation
block
adrenergic b.
affect b.
alpha b.
b. anesthesia
anodal b.
atrioventricular b.
Bier b.
cervical steroid epidural nerve b.
clonic b.
b. design
b. design subtest
b. design test
diagnostic b.
epidural b.
genetic b.
intracellular calcium b.
left bundle branch b.
mental b.
methadone b.
methylmethacrylate b.
motor conduction b.
nerve root b.
b. sampling
short-acting b. (SAB)
somatic b.

spinal b.
sugar b.
tonic b.
b. vertebra

blockade
adrenergic b.
audible speech b.
central cholinergic b.
dopamine receptor b.
emotional b.
intravenous regional sympathetic b.
muscarine b.
muscarinic receptor b.
narcotic b.
neuromuscular b.
nicotinic receptor b.
pharmacological b.
silent speech b.
thought b.

blockage
shunt b.

blocked speech
blocker
beta b.
beta-adrenergic b.
calcium channel b.
dopamine receptor b.
voltage-gated sodium channel b.

blocking
b. activity
b. agent
alpha b.
EEG alpha b.
emotional b.
b. evidence
evidence of b.
b. procedure
thought b.

Blocq disease
Blom-Singer tracheoesophageal fistula
blond, blonde
blood
b. alcohol (BA)
b. alcohol concentration
b. alcohol concentration content
(BAC)
b. alcohol level (BAL)
bad b.
b. bank
b. cell
b. component
b. count
b. crossmatch
b. donor
b. drug screen
b. dyscrasia
b. feud
b. flow
b. flow measurement
full b.
b. gas exchange
b. group
b. level
b. loss
occult b.

B

blood *(continued)*
    b. poisoning
    b. pool imaging
    b. pressure
    b. psychogenic disorder
    b. screen for drugs test
    b. smear
    b. sugar
    b. test
    b. and thunder retina
    b. transfusion
    b. type
    b. urea nitrogen (BUN)
    b. velocity
    b. vessel
    b. viscosity
    b. volume
blood-brain
    b.-b. barrier (BBB)
    b.-b. barrier disruption
    chemotherapy
    b.-b. transcytosis
blood-brain-tumor barrier (BBTB)
blood-cerebrospinal fluid barrier
blood-CSF barrier
blood-injection-injury type
blood/injection phobia
bloodless decerebration
blood-thymus barrier
blood-tissue exchange
Bloom
    B. Analogies Test
    B. disease
Blos developmental model
blot
    Southern b.
Blount laminar spreader
blow
    death b.
    lethal b.
blown pupil
blow-out fracture
BLST
    Bankson Language Screening Test
BLT-2
    Bankson Language Test-2
blue
    black and b.
    cocaine b.'s
    b. de hue
    b. edema
    flat b.'s
    French b.
    Histacryl B.
    maternity b.'s
    methylene b.
    b. nevus
    out of the b.
    paternity b.'s
    postpartum b.'s
    royal b.'s
    b. velvet syndrome
    b. vial
blue-collar worker

blue-stained
    toluidine b.-s.
Blumenau nucleus
Blumenbach clivus
blunt
    b. nerve hook
    b. spike-and-wave complex on
    EEG
    b. suction tube
blunted
    b. affect
    b. response
blunting
    affective b.
    emotional b.
    Scale for Emotional B. (SEB)
blunt-ring curette
blurred vision
blurring
    b. of vision
    visual b.
blush
    choroidal b.
    b. of dye on angiogram
BM
    basement membrane
BMI
    body mass index
B-mod
    behavior modification
B-mode
    B-m. image
    B-m. ultrasonography
BMR
    basal metabolic rate
BMT
    behavioral marital therapy
BNCT
    boron neutron capture therapy
BNDD
    Bureau of Narcotics and Dangerous
    Drugs
BNMSE
    Brief Neuropsychological Mental Status
    Examination
BNP
    brain natriuretic peptide
BO
    body odor
B&O
    belladonna and opium
    B&O Supprettes
BOA
    behavioral observation audiometry
board
    b. and care facility
    b. certified psychiatrist
    conversation b.
    direct selection communication b.
    b. eligible psychiatrist
    encoding communication b.
    gender identity b.
    Institutional Review B.
    Ouija b.
    room and b.

B

scanning communication b.
sounding b.
board-and-care home
boarders
    phantom b.
boarding-out system
bobbing
    inverse ocular b.
    ocular b.
    reverse ocular b.
Bobechko
    B. sliding barrel hook
    B. spreader
boca torcida
Bochdalek
    flower basket of B.
    B. ganglion
Bock ganglion
BOD
    braided occlusion device
Boder Test of Reading-Spelling Patterns
Bodian silver impregnation
bodily
    b. disease
    b. illusion
    b. movement
    b. orifice
body
    aortic b.
    b. appearance
    artificial vertebral b.
    b. awareness
    B. Awareness Resource Network (BARNY)
    Barr chromatin b.
    bigeminal b.
    b. boundary
    b. buffer zone
    b. build
    carotid b.
    b. cathexis
    cell b.
    b. coil
    b. composition
    b. concept-exploration maneuver
    b. conceptualization disturbance
    b. contact-exploration maneuver
    Cowdry-type intranuclear inclusion b.
    cytoid b.
    b. dipping
    b. dissatisfaction
    b. dysgnosia
    b. dysmorphic defect
    b. dysmorphic disorder (BDD)
    b. dysphoria
    b. dystonia
    b. ego
    b. ego concept
    emaciated b.
    fat b.
    b. fluid
    foreign b.
    b. of fornix
    b. functioning

geniculate b.
b. gesture
glomus b.
Herring b.
Hirano b.
hitting own b.
hookean b.
hyaline b. of pituitary
b. ideal
b. identity
b. image
b. image distortion
b. image disturbance
B. Image and Eating Questionnaire
immune b.
intraneuronal argentophilic Pick inclusion b.
juxtarestiform b.
Kelvin b.
Lafora b.
lateral geniculate b.
Lewy inclusion b.
Luys b.
mamillary b. (MB)
mammary b.
b. mass index (BMI)
b. mechanics
medial geniculate b.
b. memory
metallic foreign b.
b. monitor
b. movement
muscular b.
myelin b.
b. narcissism
nerve cell b.
newtonian b.
Nissl b.
nucleus of the mamillary b.
nucleus of medial geniculate b.
obese b.
b. odor (BO)
olivary b.
b. orifice
pacchionian b.
paraterminal b.
PAS-positive circular b.
peduncle of mamillary b.
pedunculus of pineal b.
b. percept
perception localized within the b.
perineal b.
Pick b.
pineal b.
b. position
b. posture
b. protest
psammoma b.
pseudopsammoma b.
quadrigeminal b.
restiform b.
rhinencephalic mamillary b.
b. righting reflex
b. rocking
sand b.

body *(continued)*
    b. schema
    Schwann cell b.
    B. Sensations Questionnaire
    b. shape
    B. Shape Questionnaire
    striate b.
    b. surface area
    b. swaying
    b. therapy
    b. tic
    tigroid b.
    trapezoid b.
    b. type
    Vater-Pacini b.
    Verocay b.
    b. water
    Winkler b.
    Wolf-Orton b.
body-image
    b.-i. agnosia
    b.-i. hallucination
    b.-i. perception
    b.-i. recall
body-mind dichotomy
Boehm Test of Basic Concepts
bogyphobia
bohd
Bohlman
    B. anterior cervical vertebrectomy
    B. cervical fusion technique
Bohr effect
bolasterone
boldenone
Bolgar-Fischer Word Test
Bolivian hemorrhagic fever
Bollinger
    posttraumatic apoplexy of B.
bolster
BOLT
    Basic Occupational Literacy Test
bolt
    bullet b.
    Camino microventricular b.
    Camino ventricular b.
    ICP Camino b.
    Philly b.
    Richmond b.
    subarachnoid b.
Boltzmann
    B. distribution
    B. distribution law
bolus
bombarding
bombed
bombesin
bona fide
bond
    affectional b.
    attachment b.
    emotional b.
    father-child b.
    high-energy b.
    male b.

    mother-child b.
    pair b.
    parent-offspring b.
    sibling b.
bondage
    b. and discipline
    physical b.
    sensory b.
Bondek suture
bonding
    affiliative b.
    human-pet b.
    b. in infancy
    mother-infant b.
    parent-infant b.
bone
    b. age (BA)
    b. algorithm
    allograft iliac b.
    autogenous iliac b.
    calvarial b.
    b. conduction
    b. conduction deafness
    b. curette
    b. cyst
    b. disease
    b. dissection
    b. flap
    b. graft
    b. graft collapse
    b. graft decompression
    b. graft extrusion
    b. grafting
    b. graft placement
    hyoid b.
    b. marrow suppression
    b. marrow transplantation graft-versus-host disease
    b. mineral density
    nontraumatic necrosis of b.
    occipital b.
    b. occipital malformation
    b. pain
    parietal skull b.
    b. plate
    b. plate selection
    b. pointing
    pointing of the b.
    b. punch
    b. reflex
    b. screw
    b. sensibility
    b. stock
    temporal b.
    b. tumor
    Tutoplast b.
    b. wax
    wormian b.
bone-biting rongeur
bone/ligament dissection
bone-screw interface strength
BoneSource hydroxyapatite cement
bone-window CT scan
Bonhoeffer sign
bonhomie

Bonine
Bonnet-Dechaume-Blanc syndrome
Bonnevie-Ulrich syndrome
Bonnier syndrome
Bontril
bony
    b. abnormality
    b. canal
    b. dissection
    b. dysplasia
    b. element destruction
    b. endplate
    b. exposure
    b. facet
    b. overhang
    b. purchase
booklet
    Traumatic Events B.
boost
    arousal b.
    b. irradiation technique
booster
    b. clip
    inhaled octane b.
boot
    thigh-high alternating compression
      air b.
boozer
borborygmus, pl. **borborygmi**
Borchardt olive-shaped bur
border
    b. cell
    vermilion b.
borderline
    b. behavior
    Diagnostic Interview for B.'s (DIB)
    b. dull
    b. intellectual functioning
    b. mental retardation
    b. personality
    b. personality disorder (BPD)
    b. personality organization
    b. psychosis
    b. psychosis of childhood
    b. range
    b. retardation
    Revised Diagnostic Interview
      for B.'s
    b. scale
    b. schizophrenia (BS)
    b. state
borderzone infarction
Börjeson-Forssman-Lehmann syndrome
Bornholm disease
boron neutron capture therapy (BNCT)
boronophenylalanine (BPA)
Borrelia
    B. burgdorferi
    B. hermsii
borreliosis
    Lyme b.
bossing
    occipital b.

Boston
    B. Assessment of Severe Aphasia
      (BASA)
    B. Classification System
    B. Diagnostic Aphasia Exam
      Cookie Theft Card
    B. Diagnostic Aphasia Examination
      (BDAE)
    B. Famous Faces Test
    B. LINAC
    B. Naming Test
    B. neurosurgical couch
    B. opium
    B. University Model of Psychiatric
      Rehabilitation
Bosworth spinal fusion
botanophobia
Botel Reading Inventory
Botox injection amplifier
Böttcher
    B. cell
    B. ganglion
botulinum
    b. antitoxin
    b. A toxin
    Clostridium b.
    b. toxin type A
botulism
    human b.
    infantile b.
    b. peripheral neuropathy
bouche de tapir
boufeé delirante
boulimia (*var. of* bulimia)
bound
    b. morpheme
    out of b.'s
    b. panic attack
    b. pronoun
    situationally b.
    upper b.
boundaries
    b. and gender
    b. in postanalytic supervision
    b. posttermination
    b. in psychoanalysis
boundary
    analytic b.
    body b.
    b. case
    ego b.
    external b.
    group b.
    lack of b.
    language b.
    loose b.
    loss of ego b.
    poorly defined b.
    posttermination b.
    problems with b.
    role b.
    subsystem b.
    b. violation
boundless energy
bourgeois

B

bourgeoisie
Bourneville disease
Bourneville-Pringle disease
bout of insomnia
bouton
    axonal terminal b.
    b. en passage
    synaptic b.
    terminal b.
    b. terminaux
bovarism
Bovie
    B. electrocautery
    B. electrocautery device
    B. grounding pad
bovine
    b. percardium dural graft
    b. spongiform encephalopathy
bowel
    b. control
    b. disease
    b. disorder
    b. function
    b. incontinence
    reactive b.
    stress-induced reactive b.
    b. training
Bowen
    B. Family Systems
    B. model
Bowlby
    B. developmental model
    B. theory of attachment
box
    BTE Bolt B.
    cyclin b.
    Goodman Lock B.
    jack b.
    obstruction b.
    Skinner b.
boxcar effect
boxer's
    b. dementia
    b. encephalopathy
BP
    Imagent BP
BPA
    boronophenylalanine
BPC
    Behavior Problem Checklist
BPD
    borderline personality disorder
BPI
    Basic Personality Inventory
    bipolar illness
    Bipolar Psychological Inventory
BPRS
    Brief Psychiatric Rating Scale
BPRS-C
    Brief Psychiatric Rating Scale for Children
BPS spinal angiographic catheter
BRAC
    basic rest-activity cycle

brace
    halo b.
    Hudson b.
    kyphosis b.
    Milwaukee b.
    SOMI b.
    SOMI Jr. b.
    Yale b.
brace-free ambulation
brachia (*pl. of* brachium)
brachial
    b. amyotrophy
    b. birth palsy
    b. cutaneous nerve
    b. plexus
    b. plexus avulsion
    b. plexus avulsion injury
    b. plexus exploration
    b. plexus lesion
    b. plexus neuritis
    b. plexus neuropathy
    b. radiculitis
brachial-basilar insufficiency syndrome
brachiocephalic vein
brachiocephaly
brachiofacial cortical hypesthesia
brachioradialis
    b. transfer for wrist extension
brachioradial reflex
brachium, pl. brachia
    b. colliculi inferioris
    b. colliculi superioris
    b. conjunctivum cerebelli
    b. of the inferior colliculus
    inferior quadrigeminal b.
    b. pontis
    b. quadrigeminum inferius
    b. quadrigeminum superius
    b. of superior colliculus
    superior quadrigeminal b.
brachybasia
brachycephalia
brachycephalic
brachycephalism
brachycephalous
brachycephaly
brachycranic
brachymorph
brachyskeletal
brachytherapy
    high-energy b.
    interstitial b.
    remote afterloading b. (RAB)
    b. seed implantation
    stereotactic b.
    volumetric interstitial b.
bracing
    external b.
    postoperative b.
Bracken Basic Concept Scale
Brackmann suction-irrigator
Braden flushing reservoir
bradyarthria
bradycardia
    central b.

B

bradycinesia (*var. of* bradykinesia)
bradyesthesia
bradyglossia
bradykinesia, bradicinesia
    functional b.
bradykinesia/akinesia
bradykinetic
    b. syndrome
bradykinin
bradylalia
bradylexia
bradylogia
bradyphagia
bradyphasia
bradyphemia
bradyphrasia
bradyphrenia
bradypnea
bradypragia
bradypsychia
bradyrhythmia
bradyteleocinesia, bradyteleokinesis
Bragg
    B. ionization peak
    B. peak proton beam therapy
    B. peak radiosurgery
Bragg-peak radiation
braided
    b. occlusion device (BOD)
    b. Spectra UHMWPE surgical
    cable
    b. titanium cable
braidism
Braid strabismus
braille
    B. Telecaption system
brain
    abdominal b.
    b. abnormality
    b. abscess
    b. ache
    b. age quotient
    b. aging
    archaic b.
    architecture of the b.
    b. arteriovenous malformation
    b. atrophy
    b. autopsy
    base of b.
    b. biopsy
    b. biopsy needle
    b. cell damage
    b. cicatrix
    b. clip forceps
    compression of b.
    b. concussion
    concussion of b.
    b. congestion
    contrecoup injury of b.
    b. control
    b. contusion
    b. convulsion
    b. cooling
    coup injury of b.
    b. cryolesion

    b. cyst
    b. damage language disorder
    b. death
    b. death syndrome
    b. degeneration
    b. depressant
    b. dimorphism
    b. disease organic psychosis
    dura mater of the b.
    b. dysfunction
    b. dysmorphology
    electrical activity of b.
    b. electrical activity map
    b. electrical activity mapping
    (BEAM)
    electric stimulation of the b.
    (ESB)
    b. engorgement
    enlarged b.
    b. evoked potential (BEP)
    evolution of b.
    b. fog
    b. gene therapy
    glucose metabolism in the b.
    hemangioma of the b.
    b. herniation
    b. imaging
    imaging b.
    b. imaging study
    b. infarction
    b. infection organic psychosis
    b. injury
    b. ischemia
    b. isoform
    b. laceration
    b. lesion
    b. mantle
    B. Matters Stroke Initiative
    Edinburgh Artery Study
    b. metabolism
    b. metastasis
    b. model
    b. morphometry
    b. murmur
    b. natriuretic peptide (BNP)
    nonpsychotic posttraumatic b.
    b. opioid activity
    b. pathology
    b. perfusion study
    phencyclidine mixed organic b.
    Planar Stereotaxic Atlas of the
    Human B.
    b. potential
    b. psychoorganic syndrome
    b. puncture
    B. reflex
    b. region
    b. research
    respirator b.
    b. retention
    b. retraction
    b. retractor
    b. revascularization
    b. sand
    b. scan

brain *(continued)*
  b. seizure
  b. shift
  b. spatula
  b. spatula forceps
  b. spectin
  split b.
  b. spoon
  b. stimulation
  supratentorial b.
  b. swelling
  b. synaptic membrane
  b. target
  b. test
  b. ticklers
  tight b.
  b. tissue
  b. transplantation
  b. trauma
  b. trauma organic psychosis
  b. trocar
  b. tumor
  b. tumor forceps
  B. Tumor Registry
  Virchow-Robin space of the b.
  visceral b.
  water on the b.
  b. wave activity
  b. wave complex
  b. wave cycle
  b. weight
braincase
brain-derived
  b.-d. neurotrophic
  b.-d. neurotrophic factor (BDNF)
  b.-d. neurotropic factor (BDNF)
brain-mind dichotomy
BrainSCAN
  BrainSCAN computer planning
  system
  BrainSCAN II
  BrainSCAN Linac radiosurgery
  system
brain-splitting
brainstem
  b. astrocytoma
  b. auditory evoked potential
  (BAEP)
  b. auditory evoked response
  (BAER)
  b. compression
  b. control
  b. diencephalic mapping
  b. disease
  b. displacement
  b. dysfunction
  b. edema
  b. electrical response audiometry
  b. encephalitis
  b. evoked potential
  b. function
  b. glioma
  b. hemorrhage
  b. infarction

  b. ischemia
  b. lesion
  b. reflex
  b. reticular formation
  rostral b.
  b. sign
  b. stroke
  b. syndrome
  b. tumor
brain-to-plasma ratio
brainwashing
branch
  b. artery occlusion
  callosal marginal b.
  frontal polar b.
  meningohypophyseal b.
  superior laryngeal nerve external b.
branched-chain ketoaciduria
brancher enzyme deficiency disease
branchial efferent column
branching
  anomalous b.
  b. steps in therapy
  b. tree diagram
branchiomotor nuclei
Brasdor method
brasiliensis
  Paracoccioides b.
Braun-Yasargil right-angle clip
Bravais-jacksonian epilepsy
bravura
Brawner decision
Brazelton Neonatal Behavioral
  Assessment Scale
BRDS
  Blessed-Roth Dementia Scale
BrDu
  bromodeoxyuridine
breach rhythm
breadwinner
  loss of b.
break
  acute psychotic b.
  ascending pitch b.
  psychotic b.
  b. shock
  b. state
  b. with reality
breakage
  pedicle screw b.
  screw b.
breakaway phenomenon
breakdown
  analytical b.
  myelin b.
  nervous b.
breakoff phenomenon
breakpoint
  sequencing deletion b.
breakthrough
  normal perfusion pressure b.
  (NPPB)
  perfusion pressure b.
  b. phenomenon
  b. tearfulness

breast
- b. augmentation
- b. binders
- b. complex
- b. envy
- b. feeding
- b. implant

breast-phantom phenomenon

breath
- alcohol on b. (AOB)
- b. analyzer
- b. chewing
- shortness of b.
- b. stream
- b. work

breathalyzer

breathe

breathing
- apneustic b.
- ataxic b.
- Biot b.
- Cheyne-Stokes b.
- cluster b.
- controlled b.
- crescendo-decrescendo b.
- daytime mouth b.
- diaphragmatic b.
- b. disorder
- opposition b.
- sleep disordered b. (SDB)
- b. tic

breathing-related sleep disorder

breathy
- b. dystonia
- b. voice

bredouillement

bregmocardiac reflex

Bremer
- B. AirFlo halo vest
- B. halo
- B. halo crown
- B. halo crown system
- B. halo crown traction
- B. halo crown traction set
- B. torque limiting cap

Breschet sinus

bretazenil

Brevibloc

brevis
- abductor pollicis b.

Brevital

BRI
- Basic Reading Inventory

brick gum

bridegroom's palsy

bridge region

bridging vein

brief
- B. Alcoholism Screening Test
- B. Aphasia Screening Examination (BASE)
- B. Cognitive Rating Scale (BCRS)
- b. delusional experience
- b. depressive reaction
- B. Disability Questionnaire
- B. Drinker Profile
- b. group therapy
- B. Life History Inventory (BLHI)
- B. Neuropsychological Mental Status Examination (BNMSE)
- B. Outpatient Psychopathology Scale
- b. posttraumatic stress disorder
- B. Psychiatric Rating Scale (BPRS)
- B. Psychiatric Rating Scale for Children (BPRS-C)
- b. psychotherapy
- b. psychotic disorder
- b. psychotic reaction
- b. pulse bilateral ECT
- b. pulse unilateral ECT
- b. pulse waveform
- b. reactive psychosis
- b. reactive psychosis with marked stressor
- b. situational depression
- b. stimuli technique
- b. stimulus therapy (BST)
- B. Symptom Inventory (BSI)

Brieger cachexia

Brigance Diagnostic Inventory of Early Development

Briggs law

brightness
- b. adaptation
- b. constancy
- b. contrast
- b. discrimination
- b. threshold

bright normal range

brim sign

Briquet
- B. ataxia
- B. disorder
- B. syndrome

brisk reflex

Brissaud
- B. disease
- B. infantilism
- B. reflex
- B. syndrome

Brissaud-Marie syndrome

Bristol
- B. Language Development Scale (BLADES)
- B. Social Adjustment Guides

Bristowe syndrome

British
- B. Ability Scale (BAS)
- B. Ability Scales: Spelling Scale
- B. anti-Lewisite antidote
- B. Manual of the Classification of Occupations

broad
- b. affect
- b. AO dynamic compression plate
- b. heritability
- b. phonemic transcription

Broadbent law

broadcasting
thought b.
Brobdingnagian disorder of visual perception in migraine
Broca
B. amnesia
B. aphasia
B. ataxia
B. center
B. convolution
B. diagonal band
B. dysphasia
B. field
B. fissure
B. gyrus
B. parolfactory area
B. syndrome
Brocae
area parolfactoria B.
Brodie disease
Brodmann
B. 41 area
B. area 44
B. classification
B. cortical area
B. cytoarchitectonic field
brofaromine
brofoxine
broken existing implant
bromatherapy
bromatology
bromatotherapy
bromazepam
bromfenac sodium capsule
bromide
ammonium b.
calcium b.
clidinium b.
decamethonium b.
b. hallucinosis
b. intoxication
pancuronium b.
perfluorooctyl b.
b. poisoning
potassium b.
b. psychosis
pyridostigmine b.
serum b.
sodium b.
vecuronium b.
bromidrosiphobia
bromine compound
brominism
brominized oil
bromism
bromisoval
bromisovalum
bromocriptine
b. mesylate
b. test
bromodeoxyuridine (BrDu)
bromodiphenhydramine hydrochloride
bromoglutamate
bromoiodism
bromomania

bromperidol
brompheniramine
bromzepan
bronchial
b. asthma
b. respiration
bronchodilatation, bronchodilation
bronchodilator
bronchogenic
bronchoscope
bronchospasm
Bronkosol
brontophobia
Bronx Aging Study
brooding
b. compulsion
obsessional b.
spells of doubting and b.
Brook Reaction Test (BRT)
Brooks
B. atlantoaxial arthrodesis
B. cervical fusion
B. technique
Brooks-Gallie cervical operation
Brooks-Jenkins
B.-J. atlantoaxial fusion
B.-J. cervical operation
brother complex
brotizolam
brought in by (BIB)
brow-down position
browlift
Brown
B. Assessment of Beliefs Scale
B. and Harris Life Event and Difficulty Schedule
B. Schools Behavioral Health System
B. syndrome
Brown-Adson forceps
brownian
b. motion
b. movement
Browning vein
Brown-Roberts-Wells
B.-R.-W. arc-ring assembly
B.-R.-W. arc system
B.-R.-W. base ring
B.-R.-W. computer
B.-R.-W. computerized tomography stereotaxic guidance
B.-R.-W. floor stand
B.-R.-W. head frame
B.-R.-W. headrest
B.-R.-W. head ring halo
B.-R.-W. phantom base (BRW-PB)
B.-R.-W. ring adapter
Brown-Séquard
B.-S. paralysis
B.-S. syndrome
BRP-2
Behavior Rating Profile, Second Edition
BRT
Brook Reaction Test

B

Brucella
  B. abortus
  B. melitensis
brucellosis
  cerebral b.
  b. peripheral neuropathy
Bruch membrane discontinuity
brucine
Brudzinski sign
Bruininks-Oseretsky
  B.-O. Standardized Test
  B.-O. Test
  B.-O. Test of Motor Proficiency
bruising of undetermined origin (BUO)
bruit
  aneurysmal b.
  arterial b.
  asymptomatic carotid b. (ACB)
  asymptomatic neck b.
  carotid b.
brujeria
Bruker
  B. Biospec system
  B. S 200 MR system
Brunner modified incision
Bruns
  B. ataxia
  B. gait apraxia
  B. nystagmus
  B. syndrome
brush
  Cragg thrombolytic b.
Brushfield spot
Brushfield-Wyatt disease
brusque
brute pride
bruxism
  sleep-related b.
bruxomania
BRW-PB
  Brown-Roberts-Wells phantom base
Bryant-Schwan Design Test (BSDT)
BS
  borderline schizophrenia
BSAB
  Balthazar Scales of Adaptive Behavior
BSDT
  Bryant-Schwan Design Test
BSI
  Behavior Status Inventory
  Brief Symptom Inventory
BSID
  Bayley Scales of Infant Development
BSM
  Bilingual Syntax Measure II Test
BSQ
  Behavior Style Questionnaire
BSSI
  Basic School Skills Inventory
BST
  brief stimulus therapy
BSW
  Bachelor of Social Work
BTE
  BTE Assembly Tree

BTE Bolt Box
BTE Work Simulator
B$_2$-TFn
  B$_2$-transferrin
  B$_2$-TFn assay
BTi
  biomagnetometer
B$_2$-transferrin (B$_2$-TFn)
bubble
  b. echocardiogram
  b. gum
bubo
  venereal b.
buccal
  b. frenula
  b. intercourse
  b. onanism
  b. speech
buccarum
  morsicatio b.
buccinator muscle
buccofacial apraxia
buccolingual dyskinesia
buccopharyngeal approach
Buck
  B. neurological hammer
  B. percussion hammer
buckling sign
buckthorn polyneuropathy
Bucladin-S Softab
buclizine
bucrylate
Bucy
  B. cordotomy knife
  B. laminectomy rongeur
Bucy-Frazier
  B.-F. coagulation cannula
  B.-F. suction cannula
Budde
  B. halo retractor system
  B. halo ring
  B. halo ring retractor
  B. surgical system
Budde-Greenberg-Sugita stereotactic head frame
Buddhism
  Zen B.
Budge center
budgeting
  functional b.
buffalo neck
buffer
  memory b.
  b. memory
  b. neuropathy
Bufferin
Buffex
buffoonery
  b. psychosis
  b. syndrome
bufotenin
buggery
build
  body b.
  index of body b. (IB)

building
    b. fear
    b. restriction
bulb
    auditory b.
    b. dynamometer
    end b.
    jugular b.
    Krause end b.
    b. of lateral ventricle
    olfactory b.
    b. syringe
bulbar
    b. abnormality
    b. anesthesia
    b. apoplexy
    b. cephalic pain tractotomy
    b. myelitis
    b. palsy
    b. paralysis
    b. tractotomy
bulbi (*gen. and pl. of* bulbus)
bulbocapnine
bulbocavernosus reflex
bulboid corpuscle
bulbomimic reflex
bulbonuclear
bulbopontine
bulbosacral system
bulbospinal
bulbus, gen. and pl. **bulbi**
    b. olfactorius
    phthisis bulbi
bulesis
bulging
    aneurysmal b.
bulimia, boulimia
    b. nervosa
    B. Nervosa, Nonpurging Type
    B. Nervosa, Purging Type
bulimic-anorexic spectrum
bulimic purge
bulimorexia
bulk
    b. flow transcytosis
    tumor b.
bulldog response
bullet
    b. bolt
    silver b.
bulletin
    Psychopharmacology B.
bullia capital
bullion
bull's eye deformity
bullying
bum
    skid-row b.
bumetanide
Bumex
BUN
    blood urea nitrogen
bunamiodyl
bundle
    aberrant b.

    anterior ground b.
    Arnold b.
    cingulum b.
    comma b. of Schultze
    Flechsig ground b.
    Gierke respiratory b.
    Gowers b.
    ground b.
    Held b.
    Helweg b.
    Hoche b.
    hooked b. of Russell
    Krause respiratory b.
    lateral ground b.
    Lissauer b.
    Loewenthal b.
    longitudinal pontine b.
    maculoneural b.
    medial forebrain b.
    medial longitudinal b.
    Meynert retroflex b.
    Monakow b.
    oblique b. of pons
    olfactory b.
    olivocochlear b.
    Pick b.
    posterior longitudinal b.
    precommissural b.
    predorsal b.
    Schultze b.
    Schütz b.
    solitary b.
    tumor-nerve b.
    Türck b.
    uncinate b. of Russell
    Vicq d'Azyr b.
bundle-nailing method
bundles of fibrils
Büngner band
Bunnell
    B. dissecting probe
    B. forwarding probe
Bunney-Hamburg
    B.-H. nurse rating
    B.-H. Rating Scale
bunyavirus encephalitis
BUO
    bleeding of undetermined origin
    bruising of undetermined origin
Bupap
buphthalmia, buphthalmos, buphthalmus
bupivacaine
Buprenex
buprenorphine
bupropion
    b. hydrochloride
    b. hydrochlorothiazide
bur, burr
    Adson enlarging b.
    Adson perforating b.
    Adson-Rogers cranial b.
    Albee olive-shaped b.
    barrel b.
    Borchardt olive-shaped b.
    Cushing cranial b.

B

dermabrasion b.
D'Errico enlarging drill b.
D'Errico perforating drill b.
diamond b.
Doyen cylindrical b.
Doyen spherical b.
enlarging b.
finish b.
flame tip b.
high-torque b.
b. hole
b. hole cover
b. hole drainage
b. hole neuroendoscopic fenestration
b. hole transducer
Hudson brace b.
Lindermann b.
McKenzie enlarging b.
MTM 2 b.
pear b.
perforating b.
right-ankle b.
Rosen b.
Rotablator rotating b.
round b.
Shannon b.
spherical b.
Stille b.

Burdach
B. column
B. fasciculus
B. nucleus
B. tract
Burdick Eclipse ECG machine
bureau
B. of Drug Abuse Control
(BDAC)
B. of Narcotics and Dangerous
Drugs (BNDD)
bureaucrat
Burford-Finochietto rib spreader
Burford retractor
burgdorferi
Borrelia b.
burgeoning
Burke Bariatric bed
Burkitt lymphoma
Burks Behavior Rating Scale (BBRS)
burn
napalm b.
burned-out
b.-o. anergic schizophrenia
b.-o. schizophrenic
burned rubber cement
Burnese
burning
b. feet syndrome
b. pain
b. rubber
burnout
parent b.
professional b.
b. syndrome
Burn and Rand theory
Burns/Roe Informal Reading Inventory

Buronil
burr (*var. of* bur)
Burrow
Trigant L. B.
burst
b. of delta activity
epileptogenic b.
b. fracture
b. injury
burst-suppression
electroencephalographic b.-s.
Burundanga intoxication
Buschke
B. disease
B. Free and Cued Selective
Reminding Procedure
B. Free and Cued Selective
Reminding Test
B. Selective Reminding Test
B. Short-Term Recall Test
Buschke-Fuld Selective Memory Test
bush
BuSpar patch
buspirone hydrochloride
Buss-Durkee Hostility Inventory
Busse-Buschke disease
butabarbital
b. elixir
sodium b.
b. sodium
b. sulfate
butabarbitone
butacaine sulfate
butaciamol hydrochloride
Butalan
butalbital
b. and acetaminophen
b. compound and aspirin
b. compound and codeine
butamoxane hydrochloride
butane sniffing dependence
butaperazine
butathal
butethal
butethamine hydrochloride
Butisol Sodium
butoctamide
butorphanol
b. tartrate
b. tartrate nasal spray
butoxamine hydrochloride
butriptyline hydrochloride
butter flower
butterfly
b. distribution
b. needle
b. rash
b. vertebra
**butterfly-shaped monobloc vertebral
plate**
butterfly-type glioma
button
panic b.
rubber b.
subdural b.

butyl
 b. acetate
 b. aminobenzoate
 b. chloride
 b. formate
 b. hydride
 b. nitrate
 b. nitrite
butylcholinesterase (BchE)
butyrophenone agent
butyrophenone-based neuroleptic drug
buyer
 binge b.
buying
 compulsive b.
 Minnesota Impulsive Disorder
 Interview Model for
 Compulsive B.
Buzzard maneuver
buzzing sensation
buzzword
BVMGT
 Bender Visual-Motor Gestalt Test
BVR
 basal vein of Rosenthal
BVRT
 Benton Visual Retention Test
BWAS
 Barron-Welsh Art Scale
BWM
 Bad Wildungen Metz
 BWM spine system

BWS
 battered woman syndrome
by
 brought in b. (BIB)
bypass
 AOA-MCA b.
 b. coaptation for cervical nerve
 root avulsion
 ECIC b.
 ECIC arterial b.
 extracranial-intracranial b.
 Fukushima cavernous b.
 gastric b.
 b. graft
 IC-IC b.
 STA-MCA b.
 STA-PCA b.
 STA-SCA b.
 superficial temporal artery to
 posterior cerebral artery b.
bystander
 b. dominates initial
 b. dominates initial dominant
 (BDID)
 b. effect
Bzoch-League Receptive-Expressive
Emergent Language Scale

C

C factor
C fiber
C fiber activity

C4

leukotrienes B4 and C.

C2-C3 cervical disk excision
C2 syndrome
C5b-9 complex
C6-C7 dislocation
caapi
CAAS

Children's Attention and Adjustment Survey

CAB

Comprehensive Ability Battery

cabin

c. fever
magnetic shielded c.

cable

braided Spectra UHMWPE surgical c.
braided titanium c.
coaxial c.
c. graft
SecureStrand c.
Songer c.
titanium c.
UHMWPE c.
ultra-high molecular weight polyethylene fiber c.

cabling

percutaneous c.

CABS

chronic alcoholic brain syndrome

cacation
cacesthesia
cachectic infantilism
cachexia

Brieger c.
c. hypophyseopriva
hypophysial c.
pituitary c.

cachinnation
cacodemonomania
cacoethes
cacogenesis
cacogenic
cacogeusia
cacography
cacolalia
cacophonous
cacophony
cacophoria
cacoplasty
cacosmia
cacothenics
cacotrophy
cactus

peyote c.

cacuminal

CADASIL

cerebral autosomal dominant arteriopathy with subcortical infarcts and leukoencephalopathy

cadaverous
cadence
cadherin

calcium-dependent c.

CADL

Communicative Abilities in Daily Living

CADT

Communication Abilities Diagnostic Test

caducity
Cadwell

C. 5200A somatosensory evoked potential unit
C. 5200A somatosensory evoked potential unit device

caelotherapy
cafard, cathard
Cafatine
café-au-lait (CAL)
café au lait spot
Cafergot
Cafetrate
Caffedrine
caffeine

c. abstinence
c. abuse
acetaminophen, aspirin, and c.
aspirin with butalbital, phenacetin, and c.
c. dependence
ergotamine tartrate and c.
c. intolerance
c. intoxication
orphenadrine, aspirin, and c.
c. and sodium benzoate
c. tolerance
c. withdrawal

caffeine-induced

c.-i. anxiety
c.-i. disorder

caffeinism
Caffey hyperostosis
Caffin-TD
CAGE

Ewing & Rooss four-question alcohol screening
CAGE alcohol use questionnaire

cage

population c.
Ray Threaded Fusion C.
threaded fusion c. (TFC)

CAI

Career Assessment Inventory
Cultural Attitude Inventory

Cain complex
Caine-Levine Social Competency Scale
cainophobia, cainotophobia
Cairns stupor
Cairs hemostatic forceps

Cajal
    C. cell
    nucleus of C.
CAL
    café-au-lait
calami
    lapsus c.
calamus scriptorius
Calan
calcar avis
Cal Carb-HD
calcarine
    c. artery
    c. cortex
    c. cortex infarction
    c. fasciculus
    c. fissure
    c. sulcus
Calcibind
Calci-Chew
Calciday-667
calcifediol
Calciferol
    C. Injection
    C. Oral
calcification
    basal ganglia c.
    c. of the basal ganglion
    gyriform c.
    mitral annulus c.
Calcijex
Calcimar Injection
Calci-Mix
calcinosis intervertebralis
calcinosis, Raynaud phenomenon, esophageal dysmotility, sclerodactyly, and telangiectasia (CREST)
calcitonin gene-related peptide (CGRP)
calcitriol
calcium
    c. bromide
    c. carbonate
    c. channel blocker
    c. channel blocking agent
    c. chloride
    c. citrate
    c. disodium edetate
    c. disodium versenate
    c. embolus
    fenoprofen c.
    c. glubionate
    c. gluceptate
    c. gluconate
    c. ion
    c. lactate
    c. paradox
    c. phosphate bioceramic
    c. phosphate, dibasic
    c. pyrophosphate dihydrate
      decomposition disease
    serum c.
calcium-calmodulin kinase II (CaMKII)
calcium-dependent cadherin
calculate
    ability to abstract and c.

calculation
    calendar c.
    judgment, orientation, memory, abstraction, and c.
    c. skill
    c. test
calculus, gen. and pl. calculi
    cerebral c.
Calderol
Caldwell-Luc incision
Caldwell projection
calefacient
calendar
    c. age
    c. calculation
calibrate
calibrated loop
calibration
    automated test target c. (ATTC)
    low-voltage c.
caliciform, calyciform
    c. ending
caliculus, pl. caliculi
    c. ophthalmicus
California
    C. Achievement Test (CAT)
    C. Achievement Test, Fifth Edition (CAT/5)
    C. Child Q-Set
    C. Computerized Assessment Package
    C. Critical Thinking Dispositions Inventory (CCTDI)
    C. Critical Thinking Skills Test (CCTST)
    C. encephalitis
    C. F Scale
    C. Infant Scale for Motor Development (CISMD)
    C. Life Goals Evaluation Schedule
    C. Marriage Readiness Evaluation (CMRE)
    C. Motor Accuracy Test, Southern Revised
    C. Occupational Preference Survey (COPS)
    C. Personality Inventory (CPI)
    C. Preschool Social Competency Scale (CPSCS)
    C. Psychological Inventory (CPI)
    C. Psychological Inventory Test (CPIT)
    C. Q-Sort
    C. Relative Value Studies (CRVS, CVRS)
    C. Short-Form Test of Mental Maturity (CTMM-SF)
    C. Test of Basic Skills (CTBS)
    C. Test of Mental Maturity (CTMM)
    C. Test of Mental Maturity-Short Form (CTMM-SF)
    C. Test of Mental Maturity, Short-Form

C. Test of Personality (CTP)
C. Verbal Learning Test (CVLT)
californica
    Aplysia californica
caliper
Callier-Azusa Scale
callomania
callosal
    c. agenesis
    c. apraxia
    c. area
    c. commissurotomy
    c. convolution
    c. disconnection syndrome
    c. disconnection syndrome aphasia
    c. gyrus
    c. lesion
    c. marginal branch
    c. splenium
    c. sulcus
callosomarginal
    c. artery
    c. fissure
callosotomy
    anterior c.
    corpus c.
callosum
    agenesis of corpus c.
    corpus c.
    hypogenetic corpus c.
    peduncle of corpus c.
Calman carotid clamp
calmodulin
caloric
    c. expenditure
    c. intake
    c. nystagmus
    c. stimulation test for vestibular
      function
    c. test
    c. testing
calorie
calorigenic action
calorimetry
calpain inhibitor
Cal-Plus
CALS
    Checklist of Adaptive Living Skills
Caltrate
    C. 600
    C., Jr.
calumniate
calvaria, pl. **calvariae**
calvarial
    c. bone
    c. hemangioma
    c. hook
calyciform (*var. of* caliciform)
CAM
    cell adhesion molecule
Cama Arthritis Pain Reliever
camaraderie
camazepam
Camberwell Family Interview

Cambridge
    C. Mental Disorders in Elderly
      Examination (CAMDEX)
    C. Test Battery
CAMDEX
    Cambridge Mental Disorders in Elderly
      Examination
Camelot Behavioral Checklist (CBC)
camera
    CTI-Siemens 933/08-12 PET c.
    scintillation c.
    time-of-flight positron emission
      tomographic c.
Camino
    C. fiberoptic ICP monitor
    C. intracranial catheter
    C. intracranial pressure monitoring
      system
    C. intraparenchymal fiberoptic
      device
    C. microventricular bolt
    C. OLM ICP monitor
    C. subdural screw
    C. ventricular bolt
camisole
CaMKII
    calcium-calmodulin kinase II
camouflage
cAMP
    cyclic adenosine monophosphate
campaign
    D/ART C.
    Depression: Awareness, Recognition,
      and Treatment C.
Campbell
    C. Interest and Skill Survey
      (CISS)
    C. Leadership Index (CLI)
    C. nerve root retractor
    C. Organizational Survey
camp follower
campi foreli
campotomy
camptocormia
camptocormy
camptospasm
Campylobacter jejuni
Camurati-Engelmann disease
Canadian
    C. Cognitive Abilities Test (CCAT)
    C. Neurological Scale
    C. Tests of Basic Skills (CTBS)
canal
    anal c.
    anterior vertical c.
    arachnoid c.
    auditory c.
    Bichat c.
    birth c.
    bony c.
    caudal c.
    central c.
    Cotunnius c.
    craniopharyngeal c.
    Dorello c.

C

canal *(continued)*
    Guyon c.
    haversian c.
    Hensen c.
    Hunter c.
    internal auditory c.
    intramedullary c.
    c. knife
    Löwenberg c.
    medullary c.
    neural c.
    optic c.
    c. paresis
    posterior semicircular c.
    semicircular c.
    spinal c.
    uniting c.
    c. of Vesalius
canaliculus reuniens
canalis, pl. canales
    c. centralis medullae spinae
    c. reuniens
canalization
Canavan
    C. disease
    C. leukodystrophy
    C. sclerosis
Canavan-van Bogaert-Bertrand disease
cancellation
    fat/water signal c.
    phase c.
    c. test
cancellous screw
cancer
    metastatic breast c.
    c. reaction
cancer-associated myositis
cancerophobe
cancerophobia, carcinophobia
cancerphobia
Candida **infection**
candidal
    c. meningitis
    c. microabscess
candidiasis
CANE
    computer-assisted neuroendoscopy
cane
    Thera C.
Canfield Instructional Styles Inventory
canine
    c. hysteria
    c. spasm
caninus
    risus c.
    spasmus c.
canities
cannabidiol
cannabin
cannabinoid
    cross-reacting c. (CRC)
cannabinol (CBN)
cannabis
    c. abuse

    c. and alcohol
    c. dependence
    c. equipment
    c. and heroin
    c. intoxication
    c. intoxication delirium
    c. intoxication-related disorder
    c. intoxication, with perceptual
      disturbance
    c. laced with cocaine and
      phencyclidine
    c. laced with phencyclidine
    c. mixed with insecticides
    c. and opium
    c. organic mental disorder
    c. and phencyclidine
    c. psychosis
    c. resin
    c. tablet
    c. use
    c. use disorder
cannabis,
    c. cocaine and heroin
    c. cocaine, heroin and
      phencyclidine
cannabis-induced
    c.-i. anxiety
    c.-i. anxiety disorder
    c.-i. delirium disorder
    c.-i. psychotic disorder with
      delusions
    c.-i. psychotic disorder with
      hallucinations
cannabis-related disorder, not otherwise specified
Cannabis sativa
cannibalism
cannibalistic
    c. fantasy
    c. fixation
Cannon-Bard
    C.-B. theory
    C.-B. theory of emotion
Cannon theory
cannula
    Adson brain-exploring c.
    Adson brain-extracting c.
    Bergstrom c.
    Bucy-Frazier coagulation c.
    Bucy-Frazier suction c.
    Dohrmann-Rubin c.
    Dorsey ventricular c.
    Dyonics c.
    Elsberg brain c.
    Elsberg ventricular c.
    Frazier brain-exploring c.
    Frazier ventricular c.
    Fujita suction c.
    Haynes brain c.
    large-egress c.
    McCain TMJ c.
    Portnoy ventricular c.
    Scott c.
    Sedan c.
    Sedan-Vallicioni c.

side-cutting c.
SMK C5 with a 2-mm exposed tip c.
straightening c.
c. with locking dilator
cannulated drill bit
cannulation
unilateral pedicle c.
canonical correlation
cantankerous
Cantelli sign
Canter Background Interference Procedure for the Bender Gestalt Test
cantharis, pl. **cantharides**
CAP
carotid Amytal procedure
CAP Assessment of Writing
cap
c. of the ampullary crest
Bremer torque limiting c.
capacitance
capacity
adaptive c.
channel c.
code c.
c. code
contractual c.
cranial c.
diminished c.
dissociative c.
forced vital c. (FVC)
functional residual c. (FRC)
hedonic c.
hypnotic c.
c. for independent living
intellectual c.
legal c.
measured c.
mental c.
nonverbal intellectual c.
orgasmic c.
oxygen-carrying c.
physical c.
potential intellectual c.
psychological c.
self-regulatory c.
speaking c.
testamentary c.
CAPE
Clifton Assessment Procedures for the Elderly
continuous anatomical passive exerciser
Capgras
C. phenomenon
C. syndrome
capillariomotor
capillary
c. angioma
c. fracture
c. telangiectasia
capistratus
trismus c.

CAPIT
core assessment program for intracerebral transplantation
capita (*pl. of* caput)
capital
bullia c.
C. and Codeine
c. sin
capitalize
capitation
capitis (*gen. of* caput)
capitium
Caplets
Advil Cold & Sinus C.
Bayer Select Chest Cold C.
Dimetapp Sinus C.
Dristan Sinus C.
Miles Nervine C.
Mytelase C.
TripTone C.
capnography
capnometer
MicroSpan C. 8800
Capozide
CAPP
clinical appraisal of psychosocial problems
capping
c. cardiotoxic
c. technique
CAPPS
Current and Past Psychopathology Scale
Capron
caps
Compoz Gel C.
Drixoral Cough & Sore Throat Liquid C.
Feverall Sprinkle C.
capsaicin
Capsin
capsula, gen. and pl. **capsulae**
c. externa
c. extrema
c. interna
capsular infarction
capsulatum
Histoplasma c.
capsule
Betachron E-R c.
bromfenac sodium c.
defenfluramine HCl c.
Depakote Sprinkle C.
external c.
extreme c.
gabapentin c.
Indochron E-R c.
internal c.
Kadian sustained-release morphine c.
otic c.
suprasellar c.
capsulocaudate infarction
capsulolabral complex
capsuloputaminal infarction
capsuloputaminocaudate infarction

capsulothalamic syndrome
capsulotomy
captive
    indoctrination while c.
captivus
    penis c.
captodiame
captopril and hydrochlorothiazide
capture
    IgM antibody c. (MAC EIA)
capuride
caput, gen. capitis, pl. capita
    c. cornus
    dolor capitis
    c. nuclei caudati
    semispinalis capitis
    splenius capitus
    c. succedaneum
Capzasin-P
CAQ
    Change Agent Questionnaire
    Classroom Atmosphere Questionnaire
    Clinical Analysis Questionnaire
carbachol
carbamate
    chlorphenesin c.
carbamazepine (CBZ)
carbamylcholine
carbapenem
Carbatrol
carbenicillin disodium
Carbex
Carb-HD
    Cal C.-HD
carbidopa
    levodopa and c.
carbidopa-levodopa
carbinol
    ethyl c.
Carbocaine
carbohydrate-deficient transferrin (CDT)
carbohydrate metabolism
carbon
    c. dioxide intoxication
    c. dioxide laser
    c. dioxide poisoning
    c. dioxide pressure (PCO_2)
    c. dioxide therapy
    c. disulfide intoxication
    c. monoxide (CO)
    c. monoxide intoxication
    c. monoxide poisoning
    c. tetrachloride
    c. tetrachloride poisoning
carbonate
    calcium c.
    lithium c.
    magnesium c.
carbonic
    c. acid
    c. anhydrase
    c. anhydrase inhibitor
carbonyl modification
carboplatin

carboxylase
    pyruvate c.
carboxylic acid
carboxypenicillin
carbromal
carcinogen
carcinoma, pl. carcinomas, carcinomata
    adenoid cystic c.
    leptomeningeal c.
    meningeal c.
    pancreatic c.
    c. peripheral neuropathy
carcinomatosis
    leptomeningeal c.
    meningeal c.
carcinomatosum
    coma c.
carcinomatous
    c. encephalomyelopathy
    c. myelopathy
    c. neuromyopathy
    c. neuropathy
carcinophobia (*var. of* cancerophobia)
card
    associative response to a white
      space on a c. (Ds)
    Boston Diagnostic Aphasia Exam
      Cookie Theft C.
    Mother C.
    Peabody Developmental Motor
      Scales and Activity C.'s
    Rorschach c.
    tarot c.
Cardex
    medication C.
cardiac
    c. arrest
    c. arrhythmia
    c. artifact
    c. catheterization cardiac syncope
    c. disease
    c. disorder
    c. embolism
    c. function test
    c. ganglia
    c. gating
    c. glycoside
    c. neurosis
    c. output
    c. pacemaker
    c. pacemaker artifact
    c. psychosis
    c. reaction
    c. rhythm
    c. risk index
    c. symptoms
    c. syncope
    c. wall hypokinesia
cardinal
    c. directions of gaze
    c. ocular movement
    c. sign
    c. sin
    c. trait
    c. virtue

Cardio-Conray
cardioembolic stroke
cardioexcitatory peptide
cardiogenic shock
Cardiografin
Cardiolite
    technetium-gagged C.
cardiomyopathy
    alcoholic c.
cardioneural
cardioneurosis
cardiophobia
cardiophrenia
cardiopulmonary
    c. arrest
    C. Paragon 8500 bed
    c. resuscitation
cardiopulmonary-obesity syndrome
CardioSearch sensor
cardiospasm
    psychogenic c.
CardioTec
cardiotoxic
    capping c.
cardiovascular
    c. neurosis
    c. psychogenic disorder
    c. seizure
carditis
    rheumatic c.
Cardizem
card-sorting test
care
    adoptive c.
    ambulatory c.
    ancillary c.
    clinical c.
    community c.
    continuing c.
    continuum of c.
    crisis residential c.
    custodial c.
    ethical aspects of assaultive
      client c.
    excessive need for c.
    extended c.
    family c.
    foster c.
    grossly pathogenic c.
    home c.
    hospice c.
    inappropriate dependent c.
    individual c.
    institutional c.
    K+ C.
    level of c.
    long-term c.
    managed c.
    medical c.
    need for c.
    c. organization
    pastoral c.
    pathogenic c.
    pathologic c.

    personal c.
    postoperative c.
    primary c.
    c. and protection proceeding
    respiratory c.
    c. seeker
    skilled nursing c. (SNC)
    tender loving c. (TLC)
carebaria
career
    C. Assessment Inventories: For the
      Learning Disabled
    C. Assessment Inventory (CAI)
    C. Assessment Inventory, The
      Enhanced Version
    C. Beliefs Inventory (CBI)
    c. change
    c. conference
    c. counseling
    c. counselor
    C. Decision-Making (CDM)
    c. development
    C. Development Inventory
    c. evaluation
    c. inventory
    C. Maturity Inventory (CMI)
    c. planning
    c. planning program (CPP)
    C. Problem Check List
    c. workshop
carefree
caregiver
    adoptive c.
    family c.
    primary c.
    C. Strain Index (CSI)
Caregiver's School Readiness Inventory
  (CSRI)
caretaker
    primary c.
caretaking role
carezza
cargo culture
carina, pl. **carinae**
    c. fornicis
carinatum syndrome
caring
    quality of c.
Caring Relationship Inventory (CRI)
carinii
    Litmosoides c.
    Pneumocystis c.
carisoprodol
    c. and aspirin
    c., aspirin, and codeine
Carlson Psychological Survey
C-arm
    C-a. fluoroscopic apparatus
    C-a. fluoroscopy
    reversible C-a.
carmabis
carmustine (BiCNU)
carnal knowledge

C

Carnegie
    C. Council on Adolescent
        Development
    C. Interest Inventory (CII)
carnitine
    c. palmitoyltransferase (CPT)
    c. palmitoyltransferase deficiency
L-carnitine
Carnitor
    C. Injection
    C. Oral
carnophobia
carnosine
carnosinemia aminoaciduria
carotic
caroticocavernous fistula
caroticojugular spine
caroticooculomotor membrane
caroticotympanic artery
caroticum
    rete mirabile c.
carotid
    c. ablative procedure
    c. Amytal procedure (CAP)
    c. aneurysm
    c. angiogram
    c. artery disease
    c. artery dissection
    c. artery occlusion
    c. artery stenosis with
        asymptomatic narrowing: operation
        versus aspirin (CASANOVA)
    c. artery stenosis with
        asymptomatic narrowing: operation
        versus aspirin study
    c. atherosclerosis
    c. bifurcation
    c. body
    c. body tumor
    c. bruit
    c. cave aneurysm
    c. content
    distal c.
    c. endarterectomy (CEA)
    c. ganglion
    c. plaque hematoma
    c. plexus
    c. preservation
    c. preservation technique
    c. pulsation
    c. rete
    c. ring
    c. sheath
    c. sinus massage
    c. sinus nerve
    c. sinus reflex
    c. sinus syncope
    c. sinus syndrome
    c. stenosis
    c. ultrasound test
    c. vein
carotid-basilar anastomosis
carotid-cavernous
    c.-c. fistula (CCF)
    c.-c. sinus fistula

carotid-dural fistula
carotid-ophthalmic artery aneurysm
carotid-vertebral
    c.-v. anastomosis
    c.-v. vein bypass graft
carotodynia, carotidynia
carpal tunnel syndrome
Carpenter syndrome
carphenazine
carpipramine
carpopedal
    c. contraction
    c. spasm
carpoptosis, carpoptosia
carposcope
carre-four sensitif
Carrell Discrimination Test
carrier
    insurance c.
    trait c.
    Yasargil ligature c.
Carroll Rating Scale for Depression
Carrow
    C. Elicited Language Inventory
        (CELI)
    C. Receptive Language Test
Carr-Purcell-Meiboom-Gill sequence
Carr-Purcell sequence
CARS
    Childhood Autism Rating Scale
    Children's Affective Rating Scale
Carter immobilization cushion
Cartesian coordinate representation
cartilage
    c. cranioplasty
    c. inflammation
    c. plate
    thyroid c.
    Tutoplast costal c.
cartilaginous
    c. end plate
    c. tumor
caruncula
CAS
    Child Assessment Schedule
    Concept-Specific Anxiety Scale
    Creativity Attitude Survey
    Cultural Attitude Scale
CASANOVA
    carotid artery stenosis with asymptomatic
        narrowing: operation versus aspirin
    CASANOVA study
cascade
    arachidonic acid c.
    coagulation c.
    immediate-early gene c.
case
    abuse c. (AC)
    boundary c.
    c. control study
    Dora c.
    c. ethic
    c. fatality rate
    c. finding
    c. history

c. history study
index c.
c. index
c. method
c. mix
c. register
c. report
Schreber c.
Tarasoff c.
test c.
textbook c.
c. work
caseness definition
caseous necrosis
casework
social c.
CASH
Comprehensive Assessment of Symptoms and History
Caspar
C. anterior cervical plate
C. anterior plate fixation
C. cervical retractor
C. cervical screw
C. craniotome
C. disk space spreader
C. drill
C. plating
C. retraction post
C. trapezoidal plate
caspase
CASS
computer-assisted stereotactic surgery
CASS digital read-out floorstand
CASS TrueTaper collimator
CASS whole-brain mapping system
cassava plant tropical myeloneuropathy
cassina leaf
CAST
Children of Alcoholism Screening Test
Children's Apperceptive Story-Telling Test
cast
endocranial c.
hinged c.
Risser-Cotrel body c.
Castellani-Low sign
Castilium
casting
postoperative c.
castrate
castration
anxiety c.
c. anxiety
c. complex
emotional c.
c. fear
female c.
male c.
Castroviejo eye suture forceps
CAT
California Achievement Test
Children's Apperception Test
Children's Articulation Test
Cognitive Abilities Test

College Ability Test
computerized axial tomography
CAT scanning
CAT/5
California Achievement Test, Fifth Edition
catabasia
catabolic force
catabolism
catabolite
cataclysm
cataclysmic headache
Cataflam Oral
catagelophobia, katagelophobia
catagenesis
catalepsy
epidemic c.
c. schizophrenia
schizophrenic c.
cataleptic
c. attack
c. somnambulism
cataleptiform
cataleptoid
catalexia
catalogia
catalyst
catalytic agent
catamenia
catamenial
c. migraine
c. migraine headache
c. seizure
catamite
catamnesis
catamnestic
cataphasia
cataphora
cataphoric
cataphrenia
cataplasia
cataplectic
cataplexis
cataplexy episode
Catapres Oral
cataract-oligophrenia syndrome
catastrophe theory
catastrophic
c. ancataplexy syndrome
c. anxiety
c. behavior
c. expectation
c. illness
c. migraine
c. reaction
c. response
c. schizophrenia
c. stress
catathymia
catathymic
c. amnesia
c. crisis
catatonia
deadly c.
depressive c.

C

catatonia (continued)
excited c.
lethal c.
maniac c.
c. mitis
periodic c.
c. protracts
schizophrenic c.
Stauder lethal c.
stuporous c.
catatonic, catatoniac
c. cerebral paralysis
c. dementia
c. disorder
c. disorder due to a general
medical condition
c. drug
c. excitation
c. excitement
c. feature
c. motor behavior
c. mutism
c. negativism
c. posturing
c. presentation
c. rigidity
c. schizophrenia
c. state
c. stupor
c. symptom
c. syndrome
catatonoid attitude
catatony
Catatrol
catchment area
CAT/CLAMS
Clinical Adaptive Test/Clinical Linguistic
Auditory Milestone Scale
cat-cry syndrome
catecholamine
c. hypophysis
c. neurotransmitter
catecholaminergic
catechol-O-methyltransferase (COMT)
categelophobia
categorical
c. approach
c. attitude
c. classification
c. definition
c. imperative
c. model
c. perspective
c. system
c. thinking
c. thought
categorization
symbolic c.
category
Functional Ambulation C.'s (FAC)
c. mistake
NOS c.
semantic c.

c. specific semantic impairment
syntactic c.
category-specific naming
Category Test (CT)
catelectrotonus
Catell Infant Scale
catenating
catenation
CAT-H
Children's Apperception Test-Human
cathard (var. of cafard)
catharsis
activity c.
community c.
conversational c.
emotional c.
psychodramatic c.
cathartic
c. abuse
c. method
cathectic discharge
cathepsin
c. B
c. G
catheresis
catheter
Abramson c.
Accu-Flo ventricular c.
afterloading c.
angiographic c.
Argyll ftrocar c.
balloon c.
Berenstein guiding c.
BPS spinal angiographic c.
Camino intracranial c.
cisterna magna c.
Codman ventricular silicone c.
cup c.
delivery c.
distal c.
double-lumen Swan-Ganz c.
dummy seed c.
ePTFE ventricular shunt c.
FasTRACKER-18 infusion c.
Fogarty embolectomy c.
Foley c.
Folz c.
French c.
20-gauge c.
Heplock c.
Hickman c.
HNB angiographic c.
ICP c.
ICP-T fiberoptic ICP intracranial
temperature c.
ICP-T fiberoptic ICP monitoring c.
intraventricular c.
ITC radiopaque balloon c.
Lapras c.
lumbar c.
micro-Soft Stream sidehole
infusion c.
Micro-Vac suction c.
MTC Ventcontrol ventricular c.
1505 NDSB occlusion balloon c.

nondetachable silicone balloon c.
peritoneal c.
Phoenix Anti-Blok ventricular c.
polyethylene intravenous c.
Portnoy ventricular c.
Pudenz ventricular c.
Raimondi spring c.
Raimondi ventricular c.
red rubber c.
Scott silicone ventricular c.
Seletz nonrigid ventricular c.
Shaw c.
Shiley c.
Silastic c.
Simpson c.
spinal c.
Stealth angioplasty balloon c.
Swan-Ganz c.
thin-wall introducer c.
toposcopic c.
Tracker-10 c.
Tracker-18 c.
Tracker infusion c.
transducer-tipped c.
transfemoral c.
tunnelable ventricular ICP c.
ventriculostomy c.
Ventrix SD fiberoptic subdural
  ICP c.
cathexis
affective c.
body c.
ego c.
fantasy c.
object c.
oral-sadistic c.
positive c.
word c.
cathinone
cathisophobia, kathisophobia
cathode
catochus
catoptrophobia
cat-scratch disease (CSD)
cat's-eye syndrome
Cattell
C. factorial theory of personality
C. Infant Intelligence Scale
C. Infant Scale for Intelligence
  (CISI)
C. Infant Scale Inventory (CISI)
C. Personality Factor Questionnaire
cauda, pl. **caudae**
c. equina
c. equina avulsion
c. equina compression
c. equina syndrome (CES)
c. fasciae dentatae
c. nuclei caudati
c. striati
caudal
c. canal
c. hook
c. lamina resection
c. locus ceruleus

c. neuropore
c. regression syndrome
c. to rostral
c. transtentorial herniation
caudalis
nucleus c.
pars c.
subnucleus c.
caudate
dorsolateral c.
c. nucleus
c. volume
caudatolenticular
caudatum
caudatus
nucleus c.
caudolenticular
caumesthesia
causa
trabajando la c.
causal
c. association
c. factor
c. indication
c. link
c. relationship
c. texture
causalgia
causalgic pain
causalis
indicatio c.
causality
direct c.
phenomenistic c.
presumed c.
causation
biologic c.
organismic c.
causative
c. agent
c. stress
cause
efficient c.
c. efficient
substance-related c.
cause-and-effect test
cause-effect relationship
caustic ingestion
cautery
Aesculap bipolar c.
BICAP c.
bipolar c.
Concept hand-held c.
c. hook
Mira c.
monopolar c.
right-angle bipolar c.
suction c.
cava (*pl. of* cavum)
Cavalieri direct estimator method
CAVD
completion, arithmetic, vocabulary, and
  directions
cave
Meckel c.

cavernoma
cavernoma-related epilepsy
cavernosa
    corpora c.
cavernous
    c. angioma
    c. hemangioma
    c. malformation
    c. plexus
    c. sinus
    c. sinus aneurysm
    c. sinus fistula
    c. sinus lesion
    c. sinus meningioma
    c. sinus syndrome
    c. sinus thrombophlebitis
    c. sinus thrombosis
    c. sinus tumor
cavernous-carotid aneurysm
Cavitron
    C. dissector
    C. laser
    C. ultrasonic surgical aspirator
    (CUSA)
cavity
    epidural c.
    nasal c.
    oral c.
    c. of septum pellucidum
    sinonasal c.
    subarachnoid c.
    subdural c.
    syringomyelic c.
    syrinx c.
    trigeminal c.
CAVLT-2
    Children's Auditory Verbal Learning
    Test-2
cavum, pl. cava
    c. epidurale
    inferior vena cava
    c. meckelii
    c. psalterii
    c. septi pellucidi (CSP)
    c. subarachnoideum
    c. subdurale
    c. veli interpositi (CVI)
    c. vergae
Cawthorne-Cooksey vestibular exercise
CBB
    communications in behavioral biology
CBC
    Camelot Behavioral Checklist
    child behavior characteristic
CBCL
    Child Behavioral Checklist
CBF
    cerebral blood flow
CBI
    Career Beliefs Inventory
    convergent beam irradiation
    CBI stereotactic head holder
CBN
    cannabinol

CBR
    chemical, bacteriological, radiological
CBS
    chronic brain syndrome
CBT
    cognitive behavior therapy
CBTC
    Childhood Brain Tumor Consortium
CBW
    chemical and biological warfare
CBZ
    carbamazepine
CC
    chief complaint
C1-C2
    C1-C2 cable fixation
    C1-C2 posterior arthrodesis
CCA
    common carotid artery
    CCA clamp
CCAE
    Checklist for Child Abuse Evaluation
CCAI
    Cross-Cultural Adaptability Inventory
CCAS
    Comprehensive Career Assessment Scale
CCAT
    Canadian Cognitive Abilities Test
CCD
    charge-coupled device
CCF
    carotid-cavernous fistula
CCI
    College Characteristics Index
CCK
    cholecystokinin
CCK-4
    cholecystokinin tetrapeptide
CCK-8
    cholecystokinin octapeptide
CCM
    Crime Classification Manual
CCMD-2
    Chinese Classification of Mental
    Disorders, Second Edition
CCQ
    Chronicle Career Quest
CCS
    Children's Coma Score
    concentration camp syndrome
CCSEQ
    Community College Student Experiences
    Questionnaire
CCT
    cranial computed tomography
    high-resolution CCT
CCTDI
    California Critical Thinking Dispositions
    Inventory
CCTST
    California Critical Thinking Skills Test
CCTV
    closed-circuit television
C-D
    Cotrel-Dubousset

C-D instrumentation
C-D instrumentation device
C-D instrumentation fixation
  strength
C-D instrumentation rigidity
C-D rod insertion
C-D screw modification
Cd
  color denial
CD29+ memory cell
CD34 staining
CD4+CD45RA+ cell
CD4/CD8 ratio
CD4 lymphocyte
CDC
  chemical dependency counselor
CDI
  Children's Depression Inventory
  Children's Diagnostic Inventory
CDL
  Copying Drawings with Landmarks
CDM
  Career Decision-Making
cDNA
  cyclic deoxyribonucleic acid
CDR
  Clinical Dementia Rating
    CDR Scale
CDS
  Children's Depression Scale
CDT
  carbohydrate-deficient transferrin
CD track
CEA
  carotid endarterectomy
ceaseless pacing
CEA-Tc 99m
cecocentral scotoma
CED
  convection-enhanced delivery
cefaclor
cefadroxil
cefalothin sodium
cefamandole
  c. nafate
cefazedone
cefazolin
cefotaxime
cefoxitin sodium
CEFT
  Children's Embedded Figures Test
ceftazidime
ceftizoxime
ceftriaxone
cefuroxime
ceiling
  c. age
  c. effect
Celestone
Celexa
CELI
  Carrow Elicited Language Inventory
celiac
  c. ganglia
  c. plexus

celibacy
cell
  adenohypophyseal c.
  c. adhesion molecule (CAM)
  alpha c.
  amacrine c.
  ameboid c.
  Antoni A c.
  Antoni B c.
  apolar c.
  arachnoid c.
  c. assembly
  astroglia c.
  auditory receptor c.
  basket c.
  beta c.
  Betz c.
  Bevan-Lewis c.
  36B10 glioma c.
  bipolar c.
  blood c.
  c. body
  border c.
  Böttcher c.
  Cajal c.
  CD4+CD45RA+ c.
  CD29+ memory c.
  cerebellar granule c.
  chandelier c.
  chief c.
  cochlear hair c.
  column c.
  commissural c.
  compound granule c.
  cone c. of retina
  Corti c.
  corticotroph c.
  cuboidal c.
  Deiters c.
  detention c.
  c. differentiation
  c. division
  Dogiel c.
  effector c.
  ependymal c.
  external pillar c.
  Fañanás c.
  foam c.
  fusiform c. of cerebral cortex
  ganglion c.
  gemästete c.
  gemistocytic c.
  giant pyramidal Betz c.
  gitter c.
  glial c.
  globoid c.
  globose c.
  Golgi epithelial c.
  gonadotroph c.
  granular c.
  granule c.
  gustatory c.
  gyrochrome c.
  hair c.
  hemosiderin-laden c.

C

cell *(continued)*
    Hensen c.
    heteromeric c.
    HNK c.
    horizontal c. of Cajal
    Hortega c.
    internal pillar c.
    karyochrome c.
    lactotroph c.
    Langerhans c.
    lipid-laden stromal c.
    locked c.
    lymphokine-activated killer c.
    macroglia c.
    Martinotti c.
    mastoid air c.
    Mauthner c.
    c. membrane lipid
    Merkel tactile c.
    mesoglial c.
    Meynert c.
    microglia c.
    midget bipolar c.
    mitral c.
    mononuclear c. (MNC)
    mossy c.
    motor c.
    Müller radial c.
    multipolar c.
    multipotential c.
    myxomatous c.
    Nageotte c.
    c. necrosis
    nerve c.
    neural progenitor c.
    neural tube floor plate c.
    neurilemma c.
    neuroendocrine transducer c.
    neuroepithelial c.
    neuroglia c.
    neurosecretory c.
    c. nucleus
    olfactory receptor c.
    olfactory sheathing c.
    oligodendroglia c.
    Opalski c.
    padded c.
    pallidal c.
    parenchymatous c. of corpus
      pineale
    peripheral blood mononuclear c.
      (PBMC)
    perivascular mononuclear c.
    phalangeal c.
    photoreceptor c.
    physaliphorous c.
    pillar c. of Corti
    pineal c.
    porcine dopaminergic c.
    c. proliferation
    proliferative malignant glial c.
    pseudounipolar c.
    Purkinje c.
    pyramidal c.

    reactive c.
    Renshaw c.
    rod c. of retina
    Rolando c.
    satellite c.
    C. Saver
    Schaffer collateral c.
    Schultze c.
    Schwann c.
    somatic c.
    somatotroph c.
    S phase c.
    spider c.
    spindle c.
    stellate c. of cerebral cortex
    stem serotonergic c.
    syncytiotrophoblastic giant c.
      (STGC)
    taste c.
    tau-negative nerve c.
    thymic myoid c.
    thyrotroph c.
    transducer c.
    tufted c.
    tunnel c.
    unipolar c.
    vestibular hair c.
    visual receptor c.
    wandering c.
    white blood c.
    xenogeneic chromaffin c.
cella, gen. and pl. **cellae**
    c. media
cellular
    c. brain edema
    c. immunity factor
    c. immunologic
    c. immunologic response
    c. ion homeostasis
    c. kinetics
    c. layers of cortex
cellulose
    c. acetate polymer
    oxidized regenerated c.
    c. sodium phosphate
cellulotoxic
Celontin
celsi
    alopecia c.
Celsus alopecia
celtophobia
CEM
    CUSA electrosurgical module
    CEM handswitching nosecone
cement
    BoneSource hydroxyapatite c.
    burned rubber c.
    rubber c.
Cena-K
cenesthesia, coenesthesia
cenesthesic, cenesthetic
    c. hallucination
cenesthesiopathic schizophrenia
cenesthopathic schizophrenia
cenesthopathy

Cenestin
Cenestine
Cenolate
cenophobia (*var. of* kenophobia)
cenotophobia
cenotrope
censor
    endopsychic c.
    freudian c.
    psychic c.
censorship
    dream c.
censure
census tract
center
    acoustic c.
    addiction c.
    Adult Diagnostic and Treatment C.
    anospinal c.
    C. for Anxiety and Depression
    appetitive c.
    association c.
    c. of attention
    Broca c.
    Budge c.
    ciliospinal c.
    community mental health c.
      (CMHC)
    cortical c.
    counseling c.
    crisis c.
    day treatment c. (DTC)
    Developmental Evaluation C. (DEC)
    drug information c. (DIC)
    ego c.
    C. for Epidemiologic Studies-
      Depression (CES-D)
    C. for Epidemiologic Studies-
      Depression Scale
    expiratory c.
    feeding c.
    gaze pontine c.
    higher brain c.
    inspiratory c.
    language c.
    c. median
    medullary c.
    C. for Mental Health Services
      (CMHS)
    methadone c.
    motor c.
    motor cortical c.
    motor speech c.
    pleasure c.
    pontine lateral gaze c.
    psychocortical c.
    rape crisis c.
    reflex c.
    residential treatment c. (RTC)
    respiratory c.
    satiety c.
    semioval c.
    sensory speech c.
    speech intention c.
    speech monitoring c.

    C. for Stress and Anxiety
      Disorders
    suicide prevention c.
    visual c.
    vital c.
    Wernicke c.
    word c.
centered
    child c.
    community c.
    group c.
centeredness
centering
center-surround response
centigray (cGy)
centimorgan
centophobia
centra (*pl. of* centrum)
central
    c. achromatopsia
    c. alexia
    c. amaurosis
    c. anesthesia
    c. anticholinergic toxicity
    c. aphasia
    c. apnea
    c. bradycardia
    c. canal
    c. chemosensitivity
    c. cholinergic blockade
    c. chromatolysis
    c. conflict
    c. convulsion
    c. core disease
    c. dazzle
    c. deafness
    c. direct current bright spot
    C. European encephalitis
    C. European subtype
    C. European tick-borne fever
    c. excitatory state
    c. executive component
    c. facial paresis
    c. fissure
    c. force
    c. ganglioneuroma
    c. gray
    c. gray matter (CGM)
    c. gray substance
    c. gyri
    c. hypoventilation syndrome
    c. inflammatory demyelination
    c. inhibition
    c. language disorder (CLD)
    c. language imbalance
    c. lesion
    c. lobule
    c. masking
    c. motive state
    c. motor pathways disease
    c. nervous system (CNS)
    c. nervous system hemorrhage
    c. nervous system hypersomnolence
    c. nervous system infection
    c. nervous system lymphoma

C

central *(continued)*
    c. nervous system stimulant
    c. nervous system stimulant,
      nonamphetamine
    c. neuritis
    c. neurofibromatosis
    c. neurogenic hyperventilation
    c. nystagmus
    c. pain
    c. paralysis
    c. pit
    c. pontine myelinolysis
    c. process
    c. processing dysfunction
    c. reflex time
    c. respiratory chemoreception
    c. sacral line (CSL)
    c. scotoma
    c. seizure
    c. sensory deficit
    c. sensory loss
    c. sleep apnea
    c. somatosensory conduction time
      (CSCT)
    c. sulcus
    c. tegmental fasciculus
    c. tegmental nucleus
    c. tegmental tract (CTT)
    c. tendency
    c. tendency measure
    C. Texas Veterans Health Care
      System (CTVHCS)
    c. theme
    c. trait
    c. transactional core
    c. transtentorial herniation
    c. venous channel
    c. venous pressure
    c. vision
    c. vision acuity
centralis
    ala lobuli c.
    amaurosis c.
centralist psychology
central-limit theorem
centraphose
centration
Centrax
centre médian de Luys
centrencephalic
    c. epilepsy
    c. integrating system
    c. seizure
centrencephalon
centrifugal nerve
centripetal
    c. nerve
    c. spread
centroblastic B-cell lymphoma
centrocecal visual field
centrokinesia
centrokinetic
centromedian nucleus
centromere

centronuclear myopathy
centrophenoxine
centro ritual
centrotemporal
    c. epilepsy
    c. paroxysmal focus
    c. spike
centrum, pl. **centra**
    c. medianum
    c. medullare
    c. ovale
    c. semiovale
    Vicq d'Azyr c. semiovale
    Vieussens c.
     · Willis c. nervosum
cephalad
cephalalgia, cephalgia
    histamine c.
    histaminic c.
    Horton histamine c.
    orgasmic c.
cephalea
    c. agitata
    c. attonita
    epileptic c.
cephaledema
cephalemia
cephalexin
cephalgia *(var. of* cephalalgia)
cephalgic attack
cephalhematocele
cephalhematoma *(var. of*
    cephalohematoma)
cephalhydrocele
cephalic
    c. angle
    c. aura
    c. flexure
    c. index
    c. reflex
    c. seizure
    c. tetanus
cephalitis
cephalocele
cephalocentesis
cephalodynia
cephalogenesis
cephalogyric
cephalohematocele
cephalohematoma, cephalhematoma
cephalohemometer
cephalomedullary angle
cephalomeningitis
cephalometer
    Bertillon c.
cephalometric
    c. analysis
    c. angle
cephalometrography
cephalometry
cephalomotor
Cephalonia
cephalooculocutaneous telangiectasia
cephalopalpebral reflex
cephalopathy

cephalopolysyndactyly
  Greig c.
cephaloridine
cephalorrhachidian index
cephaloskeletal dysplasia
cephalosporin
  third-generation c.
cephalostat
cephalothin
cephalotrigeminal angiomatosis
cephapirin
cephradine
Cephulac
ceptor
  chemical c.
  contact c.
  distance c.
CER
  conditioned emotional response
CERAD
  Consortium to Establish a Registry for
  Alzheimer's Disease
  CERAD Assessment Battery
ceramic vertebral spacer
ceramidase
ceramide
  c. dihexoside
  c. trihexoside
  trihexosyl c.
ceraunophobia, keraunophobia
Ceraxon
c-erbB-2-encoded oncoprotein
cercle
  arc de c.
cerea
  flexibilitas c.
  c. flexibilitas
cerebella (*pl. of* cerebellum)
cerebellar
  c. aggregation culture
  c. aggregation culture for
    teratogenicity testing
  c. arachnoid cyst
  c. artery
  c. astrocytoma
  c. ataxia
  c. attachment
  c. cortex
  c. cortical degeneration
  c. dysmetria
  c. ectopia
  c. fissure
  c. fit
  c. fits seizure
  c. folia
  c. gait
  c. gliosarcoma
  c. granule cell
  c. hematoma
  c. hemisphere
  c. hemisphere syndrome
  c. hemorrhage
  c. hemorrhage syndrome
  c. infarction
  c. malaria

  c. mass
  c. nuclei
  c. nystagmus
  c. pathway
  c. peduncle
  c. pyramid
  c. retraction
  c. retractor
  c. rigidity
  c. sign
  c. speech
  c. sulci
  c. tonsil
  c. tonsillar herniation
  c. tremor
  c. vein
  c. vermian atrophy
  c. vermis dysgenesis
  c. volume
cerebelli
  ala c.
  amygdala c.
  cortex c.
  pons c.
  tentorium c.
cerebellitis
cerebellolental
cerebellomedullaris
  cisterna c.
cerebellomedullary
  c. cistern
  c. fissure
  c. malformation syndrome
**cerebellomesoencephalic fissure Perspex
  rod**
cerebelloolivary degeneration
cerebellopontine
  c. angle
  c. angle approach
  c. angle arachnoid cyst
  c. angle cistern
  c. angle schwannoma
  c. angle syndrome
  c. angle tumor
  c. cisternography
  c. recess
cerebellorubral tract
cerebellothalamic tract
cerebellum, pl. cerebella
  Flechsig bundle in c.
  Gowers bundle in c.
  tongue of c.
cerebra (*pl. of* cerebrum)
cerebral
  c. abscess
  c. agraphia
  c. amaurosis
  c. amebiasis
  c. amyloid angiopathy
  amyloid angiopathy c.
  c. anaplastic astrocytoma
  c. anemia
  c. aneurysm
  c. angiography
  c. angiomatosis

C

cerebral *(continued)*
- c. anoxia
- c. anthrax
- c. antioxidant activity
- c. aplasia
- c. apotentiality
- c. aqueduct
- c. aqueduct compression
- c. arteriography
- c. arteriosclerosis
- c. arteriovenous oxygen content difference (AVDO₂)
- c. artery
- c. artery infarction
- c. asymmetry
- c. atherosclerosis
- c. atrophy
- c. autosomal dominant arteriopathy with subcortical infarcts and leukoencephalopathy (CADASIL)
- c. beriberi
- c. blindness
- blindness c.
- c. blood flow (CBF)
- c. blood vessel
- c. brain death
- c. brucellosis
- c. calculus
- c. cavernous angioma
- c. circulation
- c. cladosporiosis
- c. claudication
- c. commissure
- c. compromise
- c. contusion
- c. convexity
- c. convulsion
- c. cortex
- c. cortex of Ateles
- c. cortical function
- c. decompression
- c. decortication
- c. depressant
- c. diataxia
- c. digital angiogram
- c. disease
- c. disorder
- c. disorganization
- c. dominance
- c. dynamic imaging
- c. dyschromatopsia
- c. dysfunction
- c. dysplasia
- c. dysrhythmia
- c. eclipse
- c. edema
- c. electrotherapy (CET)
- c. embolus
- c. fissure
- c. flexure
- c. foreign body embolization
- c. formed-element embolism
- c. gait
- c. gaze paresis
- c. gigantism
- c. glioblastoma
- c. glioma
- c. glucose metabolic-type organic psychosis
- c. glucose metabolism
- c. gumma
- c. hemicorticectomy
- c. hemidecortication
- c. hemisphere
- c. hemodynamic variation
- c. hemorrhage
- c. hemosiderosis
- c. hernia
- c. herniation
- c. hydatid
- c. hyperesthesia
- c. hyperplasia
- c. hypertension
- c. hypoperfusion
- c. hypoplasia
- c. hypoxia
- c. impairment
- c. infarct
- c. infection
- c. injection
- c. integration
- c. intermittent claudication
- c. irritation
- c. ischemia
- c. ischemia steal
- c. laceration
- c. layer of retina
- c. lesion
- c. lipidosis
- c. localization
- c. location
- c. lymphoma
- c. mal
- c. malaria
- c. mantle
- c. mapping of apraxia
- c. metastasis
- c. microembolism
- c. neuroblastoma
- c. neurosyphilis
- c. nocardiosis
- c. outflow tremor
- c. oxygen consumption
- c. pacemaker
- c. palsy
- c. peduncle
- c. perfusion pressure (CPP)
- c. poliodystrophy
- c. porosis
- c. potential
- c. pressure autoregulation
- c. protection
- c. protective therapy
- c. ptosis
- c. radiation necrosis (CRN)
- c. revascularization
- c. salt wasting
- c. salt wasting syndrome
- c. sclerosis

c. seizure
c. sensory input
c. sign
c. sinus
c. sphingolipidosis
c. steal syndrome
c. sulcus
c. syphilis
c. tetanus
c. thrombosis (CT)
c. thumb
c. trauma
c. tuberculosis
c. vasodilating agent
c. vasoreactivity
c. vasospasm
c. vein
c. venous malformation (CVM)
c. ventricle
c. ventriculography
c. vesicle
c. voxel

cerebral-blast syndrome
cérébrale
tache c.
cerebralgia
cerebralis
adiposis c.
mycetism c.
cerebrate posturing
cerebration
unconscious c.
cerebri
anus c.
aqueductus c.
astrocytosis c.
commotio c.
contusio c.
cortex c.
falx c.
familial gliomatosis c.
fungus c.
glioblastosis c.
gliomatosis c.
lacuna c.
membrana c.
pseudotumor c.
status post commotio c.
zero cerebral pseudotumor c.
cerebritis
lupus c.
suppurative c.
cerebroatrophic hyperammonemia
cerebrocranial defect
Cerebrograph 10a
cerebrohepatorenal syndrome
cerebroma
cerebromacular
c. degeneration (CMD)
c. dystrophy
cerebromalacia
cerebromeningitis
cerebropathia
cerebropathy
cerebropsychosis

cerebroretinal angiomatosis
cerebrosclerosis
cerebroside
c. lipidosis
c. reticulocytosis
c. sulfatase
cerebrosidosis
cerebrosis
cerebrospinal
c. axis
c. convulsion
c. fever
c. fluid (CSF)
c. fluid analysis
c. fluid fistula
c. fluid leakage
c. fluid otorrhea
c. fluid pleocytosis
c. fluid protein
c. fluid rhinorrhea
c. fluid shunt
c. fluid volume
c. index
c. meningitis
c. pressure
c. seizure
c. system
cerebrospinant
cerebrotendinous
c. cholesterolosis
c. xanthomatosis (CTX)
cerebrotomy
cerebrotonia
cerebrovascular
c. accident (CVA)
c. accident dementia
c. amyloidosis
c. disease
c. disease organic psychosis
c. insufficiency
c. ischemia-type organic psychosis
c. lesion
c. malformation
c. neurosyphilis
c. regulation
c. syndrome
cerebrum, pl. **cerebra, cerebrums**
aqueduct c.
cistern of great vein of cerebrum
cistern of lateral fossa of cerebrum
lobe of c.
Cerebyx
ceremonial
c. behavior
compulsive c.
ceremonious
Ceresine
Cerestat
Ceretec imaging kit
cerium
ceroid-lipofuscinosis
ceroid lipofuscinosis
CERS
Crisis Evaluation Referral Service

C

certificate
    birth c.
    dependent adult's c.
    detention c.
    c. of incompetency
    c. of need
certified
    physician's assistant, c. (PA-C)
    c. social worker (CSW)
ceruleus
    caudal locus c.
    locus c.
ceruloplasmin
    c. deficiency
    serum c.
    c. test
cerveau isolé
cervical
    c. aortic knuckle
    c. arthrodesis
    c. carotid bifurcation
    c. collar
    c. compression syndrome
    c. cord lesion
    c. corpectomy
    c. decompression surgery
    c. discectomy
    c. disk excision
    c. disk herniation
    c. dystonia
    c. enlargement of spinal cord
    c. fibrositis
    c. flexure
    c. fusion syndrome
    c. intersegmental vein
    c. interspace
    c. intramedullary tumor
    c. laminectomy
    c. medullary junction
    c. myositis
    c. myospasm
    c. nerve
    c. nerve root injury
    c. neural foramina
    c. perivascular sympathectomy
    c. plate
    c. radiculopathy
    c. rib syndrome
    c. screw insertion technique
    c. spinal stenosis
    c. spine
    c. spine arthritis
    c. spine decompression
    c. spine injury
    c. spine internal fixation
    c. spine kyphotic deformity
    c. spine laminectomy
    c. spine posterior fusion
    c. spine posterior ligament
      disruption
    c. spine rheumatoid disease
    c. spine screw-plate fixation
    c. spine stabilization
    c. spine stabilization procedure
    c. spine trauma

    c. spondylosis
    c. spondylosis without myelopathy
    c. spondylotic myelopathy (CSM)
    c. spondylotic myelopathy fusion
      technique
    c. spondylotic myelopathy
      vertebrectomy
    c. steroid epidural nerve block
    c. sympathetic chain location
    c. tension myositis (CTM)
    c. tension syndrome
    c. vertebra
    c. vertebrectomy
    c. vessel compression
cervices (*pl. of* cervix)
cervicis (*gen. of* cervix)
cervicobrachialgia
cervicocephalic arterial dissection
cervicocollic reflex
cervicodynia
cervicogenic headache (CH)
cervicolumbar phenomenon
cervicomedullary
    c. deformity
    c. junction compression
    c. kink
cervicooccipital fusion
cervicothoracic
    c. ganglion
    c. junction
    c. junction stabilization
    c. junction surgery
    c. orthosis
    c. pedicle anatomy
    c. pedicle angle
cervix, gen. cervicis, pl. cervices
    c. of the axon
    c. columnae posterioris
    cervicis muscle
    splenius cervicis
CES
    cauda equina syndrome
    Classroom Environmental Scale
cesarean resection
CES-D
    Center for Epidemiologic Studies-
      Depression
    CES-D Scale
cesium fluoride scintillation detector
cessation
    smoking c.
Cestan-Chenais syndrome
cesticidal
CET
    cerebral electrotherapy
ceylanicum
    Ancylostoma c.
CF
    Coalition for the Family
C-factor
    cleverness factor
CFBRS
    Cooper-Farran Behavioral Rating Scale
CFE
    colony-forming efficiency

CFIDS
    chronic fatigue and immune dysfunction
        syndrome
CFIT
    Culture Fair Intelligence Test
    Culture Free Intelligence Test
c-fos
        c.-f. gene
        c.-f. protein immunoreactivity
CFQ
    Cognitive Failures Questionnaire
CFQ-for-others assessment
CFS
    chronic fatigue syndrome
CFSEI-2
    Culture-Free Self-Esteem Inventories,
        Second Edition
CFT
    Complex Figure Test
    Culture Free Test
CGAS
    Children's Global Assessment Scale
CGI
    Clinical Global Impressions
    Clinical Global Improvement
        CGI Scale
CGIC
    Clinical Global Impression of Change
CGM
    central gray matter
cGMP
    cyclic guanosine monophosphate
CGP
    Comparative Guidance and Placement
        Program
CGPS
    Current, Global, Psychiatric-Social Status
CGRP
    calcitonin gene-related peptide
CGRS
    Clinician's Global Rating Scale
cGy
    centigray
CH
    cervicogenic headache
CH50 assay
CHADD
    children and adults with attention deficit
        disorder
Chaddock
        C. reflex
        C. sign
chaetophobia
Chagas disease
chain
        aliphatic c.
        c. analysis
        c. behavior
        behavior c.
        human neurofilament light c.
        kappa light c.
        lambda light c.
        c. reflex
        c. reproduction
        respiratory c.

        c. smoker
        Sno-Traks wheelchair c.'s
chained reinforcement
chaining response
chair
        Combisit surgeon's c.
        tranquilizer c.
challenge
        neuroendocrine c.
        c. strategy
        c. test
chamber
        anechoic c.
        drip c.
        echo c.
        flush c.
        gas c.
        Sechrist monoplace hyperbaric c.
Chamberlain palatooccipital line
champagne-bottle leg
Champion Trauma Score (CTS)
CHAMPUS
    Civilian Health and Medical Program of
        the Uniformed Service
chance
        c. action
        c. difference
        c. error
        C. fracture
        c. medley
        c. response parameter
        c. variation
chancre
        hard c.
        true c.
chancroid
chancrous
chandelier cell
change
        abulic mental c.
        Adolescent-Family Inventory of
            Life Events and C.'s
        adolescent sexual c.
        affectional life c.
        affective c.
        agent of c.
        c. agent
        C. Agent Questionnaire (CAQ)
        analogic c.
        autoplastic c.
        behavioral c.
        binocular acuity c.
        biophysical life c.
        career c.
        Clinical Global Impression of C.
            (CGIC)
        compulsive c.
        conversion sensory c.
        cultural c.
        degenerative discogenic vertebral c.
        digital c.
        environmental c.
        Fairbanks c.
        Family Inventory of Life Events
            and C.'s (FILE)

C

change *(continued)*
   c. fear
   c. of heart
   job c.
   language c.
   c. of life
   life cycle c.
   major life c.
   maladaptive behavioral c.
   maladaptive psychological c.
   mental status c.
   c. in mentation
   mood c.
   c. in mood
   neuropeptide c.
   onion bulb c.
   c. of pace
   personality c.
   c. in personality characteristic
   pharmacodynamic c.
   pharmacokinetic c.
   physical c.
   c. point
   polyneuropathy, organomegaly,
     endocrinopathy, myeloma, and
     skin c. (POEMS)
   positive attitude c.
   psychological c.
   psychomotor c.
   psychophysiological c.
   reflex c.
   Schedule for Affective Disorders
     and Schizophrenia - C.
   sense of bodily c.
   sex c.
   socioeconomic life c.
   telangiectatic c.
   time-zone c.
   c. of topic
   transitional c.
   trophic c.
   unpredictable mood c.
   visual c.
changed body image
change-up
changing sleep-wake pattern
channel
   20-c. Beckman EEG instrument
   37-c. biomagnetometer
   c. capacity
   central venous c.
   c. of communication
   communication c.
   ligand-gated ion c.
   membrane ion c.
   voltage-gated calcium c. (VGCC)
   voltage-gated sodium c.
Chapman Scale
character
   acquired c.
   affectionless c.
   anal c.
   anal-aggressive c.
   c. analysis

   c. armor
   c. assassination
   c. attack
   authoritarian c.
   compulsive c.
   c. defense
   c. deficit
   dependent c.
   depressive c.
   c. development
   c. displacement
   dominant c.
   epileptic c.
   erotic c.
   exploitative c.
   genital c.
   histrionic c.
   hoarding c.
   hysterical c.
   c. impulse disorder
   impulsive c.
   masochistic c.
   narcissistic c.
   national c.
   c. neurosis
   obsessional c.
   oral c.
   oral-aggressive c.
   oral-passive c.
   oral-receptive c.
   paranoiac c.
   c. pathology
   phallic c.
   phallic-narcissistic c.
   phobic c.
   primary sex c.
   receptive c.
   c. resistance
   secondary sex c.
   sex-conditioned c.
   sex-limited c.
   sex-linked c.
   c. spectrum disorders
   c. structure
   c. trait
   c. type
   urethral c.
   c. witness
character-analytic vegetotherapy
characteristic
   c. age
   c. association
   association c.
   c. behavior
   change in personality c.
   child behavior c. (CBC)
   clang association c.
   consumer c.
   demand c.
   dominant c.
   c. feature
   c. paraphiliac focus
   c. pattern
   performance c.
   personality c.

presenting c.
primary sex c.
psychometric performance c.
receiver operating c. (ROC)
secondary sex c.
sex c.
c. sign
unique c.
c. withdrawal syndrome
characterization wit
characterological depression
CharcoAid
charcoal
Charcocaps
Charcot
C. artery
C. arthropathy
C. disease
C. gait
C. grand hysteria
C. joint
C. triad
C. vertigo
Charcot-Bouchard intracerebral aneurysm
Charcot-Marie-Tooth disease
Charcot-Weiss-Baker syndrome
charge
c. of affect
conversion sensory c.
sensory c.
charge-coupled device (CCD)
charged particle radiosurgery
Charnley suction drain
Charpentier law
chart
autobiographical life c.
Comprehensive Developmental Evaluation C.
expectancy c.
flow c.
pediatric growth c.
progress c.
Charteris Reading Test
Chaslin gliosis
Chassaignac tubercle
Chatillon dolorimeter
chatterbox effect
Chaussier line
Chavany-Brunhes syndrome
Chealamide
checkerboard
c. field
c. pattern
checking and touching rituals
checklist
Aberrant Behavior C. (ABC)
Achenbach Child Behavior C.
Achievement C. (ACL)
ACQ Behavior C.
C. of Adaptive Living Skills (CALS)
Adjective C. (ACL)
Alternative Lifestyle C. (ALC)
c. approach

Behavioral C.
Behavior Problem C. (BPC)
Camelot Behavioral C. (CBC)
C. for Child Abuse Evaluation (CCAE)
Child Behavioral C. (CBCL)
Creativity C.
Depressive Adjective C. (DAC, DACL)
Developing Skills C. (DISCUSS, DSC)
Elgin c.
Gordon Occupational C.-II (GOCL-II)
Health Problems C.
Hopkins Symptom C. (HSCL)
Hopkins Symptom C.-90 (HSCL-90)
Illness Behavior C. (IBC)
Independent Living Behavior C.
Jesness Behavior C. (JBC)
Life Experiences C. (LEC)
Louisville Behavior C.
Maastricht History and Advice C.-Revised (MAAS-R)
Mooney Problem C. (MPC, MPCL)
Multiple Affect Adjective C. (MAACL)
Normative Adaptive Behavior C.
occupational c. (OCL)
Ottawa School Behavior C. (OSBCL)
Perley-Guze Hysteria C.
Personal Problems C. (PPC)
Physical and Architectural Features C.
Problem Experiences C.
Revised Behavior Problem C.
Revised Ways of Coping C.
S-D Proneness C.
Substance Abuse Problem C.
Suicide-Depression Proneness C. (SDPC)
Symptom C.-90-Revised (SCL-90-R)
time-sample behavioral c. (TSBC)
Trauma Symptom C. for Children Ages 8–15
Young Adult Behavior C.
Chediak-Higashi syndrome
cheeking medication
cheerfulness
unnatural c.
cheese reaction headache
cheilophagia
cheiloschisis
cheimaphobia
cheimatophobia
cheirobrachialgia, chirobrachialgia
cheirognostic, chirognostic
cheirokinesthesia, chirokinesthesia
cheirokinesthetic
cheirology
cheirospasm, chirospasm
chelating agent

C

chelation
    c. therapy
Chemet
chemical
    c. abuse
    c. action
    c. addiction
    c. agent
    c. aversion therapy
    c. and biological warfare (CBW)
    c. ceptor
    c. denervation
    c. dependence
    c. dependency
    c. dependency counselor (CDC)
    endogenous c.
    exogenous c.
    c. hemostasis
    c. injury
    c. kinetics
    c. messenger
    c. neurotransmission
    c. restraint
    c. sense
    c. shift
    c. shift anisotrophy
    c. shift artifact
    c. stimulation
    c. stimulus
    c. straitjacket
    c. sympathectomy
    c. synapse
    c. transmitter
    c. warfare
    c. weapon
chemical,
    c. bacteriological, radiological (CBR)
    c. radiological, and biologic
chemically whitening cocaine
chemical-shift imaging
cheminosis
chemistry
    clinical c.
    mental c.
    psychiatric c.
    c. screening battery I (CSB I)
    c. screening battery II (CSB II)
chemoattractant
chemoceptor
chemodectoma
    petrous ridge c.
chemoneurolysis
    glycerol c.
    percutaneous retrogasserian glycerol c.
chemonucleolysis
chemopallidectomy
chemopallidothalamectomy
chemopallidotomy
chemopsychiatry
chemoreception
    central respiratory c.
chemoreceptor
    medullary c.

    peripheral c.
    c. trigger zone
    c. tumor
chemoreceptors trigger
chemoreflex
chemoresistance
chemosensitive
chemosensitivity
    central c.
chemosensory
chemosis
    orbital c.
chemothalamectomy
chemothalamotomy
chemotherapeutic
    c. agent
    c. drug
chemotherapy
    c. antiviral
    blood-brain barrier disruption c.
    combination c.
    PCV c.
chemotherapy
chemotransmitter
chemotropism
cheromania
cherophobia
Cherry
    C. brain retractor
    C. laminectomy retractor
    C. osteotome
    C. traction tongs
Cherry-Kerrison
    C.-K. laminectomy forceps
    C.-K. laminectomy rongeur
cherry-red
    c.-r. spot
    c.-r. spot myoclonus syndrome
chest
    c. discomfort
    c. pain
    c. pulse
    c. restraint
    c. roll
    c. voice
Chestnut Lodge Prognostic Scale for Chronic Schizophrenia
chevaux de frise
chewing
    c. automatism
    c. behavior
    breath c.
    c. method
chewing-speech relationship
Cheyne disease
Cheyne-Stokes
    C.-S. breathing
    C.-S. psychosis
    C.-S. respiration
CHI
    closed head injury
chi
    c. square test
    tai c.

Chiari
    C. formation
    C. III malformation
    C. II malformation
    C. II syndrome
    C. I malformation
chiasm
    cistern of c.
    glioma of optic c.
    optic c.
    prefixed c.
chiasma, pl. chiasmata
    c. opticum
    c. syndrome
chiasmal
    c. arachnoiditis
    c. compression
    c. epidermoid
    c. lesion
chiasmapexy
    transsphenoidal c.
chiasmata (*pl. of* chiasma)
chiasmatic
    c. cistern
    c. defect
    c. lesion
chiasmatic-hypothalamic pilocytic
  astrocytoma
chibih
Chicago area survey
chief
    c. cell
    c. complaint (CC)
child
    abandoned c.
    c. abuse
    abused c.
    c. abuse inventory
    C. Abuse Potential Inventory
    c. abuser
    c. abuse syndrome
    C. and Adolescent Adjustment
      Profile
    c. or adolescent antisocial behavior
    C. and Adolescent Consortium
    C. and Adolescent Fear and
      Anxiety Treatment Program
    adopted c.
    c. of alcoholic (COA)
    c. analysis
    C. Anxiety Scale
    C. Assessment Schedule (CAS)
    C. "At Risk" for Drug Abuse
      Rating Scale
    atypical c.
    autistic c.
    battered c.
    c. behavior
    C. Behavioral Checklist (CBCL)
    c. behavior characteristic (CBC)
    biologic c.
    C. Care Inventory
    c. centered
    conduct-disordered c.
    c. counselor

    c. custody
    c. depression inventory
    c. development inventory
    difficult c.
    easy c.
    exceptional c.
    c. fixation
    gifted c.
    c. group therapy
    c. guidance
    C. Health Self-Concept Scale
    c. language development
    love c.
    c. maltreatment
    mentally retarded c.
    c. molestation
    c. molester
    c. molesting
    neglect of c.
    c. neglect
    neglected c.
    C. Neuropsychological Questionnaire
      (CNQ)
    C. Personality Scale (CPS)
    physical abuse of c.
    c. pornography
    prepubertal c.
    preschool c.
    problem c.
    c. problem tic
    c. prodigy
    c. psychiatrist
    c. psychiatry (CHP, CP)
    c. psychology (CP)
    c. psychosis
    c. raising period
    scatter c.
    sexual abuse of c.
    Six-Hour Retarded C.
    c. support
    unwanted c.
    vulnerable c.
childbirth
    c. amnesia
    c. organic psychosis
    psychosis in c.
child-care
    c.-c. aide
    c.-c. facility
    c.-c. worker
child-guidance
    c.-g. clinic
    c.-g. therapy
childhood
    c. absence epilepsy
    adjustment reaction of c.
    alternating hemiplegia of c. (AHC)
    C. Antecedents Questionnaire
    c. anxiety
    anxiety disorder of c.
    c. aphasia
    c. autism
    C. Autism Rating Scale (CARS)
    avoidant disorder of c.
    behavior disorders of c.

C

childhood *(continued)*
c. benign focal epilepsy
benign partial epilepsy of c.
borderline psychosis of c.
C. Brain Tumor Consortium (CBTC)
C. Brain Tumor Consortium database
c. cross-gender behavior
dementia-aphonia syndrome of c.
developmental experimentation in c.
c. developmental stage
disinhibited-type reactive attachment disorder of infancy or c.
c. disorder
disorder of c.
early c.
emotional disturbance of c.
c. encephalopathy
c. fear
fearfulness disorder of c.
Feeding and Eating Disorders of Infancy or Early C.
c. figure
gender identity disorder of c.
hyperkinetic reaction of c.
hyperkinetic syndrome of c.
identity disorder of c.
introverted disorder of c.
lane of c.
c. motivation
c. moyamoya disease
c. muscular dystrophy
c. myositis
c. onset
oppositional disorder of c.
c. optic glioma
overanxious disorder of c.
Pediatric Examination of Educational Readiness at Middle C.
c. primitive neuroectodermal tumor
problems of c.
c. psychosis
psychosis of c.
reaction of c.
Reactive Attachment Disorder of Infancy or Early C.
relationship problems of c.
schizoid disorder of c.
c. schizophrenia
schizophrenic syndrome of c.
second c.
sensitivity reaction of c.
separation anxiety disorder of c.
shyness disorder of c.
c. social dysfunction
social withdrawal of c.
symbiotic psychosis of c.
c. Tourette syndrome
transient spasm tic disorder of c.
c. trauma
c. trauma memory
withdrawal reaction of c.

childhood-onset
c.-o. dystonia
c.-o. epilepsy
c.-o. insomnia
c.-o. pervasive
c.-o. psychosis
childish emotion
childlike silliness
child-parent fixation
child-penis wish
child-placement counseling
children
Adaptive Behavior Inventory for C. (ABIC)
c. and adults with attention deficit disorder (CHADD)
Aid to Dependent C. (ADC)
Aid to Families with Dependent C. (AFDC)
C. of Alcoholism Screening Test (CAST)
amnesia in c.
Barber Scales of Self-Regard for Preschool C.
Behavior Rating Instrument for Autistic and Other Atypical C.
bereavement in c.
Brief Psychiatric Rating Scale for C. (BPRS-C)
Council for Exceptional C.
Creativity Tests for C. (CTC)
Depression Questionnaire for C.
Diagnostic Interview Schedule for C. (DIS-C, DISC)
Early Development Scale for Preschool C.
Eating Disorder Inventory for C.
emotional maltreatment of c.
Evaluating Movement and Posture Disorganization in Dyspraxic C.
feral c.
gender identity disorder in c.
halfway c.
Hamburg-Wechsler Intelligence Test for C. (HAWIC)
Harter Self-Perception Profile for C.
It Scale for C. (ITSC)
Joint Commission on Mental Health of C. (JCMHC)
Kaufman Assessment Battery for C. (KABC)
latchkey c.
latency-age c.
Life Event Scale C.
Maxfield-Buchholz Social Maturity Scale for Blind Preschool C.
Murphy-Meisgeier Type Indicator for C. (MMTIC)
Neurological Dysfunctions of C.
Personality Inventory for C. (PIC)
Porch Index of Communicative Ability in C. (PICAC)
prepubertal c.

Reitan-Indiana Neuropsychological Test Battery for C.
Reynell-Zinkin Scales: Developmental Scales for Young Handicapped C.
Robert Apperception Test for C. (RATC)
Schedule for Affective Disorders and Schizophrenia for School-Age C. (KIDDIE-SADS, K-SADS)
Schedule for Affective Disorders and Schizophrenia for School Age C.
Schedule for Affective Disorders and Schizophrenia for School-Age C.-Epidemiologic Version (K-SADS-E)
Self-Perception Profile for C.
Short Test for Use with Cerebral Palsy C.
Stanford Hypnotic Clinical Scale and C.
State-Trait Anxiety Inventory for C. (STAIC)
Teacher and Parent Separation Anxiety Rating Scales for Preschool C.
Temperament Assessment Battery for c.
Test of Language Competence for C. (TLC-C)
Test of Learning Accuracy in C. (TLAC)
Test of Listening Accuracy in C. (TLAC)
Token Test for C.
Values Inventory for C. (VIC)
Verbal-Auditory Screen for C. (VASC)
Visual-Auditory Screen for C. (VASC)
Wechsler Intelligence Scale for C. (WISC)
Worry Scale for C.

Children's
C. Academic Intrinsic Motivation Inventory
C. Advil
C. Advil Oral Suspension
C. Affective Rating Scale (CARS)
C. Apperception Test (CAT)
C. Apperception Test-Human (CAT-H)
C. Apperceptive Story-Telling Test (CAST)
C. Articulation Test (CAT)
C. Attention and Adjustment Survey (CAAS)
C. Auditory Verbal Learning Test-2 (CAVLT-2)
C. Coma Score (CCS)
C. Depression Inventory (CDI)
C. Depression Rating Scale-Revised
C. Depression Scale (CDS)

C. Diagnostic Inventory (CDI)
C. Embedded Figures Test (CEFT)
C. Global Assessment Scale (CGAS)
C. Health Study (CHS)
C. Hospital brain spatula
C. Hospital clip
C. Hypnotic Susceptibility Scale
C. Inventory of Self-Esteem (CISE)
C. Language Battery
C. Language Processes
C. Manifest Anxiety Scale (CMAS)
C. Motrin
C. Motrin Oral Suspension
C. Perception of Support Inventory (CPSI)
C. Personality Questionnaire (CPQ)
C. Protective Service (CPS)
C. Psychiatric Rating Scale (CPRS)
C. Self-Concept Scale (CSCS)
C. Silapap
C. Version/Family Environmental Scale
C. Yale-Brown Obsessive Compulsive Scale (CY-BOCS)

chilophagia
chimeric stimulation
chin
    c. jerk
    c. reflex
Chinamania
China syndrome
Chinese Classification of Mental Disorders, Second Edition (CCMD-2)
chionomania
chionophobia
Chippaux-Smirak arch index
chirobrachialgia (*var. of* cheirobrachialgia)
Chirocaine
chirognostic (*var. of* cheirognostic)
chirokinesthesia (*var. of* cheirokinesthesia)
chirospasm (*var. of* cheirospasm)
chisel
    Adson laminectomy c.
    D'Errico lamina c.
    Freer c.
    Hajek c.
chi-square distribution
chlamydia
chloral
    c. derivative
    c. hydrate
chlorambucil
chloramphenicol sodium succinate
chlordiazepoxide
    amitriptyline and c.
    amitriptyline hydrochloride and c.
    c. hydrochloride
chlorhexidine shampoo
chloride
    ammonium c.
    amyl c.
    butyl c.

C

chloride *(continued)*
    calcium c.
    c. channel flux assay
    diphenylaminearsine c.
    edrophonium c.
    ethyl c.
    magnesium c.
    manganese c.
    methylene c.
    potassium c.
    serum c.
    sodium c.
    c. test
    ^{201}Tl c.
chlorimipramine
chlormezanone
chloroethylnitrosourea
    lipophilic c.
chloroform
chlorohydrocarbon dependence
chloroma
Chloromycetin
chloroprocaine
chloroquine
chlorothiazide
    c. and methyldopa
    c. and reserpine
chlorotic anemia
Chlorpazine
chlorphenesin carbamate
chlorpheniramine maleate
chlorphenoxamine
chlorphentermine hydrochloride
chlorproethazine
chlorpromazine hydrochloride
chlorpropamide
chlorthalidone
    atenolol and c.
    clonidine and c.
chlorthiazide
Chlor-Trimeton
chlorzoxazone and acetaminophen
Cho
    choline
chocolate ecstasy
Chodzko reflex
choice
    c. behavior
    drug of c.
    forced c.
    laxative of c. (LOC)
    narcissistic object c.
    object c.
    occupational c.
    c. point
    c. reaction
    vocational c.
choked disk
Cholac
Cholebrine
cholecystitis
cholecystokinin (CCK)
    c. octapeptide (CCK-8)

    c. test
    c. tetrapeptide (CCK-4)
Choledyl
cholelithiasis
cholera
cholera-toxin-catalyzed
    densitometry
choleric
    c. constitutional type
choleromania
cholerophobia
cholestanol storage disease
cholesteatoma
cholesterol
    c. crystal
    c. cyst
    c. embolism
    c. ester storage disease
    c. granuloma
cholesterolosis, cholesterinosis
    cerebrotendinous c.
choline (Cho)
    c. acetyltransferase
    c. magnesium trisalicylate
    c. salicylate
cholinergic
    c. crisis
    c. fiber
    c. neuron
    c. receptor
    c. side effect
    c. synapse
    c. tract
cholinesterase
    c. inhibitor
    c. inhibitory poisoning
Cholografin
Cholovue
Cho:NAA ratio
chondritis
    nasal c.
chondroblastoma
chondrocalcinosis
chondrodystrophic
    myotonia c.
    c. myotonia
chondrodystrophy
chondrohypoplasia
chondroitin sulfate proteoglycan
chondroma
    juxtacortical c.
chondromatous tumor
chondromyxoid fibroma
chondroosteodystrophy
chondrosarcoma
choo-choo phenomenon
choose
    freedom to c.
Chooz
CHOP frame
Chopper-Dixon hybrid imaging
chorda
    c. magna
    c. tympani
chordae willisii

chord length
chordoma
    clival c.
chordotomy
chorea
    acute c.
    automatic c.
    Bergeron c.
    chronic progressive c.
    c. cordis
    dancing c.
    degenerative c.
    c. dimidiata
    Dubini c.
    electric c.
    c. festinans
    fibrillary c.
    c. gravidarum
    habit c.
    hemilateral c.
    Henoch c.
    hereditary nonprogressive c.
    Huntington c. (HC)
    hysterical c.
    c. immune
    c. insaniens
    juvenile c.
    kinesigenic c.
    laryngeal c.
    c. major
    malleatory c.
    methodical c.
    mimetic c.
    c. minor
    c. mollis
    Morvan c.
    c. nutans
    oral contraceptive-induced c.
    paralytic c.
    phenytoin-induced c.
    posthemiplegic c.
    prehemiplegic c.
    procursive c.
    rheumatic c.
    rhythmic c.
    c. rotatoria
    c. sailatoria
    saltatory c.
    Schrötter c.
    senile c.
    Sydenham c.
    tetanoid c.
    thyrotoxicosis-induced c.
    unilateral c.
chorea-acanthocytosis
choreal
choreathetosis
choreic
    c. abasia
    c. ataxia
    c. dyskinesia
    c. insanity
    c. movement
    c. movement disorder
    c. syndrome

choreicus
    status c.
choreiform
    c. disorder
    c. movement
    c. syndrome
choreoacanthocytosis
choreoathetoid
    c. cerebral palsy
    c. movement
choreoathetosis
    dystonic c.
    familial paroxysmal c.
    kinesigenic c.
    paroxysmal kinesigenic c.
    phenytoin-induced c.
    psychotic c.
    thyrotoxicosis-induced c.
choreoathetotic movement
choreoid
choreomania
choreophrasia
choriocarcinoma
    pineal regional c.
choriomeningitis
    benign lymphocytic c.
    lymphocytic c.
chorionic gonadotropin
chorioretinitis
choristoma
    intrasellar
      neuroadenohyphophyseal c.
    c. nest
choroid
    c. detachment
    c. fissure
    c. glomus
    c. plexus
    c. plexus ablation
    c. plexus adenoma
    c. plexus of fourth ventricle
    c. plexus of lateral ventricle
    c. plexus papilloma
    c. plexus of third ventricle
    c. skein
    c. tela of fourth ventricle
    c. tela of third ventricle
    c. vein
choroidal
    c. blush
    lateral posterior c. (LPCh)
    medial posterior c. (MPCh)
    c. metastasis
    c. pericallosal artery
choroidal-hippocampal fissure complex
choroidectomy
choroidopathy
Chotzen syndrome
CHP
    child psychiatry
CHPM
    chronic hypertrophic pachymeningitis
chrematomania
chrematophobia
Christensen-Krabbe disease

C

Christian belief
Christmas disease
Christoferson disk bony implant
chroma
chromaffin
    c. cell transplant
    c. tumor
chromaffinoma
chromaffinopathy
chromatic
    c. audition
    c. color
    c. contrast
    c. dimming
    c. flicker
    c. granule
    c. response
    c. scale
chromaticity
chromatid
chromatin
    sex c.
chromatinolysis
chromatography
chromatolysis
    central c.
    retrograde c.
    transsynaptic c.
chromatolytic
chromatophobia, chromophobia
chromatopsia
chromesthesia
chromic
    3-0 c.
chromolysis
chromophil
    c. adenoma
    c. granule
    c. substance
chromophobia (*var. of* chromatophobia)
chromophobic adenoma
chromosomal
    c. aberration
    c. abnormality
    c. loci
    c. translocation
chromosome
    c. 4
    accessory c.
    acrocentric c.
    fragile X c.
    linear c.
    c. (9_p) monosomy
    c. number
    ring c.
    sex c.
    c. study
    c. 13 trisomy
    c. 18 trisomy
    c. 21 trisomy
    c. 21-trisomy syndrome
    c. walking
    X c.
    Y c.
chromotherapy

chromotopsia
chromotropic
chronaxia, chronaxy
chronic
    c. acquired hepatic failure
    Adjustment Disorder, C.
    c. African sleeping sickness
    c. alcohol abuse
    c. alcoholic brain syndrome (CABS)
    c. alcoholic delirium
    c. alcoholic mania
    c. alcoholism
    c. amnesia
    c. angle-closure glaucoma
    c. anorexia nervosa
    c. anterior poliomyelitis
    c. anxiety
    c. basal meningitis with cranial nerve paralysis
    c. brain syndrome (CBS)
    c. communicating hydrocephalus
    c. deficit state
    c. delusional state
    c. dementia
    c. depression
    c. disability
    C. Disease Score
    c. drinker
    c. drunkenness
    c. factitious illness
    c. familial polyneuritis
    c. fatigability
    c. fatigue
    c. fatigue and immune dysfunction syndrome (CFIDS)
    c. fatigue syndrome (CFS)
    c. feelings of emptiness
    c. habit
    c. headache
    c. hepatic failure peripheral neuropathy
    c. hypertrophic pachymeningitis (CHPM)
    c. hypomanic personality
    c. inflammatory demyelinating polyneuropathy (CIDPN)
    c. inflammatory demyelinating polyradiculopathy (CIDP)
    c. inflammatory demyelinating sensorimotor neuropathy
    c. inflammatory demyelinative neuropathy
    c. inflammatory polyradiculoneuropathy (CIP)
    c. insomnia
    c. intoxication
    c. intractable pain
    c. lead poisoning
    c. melancholia
    c. migrainous neuralgia
    c. motor tic
    c. occlusion
    pain disorder, c.

c. paranoid schizophrenic reaction (CPSR)
c. paraparesis
c. paroxysmal hemicrania
c. partial epilepsy
c. phase of stable sleep difficulty
c. posttraumatic neurosis
c. progressive chorea
c. progressive myelopathy
c. psychosis
c. relapsing polyneuropathy
c. schizophrenia
c. sleep disturbance
c. spasm tic
c. spinal epidural infection
c. spinal intradural infection
c. stress
c. stress reaction
c. subcortical encephalitis
c. thrombus
c. tissue damage
c. toxic effect
c. traumatic encephalopathy
c. trypanosomiasis
c. undifferentiated
c. undifferentiated schizophrenia
c. undifferentiated schizophrenic reaction
c. vertigo
chronica
encephalitis subcorticalis c.
chronically
c. disabling pattern
c. mentally ill (CMI)
chronicity
Chronicle Career Quest (CCQ)
chronobiological
c. disorder
c. disturbance
chronobiology
chronognosis
chronologic age
chronological
c. drinking record
c. order
c. relationship
chronology
chronometry
mental c.
chronophobia
chronotaraxis
Chronulac
CHS
Children's Health Study
chuan
chuck
T-handle Jacob c.
chum period
Churg-Strauss
C.-S. syndrome
C.-S. vasculitis
Chvostek sign
chylous leakage
Chymodiactin
chymopapain

CI
coefficient of intelligence
Cibacalcin Injection
Cibalith
Cibalith-S
CIBI
continuous intrathecal baclofen infusion
cibi
fastidium c.
cibophobia
CIC
crisis intervention clinic
cicatrices (*pl. of* cicatrix)
cicatricial alopecia
cicatrisata
alopecia c.
cicatrix, pl. cicatrices
brain c.
meningocerebral c.
CICI
Hymovich Chronicity Impact and Coping Instrument
NL CICI
normal libido, coitus, and climax
CIDP
chronic inflammatory demyelinating polyradiculopathy
CIDPN
chronic inflammatory demyelinating polyneuropathy
CIE
countercurrent immunoelectrophoresis
CIES
Correctional Institutions Environment Scale
CII
Carnegie Interest Inventory
cilazapril
cilia (*pl. of* cilium)
ciliary
c. ganglion
c. migraine
c. migraine headache
c. neuralgia
c. neurotrophic factor (CNTF)
ciliochoroid detachment
ciliospinal
c. center
c. reflex
ciliotomy
cilium, pl. cilia
cilostazol
cimetidine
CIMS
Conflict in Marriage Scale
cinanesthesia
cinchonism
cinclisis
cincture sensation
Cinderella
C. complex
C. syndrome
cinefluorography
cinefluoroscopy
cineplasty

C

cineradiography
cinerea
cinereae
    nucleus alae c.
cinereal
cinereum
    tuber c.
cineritious
cineroentgenography
cinesalgia
cineseismography
cingula (*pl. of* cingulum)
cingulate
    anterior c.
    c. convolution
    c. cortex
    c. epilepsy
    c. gyrus
    c. gyrus dysgenesis
    c. gyrus eversion
    c. herniation
    c. operation
    retrosplenial c.
    c. sulcus
cingulectomy
cinguli (*gen. of* cingulum)
cingulothalamic artery
cingulotomy
    rostral c.
    stereotactic c.
cingulum, gen. **cinguli,** pl. **cingula**
    c. bundle
cinnamedrine hydrochloride
cinnarizine
cinoxacin
cintriamide
CIP
    chronic inflammatory
      polyradiculoneuropathy
    comprehensive identification process
    critical illness polyneuropathy
ciprofloxacin
circa
circadian
    c. marker
    c. phase of sleep
    c. realignment
    c. rhythm
    c. rhythm sleep disorder
    c. rhythm sleep disorder, delayed
      sleep phase
    c. rhythm sleep disorder, jet lag
    c. rhythm sleep disorder, shift
      work
    c. system
circannual
    c. cycle
    c. rhythm
circaseptan rhythm
circle
    arterial c. of cerebrum
    Haller c.
    Ridley c.
    vascular c. of optic nerve
    vicious c.

    c. of Willis
    c. of Willis aneurysm
    Zinn vascular c.
circuit
    basal ganglia-thalamocortical
      motor c.
    convergence c.
    cortical-striatal-pallidal-thalamic
      neural c.
    divergence c.
    frontostriatal-pallidalo-thalamic c.
    frontothalamic c.
    lateral orbitofrontal c.
    limbic c.
    neuronal c.
    Papez c.
    reverberating c.
    worry c.
circuitry
    cortical language c.
circular
    c. dementia
    c. fiber
    c. insanity
    c. laminar hook with offset top
    c. nystagmus
    c. plasmid
    c. psychosis
    c. reaction
    c. sinus
    c. sulcus of Reil
    c. thinking
circular-pattern response
circulation
    cerebral c.
    collateral c.
    macro-eCVR-FV c.
    micro-eCVR-FV c.
    thalamic c.
circulatory psychosis
circulus, gen. and pl. **circuli**
    c. arteriosus cerebri
    c. arteriosus halleri
    c. vasculosus nervi optici
    c. venosus halleri
    c. venosus ridleyi
circumambulate
circumcision
    female c.
circumferentially aortofemoral graft
circumfix morpheme
circumflex
circumgemmal
circumscribed
    c. amnesia
    c. cerebral atrophy
    c. craniomalacia
    c. delusion
    c. edema
    c. lesion
    c. pyocephalus
circumscribing incision
circumscripta
    alopecia c.
    osteoporosis c.

circumscription
monosymptomatic c.
circumspect
circumstance
altered life c.
extenuating c.
inappropriate c.
other specified family c.
real-life c.
circumstantial
c. evidence
c. migraine
c. migraine headache
c. speech
c. thought process
circumventricular organ
CIRP
cooperative institutional research program
cirrhosis
alcoholic c. (AC)
Laennec c.
liver c.
syphilitic c.
toxic c.
cirrhotic liver
cirsoid aneurysm
CIS
clinically isolated syndrome
cisapride
CISE
Children's Inventory of Self-Esteem
CISI
Cattell Infant Scale for Intelligence
Cattell Infant Scale Inventory
CISMD
California Infant Scale for Motor
Development
cis-parinaric acid
cisplatin
cis-platinum
9-cis retinoic acid receptor (RXR)
CISS
Campbell Interest and Skill Survey
cissa
cistern
ambient c.
arachnoiditis of opticochiasmatic c.
cerebellomedullary c.
cerebellopontine angle c.
c. of chiasm
chiasmatic c.
crural c.
c. effacement
effacement of c.
c. of great vein of cerebrum
insular c.
interpeduncular c.
c. of lateral fossa of cerebrum
mesencephalic c.
c. of nuclear envelope
obliterated basal c.
opticochiasmatic c.
parasellar c.
perimesencephalic c.
pontine c.

prepontine c.
c. puncture
quadrigeminal c.
subarachnoidal c.
suprasellar c.
c. sylvii
trigeminal c.
cisterna, gen. and pl. **cisternae**
c. ambiens
c. basalis
c. caryothecae
c. cerebellomedullaris
c. chiasmatis
c. cruralis
c. fossae lateralis cerebri
c. fossae sylvii
c. intercruralis profunda
c. interpeduncularis
c. lumbar
c. magna
c. magna catheter
c. pontis
cisternae subarachnoideales
c. sulci lateralis
c. superioris
c. venae magnae
c. venae magnae cerebri
cisternal
c. clot
c. puncture
cisternogram
indium c.
isotope c.
radioisotope c.
cisternography
cerebellopontine c.
computed tomographic c.
isotope c.
isotopic c.
perioperative c.
radioisotope c.
radionuclide c.
cisvestism, cisvestitism
citalopram HBr
Citanest
C. Forte
C. Plain
Citelli
C. angle
C. syndrome
citicoline sodium
citolopram
Citracal
citrate
calcium c.
ethoheptazine c.
fentanyl c.
orphenadrine c.
phenyltoloxamine c.
potassium acetate, potassium
bicarbonate, and potassium c.
potassium bicarbonate, potassium
chloride, and potassium c.
sildenafil c.
citric acid cycle

C

citrullinemia
citta, cittosis
city and state test
civil
  c. commitment
  c. disobedience
  c. marriage
  c. rights
civilian-catastrophe reaction
Civilian Health and Medical Program
  of the Uniformed Service
  (CHAMPUS)
CIVRA
  continuous intravenous regional
    anesthesia
CJD
  Creutzfeldt-Jakob disease
CJ disease
c-jun gene
cladosporiosis
  cerebral c.
cladribine
claims review
clairaudience
clairsentience
clairvoyance
clairvoyant dream
clammy skin
clamp
  Bigelow calvarium c.
  Calman carotid c.
  CCA c.
  Crile c.
  Crutchfield carotid artery c.
  Dandy c.
  Diethrich bulldog c.
  Duvol lung c.
  Gardner neurosurgical skull c.
  Halifax interlaminar c.
  head c.
  interlaminar c.
  Jacobson-Potts vascular c.
  Javid carotid c.
  Kartchner carotid artery c.
  Kindt carotid c.
  Kocher c.
  Kocher-Lovelace c.
  Mayfield head c.
  Mayfield neurosurgical skill c.
  mosquito c.
  Olivecrona aneurysm c.
  Péan c.
  Poppen-Blalock carotid c.
  Roosen c.
  Salibi carotid artery c.
  Schnidt c.
  Schwartz temporary intracranial
    artery c.
  Selverstone c.
  Sugita head c.
  suture c.
  Thompson carotid c.
  three-point skull c.
  Thumb-Saver introducer c.
  Yasargil carotid c.

clamping mechanism
clang
  c. association
  c. association characteristic
Clarke
  C. column
  C. nucleus
  C. Reading Self-Assessment Survey
  C. stereotactic instrument
Clark electrode
Clarus spinescope
clash
  paradigm c.
clasp-knife
  c.-k. effect
  c.-k. phenomenon
  c.-k. response
  c.-k. rigidity
  c.-k. spasticity
clasp knife
class
  closed c.
  diagnostic c.
  c. discrimination
  c. inclusion
  c. interval
  c. limit
  Processing Word C.
  pyranocarboxylic acid c.
  skip c.
  c. word
CLASSI
  Cornell Learning and Study Skills
    Inventory
classic
  c. apraxia
  c. migraine
classical
  c. analysis
  c. conditioning
  c. depression
  c. migraine headache
  c. paranoia
  c. psychoanalytical theory
classification
  American Spinal Cord Injury
    Association c.
  Antoni-A neurinoma c.
  Brodmann c.
  categorical c.
  Daumas-Duport c.
  c. of depression
  Engel postoperative seizure c.
  Hannover c.
  Hunt-Hess aneurysm c.
  Hunt-Hess neurological c.
  Hunt and Kosnik c.
  International Working
    Formulation c.
  Kernohan system of glioma c.
  Kiel c.
  Kistler subarachnoid hemorrhage c.
  LeFort c.
  Melmon and Rosen c.
  c. method

modified Fischer c.
multiaxial c.
neo-kraepelian c.
Nordstadt c.
Ratliff avascular necrosis c.
Russell-Rubinstein cerebrovascular
    malformation c.
Spetzler-Martin c.
Sundt carotid ulceration c.
c. test
WHO astrocytoma c.
classified
Mental Disorders Due to a
    General Medical Condition Not
    Elsewhere C.
classroom
C. Atmosphere Questionnaire
    (CAQ)
C. Environmental Scale (CES)
C. Environment Index
Claude
C. hyperkinesis sign
C. syndrome
claudication
cerebral c.
cerebral intermittent c.
jaw c.
mental c.
neurogenic c.
visual c.
clausa
rhinolalia c.
clauses
disturbance between c.
disturbance within c.
claustra (*pl. of* claustrum)
claustral
c. complex
c. layer
claustrophilia
claustrophobic
claustrum, pl. **claustra**
clava
claval
clavulanic acid
clavus clinical grouping
clawed pedicle hook
clawhand deformity
clawing attack
Claybury Selection Battery
clay eating
clay-modeling
c.-m. equipment
c.-m. therapy
clay-shoveler fracture
CLCS
Comprehensive Level of Consciousness
    Scale
CLD
central language disorder
clear
c. sensorium
c. twilight state
clear-cut attachment
clearly demarcated relationship

cleft
atypical c.
pharyngeal c.
Schmidt-Lanterman c.'s
c. spine
synaptic c.
cleft-palate speech
cleidocranial dysostosis
clenching
fist c.
Cleocin
CLEP
College-Level Examination Program
General Examination
cleptomania
cleptophobia
Clerambault
C. erotomania
C. erotomania syndrome
Clerambault-Kandinsky complex
clerical
c. perception (Q)
c. response
clericorum
dysphonia c.
clerk
unit c.
ward c.
Clevenger fissure
clever
cleverness factor (C-factor)
CLI
Campbell Leadership Index
click stimulation
clidinium bromide
client-centered
c.-c. psychotherapy
c.-c. therapy
**Clifton Assessment Procedures for the
Elderly (CAPE)**
climacteric, climacterium
female c.
c. insanity
male c.
c. melancholia
c. neurosis
c. paranoid psychosis
c. paranoid reaction
c. paranoid state
c. paraphrenia
c. psychoneurosis
climate
emotional c.
group c.
climax
normal libido, coitus, and c. (NL
    CICI, NLC&C)
sexual c.
climbing fiber
clindamycin
clinging
c. behavior
c. dependency
clinic
affective disorders c. (ADC)

C

clinic *(continued)*
    child-guidance c.
    crisis intervention c. (CIC)
    mental health c. (MHC)
    mental-hygiene c.
    pain c.
    c. patient population
    Tavistock C.

clinical
    C. Adaptive Test/Clinical Linguistic Auditory Milestone Scale (CAT/CLAMS)
    c. analysis
    C. Analysis Questionnaire (CAQ)
    C. Analysis Questionnaire (Short Form)
    c. appraisal of psychosocial problems (CAPP)
    c. behavior
    c. care
    c. chemistry
    c. counseling
    c. course
    c. dementia
    C. Dementia Rating (CDR)
    C. Dementia Rating Scale
    c. depression
    c. diagnosis
    c. electromagnetic flowmeter
    c. equivalent
    c. evaluation
    C. Evaluation of Language Fundamentals-Revised
    c. experience
    c. feature
    c. finding
    C. Global Impression of Change (CGIC)
    C. Global Impressions (CGI)
    C. Global Impressions Scale
    C. Global Improvement (CGI)
    C. Global Improvement Scale
    c. immunology
    c. impression
    c. interview
    c. inventory
    c. judgment
    c. laboratory
    c. management
    c. medicine
    c. performance score (CPS)
    c. picture
    c. poverty
    c. poverty syndrome
    c. presentation
    c. profile
    c. psychiatry
    c. psychobiology
    c. psychologist
    c. psychology
    c. psychopharmacology
    C. Rating Scale (CRS)
    c. scale
    c. setting

    c. significance criterion
    c. sociology
    c. status
    c. study
    C. Support System Battery
    c. teaching
    c. training
    c. trial

clinical-facilitated intervention
clinically
    c. isolated syndrome (CIS)
    c. significant
    c. significant anxiety
    c. significant distress
    c. significant impairment

clinician
    C. Rated Anxiety Scale (CRAS)
    C. Rated Overall Life Impairment Scale

Clinician-Administered PTSD Scale
Clinician's Global Rating Scale (CGRS)
clinicopathological
clinicopathology
Clinitron air bed
clinodactyly
clinoid
    anterior c.
    c. process

clinoidal
    c. aneurysm
    c. meningioma
    c. segment (ClinSeg)

clinoidectomy
    anterior extradural c.
    extradural c.

clinomania
clinophobia
Clinoril
ClinSeg
    clinoidal segment

clip
    Acland c.
    Adson scalp c.
    aneurysm c.
    angled aneurysm c.
    c. application
    c. applier
    bayonet aneurysm c.
    Beimer-Clip aneurysm c.
    booster c.
    Braun-Yasargil right-angle c.
    Children's Hospital c.
    Codman aneurysm c.
    Cologne pattern scalp c.
    crankshaft c.
    cross-legged c.
    Delrin plastic scalp c.
    distal basilar temporary c.
    Drake fenestrated c.
    Drake-Kees c.
    Elgiloy c.
    fenestrated aneurysm c.
    ferromagnetic intracerebral aneurysm c.
    c. force meter

c. graft
heavy-duty straight c.
Heifetz c.
Heifetz-Weck c.
Housepian aneurysm c.
Ingraham-Fowler tantalum c.
Iwabuchi c.
Kerr c.
Leroy-Raney scalp c.
Ligaclip c.
c. ligation of aneurysm
L-shaped aneurysm c.
Mayfield aneurysm c.
McFadden c.
McFadden-Kees c.
McKenzie hemostasis c.
McKenzie silver c.
Michel scalp c.
microvascular c.
mini-Sugita c.
nonferromagnetic c.
Olivecrona c.
c. placement
plastic scalp c.
primary c.
Raney scalp c.
right-angle booster c.
scalp c.
Schwartz aneurysm c.
Scoville c.
Slimline c.
straight aneurysm c.
Sugita-Ikakogyo c.
Sugita side-curved bayonet c.
Sugita temporary straight c.
Sundt booster c.
Sundt-Kees encircling patch c.
Sundt-Kees graft c.
Sundt-Kees Slimline c.
Sundt straddling c.
temporary c.
titanium aneurysm c.
towel c.
Vari-Angle aneurysm c.
Weck c.
Yasargil-Aesculap spring c.
Yasargil vessel c.
Zimmer c.
clip-induced stricture
clipped speech
clipping
aneurysm c.
microsurgical neck c.
peak c.
proximal c.
shank c.
clip-reinforced cotton sling
clip-type electrode
clithrophobia
clitoral hood
clitoridectomy
clitoridis
erector c.
glans c.
clitoris

clitorism
clitoromania
clival
c. chordoma
c. meningioma
c. mucocele
clivus, pl. **clivi**
Blumenbach c.
c. canal line
lower c.
c. meningioma
mucopyocele of the c.
cloaca
cloacal theory
clobazam
clock
biologic c.
c. face test
clodanolene
Clodius dissector
clofazimine
clomethiazole
clominorex
clomipramine (CMI)
clonazepam
clone
clonic
c. block
c. cerebral palsy
c. convulsion
generalized tonic c. (GTC)
c. movement
c. seizure
c. spasm
clonicity
clonicotonic seizure
clonic-tonic-clonic seizure
clonidine
c. and chlorthalidone
c. hydrochloride
topical c.
clonism
clonogenic cell assay
clonospasm
clonus
ankle c.
persistent c.
subsultus c.
sustained ankle c.
toe c.
unsustained c.
wrist c.
cloperidone
clophenoxate
clopidogrel bisulfate
clopimozide
Clopixol depot
clorazepam
clorazepate dipotassium
clorazepic acid
clordiazepoxide
clorgyline
clorhexidine gluconate
Clorpactin

C

close
    C. Persons Questionnaire
    c. sightedness
    c. watch restriction
closed
    c. anesthesia
    c. angiography
    c. awareness
    c. class
    c. Cotrel-Dubousset hook
    c. disk space infection
    c. galea
    c. group
    c. head injury (CHI)
    c. head trauma
    c. horizon
    c. juncture
    c. place
    c. skull fracture
    c. transverse process TSRH hook
closed-chain functional assessment
closed-circuit television (CCTV)
closed-ended question
closed-loop feedback system
closet
    c. alcoholic
    c. drinker
    c. homosexual
Clostridium
    C. botulinum
    C. difficile
    C. tetani
closure
    approximating c.
    auditory c.
    law of c.
    neural tube c.
    perceptual c.
    premature c.
    c. pressure
    c. principle
    c. process
    scalp c.
    visual c.
    watertight c.
clot
    cisternal c.
clothes
    plucking at c.
    pulling of c.
clothiapine
clothixamide maleate
clotiazepam
clotrimazole
clotting disorder
clouded
    c. sensorium
    c. state
    c. state epilepsy
clouding of consciousness
clouds
    up in the c.
cloudy sensorium

cloverleaf
    c. skull
    c. skull syndrome
Cloward
    C. back fusion
    C. blade retractor
    C. bone graft impactor
    C. brain retractor
    C. cautery hook
    C. cervical arthrodesis
    C. cervical disk approach
    C. cervical dislocation reducer
    C. cervical retractor
    C. cervical vertebra spreader
    C. disk rongeur
    C. double hinge cervical retractor handle
    C. dural hook
    C. dural retractor
    C. elevator
    C. instrument
    C. lamina spreader
    C. lumbar lamina retractor
    C. nerve root retractor
    C. operation
    C. procedure
    C. skin retractor
    C. small cervical retractor
    C. spinal fusion osteotome
    C. surgical saddle
    C. technique
    C. tissue retractor
Cloward-Cone ring curette
Cloward-Cushing vein retractor
Cloward-English laminectomy rongeur
Cloward-Hoen laminectomy retractor
cloxacillin
cloxazolam
clozapine
clozapine-induced agranulocytosis
Clozaril National Registry
CLQ
    cognitive laterality quotient
CLS
    confused language syndrome
CLSM
    confocal laser scanning
clucking
    tongue c.
clumsiness syndrome
clumsy gesture
cluneal nerve
Clunis inquiry forensic psychiatry
cluster
    c. analysis
    anxious-fearful c.
    c. A personality disorder
    c. approach
    c. B personality disorder
    c. breathing
    c. characteristics in personality disorder
    c. C personality disorder
    dramatic-emotional c.
    c. headache

inner battery c.
c. marriage
c. migraine
odd-eccentric c.
c. reduction
situation c.
c. of situations
suicide c.
c. suicides
symptom c.
clustering
c. criterion
semantic c.
Clyde Mood Scale (CMS)
Clymer-Barrett Readiness Test
Clysodrast
Clytemnestra complex
CMA
Conflict Management Appraisal
CMAP
compound muscle action potential
CMAP amplitude
CMAP on electromyogram
CMAS
Children's Manifest Anxiety Scale
CMD
cerebromacular degeneration
CME
continuing medical education
CMHC
community mental health center
CMHS
Center for Mental Health Services
CMI
Career Maturity Inventory
chronically mentally ill
clomipramine
CMII
College Major Interest Inventory
CMMS
Columbia Mental Maturity Scale
CMN
cranial motor nuclei
CMP
complexity of mental process
CMRE
California Marriage Readiness Evaluation
CMS
Clyde Mood Scale
Conflict Management Survey
CMS AccuProbe 450 system
CMT
Concept Mastery Test
CMV
cytomegalovirus
CMV encephalitis
CMV meningitis
CNAP
compound nerve action potential
CNAP on electromyogram
cnidophobia
CNP
C-type natriuretic peptide
CNQ
Child Neuropsychological Questionnaire

CNR
contrast-to-noise ratio
CNS
central nervous system
CNS abnormality
CNS depressant
CNS disease group
granulomatous angiitis of the CNS
CNS insult
isolated angiitis of the CNS (IAC)
CNS lymphoma
primary angiitis of the CNS
CNS stimulant
CNS syphilis
CNS trauma
CNS vasculature
CNT
could not test
CNTF
ciliary neurotrophic factor
CNV
conative negative variation
contingent negative variation
CO
carbon monoxide
CO Dox
COA
child of alcoholic
COAB
Computer Operator Aptitude Battery
coaddiction
coagulation
bipolar c.
c. cascade
c. disorder
disseminated intravascular c. (DIC)
low current monopolar c.
monopolar c.
coagulative necrosis
coagulator
ASSI c.
bipolar c.
Concept bipolar c.
Fukushima monopolar malleable c.
Malis CMC-II bipolar c.
Malis solid state c.
Polar-Mate c.
solid state c.
coagulopathy
consumptive c.
coagulum
cryoprecipitate c.
coalesce
coalescence
coalition
confusingly fluid c.
C. for the Family (CF)
coaptation
direct end-to-end c.
coarcted personality
coarctation
aortic c.
coarse
c. nystagmus
c. tremor

C

coarticulation
    anticipatory c.
    backward c.
coast memory
coating of aneurysm
Coats disease
coaxial cable
cobalamin deficiency
cobalt
    samarium c.
    c. samarium magnet
cobalt-60
    collimated c.
Cobb
    C. method of measuring kyphosis
    C. periosteal elevator
    C. syndrome
    C. technique
cobblestone degeneration
coca
    Erythroxylum c.
    mama c.
cocaethylene assay
cocaine
    c. abuse
    c. addiction
    adulteration of c.
    C. Anonymous
    c. binge
    c. blues
    c. and cannabis use
    chemically whitening c.
    crack diluted with c.
    c. delusion
    c. delusional disorder
    c. dependence
    fake c.
    flavored c.
    c. freebase
    c. habituation
    heroin and c.
    c. hydrochloride
    c. influence
    injectable c.
    c. intoxication
    c. intoxication delirium
    c. intoxication-related disorder
    c. intoxication, with perceptual
      disturbance
    methcathinone and c.
    processed c.
    c. psychosis
    rock c.
    c. use disorder
    c. value
    c. withdrawal
cocaine,
    c. heroin and lysergic acid
      diethylamide
    c. heroin and morphine
cocaine-heroin combination
cocaine-induced
    c.-i. anxiety
    c.-i. choreoathetoid movements
    c.-i. disorder
    c.-i. psychotic disorder with
      delusions
    c.-i. psychotic disorder with
      hallucinations
    c.-i. sexual dysfunction
**cocaine-related disorder, not otherwise
  specified**
cocainism
cocainization
cocainize
cocainomania
CocAnon
coccidioidal
    c. complement fixation of
      cerebrospinal fluid
    c. meningitis
Coccidioides
    C immitis
    C infection
coccidioidomycosis
coccygeal
    c. ganglion
    c. part of spinal cord
coccygodynia
coccyx
    posterior surgical exposure of
      sacrum and c.
cochlea, pl. cochleae
    apical turn of the c.
    aqueductus c.
    membranous c.
cochlear
    c. aplasia
    c. aqueduct
    c. duct
    c. hair cell
    c. implant
    c. microphonic potential
    c. nerve
    c. nuclei
    c. part of vestibulocochlear nerve
    c. recess
    c. response time
    c. root of vestibulocochlear nerve
    c. spiral
    c. vascular supply
cochlearis
    nervus c.
cochleogram
cochleo-orbicular reflex
cochleopalpebral reflex
cochleopupillary reflex
cochleosacculotomy
cochleostapedial reflex
cochornis
Cochran-Mantel-Haenszel Test
cockalorum
Cockayne syndrome
cocktail
    lytic c.
    c. party paradigm
    Viñuela c.
coconsciousness
co-conscious personality
coconut sound

CODA
    Codependents Anonymous
coddle
code
    capacity c.
    c. capacity
    c. of ethics
    genetic c.
    imagery c.
    Model Penal C.
    moral c.
    penal c.
    professional c.
    c. test
    V c.
    Z c.
codeine
    acetaminophen and c.
    aspirin and c.
    butalbital compound and c.
    Capital and C.
    carisoprodol, aspirin, and c.
    cough preparations with c.
    c. dependence
    Empirin with c.
    Empracet with c.
    Fiorinal with c.
    glutethimide with c.
    Phenaphen with c.
    terpin hydrate with c.
    Tylenol with c.
codependency disorder
codependent personality
Codependents Anonymous (CODA)
Codman
    C. aneurysm clip
    C. anterior cervical plate system
    C. cranioblade
    C. drill
    C. neurological headrest system
    C. scissors
    C. slit valve
    C. ventricular silicone catheter
Codman-Harper laminectomy rongeur
Codman-Kerrison laminectomy rongeur
Codman-Leksell laminectomy rongeur
Codman-Medos programmable valve
Codman-Schlesinger
    C.-S. cervical laminectomy rongeur
    C.-S. laminectomy rongeur
codominance
Codoxy
coefficient
    alienation c.
    alternate forms reliability c.
    association c.
    comparable forms reliability c.
    concordance c.
    correlation c.
    c. of correlation
    equivalence c.
    c. of inbreeding
    c. of intelligence (CI)
    kappa c.
    odd-even method reliability c.

reliability c.
Spearman correlation c.
split half reliability c.
test-retest reliability c.
c. of variation (CV)
coenesthesia (*var. of* cenesthesia)
coerce
coercion
    sexual c.
coercive
    c. behavior
    c. communication
    c. persuasion
    c. philosophy
    c. treatment
coeundi
    impotentia c.
coeur
    cri de c.
coexcitation
coexistence
    c. of neurotransmitter
    peaceful c.
coexistent culture
coexisting disorder
COG
    Cognitive Observation Guide
Cogan
    C. lid twitch
    C. syndrome
cogent
    C. microillumination technology
Cogentin
COGENTLIGHT
Co-Gesic
cogitate
cognate confusion
Cognex
cognition
    being c.
    dysfunctional c.
    empiric c.
    impaired c.
    neuro c.
    paranormal c.
    Rust Inventory of Schizotypal C.
    theory of c.
    visuospatial constructive c.
cognitive
    C. Abilities Test (CAT)
    c. ability
    c. approaches to dreaming and
        repression
    c. avoidance
    c. behavior
    C. Behavior Rating Scales
    c. behavior therapy (CBT)
    c. conditioning
    c. control
    C. Control Battery
    c. decrement
    c. defect
    c. deficit
    c. derailment
    c. development

cognitive *(continued)*
    c. development stage
    c. development stages (Period I–IV)
    C. Diagnostic Battery
    c. disability
    c. disorder
    c. disorganization
    c. disruption
    c. dissonance
    c. dissonance theory
    c. distancing
    c. distortion
    c. disturbance
    c. dysfunction
    c. element
    c. factor
    C. Failures Questionnaire (CFQ)
    c. flexibility
    c. function
    c. growth
    c. impairment
    c. impairment level
    c. laterality quotient (CLQ)
    c. learning theory
    c. loss
    c. map
    c. mapping
    c. maturation
    c. mediation
    c. model
    c. need
    c. nonability
    C. Observation Guide (COG)
    c. personality trait
    c. process
    c. psychology
    c. psychotherapy
    c. rehabilitation
    c. rehearsal
    c. remediation
    c. remediation therapy
    c. research orientation
    c. reserve
    c. restitution
    c. restructuring
    c. schema
    c. science
    c. self-hypnosis training
    c. self-reinforcement
    C. Skills Assessment (CSA)
    C. Skills Assessment Battery
    c. slippage
    c. slowing
    c. stimulation
    c. strategy
    c. structure
    c. style
    c. task
    c. theory of depression
    c. theory of learning
    c. therapy
    c. triad
    c. variable

cognitive/attitudinal factor
cognitive-awareness level
cognitive-behavioral
    c.-b. intervention
    c.-b. psychotherapy
    c.-b. technique
    c.-b. treatment
cognitive-linguistic treatment
cognitive-physiological therapy
cognitivist
cognizant
cogwheel
    c. phenomenon
    c. rigidity
cohabitant
Cohen
    C. syndrome
    C. view of depressive disorder
coherence
    phase c.
coherent stream of thought
cohesion
    figural c.
    group c.
    law of c.
cohesive
    c. device
    c. family
    c. image
cohesiveness
    Inventory of Individually Perceived Group C.
    level of c.
    c. level
cohort
    c. effect
    c. study
COIB
    Crowley Occupational Interests Blank
coil
    body c.
    crossed c.
    detachable c.
    Dixon radiofrequency c.
    electrodetachable platinum c.
    c. embolization
    endovascular c.
    Golay gradient c.
    gradient c.
    Guglielmi detachable c. (GDC)
    head c.
    Helmholtz c.
    Hilal c.
    induction c.
    Ivalon wire c.
    occlusion c.
    phased-array c.
    platinum c.
    c. precision
    radiofrequency c.
    receiver c.
    RF c.
    saddle c.
    shim c.
    solenoid c.

surface c.
three axis gradient c.
thrombogenic c.
transverse gradient c.
z-gradient c.
coiled spring
coin
c. new words
c. rubbing
coinage
word c.
CO_2 inhalation test
coital
c. headache
c. orgasm
c. position
coition
coitophobia
coitus
c. analis
c. in ano
c. in axilla
c. condomatus
c. inter femora
c. interruptus
c. intra mammas
c. á la vache
oral c.
c. prolongatus
psychogenic painful c.
c. representation
c. reservatus
c. Saxonius
c. sine ejaculatione
c. á tergo
Colace
colchicine
Colclough-Scheicher laminectomy
  rongeur
cold
c. comfort
c. effect
c. fear
c. mottled insensate leg
paradoxical c.
c. shoulder
c. spot
coldness
emotional c.
cold-pack treatment
colera
coli
Escherichia c.
colic
lead c.
c. lead
colinearity
colitis
granulomatous c.
pseudomembranous c.
ulcerative c.
colla (*pl. of* collum)
collaborate
collaboration

collaborative
C. Study Psychotherapy Rating
  Scale
c. therapy
c. treatment process
collagen
intercellular c.
microfibrillar c.
collagenase inhibition
collagen-impregnated Dacron
collapse
bone graft c.
c. delirium
hemispheric c.
vertebral c.
collapsible tissue retractor
collapsing anchor
collar
Belmont c.
cervical c.
Exo-Static c.
Miami Acute Care c.
Miami J c.
Newport c.
Philadelphia c.
plastic c.
Plastizote cervical c.
collateral
c. behavior
c. blood flow
c. circulation
c. eminence
c. fissure
Schaffer c.
c. sources
c. sprouting neuron
c. sulcus
c. trigone
c. vessel
collecting mania
collection
data c.
collective
c. behavior
c. ego
c. experience
c. hypnotization
c. hysteria
c. monologue
c. neurosis
c. psychosis
c. representation
c. suicide
c. transference
c. unconscious
collector
common venous c.
college
C. Ability Test (CAT)
C. Basic Academic Subjects
  Examination
C. Characteristics Index (CCI)
c. graduate
invisible c.

college *(continued)*
 Louisiana State University
  Medical C. (LSUMC)
 C. Major Interest Inventory (CMII)
 C. Student Questionnaire (CSQ)
 Student Reactions to C. (SRC)
 C. Student Satisfaction
  Questionnaire (CSSQ)
 C. and University Environment
  Scales (CUES)
College-Level Examination Program
 General Examination (CLEP)
Collet-Sicard syndrome
collicular artery
colliculus, pl. colliculi
 anterior c.
 brachium of the inferior c.
 brachium of superior c.
 facial c.
 c. facialis
 inferior c.
 c. inferior
 c. superior
 superior c.
Collier
 C. sign
 C. tract
colligation
collimated cobalt-60
collimation
collimator
 CASS TrueTaper c.
 external c.
 c. helmet
 stereoguide c.
Collins law of survival after brain
 tumor
collision
 electron c.
 c. tumor
Collis-Romberg Mathematical Problem
 Solving Profile
collodion attachment
colloid
 c. cyst
 c. oncotic pressure (COP)
 technetium albumin c.
 technetium 99m sulfur c.
colloquial
collum, pl. colla
 c. distortum
collusion
coloboma
Cologne pattern scalp clip
Colonna shelf procedure
colony
 Gheel c.
colony-forming efficiency (CFE)
color
 achromatic c.
 c. agnosia
 c. amblyopia
 c. anomia
 c. blind

 chromatic c.
 c. constancy
 c. contrast
 c. denial (Cd)
 c. discrimination
 c. in dream
 c. dream
 flashes of c.
 flight of c.
 c. hearing
 c. mixture
 c. perception
 c. preference
 primary c.
 c. response
 c. sorting test
 c. taste
 c. theory
 c. therapy
 c. vision
 c. vision disorder
 c. vision loss
 c. weakness
 c. zone
Colorado
 C. Educational Interest Battery
 C. MicroDissection needle
 C. tick fever (CTF)
 C. tick fever viral encephalitis
color-flow
 c.-f. Doppler
 c.-f. Doppler sonography
 c.-f. imaging
Coloured Progressive Matrices
colpocephaly
Columbia Mental Maturity Scale
 (CMMS)
columella, pl. columellae
column
 anterior c. of medulla oblongata
 branchial efferent c.
 Burdach c.
 c. cell
 Clarke c.
 cortical c.
 dorsal c. of spinal cord
 forniceal c.
 c. of fornix
 general somatic afferent c.
 general somatic efferent c.
 Goll c.
 Gowers c.
 gray c.
 intermediolateral cell c. of spinal
  cord
 lateral c. of spinal cord
 ocular dominance c.
 posterior c. of spinal cord
 Rolando c.
 special somatic afferent c.
 special visceral c.
 spinal c.
 Stilling c.
 Türck c.

ventral c. of spinal cord
vertebral c.
columna, gen. and pl. **columnae**
    c. anterior
    c. fornicis
    columnae griseae
    c. lateralis
    c. posterior
    c. vertebralis
coma
    adrenocortical c.
    agrypnodal c.
    alcoholic c.
    alpha frequency c.
    apoplectic c.
    barbiturate-induced c.
    c. carcinomatosum
    diabetic c.
    hepatic c.
    hyperosmolar (hyperglycemic)
      nonketotic c.
    hypopituitary c.
    irreversible c.
    Kussmaul c.
    metabolic c.
    myxedema c.
    nonketotic hyperglycemic
      hyperosmolar c.
    pentobarbital c.
    postanoxic c.
    c. scale
    spindle c.
    c. therapy
    thyrotoxic c.
    trance c.
    c. vigil
comatose patient
combat
    c. exhaustion
    C. Exposure Scale
    c. fatigability
    c. fatigue
    c. flashback
    hors de c.
    c. hysteria
    mortal c.
    c. neurosis
    c. reaction
    single c.
    c. stress
    c. stress exposure
    c. tension
combative patient
combination
    aspirin c.
    c. chemotherapy
    cocaine-heroin c.
    fabulized c.
    frequency c.
    c. headache
    Isola spinal implant system plate-
      rod c.
    law of c.
    muscle-fascia-Gelfoam c.
    c. needle electrode

combination-drug dependence
combinative thinking
combined
    c. anesthesia
    c. anterior and posterior approach
    c. factor
    c. flexion-distraction injury and
      burst fracture
    c. low cervical and transthoracic
      approach
    c. presigmoid-transtransversarium
      intradural approach
    c. sclerosis
    c. system disease
    c. therapy
    c. transcortical aphasia
    c. transsylvian and middle fossa
      approach
combined-type
    c.-t. attention deficit hyperactivity
      disorder
    c.-t. attention-deficit/hyperactivity
      disorder
    c.-t. personality disorder
combining power test (CPT)
Combipres
Combisit surgeon's chair
Combitrans transducer
Combivir
cometophobia
comfort
    cold c.
    c. dream
    emotional c.
comitial mal
comma
    c. bundle of Schultze
    c. tract of Schultze
command
    c. auditory hallucinations
    c. automatism
    embedded c.
    c. hallucination
    c. law
    negative c.
    c. negativism
    c. style commitment
commensalism
comment
    derogatory c.
    discriminatory c.
    threatening c.
commentary
    running c.
commenting
    voices c.
comminuted skull fracture
commiserate
commissura, gen. and pl. **commissurae**
    c. alba
    c. anterior
    c. anterior grisea
    c. cinerea
    c. fornicis
    c. grisea

C

commissura *(continued)*
    c. habenularum
    c. hippocampi
    c. posterior cerebri
    c. posterior grisea
    commissurae supraopticae
    c. ventralis alba
commissural
    c. aphasia
    c. cell
    c. fiber
    c. myelotomy
    c. plate
commissure
    anterior c. (AC)
    anterior commissure-posterior c.
    (AC-PC)
    anterior white c.
    cerebral c.
    c. of cerebral hemispheres
    c. of fornix
    Ganser c.
    Gudden c.
    c. of habenulae
    habenular c.
    hippocampal c.
    Meynert c.
    posterior cerebral c.
    supraoptic c.
    Wernekinck c.
    white c.
commissurotomy
    callosal c.
    percutaneous balloon c.
commitment
    civil c.
    command style c.
    criminal c.
    ideological c.
    institutional c.
    involuntary civil c.
    laws of c.
    long-term c.
    observation c.
    sense of c.
    short-term c.
    temporary c.
    voluntary c.
committed
    legally c.
committee
    C. of International Medical
      Graduates
    C. on Family Violence and Sexual
      Abuse
    C. on History and Library
    C. on Information Systems
    C. on Psychiatric Diagnosis and
      Assessment
    C. on Quality Assurance and
      Improvement
    C. on Standards and Survey
      Procedures
    utilization review c.

common
    c. carotid artery (CCA)
    c. crus
    c. experience
    c. iliac artery injury
    c. law
    c. limb of membranous
      semicircular ducts
    c. migraine
    c. migraine headache
    c. peroneal nerve
    c. precipitant exposure
    c. sense psychiatry
    c. sense therapy
    c. shared feature
    c. theme
    c. trait
    c. venous collector
    c. venous confluence
commonality
commotio
    c. cerebri
    c. spinalis
communality
communicable hysteria
communicans
    macula c.
communicated insanity
communicating
    c. empathy
    c. epilepsy
    c. hydrocephalus
communication
    C. Abilities Diagnostic Test
      (CADT)
    C. Abilities Diagnostic Test and
      Screen
    c. ability
    augmentative c.
    c. barrier
    c. channel
    channel of c.
    coercive c.
    consummatory c.
    c. deviance
    distortion of language and c.
    c. engineering
    exaggeration of language and c.
    fragmented c.
    gestural c.
    illogical c.
    impaired effective c.
    indexical c.
    inhibited c.
    Inventory of Anger C. (IAC)
    irreverent c.
    language and c.
    c. magic
    manual c.
    c. network
    nonverbal c.
    nonvocal c.
    pathologic c.
    c. pattern
    persuasive c.

privileged c.
problem-solving c.
qualitative impairment in c.
reciprocal c.
Revised Evaluating Acquired Skills in C.
c. scale
Scale for Assessment of Thought, Language, and C.
C. Sensitivity Inventory
c. skills assessment
social c.
c. theory
therapeutic c.
c. therapy
total c.
unaided augmentative c.
c. unit
vague c.
vehicle for c.
verbal c.
visual c. (VC, VIC)
c. with adolescent
communication/cognition treatment
communications in behavioral biology (CBB)
communicative
    C. Abilities in Daily Living (CADL)
c. arson
c. competence
c. comprehension
c. disorder
c. function
c. interaction
communicatively impaired
communicology
communion principle
community
    c. assessment
c. care
c. catharsis
c. centered
C. College Student Experiences Questionnaire (CCSEQ)
c. divorce
c. feeling
homosexual c.
c. intervention
c. mental health
c. mental health center (CMHC)
C. Mental Health Centers Act
c. need
Oneida c.
c. population
c. program
c. psychiatry
c. psychology
c. resources
c. role
c. setting
c. study
c. support
therapeutic c. (TC)
community-action group

community-based treatment
community-institutional relations
Community-Oriented Programs Environment Scale (COPES)
comorbid
    c. anxiety disorder
c. Axis II diagnosis
c. personality disorder
c. tic
comorbidity
    psychiatric c.
somatopsychiatric c.
substantial c.
compacta
    pars c.
substantia nigra pars c. (Snc)
companion
    imaginary c.
phobic c.
comparable
    c. forms reliability coefficient
c. worth
comparative
    C. Guidance and Placement Program (CGP)
c. judgment
c. medicine
c. psychiatry
c. psychology
c. research
c. scanning
comparison
    factor c.
positive c.
compartment
    extradural c.
infratentorial c.
lateral sellar c.
synaptic c.
c. syndrome
COMPASS
    C. arc-quadrant stereotactic system
C. frame-based stereotactic system
compassionate
    c. feeling
c. marriage
Compass stereotactic phantom
compatibility
    ABO antigen c.
MRI c.
compatible
Compazine
compelled behavior
compelling evidence
compensable accident
compensation
    c. defense mechanism
gradient c.
c. neurosis
c. neurosis neurotic disorder
c. psychoneurosis
c. schizophrenia
synaptic c.
compensatory
    c. behavior

compensatory *(continued)*
    c. education
    c. fantasy
    c. mechanism
    c. mood swing
    c. movement
    c. scoliosis
    c. technique
    c. trait
Comperm tubular elastic bandage
competence
    apparent c.
    communicative c.
    facade of c.
    Fisher-Logemann Test of
      Articulation C. (FLTAC)
    c. knowledge
    mental c.
    c. motivation
    social c.
    Test of Language C. (TLC)
competency
    Assessing Specific C.'s
    Assessing Specific Employment
      Skill C.'s
    Assessment of Basic C.'s (ABC)
    mental c.
    c. standard
    c. to stand trial
competency-based
    c.-b. examination
    c.-b. instruction
competent
    c. decision making
    c. relational functioning
    c. relationship
competent, optimal relational
  functioning
competing theories of motivation
competition
    hemisphere c.
    intermodal c.
competitive
    c. behavior
    c. motive
complacent attitude
complain
complaining
    help-rejecting c.
complaint
    chief c. (CC)
    Frankfurt Questionnaire of C.'s
    habit c.
    pain c.
    primary c.
    sleep c.
    somatic c.
    subjective insomnia c.
complemental air
complementarity of interaction
complementary
    c. instinct
    c. role

complete
    c. amnesia
    c. aphasia
    c. birth
    c. cross-dressing
    c. genital primacy
    c. iridoplegia
    c. lateral hemilaminectomy
    c. mother
    c. Oedipus
    c. transverse myelitis
    c. visual loss
completed suicide
complete-learning method
completion
    c., arithmetic, vocabulary, and
      directions (CAVD)
    c., arithmetic, vocabulary, and
      directions test
    Horn-Hellersberg Drawing C.
    picture c. (PC)
    sentence c.
    Stein Sentence C. (SSC)
    task c.
completus
    tetanus c.
complex
    c. absence
    acoustic nerve c.
    acquired immunodeficiency
      syndrome dementia c.
    active castration c.
    AIDS dementia c. (ADC)
    AIDS-related c. (ARC)
    ALD-AMN c.
    ALS-PD c.
    amygdaloid c.
    amyotrophic lateral sclerosis-
      Parkinson dementia c.
    antigen-antibody c.
    aperiodic c.
    authority c.
    avidin-biotin peroxidase c.
    benzodiazepine-GABA-receptor c.
    brain wave c.
    breast c.
    brother c.
    Cain c.
    capsulolabral c.
    castration c.
    C5b-9 c.
    choroidal-hippocampal fissure c.
    Cinderella c.
    claustral c.
    Clerambault-Kandinsky c.
    Clytemnestra c.
    culture c.
    Dandy-Walker c.
    Diana c.
    discoligamentous c.
    dorsal vagus c.
    ego c.
    Electra c.
    c. equivalence
    Eshmun c.

father c.
femininity c.
C. Figure Test (CFT)
Friedmann c.
function c.
GABA receptor c.
God c.
grandfather c.
Griselda c.
Guam parkinsonism-dementia c.
c. hallucination
heir of the Oedipus c.
hippocampal-amygdala c.
homosexual c.
hypersexual c.
c. of ideas
immune c.
inferiority c.
Jocasta c.
K c.
kernel c.
Lear c.
c. learning process
Madonna c.
Madonna-prostitute c.
major histocompatibility c. (MHC)
martyr c.
mastoid c.
Medea c.
membrane attack c. (MAC)
c. meningioma
messiah c.
mother c.
Mother Superior c.
c. motor behavior
c. motor tic
c. multistep task
c. noise
obscenity-purity c.
occipitoatlantoaxial c.
oedipal c.
Oedipus c.
Orestes c.
organ inferiority c.
parkinsonism-dementia c.
c. partial epilepsy
c. partial seizure (CPS)
particular c.
passive castration c.
PDH c.
persecution c.
Phaedra c.
plasmin-antiplasmin c.
Polycrates c.
posttraumatic stress disorder c.
c. precipitated epilepsy
pyruvate dehydrogenase c.
Quasimodo c.
c. readiness
c. regional pain syndrome (CRPS)
c. repetitive discharge (CRD)
Rey-Osterrieth c.
robin c.
Sakoda c.
c. sentence

small penis c.
Sokoda c.
spike-and-wave c.
superiority c.
symptom c.
syringomyelia-Chiari c.
c. thematic pictures test
c. tone
c. type
urethral c.
ventrolateral nuclear c.
vertebrogenic symptom c.
c. visual perception
c. vocal tic
c. whole body movement
complexity
c. of mental process (CMP)
syntactic c.
compliance
intracranial c.
c. masking covert resistance
motor c.
overt c.
patient c.
social c.
strategic c.
compliant
complicated
c. fracture
c. grief disorder
c. migraine
c. migraine headache
complication
Isola spinal implant system c.
neurologic c.
pregnancy and birth c. (PBC)
psychosocial c.
component
articulatory loop c.
base c.
blood c.
central executive c.
hypermetabolic tumor c.
Isola spinal implant system c.
masochistic c.
signal transducing receptor c.
slave system c.
composite
c. addition technique
C. International Diagnostic
  Interview
c. person
C. Psycholinguistic Age
C. Risk Index (CRI)
total battery c.
composition
body c.
device c.
compos mentis
compound
arylcyclohexylamine c.
bromine c.
Darvon C.
dihydrocodeine c.
c. granule cell

compound *(continued)*
    lipophilic c.
    c. medicine
    c. motor action potential
    c. muscle action potential (CMAP)
    c. muscle action potential amplitude
    c. nerve action potential (CNAP)
    ovabain-like c. (OLC)
    pentazocine c.
    c. skull fracture
    Soma C.
    Talwin C.
Compoz
    C. Gel Caps
    C. Nighttime Sleep Aid
comprehension
    Assessment of Children's Language C. (ACLC)
    auditory c.
    communicative c.
    c. deficit
    language c.
    passage c.
    Progressive Achievement Tests of Listening C. (PATLC)
    c. span
    c. subtest
comprehensive
    C. Ability Battery (CAB)
    C. Assessment Program: Achievement Series
    C. Assessment of Symptoms and History (CASH)
    C. Career Assessment Scale (CCAS)
    C. Developmental Evaluation Chart
    C. Drinker Profile
    c. identification process (CIP)
    C. Level of Consciousness Scale (CLCS)
    C. Psychiatric Rating Scale (CPRS)
    C. Psychopathological Rating Scale
    c. review
    c. solution
    C. Test of Adaptive Behavior
    C. Test of Basic Skills, Forms U and V
    C. Test of Visual Functioning (CTVF)
compressed
    c. spectral analysis
    c. spectral array
compression
    c. amplifier
    c. anesthesia
    axial c.
    c. of brain
    brainstem c.
    cauda equina c.
    cerebral aqueduct c.
    cervical vessel c.
    cervicomedullary junction c.
    chiasmal c.

    c. fracture
    Harrington rod instrumentation c.
    c. instrumentation posterior construct
    c. ophthalmodynamometer
    optic chiasm c.
    optic tract c.
    c. paralysis
    percutaneous trigeminal nerve c.
    c. rod
    c. rod treatment
    spinal cord c.
    c. spring
    c. syndrome
    thecal sac c.
    c. U-rod instrumentation
    ventral medullary c.
compressive
    c. myelopathy
    c. neuropathy
    c. rod
compromise
    adenohypophyseal c.
    adrenocorticotropic c.
    cerebral c.
    c. distortion
    endocrinological c.
    c. formation
compromised function
Compton scattering
compulsion
    antisocial c.
    brooding c.
    eating c.
    c. neurosis
    c. psychoneurosis
    repetition c.
    thinking c.
compulsion-obsession
compulsive
    c. act
    c. action
    c. buying
    c. ceremonial
    c. change
    c. character
    c. cruising
    c. defense
    c. disorder
    c. disturbance
    c. drinker
    c. drug-taking behavior
    c. eating
    c. exercise
    c. fixation on an unobtainable partner
    c. gambling
    c. idea
    c. insanity
    c. laughter
    c. magic
    c. mania
    c. masturbation
    c. neurosis
    c. orderliness

c. personality
c. psychasthenia
c. psychogenic tic
c. psychoneurotic reaction
c. repetition
c. restraint
c. ritual
c. scale
c. sex
c. sexual behavior
C. Sexual Disorders Interview
c. stealing
c. substance use
c. swearing syndrome
c. symptom
c. thought
c. water drinking

computation
symbolic c.
computational process
computed
c. tomographic angioplasty (CTA)
c. tomographic cisternography
c. tomographic metrizamide myelography (CTMM)
c. tomographic myelography (CTM)
c. tomography (CT)
computer
C. Anxiety Index
biofeedback c.
Brown-Roberts-Wells c.
C. Operator Aptitude Battery (COAB)
C. Programmer Aptitude Battery (CPAB)
computer-assisted
c.-a. EEG signal analysis
c.-a. neuroendoscopy (CANE)
c.-a. speech device
c.-a. stereotactic surgery (CASS)
c.-a. volumetric stereotactic approach
computer-controlled neurological stimulation system
computerized
c. axial tomography (CAT)
c. axial tomography scanning
c. EEG signal analysis
c. infrared telethermographic imaging
C. Reaction Time Test
Comrey Personality Scale (CPS)
com score
COMT
catechol-O-methyltransferase
Comtan
conarium
conation
conative
c. appetitive striving
c. negative variation (CNV)
conatus
concatenation
concavity

concentrate
concentration
approximate lethal c. (ALC)
attention and c.
c. and attention
blood alcohol c.
c. camp syndrome (CCS)
c. deficit
c. difficulty
c. disturbance
hippocampal monoamine c.
hydrogen ion c.
impaired c.
information memory c. (IMC)
motion c.
C. Performance Test (CPT)
c. performance test
time of maximum c.
concentrica
encephalitis periaxialis c.
concentric herniation
concept
abstract c.
C. bipolar coagulator
body ego c.
Boehm Test of Basic C.'s
c. of brain function
concrete c.
conjunctive c.
critical band c.
feces-child-penis c.
c. formation
grandiose c.
C. hand-held cautery
Heidelberg c.
key c.
lexica c.
C. Mastery Test (CMT)
medicine c.
mental c.
object c.
permanence c.
psychodynamic c.
self c.
self-derogatory c.
self-role c.
three-column c.
von Monakow diaschisis c.
Winslow c.
conception
hallucination of c.
imperative c.
Concept-Specific Anxiety Scale (CAS)
conceptual
c. ability
c. disorder
c. disorganization
c. disturbance
c. learning
c. nervous system
c. skill
C. Systems Test (CST)
c. tempo
c. thinking

C

169

conceptualization
    abstract c.
    Lindamood Auditory C.
conceptualized
concern
    abandonment c.
    Inventory of Peer Influence on
      Eating C.
    sense of c.
    sexual c.
    unconscious c.
    ventilate c.
concordance
    c. coefficient
    c. rate
    twin c.
concrete
    c. abstractive ability
    c. attitude
    c. concept
    c. image
    c. intelligence
    c. operation
    c. operations period
    c. operations stage
    c. picture
    c. representation
    c. thinking
    c. thought process
concretistic thinking
concretization
    active c.
concretizing attitude
concurrent
    c. psychiatric problem
    c. reinforcement
    c. review
    c. therapy
    c. validity
concussion
    c. amnesia
    c. blindness
    brain c.
    c. of brain
    c. myelitis
    spinal cord c.
    c. syndrome
condemn
condemnation
condensation
    mitochondrial c.
    c. stimulation
condescend
condescending evaluation
condescension
condition
    abnormal pathologic c.
    amnestic disorder due to a general
      medical c.
    anxiety disorder due to a general
      medical c.
    atmospheric c.
    catatonic disorder due to a general
      medical c.
    congenital intersex c.

    craniofacial c.
    degenerative spine c.
    delirium due to a general
      medical c.
    dementia due to hepatic c.
    disorder affecting general
      medical c.
    enuresis not due to a general
      medical c.
    etiological neurological c.
    general medical c. (GMC)
    hypomyelinating c.
    illumination c.
    insomnia-type sleep disorder due to
      general medical c.
    intersex c.
    medical c.
    mental disorder due to a general
      medical c.
    mood disorder due to a general
      medical c.
    necessary c.
    neurological c.
    neuromuscular c.
    c.'s not attributable to a mental
      disorder
    not due to direct physiological
      effects of a substance or a
      general medical c.
    organic psychotic c.
    pain disorder associated with both
      psychological features and a
      general medical c.
    paranoid c.
    pathologic c.
    personality change due to a
      general medical c.
    physical c.
    physical intersex c.
    preexisting c.
    psychological factors affecting a
      mental c.
    psychologic factor affecting
      physical c.
    psychosis due to physical c.
    psychotic disorder due to a general
      medical c.
    school handicap c. (SEC)
    sexual dysfunction due to a
      general medical c.
    sexually transmitted c. (STC)
    sleep disorder due to a general
      medical c.
    test c.
    undiagnosed general medical c.
conditional
    c. arousal
    c. discharge
    c. probability
conditioned
    c. cue
    c. emotional response (CER)
    c. escape response
    c. inhibition
    c. place preference (CPP)

c. reflex
c. reinforcer
c. response
c. stimulus (CS)
c. suppression
conditioned-reflex therapy
conditioning
approximation c.
assertive c.
autonomic c.
average c.
aversion c.
aversion-covert c.
aversive c.
avoidance c.
backward c.
classical c.
cognitive c.
counter c.
cross c.
decorticate c.
escape c.
esprit de corps c.
exteroceptive c.
eyelid c.
false c.
higher order c.
instrumental c.
negative c.
operant c.
pavlovian c.
primary reward c.
respondent c.
secondary reward c.
second-order c.
skinnerian c.
c. therapy
trace c.
condom
condomatus
coitus c.
conduct
adjustment disorder with
disturbance of c.
consistent pattern of c.
disorderly c.
c. disturbance
c. disturbance adjustment disorder
c. disturbance adjustment reaction
moral c.
pattern of c.
persistent pattern of c.
solitary aggressive type c.
conductance
voltage-activated c.
conduct-disordered child
conduction
air c.
c. anesthesia
c. aphasia
bone c.
c. deafness
c. disorder
electronic c.
ephaptic c.

excitation and c.
motor nerve c.
nerve c.
saltatory c.
c. testing
conductor
Adson c.
Bailey c.
Davis c.
conduit
peripheral nerve regeneration c.
condylar
c. approach
c. hypoplasia
condyle
c. dissection
c. resection
condylectomy
mandibular c.
cone
c. cell of retina
c. fiber
growth c.
implantation c.
C. laminectomy retractor
medullary c.
retinal c.
C. ring curette
C. scalp retractor
C. skull punch
C. skull punch forceps
C. skull traction tongs
C. suction biopsy curette
C. suction tube
C. ventricular needle
C. wire-twisting forceps
Cone-Grant technique
confabulans
paraphrenia c.
confabulated
c. detail response (dD)
c. whole response (DW)
confabulation
conference
career c.
confessor
father c.
mother c.
confidence
diagnostic c.
c. interval
c. level
level of c.
confident status
configuration
Cotrel-Dubousset hook claw c.
triangular base transverse bar c.
venous lake c.
word c.
configurative culture
confinement
c. effect
c. fear
solitary c.

C

confirmed
angiographically c.
conflict
approach-approach c.
approach-avoidance c.
c. avoidance
avoidance-avoidance c.
basic c.
central c.
culture c.
emotional c.
ethical c.
extrapsychic c.
family c.
increased interpersonal c.
inferred c.
infrequent interpersonal c.
inner c.
c. of interest
intermanual c.
internal c.
interpersonal c.
intrafamilial c.
intrapersonal c.
intrapsychic c.
level of c.
c. level
c. management
C. Management Appraisal (CMA)
C. Management Survey (CMS)
marital c.
C. in Marriage Scale (CIMS)
oedipal c.
parent-child c.
psychodynamic c.
c. resolution
resolve c.
role c.
significant c.
C. Tactics Scale
unconscious c.
unresolved c.
c.'s with c.
c.'s with peers
conflicted feeling
conflict-free
c.-f. area
c.-f. function
c.-f. sphere
conflicting
c. message
c. motive
conflict-resolution strategy
conflictual
c. relationship
c. situation
confluence
common venous c.
c. method
c. of sinuses
confluens sinuum
confocal laser scanning (CLSM)
conformance
functional c.

conformity
automaton c.
conventional role c.
morality of conventional role c.
social c.
confrontation
direct c.
c. naming test
reality c.
simple c.
c. testing
confrontive
confused
c. delusion
c. language syndrome (CLS)
c. speech
confusingly fluid coalition
confusion
authority c.
bisexual c.
cognate c.
episodic c.
gender c.
gender identity c.
identity c.
identity vs. role c.
mental c.
nocturnal c.
personal identity c.
posteroperative c.
postictal c.
postoperative c.
psychogenic c.
reactive c.
c. reactive psychosis
right-left c.
role c.
time c.
c. of values
confusional
c. arousal
c. arousals from sleep
c. episode
c. insanity
c. migraine
c. migraine headache
c. psychosis
c. psychotic reaction
c. schizophreniform
c. state presenile
c. state presenile dementia
c. twilight state
congener
congenita
amyoplasia c.
amyotonia c.
aplasia cutis c.
myatonia c.
myotonia c.
paramyotonia c.
congenital
c. adrenal hyperplasia
c. aneurysm
c. anomaly
c. arachnodactyly

c. arithmetic disability
c. atonic pseudoparalysis
c. defect
c. dilation
c. dysplastic angiomatosis
c. dysplastic angiopathy
c. facial diplegia
c. hippocampal sclerosis
c. Horner syndrome
c. hydrocephalus
c. hypomyelination neuropathy
c. hypothesis
c. hypothyroidism
c. intersex condition
c. kyphosis
c. malformation
c. myasthenia gravis
c. nasal mass
c. neurosyphilis
c. nystagmus
c. ocular motor apraxia
c. paramyotonia
c. scoliosis
c. spastic paraplegia
c. sutural alopecia
c. syphilitic paralytic
c. syphilitic paralytic dementia
c. tumor
c. virilizing adrenal hyperplasia

congenitalis
alopecia c.
alopecia triangularis c.

congestion
brain c.

congestive heart failure

congophilic
c. amyloid
c. angiopathy

congruent
c. affect
mood c.

congruous hemianopia

coni (*pl. of* conus)

conjoined
c. nerve root
c. twin

conjoint
c. counseling
c. interview
c. synapse
c. therapy

conjugal
c. bereavement
c. paranoia
c. psychosis
c. visit

conjugate
c. contraversive eye movement
c. fixed gaze
c. horizontal gaze
c. nystagmus
c. palsy
c. paralysis

conjugated eye movement

conjunctive
c. concept
c. reinforcement

conjunctivitis

connectedness
family c.
impaired c.

connection
interneuronal c.

connective tissue disease

connector
adjustable pedicle c.
dual bypass c.
intrinsic transverse c.
longitudinal member to anchor c.
stepdown c.
straight c.
tandem c.
transverse c.

Conners
C. Abbreviated Symptom
  Questionnaire
C. Hyperkinesis Index, Parent
  Form
C. Hyperkinesis Index, Teacher
  Form
C. Parent Questionnaire (CPQ)
C. Parent Rating Scale
C. Parent-Teacher Rating Scale
C. Parent and Teacher Symptom
  Questionnaire
C. Preliminary Parent Report
C. Teacher Preliminary School
  Report
C. Teacher Questionnaire (CTQ)
C. Teacher Rating Scale (CRS-39,
  CTRS-28)

connexin 32 protein

Conradi syndrome

consanguineous marriage

consanguinity

conscience
authoritarian c.
humanistic c.

conscientiousness

conscious
c. avoidance
c. awareness
c. decision
c. memory
c. perception
c. process
c. resistance
c. state

consciousness
active mode of c.
altered level of c.
altered state of c. (ASC)
arousal component of c.
clouding of c.
cosmic c.
crowd c.
crude c.
declining c.
depression of c.

consciousness *(continued)*
discrimination c.
disintegration of c.
c. disturbance
disturbance of c.
c. disturbance stress reaction
double c.
effect of trauma on c.
episodic changes of c.
expanded c.
c. expansion
field of c.
fluctuating level of c.
fringe of c.
group c.
head c.
higher level of c.
higher state of c.
c. impaired
impaired c.
impairment of c.
level of c. (LOC)
loss of c. (LOC)
marginal c.
parasomniac c.
passive mode of c.
perceptual c.
reduced level of c.
social c.
state of c. (SOC)
c. state
stream of c.
subliminal c.
threshold of c.
time c.
unitary c.
consecutive insanity
consensual
c. action
c. gaze
c. reaction
c. reflex
c. response pupil
c. validation
c. validation consent
consensually
consent
age of c.
consensual validation c.
c. forms
informed c.
valid c.
Willowbrook c.
consenting
c. adult
c. partner
consequence
c. association
health-related c.
painful c.
serious c.
consequences of action
consequent
affirming the c.

conservative
c. medication
c. treatment
conservatorship
considerable external support
consideration
biologic c.
considered thought
consistency
behavioral c.
moral c.
perceptual c.
c. principle
consistent
c. irresponsibility
c. pattern of conduct
c. relationship
consociate
consolation dream
consolidated sleep
consonant blend
Consonar
consortium
Child and Adolescent C.
Childhood Brain Tumor C. (CBTC)
C. to Establish a Registry for
  Alzheimer's Disease (CERAD)
C. on Special Psychiatric Delivery
  Setting
conspiratorial
constancy
brightness c.
color c.
emotional object c.
extrinsic c.
intrinsic c.
law of c.
libidinal object c.
location c.
object c.
perceptual c.
c. phenomenon
constant
c. anger
c. current stimulator
Heinis c.
relaxation c.
time c.
T_1 relaxation c.
T_2 relaxation c.
c. worry
constantium
delirium c.
constellation
family c.
self-pitying c.
c. of signs and symptoms
Constilac
constipation
psychogenic c.
constitution
epileptic psychopathic c.
hyperadrenal c.
ideo-obsessional c.

posttraumatic psychopathic c.
psychopathic c.
constitutional
   c. bisexuality theory
   c. depression
   c. disease
   c. factor
   c. insanity
   c. psychology
   c. psychopathia inferior (CPI)
   c. psychopathic inferiority (CPI)
   c. psychopathic state (CPS)
   c. psychosis
   c. type
constraint
   morality of c.
   c. of movement
   thought c.
   c. of thought
constricted
   c. activity
   c. affect
   c. pupil
constriction
   c. of affect
   affective c.
   emotional c.
   pupillary c.
   c. of thought
construct
   anterior c.
   AO dynamic compression plate c.
   compression instrumentation
     posterior c.
   core c.
   double-rod c.
   Edwards modular system bridging
     sleeve c.
   Edwards modular system
     compression c.
   Edwards modular system
     distraction-lordosis c.
   Edwards modular system
     kyphoreduction c.
   Edwards modular system
     neutralization c.
   Edwards modular system rod-
     sleeve c.
   Edwards modular system
     scoliosis c.
   Edwards modular system
     spondylo c.
   Edwards modular system standard
     sleeve c.
   Guiot-Talairach c.
   hook-to-screw L4-S1 compression c.
   iliosacral and iliac fixation c.
   multidimensional c.
   pedicle screw c.
   personal c.
   posterior c.
   c. research
   rod-hook c.
   screw-to-screw compression c.
   segmental compression c.

single-rod c.
spondylo c.
titanium c.
TSRH double-rod c.
TSRH pedicle screw-laminar
   claw c.
upper cervical spine anterior c.
upper cervical spine posterior c.
c. validity
Wiltse system double-rod c.
Wiltse system H c.
Wiltse system single-rod c.
construction
   endocentric c.
   exocentric c.
   c. of femininity
   hierarchy c.
   mildly ungrammatical c.
   phrase c. (PC)
   visual field c.
   visuospatial c.
constructional
   c. ability
   c. apraxia
   c. dyspraxia
   c. impairment
constructive
   c. approach
   c. criticism
   c. feedback
   c. memory
Constulose
consultation
   agency-centered c.
   crisis c.
   c. liaison psychiatry
   patient-oriented c.
   c. psychiatry
   social service c.
consultation-liaison service
consulting psychologist
consumer
   c. behavior
   c. characteristic
   c. psychology
consummatory
   c. act
   c. communication
consumption
   alcohol c.
   cerebral oxygen c.
   drug c.
consumptive coagulopathy
contact
   c. behavior
   c. ceptor
   c. compressive forceps
   continuity of c.
   eye c.
   frequency of c. (FOC)
   genital sexual c.
   oral-genital c.
   sexual c.
   c. ulcer
   c. with reality

C

contagion
    emergency c.
    psychic c.
container
    drug c.
    exerciser c.
containing
    dopa-decarboxylase c.
contamination obsession
contemptuous
contendere
    nolo c.
content
    c. addressability
    c. analysis
    blood alcohol concentration c.
      (BAC)
    carotid c.
    c. of delusion
    dream c.
    grandiose c.
    c. of hallucination
    language c.
    latent c.
    manifest c.
    mood, orientation, judgment,
      affect, c. (MOJAC)
    paucity of speech c.
    positive speech c.
    poverty of c.
    c. psychology
    c. scale
    self-derogatory c.
    speech c.
    thought c.
    c. of thought
    c. thought disorder
    c. validity
context
    cultural c.
    c. reframing
contextual
    c. cue
    c. influence
    c. therapy
contiguity
    c. aphasia
    c. disorder
    c. disorder aphasia
    law of c.
    spatial c.
    temporal c.
contiguous
    c. nonoverlapping axial CT
    c. supramarginal gyrus
Contin
    MS C.
    OxyC.
continence
    fecal c.
contingency
    c. awareness
    behavioral c.
    c. contract
    c. management

    c. model
    c. reinforcement
contingent
    c. negative variation (CNV)
    c. punishment
continua
    epilepsia corticalis c.
    epilepsia partialis c.
continuation therapy
continued-stay review (CSR)
continuing
    c. care
    c. medical education (CME)
    c. petit mal seizure
continuity
    c. of attachment
    c. of contact
    sleep c.
    worse sleep c.
continuous
    c. amnesia
    c. anatomical passive exerciser
      (CAPE)
    c. bath treatment
    c. course
    c. electromyographic recording
    c. epilepsy
    c. group
    c. growth
    c. intrathecal baclofen infusion
      (CIBI)
    c. intravenous regional anesthesia
      (CIVRA)
    c. narcosis
    c. observation
    c. on-line recording
    c. panel
    C. Performance Task
    C. Performance Test (CPT)
    c. positive airway pressure (CPAP)
    c. reinforcement
    c. reinforcement schedule
    c. sleep
    c. tremor
    c. venous oximetry
    C. Visual Memory Test (CVMT)
    c. wave
continuous-sleep therapy
continuous-wave
    c.-w. Doppler
    c.-w. Doppler imaging
    c.-w. technique
continuum
    c. of care
    hypothetical c.
    introversion-extroversion c.
    c. theory
contour
    C. Emboli artificial embolization
      device
    field c.
contoured
    c. anterior spinal plate
    c. anterior spinal plate drill guide
    c. anterior spinal plate technique

contouring
Isola spinal implant system longitudinal member c.
contraception
rhythm method of c.
withdrawal method of c.
contraceptive
c. device
oral c.
contract
behavior c.
behavioral c.
contingency c.
employment c.
c. evaluation
evaluation c.
formal c.
formalized c.
group c.
informal c.
interactional c.
legal c.
marriage c.
patient c.
quasi-c.
c. review
sweetheart c.
c. therapy
contraction
carpopedal c.
lead pipe c.
maximal voluntary c. (MVC)
nonepileptic myoclonic c.
rhythmic c.
Rossolimo c.
tetanic c. (Te)
contractual
c. arrangement
c. behavior
c. capacity
c. psychiatry
c. psychotherapy
contractural diathesis
contracture
c. arachnodactyly
Dupuytren c.
functional c.
myotatic c.
organic c.
Skoog release of Dupuytren c.
Volkmann c.
contradiction
contradictory information
contrafissura
contraindication
contralateral
c. facial paralysis
c. hemianopia
c. hemiparesis
c. hemiplegia
c. loss
c. monocular nystagmus
c. neglect syndrome
c. parietal lobe
c. parietal lobe dysfunction

c. reflex
c. routing of signals (CROS)
c. routing of sound (CROS)
c. sign
c. transcallosal approach
contralesional hemifield
contrapulsion of saccades
contrasexual component of psyche
contrast
c. agent
c. angiography
brightness c.
chromatic c.
color c.
c. density
c. effect
c. enhancement
gadolinium c.
inherent c.
law of c.
maximal c.
c. media
paramagnetic c.
c. sensitivity
c. sensitivity reduction
spontaneous echo c. (SEC)
contrast-enhanced
c.-e. CT
c.-e. CT scan
c.-e. MRI
c.-e. MR image
c.-e. MR imaging
contrastimulus
contrastive
c. analysis
c. distribution
c. stress
contrast-to-noise ratio (CNR)
Contraves
C. stand
C. type floorstand
contravolition
contrecoup
c. contusion
fracture by c.
c. injury
c. injury of brain
contrectation
contributing role
contributory
c. element
c. negligence
control
aberrant autocrine c.
airway c.
c. analysis
appetite c.
attentional c.
automatic gain c.
automatic volume c.
aversive c.
balance c.
behavior c. (BC)
biologic c.
birth c. (BC)

C

control (*continued*)
  bladder c.
  bowel c.
  brain c.
  brainstem c.
  Bureau of Drug Abuse C. (BDAC)
  c. cell proliferation
  cognitive c.
  crowd c.
  degree of c.
  delusion of c.
  c. delusion
  c. device
  diffuse noxious inhibitory c.
    (DNIC)
  diminished c.
  disorder of impulse c.
  distribution of c.
  double visual c.
  3D positional c.
  ego c.
  executive c.
  experimental c.
  external force c.
  external locus of c.
  fear of losing c.
  feedback c.
  c. feedback
  FlexDial stimulus c.
  fluoroscopic c.
  c. frustration
  c. group
  idiodynamic c.
  image c.
  impaired impulse c.
  impulse c.
  in c.
  inner c.
  internal-external c.
  internal locus of c.
  interpersonal c.
  island of c.
  lack of c.
  learned autonomic c.
  locus of c. (LOC)
  locus of c.-chance (LOC-C)
  locus of c.-external (LOC-E)
  locus of c.-internal (LOC-I)
  losing c.
  loss of c.
  mental c.
  mind c.
  motor c.
  need to c.
  neurological c.
  one's own c.
  out of c. (OOC)
  outside c.
  pain c.
  parental c.
  personal locus of c. (PLC)
  poor impulse c.
  c. preoccupation
  psychooptical reflex c.

  rate c.
  reflex c.
  rigid c.
  secret c.
  social c.
  sociopolitical locus of c. (SLC)
  sphincter c.
  stimulus c.
  superego c.
  superstitious c.
  swing phase c.
  synergic c.
  taking c.
  televised radiofluoroscopic c.
  thought c.
  tonic c.
  vestibuloequilibratory c.
  voluntary c.
  weak ego c.
  worry c.
  yoked c.
controlled
  c. analgesic
  c. association
  c. attention
  c. breathing
  delusion of being c.
  c. drinking
  c. emotion
  c. environment
  c. exposure
  c. sampling
  c. substance
  C. Substances Act (CSA)
controlling
  c. external entities
  c. external spirit
  c. identity
contusio cerebri
contusion
  brain c.
  cerebral c.
  contrecoup c.
  facial c.
  scalp c.
  wind c.
conus, pl. **coni**
  c. medullaris
  c. medullaris lesion
  c. medullaris root avulsion
convalescence
convalescent dream
convection-enhanced delivery (CED)
convenience
  c. dream
  marriage of c.
conventional
  c. fractionated irradiation
  c. role conformity
  c. sign
convergence
  c. abnormality
  c. circuit
  c. nucleus of Perlia
  c. spasm

convergence-divergence **pattern**
convergence-evoked **nystagmus**
convergence-retraction **nystagmus**
convergent
    c. beam irradiation (CBI)
    c. thinking
conversational
    c. catharsis
    c. voice
conversation board
converse ocular dipping
conversing
    voices c.
conversion
    c. anesthesia
    c. aphonia
    ataxia c.
    c. ataxia
    c. blindness
    c. defense mechanism
    c. disorder
    C. Disorder, Mixed Type
    C. Disorder, Motor Type
    C. Disorder, Seizure Type
    C. Disorder, Sensory Type
    c. disorder with mixed presentation
    c. disorder with motor symptoms
      or deficit
    c. disorder with seizures or
      convulsion
    c. disorder with sensory symptom
      or deficit
    c. of emotion
    c. hysteria
    c. hysteria neurosis
    c. hysteria psychoneurosis
    c. paralysis
    c. psychoneurotic reaction
    c. seizure
    c. sensory change
    c. sensory charge
    c. symptom
    tonic-clonic c.
    c. unconsciousness
    c. V profile
conversion-type neurotic hysterical
converter
    analog to digital c.
    digital to analog c.
Convery polyarticular disability index
convexity
    cerebral c.
    cortical c.
    c. meningioma
    c. metastatic tumor
convexobasia
conviction
    delusional c.
    inferred delusional c.
convolution
    angular c.
    anterior central c.
    ascending frontal c.
    ascending parietal c.
    Broca c.

    callosal c.
    cingulate c.
    first temporal c.
    Heschl c.
    hippocampal c.
    inferior frontal c.
    inferior temporal c.
    middle frontal c.
    middle temporal c.
    posterior central c.
    second temporal c.
    superior frontal c.
    superior temporal c.
    supramarginal c.
    third temporal c.
    transitional c.
    transverse temporal c.'s
    Zuckerkandl c.
convulsant threshold
convulsion
    apoplectiform c.
    benign familial neonatal c.
    brain c.
    central c.
    cerebral c.
    cerebrospinal c.
    clonic c.
    conversion disorder with seizures
      or c.
    coordinate c.
    eclamptic c.
    epileptic c.
    epileptiform c.
    essential c.
    ether c.
    febrile c.
    GTC c.
    hysterical c.
    hysteroid c.
    immediate posttraumatic c.
    infantile c.
    jacksonian c.
    local c.
    mimetic c.
    mimic c.
    myoclonic c.
    paroxysmal c.
    psychomotor c.
    puerperal c.
    reflex c.
    repetitive c.
    salaam c.
    spasmodic c.
    spontaneous c.
    static c.
    tetanic c.
    tonic c.
    toxic c.
    uncinate c.
    uremic c.
convulsive
    c. disorder
    c. equivalent
    c. melancholia
    c. reflex

C

convulsive (*continued*)
    c. seizure
    c. shock therapy
    c. state
    c. status epilepticus
    c. syncope
    c. tic
convulsivus
    status c.
co-occurrence of depression
co-occurring
    c.-o. association
    c.-o. mental disorder
cookbook
    c. diagnosis
    c. fashion
Cook-Medley Hostility Scale
Cook stereotaxic guide
Cooley anemia
cooling
    c. of affect
    autocerebral c.
    brain c.
    c. helmet
    nasopharyngeal c.
    whole-body c.
Coombs test
cooperation
    morality of c.
cooperative
    c. behavior
    c. education
    c. institutional research program
    (CIRP)
    c. motive
    C. Primary Test (CPT)
    c. psychotherapy
    c. reward structure
    c. therapy
    c. training
    c. urban house
Cooper-Farran Behavioral Rating Scale (CFBRS)
Cooper-MacGuire Diagnostic Word Analysis Test
coordinate
    c. convulsion
    MEG sensorimotor mapping c.
    c. seizure
    Z c.
coordinated
    c. epilepsy
    c. reflex
coordination
    c. developmental delay disorder
    eye-hand c.
    fine motor c.
    motor c.
    subaverage motor c.
    visual-motor c.
coordinatus
    spasmus c.
COP
    colloid oncotic pressure

COP 1
    copolymer 1
coparental divorce
Copaxone
COPE
    Coping Operations Preference Enquiry
    Coping Orientations to Problems
    Experienced
COPES
    Community-Oriented Programs
    Environment Scale
copharmacy
cophica
    alalia c.
coping
    c. ability
    c. behavior
    ideational style of c.
    c. inventory
    c. mechanism
    C. Operations Preference Enquiry
    (COPE)
    C. Orientations to Problems
    Experienced (COPE)
    rational/cognitive c.
    C. Resources Inventory (CRI)
    c. skill
    c. strategy
    c. strategy enhancement (CSE)
    c. style
    C. with Stress Test
copodyskinesia
copolymer
    c. 1 (COP 1)
    glatirama c.-1
copper
    c. deposition
    serum c.
    c. sulfate hydrogel
    c. wire effect
copper-constantan thermocouple
coprolagnia
coprolalia
    multiple tics with c.
    tic convulsif with c.
coprolalomania
coprology
coprophagia, coprophagy
coprophagous
coprophemia disorder
coprophil, coprophilic
coprophilia
coprophobia
coprophrasia
copropraxia
coprostasophobia
COPS
    California Occupational Preference
    Survey
COPSystem Interest Inventory
copula
copulate
copulation
copulatory behavior

copy
 c. geometric designs test
 c. intersecting pentagons test
 Rey-Osterrieth Complex Figure C.
copy-cat suicide
copying
 C. Drawings with Landmarks
 (CDL)
 c. mania
coquetting
 flirting and c.
coral
 madreporic c.
 scleractinian c.
cord
 Bergmann c.
 c. bladder
 dura mater of the spinal c.
 c. embarrassment
 glioma of the spinal c.
 Lissauer tracts of spinal c.
 spinal c.
 subacute combined degeneration of
 the spinal c.
 c. syndrome
 tethered spinal c.
 vocal c.
 Weitbrecht c.
 Wilde c.
cordectomy
cordis
 chorea c.
 C. implantable drug reservoir
 device
 C. Secor implantable pump
Cordis-Hakim
 C.-H. shunt system
 C.-H. valve
cordopexy
cordotomy
 anterolateral c.
 c. hook holder
 open c.
 percutaneous c.
 posterior column c.
 spinothalamic c.
 stereotactic c.
core
 c. assessment program for
 intracerebral transplantation
 (CAPIT)
 c. body balance
 c. body temperature
 central transactional c.
 c. construct
 c. gender identity
 c. mindfulness skills
 c. sense of identity
corectopia
corencephalopathy
coreoathetoid movement
Corgard
cork the air
corkscrew dural hook

corneal
 c. anesthesia
 c. anoxia
 c. reflex
 c. respiration
 c. suffocation
Cornelia de Lange syndrome
Cornell
 C. Critical Thinking Tests, Level
 X and Level Z
 C. Depression Scale
 C. Learning and Study Skills
 Inventory (CLASSI)
 C. Medical Index
 C. Scale for Depression, Dementia
 (CSDD)
 C. Word Form (CWF)
corn-picker's pupil
cornu, gen. cornus, pl. cornua
 c. ammonis
 c. anterius
 c. inferius
 c. inferius cartilaginis thyroideae
 c. inferius hiatus saphenus
 c. inferius ventriculi lateralis
 c. laterale
 cornua of lateral ventricle
 c. posterius
 c. posterius ventriculi lateralis
 cornua of spinal cord
corollary discharge
corona, pl. coronae
 c. radiata
 Zinn c.
coronal
 c. cleft vertebra
 c. craniectomy
 c. orientation
 c. plane
 c. plane deformity
 c. plane deformity sagittal
 translation
 c. scalp incision
 c. section
 c. suture
 c. synostosis
coronary
 c. artery disease
 Global Utilization of Streptokinase
 and Tissue Plasminogen Activator
 for Occluded C. (GUSTO-1)
coronata
 Cryptococcus c.
corpectomy
 anterior c.
 cervical c.
 median c.
 c. model
 vertebral body c.
corpora (*pl. of* corpus)
corporal
 c. agnosia
 c. punishment
corporeal

C

corpulent
corpus, gen. **corporis**, pl. **corpora**
  c. amygdaloideum
  c. aorticum
  c. arenacea
  corpora arenacea
  corpora arenacea
  corpora bigemina
  c. callosal impingement
  c. callosotomy
  c. callosum
  c. callosum agenesis
  c. callosum dysgenesis
  c. callosum syndrome
  corpora cavernosa
  c. dentatum
  c. fimbriatum
  c. fornicis
  c. geniculatum externum
  c. geniculatum internum
  c. geniculatum laterale
  c. geniculatum mediale
  habeas c.
  c. luysi
  c. luysii
  c. mamillare
  c. medullare cerebelli
  c. nuclei caudati
  c. olivare
  c. paraterminale
  c. pineale
  c. pontobulbare
  corpora quadrigemina
  corpora quadrigemina
  c. quadrigeminum anterius
  c. quadrigeminum posterius
  c. restiforme
  c. spongiosum
  c. striatum
  c. trapezoideum
corpuscle
  articular c.
  axile c.
  axis c.
  bulboid c.
  Dogiel c.
  genital c.
  Golgi-Mazzoni c.
  lamellated c.
  Mazzoni c.
  Meissner c.
  Merkel c.
  oval c.
  pacchionian c.
  pacinian c.
  Purkinje c.
  Ruffini c.
  tactile c.
  terminal nerve c.
  touch c.
  Valentin c.
  Vater c.
  Vater-Pacini c.
corpusculum, pl. **corpuscula**
  corpuscula articularia

  corpuscula bulboidea
  corpuscula genitalia
  corpuscula lamellosa
  corpuscula nervosa terminalia
  c. tactus, pl. corpuscula tactus
correction
  age c.
  anterior c.
  King type IV curve posterior c.
  kyphosis c.
  mechanism of c.
  rotational c.
  surgical c.
correctional
  c. facility
  C. Institutions Environment Scale (CIES)
  C. Officers' Interest Blank
  c. psychiatry
  c. psychology
  c. transfer (CT)
corrective
  c. emotional experience
  c. feedback
  c. technique
  c. therapist
  c. therapy (CT)
correlate
  psychophysiologic c.
correlation
  canonical c.
  c. coefficient
  coefficient of c.
  image c.
  multiple c.
  negative c.
  partial c.
  positive c.
  product-moment c.
  rank c.
  rank-difference c.
  c. ratio
  c. redundancy
  c. study
  c. time
correlational method
correlative
  objective c.
correspondence
  cross c.
  point-for-point c.
corridor
  transcallosal interforniceal c.
corroborating dream
corrosive
corset, corsette
  lumbosacral c.
  Warm 'n Form lumbosacral c.
Cor-Tech guidance to stereotatic head frame
Cortef
cortex, gen. **corticis**, pl. **cortices**
  adrenal c.
  agranular c.
  allocortical c.

anterior cingulate c.
articular c.
association c.
auditory c.
calcarine c.
cellular layers of c.
cerebellar c.
c. cerebelli
cerebral c.
c. cerebri
cingulate c.
deep c.
dorsal premotor c.
dorsolateral prefrontal c.
dysgranular c.
eloquent c.
entorhinal c.
excitomotor c.
extrastriate V5/MT c.
extrinsic c.
frontal c.
granular c.
heterotypic c.
homotypic c.
inferior temporal c. (ITC)
insular c.
laminated c.
language associated c.
layer of cerebellar c.
layer of cerebral c.
limbic c.
mesial c.
mesial-frontal c.
mesial prefrontal c.
motor c.
olfactory c.
opercular c.
orbitofrontal c.
parastriate c.
parietal c.
perilesional inhibitory c.
perirolandic parietal c.
peristriate c.
perisylvian c.
piriform c.
posterior parietal c.
prefrontal c.
premotor c.
primary auditory c.
primary visual c.
pyriform c.
rolandic c.
secondary sensory c.
secondary visual c.
sensory c.
somatic sensory c.,
  somatosensory c.
striate c.
supplementary motor c.
supramarginal/angular c.
temporal cortices
temporal c.
temporoparietal intrasylvian c.
vertebral body anterior c.
visual c.

Cortexplorer cerebral blood flow monitor
Corti
C. cell
C. ganglion
organ of C.
C. organ
C. pillar
C. rod
cortical
c. alexia
c. amnesia
c. aphasia
c. apraxia
c. atrophy
c. center
c. column
c. convexity
c. deafness
c. epilepsy
c. evoked potential
c. gray matter
c. gray matter deficit
c. hamartoma
c. incision coronary dilator
c. infarction
c. language circuitry
c. lateralization
c. lesion
c. mapping
c. mapping of memory function
c. microcirulatory flow
c. myoclonus
c. network
c. neuron
c. organization
c. plate
c. psychic blindness
c. reorganization
c. resection
c. screw
c. sensibility
c. sensory loss
c. somatosensory evoked potential (CSSEP)
c. sulcus
c. syndrome
c. testing
c. thumb position
c. tissue
c. transient ischemia
c. undercutting
c. vein
c. zone
cortical-basal ganglionic degeneration
cortical-evoked response
corticalization
cortical-striatal-pallidal-thalamic neural circuit
cortical-subcortical network activity
corticectomy
frontal c.
occipital c.
parietal c.
cortices (*pl. of* cortex)

corticifugal
corticipetal
corticis (*gen. of* cortex)
corticoadrenal insufficiency
corticoafferent
corticobulbar
 c. fiber
 c. motor neuron
 c. pathway
 c. tract
corticocancellous strut
corticocerebellum
corticoefferent
corticofugal pathway
corticography
corticoid therapy
corticomedial
corticomeningeal angiomatosis
corticonuclear fiber
corticopontine
 c. fiber
 c. tract
corticoreticular fiber
corticospinal
 c. axon
 c. disease
 c. fiber
 c. motor neuron
 c. motor pathway
 c. motor system dysfunction
 c. pathway lesion
 c. tract (CST)
corticosteroid
 postoperative c.
corticothalamic
corticotomy
 Ilizarov c.
 subperiosteal c.
corticotroph cell
corticotropin
corticotropin-releasing
 c.-r. factor (CRF)
 c.-r. hormone (CRH)
cortin
cortisol
 plasma c.
 c. secretion
 c. and sodium succinate
cortisone acetate
Cortone acetate
Cortrosyn
coruscation
corybantism
Corynebacterium diphtheriae
Corzide
Cosman-Roberts-Wells (CRW)
 C.-R.-W. stereotactic frame
 C.-R.-W. stereotactic ring
 C.-R.-W. stereotactic system
Cosman telesensor
cosmetic mastoidectomy
cosmic
 c. consciousness
 c. identification
 c. sensitivity

cost
 maximum allowable c. (MAC)
costal arch reflex
Costa/McCrae factor
costaricensis
 Angiostrongylus c.
cost-benefit analysis
Costen syndrome
costocervical artery
costoclavicular syndrome
costopectoral reflex
costotransversectomy approach
costotransverse ligament
costovertebral ligament
cost-reward
 c.-r. analysis
 c.-r. model
cosyntropin
Cotard syndrome
co-therapy
cotinine
 serum c.
cotransmitter
 peptide c.
Cotrel
 C. pedicle screw
 C. pedicle screw fixation strength
 C. pedicle screw rigidity
Cotrel-Dubousset (C-D)
 C.-D. distraction system
 C.-D. dynamic transverse traction device
 C.-D. fixation
 C.-D. hook claw configuration
 C.-D. pedicle screw instrumentation
 C.-D. pedicular instrumentation
 C.-D. rod
 C.-D. rod flexibility
 C.-D. screw-rod system
 C.-D. spinal instrumentation
co-trimoxazole
cottage plan
Cotte
 C. operation
 C. presacral neurectomy
Cottle
 C. elevator
 C. knife
Cottle-Neivert retractor
cotton
 oxidized c.
 c. pad
 c. paddies
 c. pledget
 c. wool spot
 c. wrap
cottonoid pledget
cotunnii
 aqueductus c.
Cotunnius
 C. aqueduct
 C. canal
 C. disease
couch
 analytic c.

Boston neurosurgical c.
Siemens c.
couch-mounted head frame
cough
    c. headache
    c. preparations with codeine
    psychogenic c.
    c. reflex
could not test (CNT)
coulomb
Coumadin
council
    C. for Exceptional Children
    Medical Research C. (MRC)
    C. on Children, Adolescents, and
      Their Families
    C. on Psychiatric Services
counseling
    abuse c.
    adolescent c.
    alcohol c.
    career c.
    c. center
    child-placement c.
    clinical c.
    conjoint c.
    crisis c.
    divorce c.
    eclectic c.
    educational c.
    family c.
    followup c.
    genetic c.
    group c.
    individual c.
    c. interview
    c. inventory
    c. ladder
    marital c.
    marriage c.
    parent-child conflict c.
    pastoral c.
    placement c.
    premarital c.
    c. process
    c. psychologist
    c. psychology
    reevaluation c.
    reinforcement c.
    c. relationship
    c. service
    sex c.
    vocational c.
counselor
    career c.
    chemical dependency c. (CDC)
    child c.
    couples c.
    disability c.
    drug c.
    family c.
    genetic c.
    grief c.
    guidance c.
    individual c.

industrial rehabilitation c.
legal c.
Licensed Marriage Family and
    Child C. (LMFCC)
licensed professional c. (LPC)
marital c.
marriage c.
mental health c.
pastoral c.
personal c.
professional c.
rehabilitation c.
school c.
spiritual c.
substance abuse c.
youth c.
counselor-centered therapy
count
    absolute neutrophil c. (ANC)
    c. backwards from 100 test
    blood c.
    platelet c.
    reticulocyte c.
    sponge c.
counter
    c. conditioning
    over the c. (OTC)
counterculture
countercurrent
    c. immunoelectrophoresis (CIE)
    c. immunoelectrophoresis test
counterego
counterintuitive relationship
counterphobia
counterphobic attitude
Counterpoint electromyograph
countertransference
    c. behavior
    c. neurosis
counter-wish dream
counting
    c. money tremor
    c. obsession
coup injury of brain
couple member
couples
    c. counselor
    c. group therapy
    C. Pre-Counseling Inventory
    c. sex therapy
coupling
    G-protein c.
    spin-spin c.
Cournand arteriogram needle
Cournand-Grino arteriogram needle
course
    atypical c.
    clinical c.
    continuous c.
    deteriorating c.
    episodic c.
    global c.
    c. of illness
    life c.
    longitudinal c.

C

course *(continued)*
 rapid-cycling c.
 c. specifier
 c. of treatment
court
 c. of domestic relations
 juvenile c.
 c. of law
 c. order
 supreme c.
 traffic c.
 trial c.
court-mandated evaluation
courtroom psychology
courtship behavior
couvade crapulent
covariance
 analysis of c. (ANCOVA)
 multivariate analysis of c.
 (MANCOVA)
covariate
covenant
 crapulous c.
cover
 Accu-Flo polyethylene bur hole c.
 Accu-Flo silicone rubber bur
 hole c.
 bur hole c.
 titanium mini bur hole c.
covering
 titanium mini bur hole c.
covert
 c. anxiety
 c. behavior
 c. feeling
 c. hostility
 c. message
 c. modeling
 c. reinforcement
 c. resentment
 c. resistance
 c. response
 c. sensitization
 c. visuospatial attention
covetous
Covi Anxiety Scale
Cowden disease
Cowdry-type intranuclear inclusion body
CO_2-withdrawal seizure test
COX
 cytochrome c oxidase
Coxsackie encephalitis
coxsackievirus
 c. A
 c. B
 c. meningitis
CP
 child psychiatry
 child psychology
CPA
 cyproterone acetate
CPAB
 Computer Programmer Aptitude Battery

CPAP
 continuous positive airway pressure
CPI
 California Personality Inventory
 California Psychological Inventory
 constitutional psychopathia inferior
 constitutional psychopathic inferiority
CPIT
 California Psychological Inventory Test
CPK
 creatine phosphokinase
CPP
 career planning program
 cerebral perfusion pressure
 conditioned place preference
 cranial perfusion pressure
CPQ
 Children's Personality Questionnaire
 Conners Parent Questionnaire
CPRS
 Children's Psychiatric Rating Scale
 Comprehensive Psychiatric Rating Scale
CPS
 Child Personality Scale
 Children's Protective Service
 clinical performance score
 complex partial seizure
 Comrey Personality Scale
 constitutional psychopathic state
 cumulative probability of success
CPSCS
 California Preschool Social Competency
 Scale
CPSI
 Children's Perception of Support
 Inventory
CPSR
 chronic paranoid schizophrenic reaction
CPT
 carnitine palmitoyltransferase
 combining power test
 Concentration Performance Test
 Continuous Performance Test
 Cooperative Primary Test
 CPT disease
CQ
 Nicoderm CQ
CR103
 OncoScint CR103
crack
 c. craving
 c. cut with lidocaine
 c. diluted with cocaine
 c. dipped in phencyclidine
 c. equipment
 c. liquid and phencyclidine
 c. and lysergic acid diethylamide
 c. use
 c. vial
crack-like vessel
crackling
 parchment c.
craft
 c. neurosis
 c. palsy

Cragg thrombolytic brush
Craig vertebral body biopsy instrument
cramp
 accessory c.
 c. benign fasciculation
 benign fasciculation with c.
 intermittent c.
 miner's c.
 muscle c.
 musician's c.
 occupational c.
 pianist's c.
 piano player's c.
 seamstress's c.
 shaving c.
 stoker's c.
 tailor's c.
 typist's c.
 violinist's c.
 waiter's c.
 watchmaker's c.
 Wernicke c.
crania (*pl. of* cranium)
cranial
 c. aneurysm
 c. anomaly
 c. arteritis
 c. bifida
 c. bone fixation plate
 c. bone graft
 c. capacity
 c. computed tomography (CCT)
 c. cuff
 c. dermal sinus
 c. dysmorphia
 c. epidural abscess
 c. extension
 c. flexure
 c. fracture
 c. Jacobs hook
 c. motor nuclei (CMN)
 c. muscle
 c. nerve
 c. nerve abnormality
 c. nerve deficit
 c. nerve dissection
 c. nerve manipulation
 c. nerve monitoring
 c. nerve neoplasm
 c. nerve palsy
 c. neuralgia
 c. neuropathy
 c. osteomyelitis
 c. osteopetrosis
 c. osteosynthesis
 c. osteosynthesis system
 c. perforator
 c. perfusion pressure (CPP)
 c. plating system
 c. radiosurgery
 c. rongeur
 c. rongeur forceps
 c. root
 c. settling
 c. suture

 c. trauma
 c. vault
 c. venous obstruction
craniales
 nervi c.
cranialis
cranialization
craniamphitomy
craniectomy
 bilateral c.
 coronal c.
 decompressive c.
 linear c.
 metopic c.
 partial-thickness c.
 retromastoid suboccipital c.
 retrosigmoid c.
 suboccipital c.
cranii
 osteoporosis circumscripta c.
cranioblade
 Acra-Cut c.
 Codman c.
craniocardiac reflex
craniocele
craniocerebral
 c. drug trauma
 trauma c.
craniocervical
 c. junction
 c. plate
 c. region
craniofacial
 c. angle
 c. anomaly
 c. condition
 c. dysjunction
 c. dysostosis
 c. dysraphism
 c. malformation
 c. osteotomy
 c. reconstruction
 c. remodeling
 c. surgery
craniofrontonasal dysplasia
craniognomy
craniolacunia
craniology
 Gall c.
craniomalacia
 circumscribed c.
craniomaxillofacial plating system
craniomeningocele
craniometaphyseal
 dysplasia c.
 c. dysplasia
craniometry
cranioorbital
 c. deformity
 c. zygomatic craniotomy
craniopathy
craniopharyngeal canal
craniopharyngioma
 cystic c.

C

craniopharyngioma *(continued)*
    cystic papillomatous c.
    monocystic c.
cranioplasty
    acrylic c.
    alloplastic c.
    aluminum c.
    cartilage c.
    metallic c.
    methylmethacrylate c.
    c. plate
    rib c.
    tantalum c.
    vascularized split calvarial c.
craniopuncture
craniorrhachischisis
craniosacral system
cranioschisis
craniosclerosis
cranioscopy
craniosinus fistula
craniospinal
    c. meningioma
    c. space
craniostenosis
craniosynostosis
    lambdoid c.
craniotabes
craniotome
    Anspach c.
    Caspar c.
    Freiberg c.
    Hall neurosurgical c.
    Midas Rex c.
    Mira Mark V c.
    Smith air c.
craniotomy
    attached c.
    bifrontal c.
    cranioorbital zygomatic c.
    CT-assisted stereotactic c.
    c. cut
    detached c.
    endoscope-assisted c.
    c. flap
    frontal c.
    frontotemporal c.
    frontotemporoparietal c.
    open stereotactic c.
    orbital zygomatic c.
    osteoplastic c.
    parietal c.
    parietooccipital c.
    posterior fossa c.
    pterional c.
    radical decompressive c.
    retromastoid c.
    right parietal occipital vertex c.
    right temporoparietal c.
    stereotactic-guided c.
    stereotactic microsurgical c.
    subfrontal c.
    suboccipital c.
    supratentorial c.

    temporooccipital c.
    trephine c.
    Yasargil c.
craniotonoscopy
craniotrypesis
craniovertebral junction
cranium, pl. **crania**
    beaten copper c.
    bifid c.
    c. bifidum
cranium-affixed fiducial
crankshaft clip
crapulent
    couvade c.
crapulous covenant
CRAS
    Clinician Rated Anxiety Scale
crash
    depressive c.
    c. induction of anesthesia
crave
craving
    C. Analog Scale
    crack c.
    cue-elicited c.
    drug c.
    food c.
Crawford dural elevator
crazy
    fear of going c.
CRC
    cross-reacting cannabinoid
CRD
    complex repetitive discharge
    CRD on electromyogram
C-reactive
    C.-r. protein (CRP)
    C.-r. protein test
    C.-r. protein value
cream
    Zonalon Topical C.
crease
    simian c.
creatine phosphokinase (CPK)
creatinine
    urinary c.
creation
    kyphosis c.
    lordosis c.
creative
    c. self
    c. talent
    c. thinking
creativeness
creativity
    C. Assessment Packet
    C. Attitude Survey (CAS)
    C. Checklist
    c. test
    C. Tests for Children (CTC)
credence
credibility
    witness c.
credible
Creed dissector

creeping
    c. palsy
    c. substitution
creeping-crawling sensation
cremasteric reflex
cremnomania
cremnophobia
crepitance
crepuscular state
crescendo
    c. sleep
    c. transient ischemic attack
crescendo-decrescendo breathing
crescentic
    c. glomerulonephritis
    c. lobules of the cerebellum
cresomania
CREST
    calcinosis, Raynaud phenomenon,
      esophageal dysmotility, sclerodactyly,
      and telangiectasia
    CREST syndrome
crest
    acoustic c.
    acousticofacial c.
    ampullary c.
    basilar c. of cochlear duct
    cap of the ampullary c.
    falciform c.
    ganglionic c.
    neural c.
    neuroepithelium of ampullary c.
    transverse c.
    trigeminal c.
    vestibular c.
    c. of vestibule
cretin
cretinism
cretinistic
cretinoid idiocy
cretinous
Creutzfeldt-Jakob
    C.-J. disease (CJD)
    C.-J. syndrome
CRF
    corticotropin-releasing factor
CRH
    corticotropin-releasing hormone
CRI
    Caring Relationship Inventory
    Composite Risk Index
    Coping Resources Inventory
crib death
criblé
    état c.
cribriform plate
cribrosa, pl. cribrosae
    lamina c.
    macula c.
    maculae cribrosae
cribrosus
    status c.
Crichton-Browne sign
cricoarytenoid ankylosis
cricoid ring

cricopharyngeal achalasia
cricothyroid paralysis
cricothyrotomy
cri de coeur
cri-du-chat syndrome
Crigler-Najjar
    C.-N. disease
    C.-N. syndrome
Crile
    C. artery forceps
    C. clamp
    C. gasserian ganglion knife
    C. gasserian ganglion knife and
      dissector
    C. head traction
    C. hemostat
    C. needle holder
    C. nerve hook
    C. nerve hook and dissector
    C. retractor
crime
    C. Classification Manual (CCM)
    c. a deux
    heinous c.
    multiple personality c.
    c. of passion
criminal
    c. abortion
    c. act
    c. activity
    c. anthropology
    c. behavior
    c. commitment
    c. degeneracy
    habitual c.
    c. hygiene
    c. insanity
    c. irresponsibility
    c. profile
    c. psychiatry
    c. psychology
    c. response
    c. responsibility
    c. sexual psychopath (CSP)
criminally insane
crimmie
cripple
    social c.
crisis, pl. crises
    accidental c.
    adolescent c.
    adrenal c.
    bed c.
    catathymic c.
    c. center
    cholinergic c.
    c. consultation
    c. counseling
    c. effect
    emotional c.
    C. Evaluation Referral Service
      (CERS)
    existential c.
    financial c.
    gastric c.

C

crisis *(continued)*
  c. group
  c. hotline
  hypertensive c.
  identity c.
  c. intervention
  c. intervention clinic (CIC)
  laryngeal c.
  life c.
  magnetic c.
  c. management
  maturational c.
  mesmeric c.
  midlife c.
  myasthenic c.
  normative c.
  oculocephalogyric c.
  oculogyric crises
  oral c.
  parkinsonian c.
  precipitating c.
  psychogenic oculogyric c.
  psychosexual identity c.
  rapprochement c.
  c. residential care
  c. resolution
  resolution of c.
  situational c.
  spondylolisthetic c.
  suicidal c.
  tabetic c.
  c. team
  c. theory
  therapeutic c.
  c. therapy
  tumarcin c.
  tyramine-induced hypertensive c.
  unanticipated c.
  urban c.
  widowhood c.
crisis-intervention group psychotherapy
crista, pl. **cristae**
  c. ampullaris
  c. basilaris ductus cochlearis
  c. galli
  c. quarta
  c. transversa
  c. vestibuli
criteria-defined borderline personality disorder
criterion, pl. **criteria**
  C. A
  C. A2
  abuse c.
  criteria are not met for
  C. B
  Bartel criteria
  c. behavior
  behavioral c.
  C. C
  clinical significance c.
  clustering c.
  C. D
  c. data

death criteria
diagnostic criteria
c. dimension
C. E
equivalent c.
equivalent criteria
equivalent intoxication c.
equivalent withdrawal c.
evaluation of c.
c. evaluation
exclusion c.
exclusion criteria
Family History Research Diagnostic Criteria
full symptom c.
c. group
criteria have never been met for
Hunt and Hess criteria
impairment c.
method of defining c.
Mulholland and Gunn criteria
Nyquist sampling criteria
criteria of Rechtschaffen
criteria of Rechtschaffen and Kales
relevant diagnostic criteria
relevant diagnostic c.
Research Diagnostic Criteria (RDC)
criteria of Rowland
Schooler-Kane criteria
symptom criteria
C. Test of Basic Skills
theta c.
Thorndike-Lorge criteria
c. variable
Volpe criteria
von Knorring c.
White and Panjabi criteria
withdrawal criteria
criterion-referenced test
criterion-related validity
Crithidia **IFA test**
critical
  c. age
  c. analysis
  c. band concept
  c. flicker frequency
  c. illness myopathy
  c. illness polyneuropathy (CIP)
  c. judgment
  c. perfusion
  c. period
  c. point
  c. ratio
  C. Reasoning Test (CRT)
  c. region
  c. review
  c. score
  c. submodalities
  c. thinking
  c. value
critical-incident technique
Criticare
criticism
  ability to take c.
  constructive c.

destructive c.
implied c.
objective c.
overt c.
parental c.
peer c.
professional c.
criticus
status c.
critique
age c.
Crixivan
CRN
cerebral radiation necrosis
crochet
main en c.
crocidismus
Crockard
C. retractor
C. transoral clip applier
crocodile
c. tears
c. tears syndrome
Crohn disease
Crooke
C. granule
C. hyalinization
CROS
contralateral routing of signals
contralateral routing of sound
cross
c. adaptation
c. addiction
c. birth
c. conditioning
c. correspondence
c. dependence
c. dressing
c. fostering
Ranvier c.
c. sectional study
c. tolerance
c. validation
cross-bracing
spinal rod c.-b.
Wiltse system c.-b.
cross-correlation mechanism
cross-cultural
C.-c. Adaptability Inventory (CCAI)
c.-c. psychiatry
c.-c. testing
cross-culture approach
cross-dressing
c.-d. behavior
complete c.-d.
forced c.-d.
motivation for c.-d.
partial c.-d.
crossed
c. adductor jerk
c. adductor reflex
c. adductor sign
c. anesthesia
c. coil
c. dominance

c. extension reflex
c. eye
c. hemianesthesia
c. hemiplegia
c. knee jerk
c. knee reflex
c. laterality
c. paralysis
c. phrenic phenomenon
c. pyramidal tract
c. reflex of pelvis
c. spinoadductor reflex
crossed-screw fixation
cross-facial nerve graft anastomosis
cross-flow reserve
cross-gender
c.-g. behavior
forced c.-g.
c.-g. identification
c.-g. interest
cross-legged clip
crosslink
Edwards modular system rod c.
Galveston fixation with TSRH c.
Texas Scottish Rite Hospital c.
cross-linkage theory
crossmatch
blood c.
cross-modality perception
crossover
c. mirroring
c. study
cross-reacting cannabinoid (CRC)
cross-sectional
c.-s. area (CSA)
c.-s. definition
c.-s. image
c.-s. method
c.-s. prevalence
cross-sex role
crossway
sensory c.
Crouzon
C. disease
C. syndrome
CR/OV
OncoScint C.
crowd
c. behavior
c. consciousness
c. control
c. fear
crowded place
Crow-Fukase syndrome
Crowley Occupational Interests Blank (COIB)
crown
Bremer halo c.
radiate c.
Crown-Crisp Experiential Inventory
crown-rump length
CRP
C-reactive protein
CRPS
complex regional pain syndrome

CRS
Clinical Rating Scale
CRS-39
Conners Teacher Rating Scale
CRT
Critical Reasoning Test
crucial
cruciata
hemiplegia c.
cruciate ligament
crucifixion attitude
cruciform slit valve
crude
c. consciousness
c. opium
cruel
cruising
compulsive c.
crural
c. ataxia
c. cistern
c. monoplegia
c. paresis
crus, gen. cruris, pl. crura
c. anterius capsulae internae
c. cerebri
common c.
c. fornicis
c. of fornix
c. I
c. II
crura membranacea ampullaria
c. membranaceum commune ductus semicircularis
c. membranaceum simplex ductus semicircularis
crura ossea canales semicirculares
c. posterius capsulae internae
crush
c. injury
c. syndrome
crushes in adolescence
crusotomy
crutch
c. palsy
c. paralysis
Crutchfield
C. carotid artery clamp
C. drill point
C. hand drill
C. skeletal traction tongs
C. skull traction tongs
Crutchfield-Raney skull traction tongs
Cruveilhier disease
Cruz trypanosomiasis
CRVS
California Relative Value Studies
CRW
Cosman-Roberts-Wells
CRW arc system
CRW base frame
CRW head frame
CRW stereotactic system
CRx valve

cry
birth c.
epileptic c.
hue and c.
c. reflex
cryalgesia
cryanesthesia
cryesthesia
crying
c. jag
c. spell
crymodynia
cryoanalgesia
cryocooler assembly
Cryocup ice massager
cryoglobulinemia
cryohypophysectomy
transphenoidal c.
cryolesion
brain c.
cryomagnet
cryomania
cryomicrotome sectioning
cryopallidectomy
cryophobia
cryoprecipitate coagulum
cryoprobe
cryopulvinectomy
cryospasm
cryostat
cryosurgery
cryothalamectomy
cryptanamnesia
cryptesthesia
cryptic
c. arteriovenous malformation
c. depression
c. vascular malformation (CVM)
cryptococcal
granuloma c.
c. meningitis
c. spondylitis
cryptococcoma
cryptococcosis
intracranial c.
Cryptococcus
C. albicans
C. coronata
C. infection
C. neoformans
cryptogenic
c. drop attack
c. hemifacial spasm
c. infarction
c. infection
c. late-onset epilepsy
c. myoclonic epilepsy
c. seizure
c. symbolism
cryptomnesia
cryptophoric symbolism
cryptopsychic
cryptorchidism
cryptotia

crystal
cholesterol c.
c. gazing
crystalline
crystallization
crystallized
c. ability
c. grandiose delusion
c. intelligence
crystallophobia
CS
conditioned stimulus
CSA
Cognitive Skills Assessment
Controlled Substances Act
cross-sectional area
CSB I
chemistry screening battery I
CSB II
chemistry screening battery II
CSCS
Children's Self-Concept Scale
CSCT
central somatosensory conduction time
CSD
cat-scratch disease
CSDD
Cornell Scale for Depression, Dementia
CSE
coping strategy enhancement
CSF
cerebrospinal fluid
CSF outflow pathway
CSF shunt
C-shaped
C.-s. incision
C.-s. microplate
C.-s. resistive magnet
C.-s. scalp flap
CSI
Caregiver Strain Index
CSL
central sacral line
CSM
cervical spondylotic myelopathy
CSP
cavum septi pellucidi
criminal sexual psychopath
CSQ
College Student Questionnaire
CSR
continued-stay review
CSRI
Caregiver's School Readiness Inventory
CSSEP
cortical somatosensory evoked potential
CSSQ
College Student Satisfaction
Questionnaire
CST
Conceptual Systems Test
corticospinal tract
CSW
certified social worker

CT
Category Test
cerebral thrombosis
computed tomography
correctional transfer
corrective therapy
CT bone window
contiguous nonoverlapping axial CT
contrast-enhanced CT
metrizamide-enhanced CT
CT scan
serial CT
stable xenon CT
xenon CT
xenon-enhanced CT
CTA
computed tomographic angioplasty
CT-assisted stereotactic craniotomy
CTBS
California Test of Basic Skills
Canadian Tests of Basic Skills
CTC
Creativity Tests for Children
CTD
cumulative trauma disorder
CTF
Colorado tick fever
CT-guided
C.-g. biopsy
C.-g. stereotactic evacuation
CTI-Siemens 933/08-12 PET camera
CTI/Siemens 933 tomograph
CTM
cervical tension myositis
computed tomographic myelography
CTMM
California Test of Mental Maturity
computed tomographic metrizamide
myelography
CTMM-SF
California Short-Form Test of Mental
Maturity
California Test of Mental Maturity-Short
Form
CTP
California Test of Personality
CTQ
Conners Teacher Questionnaire
CTRS-28
Conners Teacher Rating Scale
CTS
Champion Trauma Score
CTT
central tegmental tract
CTVF
Comprehensive Test of Visual
Functioning
CTVHCS
Central Texas Veterans Health Care
System
CTX
cerebrotendinous xanthomatosis
C-type natriuretic peptide (CNP)

C

cubital
    c. tunnel
    c. tunnel syndrome
cuboidal cell
cuboidodigital reflex
cuddling behavior
cue
    accessing c.
    auditory distance c.
    conditioned c.
    contextual c.
    environmental c.
    c. exposure
    exposure to c.
    external c.
    eye accessing c.
    internal c.
    kinesthetic c.
    learning c.
    minimal c.
    orientation c.
    perceptual c.
    phase c.
    c. reduction
    response-produced c.
    semantic c.
    social c.
    visual c.
cued
    c. attack
    c. panic attack
    c. speech
cue-elicited craving
cueing
    semantic c.
CUES
    College and University Environment
    Scales
Cueva cranial nerve electrode
cuff
    cranial c.
    off the c.
    perivascular c.
cuffing
    perivascular c.
cuirass
    analgesic c.
    tabetic c.
Culler hook
culmen, pl. **culmina**
cult
    killer c.
    c. of personality
    personality c.
    religious c.
    satanic c.
cultural
    c. absolutism
    c. adaptability
    c. adjustment
    c. adjustment following migration
    c. anthropology
    c. area
    c. assessment
    c. assimilation

    c. attitude
    C. Attitude Inventory (CAI)
    C. Attitude Scale (CAS)
    c. background
    c. belief
    c. change
    c. context
    c. deprivation
    c. determinism
    c. disadvantage
    c. discrimination
    c. element
    c. experience
    c. factor
    c. formulation
    c. frame of reference
    c. identity
    c. inventory
    c. item
    c. lag
    C. Literacy Test
    c. norm
    c. parallelism
    c. process
    c. psychiatry
    c. reference group
    c. relativism
    c. role
    c. root
    c. shock
    c. subgroup
    c. testing
    c. training
    c. transmission
    c. variation
cultural-familial mental retardation
culturally
    c. appropriate avoidant behavior
    c. deprived
    c. different
    c. diverse population
    c. sanctioned
    c. sanctioned behavior
    c. sanctioned experience
    c. sanctioned response
    c. sanctioned symptom
    c. unsanctioned
    c. unsanctioned response
**cultural-related standards of sexual
    behavior**
culture
    adolescent c.
    cargo c.
    cerebellar aggregation c.
    coexistent c.
    c. complex
    configurative c.
    c. conflict
    drug c.
    C. Fair Intelligence Test (CFIT)
    C. Free Intelligence Test (CFIT)
    C. Free Test (CFT)
    host c.
    indigenous family c.
    individual's c.

industrialized c.
c. medium
c. of origin
person's c.
phallocentric c.
c. shock
C. Shock Inventory
street-drug c.
c. trait
youth c.
culture-bound
c.-b. belief
c.-b. syndrome
Culture-Free
C.-F. Self-Esteem Inventories for Children and Adults
C.-F. Self-Esteem Inventories, Second Edition (CFSEI-2)
culture-related feature
culture-specific
c.-s. feature
c.-s. syndrome
cumulative
c. drug action
C. Illness Rating Scale
C. Illness Rating Scale-Geriatric
c. probability of success (CPS)
c. record
c. response
c. response curve
c. scale
c. test
c. trauma disorder (CTD)
cuneate
c. fasciculus
c. funiculus
c. nucleus
cuneatus
fasciculus c. (Fc)
cunei (*pl. of* cuneus)
cuneiform lobe
cuneocerebellar tract
cuneus, pl. **cunei**
cunnilinguist
cunnilingus, cunnilinction, cunnilinctus
cunning and hiding behavior
cup
c. catheter
c. ear
c. forceps
ocular c.
optic c.
Cuprimine
cupula, pl. **cupulae**
c. cochleae
c. cristae ampullaris
cupular part
cupulate part
cupulolithiasis
cura
curandero, curanderismo
curare poisoning
curativa
indicatio c.

cure
faith c.
c. rate
talking c.
transference c.
work c.
curette, curet
blunt-ring c.
bone c.
Cloward-Cone ring c.
Cone ring c.
Cone suction biopsy c.
disk c.
downbiting Epstein c.
Epstein c.
flat back c.
Halle bone c.
Hardy c.
Hibbs spinal c.
Hibbs-Spratt spinal fusion c.
Howard spinal c.
Jansen bone c.
Malis c.
Marino transsphenoidal c.
Mayfield spinal c.
pituitary c.
Raney stirrup-loop c.
Ray pituitary c.
reverse-angled c.
Rhoton loop c.
Rhoton micro c.
Rhoton spoon c.
Richards c.
ring c.
Scoville disk c.
Scoville ruptured disk c.
secret c.
Semmes c.
straight ring c.
transsphenoidal c.
uterine c.
vertical ring c.
Yasargil micro c.
curiosity
sexual c.
curled-into-fetal-position posture
current
action c.
alternating c. (AC)
audiofrequency eddy c.
c. cognitive status
c. defense level
demarcation c.
direct c. (DC)
eddy c.
c. episode
inhibitory postsynaptic c.
c. of injury
c. night terror
C. and Past Psychopathology Scale (CAPPS)
radiofrequency eddy c.
c. tic
Current, Global, Psychiatric-Social Status (CGPS)

C

Curschmann-Steinert disease
curse
Ondine c.
cursing magic
cursiva
epilepsia c.
cursive epilepsy
Curtis
C. Completion Form
C. Interest Scale
curve
accommodation c.
bell-shaped c.
best-fit c.
cumulative response c.
distribution c.
dose-response c.
double thoracic c.
frequency dispersion c.
gaussian c.
isodose c.
Kaplan-Meier survival c.
King type I c.
King type II c.
King type III c.
King type IV c.
King type V c.
learning c.
logistic c.
low single thoracic c.
luetic c.
lumbar c.
normal c.
paretic c.
probability c.
response c.
right thoracic c.
rigid c.
severe rigid right thoracic c.
signal intensity c.
specific c.
thoracolumbar c.
time-density c.
curved
c. cannula with locking dilator
c. conventional microscissors
c. electrode
c. incision
c. knot-tying forceps
c. micro-needle holder
curved-tipped spatula
CUSA
Cavitron ultrasonic surgical aspirator
CUSA CEM system
CUSA electrosurgical module (CEM)
CUSA system 200 straight autoclavable handpiece
CUSA tip
Cushing
C. basophilia
C. bayonet forceps
C. bipolar forceps
C. bivalve retractor
C. brain forceps

C. brain spatula
C. brain spatula spoon
C. cranial bur
C. cranial perforator
C. cranial rongeur
C. decompressive retractor
C. disease
C. disk rongeur
C. dressing forceps
C. dural hook
C. dural hook knife
C. effect
C. gasserian ganglion hook
C. intervertebral disk rongeur
C. Little Joker elevator
C. monopolar forceps
C. nerve hook
C. nerve retractor
C. periosteal elevator
C. phenomenon
C. pituitary elevator
C. pituitary scoop
C. pituitary spoon
C. response
C. saw
C. saw guide
C. spatula spoon
C. staphylorrhaphy elevator
C. subtemporal retractor
C. syndrome
C. technique
C. tissue forceps
C. ulcer
C. vein retractor
C. ventricular needle
Cushing-Landolt speculum
cushingoid facies
cushion
Carter immobilization c.
custodial
c. care
c. parent
custody
Ackerman-Schoendorf Scales for Parent Evaluation of C. (ASPECT)
child c.
joint c.
parental c.
C. Quotient
c. quotient
single c.
split c.
custom
acculturation problem with expression of c.'s
foreign c.
c. implant
cut
craniotomy c.
Panama c.
visual field c.
cutaneomeningospinal angiomatosis
cutaneous
c. adenoma

c. anesthesia
c. angioma
c. experience
c. horn
c. meningioma
c. nerve
c. neurofibromatosis
c. psychogenic disorder
c. pupillary reflex
c. reaction
cut-film angiography
cutis
neuroma c.
cutter
dowel c.
Howmedica Microfixation System plate c.
Leibinger Micro System plate c.
cutting
wrist c.
CV
coefficient of variation
CVA
cerebrovascular accident
CVI
cavum veli interpositi
CVLT
California Verbal Learning Test
CVM
cerebral venous malformation
cryptic vascular malformation
CVMT
Continuous Visual Memory Test
CVRS
California Relative Value Studies
CWF
Cornell Word Form
CX-516
ampakine C.
cyad
cyamemazine
cyanide
c. antidote kit
c. poisoning
cyanoacrylate
c. glue
isobutyl-2 c.
N-butyl c.
cyanophilous
cyanopia
cyanosis
cyanotic syndrome of Scheid
cybernetic
c. theory
c. theory of aging
cybernetics
cybertherapy
Cyberware 3030RGB digitizer
CY-BOCS
Children's Yale-Brown Obsessive Compulsive Scale
cyclandelate
cyclase
adenylate c.

guanylate c.
guanylyl c.
cyclazocine
cycle
aberrant c.
c.'s of after-nystagmus
basic rest-activity c. (BRAC)
brain wave c.
circannual c.
citric acid c.
desire phase of sexual response c.
duration duty c.
estrous c.
excitement phase of sexual response c.
genesial c.
gonadal c.
late luteal phase of menstrual c.
c. length
life c.
menstrual c.
orgasmic phase of sexual response c.
perceptual c.
c.'s per second tremor
phase shift of sleep-wake c.
resolution phase of sexual response c.
sexual response c.
short c.
sleep c.
sleep-wake c.
urea c.
vicious c.
cycler
rapid c.
cyclic
c. abulia
c. adenosine monophosphate (cAMP)
c. deoxyribonucleic acid (cDNA)
c. endoperoxide
c. ether
c. guanosine monophosphate (cGMP)
c. headache
c. history
c. illness
c. insanity
c. medication
c. mood disorder
c. mood swing
c. schizophrenia
c. vomiting
cyclical
c. depression
c. pattern of symptoms
cyclin box
cyclin-dependent kinase inhibitory protein
cycline
cycling
futile c.
mood disorder with rapid c.

C

cycling *(continued)*
    phase c.
    rapid c.
cyclizine
cyclobarbital
cyclobenzaprine hydrochloride
cycloid
    c. personality
    c. psychosis
cyclooxygenase
    c. inhibitor
Cyclopan
cyclopentolate
cyclophenazine
cyclophosphamide
cyclophrenia
cycloplegia
cyclops lesion
cycloserine
cyclosporin A
cyclosporine
cyclothyme
cyclothymia
cyclothymiac, cyclothymic
    c. personality
    c. personality disorder
cyclothymic-depressive behavior
cyclothymosis
cycrimine hydrochloride
cyesis
Cylert
cylinder
    axis c.
cylindraxis
cylindroma
cymophobia
cynanthropy
cynic spasm
cynobex hebetis
cynomania
cynophobia
cynorexia
Cyon nerve
cyophoria
cypenamine
cyprazepam
cypridophobia, cypriphobia
cyprodenate
cyproheptadine hydrochloride
cyprolidol
cyproterone acetate (CPA)
cyproximide
cyst
    aneurysmal bone c.
    apoplectic c.
    arachnoid c.
    bilateral arachnoid c.
    bilateral choroid plexus c.
    bone c.
    brain c.
    cerebellar arachnoid c.
    cerebellopontine angle arachnoid c.
    cholesterol c.
    colloid c.

    Dandy-Walker c.
    daughter c.
    dermoid c.
    enteric c.
    enterogenous c.
    ependymal c.
    epidermoid c.
    extradural c.
    c. fenestration
    foramen magnum c.
    frontoparietal convexity c.
    giant sacral perineural c.
    glial parenchymal c.
    hydatid c.
    interhemispheric c.
    intracerebral hydatid c.
    intracranial arachnoid c.
    intradiploic epidermoid c.
    intramedullary epidermoid c.
    intraneural ganglion c.
    intraparenchymal c.
    intrasellar Rathke cleft c.
    leptomeningeal c.
    lumbar synovial c.
    middle cranial fossa c.
    nasopharyngeal mucus retention c.
    neural c.
    neuroenteric c.
    neuroepithelial c.
    nonenteric c.
    paraphysial c.
    paraventricular c.
    perineurial c.
    pineal c.
    pontine hydatid c.
    pontomedullary epidermoid c.
    porencephalic c.
    posttraumatic leptomeningeal c.
    primary epidural c.
    quadrigeminal arachnoid c.
    Rathke cleft c.
    Rathke pouch c.
    recurrent enteric c.
    retinal c.
    sacral nerve root c.
    sellar c.
    solitary hydatid c.
    spinal canal hydatid c.
    spinal endodermal c.
    spinal neurenteric c.
    spindle-shaped c.
    subperiosteal c.
    suprasellar c.
    synovial c.
    Tarlov c.
    temporal arachnoid c.
    xanthogranulomatous c.
    xanthomatous Rathke cleft c.
cystadenoma
    apocrine c.
    cystine c.
    eccrine c.
cystathionine synthetase deficiency
cystathioninuria aminoaciduria
cysteine proteinase

cystic
- c. craniopharyngioma
- c. encephalomalacia
- c. fibrosis
- c. hydroma
- c. intraparenchymal meningioma
- c. lacunar infarct
- c. medial necrosis
- c. microadenoma
- c. myelomalacia
- c. papillomatous craniopharyngioma
- c. periventricular leukomalacia

cystica
- spina bifida c.

cysticercal infection

cysticerci
- subarachnoid c.

cysticercosis

cysticerotic arachnoiditis

cystine cystadenoma

cystoatrial shunt

Cystografin

Cystokon

cystoma
- papilliferous c.

cystoscope
- Olympus neonatal c.

cytoarchitectonic abnormality

cytoarchitectonics

cytoarchitectural
- c. asymmetry
- c. organization

cytoarchitecture
- neural c.

cytochrome
- c. c oxidase (COX)
- c. oxidase defect
- c. P-450 2E1
- c. P450 metabolic enzyme

cytochrome-c oxidase deficiency

cytogenetics

cytogenic

cytoid body

cytokeratin
- c. immunostain
- low molecular weight c.

cytokine
- c. inhibitor
- interacting c.

cytology

cytolysis

cytomegalic inclusion disease

cytomegalovirus (CMV)

Cytomel

cytometry
- flow c.

cyton

cytopathy
- mitochondrial c.

cytophotometry
- Feulgen c.

cytoplasm

cytoplasmic microtubule

cytoprotective

cytoreduction

cytoreductive surgery

cytosine

cytoskeletal
- c. abnormality
- c. degradation
- c. protein

cytoskeletal-membrane event

cytotoxic
- c. drug
- c. edema

Cytoxan
- C. Injection
- C. Oral

Czerny suture

C

2D
two-dimensional
2D graphic localization
3D
three dimensional
3D positional adjustability
3D positional control
3D relationship analysis
3D titanium mini bone plate
/d
per day
δ-9-THC
delta-9-tetrahydrocannabinol
DAB-2
Diagnostic Achievement Battery, Second
Edition
DABS
Derogatis Affects Balance Scale
DAC
Depressive Adjective Checklist
DACA
Drug Abuse Control Amendments
dacarbazine
d'accoucheur
main d.
DACL
Depressive Adjective Checklist
DaCosta syndrome
Dacron
collagen-impregnated D.
dacryoadenitis
dacryocystic epilepsy
dacryocystitis
dactinomycin
dactylology
dactylophasia
dactylospasm
dad
deadbeat d.
DAF
dural arteriovenous fistula
DAG
diacylglycerol
dianhydrogalactitol
Dahlgren cranial rongeur
DAI
diffuse axonal injury
daily
d. dose
d. living
d. symptom rating
daily-living aids
Dalalone
DALE
Developmental Assessment of Life
Experiences
DALE System
Dale law
Dalgan
DALI
Dartmouth Assessment of Lifestyle
Instrument

Dalmane
DALYs
Disability Adjusted Life Years
DAMA
discharged against medical advice
damage
anoxic d.
anterior cervical surgery vocal
cord d.
brain cell d.
chronic tissue d.
hippocampal d.
Hunt-Minnesota Test for Organic
Brain D.
hypoxic brain d.
hypoxic-ischemic brain d.
ischemic brain d.
minimal brain d.
retraction-induced cerebral d.
Damasio and Damasio template
Damason-P
dammed-up
d.-u. emotion
d.-u. feeling
d.-u. libido
dammin
damn
damnable
damnify
damning
dampened waveform
d-amphetamine
damping effect
Dana
D. operation
D. posterior rhizotomy
danaparoid sodium
danazol
dance
d. education
d. fever
Saint Anthony's d.
Saint John's d.
Saint Vitus d.
shadow d.
song and d.
d. therapy
dancing
d. chorea
d. disease
d. eye
d. mania
d. spasm
Dandy
D. clamp
D. maneuver
D. myocutaneous scalp flap
D. nerve hook
D. neurological scissors
D. neurosurgical scissors
D. operation
D. probe

D

Dandy *(continued)*
 D. scalp hemostatic forceps
 D. suction tube
 D. trigeminal nerve scissors
 D. ventricular needle
Dandy-Walker
 D.-W. complex
 D.-W. cyst
 D.-W. malformation
 D.-W. syndrome
danger
 focus of anticipated d.
 future d.
 d. to others/self
dangerous
 d. behavior reaction
 d. drug
 d. to one's self
 d. to others
 d. patient
dangerousness
 acute d.
 prediction of d.
Danielssen-Boeck disease
Danielssen disease
Danocrine
Dantomania
Dantrium
dantrolene sodium
DAP
 Diversity Awareness Profile
 Draw-a-Person
 DAP Test
DAPP-BQ
 Dimensional Assessment of Personality
 Pathology-Basic Questionnaire
dapsone
DAP:SPED
 Draw A Person Screening Procedure for
 Emotional Disturbance
DAR
 Diagnostic Assessments of Reading
Daraprim
DARE
 Drug Abuse Resistance Education
dare
daredevil
dark
 d. adaptation
 d. environment
darkening vision
Darkschewitsch
 nucleus of D.
Dark Warrior epilepsy
D/ART
 Depression: Awareness, Recognition, and
 Treatment
 D/ART Campaign
**Dartmouth Assessment of Lifestyle
 Instrument (DALI)**
Darvocet
 D.-N
 D.-N 100
 D.-N 50

Darvon
 D. Compound
 D. Compound-65 Pulvules
 D. with ASA
Darvon-N
darwinian reflex
darwinism
 social d.
DAS
 Death Anxiety Scale
DASE
 Denver Articulation Screening Evaluation
Dasein analysis
DASI
 Developmental Activities Screening
 Inventory
DAT
 dementia of Alzheimer type
 Developmental Articulation Test
 Differential Aptitude Test
 DAT for PCA
data
 d. acquisition bandwidth
 d. acquisition system
 d. base
 biographical d.
 biologic d.
 d. collection
 criterion d.
 empirical d.
 epidemiological d.
 evaluability-assessment d.
 field d.
 historical d.
 identifying d.
 laboratory d.
 long-term d.
 NIMH d.
 normative d.
 paucity of d.
 Q d.
 d. reanalysis strategy
 reanalyzed d.
 d. set
 d. snooping
 survey d.
database
 Childhood Brain Tumor
 Consortium d.
 whole-brain mapping d.
date
 anniversary d.
 bind analysis d.
 birth d.
 d. of birth
 personnel d.
 d. rape
 d. rape drug
Datex infrared CO_2 monitor
dating bar
Datril
DATTA
 Diagnostic and Therapeutic Technology
 Assessment
Datura arobrea

dauernarkose
Dauerschlaf
daughter
    d. abscess
    d. cyst
    d. language
Daumas-Duport
    D.-D. classification
    D.-D. system
daunosamine residue
dauntless
Davidoff age stratification
Davidoff-Dyke-Masson syndrome
Davis
    D. brain retractor
    D. brain spatula
    D. coagulating forceps
    D. conductor
    D. dura dissector
    D. dural separator
    D. monopolar forceps
    D. nerve separator
    D. nerve separator-spatula
    D. nerve spatula
    D. percussion hammer
    D. rib spreader
    D. saw guide
    D. scalp retractor
dawamesk
DAWN
    Drug Abuse Warning Network
Dawson encephalitis
Daxolin
day
    D. Barb
    d. care residential treatment
    d. dream
    every d.
    every other d.
    four times a d.
    d. hospital
    d. of month test
    packs per d. (PPD, Ppd)
    per d. (/d)
    d. residue
    d. school
    d. terror
    three times a d.
    d. treatment center (DTC)
    d. treatment unit
    twice a d.
daydream
    hero d.
    suffering-hero d.
daymare
Daypro
daytime
    d. fatigability
    d. mouth breathing
    d. sedation
    d. sleep episode
    d. sleepiness
    d. somnolence
day-to-day function
dazadrol maleate

Dazamide
dazoxidine
dazzle
    central d.
db
    decibel
3DBCT
    Three-Dimensional Block Construction
    Test
DBD Scale
DBH
    dopamine-beta hydroxylase
    plasma dopamine beta-hydroxylase
DBI
    diffuse brain injury
DBS
    deep brain stimulation
    direct brain stimulation
        DBS electrode
        DBS electrode implantation
DBSL
    dorsal brain stem lipoma
DC
    direct current
        DC SQUID sensor
DCA
    directional coronary atherectomy
DCD
    Dennis Test of Child Development
DCS
    dorsal column stimulator
    dorsal cord stimulation
DCT
    dynamic computed tomography
D-cycloserine
Dd
    unusual detail response
dD
    confabulated detail response
DDD
    Division of Developmental Disabilities
D-dimer
DDNOS
    dissociative disorder not otherwise
    specified
DDS
    disability determination service
DDST
    Denver Developmental Screening Test
DdW
    detail response elaborating the whole
de
    D. Andrade-McNab occipito-cervical
    arthrodesis
    d. Clerambault syndrome
    d. Lange syndrome
    d. lunatico d.
    D. Mayo two-point discrimination
    device
    D. Monte grading
    d. Morsier syndrome
    d. novo
    d. novo aneurysm
    d. novo appearance
    d. novo development

D

de (continued)
    d. pensós echo
    d. Quervain disease
    d. retour age
    D. Sanctis-Cacchione syndrome
DEA
    Drug Enforcement Administration
dead
    desire to be d.
    d. on arrival (DOA)
    playing d.
    d. room
    d. space
deadbeat dad
deadly
    d. catatonia
    d. nightshade poisoning
    d. sin
deadness
    emotional d.
deaf
deaf-blind
deafferentation
    hemispherical d.
    d. pain
    d. pain syndrome
deafness
    acoustic trauma d.
    air conduction d.
    Alexander d.
    bone conduction d.
    central d.
    conduction d.
    cortical d.
    developmental word d.
    exposure d.
    functional d.
    high frequency d.
    hysterical d.
    infantile X-linked d.
    midbrain d.
    music d.
    nerve d.
    neural d.
    occupational d.
    organic d.
    perceptive d.
    prelingual d.
    psychic d.
    psychogenic d.
    pure word d.
    retrocochlear d.
    selective d.
    sensorineural d.
    temporary d.
    tone d.
    toxic d.
    word d.
deaggressivization
dealer of bogus drug
dealing
    drug d.
dealkylation

3′-deamino-3′-morpholino-13-deoxo-10-hydroxycarminomycin (MX2)
deanalize
deanol acetaminobenzoate
deaquation
Dear John letter
death
    accidental d.
    d. anxiety
    D. Anxiety Scale (DAS)
    apparent d.
    attitude to d.
    autopsy-negative d.
    barbiturate-induced d.
    black d.
    d. blow
    brain d.
    cerebral brain d.
    crib d.
    d. criteria
    exhaustion d.
    expectation of d.
    d. expectation
    expected d.
    fear of d.
    d. feigning
    fetal d.
    functional d.
    hypoxyphilia-caused d.
    impending d.
    d. instinct
    intentional d.
    d. by lethal injection
    living d.
    d. mask
    nerve cell d.
    neuronal d.
    d. neurosis
    D. Personification Exercise (DPE)
    premature d.
    d. preoccupation
    preoccupation with d.
    programmed cell d.
    d. rate
    d. rattle
    reaction to d.
    d. row
    d. sentence
    sniffing d.
    sudden d. (SD)
    suffering d.
    survivor of d.
    d. theme
    thoughts of d.
    threat of d.
    timely d.
    d. trance
    d. trap
    d. trend
    unintentional d.
    untimely d.
    violent d.
    voodoo d.
    d. warrant
Deaver retractor

DeBakey
    D. endarterectomy scissors
    D. forceps
    D. rib spreader
DeBastiani
    D. distractor
    D. external fixator
    D. frame
debauchee
debauchery
debilitate
debilitating anxiety
debility
    nervous d.
debonair, debonaire
Debrancher enzyme deficiency
Debré-Sémélaigne pseudomyotonia
debriefing
    psychological d.
debris
    word d.
debulk
debulking procedure
DEC
    Developmental Evaluation Center
decadence
Decadron
decamethonium bromide
decanoate
    fluphenazine d.
    Haldol D.
    haloperidol d.
    nandrolone d.
    Prolixin D.
decarboxylase
    dopa d.
    glutamate d. (GAD)
    glutamic acid d.
    ornithine d.
decarceration
decathexis
decay
    free induction d. (FID)
    reflex d.
    d. theory
deceit
    biology of d.
    determinants of d.
    facial d.
    technological detection of d.
deceitfulness
deceive
    intention to d.
deceleration injury
decentralization
deception
    effects of d.
    d. style
decerebrate
    decorticate and d.
    d. plasticity
    d. posture
    d. posturing
    d. rigidity

decerebration
    bloodless d.
decerebrize
decibel (db)
decimate
decinormal
decision
    Brawner d.
    Career D.-Making (CDM)
    conscious d.
    Durham d.
    Gault d.
    Inquiry Mode Questionnaire: A Measure of How You Think and Make D.'s (INQ)
    d. making
    D. Making Inventory
    Management Inventory on Leadership, Motivation and D.-Making (MILMD)
    Parham d.
    d. support
    d. support system
    Tarasoff d.
    d. theory
    d. tree
    unilateral d.
decision-making
    d.-m. Organizer
    d.-m. process
    d.-m. skill
Decker
    D. alligator forceps
    D. alligator scissors
    D. microsurgical forceps
    D. microsurgical scissors
declaration
    dying d.
declassify
decline
    d. in academic functioning
    age-related cognitive d.
    Rating Scale of Communication in Cognitive D. (RSCCD)
declining consciousness
declive
declivis
decode
decoding
    d. skill
    D. Skills Test
decompensation
    impending d.
decompensative neurosis
decomposition
    d. in dreams
    ego d.
    d. of ego
    d. of movement
decompress
decompression
    anterior d.
    bone graft d.
    cerebral d.
    cervical spine d.

D

decompression *(continued)*
    d. equipment
    extensive posterior d.
    foramen magnum d. (FMD)
    foraminal d.
    hindbrain d.
    interlaminar d.
    internal d.
    lumbar spine d.
    microvascular d. (MVD)
    nerve d.
    d. operation
    orbital d.
    posterior d.
    sacral spine d.
    d. sickness
    simple d.
    spinal d.
    suboccipital d.
    subtemporal d.
    surgical d.
    thoracic spine d.
    thoracolumbar spine d.
    timing of d.
    transantral ethmoidal orbital d.
    trigeminal d.
    vascular d.
    ventricular d.
    vertebral body d.
decompressive
    d. craniectomy
    d. laminectomy
    d. surgery
deconditioning
decontaminate
decoration scruple
decorticate
    d. conditioning
    d. and decerebrate
    d. posturing
    rigidity d.
    d. rigidity
decortication, decortization
    cerebral d.
    reversible d.
    d. technique
decreased
    d. arm swing
    d. interest
    d. memory
    d. motivation
decreasing-decrement
decree
    divorce d.
decrement
    cognitive d.
    work d.
decremental procedure
decrepitude
decrescendo discharge
decriminalize
decrudescence

decubitus
    d. paralysis
    d. ulcer
decussate
decussatio, pl. decussationes
    d. brachii conjunctivi
    d. fontinalis
    d. lemniscorum
    d. motoria
    d. nervorum trochlearium
    d. pedunculorum cerebellarium
      superiorum
    d. pyramidum
    d. sensoria
    decussationes tegmenti
decussation
    d. of brachia conjunctiva
    dorsal tegmental d.
    d. of the fillet
    Forel d.
    fountain d.
    Held d.
    d. of medial lemniscus
    Meynert d.
    motor d.
    optic d.
    pyramidal d.
    rubrospinal d.
    sensory d. of medulla oblongata
    d. of superior cerebellar peduncles
    tectospinal d.
    tegmental d.
    d. of trochlear nerves
    ventral tegmental d.
    Wernekinck d.
dedifferentiation
dedolation
deduction
deductive reasoning
deefferentation
deep
    d. abdominal reflex
    d. brain extension
    d. brain lead
    d. brain stimulation (DBS)
    d. cerebellar nucleus
    d. cortex
    d. depression
    d. hypothermic circulatory arrest
    d. middle cerebral vein
    d. origin
    d. retractors
    d. sensibility
    d. sleep
    d. structure
    d. tendon reflex (DTR)
    d. trance
    d. trance identification
    d. transitional gyrus
    d. venous thrombosis (DVT)
    d. white matter lesion (DWML)
deep-pressure sensitivity
de-erotize
de-escalate
de-escalating aggressive behavior

defalcate
defamation
defatigation
defaulter
    drug d.
defeat
defeatist attitude
defecalgesiophobia
defecate
defecation reflex
defect
    activation d.
    afferent pupillary d.
    alcohol-related birth d. (ARBD)
    arcuate visual field d.
    arousal d.
    awareness d.
    birth d.
    body dysmorphic d.
    cerebrocranial d.
    chiasmatic d.
    cognitive d.
    congenital d.
    cytochrome oxidase d.
    developmental d.
    exaggerated d.
    excessive concern for d.
    extradural d.
    field d.
    focal plaquelike d.
    galactosidase d.
    genetic d.
    glycosphingolipid metabolic d.
    high-grade d.
    imagined d.
    learning d.
    memory d.
    mental d.
    metabolic d.
    midline fusion d.
    neural tube d. (NTD)
    neurological d.
    nonhomonymous field d.
    organic d.
    partial homonymous field d.
    perceptual d.
    physical d.
    polytrophic d.
    polytropic d.
    postoperative skull d.
    d. preoccupation
    preoccupation with d.
    protrusio d.
    pursuit d.
    relative afferent pupillary d.
    residual dense nasal d.
    retention d.
    sensory d.
    slight d.
    smooth pursuit d.
    teratological d.
    d. theorist
    visual field d.
    visuoperceptive d.
defected eye

defective
defeminization
defend
defenestrated
defenfluramine HCl capsule
defense
    attitude d.
    d. attitude
    character d.
    compulsive d.
    ego d.
    egomechanism of d.
    d. hysteria
    hysterical character d.
    hysteroid d.
    insanity d.
    d. interpretation
    d. level
    masochistic character d.
    mature d.
    d. mechanism
    D. Mechanism Inventory (DMI)
    d. organization
    perceptual d.
    d. psychoneurosis
    d. reaction
    d. reflex
    screen d.
    stormed d.
    d. strategy
defensible space
defensive
    d. adultomorphic stance
    d. behavior
    d. dysregulation
    d. dysregulation level
    d. emotion
    d. functioning axis
    D. Functioning Scale (DFS)
    d. reaction
defensiveness
    Personal Experience Inventory D.
defer
deference
deferoxamine, desferrioxamine
deferred
    diagnosis or condition d. on axis
      I
    diagnosis d. on axis II
    d. obedience
    d. reaction
    d. shock
defiance
defiant
    d. behavior
    d. rage
defiantrage
deficiency
    acid maltase d. (AMD)
    adult acid maltase d.
    aldosterone d.
    aminoaciduria d.
    antithrombin III d.
    aqueous humor d.
    arginase d.

D

deficiency *(continued)*
 autoimmune d.
 bioenergetic d.
 carnitine palmitoyltransferase d.
 ceruloplasmin d.
 cobalamin d.
 cystathionine synthetase d.
 cytochrome-c oxidase d.
 Debrancher enzyme d.
 dementia due to vitamin d.
 environmental d.
 factor VIII d.
 factor XII d.
 familial d.
 folate d.
 glucuronidase d.
 glutathione synthetase d.
 hereditary d.
 hexosaminidase d.
 idiopathic growth hormone d.
 immune d.
 infantile acid maltase d.
 iron d.
 d. love
 mental d.
 moral d.
 d. motivation
 d. motive
 myopathic carnitine d.
 myophosphorylase d.
 niacin d.
 nicotinic acid d.
 nutritional d.
 orgasmic d.
 oxygen d.
 phosphorylase d.
 platelet glycoprotein Ia/IIa d.
 protein C d.
 protein S d.
 pyruvate carboxylase d.
 secondary mental d.
 sulfatase A d.
 thiamine d.
 vitamin B1 d.
 vitamin B6 d.
 vitamin B12 d.
 vitamin D d.
 vitamin E d.

deficiens
 ejaculatio d.
 orgasmus d.

deficient
 mentally d. (MD)
 d. sexual desire
 d. spinous process

deficit
 attention d.
 auditory transfer d.
 awareness d.
 bimanual coordination d.
 central sensory d.
 character d.
 cognitive d.
 comprehension d.

 concentration d.
 conversion disorder with motor symptoms or d.
 conversion disorder with sensory symptom or d.
 cortical gray matter d.
 cranial nerve d.
 delayed ischemia d. (DID)
 delayed ischemic neurological d. (DIND)
 emotional d.
 expressive language d.
 focal neurologic d.
 gaze d.
 global cognitive d.
 gross motor d.
 gross neurologic d.
 gross sensory d.
 hearing d.
 information processing d.
 interpersonal relationship d.
 ipsilateral d.
 language d.
 memory d.
 mental d.
 mesocortical dopaminergic system d.
 motor d.
 multiple cognitive d.'s
 neural d.
 neurocognitive d.
 neurolinguistic d.
 neurological d.
 neuropsychologic d.
 osteoporosis with vertebral collapse and neurologic d.
 parietotemporal perfusion d.
 perception d.
 perceptual d.
 perfusion d.
 perseveration d.
 pixelated parietotemporal perfusion d.
 presynaptic functional d.
 primary motor d.
 proprioception d.
 proprioceptive sensory d.
 radicular d.
 radicular motor d.
 d. reversal
 reversible ischemic neurological d. (RIND)
 sensory d.
 serotonergic d.
 social skills d.
 speech-motor d.
 d. symptom
 d. syndrome
 tactile transfer d.
 temporal integration d.
 transfer d.
 vigilance d.
 visual field d.
 visual perceptual d.

defile

definition
  AVM nidus d.
  caseness d.
  categorical d.
  cross-sectional d.
  nidus d.
  operational d.
  three-dimensional target d.
definitive
deflazacort
deflected eye
deflection
  d. force
  high-voltage d.
  initial upward d.
deformans
  dystonia musculorum d.
  osteitis d.
  recessive dystonia musculorum d.
  spondylitis d.
deformation
  d. of self
  shear-strain d.
  trefoil tendon d.
deformity
  d. analysis
  Arnold-Chiari d.
  bull's eye d.
  cervical spine kyphotic d.
  cervicomedullary d.
  clawhand d.
  coronal plane d.
  cranioorbital d.
  flat back d.
  hand d.
  hindbrain d.
  J-sella d.
  kyphotic d.
  lumbar spine kyphotic d.
  posttraumatic spinal d.
  saddle nose d.
  sagittal d.
  skeletal d.
  spinal d.
  spinal coronal plane d.
  swan neck d.
  thoracic spine scoliotic d.
deformity/instability
  spinal d./i.
defuse
defusion
deganglionate
degeneracy
  criminal d.
  d. theory
degeneration
  acquired hepatocerebral d.
  adiposogenital d.
  alcohol acquired (non-wilsonian)
    chronic hepatocerebral d.
  alcohol cerebellar d.
  Alzheimer neurofibrillary d.
  ascending d.
  axonal d.
  axoplasm d.

  brain d.
  cerebellar cortical d.
  cerebelloolivary d.
  cerebromacular d. (CMD)
  cobblestone d.
  cortical-basal ganglionic d.
  dentatorubral d.
  descending d.
  end-organ d.
  fascicular d.
  fibrinoid d.
  focal d.
  Gombault d.
  granulovacuolar d.
  gray d.
  hepatocerebral d.
  hepatolenticular d.
  Holmes cerebellar d.
  Holmes cortical cerebellar d.
  hypertrophic olivary d.
  infantile neuronal d.
  lattice d.
  lenticular progressive d.
  Marchi d.
  Menzel olivopontocerebellar d.
  neurofibrillary d.
  neurofibrillatory d. (NFD)
  neuronal d.
  Nissl d.
  olivary d.
  olivopontocerebellar d.
  orthograde d.
  oxidative d.
  pallidal d.
  paraneoplastic cerebellar d.
  parenchymatous cerebellar d.
  paving stone d.
  primary neuronal d.
  primary progressive cerebellar d.
  d. psychosis
  Ramsay Hunt type of inherited
    dentatorubral d.
  reaction of d. (RD)
  retinal d.
  retrograde d.
  secondary d.
  senile d.
  spinocerebellar d.
  spinopontine d.
  spongy d.
  striatonigral d.
  subacute cerebellar d.
  subacute combined d. of the spinal
    cord
  synaptic d.
  transsynaptic d.
  Türck d.
  wallerian d.
  Wilson hepatolenticular d.
degenerative
  d. arthritis
  d. brain disease
  d. cervical disk disease
  d. chorea
  d. dementia

D

degenerative *(continued)*
    d. discogenic end-plate disease
    d. discogenic vertebral change
    d. disk disease
    d. disorder
    d. encephalopathy
    d. hypothesis
    d. insanity
    d. lumbar scoliosis
    d. lumbar spine fusion
    d. narrowing
    d. primary dementia
    progressive d.
    d. psychosis
    d. spine condition
    d. spondylolisthesis
    d. spondylosis
    d. spondylosis decompression and
      fusion
    d. status
    d. subluxation
degenerativus
    status d.
degenitalize
degloving
    midface d.
deglutition
    d. paralysis
    d. reflex
Degos disease
degradation
    cytoskeletal d.
    elastin d.
    myelin d.
degrading ritual
degree
    d. of amnesia
    d. of control
    d. of disability
    d. of freedom
    d. of impairment
    d. of pain
degustation
dehumanization
dehumanizing
dehydration
    d. reaction
    voluntary d.
dehydroepiandrosterone (DHEA)
    d. sulfate (DHEA-S)
dehydrogenase
    alcohol d. (ADH)
    aldehyde d.
    lactate d. (LHD)
    pyruvate d. (PDH)
dehydromorphine
dehypnotize
deicide
deictic
deify
deindividualism
deinstitutionalization
deinstitutionalize
deipnophobia

deism
deiterospinal tract
Deiters
    D. cell
    D. nucleus
    D. process
deity
    spectral relationship to d.
deixis
    person d.
    place d.
    time d.
déjà
    d. entendu
    d. eprouve
    d. pensé
    d. vu
    d. vu aura
    d. vu phenomenon
dejected mood
dejection
Dejerine
    D. anterior bulb syndrome
    D. disease
    D. hand phenomenon
    D. onion peel sensory loss
    D. percussion hammer
    D. peripheral neurotabes
    D. reflex
    D. sign
Dejerine-Davis percussion hammer
Dejerine-Klumpke
    D.-K. palsy
    D.-K. paralysis
Dejerine-Lichtheim phenomenon
Dejerine-Roussy syndrome
Dejerine-Sottas
    D.-S. disease
    D.-S. peripheral neuropathy
Delatestryl
delavirdine
delay
    developmental d.
    global d.
    inhibition of d.
    macrocephaly with somatic and
      genital growth d.
    patient d.
    phase d.
    readout d.
    specific d.
    d. therapy
delayed
    d. apoplexy
    d. auditory feedback
    d. axotomy
    d. cerebral vasospasm
    d. computed tomographic
      myelography
    d. depolarization
    d. development
    d. discharge
    d. ejaculation
    d. gratification
    d. grief

d. hydrocephalus
d. hypersensitivity reaction
d. ischemia deficit (DID)
d. ischemic deterioration (DID)
d. ischemic neurological deficit (DIND)
d. language
d. memory
d. postanoxic encephalopathy
d. postischemic hypoperfusion
d. posttraumatic stress disorder
d. reaction experiment
d. recall
d. reflex
d. reinforcement
d. response
d. reward
d. sensation
d. shock
d. sleep phase syndrome
d. speech
d. therapy
d. toilet training
d. traumatic intracerebral hemorrhage (DTICH)

delayed-alteration test
delayed-matching test
delayed-onset postherpetic neuralgia
delectation
deleterious
deletion
d. mutation
thought d.
deliberate
d. fire-setting
d. self-harm (DSH)
d. therapy
delicto
flagrante d.
Delilah syndrome
delimitation
delineate
delineation
delineator
Gregorc Style D.
delinquency
adaptive d.
adolescent neurotic d.
geriatric d.
group d.
juvenile neurotic d.
neurotic d.
recovery from d.
socialized d. (SD)
delinquent
d. adolescent
d. behavior
juvenile d.
deliquium
delirante
boufeé d.
deliria (*pl. of* delirium)
deliriant
delirifacient

delirio
delirium sine d.
sine d.
deliriosa
schizophrenia d.
delirious
d. mania
d. reaction
d. shock
d. transient organic psychosis
delirium, pl. deliria
abstinence d.
active d.
acute alcoholic d.
alcohol d.
d. alcoholicum
d. alcoholism
ammonium chloride d.
amphetamine d.
anticholinergic d.
anxiolytic d.
anxious d.
d. arteriosclerotic dementia
asthenic d.
cannabis intoxication d.
chronic alcoholic d.
cocaine intoxication d.
collapse d.
d. constantium
digitalis-induced d.
drug-induced d.
d. due to a general medical condition
d. due to multiple etiologies
eclamptic d.
ecmnesiac d.
d. epilepticum
d. e potu
exhaustion d.
febrile d.
d. ferox
focused d.
frank d.
full-blown d.
grandiose d.
grave d.
d. grave
hallucinogen intoxication d.
hypnotic d.
hypoglycemic d.
hysterical d.
d. hystericum
inhalant-induced d.
inhalant intoxication d.
intoxication d.
lingual d.
low d.
macromaniacal d.
manic d.
marijuana d.
melancholia with d.
micromaniacal d.
microptic d.
d. mite
d. mussitans

D

delirium *(continued)*
    muttering d.
    d. of negation
    occupational d.
    oneiric d.
    opioid-induced d.
    opioid intoxication d.
    organic d.
    d. palingnosticum
    panic d.
    partial d.
    PCP intoxication d.
    d. of persecution
    phencyclidine intoxication d.
    posttraumatic d.
    d. in presenile dementia
    psychasthenic d.
    psychoactive substance d.
    puerperal d.
    rhyming d.
    d. schizophrenoides
    sedative d.
    senile d.
    d. in senile dementia
    d. sine delirio
    d. state drug psychosis
    subacute d.
    substance-induced d.
    superimposed d.
    sympathomimetic d.
    thyroid d.
    toxic d.
    d. transient organic
    d. transient organic psychosis
    trauma-induced d.
    traumatic d.
    d. tremens (DT)
    d. tremens alcoholic psychosis
    unfocused d.
    vascular dementia with d.
    d. verborum
    withdrawal d.
Delirium, Dementia, and Amnestic and Other Cognitive Disorders
delirium-like state
delirium-related mental disorder
delitescence
delivery
    d. catheter
    convection-enhanced d. (CED)
    d. guidewire
    intraarterial drug d.
    method of d.
delorazepam
Delrin
    D. plastic scalp clip
    D. rod
Del Rio Language Screening Test (DRLST)
delta
    d. activity
    d. alcoholism
    d. fornicis
    d. index

    d. level
    monorhythmic frontal d. (MFD)
    d. opiate receptor
    d. rhythm
    d. sleep-inducing peptide
    D. valve
    d. wave
Delta-Cortef Oral
Deltasone
delta-9-tetrahydrocannabinol (δ-9-THC)
delta-wave sleep
deltoid-splitting incision
delusion
    affect-laden d.
    alcohol-induced psychotic disorder with d.'s
    allopsychic d.
    amphetamine-induced psychotic disorder with d.'s
    anxiolytic-induced psychotic disorder with d.'s
    autochthonous d.
    autopsychic d.
    d. of being controlled
    bizarre d.
    cannabis-induced psychotic disorder with d.'s
    circumscribed d.
    cocaine d.
    cocaine-induced psychotic disorder with d.'s
    confused d.
    content of d.
    control d.
    d. of control
    crystallized grandiose d.
    depressive d.
    disorganized d.
    dysmorphic d.
    encapsulated d.
    erotic d.
    erotomanic d.
    established d.
    expansive d.
    expressive d.
    first rank symptoms of d.
    fixed d.
    fleeting d.
    fragmentary d.
    d. of grandeur
    grandeur d.
    grandiose d.
    hallucinogen-induced psychotic disorder with d.'s
    hypnotic-induced psychotic disorder with d.'s
    infestation d.
    infidelity d.
    d. of infidelity
    d. of influence
    influence d.
    inhalant-induced psychotic disorder with d.'s
    interpretation d.
    isolated d.

jealous-type d.
Mignon d.
d.'s of mind reading
mixed-type d.
mood-congruent d.
mood-incongruent d.
multiple d.'s
d. of negation
negation d.
negative d.
nihilistic d.
nonbizarre d.
nonsystematized d.
object of a d.
observation d.
d. of observation
opioid-induced psychotic disorder
  with d.'s
d. of orientation
paranoid grandiose d.
partial d.
d. of passivity
passivity d.
pejorative d.
persecution d.
d. of persecution
persecutory d.
persistent d.
phencyclidine-induced psychotic
  disorder with d.'s
poorly systematized d.
poverty d.
d. of poverty
primordial d.
psychotic d.
psychotic disorder with d.'s
d. of reference
referential d.
reformist d.
religious d.
schneiderian d.
sedative-induced psychotic disorder
  with d.'s
d. of self-accusation
sexual d.
somatic d.
d. stupor
d. symptom
systematized d.
thought broadcasting d.
thought insertion d.
unspecified-type d.
unsystematized d.
vascular dementia with d.'s
well-formed d.

delusional
d. behavior
d. belief
d. conviction
d. depression
d. equivalent
d. feature
floridly d.
d. insanity
d. intensity

d. jealousy
d. loving
d. network
d. paranoid disorder
d. projection
d. proportion
d. syndrome
d. syndrome drug psychosis
d. system
d. thinking
d. thought
d. thought pattern
d. transient organic
d. transient organic psychosis
delusive
Demadex
demagogue
demand
d. characteristic
role d.
d.'s of society
unreasonable d.
demanding behavior
demarcated relationship
demarcation
d. current
d. potential
d. in sensory testing
demarche
DeMarneffe meniscotomy knife
DeMartel
D. scalp flap forceps
D. wire saw
demasculinization
demeanor
demented
dementia
acquired d.
acute d.
acute confusional state
  arteriosclerotic d.
acute primary d.
advanced d.
alcohol-associated d.
alcoholic d.
alcohol-induced persisting d.
alcoholism associated with d.
Alzheimer atrophic d.
Alzheimer-like senile d. (ALSD)
D. of the Alzheimer's Type
d. of Alzheimer type (DAT)
d. of the Alzheimer type, with
  early onset
d. of the Alzheimer type, with
  late onset
amyotrophic lateral sclerosis-
  Parkinson d. (ALS-PD)
anxiolytic-induced persisting d.
apoplectic d.
d. apoplectica
Arizona Battery for Communication
  Disorders of D. (ABCD)
arteriosclerotic d.
d. associated with alcoholism
atrophic d.

D

dementia *(continued)*
   beclouded d.
   d. behavior disturbance
   D. Behavior Disturbance Scale
   Binswanger d.
   boxer's d.
   catatonic d.
   cerebrovascular accident d.
   chronic d.
   circular d.
   clinical d.
   confusional state presenile d.
   congenital syphilitic paralytic d.
   Cornell Scale for Depression, D.
    (CSDD)
   degenerative d.
   degenerative primary d.
   delirium arteriosclerotic d.
   delirium in presenile d.
   delirium in senile d.
   depressive d.
   developmental d.
   dialysis d.
   dialytica d.
   driveling d.
   drug-induced d.
   d. due to Creutzfeldt-Jakob disease
   d. due to head trauma
   d. due to hepatic condition
   d. due to multiple etiologies
   d. due to traumatic brain injury
   d. due to vitamin deficiency
   early phase of d.
   end-stage d.
   d. in epilepsy
   epileptic d.
   ethical aspects of d.
   d. evaluation
   exhaustion senile d.
   familial d.
   frontal lobe d.
   frontosubcortical d.
   global d.
   hallucinatory d.
   hebephrenic d.
   Heller d.
   hereditary d.
   higher d.
   HIV-based d.
   hydrocephalic d.
   hypnotic-induced persisting d.
   impairment of d.
   infantile d.
   d. infantilis
   infarct d.
   inhalant-induced persisting d.
   ischemic vascular d.
   juvenile paralytic d.
   lacunar d.
   language disorder in d.
   Lewy body d.
   D. Mood Assessment Scale
    (DMAS)
   multi-infarct d.

multiple sclerosis d.
d. myoclonica
non-Alzheimer frontal lobe type d.
old-age d.
organic d.
paralytic d.
d. paralytica
d. paralytica juveniles (DPJ)
paranoid d.
d. paranoides
d. paranoides gravis
d. paranoides mitis
paraphrenic d.
paretic d.
pellagra d.
persisting d.
d. phase
Pick disease d.
polyarteritis nodosa d.
postfebrile d.
posttraumatic d.
d. praecocissima
d. praecox
preexisting d.
presenile d.
d. presenilis
primary degenerative d. (PDD)
primary senile d.
d. process
profound d.
progressive d.
psychoactive substance d.
psychobiological process of d.
puerperal d.
d. pugilistica
D. Rating Scale
relative d.
remitting d.
repeated infarct d.
d. reversible
schizophrenic d.
secondary d.
sedative, hypnotic, or anxiolytic-
  induced persisting d.
sedative-induced persisting d.
d. sejunctiva
semantic d.
senile d. (SD)
severe d.
simple depressive d.
simple senile d.
socialized d. (SD)
d. stage
d. state drug psychosis
static d.
subcortical d.
substance-abuse persisting d.
substance-induced persisting d.
superimposed d.
syphilitic d.
syphilitic paralytic d.
syphilitic progressive d.
tabetic form paralytic d.
tardive d.
terminal d.

thalamic d.
toxic d.
transmissible virus d. (TVD)
traumatic d.
vascular d.
vitamin B12 deficiency d.
Wernicke d.
Wilson disease d.
dementia-aphonia
d.-a. syndrome
d.-a. syndrome of childhood
dementia-related
d.-r. behavior
d.-r. mental disorder
d.-r. psychiatric syndrome
dementing process
Demerol
demigod
demise
untimely d.
demissio animi
demiurge
democratic leadership pattern
demodulator
demography
dynamic d.
static d.
demomania
demoniac
demonic possession
demonolatry
demonology
demonomania
démonomaniaque
folie d.
demonopathy
demonophobia
demonstration
Ames d.
demoralization
personal d.
demorphinization
demotivate
demulcent
demutization
demyelinating
d. disease
d. encephalopathy
d. lesion
d. neuropathy
d. polyradiculoneuropathy
demyelination, demyelinization
central inflammatory d.
multifocal subcortical d.
demyelinative
d. disorder
d. spinal fluid profile
demystify
denarcissism
denarcotize
denarcotized opium
dendraxon
dendriform
dendrite
apical d.

dendritic
d. process
d. spine
d. thorn
d. tuft
dendrodendritic synapse
dendroid
dendron
dendrophilia, dendrophily
dendrophobia
dendrotomy
denegation
denervate
denervation
autonomic d.
chemical d.
Krause d.
law of d.
d. level
d. pain syndrome
deneutralization
dengue
d. fever
d. viral encephalitis
d. virus
denial
d. of amotivation
d. of anergy
d. of anhedonia, amotivation or anergy
color d. (Cd)
d. defense mechanism
d. of external reality
psychotic d.
reality d.
d. visual hallucination syndrome
denicotinize
denied grief
denigrated self-esteem
denigration
Denis
D. Browne, Foley syndrome
D. Browne neuropathy
D. Browne syndrome
Dennie-Marfan syndrome
Dennis Test of Child Development (DCD, DTCD)
denomination
denotation
denounce
denovo
dens, pl. **dentes**
d. anterior screw fixation
densa
macula d.
densate focus
dense
d. hemianopia
d. hemiparesis
d. hemiplegia
d. scotoma
d. sensory loss
densitometric analysis

D

densitometry
    cholera-toxin-catalyzed
        d.
    optical d.
density
    bone mineral d.
    contrast d.
    frontal lobe neuronal d.
    inside d.
    lumbosacral junction bone d.
    outside d.
    population d.
    proton d.
    receptor d.
    REM d.
    spectral d.
    spin d.
    striatal dopamine transporter d.
dental
    d. anxiety
    d. erosion
    d. infection
    d. jurisprudence
    d. nerve
dental-patient reaction
dentata
    vagina d.
dentate
    d. fascia
    d. fissure
    d. gyrus
    d. ligament
    d. nucleus of cerebellum
dentatectomy
dentated serration
dentato-olivary pathway
dentatorubral
    d. atrophy
    d. degeneration
dentatorubropallidoluysian atrophy
dentatothalamic
    d. tract
dentatum
dentes (*pl. of* dens)
denticola
    Treponema d.
denticulate ligament
dentinogenesis imperfecta
dentoliva
denuding
    hair d.
denunciation
denutrition
Denver
    D. Articulation Screening
      Evaluation (DASE)
    D. Articulation Screening
      Examination
    D. Developmental Screening Test
      (DDST)
    D. hydrocephalus shunt
    D. II test
    D. valve
deodoratum
    opium d.

deodorized opium
deontology
deoppilant
deorality
deoxygenation
deoxyhemoglobin
    intracellular d.
deoxynucleside triphosphates
deoxyribonucleic acid (DNA)
Depacon
Depade
Depakene
Depakote
    D. Sprinkle Capsule
    D. Tablets
depalatalization
department
    D. of Health and Human Services
      (DHHS)
    D. of Mental Health (DMH)
depatterning
dependence
    absinthe addiction or d.
    aerosol spray d.
    airplane glue d.
    alcohol d.
    amphetamine d.
    anxiolytic d.
    barbiturate d.
    benzodiazepine d.
    butane sniffing d.
    caffeine d.
    cannabis d.
    chemical d.
    chlorohydrocarbon d.
    cocaine d.
    codeine d.
    combination-drug d.
    cross d.
    d. disorder
    drug d.
    emotional d.
    ethanol d.
    ether d.
    field d.
    hallucinogen d.
    hypnotic d.
    inhalant d.
    instrumental d.
    laxative d.
    lighter fluid d.
    LSD d.
    marijuana d.
    methadone d.
    methamphetamine d.
    morning glory seeds d.
    morphine d.
    narcotic d.
    nicotine d.
    nitrous oxide d.
    d. on pornography
    d. on therapy
    opioid d.
    opium d.
    oral d.

d. organic psychosis
peyote d.
phencyclidine d.
physical d.
physiological d.
polysubstance d.
pornography d.
propoxyphene d.
psilocybin d.
psychedelic agent d.
psychic d.
psychoactive substance d.
psychostimulant d.
psychotomimetic agent d.
reward d.
sedative d.
social d.
solvent (inhalation) d.
soporific drug d.
state d.
substance abuse and d.
d. syndrome
synthetic drug d.
synthetic heroin d.
Task Force on Nicotine D.
d. tendency
tetrahydrocannabinol d.
THC d.
therapeutic dose d.
tobacco d.
tranquilizer drug d.
unspecified substance d.
dependence-independence
field d.-i.
dependence-type organic psychosis
dependency
chemical d.
clinging d.
drug d.
hypnotic d.
interpersonal d.
long-term d.
morbid d.
d. need
passive d.
dependent
d. adult's certificate
d. behavior
d. character
d. edema
d. neurotic personality disorder
d. patient role
d. personality
d. scale
trait d.
d. variable
dependent-passive personality disorder
depersonalization
d. episode
d. experience
d. neurosis
d. neurotic disorder
neurotic state with d.
d. psychoneurosis
d. psychoneurotic

d. psychoneurotic reaction
recurrent d.
d. syndrome
depersonalize
depletion
metabolic volume d.
depMedalone Injection
Depoject Injection
depolarization
delayed d.
depolarizing muscle relaxant
Depo-Medrol Injection
Depopred Injection
Depo-Provera
deposition
amyloid d.
copper d.
hemosiderin d.
depot
Clopixol d.
fat d.
Fluanxol D.
d. medication
d. medication injection
d. medication injection therapy
Piportil D.
Depo-Testosterone
depravation
depravity
deprecatory
depreciated subsystem
deprementia
deprenyl
depressant
brain d.
cerebral d.
CNS d.
motor d.
depressed
d. affect
d. bipolar affective psychosis
d. mood
d. mood adjustment disorder
d. mood adjustment reaction
d. mood episode
d. mood theme
d. reflex
d. schizoaffective schizophrenia
d. skull fracture
d. state
d. tone
d. ventilatory response to hypercarbia
depressiform
depressiogenic effect
depression
acute anxiety d.
acute situational d.
adolescent d.
agitated d.
akinetic d.
anaclitic d.
anancastic d.
anergic d.
anxiety d.

D

depression *(continued)*
    anxious d.
    arteriosclerotic d.
    atypical d.
    autogenous d.
    autonomous d.
    aversion d.
    D.: Awareness, Recognition, and
        Treatment (D/ART)
    D.: Awareness, Recognition, and
        Treatment Campaign
    Bellevue Index of D.
    bereavement-related d.
    biologic sign d.
    bipolar d.
    brief situational d.
    Carroll Rating Scale for D.
    Center for Anxiety and D.
    characterological d.
    chronic d.
    classical d.
    classification of d.
    clinical d.
    cognitive theory of d.
    d. of consciousness
    constitutional d.
    co-occurrence of d.
    cryptic d.
    cyclical d.
    deep d.
    delusional d.
    depression sine d. (DSD)
    double d.
    endogenomorphic d.
    endogenous d.
    d. in epilepsy
    exogenous d.
    d. history
    holiday d.
    hypersomnia associated with d.
    hyposomnia associated with d.
    hysterical delirium hysterical d.
    ictal d.
    insomnia associated with d.
    d. inventory
    Inventory to Diagnose D.
    involutional d.
    Leeds Scales for the Self-
        Assessment of Anxiety and D.
    light treatment for winter d.
    major d.
    manic d.
    marked d.
    masked d.
    maternal d.
    melancholic d.
    menopausal d.
    mental d.
    mild d.
    moderate d.
    monopolar d.
    nervous d.
    neurotic d.
    d. neurotic disorder

    nonmajor d.
    nonpsychotic unipolar d.
    nonreactive d.
    opticochiasmatic d.
    overwhelming d.
    Peer Nomination Inventory of D.
    d. period
    physiogenetic d.
    postdivorce d.
    postdormital d.
    posthysterectomy d.
    postictal d.
    postinfectious d.
    postnatal d.
    postpartum major d.
    postpsychotic d.
    poststroke d.
    Prevention and Treatment of D.
        (PTD)
    prolonged situational d.
    pseudodementia of d.
    psychogenic d.
    psychoneurotic d.
    psychotic d. (PD)
    d. questionnaire
    D. Questionnaire for Children
    D. Rating Scale
    reactive psychotic d.
    recurrent episode psychotic d.
    resistant d.
    retarded d.
    d. risk
    d. scale
    secondary d.
    Self-Assessment D. (SAD)
    self-blaming d.
    senile d.
    severe d.
    sign d.
    simple affective d.
    single-episode psychotic d.
    situational d.
    somatic treatment for d.
    somatizing clinical d.
    spreading d. (SD)
    D. Status Inventory (DSI)
    stuporous d.
    d. symptom
    syndromal d.
    D. Test of Visual Perception
        (DTVP)
    unipolar d.
    vascular d.
    winter d.
depression-related
    d.-r. mental disorder
    d.-r. psychiatric syndrome
depressive
    D. Adjective Checklist (DAC,
        DACL)
    d. affect
    d. catatonia
    d. character
    d. crash
    d. delusion

d. dementia
d. disorder
d. episode
d. equivalent
d. experience
D. Experiences Questionnaire (DEQ)
d. feature
d. hallucination
manic d.
d. neurosis
d. personality
d. phase
d. position
psychological trauma d.
d. psychosis
d. reaction
d. spectrum disorder (DSD)
d. state
d. stupor
d. symptomatology
depressive-type
d.-t. psychoneurosis
d.-t. psychoorganic syndrome
depressogenic
depressomotor
depressor
d. fiber
d. nerve of Ludwig
deprivation
activity d.
cultural d.
early parental d.
emotional d.
environmental d.
food d.
masked d.
maternal d.
oxygen d.
paternal d.
perceptual d.
psychological d.
psychosocial d.
role d.
sensory d.
severe environmental d.
sleep d.
social d.
d. syndrome
thought d.
water d.
deprived
culturally d.
educationally d.
Deprol
depth
analysis in d.
d. guard
d. of mood
d. perception
d. psychology
d. recording
skin d.
d. of sleep

d. therapy
wire penetration d.
DePuy nerve hook
DEQ
Depressive Experiences Questionnaire
derailment
actual d.
cognitive d.
frequent d.
speech d.
thought d.
d. of volition
deranged
mentally d.
derangement
mental d.
metabolic d.
derby hat fracture
derealization
dereism
dereistic thinking
derelict
skid-row d.
dereliction
deride
derision
derivation
source d.
derivative
alcohol d.
chloral d.
ergot d.
hematoporphyrin d.
indole d.
phenothiazine d.
piperidine d.
piperidyl d.
thioxanthene d.
tryptamine d.
valproic acid and d.'s
dermabrasion bur
Dermaflex Gel
dermal meningioma
DermaTemp infrared thermographic sensor
dermatica
zona d.
dermatitidis
Blastomyces d.
dermatitis
psychogenic d.
dermatofibrosarcoma protuberans
dermatogenic torticollis
dermatoglyphic
abnormal d.
dermatome
dermatomyositis (DM)
juvenile d.
dermatomyotome
dermatoneurosis
dermatopathophobia, dermatophobia, dermatosiophobia
dermatosensory evoked potential
dermatosiophobia
dermatothlasia

D

dermenchysis
dermis
dermoid
    d. cyst
    nasal d.
    d. tumor
dermoneurosis
derogate
Derogatis Affects Balance Scale (DABS)
derogatory
    d. comment
    d. remark
D'Errico
    D. bayonet pituitary forceps
    D. brain spatula
    D. enlarging drill bur
    D. hypophyseal forceps
    D. lamina chisel
    D. nerve root retractor
    D. perforating drill
    D. perforating drill bur
    D. periosteal elevator
    D. pituitary forceps
    D. skull trephine
    D. tissue forceps
    D. ventricular needle
D'Errico-Adson retractor
dervish
DES
    diethylstilbestrol
    Dissociative Experience Scale
desacralize
desamino-D-arginine vasopressin
desanimania
DESBRS-II
    Devereux Elementary School Behavior
    Rating Scale II
descendens
    d. cervicalis
    d. hypoglossi
descending
    d. degeneration
    d. dyscontrol
    d. dyscontrol durable
    d. neuritis
    d. nucleus of the trigeminus
    d. technique
    d. tract of trigeminal nerve
description
    D. of Body Scale
    graphic d.
    d. questionnaire
    Supervisory Behavior D. (SBD)
    textual d.
descriptive
    d. approach
    d. detail
    d. feature
    d. psychiatry
    d. statistics
    d. validity
descriptor
    Preschool and Kindergarten
    Interest D.

desensitization
    imaginal d.
    phobic d.
    psychologic d.
    reciprocal inhibition and d.
    systematic d.
    systemic d.
deserpidine
    methyclothiazide and d.
desertion
    d. anxiety
    maternal d.
    paternal d.
Desert Storm Trauma Questionnaire
deserved
    d. punishment
    d. punishment theme
desexualize
Desferal Mesylate
desferrioxamine (*var. of* deferoxamine)
desflurane
desiccant
desiccate
desiccated thyroid
design
    A/B/A d.
    block d.
    environmental d.
    equipment d.
    experimental d.
    factorial d.
    geometric d.
    hook hollow-ground connection d.
    hook V-groove connection d.
    interdisciplinary environmental d.
    Isola spinal implant system d.
    job d.
    Kohs Block D.
    mechanical plate d.
    memory for d. (MFD)
    mixed d.
    multiple baseline d.
    pedicle screw linkage d.
    quasi-experimental d.
    randomized group d.
    Rey-Osterrieth Complex Figure D.
    spinal implant d.
    study d.
    time-series d.
    transpedicular fixation system d.
    V-groove hollow-ground
      connection d.
designer drug
designs
    d. for vision frame
    d. for vision side shield
desipramine
    d. hydrochloride
desirability
    Marlowe-Crowne Scale of
      Social D.
    social d. (SD)
desire
    absent sexual d.
    active d.

d. to be dead
deficient sexual d.
disturbance in sexual d.
hyperactive sexual d.
hypoactive sexual d.
impaired sexual d.
incestuous d.
inhibited sexual d.
intense d.
irrational d.
d. level
low sexual d.
morbid d.
d. for personal gain
d. phase of sexual response cycle
d. for revenge
situational hypoactive sexual d.
stated d.
desired effect
desirous
desmethylclomipramine
desmethyldiazepam (DMDZ)
desmethylimipramine
desmin tumor marker
desmocytoma
desmodynia
desmoplastic
d. infantile ganglioglioma
d. medulloblastoma
desmopressin acetate
desomorphine
Desormaux endoscope
desoxycorticosterone acetate
desoxymorphine
Desoxyn
desoxyphenobarbital
despair
ego integrity versus d.
integrity versus d.
despeciation
despondent
destiny
manifest d.
destruction
bony element d.
nerve cell d.
d. of property
destructive
d. aggression
d. behavior
d. criticism
d. drive
d. instinct
d. interference technique
d. obedience
d. relationship
d. tendency
destructiveness
withdrawal d.
destrudo
desynchronization
d. activity
event-related d. (ERD)
desynchronous
Desyrel

detachable
d. balloon
d. coil
detached
d. cranial section
d. craniotomy
d. manner
detachment
choroid d.
ciliochoroid d.
dural d.
emotional d.
feeling of d.
d. from social relationship
pattern of d.
retinal d.
sense of d.
social d.
somnolent d.
detail
descriptive d.
minimization of emotional d.
d.'s preoccupation
preoccupation with d.
d. response elaborating the whole (DdW)
detailed
d. dream
d. history
DeTakats-McKenzie brain clip forceps
detectability threshold
detection
arousal d.
lie d.
d. threshold
detector
cesium fluoride scintillation d.
lie d.
phase-sensitive d.
quadrature d.
detention
d. cell
d. certificate
d. facility
d. home
deteriorated
d. affective disorder
d. bipolar disorder
deteriorating
d. course
d. function
deterioration
age-related d.
alcoholic d.
appearance d.
delayed ischemic d. (DID)
d. effect
emotional d.
end-of-dose d.
d. epilepsy
epileptic d.
functioning d.
global d.
grooming d.
habit d.

D

deterioration *(continued)*
    hygiene d.
    d. index (DI)
    intellectual d.
    irradiation-induced mental d.
    language function d.
    manners d.
    mental d.
    mood d.
    motivation d.
    neurologic d.
    personality d.
    posttraumatic d.
    progressive d.
    prominent d.
    d. quotient
    radiation-induced mental d.
    reaction-type d.
    d. reaction type
    d. scale
    senile d.
    significant d.
    simple d.
    social skills d.
    status d.
    stepwise d.
    uniformly progressive d.

determinant
    behavior d.
    d.'s of deceit
    dominant d.
    dream d.
    environmental d.

determination
    forensic d.
    fusion limit d.
    legal d.
    serum enzyme d.
    sex d.

determining quality

determinism
    biologic d.
    biosocial d.
    cultural d.
    linguistic d.
    psychic d.
    reciprocal d.

deterrent therapy

detestable

detiria

detoxification
    alcohol d.
    drug used for d.
    narcotic d.

detoxified alcoholic

detract

d'être
    raison d.

detrimental

Detroit
    D. Test of Learning Aptitude
    (DTLA)
    D. Test of Learning Aptitude-Adult
    (DTLA-A)

    D. Test of Learning Aptitude -
    Primary, Second Edition (DTLA-
    P:2)
    D. Test of Learning Aptitude,
    Third Edition (DTLA-3)

detrusor
    d. areflexia
    d. reflex

detumescence

deutencephalon

deuteropathy

deux
    A d.
    crime a d.
    egoïsme à d.
    folie à d.
    semiobsession à d.

devaluation

devalue

devascularized

develop
    failure to d.

developing
    d. psychotic disorganization
    D. Skills Checklist (DISCUSS,
    DSC)

development
    abnormal d.
    Adapted Sequenced Inventory of
    Communication D. (A-SICD)
    anal stage psychosexual d.
    arrest of d.
    arrested d.
    Assessment of Career D. (ACD)
    atypical d.
    Bayley Scales of Infant D. (BSID)
    behavioral d.
    Brigance Diagnostic Inventory of
    Early D.
    California Infant Scale for
    Motor D. (CISMD)
    career d.
    Carnegie Council on Adolescent D.
    character d.
    child language d.
    cognitive d.
    delayed d.
    Dennis Test of Child D. (DCD,
    DTCD)
    de novo d.
    deviant pathway of d.
    ego d.
    emotional d.
    expressive language d.
    fetal d.
    gender identity psychosexual d.
    Houston Test for Language D.
    impaired d.
    intellectual d.
    d. inventory
    Inventory for Counseling and D.
    (ICD)
    Inventory of Psychosocial D. (IPD)
    language d.
    d. language scale

latency period psychosexual d.
late speech d.
learning d.
level of d.
libidinal d.
life-span d.
Measurement of Language D.
Measures of Psychosocial D.
  (MPD)
mental d.
moral d.
motor d.
normal childhood d.
optimal d.
oral stage psychosexual d.
Ordinal Scales of Psychological D.
perinatal d.
personal d.
personality d.
pervasive impairment of d.
phallic stage psychosexual d.
postnatal d.
prenatal d.
d. profile
d. program
Progress Assessment Chart of
  Social and Personal D. (PAC)
d. psychobiology
psychomotor d.
psychosexual d.
psychosocial d.
d. questionnaire
Quick Screening of Mental D.
receptive language d.
retarded d.
Ring and Peg Tests of
  Behavior D.
d. scale
Scale of Social D.
Screening Kit of Language D.
  (SKOLD)
sensorimotor d.
Sequenced Inventory of
  Communication D. (SICD)
Sequenced Inventory of
  Language D. (SILD)
sexual d.
Skill Scan for Management D.
slow rate of language d.
social d.
subsequent d.
Tasks of Emotional D. (TED)
d. test
Test of Early Language D.
  (TELD)
Test of Early Language D.,
  Second Edition (TELD-2)
Test of Language D. (TOLD)
Test of Language D. -
  Intermediate, Second Edition
  (TOLD-I:2)
Test of Language D. - Primary,
  Second Edition (TOLD-P:2)
Utah Test of Language D.
  (UTLD)

developmental
D. Activities Screening Inventory
  (DASI)
d. age
d. agraphia
d. aphasia
D. Articulation Test (DAT)
d. articulatory apraxia
D. Assessment of Life Experiences
  (DALE)
d. defect
d. delay
d. dementia
d. disability
d. disorder
d. disorder associated with
  hyperkinesis
d. dyslexia
d. dysphasia
D. Evaluation Center (DEC)
d. experimentation in childhood
d. expressive writing
d. hand-function test (DHFT)
d. hyperactivity
d. idiocy
d. imbalance
d. impact
D. Indicators for Assessment of
  Learning (DIAL)
D. Indicators for Assessment of
  Learning, Revised/AGS Edition
  (DIAL-R)
d. landmark
d. learning problem (DLP)
d. level
d. malformation
d. milestone
d. pattern
d. period
d. phase
d. psychology
d. retardation
d. root
d. scale
d. schedule
d. screening
D. Sentence Analysis
D. Sentence Scoring Test
d. skills
d. stage
D. Test of Visual Motor
  Integration (DVMI)
D. Test of Visual-Motor
  Integration, Third Edition
D. Test of Visual Perception,
  Second Edition (DTVP-2)
d. theory
d. word blindness
d. word deafness
developmentally
d. appropriate avoidant behavior
d. appropriate self-stimulatory
  behaviors in the young
d. appropriate shy behavior
d. cumulative alcoholism

D

developmentally *(continued)*
    d. disabled
    d. inappropriate social relatedness
    d. limited alcoholism
Devereux
    D. Adolescent Behavior Rating
      Scale
    D. Elementary School Behavior
      Rating Scale II (DESBRS-II)
deviance
    communication d.
    psychiatric d.
    psychopathic d.
    role d.
    secondary d.
    sexual d.
    social d.
deviant
    d. belief
    d. language
    d. pathway of development
    d. political behavior
    d. religious behavior
    sex d.
deviate
    psychopathic d. (PD)
deviation
    alternating skew d.
    disconjugate eye d.
    ego d.
    d. from physiological norm
    ipsilateral tonic d.
    mean d.
    ocular d.
    personality d.
    population standard d.
    primary sexual d.
    quartile d. (q)
    d. quotient
    response d.
    sample standard d.
    sexual d.
    skew d.
    standard d. (SD)
    statistical d.
    wrong-way d.
Devic
    D. aminoaciduria
    D. disease
device
    anterior internal fixation d.
    antisiphon d. (ASD)
    assistive technology d. (ATD)
    Bassett electrical stimulation d.
    Bovie electrocautery d.
    braided occlusion d. (BOD)
    Cadwell 5200A somatosensory
      evoked potential unit d.
    Camino intraparenchymal
      fiberoptic d.
    C-D instrumentation d.
    charge-coupled d. (CCD)
    cohesive d.
    d. composition

computer-assisted speech d.
Contour Emboli artificial
    embolization d.
contraceptive d.
control d.
Cordis implantable drug
    reservoir d.
Cotrel-Dubousset dynamic transverse
    traction d.
De Mayo two-point
    discrimination d.
DeWald spinal d.
Dunn d.
Dwyer d.
dynamic transverse traction d.
Edwards modular system sacral
    fixation d.
Edwards sacral fixation d.
Egemen keyhole suction-control d.
ferromagnetic monitoring d.
Fischer-Leibinger bur hole-mounted
    fixation d.
fixation d.
fracture fixation d.
Galtac d.
Harrington rod instrumentation
    distraction outrigger d.
head fixation d.
Heyer-Schulte antisiphon d.
In-Exsufflator respiratory d.
interrupter d.
intravascular d.
JACE-STIM electrotherapy
    stimulation d.
Kaneda anterior spine stabilizing d.
Kostuik-Harrington d.
language acquisition d. (LAD)
Leksell adapter to Mayfield d.
malleable microsurgical suction d.
manipulative d.
Mayfield/ACCISS stereotactic d.
Medelec five-channel
    neurophysiological d.
MurphyScope neurologic d.
Neuromed Octrode implantable d.
newer-generation d.
Nicolet Pathfinder I recording d.
noise reduction d.
Novo-10a CBF measuring d.
optical d.
Portnoy DPV d.
Prosthetic Disc Nucleus d.
Quartzo d.
Roeder manipulative aptitude
    test d.
safety d.
sequential compression d. (SCD)
Silastic d.
Sofamor spinal instrument d.
Somanetics INVOS cerebral
    oximeter d.
SomaSensor d.
Sono-Stat Plus sound d.
SynchroMed drug administration d.

TACTICON peripheral neuropathy screening d.
Taylor halter d.
Texas Scottish Rite Hospital corkscrew d.
Texas Scottish Rite Hospital mini-corkscrew d.
d. for transverse traction (DTT)
ultrasonic aspirating d.
Viking II nerve monitoring d.
DeVilbiss
D. cranial rongeur
D. rongeur forceps
D. skull trephine
devil-may-care attitude
devil's pact
devil worship
Devine Inventory
devious manner
devitalize
devotion
devour
devout
DeWald spinal device
Dewar posterior cervical fixation procedure
DEXA
dual-energy x-ray absorptiometry
dexamethasone
high-dose d. (hdDXM)
d. suppression test (DST, DXM)
dexamisole
dexamphetamine
dexanabinol
Dexasone L.A.
Dexatrim
dexciamol hydrochloride
Dexedrine
dexfenfluramine hydrochloride
deximafen
Dexone LA
Dexoval
dexterity
manual d.
dexterous
dextral
dextrality
dextrality-sinistrality
dextramethasone nonsuppression
dextran
dextroamphetamine
d. and amphetamine
d. phosphate
d. saccharate
d. sulfate
dextrocerebral
dextromanual
dextromethorphan
acetaminophen and d.
dextropedal
dextrophobia
dextropropoxyphene
dextrorotoscoliosis
dextroscoliosis

dextrose
tetracaine and d.
dextrosinistral
Dextrostix Uristix
Deyerle sciatic tension test
dezocine
DFMO
dl-alpha-difluoromethylornithine
DFS
Defensive Functioning Scale
2DFT
two-dimensional Fourier transform
2DFT gradient-echo imaging
2DFT GRASS
2DFT time-of-flight MR angiography
3DFT
three-dimensional Fourier transform
anisotropic 3DFT
3DFT gradient-echo imaging
3DFT gradient-echo MR imaging
3DFT GRASS
isotropic 3DFT
DFTT
Digital Finger Tapping Test
DHC Plus
DHEA
dehydroepiandrosterone
DHEA-S
dehydroepiandrosterone sulfate
D.H.E. 45 Injection
DHFT
developmental hand-function test
DHHS
Department of Health and Human Services
DI
deterioration index
drug information
drug interaction
diabetes
gestational d.
d. insipidus
d. mellitus
diabetic
d. amyotrophy
d. arthropathy
d. coma
d. ketoacidosis
d. myelopathy
d. neuropathy
d. neuropathy neuralgia pain
d. polyradiculopathy
d. pseudotabes
d. puncture
d. sensorimotor polyneuropathy
d. third nerve palsy
diabetica
tabes d.
diabetophobia
Diabinese
diablerie
diabolepsy
diabolism
diacele

D

diacetylmorphine hydrochloride
diachorema
diachoresis
diachronic study
diacrisis
diacritic
diacylglycerol (DAG)
diadem
diadochokinesia rate
diadochokinesis
Diaginol
diagnosis, pl. **diagnoses (DX, Dx)**
    admitting d. (AD)
    alternative d.
    clinical d.
    comorbid Axis II d.
    d. or condition deferred on axis I
    cookbook d.
    d. deferred on axis II
    differential d.
    DSM-IV d.
    dual d.
    equivalent d.
    d. by exclusion
    d. ex juvantibus
    false-negative d.
    false-positive d.
    final d.
    geriatric d.
    intrauterine sonographic d.
    laboratory d.
    negative d.
    neurologic d.
    noninvasive d.
    pathologic d.
    prenatal d.
    primary d.
    principal d.
    proband d.
    provisional d.
    provocative d.
    psychiatric d.
    serum d.
    social d.
    structural d.
    wastebasket d.
diagnosis-related group (DRG)
diagnostic
    D. Achievement Battery, Second
      Edition (DAB-2)
    D. Achievement Test for
      Adolescents
    d. algorithm
    d. anesthesia
    d. apraxia
    D. Assessments of Reading (DAR)
    Basic School Skills Inventory - D.
    d. battery
    d. block
    D. Checklist for Behavior-Disturbed
      Children Form E-2
    d. class
    d. confidence
    d. criteria
    D. Employability Profile

    d. feature
    d. interview
    D. Interview for Borderline
      Patients
    D. Interview for Borderlines (DIB)
    D. Interview for Children and
      Adolescents
    D. Interview for Children and
      Adolescents-Child Version (DICA-
      C)
    D. Interview for Children and
      Adolescents-Parent Version
      (DICA-P)
    D. Interview for Children and
      Adolescents-Revised (DICA-R)
    D. Interview Schedule (DIS)
    D. Interview Schedule for Children
      (DIS-C, DISC)
    d. inventory
    d. judgment
    d. laboratory
    D. Mathematics Inventory (DMI)
    D. Mathematics Profile
    d. overshadowing
    d. procedure
    Process D. (PD)
    D. Questions for Early or
      Advanced Alcoholism
    d. related group (DRG)
    D. Skills Battery
    D. and Statistical Manual of
      Mental Disorders (DSM)
    D. and Statistical Manual of
      Mental Disorders-3rd Edition
      (DSM-III)
    D. and Statistical Manual of
      Mental Disorders-3rd Edition
      Revised (DSM-III-R)
    D. and Statistical Manual of
      Mental Disorders-4th Edition
      (DSM-IV)
    d. subtype
    D. Symptom Questionnaire
    d. teaching
    Test of Articulation Performance -
      D. (TAP-D)
    D. Tests and Self-Helps in
      Arithmetic
    D. and Therapeutic Technology
      Assessment (DATTA)
    d. therapy
    d. use of hypnosis
diagnostician
diagonal nystagmus
diagram
    branching tree d.
    pulse timing d.
    scatter d.
    vector d.
DIAL
    Developmental Indicators for Assessment
      of Learning
Dial Away Pain 400 electrotherapy unit
dialectic

dialectical
    d. behavior therapy
    d. dilemma
dialogue
DIAL-R
    Developmental Indicators for Assessment
    of Learning, Revised/AGS Edition
dialysis
    d. dementia
    d. dysequilibrium syndrome
    d. encephalopathy syndrome
dialytica dementia
diamagnetism
diambista
diameter
    effective pedicle d.
    effective thread d.
    horizontal pedicle d.
    lumbar spine pedicle d.
    pedicle d.
    sagittal pedicle d.
    thoracic spine pedicle d.
    transcerebellar d. (TCD)
    transpedicular fixation effective
      pedicle d.
    transverse pedicle d.
    vertical pedicle d.
diametrically opposed
diamond
    d. bur
    d. high-speed air drill
    d. knife
diamorphine
Diamox challenge testing
Dianabol
Diana complex
dianhydrogalactitol (DAG)
dianoetic
diaphemetric
diaphoresis
diaphragma, pl. **diaphragmata**
    d. sellae
diaphragmatic breathing
diaphragm of sella
Diapid
diaplexus
diarrhea
    emotional d.
    nocturnal d.
    psychogenic d.
diary
    symptom d.
diaschisis
Diasonics magnetic resonance imaging
diasostic
diastasis
    suture d.
diastatic skull fracture
Diastat Rectal Delivery System
diastematocrania
diastematomyelia
diastole-phased pulsatile infusion
diataxia
    cerebral d.
diatela

diathesis
    asthenic d.
    biologic d.
    contractural d.
    epileptic d.
    neuropathic d.
    panic d.
    psychopathic d.
    spasmodic d.
    spasmophilic d.
    stress-driven d.
    traumatophilic d.
diathesis-stress
    d.-s. paradigm
    d.-s. theory of schizophrenia
diatribe
diatrizoate
    meglumine d.
    d. meglumine
diatrizoic acid
Diazemuls Injection
diazepam (DZP)
    D. Intensol
    d. rectal gel
diazoxide
DIB
    Diagnostic Interview for Borderlines
dibasic
    d. calcium phosphate
    calcium phosphate, d.
dibenzepin
    d. benzothiazine
    d. hydrochloride
dibenzodiazepine
dibenzothiazepine
dibenzoxazepine
    tricyclic d.
dibenzoxozepine agent
Dibenzyline
dibromodulcitol
dibucaine hydrochloride
DIC
    disseminated intravascular coagulation
    drug information center
DICA-C
    Diagnostic Interview for Children and
      Adolescents-Child Version
DICA-P
    Diagnostic Interview for Children and
      Adolescents-Parent Version
DICA-R
    Diagnostic Interview for Children and
      Adolescents-Revised
Dicarbosil
dichloralphenazone
    acetaminophen, isometheptene,
      and d.
dichlorodifluoromethane and
   trichloromonofluoromethane
dichlorotetrafluoroethane
    ethyl chloride and d.
dichotic
    d. listening task
    d. message
dichotomization of score

D

dichotomized MMPI subscale
dichotomous
  d. scale
  d. thinking
dichotomy
  body-mind d.
  brain-mind d.
dichromatic
dichromatopsia
Dick AO fixateur interne
Dickman
  method of D.
diclofenac
dicloxacillin
dicoumarol
dictatorial
diction
dictum
dicyclic
dicyclomine
DID
  delayed ischemia deficit
  delayed ischemic deterioration
  dissociative identity disorder
didactic
  d. analysis
  d. group psychotherapy
didanosine
didaskaleinophobia
dido
Didrex
Didronel
diehard personality
diencephala (*pl. of* diencephalon)
diencephalic
  d. astrocytoma
  d. epilepsy
  d. membrane
  d. seizure
  d. stupor
  d. syndrome of infancy
  d. transition area
  d. vein
diencephalohypophysial
diencephalon, pl. **diencephala**
  ventricle of d.
diestrus
  gestational d.
  lactational d.
diet
  absolute d.
  ADA d.
  adequate d.
  aspartame-restricted d.
  balanced d.
  Banting d.
  basal d.
  basic d.
  Baylorfast d.
  bland d.
  dietetic d.
  elemental d.
  elimination d.
  fad d.
  Feingold d.

high-calorie d.
high-fat d.
high-fiber d.
high-protein d.
improper d.
Jenny Craig d.
ketogenic d.
lactoovovegetarian d.
lactovegetarian d.
light d.
limited d.
liquid d.
low-calorie d.
low-fat d.
low-salt d.
low-tyramine d.
macrobiotic d.
d. management
Nutri/System d.
Optifast d.
optimal d.
Pritikin d.
reduced sodium diet restricted d.
regular d.
restricted d.
salt-free d.
soft d.
subsistence d.
d. treatment
unrestricted d.
vegan d.
vegetarian d.
Weight Watchers d.
dietary
  d. amenorrhea
  d. chaos syndrome
  d. excess
  d. states
  d. theory
  d. toxin
dietetic diet
Diethrich bulldog clamp
diethylamide
  cocaine, heroin and lysergic
    acid d.
  crack and lysergic acid d.
  lysergic acid d. (LSD)
diethylenetriamine-penta-acetate
  gadolinium d.-p.-a.
diethylenetriamine penta-acetic acid
  (DTPA)
diethylmalonylurea
diethylpropion hydrochloride
diethylstilbestrol (DES)
diethyltryptamine
dietitian
dietotherapy
dietotoxicity
Differante disease
difference
  cerebral arteriovenous oxygen
    content d. $(AVDO_2)$
  chance d.
  gender d.
  group d.

individual d.
interear d.
interindividual d.'s
just noticeable d. (JND)
d. limen
mean consecutive d. (MCD)
mean sorted d. (MSD)
phase d.
qualitative d.
significant d.
standard error of d.
different
culturally d.
differentia
differential
D. Ability Scale
D. Aptitude Test (DAT)
D. Aptitude Test for Personnel
and Career Assessment
d. diagnosis
d. display of messenger ribonucleic
acid
d. equation
d. extinction
d. function
d. prevalence
d. reinforcement
d. reinforcement of other behavior
(DRO)
d. relaxation
d. response
semantic d.
D. Test of Conduct and Emotional
Problems (DT/CEP)
d. therapeutics
threshold d.
d. threshold
differentiation
cell d.
neuronal d.
regional d.
retrogressive d.
Schwann cell d.
sex d.
difficile
Clostridium d.
difficult child
difficulty, pl. difficulties
academic d.
d. in changing response set
chronic phase of stable sleep d.
concentration d.
d. controlling anger
Durrell Analysis of Reading D.:
Third Edition
emotional d.
emotional and behavioral difficulties
(EBD)
interpersonal d.
item d.
language d.
learning d.
d. level
life d.
memory d.

moderate d.
multiple life d.
protracted d.
school d.
sensory d.
speech d.
stable sleep d.
sublimation d.
tactile sensory d.
word-finding d.
diffident
diffusa
encephalitis periaxialis d.
diffuse
d. anxiety
d. axonal injury (DAI)
d. brain dysfunction
d. brain injury (DBI)
d. cerebral histiocytosis
d. cerebral sclerosis
d. disseminated atheroembolism
d. distribution of activity
d. encephalopathy
d. fibrillary astrocytic tumor
d. function
d. idiopathic skeletal hyperostosis
d. infantile familial sclerosis
d. intrinsic brainstem tumor
d. Lewy body disease
d. necrotizing leukoencephalopathy
d. noxious inhibitory control
(DNIC)
d. phoneme
d. pontine glioma
d. pontine lesion
d. slowing of EEG
d. white matter shearing injury
diffused reflex
diffusion
identity versus role d.
d. imaging
normoxic d.
d. respiration
role d.
d. transmission
diffusional state
diffusion-weighted scanning
diffusum
angiokeratoma corporis d.
diflavin free radical
diflunisal
difluoromethylornithin
digamy
digastric
d. line
d. muscle
digestible
digestive
d. epilepsy
d. psychogenic disorder
digit
d. recall
d. repetition test
d. reversal test
d. span (DS)

D

digit *(continued)*
 D. Span Distractibility Test
 d. span subtest
 d. stamp
 d. symbol (DS)
 D. Symbol Test
digital
 d. to analog converter
 d. angiography
 d. change
 D. Finger Tapping Test (DFTT)
 d. intravenous angiography
 d. nerve
 d. reflex
 d. signal analysis
 d. subtraction angiogram
 d. subtraction angiography (DSA)
 d. subtraction venography
 d. subtraction venous angiography
 d. subtraction venous angiography
  slice
 d. temple massage
 d. vascular imaging (DVI)
 d. vernier scale
digitalgia paresthetica
digitalis-induced delirium
digitized
 d. instrument
 d. spinography
digitizer
 AdVans three dimensional d.
 Cyberware 3030RGB d.
 three-dimensional sonic d.
digitoxin
digits test
Digit-Symbol and Incidental Memory
diglossia
digoxin
digraph
digress
dihexoside
 ceramide d.
dihybrid
dihydrochloride
 triethylene tetramine d.
 zuclopenthixol d.
dihydrocodeine
 d. bitartrate
 d. compound
dihydrocodeinone bitartrate
dihydroergotamine
 d. mesylate
 d. mesylate nasal spray
dihydroindolone
dihydrolone
dihydromorphinone hydrochloride
dihydromorphone
dihydrotachysterol
dihydroxyphenylalanine
3,4-dihydroxyphenylalanine (DOPA,
 Dopa, dopa)
DIL
 drug information log

Dilantin
 D. Infatab
 D. Kapseals
dilantinization
dilatation *(var. of* dilation)
dilate
dilated
 d. intercavernous sinus
 d. pupils
 d. ventricle
dilation, dilatation
 aneurysmal d.
 arachnoid nerve root sheath d.
 congenital d.
 episcleral vascular d.
 junctional d.
 progressive ventricular d.
dilator
 cannula with locking d.
 cortical incision coronary d.
 curved cannula with locking d.
 Eder-Puestow metal olive d.
 straight cannula with locking d.
dilatory nature
Dilaudid
 D.-5
 D.-HP
dildo
dilemma
 dialectical d.
 need-fear d.
 organic-functional d.
diligence
diligent
dillydally
Dilocaine
Dilone
diltiazem
dilution
 transference d.
DiMauro syndrome
dimeglumine
 gadopentetate d.
dimenhydrinate
dimension
 criterion d.
 D.'s of Delusional Experience
  Scale
 group d.
 hyperactivity-impulsivity d.
 inattention d.
 Isola spinal implant system d.
 job d.'s
 pedicle d.'s
dimensional
 d. approach
 D. Assessment of Personality
  Pathology-Basic Questionnaire
  (DAPP-BQ)
 d. model
 3-d. reconstruction wand
 d. setting
 d. system
dimensionality
 three d.

Dimensyn
dimercaprol
dimerization
    receptor d.
Dimetabs Oral
Dimetane
Dimetapp Sinus Caplets
2,5-dimethoxy-4-methylamphetamine
dimethoxyquinazoline
dimethylaminoethyl methacrylate
dimethyl sulfoxide (DMSO)
N,N-dimethyltryptamine
dimethyltryptamine
dimidiata
    chorea d.
diminish
diminished
    d. capacity
    d. control
    d. effect
    d. libido
    d. pleasure in everyday activities
    d. reality testing
    d. recall
    d. reflex
    d. response to pain
    d. responsibility
    d. responsiveness
    d. sensation
    d. sexual interest
diminution
    d. of affect
    d. of goal-directed behavior
    d. of thought
diminutive
dimming
    chromatic d.
dimorphic
    sexually d.
dimorphism
    brain d.
    sexual d.
dimple
    acromial d.
    sacral d.
DIMS
    disorder of initiating and maintaining
      sleep
Dinate Injection
DIND
    delayed ischemic neurological deficit
ding-dong theory
Dingman
    D. mouth gag
    D. oral retraction system
dinitrate
    isosorbide d.
dinitrophenol peripheral neuropathy
dinomania
dinophobia
dinucleotide
    flavin adenine d. (FAD)
dioctyl sodium sulfosuccinate
diode
    light-emitting d. (LED)

diodine
diodone
Diodrast
diogenism
Dionosil
dionysian attitude
diotic
    d. listening
    d. message
dioxide
    partial arterial gas tension of
      carbon d. (PaCO2)
    thorium d.
dioxyamphetamine
    methylene d.
dip
diphasic milk fever
Diphenhist
diphenhydramine
    acetaminophen and d.
    d. hydrochloride
diphenylaminearsine chloride
Diphenylan Sodium
diphenylbutyl
diphenylbutylpiperidine
diphenylchlorarsine
diphenylhydantoin
diphosphate
    guanosine d. (GDP)
diphtheriae
    Corynebacterium d.
diphtheria peripheral neuropathy
diphtheria, tetanus toxoids, and
  pertussis vaccine (DTP)
diphtheritic
    d. neuropathy
    d. paralysis
diphtheroid
dipipanone hydrochloride
diplacusis dysharmonica
diplegia
    ataxic d.
    congenital facial d.
    facial d.
    infantile d.
    masticatory d.
    spastic d.
diplegic idiocy
diploë
diploic vein
diploid
diplomacy
Diploma in Psychological Medicine
  (DPM)
diplomyelia
diplopia
diplopiaphobia
diploscope
dipole
    d. field
    d. localization
    magnetic d.
    d. tracing (DT)

D

dipole-dipole
    d.-d. interaction
    d.-d. relaxation
dipotassium
    clorazepate d.
dipping
    body d.
    converse ocular d.
    ocular d.
dippoldism
Diprivan
dipropyltryptamine
Diprotrizoate
dipsesis
dipsetic
dipsomania
dipsophobia
dipsosis
dipyridamole
DIR
    disturbed interpersonal relationships
direct
    D. Assessment of Functional Status
      Scale
    d. association
    d. auditory compound actional
      potential
    d. brain stimulation (DBS)
    d. causality
    d. causative pathophysiological
      mechanism
    d. confrontation
    d. current (DC)
    d. embolectomy
    d. end-to-end coaptation
    d. fracture
    d. image
    d. interview
    d. motor system
    d. multiplanar imaging
    d. observation
    d. physiological effect
    d. pyramidal tract
    d. screw fixation technique
    d. selection communication board
    d. self-destructive behavior (DSDB)
    d. suggestion under hypnosis
      (DSUH)
directed
    d. group therapy
    inner d.
    other d.
    d. thinking
    tradition d.
Directin
direction
    completion, arithmetic, vocabulary,
      and d.'s (CAVD)
    flow d.
    phase-encoding d.
    d. prognosis
    psychotic d.
directional coronary atherectomy (DCA)
directionality

directive
    genetic d.
    d. psychotherapy
directivity
direful situation
dirigation
dirigomotor
dirt eating
dirtiness
    feelings of d.
dirty
    d. needle
    d. pool
    d. urine
    d. words
DIS
    Diagnostic Interview Schedule
disability
    abstracting d.
    D. Adjusted Life Years (DALYs)
    associated d.
    chronic d.
    cognitive d.
    congenital arithmetic d.
    d. counselor
    degree of d.
    d. determination service (DDS)
    developmental d.
    Division of Developmental D.'s
      (DDD)
    drawing d.
    emotional d.
    functional d.
    general language d.
    language d.
    learning d. (LD)
    d. level
    long-term d. (LTD)
    manifested d.
    memory d.
    mental d.
    mild d.
    mobility d.
    motor d.
    National Information Center for
      Children & Youth with D.'s
    neurologic d.
    observable d.
    output d.
    partial permanent d.
    perceptual d.
    perceptual-motor d.
    permanent d.
    posttraumatic chronic d.
    progressive d.
    psychiatric d.
    Pupil Rating Scale: Screening for
      Learning D.'s
    reading d.
    residual d.
    reversible ischemic neurologic d.
      (RIND)
    Screening for Learning D.'s

SEARCH: A Scanning Instrument for the Identification of Potential Learning D.
sequencing d.
service-connected d. (SCD)
severe d. (SD)
social d.
Social Security D. (SSD)
speech d.
d. status scale (DSS)
temporary d.
total d.
work d.
writing d.

disabled
Career Assessment Inventories: For the Learning D.
developmentally d.
emotionally disturbed/learning d. (ED/LD)
learning d.
partially d.
psychiatrically d.
temporarily d.
totally d.
Weller-Strawser Scales of Adaptive Behavior for the Learning D.

disabling
d. headache
d. stress

disaccharide malabsorption
disadvantage
cultural d.
economic d.
educational d.

disaggregation
Disalcid
disappointment
disapproval
fear of d.

disarray
myofibrillary d.

disassimilation
disassociate
disassociation (*var. of* dissociation)
disastrous
disavowal level
DIS-C, DISC
Diagnostic Interview Schedule for Children

disc (*var. of* disk)
Disease
discectomy, diskectomy
anterior d.
automated percutaneous lumbar d. (APLD)
cervical d.
lumbar d.
microlumbar d.
microsurgery d.
Robinson anterior cervical d.
thoracic d.
transthoracic d.

discernible

discharge
affective d.
anxiety d.
bad conduct d. (BCD)
bilateral independent periodic lateralizing epileptiform d. (BIPLED)
cathectic d.
complex repetitive d. (CRD)
conditional d.
corollary d.
decrescendo d.
delayed d.
dishonorable d.
early d.
EEG anteromesial temporal d.
epileptiform d.
epileptiform burst d.
focal epileptiform d.
honorable d.
ictal focal epileptiform d.
Intensity, Severity, and D. (ISD)
interference pattern of d.
interictal focal epileptiform d.
interictal generalized spike-and-wave d.
interictal spike d.
InterQual Intensity, Severity, and D.
involuntary d.
medical d.
myokymic d.
myotonic d.
neuromyotonic d.
periodic lateralizing epileptiform d. (PLED)
polyspike-and-wave d.
psuedoperiodic d.
rhythmical midtemporal d. (RMTD)
rolandic epileptiform d.
spike d.
waning d.

discharged against medical advice (DAMA)
discharging lesion
dischronation
disci (*pl. of* discus)
disciplinarian
disciplinary
d. problem
d. segregation

discipline
bondage and d.
formal d.
harsh d.
inadequate d.
inconsistent parental d.
mental d.

discission knife
discitis, diskitis
iatrogenic d.
intervertebral d.
pyogenic d.

disclaim
disclose

D

disclosure
    truth d.
discogenic, diskogenic
    d. sclerosis
discogram, diskogram
discography, diskography
discoid
    d. marker
    d. skin lesion
discoligamentous
    d. complex
    d. injury
discomfort
    abdominal d.
    chest d.
    gender role persistent d.
    d. level
    persistent d.
    threshold of d. (TD)
    d. threshold
    d. with emotion
    d. with gender role
discommodity
disconjugate eye deviation
disconnected
    d. idea
    d. thought
disconnection
    d. apraxia
    d. hypothesis
    social d.
    d. syndrome
    d. thought disorder
    d. with reality
disconnect speech
discontinuity
    Bruch membrane d.
    facial nerve d.
    nerve d.
discontinuous activity
discopathy
    traumatic cervical d.
discord
    marital d.
discordant
    d. behavior
    d. facial expression
discoscope
    percutaneous d.
discotomy
discourse
    spontaneous narrative d.
    Test of Word Finding in D.
      (TWFD)
discrepancy scale
discrepant intellectual function
discrete period
discriminant
    d. analysis
    d. validity
discrimination
    age d.
    auditory d.
    brightness d.
    class d.

    color d.
    d. consciousness
    cultural d.
    form d.
    gender d.
    index of d.
    d. learning
    loss d.
    pattern d.
    pitch d.
    pure tone d.
    racial d.
    reverse d.
    right-left d.
    score d.
    sensory d.
    sexual d.
    Sweet two-point d.
    Test of Auditory D. (TAD)
    Testing-Teaching Module of
      Auditory D. (TTMAD)
    Test of Nonverbal Auditory D.
      (TENVAD, TNVAD)
    training d.
    visual d.
    weight d.
    Wepman Test of Auditory D.
discriminative stimulus
discriminatory
    d. behavior
    d. comment
discursive
discus, pl. disci
    d. lentiformis
DISCUSS
    Developing Skills Checklist
discussion
    leaderless group d. (LGD)
discutient
disdiadochokinesia
disease
    Acosta d.
    Adams-Stokes d.
    adaptation d.
    d. adaptation
    Addison d.
    advanced cortical d.
    affective d.
    Akureyri d.
    Albright d.
    alcoholic liver d. (ALD)
    Alexander d.
    Alpers d.
    altitude d.
    Alzheimer d. (AD)
    Andes d.
    anterior horn cell d.
    antiepileptic drug-induced bone d.
    aortocranial d.
    Aran-Duchenne d.
    arterial occlusive d.
    arteriosclerotic brain d.
    arteriosclerotic cardiovascular d.
      (ASCVD)
    association d.

atheromatous d.
atherosclerotic d.
atherosclerotic heart d.
atypical bipolar d.
Australian X d.
autoimmune d.
aviator's d.
Ayala d.
Azorean d.
Azorean-Joseph-Machado d.
Ballet d.
Baló d.
Bamberger d.
Bannister d.
barbed-wire d.
basilar-vertebral artery d.
Bassen-Kornzweig d.
Batten d.
Batten-Mayou d.
Baxter d.
Bayle d.
Beard d.
Bechterew d.
Begbie d.
Behavioral Pathology in
  Alzheimer D. (BEHAVE-AD)
Behçet d.
Bell d.
Bergeron d.
Bernard-Soulier d.
Bernhardt d.
Bielschowsky d.
Bielschowsky-Jansky d.
Biemond d.
Binswanger d.
biology of affective d.
Blocq d.
Bloom d.
bodily d.
bone d.
bone marrow transplantation graft-
  versus-host d.
Bornholm d.
Bourneville d.
Bourneville-Pringle d.
bowel d.
brainstem d.
brancher enzyme deficiency d.
Brissaud d.
Brodie d.
Brushfield-Wyatt d.
Buschke d.
Busse-Buschke d.
calcium pyrophosphate dihydrate
  decomposition d.
Camurati-Engelmann d.
Canavan d.
Canavan-van Bogaert-Bertrand d.
cardiac d.
carotid artery d.
cat-scratch d. (CSD)
central core d.
central motor pathways d.
cerebral d.
cerebrovascular d.

cervical spine rheumatoid d.
Chagas d.
Charcot d.
Charcot-Marie-Tooth d.
Cheyne d.
childhood moyamoya d.
cholestanol storage d.
cholesterol ester storage d.
Christensen-Krabbe d.
Christmas d.
CJ d.
Coats d.
combined system d.
connective tissue d.
Consortium to Establish a Registry
  for Alzheimer's D. (CERAD)
constitutional d.
coronary artery d.
corticospinal d.
Cotunnius d.
Cowden d.
CPT d.
Creutzfeldt-Jakob d. (CJD)
Crigler-Najjar d.
Crohn d.
Crouzon d.
Cruveilhier d.
Curschmann-Steinert d.
Cushing d.
cytomegalic inclusion d.
dancing d.
Danielssen d.
Danielssen-Boeck d.
degenerative brain d.
degenerative cervical disk d.
degenerative discogenic end-plate d.
degenerative disk d.
Degos d.
Dejerine d.
Dejerine-Sottas d.
dementia due to Creutzfeldt-
  Jakob d.
demyelinating d.
de Quervain d.
Devic d.
Diferrante d.
diffuse Lewy body d.
disturbance associated with organic
  mental d.
Down d.
drug d.
Dubini d.
Duchenne d.
Duchenne-Aran d.
dynamic d.
Eales d.
early-onset familial Alzheimer d.
Economo d.
Emery-Dreifuss d.
emotional d.
Engelmann d.
enterococcal d.
epidural hemorrhage epidural
  metastatic d.
Erb d.

D

disease *(continued)*
Erb-Charcot d.
Erichsen d.
Escobar d.
Eulenburg d.
exophytic joint d.
extracranial carotid occlusive d.
extracranial occlusive vascular d.
extrapyramidal d.
Fabry d.
Fahr d.
familial Alzheimer d. (FAD)
familial paroxysmal
    choreoathetosis d.
familial pure depressive d. (FPDD)
Farber d.
fatigue d.
feared d.
Feer d.
Flatau-Schilder d.
flight into d.
Foix-Alajouanine d.
Folling d.
Forbes d.
Forbes-Cori d.
Forestier d.
Fothergill d.
Freiberg-Kohler d.
d. frequency
Friedmann d.
Friedreich d.
Fuerstner d.
Fukuyama d.
functional d.
Gairdner d.
Gaucher d.
genetic d.
genetotrophic d.
Gerhardt d.
Gerlier d.
Gerstmann-Straussler-Scheinker d.
Gilles de la Tourette d.
Glanzmann d.
glial d.
glycogen storage d.
Goldflam d.
Gowers d.
Graefe d.
graft-versus-host d. (GVHD)
Graves d.
Greenfield d.
Guinon d.
Haglund d.
Hallervorden-Spatz d.
Hammond d.
hand-foot-and-mouth d.
Hand-Schüller-Christian d.
Hansen d.
Hartnup d.
Hashimoto d.
heart d.
Heidenhain d.
Heller d.
hepatocerebral d.

hepatolenticular d.
hereditary striatopallidal d.
heterogeneous system d.
Hippel d.
Hippel-Lindau d.
Hirschsprung d.
HIV d.
Hodgkin d.
Holmes cerebellar degeneration d.
Hoppe-Goldflam d.
Horton d.
human prion d.
Hunt d.
Hunter d.
Huntington d. (HD)
Hurler d.
Hurler-Scheie d.
Hurst d.
hydatid d.
iatrogenic d.
Iceland d.
idiopathic Parkinson d.
infectious d.
inflammation bowel d.
inflammatory demyelinating d.
inherited progressive degenerative d.
International Classification of D.'s
    (ICD)
International Classification of D.'s
    and Related Health Problems,
    10th Edition (ICD-10)
International Classification of D.'s,
    9th edition (ICD-9)
International Classification of D.'s,
    9th Edition, Clinical Modification
    (ICD-9-CM)
interstitial lung d. (ILD)
intradural inflammatory d.
intraneuronal inclusion d.
intrinsic d.
ischemic d.
ischemic heart d. (IHD)
Jakob-Creutzfeldt d.
Janet d.
Jansky-Bielschowsky d.
Jeep driver's d.
Joseph d.
jumper d. of Maine
juvenile nonneuropathic Niemann-
    Pick d.
Kanner d.
Kearns-Sayre d.
Kempf d.
Kennedy-Fischbeck d.
kinky-hair d.
Kinnier-Wilson d.
kissing d.
Klippel d.
Korsakoff d.
Krabbe d.
Krabbe-Weber-Dimitri d.
Kraepelin d.
K's d.
Kufs d.
Kugelberg-Welander d.

labyrinthine d.
Lafora d.
Landouzy-Dejerine d.
Lasègue d.
laughing d.
L4-5 disk d.
Leber d.
Legg d.
Leigh d.
leptomeningeal d.
Lesch-Nyhan d.
Letterer-Siwe d.
Lewy body variant of
  Alzheimer d.
Lhermitte-Duclos d.
Lichtheim d.
life-threatening d.
Lindau d.
Little d.
liver d.
Lou Gehrig d.
L5-S1 disk d.
Luft d.
lumbar disk d.
lumbar facet d.
Lyme d.
Lyodura-associated Creutzfeldt-
  Jakob d.
lysosomal storage d.
Lytico-Bodig d.
Machado-Joseph d.
maple syrup urine d. (MSUD)
Marateaux-Lamy d.
Marchiafava-Bignami d.
Marie-Foix-Alajouanine d.
Marie-Strümpell d.
Maroteaux-Lamy d.
Meige d.
Ménière d.
Menkes d.
mental d.
Merzbacher-Pelizaeus d.
metastatic d.
Milton d.
Minamata d.
Mitchell d.
mixed connective tissue d.
  (MCTD)
Möbius d.
Morel-Kraepelin d.
Morgagni d.
Morquio d.
Morvan d.
motor neuron d.
motor pathways d.
moyamoya d.
multicore d.
myelinoclastic d.
National Institute of Allergy and
  Infectious D. (NIAID)
Neftel d.
neoplastic d.
nervous d.
neuro-Behçet d.
neurodegenerative d.

neurologic d.
Niemann-Pick d. (type A, B, C)
nonneoplastic d.
oasthouse urine d.
occlusive cerebrovascular d.
occupational d. (OD)
oculocraniosomatic d.
Ollier d.
Oppenheim d.
organic brain d. (OBD)
other neurological d. (OND)
Paget d.
Parkinson d. (PD)
Parry-Romberg d.
Parsonage-Turner d.
pediatric moyamoya d.
Pelizaeus-Merzbacher d.
periatrial d.
peripheral nerve d.
peripheral vascular d.
periventricular d.
peroxisomal d.
Pette-Döring d.
Peyronie d.
d. phobia
Pick d.
pink d.
Pompe d.
Portuguese-Azorean d.
Pott d.
primary Parkinson d.
Pringle d.
prion d.
d. process
progressive d.
progressive degenerative d.
pseudomyotonia d.
psychiatric d.
psychotic d.
pulseless d.
Quincke d.
Rabot d.
Ragin' Cajun d.
Recklinghausen d.
rectal d.
Refsum d.
Rendu-Osler-Weber d.
reversible motor neuron d.
rheumatic heart d.
rheumatoid d.
Romberg d.
Roth d.
Roth-Bernhardt d.
Roussy-Lévy d.
Rust d.
Saint Dymphna d.
Saint Martin d.
Saint Mathurin d.
Salla d.
sanatorium d.
Sander d.
Sandhoff d.
Sanfilippo d.
Santavuori d.
Santavuori-Haltia d.

D

disease *(continued)*
Santavuori-Haltia-Hagberg d.
Schaumberg d.
Scheie d.
Scheuermann d.
Schilder d.
Schmitt d.
Scholz d.
Seitelberger d.
Selter d.
severe degenerative disk d.
sexually transmitted d. (STD)
sickle cell d.
Siemerling-Creutzfeldt d.
skin d.
Sly d.
social d.
Spielmeyer-Sjögren d.
Spielmeyer-Vogt d.
Spielmeyer-Vogt-Sjögren d.
spinal cord d.
spinal metastatic d.
sporadic depressive d. (SDD)
startle d.
Steele-Richardson-Olszewski d.
Steinert d.
Stokes-Adams d.
Strümpell d.
Strümpell-Lorrain d.
Strümpell-Marie d.
Strümpell-Westphal d.
student's d.
Sturge d.
Sturge-Weber d.
suspected d.
Sydenham d.
Takayasu d.
Talma d.
Tangier d.
Tay-Sachs d.
d. theme
Thomsen d.
thoracolumbar degenerative d.
Thornton-Griggs-Moxley d.
Tourette d.
Trevor d.
Unverricht d.
Unverricht-Lafora d.
Unverricht-Lundborg d.
Urbach-Wiethe d.
van Bogaert d.
van Bogaert-Canavan d.
venereal d. (VD)
venous occlusive d.
venous thromboembolic d. (VTED)
vertebrobasilar d.
Virchow d.
vitreous d.
Vogt d.
Vogt-Spielmeyer d.
von Economo d.
von Eulenberg d.
von Gierke d.
von Hippel-Lindau d.

von Recklinghausen d.
Weber-Christian d.
Welander d.
Werdnig-Hoffmann d.
Wernicke d.
Westphal d.
Whipple d.
white matter d.
Wilson hepatolenticular
  degeneration d.
Winkelman d.
Wohlfart-Kugelberg-Welander d.
Wolman d.
Ziehen-Oppenheim d.
disease-oriented/medical model approach
disembody
disenfranchise
disengagement mechanism
disentangle
disequilibrium *(var. of* dysequilibrium)
disfigurement
  facial d.
disfluency
  d. dyskinesia
  speech d.
disgust
  feeling of d.
disharmony
  affective d.
disheveled appearance
dishonorable discharge
dishpan fracture
disialyl ganglioside
disinhibited
  d. behavior
  d. type of passive developmental
    disorder
disinhibited-type reactive attachment
  disorder of infancy or childhood
disinhibition
  emotional d.
  motor d.
  d. psychiatric syndrome
disintegrate
disintegration
  d. of consciousness
  personality d.
disintegrative
  d. childhood psychosis
  d. disorder
disk, disc
  Bardeen d.
  choked d.
  d. curette
  embryonic d.
  frayed d.
  free fragment d.
  herniated cervical d.
  herniated intervertebral d. (HID)
  d. herniation
  injury of intervertebral d.
  intervertebral d.
  intraspinal herniated d.
  magnetic d.
  d. matrix proteoglycan

Merkel tactile d.
optic d.
protruded d.
d. punch
Ranvier d.
d. rongeur
ruptured d.
Schiefferdecker d.
sequestrated d.
d. space
d. space infection
d. syndrome
tactile d.
vacuum d.
diskectomy (*var. of* discectomy)
diskiform
diskitis (*var. of* discitis)
diskogenic (*var. of* discogenic)
diskogram (*var. of* discogram)
diskography (*var. of* discography)
dislocation
atlantoaxial d.
C6-C7 d.
fracture d.
temporomandibular joint d.
dislodgement
hook d.
dismutase
superoxide d. (SOD)
Dismutec
disobedience
civil d.
disobedient behavior
disodium
carbenicillin d.
edetate d.
edetate calcium d.
etidronate d.
d. etidronate
moxalactam d.
disofenin
technetium 99m d.
disopyramide phosphate
disorder
abnormal involuntary movement d.
(AIMD)
Abraham view of depressive d.
academic skills d.
academic underachievement d.
accommodation d.
acquired-type d.
acute stress d. (ASD)
addictive d.
adjustment interface d.
adjustment reaction conduct d.
adolescent-onset conduct d.
adrenal d.
d. of affect
d. affecting general medical
condition
affective bipolar d.
affective determined d.
affective neurotic personality d.
affective spectrum d.
aggressive d.

agoraphobia without history of
panic d.
alcohol amnestic d.
alcoholic organic mental d.
alcohol intoxication-related d.
alcohol-related use d., not
otherwise specified
alcohol use d.
allergic psychogenic d.
alpha-methyldopa-induced mood d.
alternating bipolar d.
alternative criterion B for
dysthymic d.
American Academy of Stress D.'s
amitriptyline-induced mood d.
amnestic d.
amphetamine delusional d.
amphetamine-related d.
amphetamine use d.
anorexia nervosa and
associated d.'s (ANAD)
antisocial personality d. (ASPD)
anxiety adjustment d.
anxiety-avoiding personality d.
anxiety-related mental d.
anxiety state neurotic d.
anxiolytic amnestic d.
anxiolytic use d.
apathetic-type personality d.
aphasia d.
apperceptive d.
appetite psychogenic d.
apraxic d.
arithmetic d.
arithmetical developmental delay d.
arousal d.
arteriosclerotic brain d.
articulation developmental delay d.
artificial d.
Asperger d.
associated d.
asthenic personality d.
attachment d.
attachment-separation d.
attention deficit d. (ADD)
attention deficit hyperactivity d.
(ADHD)
attention-deficit/hyperactivity d.
attention deficit hyperactivity d.-
predominantly inattentive (ADHD-
PI)
auditory d.
autistic d.
autoimmune obsessive-compulsive
tic d.
autonomic d.
avoidant neurotic personality d.
Axis I d.
Axis II d.
balance d.
Beck view of depressive d.
behavioral d.
bereavement d.
Bibring view of depressive d.
binge-eating d.

D

disorder *(continued)*

bipolar affective d.
bipolar depression d.
bipolar I d.
bipolar II d.
bipolar type schizoaffective d.
bizarre behavior/formal thought d.
bleeding d.
blood psychogenic d.
body dysmorphic d. (BDD)
borderline personality d. (BPD)
bowel d.
brain damage language d.
breathing d.
breathing-related sleep d.
brief posttraumatic stress d.
brief psychotic d.
Briquet d.
caffeine-induced d.
cannabis-induced anxiety d.
cannabis-induced delirium d.
cannabis intoxication-related d.
cannabis organic mental d.
cannabis-related d., not otherwise
  specified
cannabis use d.
cardiac d.
cardiovascular psychogenic d.
catatonic d.
Center for Stress and Anxiety D.'s
central language d. (CLD)
cerebral d.
character impulse d.
character spectrum d.'s
childhood d.
d. of childhood
children and adults with attention
  deficit d. (CHADD)
Chinese Classification of
  Mental D.'s, Second Edition
  (CCMD-2)
choreic movement d.
choreiform d.
chronobiological d.
circadian rhythm sleep d.
clotting d.
cluster A personality d.
cluster B personality d.
cluster characteristics in
  personality d.
cluster C personality d.
coagulation d.
cocaine delusional d.
cocaine-induced d.
cocaine intoxication-related d.
cocaine-related d., not otherwise
  specified
cocaine use d.
codependency d.
coexisting d.
cognitive d.
Cohen view of depressive d.
color vision d.

combined-type attention deficit
  hyperactivity d.
combined-type attention-
  deficit/hyperactivity d.
combined-type personality d.
communicative d.
comorbid anxiety d.
comorbid personality d.
compensation neurosis neurotic d.
complicated grief d.
compulsive d.
conceptual d.
conditions not attributable to a
  mental d.
conduct disturbance adjustment d.
conduction d.
content thought d.
contiguity d.
conversion d.
convulsive d.
co-occurring mental d.
coordination developmental delay d.
coprophemia d.
criteria-defined borderline
  personality d.
cumulative trauma d. (CTD)
cutaneous psychogenic d.
cyclic mood d.
cyclothymic personality d.
degenerative d.
delayed posttraumatic stress d.
Delirium, Dementia, and Amnestic
  and Other Cognitive D.'s
delirium-related mental d.
delusional paranoid d.
dementia-related mental d.
demyelinative d.
dependence d.
dependent neurotic personality d.
dependent-passive personality d.
depersonalization neurotic d.
depressed mood adjustment d.
depression neurotic d.
depression-related mental d.
depressive d.
depressive spectrum d. (DSD)
deteriorated affective d.
deteriorated bipolar d.
developmental d.
Diagnostic and Statistical Manual
  of Mental D.'s (DSM)
Diagnostic and Statistical Manual
  of Mental D.'s-3rd Edition
  (DSM-III)
Diagnostic and Statistical Manual
  of Mental D.'s-3rd Edition
  Revised (DSM-III-R)
Diagnostic and Statistical Manual
  of Mental D.'s-4th Edition
  (DSM-IV)
digestive psychogenic d.
disconnection thought d.
disinhibited type of passive
  developmental d.
disintegrative d.

disorganized-type schizophrenic d.
displacement d.
disruptive behavior d.
dissociative d.
dissociative identity d. (DID)
dissociative d. not otherwise
  specified (DDNOS)
dissociative trance d.
dream anxiety d.
drug-induced mental d.
drug-related d.
d. due to combined factors
dysmorphic somatoform d.
dyspneic psychogenic d.
dyssocial personality d.
dysthymic neurotic d.
early trauma hypothesis of
  autistic d.
eating d.
ejaculation d.
electroconvulsive therapy-induced
  mood d.
elimination d.
emaciation d.
emancipation d.
emancipatory d.
emotional disturbance adjustment d.
emotional instability personality d.
emotionally unstable character d.
  (EUCD)
endocrine psychogenic d.
epileptic d.
epileptoid personality d.
episodic d.
erectile arousal d.
erythrocyte d.
esophagus psychogenic d.
evidence of dissociation d.
d. of excessive sleepiness
d.'s of excessive somnolence
  (DOES)
experimental d.
explosive d.
expressive language development d.
expressive writing development d.
extractive d.
extrapyramidal d.
eye movement d.
eye psychogenic d.
factitious d., combined type
factitious interface d.
factitious d., physical type
factitious d., psychological type
factitious-type neurotic hysteric d.
false role d.
familial d.
feeding and eating d.
feeding psychogenic d.
female hypoactive sexual desire d.
fluency d.
food intake d.
formal thought d.
Freud view of depressive d.
frontal gait d.
frontal perceptual d.

functional d.
gait d.
gastric psychogenic d.
gastrointestinal d.
gender identity d. (GID)
generalized anxiety d. (GAD)
genetic d.
genitourinary psychogenic d.
geriatric depressive d.
glycoprotein storage d.
Grid Test of Schizophrenic
  Thought D. (GTSTD)
group-type conduct d.
habit d.
hallucinogen-affective d.
hallucinogen-delusional d.
hallucinogen-induced delirium and
  anxiety d.
hallucinogen persisting perception d.
hallucinogen-related d., not
  otherwise specified
hallucinogen use d.
Hartnup d.
Haws Screening Test for
  Functional Articulation D.'s
hearing d.
heart d.
hereditary d.
histrionic neurotic personality d.
histrionic personality d.
homosexual conflict d.
hyperactive d.
hyperactive-impulse attention-
  deficit/hyperactivity d.
hyperactivity d.
hyperkinetic d.
hypersomnia d.
hypersomnia-type sleep d.
hypersomnolence d.
hyperthymic personality d.
hypnotic-induced d.
hypnotic use d.
hypoactive sexual desire d.
hypochondriacal psychogenic d.
hypochondriasis neurotic d.
hypomanic d.
hypothermic d.
hypothymic personality d.
hysteria neurotic d.
hysterical gait d.
iatrogenic d.
identity d.
immature personality d.
immune d.
d. of impulse control
impulse control d. (ICD)
impulse control conduct d.
inadequate personality d.
inattentive-type attention-
  deficit/hyperactivity d.
induced paranoid d.
induced psychotic d.
d. of infancy, childhood, or
  adolescence
inhalant-induced d.

D

disorder *(continued)*

inhalant-related d.
inhalant use d.
inherited global
  neurodegenerative d.
inhibited-type reactive attachment d.
inhibited-type reactive attachment d.
  of infancy or early
d. of initiating and maintaining
  sleep (DIMS)
insomnia d.
insomnia related to another
  mental d.
insomnia-type substance-induced
  sleep d.
intelligence d.
intermittent explosive d.
International Classification of
  Sleep D.'s
intersensory d.
intersexual d.
intracranial d.
introverted personality d.
intrusive sexual d.
isolated explosive d.
Jacobson view of depressive d.
joint d.
Klein view of depressive d.
labile personality d.
labyrinthine d.
language developmental delay d.
language and speech d.
late luteal phase dysphoric d.
  (LLPDD)
learning developmental d.
less pervasive d.
lifelong-type d.
light-therapy-induced mood d.
limbic system d.
limb movement d.
lipid metabolism d.
logicogrammatical d.
lung d.
lymphoproliferative d.
major depressive d. (MDD)
male dyspareunia male erectile d.
male hypoactive sexual desire d.
malingering d.
manic bipolar d.
manic-depressive d.
marijuana delusional d.
masochistic personality d.
mastication d.
mathematics d.
medical/neurological d.
medical/psychiatric sleep d.
medication-induced movement d.,
  not otherwise specified
memory d.
menstrual d.
mental psychoneurotic d.
mental subnormality d.
metabolic d.
micturition d.

mild neurocognitive d.
minor depressive d.
Mississippi Scale for Combat-
  Related Posttraumatic Stress D.
mitral valve d.
mixed anxiety depression d.
  (MADD)
mixed bipolar d.
mixed conduct/emotional disturbance
  adjustment d.
mixed conduct/emotions conduct d.
mixed development developmental
  delay d.
mixed receptive-expressive
  language d.
mixed specific developmental d.
monogenetic d.
monoplegic d.
mood d.
mood-cyclic d.
moral deficiency personality d.
motility d.
motor retardation developmental
  delay d.
motor skills d.
motor tic d.
motor-verbal tic d.
motor-vocal tic d.
mouth d.
movement d.
multiple personality d. (MPD)
muscle d.
musculoskeletal d.
myeloproliferative d.
narcissistic neurotic personality d.
National Institute on Deafness &
  Other Communication D.'s
negativistic personality d.
neoplastic d.
neurasthenia neurotic d.
neurocirculatory psychogenic d.
neurocognitive d.
neurodevelopmental d.
neurogenic d.
neuroleptic-induced acute
  movement d.
neuroleptic treatment of childhood
  conduct d.
neurologic d.
neurological d.
neurometabolic d.
neuromuscular d.
neuronal lysosomal storage d.
neuropsychiatric movement d.
neuropsychologic d.
neurotic hysteric d.
nicotine-induced d.
nicotine organic brain d.
nicotine-related d., not otherwise
  specified
nicotine use d.
nightmare d.
nonorganic steep d.
nonpsychotic mental d.
non-substance-induced mental d.

nontranssexual cross-gender d.
nutritional deficiency d.
obsessional d.
obsessive d.
obsessive-compulsive d. (OCD)
obsessive psychogenic d.
occupational d.
opioid-induced d.
opioid use d.
oppositional defiant d. (ODD)
oppression-artifact d.
optokinetic d.
organic d.
organic brain d. (OBD)
organic mental d. (OMD)
orgasmic d.
orientation d.
other type personality d.
overanxious d.
overconscientious personality d.
overreactive d.
over-the-counter drug-related d.
pain prone d.
pain somatoform d.
panic d. (PD)
paralytic d.
paranoid neurotic personality d.
paranoid-schizotypal personality d.
paraphiliac coercive d.
parasomnia-type sleep d.
parasomnia-type substance-induced
  sleep d.
parathyroid d.
paroxysmal sleep d.
passive-aggressive neurotic
  personality d.
PCP-induced anxiety d.
PCP-related d., not otherwise
  specified
PCP use d.
perception d.
perceptual d.
periluteal phase dysphoric d.
periodic limb movement d.
permissive hypothesis of
  affective d.'s
persecutory delusional d.
persistent vegetative state d.
persisting d.
personality neurotic d.
pervasive developmental d. (PDD)
pervasive disinhibited type of
  developmental d.
phencyclidine delusional d.
phencyclidine-induced d.
phencyclidine-related d.
phencyclidine use d.
phenylalanine d.
phobic d.
phonological d.
physical d.
pica d.
platelet d.
polysubstance-related d.
positive thought d.

possession/trance d.
postconcussion d.
posthallucinogen perception d.
postpsychotic depressive d.
posttraumatic stress d. (PTSD)
potential cumulative trauma d.
predominantly hyperactive-impulse
  attention deficit hyperactivity d.
predominantly inattentive-type
  attention deficit hyperactivity d.
preexisting mental d.
premenstrual dysphoric d.
prescription drug-related d.
presenile mental d.
primary affective d. (PAD)
primary anxiety d.
primary behavior d.
Primary Care Evaluation of
  Mental D.'s (PRIME-MD)
processing d.
prolonged posttraumatic stress d.
pruritic d.
pseudosocial personality d.
psychiatric system interface d.
psychic d.
psychoactive d.
psychoaffective d. (PAD)
psychogenic d.
psychomotor d.
psychoneurotic mental d.
psychophysiological d.
psychosexual d.
psychosomatic d.
psychotic d.
pyromania d.
Rado view of depressive d.
rapid-cycling bipolar d.
reactive d.
reactive attachment d.
reading developmental delay d.
receptive language d.
rectal psychogenic d.
recurrent brief depressive d.
reflex d.
related sleep d.
REM behavior d. (RBD)
REM sleep behavior d.
repetitive impulse d.
residual type schizophrenic d.
resonance d.
respiratory impairment sleep d.
retardation developmental delay d.
Rett d.
rheumatic d.
rheumatoid d.
rumination d.
sadistic personality d.
sadomasochistic personality d.
Sandler view of depressive d.
Scale for the Assessment of
  Unawareness of Mental D.
  (SUMD)
schizoaffective d.
schizoid d.
schizoid personality d.

D

disorder *(continued)*
schizoid-schizotypal personality d. (SSPD)
schizophrenic d.
schizophreniform d.
schizotypal personality d.
Screen for Child Anxiety Related Emotional D.'s
seasonal affective d. (SAD)
seasonal mood d.
secondary sleep d.
sedative, hypnotic, or anxiolytic-induced anxiety d.
sedative-induced d.
sedative use d.
seductive personality d.
self-defeating personality d.
Seligman view of depressive d.
Selz and Reitan rules to assess learning d.'s
semantic pragmatic d.
semantogenic d.
senile gait d.
senile psychotic mental d.
separation anxiety d. (SAD)
sexual d.
sexual aversion d.
sexual desire d.
sexual deviance d.
sexual deviation neurotic d.
sexual and gender identity d.
sham d.
shamanistic thought d.
shared paranoid d.
shared psychotic d.
simple deteriorative d.
situational-type d.
situational-type female orgasmic d.
situational-type female sexual arousal d.
sleep d.
sleep behavior d.
sleep-wake schedule d.
sleepwalking d.
smell d.
social anxiety d.
socialized conduct d.
sociopathic personality d. (SPD)
solitary aggressive-type conduct d.
somatic paranoid d.
somatization neurotic d.
somatizing d.'s
somatoform interface d.
somatoform pain d.
somatopsychic d.
specific developmental d. (SDD)
speech d.
speech developmental delay d.
speech and language d.
Standardized Assessment of Depressive D.'s (SADD)
stereotypic movement d. (SMD)
stereotypy and habit d.
stomach psychogenic d.

stress d.
stress-related d.
Structured Clinical Interview for DSM-III-R Dissociative D.'s (SCID-D)
Structured Clinical Interview for DSM-III-R Psychotic D.'s (SCID-PD)
Structured Clinical Interview for DSM-IV Axis II Personality D.'s (SCID-II)
Structured Clinical Interview for DSM-IV Dissociative D.'s (SCID-D, SCID-IV)
Structured Composite International Diagnostic Interview for Psychological D.'s
substance abuse and dependence d.
substance-induced d.
substance-related d.
substance use d.
substantia nigra d.
substitution d.
subsyndromal thought d.
swallowing d.
sympathomimetic delusional d.
systemic giant cell d.
tactile-perceptual d.
taste d.
temporal-perceptual d.
thinking d.
thought process d.
thyroid d.
tic d.
time and rhythm d.
tobacco use d.
Tourette d.
toxic d.
trance-possession d.
transient situational personality d.
transient tic d.
traumatic d.
unaggressive conduct d.
underachievement d.
undersocialized d.
undifferentiated attention-deficit d.
unhappiness and misery d.
unipolar d.
unitary d.
unknown substance-induced mood d.
unsocialized d.
urea cycle d.
use d.
vestibular d.
visceral d.
visual image movement d.
visuospatial d.
vocal, chronic motor, or tic d.
voice d.
wakefulness d.
withdrawal d.
withdrawal-related mood d.
writing d.
d. of written expression

x-linked cortical migration d.
Yale Schedule for Tourette
Syndrome and Other
Behavioral D.'s
disordered
d. mentally
d. mental status
d. personality
d. relating
d. thinking
disorderly
d. conduct
drunk and d.
disorganization
autonomic d.
background d.
cerebral d.
cognitive d.
conceptual d.
developing psychotic d.
d. dimension of positive
schizophrenic symptoms
EEG background d.
linguistic d.
mental d.
psychotic d.
segmental arterial d.
spatial d.
d. syndrome
thought d.
disorganized
d. behavior
d. delusion
d. factor
d. factor in schizophrenia
d. speech
d. speech assessment
d. speech in schizophrenia
d. state
d. subtype
d. thinking
disorganized-type
d.-t. schizophrenia
d.-t. schizophrenic
d.-t. schizophrenic disorder
disorient
disorientation
auditory d.
autopsychic d.
graphic d.
posttraumatic d.
right-left d.
spatial d.
speech d.
thought d.
time d.
topographical d.
visuospatial d.
disoriented patient
Disotate
disparity
phase d.
vision d.
dispersion
intravoxel phase d.

nuclear magnetic relaxation d.
response d.
displaceability of libido
displaced
d. child syndrome
d. person
displacement
activity d.
d. of affect
affect d.
brainstem d.
character d.
d. defense mechanism
d. disorder
dream d.
geographic d.
guilt d.
d. of interhemispheric fissure
retroactive d.
significant d.
spondylolisthesis with significant d.
d. substitute
symbolic d.
traumatic d.
d. wit
display
affect d.
emotional d.
facial d.
Virtual Vision heads-up d.
**disposable Doppler-constant
thermocouple sensor**
disposition
personal d.
placid d.
polymorphous perverse d.
d. system
volatile d.
dispositional
d. attribution
d. tolerance
disproportionate impairment
disregard for rules
disreputable
disrupted
d. relationship
d. sleep organization
**disrupted, dysfunctional relational
functioning**
disruption
anterior column d.
behavior d.
cervical spine posterior ligament d.
cognitive d.
family d.
marital d.
pedicle cortex d.
sleep d.
disruptive
d. behavior
d. behavior disorder
d. emotion
d. family functioning

D

dissatisfaction
    body d.
    marital d.
dissectible cognitive operation
dissecting
    d. aneurysm
    d. forceps
    d. hook
dissection
    bone d.
    bone/ligament d.
    bony d.
    carotid artery d.
    cervicocephalic arterial d.
    condyle d.
    cranial nerve d.
    familial cervicocephalic arterial d.
    flank d.
    hard palate d.
    incisural d.
    intradural d.
    jugular vein d.
    middle fossa floor/petrous d.
    muscle d.
    nasal d.
    neck d.
    parotid d.
    soft tissue d.
    subperiosteal d.
    subtemporal d.
    suction d.
    sylvian d.
    vertebral d.
dissector
    aneurysm neck d.
    Angell James d.
    Cavitron d.
    Clodius d.
    Creed d.
    Crile gasserian ganglion knife
      and d.
    Crile nerve hook and d.
    Davis dura d.
    Effler-Groves d.
    endarterectomy d.
    Fager pituitary d.
    Field suction d.
    Freer d.
    golf-stick d.
    Hajek-Ballenger d.
    Hardy d.
    hockey-stick d.
    Jannetta aneurysm neck d.
    joker d.
    Kennerdell-Maroon d.
    Kneerdell-Maroon d.
    Kocher d.
    MacDonaldd d.
    Malis d.
    Marino transsphenoidal d.
    Maroon-Jannetta d.
    Milligan d.
    needle d.
    neural d.
    Oldberg d.

    Olivecrona dura d.
    Penfield d.
    Rayport dural and knife d.
    Rhoton ball d.
    Rochester lamina d.
    Schmieden-Taylor d.
    Scoville d.
    Smithwick d.
    spatula d.
    teardrop d.
    tissue plane d.
    Toennis-Adson d.
    Toennis dura d.
    ultrasonic d.
    Yasargil d.
    Yasargil micro d.
disseminate
    alopecia d.
disseminated
    d. CNS histoplasmosis
    d. encephalomyelitis
    d. intravascular coagulation (DIC)
    d. leiomyosarcoma
    d. sclerosis
dissemination
    evaluation d.
dissidence
dissident
dissimilation rule
dissimulator
dissociable
dissociated
    d. anesthesia
    d. learning
    d. nystagmus
    d. sensory loss
    d. state
dissociate-dysmnesic
    d.-d. substitution
    d.-d. substitution reaction
dissociation, disassociation
    albuminocytologic d.
    d. defense mechanism
    d. of learning
    peritraumatic d.
    semantic d.
    d. sensibility
    sensory d.
    sleep d.
    d. syndrome
    syringomyelic d.
    tabetic d.
dissociative
    d. amnesia
    d. anesthesia
    d. capacity
    d. disorder
    d. disorder not otherwise specified
      (DDNOS)
    d.'s Disorders Interview Scale
    d.'s Disorders Interview Schedule
    d. episode
    d. episode experience
    d.'s Experience Scale (DES)
    d. fugue

d. hysteria
d. hysteria psychoneurosis
d. identity disorder (DID)
d. paranoia
d. phenomenon
d. reaction
d. state
d. symptom
d. trance
d. trance disorder
dissociative-type
d.-t. hysterical neurosis
d.-t. neurotic hysterical
dissolution
dissonance
cognitive d.
dissonant
dissuasive
distal
d. anterior cerebral artery aneurysm
d. basilar temporary clip
d. carotid
d. catheter
d. catheter lengthening
d. distinctive feature analysis
d. motor latency
d. motor paresis
d. myopathy
d. neuropathy
d. occlusion
d. part of anterior lobe of
  hypophysis
d. polyneuropathy
d. stimulation generator
d. sympathetic stump
d. tingling on percussion (DTP)
distance
d. ceptor
functional d.
internodal d. (IND)
interpedicular d.
interuncal d.
optimal interpersonal d.
d. perception
professional d.
d. receptor
social d.
sociometric d.
distancing
cognitive d.
distant metastasis
distensae
striae d.
distensible tissue
distinctive feature analysis
distorted
d. body image
d. communication in schizophrenia
d. grief
d. inferential thinking
d. language in schizophrenia
d. perception
distortion
apperceptive d.
auditory d.

body image d.
cognitive d.
compromise d.
ego d.
figure-ground d.
inferential behavioral monitoring d.
d. of inferential behavioral
  monitoring
inferential perception d.
d. of inferential thinking
d. of interpretation
intrapsychic d.
d. of language and communication
language and communication d.
local field d.
memory d.
metonymic d.
nonlinear d.
paratactic d.
parataxic d.
perceptual d.
psychological d.
psychotic d.
significant subjective d.
social avoidance and d.
spatial d.
time d.
transient d.
visual d.
visual-spatial d.
distortum
collum d.
distractibility
easy d.
distractible
easily d.
d. speech
distracting stimuli
distraction
apical d.
d. bar
d. force
Harrington d.
d. instrumentation
d. instrumentation biomechanics
d. rod
distraction/compression scoliosis
  treatment
distractor
DeBastiani d.
distress
clinically significant d.
emotional d.
event-related d.
fetal d.
intense psychological d.
intrapsychic d.
menopausal d.
no acute d. (NAD)
present d.
psychological d.
separation d.
sexual orientation d.
social avoidance and d. (SAD)
subjective d.

D

distressing
    d. dream
    d. thought
distributed
    d. effort
    d. memory
    d. processing
distribution
    bimodal d.
    binomial d.
    Boltzmann d.
    butterfly d.
    chi-square d.
    contrastive d.
    d. of control
    d. curve
    frequency d.
    gaussian d.
    nervous d.
    noncontrastive d.
    normal d.
    Poisson d.
    d. of power
    d. of responsibility
    sensory d.
    skew d.
    stocking-glove d.
    unequal d.
distributive
    d. analysis
    d. analysis and synthesis
distrust
    interpersonal d.
    malevolent d.
    pervasive d.
disturbance
    acid-base d.
    activity and attention d.
    acute situational d.
    adjustment reaction d.
    affective d.
    amphetamine intoxication, with
      perceptual d.
    analyzing new information d.
    anxiety d.
    aphasic d.
    appetite d.
    Appraisal of Language D.'s (ALD)
    assimilating information d.
    d. associated with conversion
      phenomenon
    d. associated with organic mental
      disease
    d. of attention
    attentional d.
    behavioral d.
    behavioral set of d.'s
    d. between clauses
    body conceptualization d.
    body image d.
    cannabis intoxication, with
      perceptual d.
    chronic sleep d.
    chronobiological d.

    cocaine intoxication, with
      perceptual d.
    cognitive d.
    compulsive d.
    concentration d.
    conceptual d.
    conduct d.
    d. of consciousness
    consciousness d.
    d. in content of thought
    dementia behavior d.
    domestic d.
    dopamininergically modulated
      prefrontal d.
    Draw A Person Screening
      Procedure for Emotional D.
      (DAP:SPED)
    eating d.
    electrolyte d.
    emotional d.
    executive functioning d.
    explosive d.
    fluctuating mood d.
    fluency d.
    fluid d.
    focal neurologic d.
    d. in form of thinking
    frequency d.
    functioning d.
    gait d.
    global assessment of sensory d.
    habit d.
    high-level perceptual d.
    hyperkinetic d.
    identity d.
    infancy and early childhood d.
    intermittent explosive d.
    isolated explosive d.
    language d.
    learning new information d.
    linguistic d.
    d. of memory
    memory d.
    mental d.
    metabolic d.
    mixed conduct/emotional d.
    mixed symptom picture with
      perceptual d.
    mood d.
    motor skill d.
    neurologic d.
    oculomotor d.
    opioid intoxication, with
      perceptual d.
    perception d.
    d. of perception
    perceptual d.
    perceptual motor abilities d.
    d. in perceptual motor ability
    personality d.
    personality pattern d.
    personality trait d.
    phencyclidine intoxication, with
      perceptual d.
    planning d.

posttraumatic d.
predominant mood d.
psychiatric d.
psychic d.
psychographic d.
psychomotor d.
psychotic d.
rate of fluency d.
reasoning d.
recalling new information d.
sensory d.
sexual desire d.
d. in sexual desire
sexual orientation d.
situational d.
sleep continuity d.
socialized d.
social relatedness d.
sociopathic personality d. (SPD)
d. in speech
speech d.
speed of information processing d.
stress-related d.
d. in suggestibility
superego d.
thought d.
transient situational d.
undersocialized socialized d.
visual d.
visual field d.
d. of the will
will d.
d. within clauses
word-finding ability d.

disturbed
d. body image
d. eating behavior
d. home environment
d. interpersonal relationships (DIR)
d. orientation
d. person
d. personality
d. sense of self
d. sleep pattern
d. social relatedness
d. ward

disturbing
d. experience
d. feeling
d. thought

disulfide
tetraethylthiuram d.

disulfiram
disuse
d. osteoporosis
d. principle

Ditropan
Ditthomska syndrome
Diucardin
diuresis
diuretic
loop d.
osmotic d.
potassium sparing d.
thiazide d.

Diurigen
Diuril
diurnal
d. enuresis
d. epilepsy
d. variation

diurnus
pavor d.

divagate
divagation
divalproex sodium
divergence
d. circuit
synergistic d.

divergent
d. production
d. thinking

diverse group
diversional therapy
diversionary
diversity
D. Awareness Profile (DAP)
group d.

diversive exploration
diverticula
meningeal d.

diving reflex
division
cell d.
D. of Developmental Disabilities
(DDD)
lobar d.

divorce
community d.
coparental d.
d. counseling
d. decree
economic d.
emotional d.
legal d.
psychic d.
d. rate
d. therapy

divorcee
Divry-van Bogaert familial
corticomeningeal angiomatosis
Dix-Hallpike
D.-H. maneuver
D.-H. test

Dixon
D. method opposed imaging
D. radiofrequency coil

dixyrazine
Dizac Injectable Emulsion
Dizmiss
dizygotic (DZ)
d. twin

dizziness
dizzy spell
dl-alpha-difluoromethylornithine
DLP
developmental learning problem

DM
dermatomyositis

D

DMAS
  Dementia Mood Assessment Scale
DMD
  Duchenne muscular dystrophy
    DMD gene
    DMD phenotype
DMDZ
  desmethyldiazepam
D-Med Injection
DMH
  Department of Mental Health
DMI
  Defense Mechanism Inventory
  Diagnostic Mathematics Inventory
DMSO
  dimethyl sulfoxide
DNA
  deoxyribonucleic acid
    DNA analysis
    double-stranded DNA (dsDNA)
    DNA marker
    mitochondrial DNA
    DNA repletion syndrome
    DNA transcription factor
    DNA virus
DNIC
  diffuse noxious inhibitory control
DNR
  do not resuscitate
DNT
  dysembryoplastic neuroepithelial tumor
DOA
  dead on arrival
Doan's
    Extra Strength D.
Doan's, Original
dobutamine
Dobutrex
d'Ocagne nomogram
docosahexanoic acid
doctor
    hex d.
    root d.
    witch d.
doctor-patient relationship
doctrine
    Flourens d.
    neuron d.
    parental right d.
documented pseudarthrosis
Dodd Test of Time Estimation
DOES
  disorders of excessive somnolence
dog-eat-dog attitude
Dogiel
    D. cell
    D. corpuscle
Dohn-Carton brain retractor
Dohrmann-Rubin cannula
doing
    learning by d.
Dolacet
dolce far niente
doldrums
doleful

Dolenc technique
Dolene
Dole-Nyswauder program
Dole Vocational Sentence Completion Blank
dolichocephaly
dolichoectasia
    intracranial arterial d.
dolichoectatic
    d. aneurysm
    d. artery
dolicoectatic internal carotid artery
doll
    amputation d.
doll's
    d. eye maneuver
    d. eye reaction
    d. eye reflex
    d. eye sign
    d. eyes phenomenon
    d. head anesthesia
    d. head phenomenon
Dolobid
Dolophine
Dolorac
dolor capitis
dolore
    angina pectoris sine d.
dolorific
dolorificus
    trismus d.
dolorimeter
    Chatillon d.
dolorimetry
dolorogenic zone
dolorology
dolorosa
    analgesia d.
    anesthesia d.
    facies d.
    hypalgesia d.
    paraplegia d.
dolorosum
    punctum d.
dolorous
domain
    adaptive skill d.
    analog d.
    microtubule-binding d.
    outcome d.
    particle d.
domatophobia
dome
    d. of aneurysm
    aneurysmal d.
    double d.
Domen laminoplasty
domestic
    d. aggression
    d. disturbance
    d. environment
    d. fight
    d. medicine
    d. violence (DV)
domesticated pride

domex
domicile
domiciliary
    d. care home
dominance
    cerebral d.
    crossed d.
    eye d.
    Harris Tests of Lateral D.
    d. hierarchy
    lack of clear-cut cerebral d.
    lateral d.
    left hemisphere d.
    left/right hemisphere d.
    manual d.
    Miles ABC Test of Ocular D.
    mixed cerebral d.
    right hemisphere d.
    social d.
    territorial d.
    d. test
    theory of social d.
    time d.
    X-linked d.
dominance-subordination
dominant
    d. association
    autosomal d.
    bystander dominates initial d.
    (BDID)
    d. character
    d. characteristic
    d. delusional belief
    d. determinant
    d. feature
    d. gene
    d. genotype
    d. hand
    hand d.
    d. hemisphere
    d. hemisphere infarction
    d. hemisphere lesion
    d. idea
    d. language
    d. laterality
    left-hand d.
    d. mentality
    mixed foot d.
    d. person
    d. personality
    right-hand d.
    d. spouse
    d. trait
    d. waking frequency
dominant-subordinate behavior
domination
    sexual d.
dominatrix
domperidone
Don
    D. Juan
    D. Juan syndrome
    D. Juan type
    D. Quixote

Dona
    D. Juana
    D. Juanita
Donaghy angled suture needle holder
donepezil
    d. HCl
    d. hydrochloride
donna
    prima d.
donor
    blood d.
do-not-care attitude
do not resuscitate (DNR)
doom
    impending d.
    sense of impending d.
doomsayer
doomsday
door-in-the-face effect
Doose syndrome
DOPA, Dopa, dopa
    3,4-dihydroxyphenylalanine
dopa
    d. decarboxylase
    methyl d.
dopa-decarboxylase
    d.-d. containing
dopamine
    d. agonist
    d. hydrochloride
    d. hypothesis
    mesolimbic d.
    d. metabolite
    d. ratio
    d. receptor
    d. receptor blockade
    d. receptor blocker
    d. receptor sensitivity
    d. reuptake
    striatal d.
dopamine-beta hydroxylase (DBH)
dopaminergic
    d. activity
    d. drug
    d. hyperactivity
    d. medication-induced postural
    tremor
    d. pathway
    d. synapse
    d. tract
dopaminergic-cholinergic balance
dopaminergically modulated prefrontal
    disturbance
Dopar
Dopascan injection
dope
dopium
Doppler
    color-flow D.
    continuous-wave D.
    D. effect
    D. flowmetry
    D. frequency spectrum
    D. imaging
    Mizuho surgical D.

D

Doppler *(continued)*
    D. monitoring
    Neuroguard transcranial D.
    D. phenomenon
    D. precordial end-tidal carbon
      dioxide monitoring
    D. probe
    D. pulsatility index
    pulsed D.
    pulse wave D.
    D. shift
    D. sonography
    transcranial D. TCD
    D. ultrasonography
    D. ultrasound
    D. ultrasound monitor
Dora case
Doral
doramania
doraphobia
Dorcol
Dorello canal
Dorian love
Doriden
Doriglute
Dormalin
Dormarex Oral
dormido
    sangue d.
dormifacient
Dormin Oral
dormitory
doromania
dorsal
    d. accessory olivary nucleus
    d. aponeurotic expansion hood
    d. brain stem lipoma (DBSL)
    d. cochlear nucleus
    d. column of spinal cord
    d. column stimulation
    d. column stimulator (DCS)
    d. cord stimulation (DCS)
    d. enteric fistula
    d. funiculus
    d. gray matter
    d. horn
    d. horn neuronal response
    d. longitudinal fasciculus
    d. mesencephalic syndrome
    d. midbrain syndrome
    d. motor nucleus of vagus
    d. nucleus of vagus
    d. part of pons
    d. plate of neural tube
    d. premotor cortex
    d. rami
    d. raphe
    d. raphe nuclei
    d. reflex
    d. rhizotomy
    d. root
    d. root entry zone (DREZ)
    d. root entry zone lesion
    d. root entry zone lesioning

    d. root ganglion (DRG)
    d. scapular nerve
    d. spine
    d. spinocerebellar tract
    d. subcutaneous space
    d. tegmental decussation
    d. vagus complex
dorsalis
    hypertrophic pachymeningitis d.
    tabes d.
    tetanus d.
Dorsey
    D. dural separator
    D. ventricular cannula
dorsiflex
dorsocuboidal reflex
dorsolateral
    d. caudate
    d. convexity syndrome
    d. fasciculus
    d. pathway
    d. prefrontal cortex
    d. prefrontal syndrome
    d. region
    d. tract
dorsomedial
    d. hypothalamic nucleus
    d. mesencephalic syndrome
dorsum
    d. of foot reflex
    d. pedis reflex
    d. sellae atrophy
    d. sella erosion
dosage
    equivalent d.
dose
    daily d.
    effective d.
    equivalent d. (ED)
    lethal d. (LD)
    low d.
    maintenance d.
    maximum permissible d.
    maximum recommended human d.
      (MRHD)
    maximum tolerated d. (MTD)
    measured d.
    minimum d.
    nominal standard d. (NSD)
    optimum d.
    periphery d.
    permissible d.
    therapeutic d.
    tolerance d.
    toxic d.
dose-dependent effect
dose-response curve
dosimeter
    thermoluminescent d.
dosimetric medicine
dosimetry
Dospan
    Tenuate D.
dot
    line frequency noise d.

dothiepin
double
    d. antihelix
    d. assimilation
    d. bind
    d. bind theory of schizophrenia
    d. blind
    d. blind theory
    d. compartment hydrocephalus
    d. congenital athetosis
    d. consciousness
    d. depression
    d. dome
    d. entendre
    d. fishhook retractor
    d. fragment sign
    d. hemiplegia
    illusion of d.'s
    d. insanity
    d. major curve pattern
    d. major curve scoliosis
    d. meaning
    d. orientation
    d. personality
    d. simultaneous stimulation (DSS)
    d. spring ball valve
    d. standard
    subjective d.'s
    d. superego
    d. thoracic curve
    d. thoracic curve scoliosis
    d. vision
    d. visual control
    d. yoke
    d. Zielke instrumentation
double-action rongeur
double-bind
    unipolar d.-b.
double-blind study
double-L spinal rod
double-lumen Swan-Ganz catheter
double-point threshold
double-pore vent system
double-rod
    d.-r. construct
    d.-r. technique
double-stranded DNA (dsDNA)
double-vector
    d.-v. blade
    d.-v. brain spatula
doubt
    autonomy vs. shame and d.
    d.'s of loyalty
    morbid d.
    obsessive d.
    d.'s of trustworthiness
doubting
    d. insanity
    d. mania
    d. spell
douloureux
    tic d.
Dover powder
dowel cutter

Dowling
    D. intracranial cyst removal
    D. intracranial cyst removal
      technique
down
    D. disease
    d. from overdose
    d. gaze
    D. syndrome
    d.'s syndrome proband
downbeat nystagmus
downbiting Epstein curette
Downing retractor
downsized circular laminar hook
downward
    d. drift
    d. gaze paresis
Dox
    CO D.
doxefazepam
doxepin hydrochloride
Doxised
doxogenic
doxorubicin hydrochloride
doxycycline
doxylamine
Doyen
    D. cylindrical bur
    D. rib spreader
    D. spherical bur
Doyère eminence
DPE
    Death Personification Exercise
d-penicillamine
D-penicillamine treatment
DPI
    Dynamic Personality Inventory
DPJ
    dementia paralytica juveniles
DPM
    Diploma in Psychological Medicine
DPP
    Dropout Prediction and Prevention
Dr
    rare detail response
dr
    unusual rare detail response
dracunculiasis
Drager MTC transducer
Dragons
    Dungeons and D.
drain
    Charnley suction d.
    Hemovac Hydrocoat d.
    Heyer-Schulte wound d.
    Jackson-Pratt d.
    Penrose d.
    Shirley d.
    subgaleal d.
    Surgivac d.
    Wound-Evac d.
drainage
    bur hole d.
    epidural venous d.
    external ventricular d.

D

drainage *(continued)*
  lumbar d.
  serial percutaneous needle d.
  Spetzler-Martin Grade III medium-size lesion with deep venous d.
  Spetzler-Martin Grade II small lesion with deep venous d.
  spinal d.
  stereotactic catheter d.
  syrinx d.
  ventricular d.
draining vein
Drake
  D. fenestrated clip
  D. tandem clipping technique
  D. tourniquet
Drake-Kees clip
drama affect
Dramamine
  D. II
  D. Oral
dramatic
  d. affect
  d. interpersonal style
  d. play
  d. speech
dramatic-emotional cluster
dramatism
dramatization
dramatize
dramatogenic
drape
  NeuroDrape surgical d.
  OpMi microscopic d.
draped
  prepared and d.
drapetomania
Draw-A-Bicycle Test
Draw-A-Clock-Face Test
Draw-A-Family Test
Draw-A-Flower Test
Draw-A-House Test
Draw-A-Man Test
Draw-a-Person (DAP)
Draw A Person Screening Procedure for Emotional Disturbance (DAP:SPED)
Draw-A-Person Test
Draw-A-Picture-From-Memory Test
drawing
  d. ability
  automatic d.
  Bender Visual Gestalt d.
  d. disability
  Human Figure D. (HFD)
  Kinetic Family D.'s (KFD)
  mirror d.
  pain d.
  d. test
drawn laughter
dread
  feeling of d.
  d. of insanity
  talion d.

dreaded situation
dream, dreamer
  American d.
  anxiety d.
  d. anxiety attack
  d. anxiety disorder
  artificial d.
  d. association
  bad d.
  d. censorship
  clairvoyant d.
  color d.
  color in d.
  comfort d.
  consolation d.
  d. content
  convalescent d.
  convenience d.
  corroborating d.
  counter-wish d.
  day d.
  decomposition in d.'s
  detailed d.
  d. determinant
  d. displacement
  distressing d.
  dream within a d.
  d. ego
  d. embarrassment
  embarrassment d.
  erotic d.
  examination d.
  exhibition d.
  d. experience
  frustration d.
  d. function
  d. gum
  d. illusion
  d. induction
  insomnium d.
  d. interpretation
  made-to-order d.
  manifest d.
  masochistic wish d.
  d. pain
  paired d.'s
  parallel d.
  perennial d.
  prophetic d.
  punishment d.
  d. recall
  reconstruction d.
  recurrent d.
  recurring d.
  d. screen
  secondary elaboration of d.
  Sisyphus d.
  speech in d.
  d. state
  d. stimulus
  d. symbolism
  telepathic d.
  terror d.
  d. time
  veridical d.

vivid d.
wet d.
wish d.
d. work
dreaming
amnesia for sleep and d.
dreamless sleep
dreamlike
d. hallucination
d. state
dreamy state
dredge
dress
Dressinet netting bandage
dressing
4 × 4 d.
Allevyn d.
d. apraxia
cross d.
dry sterile d.
DuoDerm d.
Fabco gauze d.
Flexinet d.
d. forceps
hour-glass d.
Inerpan flexible burn d.
Kaltostat d.
Kerlix d.
Mills d.
modified Robert Jones d.
Mother Jones d.
NeoDerm d.
OpSite d.
Owen gauze d.
Reston d.
Sof-Rol d.
Sof-Wick d.
Stimson d.
surgical d.
Surgicel Nu-Knit d.
Telfa d.
Tubex gauze d.
DREZ
dorsal root entry zone
DREZ lesioning
DREZ procedure
DREZ surgery
DREZotomy
microsurgical D.
DRG
diagnosis-related group
diagnostic related group
dorsal root ganglion
DRI
Driver Risk Inventory
drift
downward d.
EEG amplifier d.
genetic d.
genic d.
d. hypothesis
mesenchymal d.
observer d.
drill
acorn d.

Acra-Cut wire pass d.
air d.
air-powered d.
Anspach d.
Anspach 65K d.
Caspar d.
Codman d.
Crutchfield hand d.
D'Errico perforating d.
diamond high-speed air d.
electric d.
Fisch d.
d. guide
d. guide with drill bit
Hall Surgairtome II d.
Hall UltraPower d.
Hall Versipower d.
high-speed air d.
Hudson d.
McKenzie perforating twist d.
Midas Rex d.
Mira Mark III cranial d.
Phoenix cranial d.
power d.
right-angle d.
Stryker d.
twist d.
drilling technique
drinker
binge d.
chronic d.
closet d.
compulsive d.
evening d.
incurable problem d. (IPD)
jag d.
periodic d.
problem d. (PD)
repeated heavy d.
social d.
D. tank respirator
weekend d.
drinking
aftereffect of d.
air d.
alcohol d.
d. behavior
binge d.
compulsive water d.
controlled d.
dyssocial d.
early onset d.
escape d.
evening d.
d. history
inveterate d.
jag d.
light d.
morning d.
nonproblematic d.
occupational d.
paroxysmal d.
periodic d.
recreational d.
social d.

D

drinking *(continued)*
    somatopathic d.
    state markers of heavy d.
    thymogenic d.
    volitional d.
    water d.
    weekend d.
drip
    d. chamber
    perfusate d.
Drisdol Oral
Dristan Sinus Caplets
drive
    absent d.
    achievement d.
    acquired d.
    activity d.
    affectional d.
    affiliative d.
    aggressive d.
    appetitive d.
    aversive d.
    biologic d.
    destructive d.
    ego d.
    elimination d.
    erotic d.
    exploration d.
    exploratory d.
    fear d.
    hedonic d.
    homonomy d.
    hunger d.
    innate d.
    internal d.
    kinetic d.
    learned d.
    manipulative d.
    maternal d.
    obstruction d.
    paternal d.
    physiological d.
    primary d.
    d. reduction
    d. reduction theory
    repressed instinctual d.
    secondary d.
    sex d.
    sexual d.
    stimulus d. (Sd)
    subjective d.
    thirst d.
driveling dementia
driven
    d. motor behavior
    treatment d.
drivenness
    organic d.
driver
    drunk d.
    D. Risk Inventory (DRI)
    slave d.

driver's
    d. rage
    d. thigh
driving
    d. behavior
    Mothers Against Drunk D.
      (MADD)
    d. phobia
    photic d.
    Students Against Drunk D.
      (SADD)
    d. under the influence (DUI)
    d. while intoxicated (DWI)
Drixoral Cough & Sore Throat Liquid
    Caps
DRLST
    Del Rio Language Screening Test
DRO
    differential reinforcement of other
      behavior
dromedary gait
dromica
    epilepsia d.
dromolepsy
dromomania
dromophobia
dronabinol
droning speech
drooping eyelid
drop
    d. attack
    d. foot
    d. hand
    d. metastasis
    toe d.
    wrist d.
drop-entry (closed body) hook
droperidol
    d. and fentanyl
drop-out
    school d.-o.
Dropout Prediction and Prevention
    (DPP)
Dropouts Anonymous
dropped foot
drops
    nose d.
drowsiness
    pathologic d.
drowsy
DR or RD
drug
    abreactive d.
    d. abstinence
    d. abstinence syndrome
    d. abuse
    D. Abuse Control Amendments
      (DACA)
    abused d.
    abuse of nonprescribed d.
    d. abuser
    d. abuse rehabilitation program
    D. Abuse Resistance Education
      (DARE)
    d. abuse scale

D. Abuse Warning Network (DAWN)
d. addict
addicting d.
d. addiction
addictive d.
addictive potential of d.
adulterate d.
all-American d.
alpha adrenergic blocking d.
alpha adrenergic stimulating d.
anticholinergic d.
anticonvulsant d.
antidote d.
antiepileptic d. (AED)
anti-inflammatory d.
antimuscarinic d.
antiseizure d.
anxiolytic d.
d. assay
ataractic d.
atypical antipsychotic d.
autonomic sympathomimetic d.
beta-adrenergic blocking d.
d. binge
Bureau of Narcotics and Dangerous D.'s (BNDD)
butyrophenone-based neuroleptic d.
catatonic d.
chemotherapeutic d.
d. of choice
d. consumption
d. container
d. counselor
d. craving
d. culture
cytotoxic d.
dangerous d.
date rape d.
dealer of bogus d.
d. dealing
d. defaulter
d. dependence
d. dependency
designer d.
d. disease
dopaminergic d.
d. education
D. Enforcement Administration (DEA)
d. equipment
experimental d.
d. fever
gateway d.
God's d.
d. habit
hallucinatory d.
hallucinogenic d.
heterocyclic antidepressant d.
high-dose d.
d. holiday
hypnotic d.
hypnotic-sedative d.
illegal d.
illicit d.

D. Induced Rape Prevention and Punishment Act
d. influence
d. information (DI)
d. information center (DIC)
d. information log (DIL)
d. infusion pump
d. ingestion
inhalation of d.
d. injection
d. insanity
d. interaction (DI)
d. intolerance
d. level
low-quality d.
maintenance d.
d. maintenance
d. maintenance treatment
d. management
mind-altering d.
mood-altering d.
mood-elevating d.
movie star d.
narcotic agonist d.
narcotic antagonist d.
narcotic blocking d.
neuroleptic d.
nonprescription d.
nonpsychotropic d.
nonsteroidal anti-inflammatory d. (NSAID)
noradrenergic d.
nosotropic d.
orphan d.
OTC d.
d. overdose
over-the-counter d.
d. paraphernalia
parasympathomimetic d.
parenteral d.
d. party
d. pathological intoxication
personal supply of d.
poor quality d.
d. possession
prescription d.
psychoactive d.
psychodysleptic d.
psychogenic d.
d. psychosis
d. psychosis hallucinatory state
psychostimulant d.
psychotherapeutic d.
psychotomimetic d.
psychotropic d. (PTD)
purchase d.
purchase fake d.
Q&Q d.
quality d.
d. quantity
d. reaction
recreational d.
d. related
d. resistance plasmid
schedule d.

D

drug *(continued)*
    d. screen
    sedative d.
    sedative-hypnotic d.
    self-administration of
      psychoactive d. (SAPD)
    street d.
    d. supply
    sympatholytic d.
    sympathomimetic d.
    tertiary amine tricyclic
      antidepressant d.
    d. tetanus
    d. therapy
    d. tolerance
    d. toxicity
    tricyclic antidepressant d. (TCAD)
    d. use
    d. used for detoxification
    D. Use Index
    d. use review (DUR)
    d. vial
    d. withdrawal
    d. withdrawal seizure
    d. withdrawal syndrome
    wonder d.
drug-buying area
drug-dependent insomnia
drug-induced
    d.-i. anemia
    d.-i. confusional state
    d.-i. delirium
    d.-i. dementia
    d.-i. floating sensation
    d.-i. hallucination
    d.-i. hallucinosis
    d.-i. mental disorder
    d.-i. nystagmus
    d.-i. parkinsonism
    d.-i. psychosis
    d.-i. seizure
drug-injecting equipment
drugmaker
drug-negative urine
drug-related
    d.-r. disorder
    d.-r. insomnia
    d.-r. violence
drug-seeking behavior
Drummond
    D. spinous wiring technique
    D. wire
drunk
    blind d.
    d. and disorderly
    d. driver
    dry d.
    legally d.
    punch-d.
drunkard
drunkenness
    acute d.
    alcoholic d.
    chronic d.

    ether d.
    maudlin d.
    pathologic d.
    public d.
    simple d.
    simple alcoholic d.
    sleep d.
    sleeping d.
drunkometer
drusen
dry
    d. beriberi
    d. drunk
    d. eye syndrome
    d. leprosy
    d. mouth
    d. orgasm
    d. sterile dressing
DS
    digit span
    digit symbol
    Tolectin DS
Ds
    associative response to a white space on
    a card
DSA
    digital subtraction angiography
DSC
    Developing Skills Checklist
    Parafon Forte DSC
DSD
    depression sine depression
    depressive spectrum disorder
DSDB
    direct self-destructive behavior
dsDNA
    double-stranded DNA
D$_2$-selective dopamine agonist
DSH
    deliberate self-harm
DSI
    Depression Status Inventory
DSM
    Diagnostic and Statistical Manual of
    Mental Disorders
DSM-III
    Diagnostic and Statistical Manual of
    Mental Disorders-3rd Edition
DSM-III-R
    Diagnostic and Statistical Manual of
    Mental Disorders-3rd Edition Revised
    Structured Clinical Interview for
    DSM-III-R (SCID)
DSM-IV
    Diagnostic and Statistical Manual of
    Mental Disorders-4th Edition
    DSM-IV diagnosis
    Structured Clinical Interview for
    DSM-IV (SCID)
    Structured Clinical Interview for
    DSM-IV Patient Edition
DSS
    disability status scale
    double simultaneous stimulation

DST
   dexamethasone suppression test
DSUH
   direct suggestion under hypnosis
DT
   delirium tremens
   dipole tracing
   duration tetany
DTC
   day treatment center
DTCD
   Dennis Test of Child Development
DT/CEP
   Differential Test of Conduct and
     Emotional Problems
DTICH
   delayed traumatic intracerebral
     hemorrhage
DTLA
   Detroit Test of Learning Aptitude
DTLA-3
   Detroit Test of Learning Aptitude, Third
     Edition
DTLA-A
   Detroit Test of Learning Aptitude-Adult
DTLA-P:2
   Detroit Test of Learning Aptitude -
     Primary, Second Edition
DTP
   diphtheria, tetanus toxoids, and pertussis
     vaccine
   distal tingling on percussion
DTPA
   diethylenetriamine penta-acetic acid
     gadolinium DTPA
DTR
   deep tendon reflex
DTT
   device for transverse traction
     DTT implant
DTVP
   Developmental Test of Visual Perception
DTVP-2
   Developmental Test of Visual Perception,
     Second Edition
dual
   d. ambivalence
   d. bypass connector
   d. compression scoliosis treatment
   d. diagnosis
   d. diagnosis patient
   d. diagnosis program
   d. leadership
   d. octapolar lead
   d. personality
   d. quadrapolar lead
   D. Quattrode spinal cord
     stimulation system
   d. therapy
   d. transference therapy
dual-arousal model
dual-energy x-ray absorptiometry
  (DEXA)
dual-instinct theory

dualism
   mind/body d.
   psychic d.
dual-isotope SPECT
dual-process theory
dual-sex therapy
Duane retraction syndrome
Dubini
   D. chorea
   D. disease
Dubois method
Dubowitz syndrome
Duchenne
   D. disease
   D. muscular dystrophy (DMD)
   D. paralysis
   D. sign
   D. syndrome
Duchenne-Aran
   D.-A. disease
   D.-A. spinal muscular atrophy
Duchenne-Erb paralysis
duck-billed anodized spatula
Duckworth phenomenon
duct
   cochlear d.
   ejaculatory d.
   endolymphatic d.
   Hensen d.
   lacrimal d.
   parotid d.
   perilymphatic d.
   semicircular d.
   Stensen d.
   uniting d.
   utriculosaccular d.
ductus, gen. and pl. **ductus**
   d. cochlearis
   d. endolymphaticus
   d. perilymphaticus
   d. reuniens
   d. semicirculares
   d. semicircularis anterior
   d. semicircularis lateralis
   d. semicircularis posterior
   d. utriculosaccularis
due process
DUI
   driving under the influence
Duke
   D. Religion Index
   D. Severity of Illness Scale
dulcify
dull
   d. affect
   borderline d.
   d. headache
   d. normal range
dullard
dullness
   emotional d.
Dumbach cranial titanium mesh
dumbbell
   d. ganglioneuroma

D

dumbbell *(continued)*
    d. neurofibroma
    d. tumor
dumbbell-shaped
    d.-s. neurinoma
    d.-s. spinal cavernous hemangioma
dumbbell-type neuroblastoma
dumbness
    word d.
dummy seed catheter
Duncan
    D. syndrome
    D. ventricle
Dunedin Multidisciplinary Health and Development Study
Dungeons and Dragons
Dunn device
Dunnett test
DuoCet
Duo-Cline bed wedge
duodenal ulcer
DuoDerm dressing
Duografin
Duphalac
duplex
    d. scanning
    d. transmission
duplication
    d. anomaly
    d. of ego
duplicative reaction
duplicity
Dupuytren contracture
DUR
    drug use review
dura
    endosteal d.
    freeze-dried cadaveric d.
    d. hook
    lyophilized d.
    lyophilized cadaveric d.
    d. mater
    d. mater of the brain
    d. mater encephali
    d. mater of the spinal cord
    d. mater spinalis
    d. propria
    d. protecting forceps
    Tutoplast D.
durable
    descending dyscontrol d.
durabolin
Duract
Duragesic Transdermal
Dura-Kold ice wrap
dural
    d. arteriovenous fistula (DAF)
    d. arteriovenous malformation
    d. attachment
    d. detachment
    d. ectasia
    d. fibrosis
    d. graft
    d. graft matrix

    d. hematoma
    d. incision
    d. margin
    d. metastasis
    d. punch
    d. retractor
    d. ring
    d. sac effacement
    d. scissors
    d. separator
    d. sheath
    d. sinus occlusion
    d. sinus thrombosis
    d. tack-up suture
    d. tail
    d. venous fistula
    d. venous sinus
Duralone Injection
dura mater
duramatral
Duramorph Injection
duraplasty
duration
    d. of drug action
    d. duty cycle
    emergency dyscontrol d.
    d. of mood
    short sleep d.
    stimulus d.
    d. tetany (DT)
Dürck node
duress
    episodic dyscontrol d.
Duret
    D. hemorrhage
    D. lesion
Durham
    D. decision
    D. rule
    D. test
Durkan CTS gauge
Durkheim theory of suicide
durocutaneous fistula
Durog
Duroliopaque
Duros
durotomy
    paramedian d.
Durrax
Durrell Analysis of Reading Difficulty: Third Edition
duteous
dutiful
duty
    line of d.
    neglect of d.
    omission of d.
    d. to warn
Duvol lung clamp
DV
    domestic violence
DVI
    digital vascular imaging

DVMI
 Developmental Test of Visual Motor
 Integration
DVT
 deep venous thrombosis
DW
 confabulated whole response
dwarf
dwarfism
 achondroplastic d.
 pituitary d.
 psychosocial d.
 tryptophanuria with d.
DWI
 driving while intoxicated
DWML
 deep white matter lesion
Dwyer
 D. device
 D. instrument
 D. instrumentation biomechanics
DX, Dx
 diagnosis
DXM
 dexamethasone suppression test
dyad
 parent-child d.
 social d.
dyadic
 D. Adjustment Scale
 D. Parent-Child Interaction Coding
 System
 d. psychotherapy
 d. session
 d. symbiosis
Dyazide
dybbuk
dying-back
 d.-b. neuropathy
 d.-b. polyneuropathy
dying declaration
Dymelor
Dymenate Injection
dymethzine
Dynafed IB
DYNA-LOC anterior fixation system
dynamic
 adaptational d.'s
 d. ambulatory balance
 d. aphasia
 d. bed
 behavioral d.'s
 d. compression plate instrumentation
 d. computed tomography (DCT)
 d. demography
 d. disease
 d. entrapment of vertebral artery
 d. equilibrium
 family d.'s
 flow d.'s
 group d.'s
 infantile d.'s
 D. mesh pre-angled connecting bar
 personality d.'s
 d. personality

 D. Personality Inventory (DPI)
 d. physical activity
 d. principle
 d. psychiatry
 d. psychology
 d. psychotherapy
 d. range
 d. reasoning
 d. referencing
 d. single photon emission
 computed tomography
 d. standing balance
 d. transverse traction device
dynamica
 alopecia d.
dynamism
 lust d.
 mental d.
dynamo
dynamometer
 bulb d.
dynamopsychism
dynamorphany
Dynapen
dyne
dynorphin
Dyonics
 D. cannula
 D. rod-lens endoscope
Dyrenium
dysacusis
dysanagnosia
dysangiogenesis
 hemorrhagic d.
dysantigraphia
dysaphia
dysaphic
dysarthria
 apraxic d.
 ataxic d.
 athetoid d.
 athetosic d.
 flaccid d.
 hyperkinetic d.
 hypokinetic d.
 labial d.
 laryngeal d.
 d. literalis
 parkinsonian d.
 peripheral d.
 progressive d.
 sensual d.
 somesthetic d.
 spastic d.
 d. syllabaris spasmodica
dysarthria-clumsy hand syndrome
dysarthric
 d. behavior
 d. speech
dysarthrosis
dysautonomia
 familial d.
dysautonomic illness
dysbasia lordotica progressiva
dysbasis

D

dysbulia, dysboulia
dysbulic
dyscalculia
dyscheiral, dyschiral
dyscheiria, dyschiria
dyschezia
dyschiral (*var. of* dyscheiral)
dyschromatopsia
    cerebral d.
dyschronism
dyscinesia (*var. of* dyskinesia)
dyscoimesis
dysconjugate
    d. gaze
    d. movement
dyscontrol
    affective d.
    behavioral d.
    descending d.
    emergency d.
    emotional d.
    episodic d.
    impulsive d.
    instinctual d.
    organic d.
    seizure d.
    temper d.
dyscrasia
    blood d.
    plasma cell d.
dysdiadochokinesia, dysdiadochocinesia
dysembryoplastic neuroepithelial tumor
  (DNT)
dyseneia
dysequilibrium, disequilibrium
    frontal d.
    d. state
    subcortical d.
    subcortical d.
dyserethesia
dyserethism
dysergastic reaction
dysergia
dysesthesia
dysesthesic sensation
dysesthetic
dysfibrous layer
dysfluency
    avoidance of speech d.
    d. dyskinesia
dysfunction
    acquired sexual d.
    adult social d.
    alcohol-induced sexual d.
    amphetamine-induced sexual d.
    anorectal physiological d.
    anxiolytic-induced sexual d.
    arousal d.
    attentional/executive system d.
    atypical psychosexual d.
    autonomic d.
    behavioral d.
    bilateral hemisphere d.
    biologic d.
    brain d.

brainstem d.
central processing d.
cerebral d.
childhood social d.
cocaine-induced sexual d.
cognitive d.
contralateral parietal lobe d.
corticospinal motor system d.
diffuse brain d.
educational d.
ejaculatory d.
emotional d.
erectile d.
executive d.
focal d.
focal/lateralized d.
frontal lobe d.
functional d.
functional dyspareunia
  psychosexual d.
functional vaginismus
  psychosexual d.
generalized sexual d.
hemispheral d.
hemispherical d.
higher cerebral d. (HCD)
higher cortical d.
hypnotic-induced sexual d.
hypothalamic-pituitary d.
hypothalamic-pituitary axis d.
interpersonal d.
lacrimal gland d.
language d.
lateralized d.
life-long sexual d.
lingual airway d.
lobe d.
male erectile d.
mental d.
midbrain d.
minimal brain d. (MBD)
neurodevelopmental d.
neurological d.
oculosympathetic d.
opioid-induced sexual d.
organic brain d.
orgasmic d.
parietal lobe d.
perceptual motor d.
pituitary d.
posttraumatic cortical d.
premature ejaculation
  psychosexual d.
primary orgasmic d.
psychological d.
psychosexual d.
salivary gland d.
school d.
sedative, hypnotic, or anxiolytic-
  induced sexual d.
self-care d.
severe diffuse brain d.
sexual d.
situational sexual d.
sleep d.

social d.
speech d.
substance-induced sexual d.
sympathetic d.
work d.
dysfunctional
d. cognition
d. family
d. personality style
d. relational functioning
d. relationship
dysgenesis
cerebellar vermis d.
cingulate gyrus d.
corpus callosum d.
gonadal d.
ovarian d.
dysgenic
dysgenitalism
dysgerminoma
parasellar d.
dysgeusia
dysgnosia
auditory-verbal d.
body d.
number d.
visual letter d.
visual number d.
dysgonesis
dysgrammatism
dysgranular cortex
dysgraphia
dysgraphicus
status d.
dysharmonica
diplacusis d.
dysidentity
dysimmune polyneuropathy
dysjunction
craniofacial d.
personal d.
dysjunctive
d. gaze
d. nystagmus
dyskinesia, dyscinesia
d. algera
belly dancer d.
biliary d.
buccolingual d.
choreic d.
disfluency d.
dysfluency d.
extrapyramidal d.
faciobuccolingual d.
levodopa-induced d.
medication-induced tardive d.
neuroleptic-induced tardive d.
ocular d.
oral d.
oral-buccal-lingual d.
orobuccal d.
orofacial d.
orolingual-buccal d.
d. paroxysmal
paroxysmal d.

peak-dose d.
spontaneous d.
tardive d.
tardive oral d.
tardive orobuccal d.
withdrawal d.
dyskinetic
d. cerebral palsy
d. movement
dyskoimesis
dyslalia
dyslexia
acquired d.
D. Determination Test
developmental d.
D. Screening Survey
dyslogia
dyslogistic
dyslysis
dysmegalopsia
dysmenorrhea
psychogenic d.
dysmentia
dysmetria
cerebellar d.
lower limb d.
ocular d.
truncal d.
dysmetric hand movement
dysmetropsia
dysmimia
dysmnesia
dysmnesic
d. psychosis
d. syndrome
dysmorphia
cranial d.
dysmorphic
d. delusion
d. somatoform disorder
dysmorphogenesis
dysmorphology
brain d.
dysmorphomania
dysmorphophobia
dysmorphopsia
dysmyelination
dysmyelinisatus
status d.
dysmyotonia
dysnisophrenia
dysnomia
amnestic d.
autonomic d.
dysnystaxis
dysorexia
dysorthographia
dysorthography
dysosmia
dysostosis
cleidocranial d.
craniofacial d.
mandibulofacial d.
d. multiplex
dyspallia

D

dyspareunia
    acquired-type d.
    female d.
    female dyspareunia-male d.
    functional d.
    generalized-type d.
    lifelong-type d.
    male d.
    psychogenic d.
    situational-type d.
dyspepsia
    psychogenic d.
dysperception
    metabolic d.
dysphagia
    d. globosa
    d. nervosa
    neurogenic d.
    receptive d.
dysphasia
    Broca d.
    developmental d.
    expressive d.
    receptive d.
dysphemia
dysphonia
    adductor spasmodic d.
    d. clericorum
    hyperkinetic d.
    spastic d.
    d. spastica
    ventricular d.
dysphoretic
dysphoria
    body d.
    gender d.
    hysteroid d.
    intense episodic d.
    d. nervosa
    neuroleptic-induced d.
dysphoriant
dysphoric
    d. affect
    d. mood
    d. response
dysphrasia
dysphrenia
dysphylaxia
dysplasia
    bony d.
    cephaloskeletal d.
    cerebral d.
    craniofrontonasal d.
    d. craniometaphyseal
    craniometaphyseal d.
    fibromuscular d.
    fibrous d.
    focal cortical d.
    mullerian duct aplasia, renal
      aplasia, cervicothoracic somite d.
      (MURCS)
    odontoid d.
    septooptic d.
    sphenoid wing d.

dysplastic
    d. constitutional type
    d. gangliocytoma
dyspnea
    functional d.
    d. response
    sighing d.
dyspneic psychogenic disorder
dysponderal amenorrhea
dysponesis
dyspractic movement
dyspragia
dyspraxia
    constructional d.
    ideomotor d.
    innervatory d.
    limb-kinetic d.
    speech d.
    spelling d.
    d. syndrome
dysprosium-DTPA
dysprosody
dysraphia
dysraphicus
    status d.
dysraphism
    craniofacial d.
    occult spinal d.
    spinal d.
dysreactivity
    autonomic d.
dysreflexia
dysregulation
    affective d.
    anger d.
    autonomic d.
    defensive d.
    endocrine d.
    level of defensive d.
    limbic d.
    prefrontal cortical activity d.
dysrhaphic
dysrhythmia
    cerebral d.
    electroencephalographic d.
    paroxysmal cerebral d.
dysrhythmic
    d. aggressive behavior
    d. movement
    d. speech
dyssocial
    d. behavior
    d. drinking
    d. personality
    d. personality disorder
    d. reaction
dyssombole
dyssomnia
    jet lag-type d.
    shift work-type d.
    sleep phase d.
    unspecified-type d.
dysspondylism
dysstasia
dyssymbiosis

dyssymbolia
dyssymboly
dyssynergia
   d. cerebellaris myoclonica
   d. cerebellaris progressiva
dystasia
   hereditary areflexic d.
   Roussy-Lévy hereditary areflexic d.
dystaxia
dysteleology
dysthymia
   primary d.
   d. scale
   subaffective d.
dysthymic
   d. adjustment reaction
   d. neurotic disorder
dystonia
   action d.
   adult-onset d.
   arm d.
   athetosic d.
   body d.
   breathy d.
   cervical d.
   childhood-onset d.
   facial d.
   idiopathic d.
   d. lenticularis
   d. musculorum deformans
   neuroleptic-induced acute d.
   nocturnal paroxysmal d.
   nuchal d.
   oropharyngeal d.
   paroxysmal d.
   pathogenic d.
   psychogenic d.
   spastic d.
   substance-induced d.
   symptomatic d.
   tardive d.
   torsion d.
   whispering d.
   withdrawal d.
dystonic
   d. amyotrophy
   d. cerebral palsy
   d. choreoathetosis
   d. movement
   d. posturing
   d. reaction
   d. torticollis
   d. tremor
dystopia
   orbital d.
dystrophia
   adiposogenital d.
   d. adiposogenitalis
   d. myotonica
dystrophica
   myotonia d.

dystrophic neurit
dystrophin
dystrophinopathy
dystrophoneurosis
dystrophy
   adiposogenital d.
   adult pseudohypertrophic
    muscular d.
   Barnes d.
   Becker-Kiener d.
   Becker muscular d.
   Becker-type tardive muscular d.
   Becker variant of Duchenne d.
   benign X-linked recessive
    muscular d.
   cerebromacular d.
   childhood muscular d.
   Duchenne muscular d. (DMD)
   Emery-Dreifuss muscular d.
   Erb muscular d.
   fascioscapulohumeral d.
   FSH d.
   Fukuyama congenital muscular d.
   Gowers muscular d.
   humeroperoneal muscular d.
   infantile neuroaxonal d.
   Kiloh-Nevin ocular form or
    progressive muscular d.
   Landouzy-Dejerine d.
   Leyden-Möbius muscular d.
   limb-girdle muscular d.
   muscular d.
   myotonic muscular d.
   neuroaxonal d.
   oculogastrointestinal muscular d.
    (OGIMD)
   oculopharyngeal muscular d.
    (OPMD)
   pelvofemoral muscular d.
   progressive muscular d.
   pseudohypertrophic muscular d.
   reflex sympathetic d. (RSD)
   scapuloperoneal muscular d.
   severe childhood autosomal
    recessive muscular d. (SCARMD)
   Steinert myotonic d.
   sympathetic reflex d.
   Thomsen d.
   Welander muscular d.
   X-linked recessive muscular d.
dystropy
   myotonic d.
dystychia
dysuria
   psychogenic d.
DZ
   dizygotic
DZP
   diazepam

D

E

E scale
E trisomy

E-2

Diagnostic Checklist for Behavior-
Disturbed Children Form E-2
Occupational Environment Scales,
Form E-2

2E1

cytochrome P-450 2E1

EA

educational age

EA-2

episodic ataxia type 2

EAA

excitatory amino acid

EAE

experimental allergic encephalitis
experimental allergic encephalomyelitis

eagerness

Eagle

E. minimum essential medium
E. syndrome

Eales disease

EAP

Employee Assistance Program

ear

e. anomaly
e. cartilage inflammation
cup e.
e. forceps
glue e.
listening with the third e.
e. pulling
third e.
wet behind the e.'s

Earle salts

early

e. adolescence
e. adulthood
E. Child Development Inventory
e. childhood
e. component waveform
E. Coping Inventory
E. Development Scale for
Preschool Children
e. discharge
e. full remission
e. genital primacy
e. infantile autism
E. Language Milestone Scale
e. latency potential
e. onset drinking
e. parental deprivation
e. and periodic screening,
diagnosis, and treatment (EPSDT)
e. phase of dementia
e. posttraumatic epilepsy
e. relationship
E. School Assessment (ESA)
E. School Personality Questionnaire
(ESPQ)

E. Screening Inventory
E. Social Communication Scale
(ESCS)
E. Speech Perception Test (ESP)
e. trauma hypothesis of autistic
disorder
e. traumatic epilepsy
e. treatment
E. Years Easy Screen (EYES)

early-onset

e.-o. ataxia
e.-o. familial Alzheimer disease
e.-o. schizophrenia

earphone

intrameatal e.

earth eating

ease of fatigue

easily

e. distractible
e. disturbed sleep

Easprin

East

E. African
E. African sleeping sickness
E. African trypanosomiasis

eastern

e. equine encephalomyelitis (EEE)
e. equine viral encephalitis
E. subtype

easy

e. child
e. distractibility
e. fatigability
e. virtue

**EasyGuide Neuro image-guided surgery
system**

EAT

Edinburgh Articulation Test
Education Apperception Test

eating

e. aids
E. Attitudes Test
e. behavior
e. binge
binge e.
clay e.
e. compulsion
compulsive e.
dirt e.
e. disorder
E. Disorder Examination
E. Disorder Inventory (EDI)
E. Disorder Inventory for Children
E. Disorder Inventory, 2nd edition
(EDI-2)
e. disturbance
earth e.
e. epilepsy
e. fear
e. habit
e. hair
E. Inventory

E

eating *(continued)*
    e. and purging
    starch e.
    e. without satiation
Eaton-Lambert syndrome
Ebbinghaus curve of retention test
EBD
    emotional and behavioral difficulties
Ebonics
EBPS
    Emotional and Behavior Problem Scale
EBV
    Epstein-Barr virus
    EBV encephalitis
Eby Elementary identification Instrument
ECA
    external carotid artery
ECA-PCA bypass surgery
eccentric
    e. arteriosclerosis
    e. behavior
    e. paranoia
    e. personality
    e. projection
    e. thinking
ecchordosis physaliformis
ecchymosis
    periorbital e.
    posterior e.
ecclesiasticism
ecclesiophobia, ecclesiaphobia
eccrine
    e. angiomatous hamartoma
    e. cystadenoma
    e. gland
ecdemiomania
ecdemonomania
ecdysiasm
ECES
    Education and Career Exploration System
ECG
    electrocardiogram
echelon
    higher e.
echinococcosis
echinomycosis lymphocytic meningitis
Echlin laminectomy rongeur
Echlin-Luer rongeur
ECHO, pl. echoes
    enteric cytopathic human orphan
    ECHO virus
echo
    e. chamber
    de pensós e.
    e. des penses
    gradient e.
    Hahn e.
    e. phenomenon
    e. planar imaging
    e. principle
    radiofrequency-induced e.
    e. reaction
    e. sign

    e. speech
    spin e.
    e. time (TE)
    T1-weighted spin e.
    T2-weighted spin e.
echoacousia
echocardiogram
    bubble e.
echocardiograph
    Siemens Sonoline SL-2 e.
echocardiography
    transesophageal e.
echodensity
    intraparenchymal periventricular e.
echoencephalography
echoes *(pl. of* ECHO)
echographia
echoic memory
echoing
    thought e.
echokinesis, echokinesia
echolalia
    immediate e.
    mitigated e.
    unmitigated e.
echolalus
echolocation
Echols retractor
echomatism, echomotism
echomimia
echopalilalia
echopathy
echophobia
echophotony
echophrasia
echopraxia
echopraxis
echovirus
    e. infection ataxia
    e. meningitis
Echovist
echul
ECI
    electrocerebral inactivity
ECIC, EC-IC
    extracranial-intracranial
    ECIC arterial bypass
    ECIC bypass
eclactisma
eclampsia
    puerperal e.
eclamptic
    e. amentia
    e. convulsion
    e. delirium
    e. idiocy
    e. seizure
    e. symptoms
eclamptogenic, eclamptogenous
eclectic
    e. behaviorism
    e. counseling
eclipse
    cerebral e.

mental e.
E. TENS unit
ECM
endoscope-controlled microsurgery
erythema chronicum migrans
external chemical messenger
extracellular matrix
ecmnesia
ecmnesiac delirium
ECoG
electrocorticogram
electrocorticography
ECoG monitoring
ecogenetics
ecological
e. perception
e. psychiatry
e. study
e. systems model
e. validity
ecology
human e.
ecomania
economic
e. advantage
e. approach
e. disadvantage
e. divorce
e. principle
Economo
E. disease
E. encephalitis
economy
token e.
ecopharmacology
ecophobia (*var. of* oikophobia)
ecopsychiatry
ecopsychology
Ecotrin Low Adult Strength
ecouteur
ecouteurism
ecphoria
ecphorize
ECR
evoked cortical response
ECS
electrocerebral silence
electroconvulsive shock
epileptic confusional state
extracellular space
E2CS
Edinburgh 2 Coma Scale
ECST
electroconvulsive shock therapy
electroconvulsive shock treatment
ecstasy
chocolate e.
Herbal E.
Liquid E.
religious e.
ecstatic
e. behavior
e. pain
e. trance

ECT
electroconvulsive therapy
electroconvulsive treatment
electroshock therapy
bilateral ECT
brief pulse bilateral ECT
brief pulse unilateral ECT
sine wave unilateral ECT
suprathreshold ECT
unilateral brief pulse ECT
unilateral nondominant-hemisphere ECT
unilateral sine wave ECT
ectal origin
ectasia
basilar e.
dural e.
ectimia
ectoderm
embryonic neural e.
neural e.
ectodermogenic neurosyphilis
ectomorph
ectomorphic constitutional type
ectopia
cerebellar e.
e. lentis
posterior pituitary gland e.
ectopic
e. ACTH syndrome
e. hormone
e. intracranial retinoblastoma
e. pinealoma
ectoplasm
ectoretina
ectropion
ectype
ecumenics
eCVR
estimated cerebrovascular resistance
eczema
psychogenic e.
ED
equivalent dose
EDAMS
encephaloduroarteriomyosynangiosis
EDAS
encephaloduroarteriosynangiosis
EDAS procedure
eddy, pl. **eddies**
e. current
e. current heating
Edecrin
edema
airway e.
alimentary e.
angioneurotic e.
blue e.
brainstem e.
cellular brain e.
cerebral e.
circumscribed e.
cytotoxic e.
dependent e.
granulocytic brain e.

E

edema *(continued)*
    hereditary angioneurotic e. (HANE)
    holohemispheric vasogenic e.
    hunger e.
    interstitial hydrocephalic e.
    intraneural e.
    ipsilateral vasogenic e.
    ischemic brain e.
    meningioma-associated cerebral e.
    nerve root e.
    neurogenic pulmonary e. (NPE)
    nutritional e.
    perifocal e.
    periodic e.
    peritumoral brain e.
    perocephalic e.
    pitting e.
    pulmonary e.
    Quincke e.
    retroauricular e.
    toxic e.
    vasogenic e.

EDEN
    Evaluation Disposition (toward the)
    Environment

edeomania

Eder-Puestow metal olive dilator

edetate
    calcium disodium e.
    e. calcium disodium
    e. disodium

edge enhancement

EDI
    Eating Disorder Inventory

EDI-2
    Eating Disorder Inventory, 2nd edition

Edinburgh
    E. Articulation Test (EAT)
    E. 2 Coma Scale (E2CS)
    E. Handedness Inventory
    E. Picture Test
    E. Postnatal Depression Scale
    E. Reading Test
    E. Rehabilitation Status Scale

Edinger-Westphal nucleus

edipism

EdiT
    electric differential therapy

ED/LD
    emotionally disturbed/learning disabled

Edmonton extension tongs

EDPA
    Erhardt Developmental Prehension
    Assessment

EDR
    electrodermal response
    electrodermal response biofeedback

EDRF
    endothelium-derived relaxing factor

Edronax

edrophonium
    e. chloride
    e. chloride test

EDS
    Ego Development Scale
    excessive daytime sleepiness

EDTA
    ethylenediaminetetraacetic acid

educable mentally retarded (EMR)

education
    E. Apperception Test (EAT)
    E. and Career Exploration System
    (ECES)
    compensatory e.
    continuing medical e. (CME)
    cooperative e.
    dance e.
    drug e.
    Drug Abuse Resistance E. (DARE)
    environmental e.
    Personal Assessment for
    Continuing E. (PACE)
    progressive e.
    psychiatric e.
    e. quotient (EQ)
    sex e.
    special e.
    vocational rehabilitation and e.
    (VR&E)

educational
    e. acceleration
    e. achievement
    e. achievement battery
    e. age (EA)
    e. counseling
    E. Development Series
    e. disadvantage
    e. dysfunction
    e. functioning
    e. history
    e. information
    e. level
    e. measurement
    e. opportunity
    e. program
    e. psychology
    e. psychotherapy
    e. quotient (EQ)
    e. setting
    e. situation
    e. test
    E. Testing Service (ETS)
    e. therapist
    e. treatment
    e. value

educationally
    e. deprived
    e. mentally handicapped (EMH)
    e. mentally retarded (EMR)
    e. subnormal (ESN)

educational-socialization model

educative intervention

educe

eduction

EDVA
    Erhardt Developmental Vision
    Assessment

Edwards
  E. instrumentation
  E. modular system
  E. modular system bridging sleeve
    construct
  E. modular system compression
    construct
  E. modular system construct
    selection
  E. modular system distraction-
    lordosis construct
  E. modular system dynamic
    loading
  E. modular system kyphoreduction
    construct
  E. modular system load sharing
  E. modular system neutralization
    construct
  E. modular system rod crosslink
  E. modular system rod-sleeve
    construct
  E. modular system sacral fixation
    device
  E. modular system scoliosis
    construct
  E. modular system spinal rod-
    sleeve
  E. modular system spondylo
    construct
  E. modular system standard sleeve
    construct
  E. modular system universal rod
  E. Personal Preference Schedule
    (EPPS)
  E. sacral fixation device
  E. sacral screw
  E. syndrome
Edwards/Barbaro syringo-peritoneal
  shunt
Edwards-Levine rod
EE
  expressed emotion
EEE
  eastern equine encephalomyelitis
EEF probe
EEG
  electroencephalogram
  electroencephalograph
  electroencephalography
    abnormal EEG
  EEG activating procedure
  EEG activation
  EEG activity measurement
  EEG alpha blocking
  EEG alpha pattern
  EEG alpha rhythm
  EEG alpha spindle
  EEG alpha wave
  EEG amplifier drift
  EEG anachronism
  EEG anteromesial temporal
    discharge
  attenuation of alpha rhythm on
    EEG
  EEG background disorganization

Bancaud phenomenon on EEG
beta pattern on EEG
beta rhythm on EEG
beta wave on EEG
EEG biofeedback
BIPLED on EEG
blunt spike-and-wave complex on
  EEG
diffuse slowing of EEG
frontal intermittent rhythmic delta
  activity on EEG
ictal pattern on EEG
nonspecific abnormality on EEG
phase lag on EEG
phase spike on EEG
EEG potential
scattered dysrhythmic slow activity
  on EEG
sleep deprived EEG
sleep spindle on EEG
theta wave on EEG
EEG tracing
waking EEG
EEG with NP lead
EEG-electrogenesis
efavirenz
EFF
  electromagnetic focusing field
effacement
  cistern e.
  e. of cistern
  dural sac e.
  nerve root sheath e.
  sulcus e.
  ventricle e.
effect
  adverse side e.
  age e.
  air pressure e.
  alerting e.
  antiadrenergic e.
  anticholinergic side e.
  antiserotonergic e.
  anxiolytic e.
  aspirin e.
  assimilation e.
  asymmetry and order e.
  atmosphere e.
  autokinetic e.
  autonomic side e.
  Barnum e.
  blast e.
  Bohr e.
  boxcar e.
  bystander e.
  ceiling e.
  chatterbox e.
  cholinergic side e.
  chronic toxic e.
  clasp-knife e.
  cohort e.
  cold e.
  confinement e.
  contrast e.
  copper wire e.

E

effect *(continued)*
    crisis e.
    Cushing e.
    damping e.
    e.'s of deception
    depressiogenic e.
    desired e.
    deterioration e.
    diminished e.
    direct physiological e.
    door-in-the-face e.
    Doppler e.
    dose-dependent e.
    effect expectancy e.
    electrocardiographic e.
    enlightenment e.
    environmental e.
    ether e.
    euphorigenic e.
    experimenter e.
    experimenter-expectancy e.
    extrapyramidal medication side e.
    Féré e.
    fetal alcohol e. (FAE)
    first-pass e.
    flow e.
    flow-induced influx e.
    Glick e.
    e. gradient
    Halloween e.
    hallucinogen toxic e.
    halo e.
    hangover e.
    head shadow e.
    heat e.
    humidity e.
    idiosyncratic side e.
    inflow e.
    interaction e.
    interviewer e.
    isolation e.
    kindling e.
    law of e.
    e. law
    less than maximal e.
    long-hot-summer e.
    long-term e.
    loss of e.
    magnetohydrodynamic e.
    maximal e.
    Mellanby e.
    mere-exposure e.
    misinformation e.
    missile e.
    movement disorder e.
    muscarinic side e.
    off e.
    on e.
    Orbeli e.
    panicogenic e.
    paradoxical e.
    parkinsonism-like e.
    partial-reinforcement e. (PRE)
    passing stranger e.

    peripheral sympathomimetic e.
    Perky e.
    personal e.'s
    phase e.
    phase-shift e.
    physiological e.
    placebo e.
    potential adverse e.
    practice e.
    psychoactive e.
    Pygmalion e.
    radiation e.
    secure base e.
    sedative e.
    side e.
    stimulant e.
    Stroop e.
    suggestibility e.
    susceptibility e.
    sympathectomy e.
    sympathomimetic e.
    temperature e.
    therapeutic e.
    Thorndike law of e.
    time-of-flight e.
    toxic e.
    Transylvania e.
    e. of trauma on consciousness
    unintended e.
    Vulpian e.
    washboard e.
    Wever-Bray e.
    wind e.
    Zeigarnik e.
effectance motive
effected pain
effective
    e. action
    e. dose
    e. ego
    e. masking
    occupationally e.
    e. pedicle diameter
    E. Reading Test
    E. School Battery (ESB)
    socially e.
    e. stimulus
    e. thread diameter
effective-habit strength
effectiveness
    relative biological e. (RBE)
effective-reaction potential
effector
    e. cell
    e. operation
effectual
effeminacy
effeminate
    e. homosexuality
    e. man
efferent
    e. feedback
    gamma e.
    e. motor aphasia
    e. motor unit

e. nerve
e. sympathetic activity
Effer-K
effervescent
    K+ Care E.
    K-Electrolyte E.
    K-Gen E.
    Klorvess E.
    K-Lyte E.
    potassium bicarbonate and
      potassium chloride, e.
    potassium bicarbonate and
      potassium citrate, e.
Effexor-XR
efficacy, pl. **efficacies**
    e. study
efficiency
    colony-forming e. (CFE)
    good sleep e.
    masking e.
    neural e.
    REM sleep e.
    sleep e.
efficient
    cause e.
    e. cause
Effler-Groves dissector
effort
    distributed e.
    e. level
    new-work e.
    e. syndrome
effort-reward imbalance
effort-shape technique
effusion ego egocentric
E-F scale
EFT
    Embedded Figures Test
    extended family therapy
egalitarianism
Egemen keyhole suction-control device
egerism
egersis
EGFR
    epidermal growth factor receptor
eggcrate mattress
ego
    e. alien
    alter e.
    e. alter theory
    e. analysis
    antilibidinal e.
    e. anxiety
    auxiliary e.
    body e.
    e. boundary
    e. boundary loss
    e. cathexis
    e. center
    collective e.
    e. complex
    e. control
    e. decomposition
    decomposition of e.
    e. defense

e. defense mechanism
e. development
E. Development Scale (EDS)
e. deviation
e. distortion
dream e.
e. drive
duplication of e.
e. dystonic homosexuality
e. dystonic pseudohallucination
effective e.
e. erotism
escape from the e.
extinction of e.
e. formation
fragmentation of e.
e. function
E. Function Assessment
id e.
e. ideal
ideal e.
e. identity
e. instinct
e. integration
e. integrity
e. integrity versus despair
e. involvement
e. libido
loss of boundaries of e.
e. maximation
mental e.
e. model
motor control of the e.
e. narcissism
negation of the e.
e. neurosis
e. nucleus
oral e.
perception e.
pleasure e.
preschizophrenic e.
e. proper
e. psychology
e. psychotherapy
purified pleasure e.
reality e.
reality life of e.
reasonable e.
e. resistance
e. restriction
e. retrenchment
safety of e.
split in the e.
e. splitting
stability of e.
e. state
E. State Inventory (ESI)
e. strength (ES)
e. strength scale
e. stress
e. structure
e. subject
e. substance
e. suffering
supportive e.

E

ego *(continued)*
    surface e.
    e. syntonic
    e. transcendence
    weak e.
    e. weakness
egocentric
    effusion ego e.
    e. language
    e. speech
    e. thinking
    e. thought process
egocentricity
    E. Index
egocentrism
ego-coping skill
egodystonia
ego-dystonic
    e.-d. behavior
    e.-d. intrusion
    e.-d. orientation
    e.-d. promiscuity
egodystonicity
Ego-Ideal and Conscience Development Test (EICDT)
egoism
egoïsme à deux
egoistic
egoity
egology
egomania
egomechanism of defense
egometer
egomorphism
egonomics
egopathy
egopathyegotism
egophobia
egostate
    parent e.
ego-state therapy
egosyntonia
egosyntonic
    e. behavior
    e. trait
egosyntonicity
egotheism
egotism
egotistical
egotistic suicide
egotropic
egotropy
egregorsis
EH
    emotional handicap
    epithelial hemangioendothelioma
    epithelioid hemangioendothelioma
E&H
    environment and heredity
Ehlers-Danlos syndrome
Ehrenritter ganglion
Ehret syndrome

EIA
    MAC EIA
        IgM antibody capture
EICDT
    Ego-Ideal and Conscience Development Test
Eichhorst neuritis
eicosanoid
eicosapentaenoic acid
eidetic
    e. ability
    e. image
    e. imagery
    E. Parents Test (EPT)
    e. personification
    e. type
eidolon
eidoptometry
eight
    e. stages of man
    E. State Questionnaire
eight-ball hemorrhage
eighth
    e. cranial nerve
    e. nerve herpetic neuritis
    e. nerve tumor
eighth-month anxiety
EIO
    exploratory insight-oriented psychotherapy
Eisenlohr syndrome
eisodic
eisoptrophia
eisoptrophobia
either-or
    e.-o. situation
    e.-o. thinking
ejaculatio
    e. deficiens
    e. praecox
    e. retardate
ejaculation
    delayed e.
    e. disorder
    female e.
    immediate e.
    e. physiology
    premature e.
    primary retarded e.
    e. reflux
    retarded e.
    retrograde e.
    secondary retarded e.
ejaculatione
    coitus sine e.
ejaculatory
    e. duct
    e. dysfunction
    e. impotence
    e. incompetence
    e. pain
    e. reflex
ejection fraction
Ekbom syndrome
ekistics

ekphorize
EL
  elopement
elaborate dream sequence
elaboration
  secondary e.
  symbolic e.
Elan-E electronic motor system
elantrine
elastase
  myeloid e.
  plasma e.
Elastica-Masson stain
Elastica van Gieson stain
elasticity
elasticum
  pseudoxanthoma e.
elastin
  e. degradation
  e. gene
elated affect
Elavil
elbow
  e. jerk
  e. reflex
Eldepryl
elder
  e. abuse
  e. adult neglect
  e. maltreatment
elderly
  Clifton Assessment Procedures for
    the E. (CAPE)
  Kendrick Cognitive Tests for
    the E.
ELDH
  extraforaminal lumbar disc herniation
eldritch
electicism
elective
  e. abortion
  e. admission
  e. anorexia
  e. mutism
  e. mutism adjustment reaction
  e. sterility
  e. therapy
Electra complex
electric
  e. anesthesia
  e. auditory
  e. aura
  e. chorea
  e. differential therapy (EdiT)
  e. drill
  e. field
  e. irritability
  e. knife
  E. Kool Aid
  e. shock therapy (EST, est)
  e. shock treatment (EST, est)
  e. skin shock
  e. sleep
  e. stimulation of the brain (ESB)

electrical
  e. activity of brain
  e. current brain trauma organic
    psychosis
  e. habituation
  e. injury
  e. intracranial stimulation
  e. potential
  e. shock
  e. stimulation mapping
  e. synapse
  e. transcranial stimulation (ETS)
electricity
  feeling of e.
Electri-Cool cold therapy system
electroanalgesia
electroanalysis
electroanesthesia
electroaxonography
electrobasograph
electroblotting isoproterenol
electrocardiogram (ECG)
electrocardiographic effect
electrocautery
  Aspen e.
  bipolar e.
  Bovie e.
  monopolar e.
electrocerebral
  e. activity
  e. inactivity (ECI)
  e. silence (ECS)
electrocoagulation
  RF e.
electrocoagulator
electrocochleogram
electrocoma
electrocontractility
electroconvulsive
  e. shock (ECS)
  e. shock therapy (ECST)
  e. shock treatment (ECST)
  e. therapy (ECT)
  e. therapy-induced mood disorder
  e. treatment (ECT)
electrocorticogram (ECoG)
electrocorticography (ECoG)
electrode
  active surface e.
  Adtech Spencer platinum depth e.
  A-frame e.
  Aspen laparoscopy e.
  Clark e.
  clip-type e.
  combination needle e.
  Cueva cranial nerve e.
  curved e.
  DBS e.
  El-Naggar-Nashold right-angled
    nucleus caudalis DREZ e.
  epidural peg e.
  flexible wire e.
  Goldmann-Offner reference of e.
  ground e.
  e. impedance

E

electrode *(continued)*
    intracerebral depth e.
    intrameatal e.
    Levin thermocouple cordotomy e.
    metal e.
    e. migration
    monopolar e.
    Nashold TC e.
    needle e.
    Nichrome cylindrical e.
    noncephalic e.
    percutaneous epidural e.
    Pices e.
    Pisces e.
    e. placement
    reference e.
    Resume e.
    self-adhering e.
    self-attaching e.
    Silverman placement of e.
    Sluyter-Mehta thermocouple e.
    Somatics monitoring e.
    Spencer probe depth e.
    spring-loaded e.
    Stephenson-Gibbs reference e.
    straight needle e.
    subdural grid e.
    subdural strip e.
    temporary percutaneous SCS e.
    Thymapad stimulus e.
    trigeminal e.
    Wolfram needle e.
    Wyler cylindrical subdural e.
electrodecremental seizure
electrode-popping artifact
electrodermal
    e. response (EDR)
    e. response biofeedback (EDR)
electrodetachable
    e. balloon
    e. platinum coil
electrodiagnosis
electrodiagnostic
    e. study
    e. testing
electroencephalogram (EEG)
    alerting maneuver on e.
    alerting stimulus on e.
    aliasing on e.
    audiovisual e. (AVEEG)
    Bancaud phenomenon on e.
    flat e.
    HFF on e.
    IRDA on e.
    isoelectric e.
    Janz response on e.
    Laplacian montage on e.
    LFF on e.
    MFD waves on e.
    MSLT with e.
    OIRDA on e.
    PDA on e.
    POSTS on e.
    quantitative e. (QEEG)

    RMTD on e.
    SLEM on e.
    SREDA on e.
    SSS on e.
    stereotactic e. (SEEG)
    stereotactic depth e. (SDEEG)
electroencephalograph (EEG)
electroencephalographic
    e. burst-suppression
    e. dysrhythmia
electroencephalography (EEG)
    intracranial e. (ICEEG)
    quantitative e. (QEEG)
    scalp e.
    scalp-sphenoidal e. (SSEEG)
electrographic seizure activity
electrogustometry
electrokinetic
electrolepsy
electrolyte
    e. abnormality
    e. balance
    e. disturbance
    e. imbalance
    e. replacement
    E. Supplement
electromagnetic
    e. flowmeter
    e. flow probe
    e. focusing field (EFF)
    e. focusing field probe
    e. radiation
    e. wave
electromagnetoencephalograph (EMEG)
electromicturition
electromigratory
electromotive force
electromuscular sensibility
electromyelogram (EMG)
electromyelography
electromyogram (EMG)
    CMAP on e.
    CNAP on e.
    CRD on e.
    Erb point stimulation on e.
    MUAP on e.
    SNAP on e.
    SSR on e.
electromyograph (EMG)
    Counterpoint e.
electromyographic (EMG)
    e. feedback
    e. incomplete interference pattern
    needle e.
    e. perineometer
    e. potential
    e. response
electromyography (EMG)
    e. biofeedback
    facial e.
    needle e.
    single-fiber e. (SFEMG)
electron
    e. collision
    e. micrograph

e. microscopy
unpaired e.
electronarcosis (EN)
electron-coupled nuclear spin-spin interaction
electroneurogram (ENoG)
electroneurography
facial e.
electroneurolysis
electroneuromyography
electronic
e. aid
e. conduction
electronystagmography (ENG)
electrooculogram (EOG)
electrooculographic
e. activity
e. analysis
electrooculography (EOG)
electroolfactogram (EOG)
electropathology
electrophobia
electrophoresis
agarose gel e.
protein e.
pulsed-field gel e.
sodium dodecyl sulfate-polyacrylamide gel e. (SDS-PAGE)
thin-layer agarose gel e.
electrophrenic respiration
electrophysiological
e. battery
e. guidance
e. mapping
e. stimulation
electrophysiologic integrity
electrophysiology
electroplexy
electroretinogram (ERG)
electroretinography
electroshock
maximal e. (MES)
e. therapy (ECT, EST, est)
e. treatment (EST, est)
electroshock-induced
e.-i. psychotic
e.-i. psychotic syndrome
electrosleep therapy (ETS)
electrospectrography
electrospinogram
electrospinography
electrostimulation
electrostriatogram
electrosynthesis
electrotherapeutic
e. sleep
e. sleep therapy
electrotherapist
electrotherapy
cerebral e. (CET)
transcerebral e. (TCET)
electrothrombosis

electrotonic
e. junction
e. synapse
electrotonus
electrovibratory massage
Elekta
E. Leksell rongeur
E. stereotactic head frame
E. viewing wand
element
cognitive e.
contributory e.
cultural e.
glioneuronal e.
identical e.
thyroid response e. (TRE)
elemental diet
elementarism
elementary
e. anxiety
e. hallucination
e. manner
e. partial seizure
e. process
elephantiasis
e. neuromatosa
elephantiasis neuromatosa
elephantine
eleutheromania
eleutherophobia
elevated
e. mood
e. risk
elevation
flap e.
e. paresis
elevator
Adson e.
Cloward e.
Cobb periosteal e.
Cottle e.
Crawford dural e.
Cushing Little Joker e.
Cushing periosteal e.
Cushing pituitary e.
Cushing staphylorrhaphy e.
D'Errico periosteal e.
Frazier dural e.
Freer septal e.
Hajek-Ballenger septal e.
Jannetta duckbill e.
Jarit periosteal e.
Kennerdell-Maroon e.
Key e.
Langenbach e.
Langenbeck periosteal e.
Malis e.
mood e.
periosteal e.
round-tipped periosteal e.
Yasargil e.
elevatus
iatrogenic e.
eleventh cranial nerve
elfin facies

E

Elgiloy
    E. clip
    E. clip material
Elgin checklist
ELI
    Environmental Language Inventory
elicited
    e. behavior
    e. imitation
Elihorn Maze Test
elimination
    e. diet
    e. disorder
    e. drive
    process of e.
ELISA
    enzyme-linked immunosorbent assay
    ELISA test
elision
Elithorn maze
elixir
    amobarbital e.
    aprobarbital e.
    butabarbital e.
    high-alcoholic e.
    potassium chloride e.
    terpin hydrate e.
    three bromides e.
**Elizur Test of Psycho-Organicity:
    Children and Adults**
ellipsis wit
elliptical
    e. incision
    e. nystagmus
**El-Naggar-Nashold right-angled nucleus
    caudalis DREZ electrode**
elopement (EL)
    e. ideation
    e. status (ES)
eloquent cortex
ELP
    estimated learning potential
Elpenor syndrome
ELS
    endolymphatic sac
Elsberg
    E. brain cannula
    E. ventricular cannula
**El Senoussi Multiphasic Marital
    Inventory**
elucidation
elurophobia
elusion
elusive syndrome
emaciated body
emaciation disorder
emanate
emanative
emancipated minor
emancipation
    e. disorder
    e. disorder of adolescence
emancipatory
    e. disorder
    e. striving

emarginate
EMAS
    Endler Multidimensional Anxiety Scale
emasculate
embarrass
embarrassment
    cord e.
    dream e.
    e. dream
    nerve root e.
    e. psychosis
    respiratory e.
embedded
    e. command
    E. Figures Test (EFT)
embedding
    paraffin e.
embody
embolalia, embololalia
embolectomy
    direct e.
emboli (*pl. of* embolus)
embolic
    e. apoplexy
    e. infarction
    e. stroke
emboliform nucleus
emboligenic
embolism
    air e.
    artery-to-artery e.
    cardiac e.
    cerebral formed-element e.
    cholesterol e.
    fat e.
    paradoxical air e. (PAE)
    paradoxical cerebral e.
    pulmonary e.
    retinal e.
    therapeutic e.
    venous e.
embolization
    cerebral foreign body e.
    coil e.
    flow-directed e.
    histoacryl e.
    particulate e.
    percutaneous intraarterial e.
    percutaneous transvenous coil e.
    selective e.
    staged e.
    superselective e.
    therapeutic e.
    transarterial platinum coil e.
    transtorcular e.
    venous-side e.
embololalia (*var. of* embolalia)
embolophasia
emboloplasia
embolotherapy
embolus, pl. emboli
    air e.
    calcium e.
    cerebral e.
    fat e.

fibrin-platelet-fibrin e.
Gelfoam powder emboli
organism e.
platelet-fibrin e.
septic e.
Embolyx liquid embolic system
embouchment
embracing behavior
embryogenesis
embryological pathogenetic factor
embryology
embryonic
e. cervical somite
e. disk
e. implant
e. isoform
e. neural ectoderm
EMC
encephalomyocarditis
EMC encephalitis
EMDR
eye movement desensitization and
reprocessing
EMEG
electromagnetoencephalograph
emergency
e. care facility
e. contagion
e. dyscontrol
e. dyscontrol duration
e. emotion
e. intervention
e. medical technician (EMT)
e. medicine
opiate-induced e.
psychiatric e.
e. psychotherapy
e. room (ER)
e. theory
e. theory of emotion
emergent
emergent evolution
treatment emergent
emerogene
Emery-Dreifuss
E.-D. disease
E.-D. muscular dystrophy
emetatrophia
emetine peripheral neuropathy
emetocathartic
emetomania
emetophobia
EMG
electromyelogram
electromyogram
electromyograph
electromyographic
electromyography
EMG biofeedback
Nomad-LE EMG
EMG stimulator
EMH
educationally mentally handicapped
emigrant

eminence
arcuate e.
collateral e.
Doyère e.
facial e.
hypoglossal e.
malar e.
medial e.
median e.
olivary e.
restiform e.
round e.
thenar e.
eminentia, pl. eminentiae
e. abducentis
e. collateralis
e. facialis
e. hypoglossi
e. medialis
e. mediana
e. restiformis
e. teres
emissary
e. foramina
e. vein
emission
e. computed tomography
nocturnal e.
e. tomography scan
Emitrip
emitted behavior
EMLA
eutectic mixture of local anesthetics
emotiomotor
emotiomuscular
emotion
activation theory of e.
adjustment disorder with mixed
disturbance of e.'s
Cannon-Bard theory of e.
childish e.
controlled e.
conversion of e.
dammed-up e.
defensive e.
discomfort with e.
disruptive e.
emergency e.
emergency theory of e.
expressed e. (EE)
ictal e.
James-Lange theory of e.
negative e.
Papez theory of e.
pervasive e.
positive e.
E.'s Profile Index
public display of e.
recall-generated e.
roller-coaster e.
sustained e.
uncanny e.
welfare e.
emotional
e. abandonment

E

emotional *(continued)*
- e. abuse
- e. acrescentism
- e. activity
- e. adjustment
- e. age
- e. agitation
- e. amalgam
- e. amenorrhea
- e. amnesia
- e. anesthesia
- e. atmosphere
- e. attachment/commitment
- e. attainment
- e. attitude
- e. awareness
- e. beggar
- e. and behavioral difficulties (EBD)
- E. and Behavior Problem Scale (EBPS)
- e. bias
- e. blackmail
- e. blockade
- e. blocking
- e. blunting
- e. bond
- e. castration
- e. catharsis
- e. cause of seizure
- e. climate
- e. coldness
- e. comfort
- e. conflict
- e. conflicts or reaction
- e. constriction
- e. crisis
- e. deadness
- e. deficit
- e. dependence
- e. deprivation
- e. detachment
- e. deterioration
- e. development
- e. diarrhea
- e. difficulty
- e. disability
- e. disease
- e. disinhibition
- e. display
- e. distress
- e. disturbance
- e. disturbance adjustment disorder
- e. disturbance adjustment reaction
- e. disturbance of adolescence
- e. disturbance of childhood
- e. disturbance stress reaction
- e. divorce
- e. dullness
- e. dyscontrol
- e. dysfunction
- e. emptiness
- e. excitability
- e. experience
- e. explosivity
- e. expression
- e. fatigue
- e. fatigue study
- e. flatness
- e. flooding
- e. handicap (EH)
- e. health
- e. illness
- e. immaturity
- e. impairment
- e. incontinence
- e. inhibition
- e. inoculation
- e. insanity
- e. insight
- e. instability personality disorder
- e. insulation
- e. investment
- e. lability
- e. leukocytosis
- e. maltreatment of children
- e. manipulation
- e. maturity
- e. modulation
- e. monomania
- e. need
- e. numbing
- e. nutriment
- e. object constancy
- e. overinvolvement
- e. overlay
- e. overreaction
- e. personality
- e. problem
- e. range
- e. reaction
- e. reciprocity
- e. reeducation
- e. reenactment
- e. release
- e. repression
- e. response
- e. responsiveness
- e. scar
- e. security
- e. shading
- e. speech
- e. stability
- e. state
- e. stimulus
- e. storm
- e. stress
- e. stress depressive psychosis
- e. stress precipitating tremor
- e. stupor
- e. supply
- e. support
- e. symptom
- e. tension
- e. thought
- e. tone
- e. trauma
- e. turmoil
- e. undercontrol
- e. vulnerability

emotional/activation factor
emotionality
    excessive e.
    labile e.
    negative e.
    pathologic e.
    positive e.
emotionally
    e. disturbed/learning disabled
    (ED/LD)
    handicapped e.
    e. impaired
    e. inhibited
    e. isolated
    e. laden topic
    e. provoking stimulus
    e. ungiving
    e. unstable
    e. unstable character disorder
    (EUCD)
    e. unstable immaturity
    e. unstable immaturity reaction
    e. unstable personality
    e. upset
emotional-object amalgam
emotion-cognition interface
emotion-laden situation
emotion-related feedback stimulus
emotions-conduct adjustment reaction
emotiovascular
emotive
    e. energy
    e. imagery
    e. language
    e. process
    e. speech
    e. therapy
empathic
    e. behavior
    e. identification
    e. index
empathize
empathy
    accurate e. (AE)
    communicating e.
    failure to develop e.
    generative e.
emphatic speech
emphrensy
emphysema
    subgaleal e.
empiric
    e. cognition
    e. drug treatment
    e. risk
empirical
    e. data
    e. evidence
    e. formula
    e. law
    e. process
    e. review
    e. self
    e. support

    systematic, complete, objective,
    practical, e. (SCOPE)
    e. test
    e. validity
empirical-criterion keying
empirical-rational strategy
empiricism
empiricist theory
empiric-risk figure
Empirin with codeine
empleomania
Employability Inventory
employed
    gainfully e.
employee
    E. Aptitude Survey Test
    E. Assistance Program (EAP)
    E. Attitude Inventory
    E. Effectiveness Profile
    e. evaluation
    E. Reliability Inventory (ERI)
    E. Retirement Income Security Act
    (ERISA)
employment
    e. contract
    e. interview
    e. inventory
    e. profile
    e. workshop
empowered family
empowerment
Empracet with codeine
emprosthotonos
emptiness
    e. of affect
    chronic feelings of e.
    emotional e.
    e. fear
empty
    e. delta sign
    e. nest
    e. nest syndrome
    e. organism
    e. sella
    e. sella sign
    e. sella syndrome
    e. stare
    e. triangle sign
    e. word
empty-chair technique
emptying reflex
empyema
    subdural e.
EMR
    educable mentally retarded
    educationally mentally retarded
EMS
    encephalomyosynangiosis
    eosinophilia-myalgia syndrome
EMT
    emergency medical technician
emulsion
    Dizac Injectable E.
    polyvinyl acetate e.

E

EMV
eye-motor-verbal
eyes, motor, voice/verbal
emylcamate
EN
electronarcosis
en
e. bloc
e. masse
e. passage feeder artery
e. plaque meningioma
e. rapport
enactive
e. mode
e. period
enactment
enalapril and hydrochlorothiazide
enanthate
fluphenazine e.
Prolixin e.
testosterone e.
enantiodromia
enantiolalia
enantiopathic
encapsulated
e. brain abscess
e. delusion
e. end organ
encephala (*pl. of* encephalon)
encephalalgia
encephalasthenia
encephalatrophic
encephalatrophy
encephalauxe
encéphale isolé
encephalemia
encephali
dura mater encephali
pia mater encephali
encephalic
e. angioma
e. vesicle
encephalitis, pl. **encephalitides**
e. A
acute hemorrhagic e.
acute necrotizing e.
Australian X e.
benign myalgic e.
Bickerstaff e.
Binswanger e.
biundulant viral e.
brainstem e.
bunyavirus e.
California e.
Central European e.
chronic subcortical e.
CMV e.
Colorado tick fever viral e.
Coxsackie e.
Dawson e.
dengue viral e.
eastern equine viral e.
EBV e.
Economo e.
EMC e.

enteroviral e.
epidemic e.
equine e.
experimental allergic e. (EAE)
Far East Russian e.
fulminant necrotizing e.
Hayem e.
e. hemorrhagica
herpes simplex virus e. (HSVE)
herpesvirus e.
herpetic e.
HSV e.
hyperergic e.
Ilhéus e.
inclusion body e.
Japanese e. (JE)
Japanese B e.
e. japonica
La Crosse e.
Langat viral e.
lead e.
Leichtenstern e.
e. lethargica
limbic e.
lymphogranuloma venereum e.
measles e.
Mengo e.
metabolic e.
mumps e.
Murray Valley e.
Mycoplasma pneumoniae e.
myoclonic e.
necrotizing e.
e. neonatorum
paraneoplastic limbic e.
e. periaxialis concentrica
e. periaxialis diffusa
postvaccinal e.
Powassan e.
psittacosis e.
purulent e.
e. pyogenica
rabies e.
Rasmussen e.
Russian autumn e.
Russian spring-summer e. (Eastern
or Western subtype)
Russian tick-borne e.
Saint Louis e.
Schilder e.
sclerosing e.
secondary e.
slow-acting viral e.
Strümpell-Leichtenstern e.
subacute inclusion body e.
subacute measles e.
e. subcorticalis chronica
subcorticalis chronica e.
suppurative e.
tick-borne e. (Central European or
Eastern subtype)
toxoplasmic e.
traumatic e.
van Bogaert e.
varicella e.

Venezuelan equine e.
vernal e.
viral e.
von Economo e.
Western equine e. (WEE)
West Nile e.
woodcutter's e.
yellow fever e.
encephalitogen
encephalitogenic
encephalization
encephalocele
anterior basal e.
frontoethmoidal e.
frontosphenoidal e.
nasoethmoidal e.
nasofrontal e.
nasoorbital e.
occipital e.
orbital e.
parietal e.
sphenoethmoidal e.
sphenoid e.
sphenomaxillary e.
sphenoorbital e.
suboccipital e.
transethmoidal e.
transsphenoidal e.
encephalociastic
encephaloclastic microcephaly
encephalocystocele
encephalodialysis
encephaloduroarteriomyosynangiosis
(EDAMS)
encephaloduroarteriosynangiosis (EDAS)
encephaloduromyosynangiosis
ribbon e.
encephalodynia
encephalodysplasia
encephalogram
isoelectric e.
encephalography
encephaloid
encephaloleukopathia scleroticans
encephalolith
encephalology
encephaloma
encephalomalacia
cystic e.
end-stage ischemic e.
multicystic e.
subcortical e.
encephalomeningitis
encephalomeningocele
encephalomeningopathy
encephalometer
encephalomyelitis
acute disseminated e. (ADE, ADEM)
allergic e.
benign myalgic e.
disseminated e.
eastern equine e. (EEE)
epidemic myalgic e.
experimental allergic e. (EAE)

granulomatous e.
Leigh subacute necrotizing e.
necrotizing e.
post infectious disseminated e.
postparainfectious e.
toxoplasmic e.
Venezuelan equine e. (VEE)
virus e.
Western equine e. (WEE)
zoster e.
encephalomyelocele
encephalomyeloneuropathy
nonspecific e.
encephalomyelonic axis
encephalomyelopathy
carcinomatous e.
epidemic myalgic e.
mitochondrial e.
necrotizing e.
paracarcinomatous e.
encephalomyeloradiculitis
encephalomyeloradiculopathy
encephalomyocarditis (EMC)
encephalomyopathy
mitochondrial e.
mitochondrial
neurogastrointestinal e. (MNGIE)
encephalomyosynangiosis (EMS)
encephalon, pl. **encephala**
encephalonarcosis
encephalopathia
e. addisonia
encephalopathia addisonia
encephalopathy
acute toxic e.
AIDS e.
air e.
alcoholic pellagra e.
alcoholic possible pancreatic e.
allergic e.
amyotrophic type of spongiform e.
anoxic e. (AE)
bilirubin e.
Binswanger e.
bovine spongiform e.
boxer's e.
childhood e.
chronic traumatic e.
degenerative e.
delayed postanoxic e.
demyelinating e.
diffuse e.
epileptogenic e.
familial e.
fulminant hepatic e.
Heidenhain type of spongiform e.
hepatic e. (HE)
hyperkinetic e.
hypernatremic e.
hypertensive e.
hypoglycemic e.
hyponatremic e.
hypoparathyroid e.
hypoxic e.
hypoxic-ischemic e. (HIE)

E

encephalopathy *(continued)*
  idiopathic e.
  infantile e.
  ischemic-hypoxic e.
  lead e.
  Leigh necrotizing e.
  mercury e.
  metabolic e.
  mitochondrial e.
  myoclonic e.
  myo-neuro-gastrointestinal e.
    (MNGIE)
  neoplastic e.
  Nevin-Jones subacute spongiform e.
  painter's e.
  palindromic e.
  pancreatic e.
  portal systemic e. (PSE)
  postanoxic e.
  postcontusion syndrome e.
  posttraumatic e.
  progressive multifocal leuko-J e.
    (PMJ)
  progressive subcortical e.
  progressive traumatic e.
  pulmonary e.
  punch-drunk e.
  recurrent e.
  saturnine e.
  spongiform virus e.
  static e.
  subacute necrotizing e.
  subacute spongiform e.
  subcortical arteriosclerotic e.
  subcortical vascular e.
  thiamine deficiency e. (TDE)
  thyrotoxic e.
  toxic e.
  toximetabolic e.
  transmissible spongiform viral e.
  traumatic progressive e.
  uremic e.
  viral e.
  Wernicke fluent e.
  Wernicke-Korsakoff e.
encephalopsy
encephalopsychosis
encephalopuncture
encephalopyosis
encephaloradiculitis
encephalorrhachidian
encephalorrhagia
encephaloschisis
encephalosclerosis
encephaloscope
encephalosepsis
encephalosis
encephalospinal
encephalothlipsis
encephalotome
encephalotrigeminal
  e. angiomatosis
  e. angiomatosis seizure
  e. vascular syndrome

encephalotrophy
enciprazine
enclosed macroadenoma
encoding
  e. communication board
  frequency e.
  memory e.
  phase e.
  e. skill
  velocity e.
encopresis
  functional e.
  overflow e.
  primary e.
encopresis,
  e. with constipation and overflow
    incontinence
  e. without constipation and
    overflow incontinence
encotretic
encounter
  e. group
  indiscriminate sexual e.
  marriage e.
  e. movement
encroachment
  foraminal e.
end
  e. bulb
  e. organ
  e. plate
  e. point
  e. point tremor
  e. product
  e. spurt
  e. state
endamage
endangered
  physically e.
endarterectomy
  carotid e. (CEA)
  e. dissector
endbrain
endemic
  e. neuritis
  e. paralytic vertigo
endemica
  panneuritis e.
endergonic
endermic
end-gaze physiologic nystagmus
ending
  act e.
  annulospiral e.
  caliciform e.
  epilemmal e.
  flower-spray e.
  free nerve e.
  grape e.
  hederiform e.
  nerve e.
  sole-plate e.
  synaptic e.
Endler Multidimensional Anxiety Scale
  (EMAS)

endo
endoaneurysmoplasty
endoaneurysmorrhaphy
Endobile
endocarditis
    bacterial e.
    infective e.
    marantic e.
    nonbacterial thrombotic e.
endocathection
endoceliac
endocentric construction
endocept
endocranial cast
endocranium
endocratic power
endocrine
    e. axes
    e. disease organic psychosis
    e. dysregulation
    e. gland
    e. obesity
    e. psychogenic disorder
    e. system
    e. therapy
endocrine-inactive pituitary adenoma
endocrinologic
endocrinological compromise
endocrinology
    behavioral e.
endocrinopathy
endoderm
endodermal sinus
end-of-dose deterioration
endogamy
endogenesis
endogenetic
endogenic
endogenomorphic
    e. depression
    e. syndrome
endogenous
    e. abnormality
    e. chemical
    e. chromosomal promoter
    e. circadian pacemaker
    e. circadian period
    e. circadian rhythm phase
    e. depression
    e. factor
    e. fiber
    e. negativity
    e. obesity
    e. opioid
    e. pain
    e. rhythm
    e. smile
    e. stimulation
    e. thyrotoxicosis
    e. Zeitgeber
endogenously produced substance
endogeny
endoglycosidase
Endografin

Endolor
endolymph
endolymphatic
    e. duct
    e. hydrops
    e. sac (ELS)
endomeninx
endometrium
endomorph
endomorphic constitutional type
endomusia
endoneural tube
endoneurial fluid
endoneuritis
endoneurium
endonuclease
    restriction e.
endoperineuritis
endoperoxide
    cyclic e.
endoplasmic reticulum
endopredator
endopsychic
    e. censor
    e. perception
    e. structure
endoreactive
end organ
end-organ degeneration
endorphin
    beta e.
endorphinergic
endorrhachis
endorsement of deviant thoughts and beliefs
endosaccular coil placement
endoscope
    Desormaux e.
    Dyonics rod-lens e.
    Gaab e.
    malleable e.
    percutaneous spinal e.
    Wolf e.
endoscope-assisted craniotomy
endoscope-controlled microsurgery (ECM)
endoscopic
    rectosigmoidal e.
    e. sinus surgery
    e. sphenoidal biopsy
    e. visualization
endoscopy
    heads-up adjunctive e.
    intraventricular e.
    laser-assisted spinal e. (LASE)
endosteal dura
endosymbiosis
endothelial
    e. injury
    e. nitric oxide synthase (eNOS)
endothelin
endothelin-1 platinum-Dacron microcoil
endotheliomatous meningioma

E

endothelium
tight junctioned e.
endothelium-derived relaxing factor (EDRF)
endotracheal tube
endovascular
e. balloon occlusion
e. coil
e. technique
e. therapy
e. treatment
endovasculoscopy
endowment
genetic e.
endplate, end-plate
bony e.
motor e.
e. potential (EPP)
Endrate
end-stage
e.-s. dementia
e.-s. ischemic encephalomalacia
end-tidal nitrogen monitoring
end-to-end anastomosis
endurance level
enduring
e. pattern
e. pattern of inflexibility
Enduron
Enduronyl Forte
endyma
end-zone pain
enelicomorphism
enema
e. addiction
e. drug administration
nutritive e.
enemator
energizer
psychic e.
energy
acoustic e.
active displacement of emotive e.
affect e.
e. affect
e. balance
boundless e.
emotive e.
increased e.
kinetic e.
lack of e.
e. level
libidinal e.
life e.
loss of e.
low e.
mental e.
metabolic e.
e. output
potential e.
psychic e.
e. requirement
sexual e.
e. swing
vital e.

enervate
enervation
enetophobia
enfant terrible
enfeedable
enflurane
enforced treatment
ENG
electronystagmography
engagement level
Engelmann disease
Engel postoperative seizure classification
engineering
biomedical e.
communication e.
genetic e.
human e.
microsocial e.
e. psychologist
e. psychology
social e.
English
African American vernacular E.
E. as a second language (ESL)
Black E.
TOEFL Test of Written E.
engorgement
brain e.
engrafted schizophrenia
engram
function e.
engraphia
engrossment
engulfment
enhancement
contrast e.
coping strategy e. (CSE)
edge e.
flow-related e.
gadolinium e.
MR imaging with gadolinium e.
nodular e.
paramagnetic contrast e.
relaxation rate e.
selective relaxation e.
vertebral end-plate e.
enhancing
e. exophytic tumor
e. ring
enhexymal
enigma
enkephalinergic
enkephalins
Enker brain retractor
enlarged brain
enlargement
cervical e. of spinal cord
job e.
lumbar e. of spinal cord
moyamoya collateral e.
sulcal e.
enlarging bur
enlightenment
e. effect
enlisted man

Enlon Injection
enmeshment
ennui
ENoG
    electroneurogram
enolase
    neuron-specific e. (NSE)
enoltestovis
enomania
enophthalmos
eNOS
    endothelial nitric oxide synthase
enosimania
enosiophobia
Enovil
enoxaparin
enquiry
    Coping Operations Preference E.
    (COPE)
    Life Interpersonal History E.
    (LIPHE)
enriched environment
enrichment
    environmental e.
    job e.
    e. program
entacapone
entactin
entailment
ental origin
Entamoeba
    E. histolytica
    E. histolytica cerebral amebiasis
entangle
entasia, entasis
entatic
entelechy
entendre
    double e.
entendu
    déjà e.
enteral alimentation
enteric
    e. cyst
    e. cytopathic human orphan
    (ECHO)
    e. cytopathic human orphan virus
    e. virus infection
entering root
enteritis
    regional e.
enterococcal disease
enterocolitica
    Yersinia e.
enterogastric reflex
enterogenous cyst
enteropathic arthritis
enteroptosis
enteroviral encephalitis
enterovirus
    e. infection
    e. meningitis
entheomania
enthesitis
enthesopathy

enthlasis
enthrall
enthymeme
entitlement
    e. program
    sense of e.
entity, pl. entities
    controlling external entities
    external e.
entity locative
entoderm
entomomania
entomophobia
entopic vision
entoretina
entorhinal
    e. area
    e. cortex
entorhinal-hippocampal system
entourage
entrainment
entrance
    e. event
    sellar e.
entrapment
    median nerve e.
    e. mononeuropathy
    nerve e.
    e. neuropathy
    PIN e.
    suprascapular nerve e.
    ulnar nerve e.
entrapy
entropion
entropy
entry
    e. behavior
    e. point
    e. zone
    e. zone lesion
enucleation
    eye e.
    tumor e.
enucleator
    Hardy microsurgical e.
    Marino transsphenoidal e.
Enulose
enuresis
    diurnal e.
    functional e.
    e. nocturna
    nocturnal e.
    e. not due to a general medical
      condition
    primary nocturnal e.
    psychogenic e.
enuretic
    e. absence
    e. event
envelope
    cistern of nuclear e.
    nuclear e.
envious behavior
environment
    academically understimulating e.

E

environment *(continued)*
    barrier-free e.
    controlled e.
    dark e.
    disturbed home e.
    domestic e.
    enriched e.
    Evaluation Disposition (toward the) E. (EDEN)
    free-access e.
    e. and heredity (E&H)
    home e.
    Home Observation for Measurement of the E.
    immediate e.
    impoverished early e.
    inadequate school e.
    institutional e.
    invalidating e.
    low sensory e.
    low stimulation e.
    e. modification
    multicultural e.
    natural e.
    nurturing e.
    permissive e.
    physical e.
    planned learning e.
    polluted e.
    respond to e.
    response to e.
    E. Scale
    Scales of Creativity and Learning E. (SCALE)
    secondary e.
    secure e.
    sensory e.
    social e.
    socially disruptive e.
    stimulating e.
    therapeutic e.
    unawareness of e.
    uteroplacental e.
    working e.
environmental
    e. approach
    e. assessment
    e. attribution
    e. awareness
    e. change
    e. cue
    e. deficiency
    e. deprivation
    e. design
    e. determinant
    e. disturbance of sleep
    e. education
    e. effect
    e. enrichment
    e. experimentation
    e. factor
    e. hazard
    interdisciplinary e.
    e. inventory

    E. Language Inventory (ELI)
    e. learning theory
    e. load theory
    e. manipulation
    e. medicine
    e. modification
    e. mold trait
    e. neurology
    e. neurosis
    E. Pre-Language Battery
    e. pressure
    e. problem
    e. psychologist
    e. psychology
    E. Response Inventory (ERI)
    e. stimulation
    e. stimulus
    e. stress
    e. stress theory
    e. support
    e. therapy
environmentally
    e. aesthetic
    e. induced anxiety
environment-centered service
envy
    breast e.
    penis e.
    phallus e.
    vaginal e.
    womb e.
enzygotic
enzyme
    e. activation
    e. autoinduction
    cytochrome P450 metabolic e.
    e. deficiency syndrome
    e. gene
    Hind III e.
    e. induction
    neurotransmitter synthesizing e.
    porphyria synthesizing e.
enzyme-linked immunosorbent assay (ELISA)
E&O
    evaluation and observation
EOG
    electrooculogram
    electrooculography
    electroolfactogram
eonism
eosinopenia
eosinophil adenoma
eosinophilia
eosinophilia-myalgia syndrome (EMS)
eosinophilic
    e. granuloma
    e. granulomatosis
    e. leukocyte
    e. meningitis
    e. meningoencephalitis
    e. myositis
eosophobia

EP
    evoked potential
        EP trending
EPAQ
    Extended Personal Attributes
    Questionnaire
ependyma
    ventricular e.
ependymal
        e. cell
        e. cyst
        e. layer
        e. zone
ependymitis
    granular e.
        e. granularis
ependymoblastoma
ependymocyte
ependymoma
    anaplastic e.
    exophytic e.
    intramedullary e.
        e. intramedullary
    myxopapillary e.
    sacrococcygeal myxopapillary e.
    spinal e.
    subcutaneous sacrococcygeal
        myxopapillary e.
    supratentorial lobar e.
ephapse
ephaptic
        e. conduction
        e. transmission
epharmony
ephebiatrics
ephebic
ephebogenesis
ephebology
ephedra
ephedrine sulfate
ephedrone
ephemeral mania
EPI
    extrapyramidal involvement
    Eysenck Personality Inventory
epicanthus
epicondylectomy
    medial e.
epicortical lesion
epicranium
epicrisis
epicritic
        e. sensation
        e. sensibility
        e. system
epicure
epidemic
        e. catalepsy
        e. cerebrospinal meningitis
        e. encephalitis
        e. hysteria
        e. myalgic encephalomyelitis
        e. myalgic encephalomyelopathy
        e. neuromyasthenia

        e. tetany
        e. vertigo
epidemica
    tetania e.
epidemiologic
epidemiological
        E. Catchment Area Study
        e. data
epidemiologist
epidemiology
    Multi-Institutional Research in
        Alzheimer Genetic E. (MIRAGE)
epidermal
        e. growth factor
        e. growth factor receptor (EGFR)
        e. necrolysis
epidermidis
    Staphylococcus e.
epidermoid
    chiasmal e.
        e. cyst
        e. lipoma
        e. tumor
epidural
        e. abscess
        e. abscess evacuation
        e. angiolipoma
        e. block
        e. cavernous hemangioma
        e. cavity
        e. fat
        e. hematoma
        e. hemorrhage
        e. hemorrhage epidural metastatic
        disease
        e. implant
        e. infection
        e. meningioma
        e. meningitis
        e. needle
        e. peg electrode
        e. pneumatosis
        e. pneumocephalus
        e. space
        e. steroid injection
        e. tumor
        e. tumor evacuation
        e. venography
        e. venous drainage
        e. venous plexus
epidurography
epigastric
        e. aura
        e. reflex
epigenesis
epigenetic
        e. principle
        e. theory
epilation
    permanent e.
    temporary e.
epilemma
epilemmal ending
epilepsia
        e. arithmetica

E

epilepsia *(continued)*
  e. corticalis continua
  e. cursiva
  e. dromica
  e. gravior
  e. major
  e. minor
  e. mitior
  e. mitis
  e. nutans
  e. partialis continua
  e. partialis continua seizure
  e. tarda
  e. vertiginosa
epilepsy
  abdominal e.
  absence e.
  acousticomotor e.
  acquired e.
  activated e.
  adolescent-onset e.
  adult-onset e.
  affective prodrome of e.
  akinetic e.
  alcoholic e.
  alcohol-precipitated e.
  amygdalar e.
  anosognosic e.
  anterior polar-amygdalar e.
  atonic e.
  audiogenic e.
  automatic e.
  autonomic e.
  Baltic myoclonus e.
  benign familial myoclonic e.
  benign focal of childhood e.
  benign rolandic e.
  Bravais-jacksonian e.
  cavernoma-related e.
  centrencephalic e.
  centrotemporal e.
  childhood absence e.
  childhood benign focal e.
  childhood-onset e.
  chronic partial e.
  cingulate e.
  clouded state e.
  communicating e.
  complex partial e.
  complex precipitated e.
  continuous e.
  coordinated e.
  cortical e.
  cryptogenic late-onset e.
  cryptogenic myoclonic e.
  cursive e.
  dacryocystic e.
  Dark Warrior e.
  dementia in e.
  depression in e.
  deterioration e.
  diencephalic e.
  digestive e.
  diurnal e.

early posttraumatic e.
early traumatic e.
eating e.
erotic e.
essential e.
extrapyramidal e.
extrinsic e.
familial progressive myoclonic e.
e. fear
focal e.
frontal lobe e.
gelastic e.
generalized flexion e.
generalized tonic-clonic e.
genuine e.
gestational e.
grand mal e.
hallucinatory e.
haut mal e.
hemiconvulsions, hemiplegia, and e.
  (HHE)
hippocampal e.
hysterical e.
idiopathic generalized e.
e. implant
impulsive petit mal e.
inhibition e.
inhibitory e.
insular e.
intractable e.
Jackson e.
jacksonian e.
juvenile myoclonic e.
Kojewnikoff e.
Koshevnikoff e.
Lafora familial myoclonic e.
larval e.
larvated e.
laryngeal e.
late e.
latent e.
late traumatic e.
limbic e.
local e.
localized e.
Lundborg myoclonic e.
major e.
masked e.
matutinal e.
mesiobasal limbic e.
minor e.
mixed type e.
musicogenic e.
myoclonic astatic e.
myoclonus e.
Nintendo e.
nocturnal e.
opercular e.
orbitofrontal e.
organic e.
e. organic psychosis
parasympathetic e.
partial e.
pattern-induced e.
pattern sensitive e.

perceptive e.
peripheral e.
petit mal e.
photic e.
photogenic e.
photosensitive e.
postanoxic e.
posttraumatic e.
precipitating of e.
primary generalized e.
primary rhinencephalic
  psychomotor e.
procursive e.
psychic e.
psychomotor e.
psychopathology of e.
psychosensory e.
quiritarian e.
reactive e.
reading e.
reflex inhibition of e.
regional e.
retropulsive e.
rolandic e.
secondary generalized e.
seizure e.
senile e.
sensorial e.
sensory-induced e.
sensory precipitated e.
serial e.
short stare e.
situation-related e.
sleep e.
sleep-related e.
somatomotor e.
somatosensory e.
somnambulic e.
startle e.
status e.
supplementary motor e.
e. surgery
surgical e.
sympathetic e.
symptomatic e.
tardy e.
television-induced e.
temporal lobe e. (TLE)
temporolimbic e.
tetanoid e.
thalamic e.
tonic e.
tornado e.
traumatic e.
true e.
twilight e.
uncinate e.
Unverricht-Lundborg myoclonus e.
Unverricht myoclonus e.
vasomotor e.
vasovagal e.
vertiginous e.
vestibulogenic e.
visceral e.
visual e.

epileptic
  e. absence
  e. aura
  e. automatism
  e. automatism syndrome
  e. cephalea
  e. character
  e. confusional state (ECS)
  e. convulsion
  e. cry
  e. dementia
  e. deterioration
  e. diathesis
  e. disorder
  e. drop attack
  e. equivalent
  e. focus
  e. fugue
  e. furor
  e. idiocy
  e. mania
  e. neuron
  e. neuronal aggregate
  e. personality
  e. prodrome
  e. psychopathic constitution
  e. seizure
  e. stupor
  e. swindler
  e. transient organic psychosis
  e. variant
  e. vertigo
epileptica
  absentia e.
  e. absentia
epilepticum
  delirium e.
epilepticus
  convulsive status e.
  focal status e.
  furor e.
  globus e.
  ictus e.
  nonconvulsive status e.
  refractory status e. (RSE)
  status e.
epileptiform
  e. activity
  e. burst discharge
  e. convulsion
  e. discharge
  e. neuralgia
  e. seizure
epileptogenesis
epileptogenic, epileptogenous
  e. burst
  e. encephalopathy
  e. foci
  e. focus
  e. stimulation
  e. stimulus
  e. temporal lesion
  e. zone
epileptogenicity

E

epileptoid
    e. amaurosis
    orthostatic e.
    e. personality
    e. personality disorder
epileptology
epileptosis
epiloia
epinephrine
    lidocaine and e.
    Xylocaine with e.
epinephrine-anesthetic mixture
epineural
epineurectomy
epineurial neurorrhaphy
epineurium
epineurolysis
epinosic gain
epinosis
epiphenomenalism
epiphenomenon
epiphora
epiphyseal
epiphysiopathy
epiphysis, pl. **epiphyses**
    e. cerebri
epipial
episcleral vascular dilation
episcleritis
episode
    absence e.
    acute schizophrenic e.
    amnestic e.
    antidepressant treatment-induced
      manic e.
    aphonic e.
    bipolar I disorder, single manic e.
    cataplexy e.
    confusional e.
    current e.
    daytime sleep e.
    depersonalization e.
    depressed mood e.
    depressive e.
    dissociative e.
    florid e.
    gray-out e.
    hypomanic e.
    hypomanic mood e.
    intoxication e.
    length of e.
    major depressive e. (MDE)
    major depressive disorder, single e.
    manic e.
    manic-like e.
    manic mood e.
    micropsychotic e.
    mitochondrial encephalomyopathy
      with lactic acidosis and
      strokelike e. (MELAS)
    mixed mood e.
    mood e.
    neurotic state with
      depersonalization e.
    nocturnal sleep e.

    prodromal e.
    prolonged nocturnal sleep e.
    psychoepileptic e.
    psycholeptic e.
    psychotic schizophrenic e.
    recurrent e.
    Schedule for Affective Disorders
      and Schizophrenia for School-Age
      Children-Present E. (K-SADS-P)
    schizoaffective e.
    schizophrenic e.
    single e.
    sleep-onset e.
    sleep terror e.
    substance-induced manic e.
    unintentional daytime sleep e.
    uninterrupted e.
    unspecified mood e.
    untreated e.
    e. version
episodic
    e. amnesia
    e. apnea
    e. ataxia type 2 (EA-2)
    e. bilateral loss of muscle tone
    e. changes of consciousness
    e. confusion
    e. course
    e. disorder
    e. dyscontrol
    e. dyscontrol duress
    e. dyscontrol syndrome
    e. memory
    e. paroxysmal hemicrania
    e. tension-type headache (ETTH)
    e. vertigo
epispinal
epistaxis
epistemic
epistemology
    genetic e.
epistemophilia
epithalamus
epithelial
    e. choroid layer
    e. hemangioendothelioma (EH)
    e. lamina
    e. membrane antigen tumor marker
epithelioid
    e. hemangioendothelioma (EH)
    e. histiocyte
epithelioma
epitheliopathy
    multifocal placoid pigment e.
    placoid pigment e.
    retinal pigment e.
epithelioserosa
    zona e.
epithelium
    olfactory e.
    retinal pigment e.
epithet
    national e.
Epitol
epitonic

epitonos
epitope
    surface e.
Epivir
epochal amnesia
epochs
    wakefulness e.
EPP
    endplate potential
EPPS
    Edwards Personal Preference Schedule
EPQ
    Eysenck Personality Questionnaire
EPR
    evoked potential response
eprouve
    déjà e.
EPS
    exhaustion syndrome
    extrapyramidal symptom
    extrapyramidal syndrome
    extrapyramidal system
EPSDT
    early and periodic screening, diagnosis,
    and treatment
epsilon
    e. alcoholism
    e. movement
    e. opiate receptor
epsilon-aminocaproic acid
EPSP
    excitatory postsynaptic potential
Epstein
    E. curette
    E. neurological hammer
    E. staging system
    E. symptom
Epstein-Barr
    E.-B. syndrome
    E.-B. virus (EBV)
EPT
    Eidetic Parents Test
ePTFE
    expanded polytetrafluoroethylene
        ePTFE ventricular shunt catheter
EQ
    educational quotient
    education quotient
equable
Equagesic
equal
    e. employment opportunity
    e. potential
equal-and-unequal-cases method
equal-appearing-intervals method
equal-interval scale
equality
    law of e.
    e. law
    point of subjective e. (PSE)
    e. stage
    subjective e.
equalization of excitation
Equanil
equanimity

equation
    Bloch e.
    differential e.
    Larmor e.
    personal e.
    Poiseuille e.
    Solomon-Bloembergen e.
equatorial phase
equicaloric
equidominant
Equilet
equilibration
    hanging-drop e.
equilibratory
    e. ataxia
    e. sense
equilibrist
equilibrium
    dynamic e.
    genetic e.
    Hardy-Weinberg e.
    homeostatic e.
    narcissistic e.
    nutritive e.
    sense of e.
equina
    cauda e.
equine
    e. encephalitis
    e. gait
equinophobia
Equinox EEG neuromonitoring system
equipment
    adaptive e.
    cannabis e.
    clay-modeling e.
    crack e.
    decompression e.
    e. design
    drug e.
    drug-injecting e.
    insertion e.
    stainless steel e.
    Vitallium e.
equiponderant
equipotential
equipotentiality law
equitable
equity
    e. stage
    e. theory
equivalence
    e. coefficient
    complex e.
equivalent
    age e. (AEq)
    arithmetic grade e.
    clinical e.
    convulsive e.
    e. criteria
    e. criterion
    delusional e.
    depressive e.
    e. diagnosis
    e. dosage

E

equivalent *(continued)*
    e. dose (ED)
    epileptic e.
    e. form
    e. form reliability
    grade e.
    grammatical e.
    e. group
    e. intoxication criterion
    masturbation e.
    e. method
    pharmaceutical e.
    psychic e.
    reading grade e.
    spelling grade e.
    e. symptom
    e. symptomatic presentation
    e. withdrawal criterion
equivocate
ER
    emergency room
    evoked response
era
    juvenile e.
    neo-myerian e.
eradicate
ERB
    ethnic relational behavior
Erb
    E. atrophy
    E. disease
    E. injury
    E. muscular dystrophy
    E. palsy
    E. point
    E. point stimulation on
      electromyogram
    E. sign
    E. spastic paraplegia
    E. spinal paralysis
Erb-Charcot disease
Erb-Duchenne-Klumpke
    E.-D.-K. injury
    E.-D.-K. injury to brachial plexus
Erb-Duchenne syndrome
Erb-Westphal sign
Ercaf
ERD
    event-related desynchronization
Erdheim tumor
erectile
    e. arousal disorder
    e. disorder due to combined
      factors
    e. disorder due to psychological
      factors
    e. dysfunction
    e. impotence
erection
    psychogenic painful e.
    sleeping e.
erective impotence

erector
    e. clitoridis
    e. penis
erector-spinal reflex
eremiomania
eremiophobia
eremite
eremophilia
eremophobia
erethism
    e. mercurialis
    sexual e.
erethismic, erethistic, erethitic
    e. idiocy
    e. idiot
    e. shock
erethisophrenia
ereuthophobia (*var. of* erythrophobia)
ERG
    electroretinogram
    ERG theory
erg
ergasia
ergasiatry
ergasiology
ergasiomania
ergasiophobia
ergasthenia
ergastic
ergic trait
ergocalciferol
ergodialeipsis
ergogenic
ergograph
ergoloid mesylate
ergomania
Ergomar
ergometer
ergonomic
ergonovine
ergophobia
Ergostat
ergot
    e. alkaloid
    e. derivative
    e. mesylate
ergotamine
    Medihaler e.
    e. tartrate
    e. tartrate and caffeine
ergotherapy
ergotica
    tabes e.
ergotism
ergotropic
    e. process
    e. system
Erhard Seminar Training (EST, est)
Erhardt
    E. Developmental Prehension
      Assessment (EDPA)
    E. Developmental Vision
      Assessment (EDVA)

ERI
 Employee Reliability Inventory
 Environmental Response Inventory
Erichsen disease
Erickson
 E. developmental model
 E. theory of latency
erigendi
 impotentia e.
Erikson eight stages of man
ERISA
 Employee Retirement Income Security
  Act
Erispan
eristic
ermitophobia
erogeneity
erogenous zone
eromania
eros
erosion
 dental e.
 dorsum sella e.
 vascular e.
erosive sphenoid mucocele
erotic
 e. arousal
 e. behavior
 e. character
 e. delusion
 e. dream
 e. drive
 e. epilepsy
 e. fantasy
 e. instinct
 e. obsession
 organ e.
 e. paranoia
 e. pyromania
 e. seizure
 e. stimulus
 e. transference
 e. type
 e. zoophilism
erotica
erotic-arousal pattern
eroticism (*var. of* erotism)
eroticize
eroticized
 e. behavior
 e. fantasy
eroticomania
eroticophobia
erotism, eroticism
 anal e.
 ego e.
 genital e.
 lip e.
 muscle e.
 olfactory e.
 oral e.
 organ e.
 paranoid e.
 skin e.

 temperature e.
 urethral e.
erotization
erotized
 e. anxiety
 e. hanging
erotocrat
erotogenesis
erotogenic
 e. masochism
 e. zone
erotographomania
erotolalia
erotology
erotomania
 Clerambault e.
erotomanic
 e. delusion
 e. delusional state
 E. Type
erotopathy
erotophobia
erotopsychic
erotosexual
ERP
 event-related potential
errant thought
erratic
 e. behavior
 e. mood
 e. parenting
 e. speech rhythm
 e. thinking
erroneous
 e. belief
 e. impression
error
 accidental e.
 alpha e.
 e. analysis
 anomic e.
 anticipatory e.
 aphasic e.
 attribution e.
 e. attribution
 best registration e.
 beta e.
 chance e.
 experimental e.
 frequency e.
 fundamental attribution e.
 genetic e.
 line bisection e. (LBE)
 e. of measurement
 motivated e.
 paraphasic e.
 perseverative e.
 probable e. (PE)
 registration e.
 root mean square e.
 standard e. (SE)
 subjective e.
 target localization e.
 time e.
 trial and e.

E

error *(continued)*
 type I e.
 type II e.
 e. variance
 vicarious trial and e. (VTE)
ERT
 estrogen replacement therapy
eructation
erythema
 e. chronicum migrans (ECM)
 e. multiforme
 e. multiforme-like
erythematosus
 lupus e. (LE)
 neuropsychiatric systemic lupus e. (NP-SLE)
 systemic lupus e. (SLE)
erythermalgia
erythralgia
erythredema polyneuritis
erythrism
erythroblastosis fetalis
erythrocyte
 e. disorder
 e. sedimentation rate (ESR)
erythrocytosis
erythroderma
erythromania
erythromelalgia
erythromycin
erythrophobia, ereuthophobia
erythroprosopalgia
Erythroxylum coca
ES
 ego strength
 elopement status
 Vicodin ES
ESA
 Early School Assessment
ESB
 Effective School Battery
 electric stimulation of the brain
escalative process
escapade
 sexual e.
escape
 e. behavior
 e. conditioning
 e. drinking
 e. from the ego
 e. from freedom
 e. from reality
 e. into illness
 e. learning
 e. mechanism
 e. phenomenon
 e. reaction
 e. training
escapism
escapology
eschar
eschatology
Escherichia coli
Escherich sign

eschrolalia
Escobar
 E. disease
 E. syndrome
ESCS
 Early Social Communication Scale
escutcheon
ESEP
 extreme somatosensory evoked potential
Esgic Plus
Eshmun complex
ESI
 Ego State Inventory
Esidrix
Eskalith-CR
ESL
 English as a second language
esmolol
ESN
 educationally subnormal
esodeviation
esodic nerve
esoethmoiditis
esophageal
 e. achalasia
 e. airway
 e. neurosis
 e. perforation
 e. voice
esophagosalivary reflex
esophagus psychogenic disorder
esophoria
esoteric
esotropia
ESP
 Early Speech Perception Test
 extrasensory perception
espanto
espiritismo
Espocan combined spinal/epidural needle
ESPQ
 Early School Personality Questionnaire
esprit de corps conditioning
ESR
 erythrocyte sedimentation rate
essay test
essential
 e. alcoholism
 e. amino acid
 e. anosmia
 e. blepharospasm
 e. convulsion
 e. epilepsy
 e. feature
 e. headache
 e. hypertension
 e. hypotonia
 e. seizure
 e. thrombocytosis
 e. tremor (ET)
 e. vertigo
Essex-Lopresti axial fixation
ESSF
 external spinal skeletal fixator
Essick cell band

EST, est
electric shock therapy
electric shock treatment
electroshock therapy
electroshock treatment
Erhard Seminar Training
established delusion
estate
A Sales Potential Inventory for Real E. (ASPIRE)
estazolam
esteem-enhancing
esteem need
esterase
acetylcholine e.
Esterom
esthematology
esthesia
esthesic
esthesiodic system
esthesiogenesis
esthesiogenic
esthesiography
esthesiology
esthesiomania
esthesiometer
Semmes-Weinstein e.
Weber e.
esthesiometry
esthesioneuroblastoma
olfactory e.
esthesioneurocytoma
esthesioneurosis
esthesionosus
esthesiophysiology
esthesioscopy
esthesodic
esthetic (*var. of* aesthetic)
estimated
e. cerebrovascular resistance (eCVR)
e. learning potential (ELP)
e. length of stay
estimation
Dodd Test of Time E.
estradiol
ethinyl e.
estrangement
feelings of e.
inner e.
Estridge biopsy needle
estrin
estriol
estrogen replacement therapy (ERT)
estromania
estrone
estrous
e. behavior
e. cycle
estrual
estrus
estuffa
esurience
esurient

ET
essential tremor
alpha ET
état
e. criblé
e. lacunaire
etazolate hydrochloride
eternal suckling
eternity fear
eternus
puer e.
eterobarb
ethacrynic acid
ethambutol
ethamivan
ethanol
e. abuse
e. dependence
e. intoxication
e. treatment
e. withdrawal
ethanolism
ethaverine hydrochloride
ethchlorvynol
ether
e. base
e. convulsion
cyclic e.
e. dependence
e. drunkenness
e. effect
ethyl e.
hexafluorodiethyl e.
e. screen
e. spirit
etherize
etheromania
ethic
case e.
work e.
ethical
e. approach
e. aspects of assaultive client care
e. aspects of dementia
e. behavior
e. conflict
e. highbrow
e. imperative
e. risk hypothesis
e. self
Ethicon Ligaclip
ethics
achievement e.
code of e.
medical e.
normative e.
professional e.
situational e.
ethinamate
ethinyl estradiol
Ethiodane
ethiodized oil
Ethiodol

E

ethmoidal
e. meningoencephalocele
e. osteotomy
ethmoidectomy
ethmoid sinus
ethnic
e. background
e. factor
e. prejudice
e. reference group
e. relational behavior (ERB)
ethnicity
ethnocentrism scale
ethnocultural
ethnographic approach
ethnography
ethnology
ethnomethodology
ethnopsychiatry
ethnopsychology
ethnopsychopharmacology
ethnoscience
ethnosemantic
ethogram
ethoheptazine citrate
ethological
e. models of personal space
e. study
ethology
ethomoxane hydrochloride
ethopharmacology
ethopropazine hydrochloride
ethos
ethosuximide
ethotoin
ethybenztropine
ethyl
e. alcohol
e. alcohol addiction
e. alcohol peripheral neuropathy
e. carbinol
e. chloride
e. chloride and
dichlorotetrafluoroethane
e. ether
e. loflazepate
e. nitrite
e. salicylate
ethylamine
ethylene
e. glycol poisoning
e. vinyl alcohol copolymer liquid
ethylenediaminetetraacetic acid (EDTA)
ethyliodophenylundecyl
ethylism
ethyltryptamine
alpha e.
etidocaine
etidronate
disodium e.
e. disodium
technetium e.
etifoxine
etiolate

etiological
e. agent
e. association
e. factor
e. neurological condition
e. relationship
e. validity
etiology, pl. etiologies
delirium due to multiple etiologies
dementia due to multiple etiologies
Four-Factor Theory of E.
general medical e.
medical e.
presumed e.
substance-induced e.
etiopathogenesis
etiopathogenic
etiopathology
etiotropic
etizolam
etodolac
etodroxizine
ETOH, EtOH
etomidate injection
Etomidate-Lipuro
etomidate-propylene glycol infusion
etoperidone
etoposide (ETP)
etoxadrol hydrochloride
ETP
etoposide
Etrafon
E.-A
E.-Forte
ETS
Educational Testing Service
electrical transcranial stimulation
electrosleep therapy
ETTH
episodic tension-type headache
etymology
EU
expected utility
eubiotics
eucaine
EUCD
emotionally unstable character disorder
euchromatopsy
eucodal
eucrasia
eudemonia
affective e.
euergasia
euesthesia
eugenicist
eugenics
negative e.
positive e.
eugenic sterilization law
eugnathia
eugnosia
euhemerism
eukaryotic messenger
eukinesia
eukinetic

Eulenburg disease
eulogize
eumetria
eumorphic
eunoia
eunuch
eunuchism
    pituitary e.
eunuchoidism
    female e.
eunuchoid voice
euosmia
eupeptic
euphenics
euphonia
euphonic
euphoretic
euphoria
    event-related e.
    false e.
    indifferent e.
    postcoital e.
euphoric
    e. affect
    e. apathy
    e. mood
    e. speech
euphorigenic effect
euphorohallucinogen
eupnea
eupraxia
Eurasian
eurotophobia
eurycephalic, eurycephalous
eurymorph
euryplastic
eurythmic
eurythmy
eurytopic
eusitia
eusthenia
eusthenic
eustress
eutectic mixture of local anesthetics
    (EMLA)
eutelegenesis
euthanasia
    active e.
    passive e.
    voluntary e.
euthenic
eutherapeutics
euthymia
euthymic
    e. mood
    e. state
euthyroid
eutonia sclerotica
eutonic
Eutron
eutrophia
eutropic
eutychian
evacuant

evacuation
    CT-guided stereotactic e.
    epidural abscess e.
    epidural tumor e.
    hematoma e.
    transsphenoidal e.
evacuator
evagination
Evalose
evaluability
evaluability-assessment data
evaluating
    E. Educational Programs for
      Intellectually Gifted Students
    E. Movement and Posture
      Disorganization in Dyspraxic
      Children
    E. the Participant's Employability
      Skills
evaluation
    e. of adolescent
    Bay Area Functional
      Performance E., Second Edition
    California Marriage Readiness E.
      (CMRE)
    career e.
    Checklist for Child Abuse E.
      (CCAE)
    clinical e.
    condescending e.
    e. contract
    contract e.
    court-mandated e.
    e. of criterion
    criterion e.
    dementia e.
    Denver Articulation Screening E.
      (DASE)
    E. Disposition (toward the)
      Environment (EDEN)
    e. dissemination
    employee e.
    event-related potentials e.
    false e.
    family e.
    Fuld Object-Memory E.
    Grassi Basic Cognitive E. (GBCE)
    home e.
    in-house e.
    e. interview
    job e.
    Kenny Self-Care E.
    Leadership Ability E.
    Longitudinal Interval Follow-up E.
    Marital Attitudes E. (MATE)
    medical care e. (MCE)
    mental capacity e.
    Mother-Child Relationship E.
      (MCRE)
    multiaxial e.
    myasthenia gravis e.
    negative e.
    neurologic e.
    neurological e.
    Neurometer CPT/C for nerve e.

E

evaluation *(continued)*
    neuropsychologic e.
    Nurses' Observation Scale for
      Inpatient E. (NOSIE)
    e. and observation (E&O)
    operational e.
    pedicle e.
    Phobic Attitude E.
    preoperative e.
    psychiatric e.
    psychoeducational e.
    psychological e.
    psychometric e.
    Psychosocial Factor E.
    rehabilitation e.
    e. research
    Rule Eleven Psych E.
    social e.
    symptoms e.
    testing and e. (T&E)
    e. of training
    transactional e.
    e. utilization
    vocational e.
evaluative
    e. rating
    e. reasoning
evaluator bias
evaluator/clinician
evaluee/patient
evanescent
Evans
    E. index
    E. ratio
evasion
evasive
    e. behavior
    e. tendency
evasiveness
even-echo rephasing
evening
    e. drinker
    e. drinking
    e. headache
event
    amnesia for sleep-terror e.
    antecedent e.
    cytoskeletal-membrane e.
    entrance e.
    enuretic e.
    exit e.
    external e.
    independent e.
    life e.
    milestone e.
    negative life e.
    neuroleptic-related e.
    past e.
    positive e.
    potential positive e.
    precipitating e.
    psychosocial e.
    recent life e. (RLE)
    reexperienced traumatic e.

    sequence of e.'s
    sleep-terror e.
    Systematic Assessment for
      Treatment of Emergent E.'s
      (SAFTEE)
    totality of possible e.'s
    transient focal neurologic e.
      (TFNE)
    traumatic e.
    triggering e.
event-related
    e.-r. desynchronization (ERD)
    e.-r. distress
    e.-r. euphoria
    e.-r. potential (ERP)
    e.-r. potentials evaluation
Evers diet for multiple sclerosis
Evershears surgical instrument
eversion
    cingulate gyrus e.
    e. theory of aging
every (q)
    e. day
    e. night
    e. other day
everyday
    e. memory questionnaire
    E. Worries Scale
evidence
    admissible e.
    e. of amnesia
    amnesia e.
    e. of blocking
    blocking e.
    circumstantial e.
    compelling e.
    e. of dissociation disorder
    empirical e.
    incontrovertible e.
    indirect e.
    e. of interruption
    e. of intrusion of idiosyncratic
    e. of intrusion of idiosyncratic
      material
    e. of intrusion of private material
    rules of e.
evidence-based process
evil
    e. eye
    e. influence
eviration
evisceroneurotomy
EVM grading of Glasgow Coma Scale
evoked
    e. cortical response (ECR)
    e. potential (EP)
    e. potential response (EPR)
    e. potential trending
    e. response (ER)
    e. somatosensory response
evolution
    e. of brain
    emergent e.
    mental e.

saltatory e.
e. theory
evolutionary intervention
evolving hematoma
evulsion
Ewald-Hudson forceps
EWI
Experiential World Inventory
Ewing
E. & Rooss four-question alcohol
screening (CAGE)
E. sarcoma
E.X.
Extra Strength Dynafed E.X.
ex
e. post facto
e. post facto research
exacerbated symptoms
exacerbation
acute e.
pain e.
psychotic e.
schizophrenic e.
ex-addict
exaggerated
e. achievement
e. belief
e. communication in schizophrenia
e. defect
e. expression
e. feeling
e. inferential thinking in
schizophrenia
e. negative quality
e. perception
e. positive quality
e. startle response
exaggeration
e. of inferential behavioral
monitoring
e. of language and communication
e. in wit
exaltation
reactive e.
exalted paranoia
exam
Parkland Rapid E. (PRE)
Scholastic Level E. (SLE)
examination
Adult Basic Learning E. (ABLE)
Advanced Placement E. (APE)
alpha e.
e. anxiety
Boston Diagnostic Aphasia E.
(BDAE)
Brief Aphasia Screening E.
(BASE)
Brief Neuropsychological Mental
Status E. (BNMSE)
Cambridge Mental Disorders in
Elderly E. (CAMDEX)
College Basic Academic
Subjects E.
College-Level Examination Program
General E. (CLEP)

competency-based e.
Denver Articulation Screening E.
e. dream
Eating Disorder E.
flexible nasopharyngeal e.
followup e.
Folstein Mini-Mental Status E.
Graduate Record E. (GRE)
Hertel exophthalmometry e.
Lateral Dominance E. (LDE)
longitudinal mental status e.
mental status e. (MSE)
Mini-Mental State E. (MMSE)
Multilingual Aphasia E. (MAE)
Neurobehavioral Cognitive Status E.
neurological e.
Neuropsychological Screening E.
Neuropsychological Status E.
objective e.
ocular motility e.
Pediatric Early Elementary E.
peripheral e.
Personality Disorder E.
e. phobia
physical e. (PE)
Present State E. (PSE)
Professional and Administrative
Career E. (PACE)
psychiatric e.
psychological e.
Reitan-Klove Lateral Dominance E.
Reitan-Klove Sensory Perceptual E.
screening e.
Sensory Perceptual E. (SPE)
sexological e.
status e.
e. stupor
tangent screen e.
examiner
medical e.
National Board of Medical E.'s
trial e.
Examining for Aphasia Test
exanthema, exanthem
pruritic e.
exasperate
Excedrin
E. IB
E. PM
Excedrin, Extra Strength
Excegran
exceptional
e. child
e. stress
Excerpta Medica
excess
dietary e.
excessive
e. admiration
e. concern for defect
e. daytime sleepiness (EDS)
e. diffuse low and medium wave
beta activity
e. emotionality
e. fatigability

E

excessive *(continued)*
    e. motor activity
    e. need
    e. need for care
    e. pride
    e. rigidity
    e. social anxiety
    e. somnolence
    e. stress
    e. volubility
    e. worry
excessively
    e. impressionistic speech
    e. loud speech
    e. soft speech
    e. upset
exchange
    angry word e.
    blood gas e.
    blood-tissue e.
    fetal-maternal e.
    e. force
excipient
excision
    C2-C3 cervical disk e.
    cervical disk e.
    extratemporal e.
    retropulsed bone e.
excitability
    emotional e.
    e. of neuron
    e. test
excitable
    e. area
    e. behavior
excitation
    catatonic e.
    e. and conduction
    equalization of e.
    e. gradient
    number of e.'s (NEX)
    psychogenic e.
    e. psychotic reaction
    reactive e.
    selective e.
    subliminal e.
excitation-contraction
excitative psychosis
excitative-type nonorganic psychosis
excitatory
    e. agent
    e. amino acid (EAA)
    e. amino acid receptor
    e. field
    e. impulse
    e. irradiation
    e. lesion
    e. neurotransmitter
    e. postsynaptic potential (EPSP)
    e. pyramidal neuron
    e. synapse
excitatory-inhibitory process
excited
    e. catatonia

    e. catatonic schizophrenia
    e. schizoaffective schizophrenia
    e. state
excitement
    anniversary e.
    catatonic e.
    inhibited sexual e. (ISE)
    manic e.
    mental e.
    e. phase
    e. phase of sexual response cycle
    psychomotor e.
    reactive e.
    reactive mental e.
    schizophrenic e.
    sexual e.
excitement-seeking tendency
excitomotor cortex
excitomuscular
excitonutrient
excitoreflex nerve
excitor nerve
excitotoxicity
    glutamate e.
    glutamatergic e.
excitotoxic neurotransmitter antagonist
excitotoxins
exclamation theory
exclusion
    e. criteria
    e. criterion
    diagnosis by e.
exclusive
    mutually e.
excogitate
excoriation
    neurotic e.
    psychogenic e.
excrement fear
excrescence
excretory perversion
excursive
excyclotorsion
executant ego function
executive
    e. aphasia
    e. aspect
    e. control
    e. dysfunction
    e. ego function
    e. functioning
    e. functioning disturbance
    e. language
    e. (or frontal) deficit transient global amnesia
    e. organ
    E. Profile Survey
    e. speech
    e. stress
exegesis
    analytic e.
Exelon
exencephalia
exencephalic
exencephalocele

exencephalous
exencephaly
exenteration
exercise
    Cawthorne-Cooksey vestibular e.
    compulsive e.
    Death Personification E. (DPE)
    holding e.
    intergroup e.
    journaling e.
    law of e.
    e. law
    mirror e.
    modeling e.
    patterning e.
    PNF e.
    therapeutic e.
    e. therapy
    e. treatment
exerciser
    e. container
    continuous anatomical passive e.
    (CAPE)
exertional headache
exhaustion
    combat e.
    e. death
    e. delirium
    heat e.
    Maastricht Interview for Vital E.
    e. management
    mental e.
    nervous e.
    e. paralysis
    postactivation e.
    e. postactivation
    e. psychosis
    e. senile dementia
    stage of e.
    e. stage
    e. state
    e. syndrome (EPS)
exhaustive
    e. psychosis
    e. stupor
exhibition
    e. dream
    sexual e.
    e. wit
exhibitionism
    e. paraphilia
    shock e.
exhibitionistic behavior
exhibitionist need
exifone
existence need
existence, relatedness, and growth
  theory
existential
    e. analysis
    e. anguish
    e. anxiety
    e. crisis
    e. ego function
    e. living

    e. neurosis
    e. phenomenology
    e. psychiatry
    e. psychoanalysis
    e. psychology
    e. psychotherapy
    e. school
    e. vacuum
existential-humanistic therapy
exit
    e. event
    e. interview
exiting segment
Ex-Lax
Exner
    E. plexus
    E. Scoring System
exocathection
exocentric construction
exocytosis
exodic nerve
exogamy
exogenesis
exogenetic
exogenous
    e. chemical
    e. depression
    e. factor
    e. fiber
    e. obesity
    e. psychosis
    e. reaction
    e. smile
    e. stimulation
    e. stress
    e. Zeitgeber
exonerative moral reasoning
exon splicing
exophoria
exophthalmometer
    Hertel e.
exophthalmos
exophytic
    e. ependymoma
    e. joint disease
exopsychic
exorcism
exosomatic method
Exo-Static collar
exostosis
exotic
    e. bias
    e. psychosis
exoticism
exotoxin
    Pseudomonas e.
exotropia
    paralytic pontine e.
expanded
    e. consciousness
    e. polytetrafluoroethylene (ePTFE)
expansion
    consciousness e.
    field e.
    perceptual e.

E

expansion *(continued)*
    trinucleotide repeat e.
    volume e.
expansiva
    paraphrenia e.
expansive
    e. delusion
    e. idea
    e. mood
    e. solution
expansiveness
    grandiose e.
expectancy
    e. chart
    life e.
    lifetime e.
    quality-adjusted life e. (QALE)
    e. theory
expectant analysis
expectation
    anxious e.
    apprehension e.
    catastrophic e.
    death e.
    e. of death
    internal world of e.
    e. of life
    e. neurosis
expected
    e. death
    e. frequency
    e. level of achievement
    e. utility (EU)
    e. weight gain
expenditure
    caloric e.
    resting energy e.
experience
    accidental e.
    Adolescent-Coping Orientation for
      Problem E.'s
    affective e.
    atypical delusional e.
    bad PCP e.
    brief delusional e.
    clinical e.
    collective e.
    common e.
    corrective emotional e.
    cultural e.
    culturally sanctioned e.
    cutaneous e.
    depersonalization e.
    depressive e.
    Developmental Assessment of
      Life E.'s (DALE)
    dissociative episode e.
    disturbing e.
    dream e.
    emotional e.
    external world e.
    false sensory e.
    fantasized sexual e.
    group e.

    human therapeutic e.
    immediate e.
    inner e.
    job-sample e.
    Learning Inventory of
      Kindergarten E.'s (LIKE)
    life e.
    loss e.
    mystical e.
    narcolepsy e.
    openness to e.
    out-of-body e. (OBE)
    outside the range of normal
      human e.
    paradigmatic stress from life e.
    past e.
    peak e.
    physical e.
    pleasure e.
    Profile of Out-of-Body E.'s
      (POBE)
    psychic e.
    Psychosocial Assessment of
      Childhood E.'s (PACE)
    repeated painful e.
    e.'s scale
    Schedule of Recent E. (SRE)
    self e.
    sensory e.
    sexual e.
    social phobia e.
    spiritual possession e.
    stimulating e.
    stress from life e. (SFLE)
    stressful life e.
    subjective e.
    success e.
    syntaxic mode of e.
    terrifying e.
    tests of basic e. (TOBE)
    transient hallucinatory e.
    traumatic e.
    troubling e.
experienced
    Coping Orientations to Problems E.
      (COPE)
experiential
    e. group
    e. psychotherapy
    e. therapy
Experiential World Inventory (EWI)
experiment
    analog e.
    delayed reaction e.
    factorial e.
    field e.
experimental
    e. allergic encephalitis (EAE)
    e. allergic encephalomyelitis (EAE)
    e. analysis of behavior
    e. bias
    e. control
    e. design
    e. disorder
    e. drug

e. error
e. game
e. group
e. hypothesis
e. marriage
e. medication
e. medicine
e. method
e. neurasthenia
e. neurosis
e. psychiatry
e. psychology
e. realism
e. series
e. therapy
e. variable
experimentation
environmental e.
pharmacological e.
role e.
experimenter
e. bias
e. effect
experimenter-expectancy effect
expert
e. system
e. testimony
e. witness
expertise
expiatory
e. punishment
e. self-punishment
expiratory center
explanation
reassuring e.
explicit
e. behavior
e. memory
e. process
e. role
e. type
exploitation
interpersonal e.
exploitative
e. character
e. orientation
e. personality
exploitative-manipulative behavior
exploiter
professional e.
exploiting type
exploration
brachial plexus e.
diversive e.
e. drive
Individual Career E. (ICE)
stereotactic biopsy e.
transcranial orbital e.
exploratory
e. behavior
e. drive
e. incision
e. insight-oriented

e. insight-oriented psychotherapy (EIO)
e. therapy
explorer
Occupational Interests E. (OIE)
explosion readiness
explosive
e. aggressive behavior
e. disorder
e. disturbance
e. outburst
e. personality
e. rage
e. speech
explosivity
emotional e.
exposition attitude
exposure
anterior surgical e.
bony e.
combat stress e.
common precipitant e.
controlled e.
e. to cue
cue e.
e. deafness
exteroceptive e.
extradural e.
graded e.
half-and-half e.
e. hierarchy
imaginal e.
indecent e.
interoceptive e.
e. keratopathy
middle fossa e.
midline e.
occupational e.
e. of person
e. and response prevention
self-directed e.
surgical e.
thoracolumbar junction surgical e.
thoracolumbar spine anterior e.
toxic e.
toxin e.
e. to toxins
e. to trigger
upper cervical spine anterior e.
vertebral e.
e. in vivo
in vivo situational e.
exposure-based cognitive behavior therapy
expressed
e. emotion (EE)
e. motivation
e. skull fracture
expressible
expression
abstract e.
affective e.
discordant facial e.
disorder of written e.
emotional e.

E

expression *(continued)*
exaggerated e.
facial e.
lines of e.
e. method
neurofilament e.
neurotrophic factor e.
nontoxic gene e.
nonverbal e.
parenthetical e.
passivity in anger e.
phenotypic e.
restricted range of emotional e.
RNA e.
sexual e.
shallow e.
staring facial e.
unassertive e.
verbal e.
e. with feeling
written e.
expressionism factor
expressive
e. amimia
e. amusia
e. aphasia
e. delusion
e. dysphasia
e. function
e. language
e. language deficit
e. language development
e. language development disorder
e. language quotient
e. language skill
e. movement
E. One Word Picture Vocabulary Test
E. One-Word Picture Vocabulary Test, Upper Extension
e. pattern
e. therapy
e. writing development disorder
expressive-receptive aphasia
Extencaps
Micro-K 10 E.
extended
e. ADL
e. care
e. family
e. family therapy (EFT)
e. jargon paraphasia
E. Merrill-Palmer Scale
E. Personal Attributes Questionnaire (EPAQ)
e. phenytoin sodium capsules, USP
e. play
e. sector ultrasonic probe
e. sick leave
e. subfrontal approach
extended-care
e.-c. facility
e.-c. review
extended-stay review

extension
brachioradialis transfer for wrist e.
cranial e.
deep brain e.
extrameatal tumor e.
e. injury
e. injury posterior atlantoaxial arthrodesis
intrasellar e.
neurite e.
Orascoptic loupe e.
paraplegia in e.
radiolucent operating room table e.
e. semantics
subependymal e.
suprasellar e.
tumor e.
extension-type cervical spine injury
extensive
e. neoplasm
e. posterior decompression
extensor
e. plantar response
e. rigidity
e. tetanus
e. thrust
extent prognosis
extenuating circumstance
exterior band of Baillarger
exteriorization
exteriorize
externa
glia limitons e.
globus pallidus e.
hematorrhachis e.
ophthalmoplegia e.
pachymeningitis e.
external
e. acoustic meatus
e. arcuate fiber
e. boundary
e. bracing
e. capsule
e. carotid artery (ECA)
e. chemical messenger (ECM)
e. collimator
e. cue
e. cuneate nucleus
e. entity
e. event
e. force
e. force control
e. genitalia
e. hydrocephalus
e. incentive motivation
e. inhibition
e. intercostal muscle
internal versus e. (I-E)
e. locus of control
e. malleolar sign
e. memory aid
e. meningitis
e. oblique reflex
e. pillar cell
e. popliteal nerve

e. pyocephalus
e. reality
e. reward
e. rhinoplasty
e. sense
e. spinal fixation
e. spinal skeletal fixator (ESSF)
e. spirit
e. stigmata
e. stimulation
e. stimulus
e. stressor
e. structure
e. support
e. validity
e. ventricular drainage
e. world
e. world experience
externalization
externalize blame
externalizing behavior
externalizing/internalizing
exteroceptive
e. conditioning
e. exposure
exteroceptor
exterofective system
exteropsychic
extinction
differential e.
e. of ego
order of e.
perceptual e.
e. phenomenon
e. ratio
sensory e.
tactile e.
visual e.
extinction-type pattern
extinguish
extirpation
tumor e.
extra
fecundatio ab e.
E. Strength Adprin-B
E. Strength Bayer Enteric 500 Aspirin
E. Strength Bayer Plus
E. Strength Doan's
E. Strength Dynafed E.X.
extraaxial
e. cavernous hemangioma
e. lesion
extracanicular acoustic neuroma
extracellular
e. acidosis
e. calcium activity
e. matrix (ECM)
e. space (ECS)
extraception
extracerebral
e. activity
e. aneurysm
e. cavernous angioma
e. hematoma

extrachromosomal
extracorporeal membrane oxygenation
extracranial
e. aneurysm
e. carotid occlusive disease
e. mass lesion
e. meningioma
e. occlusive vascular disease
e. pneumatocele
e. pneumocele
e. radiosurgery
extracranial-intracranial (ECIC, EC-IC)
e.-i. bypass
e.-i. bypass surgery
extracranial-to-intracranial bypass procedure
extractive disorder
extradural
e. abscess
e. anastomosis
e. clinoidectomy
e. compartment
e. cyst
e. defect
e. exposure
e. hematoma
e. hematorrhachis
e. hemorrhage
e. infection
e. injection
e. meningioma
e. phase
e. space
e. spinal metastasis
e. tumor
e. vertebral artery
extraforaminal
foraminal e.
e. lumbar disc herniation (ELDH)
extraindividual behavior
extrajection
extralemniscal myelotomy
extramarital
e. affair
e. behavior
e. intercourse
e. relations
e. sex
extrameatal
e. intracapsular tumor
e. tumor extension
extramedullary
e. hemangioma
e. spinal cord tumor
extraneous
e. movement
e. noise
extraocular
e. muscle involvement
e. muscle palsy
e. muscle paresis
e. paralysis
extrapersonal space
extrapineal pinealoma
extrapolate

E

extrapsychic conflict
extrapunitive
extrapyramidal
    e. cerebral palsy
    e. disease
    e. disorder
    e. dyskinesia
    e. epilepsy
    e. involvement (EPI)
    e. medication side effect
    e. nucleus
    e. structure
    e. symptom (EPS)
    E. Symptom Rating Scale
    e. symptom-sparing
    e. syndrome (EPS)
    e. system (EPS)
    e. tract
extrasensory
    e. perception (ESP)
    e. thought transference
extraspective perspective
extraspinal leiomyoma
extrastriatal dopamine transmission
extrastriate V5/MT cortex
extrasynaptic receptor
extratemporal excision
extratensive personality style
extratransference issue
extraversion (*var. of* extroversion)
extravert (*var. of* extrovert)
extravisual
extreme
    e. agitation
    e. anxiety
    e. capsule
    e. lateral inferior transcondylar
      approach
    e. lateral transcondylar approach
    e. narrowing limit
    e. negativism
    e. somatosensory evoked potential
      (ESEP)
    e. stressor
    e. trauma
extremis
    in e.
extremity
    anterior e. of caudate nucleus
    phantom e.
extricate
extrinsic
    e. asthma
    e. constancy
    e. cortex
    e. epilepsy
    e. motivation
    e. reward
extroceptor
extroversion, extraversion
extrovert, extravert
extroverted
    e. personality
    e. type

extrusion
    bone graft e.
    wire e.
extubation
    postoperative e.
eye
    e. accessing cue
    e. blink artifact
    e. blinking
    e. contact
    crossed e.
    dancing e.
    defected e.
    deflected e.
    e. dominance
    e. enucleation
    evil e.
    glassy e.
    e. gouging
    lusterless e.
    e. memory
    mind's e.
    e. movement
    e. movement abnormality
    e. movement artifact
    e. movement desensitization and
      reprocessing (EMDR)
    e. movement disorder
    e. muscle weakness
    e. opener
    e. preference
    e. psychogenic disorder
    raccoon e.
    redness of e.
    e. scan
    e. scanning
eyeblind
    black e.
eye-closure reflex
eye-hand coordination
eyelash sign
eyelid
    e. conditioning
    drooping e.
    insufficiency of e.
eye-motor-verbal (EMV)
    e.-m.-v. profile
eye-roll sign
EYES
    Early Years Easy Screen
eyes, motor, voice/verbal (EMV)
eye-to-eye
eye-voice span
Eysenck
    E. Personality Inventory (EPI)
    E. Personality Questionnaire (EPQ)
E-Z
    E.-Z. Flap cranial bone plate
    E.-Z. flap cranial flap fixation
      system
Ezide

F
  form response
    F response
F+
  good form response
F$_7$
f
  frequency
FaAct
  Foundation for Accountability
Fabco gauze dressing
fables test
Fabry disease
fabulation
fabulized
    f. combination
    f. response
FAC
  Functional Ambulation Categories
facade of competence
face
    about f.
    anthropomorphic f.
    staring f.
    f. validity
Face-Hand Test
face-saving behavior
FACES III
  Family Adaptability and Cohesion
    Evaluation Scale III
facet, facette
    bony f.
    f. excision technique
    f. fracture stabilization wiring
    f. hypertrophy
    f. joint
    f. joint preparation
    locked f.
    f. replacement
    f. rhizotomy
    f. subluxation stabilization wiring
    f. syndrome
facetectomy
    partial f.
facetious
facette (var. of facet)
facial
    F. Action Coding System (FACS)
    f. affect
    f. agnosia
    f. apraxia
    f. artery
    f. asymmetry
    f. colliculus
    f. contusion
    f. deceit
    f. diplegia
    f. disfigurement
    f. display
    f. dystonia
    f. electromyography
    f. electroneurography

    f. eminence
    f. expression
    f. expression automatism
    f. fracture
    f. genu
    f. grimace
    f. habit spasm
    f. hematoma
    f. hemiatrophy
    f. hemiplegia
    f. hemispasm
    f. hillock
    f. identification
    f. migraine
    f. motor nucleus
    f. myokymia
    f. nerve
    f. nerve discontinuity
    f. neuralgia
    f. neuroma
    f. neuropathy
    f. osteosynthesis
    f. pain
    f. palsy
    f. paralysis
    f. paresis
    f. perception
    f. reanimation
    f. recognition
    F. Recognition Test
    f. reflex
    f. responsiveness
    f. root
    f. sensation
    f. tic
    f. tremor
    f. trophoneurosis
    f. twitch
    f. vision
facialis
    nervus f.
    f. phenomenon
facies, pl. facies
    birdlike f.
    cushingoid f.
    f. dolorosa
    elfin f.
    hatchet f.
    Hutchinson f.
    f. inferior cerebri
    f. inferior hemispherii cerebelli
    masked f.
    masklike f.
    f. medialis cerebri
    moon f.
    myasthenic f.
    myopathic f.
    myotonic f.
    Parkinson f.
    parkinsonian f.
    f. superior hemispherii cerebelli
    f. superolateralis cerebri

F

facilitation
    associative f.
    behavioral f.
    postactivation f.
    postspike f.
    proprioceptive neuromuscular f.
    (PNF)
    reproductive f.
    social f.
    Wedensky f.
facility
    board and care f.
    child-care f.
    correctional f.
    detention f.
    emergency care f.
    extended-care f.
    health-related f.
    intermediate-care f.
    long-term care f.
    rehabilitation f.
    residential treatment f.
    short-term care f.
    treatment f.
facioauriculovertebral (FAV)
faciobuccolingual dyskinesia
faciocephalalgia
faciocephalic pain
faciofacial nerve anastomosis
faciohypoglossal anastomosis
faciolingual
facioplegia
facioplegic
    f. migraine
    f. migraine headache
facioscapulohumeral (FSH)
    f. atrophy
faciostenosis
FACS
    Facial Action Coding System
FACT
    Flanagan Aptitude Classification Test
fact
    f. finding
    f. giver
    f. of life
    matter of f.
    f. seeker
faction
    time f.
factitial
factitious
    f. attack
    f. disorder, combined type
    f. disorder, physical type
    f. disorder by proxy
    f. disorder, psychological type
    f. illness
    f. interface disorder
factitious-type neurotic hysteric disorder
facto
    ex post f.
factor
    alpha f.
    f. analysis

arousability f.
basal endothelium-derived
  relaxing f.
basic fibroblast growth f. (bFGF)
biologic f.
biomechanical f.
brain-derived neurotrophic f.
  (BDNF)
brain-derived neurotropic f. (BDNF)
C f.
causal f.
cellular immunity f.
ciliary neurotrophic f. (CNTF)
cleverness f. (C-factor)
cognitive f.
cognitive/attitudinal f.
combined f.
f. comparison
f. comparison method
constitutional f.
corticotropin-releasing f. (CRF)
Costa/McCrae f.
cultural f.
3-f. dimensional model of
  schizophrenia
disorder due to combined f.'s
disorganized f.
DNA transcription f.
embryological pathogenetic f.
emotional/activation f.
endogenous f.
endothelium-derived relaxing f.
  (EDRF)
environmental f.
epidermal growth f.
erectile disorder due to
  combined f.'s
erectile disorder due to
  psychological f.'s
ethnic f.
etiological f.
exogenous f.
expressionism f.
familial f.
father f.
feedback inhibition f. (FIF)
Fiblast trafermin growth f.
fibroblast growth f. receptor 2
  (FGFR2)
fiddle f.
filling f.
fork head response f.
Frankenstein f.
Frohman f.
G f.
general f.
geriatric f.
gestalt f.
glial-cell-line derived
  neurotrophic f. (GDNF)
growth f.
growth hormone-release inhibiting f.
  (GHRIF)
growth hormone-releasing f.
Hageman f.

hedonic-tone f.
helix-loop-helix response f.
HLH f.
human growth f. (HGF)
insulin growth f.
insulin-like growth f. (IGF)
interest f.
International Primary F.'s (IPF)
known organic f.
lethal f.
leukemia inhibitory f. (LIF)
f. loading
f. matrix
mauve f.
melanocyte-inhibiting f.
method f.
motivational f.
motivational/behavioral f.
negative f.
nerve growth f. (NGF)
neural growth f.
neurobiological f.
noise f.
organic f.
perpetuating f.
physiological f.
plasma f.
platelet activating f.
platelet-derived growth f.
precipitating f.
predisposing f.
pregenital f.
pre-oedipal f.
primary f.
prolactin-inhibiting f. (PIF)
prolactin-releasing f. (PRF)
protection f.
psychic f.
psychological f.
psychosexual f.
psychosocial f.
psychotic f.
quality f.
f. reflection
religious orthodoxy f.
rheumatoid f.
risk f.
f. rotation
S f.
schizophrenic f.
significant risk f.
spiritual f.
Stuart-Power f.
subjectivism f.
suicide-risk f.
synthetic corticotropin-releasing f.
f. theory
f. theory of personality
thinking disturbance f. (TDF)
trait f.
tumor necrosis f. (TNF)
uncertainty f.
uncertainty-arousal f.
unconscious f.
unspecified psychological f.

V f.
vascular endothelial growth f.
  (VEGF)
verbal comprehension f.
F. VIII antigen tumor marker
f. VIII deficiency
will f.
f. XII deficiency
factor-α, factor-alpha
recombinant human tumor
  necrosis f.
tumor necrosis f.
factorial
f. design
f. experiment
f. invariance
f. validity
faculty
fusion f.
f. fusion
intellectual f.
language f.
mental f.
f. psychology
FAD
familial Alzheimer disease
flavin adenine dinucleotide
fad diet
faddism
food f.
fading
stimulus f.
FAE
fetal alcohol effect
Fager pituitary dissector
Fagerstrom
F. Nicotine Addiction Scale
F. Tolerance Questionnaire
Fahr
F. disease
F. syndrome
failed
f. back surgery syndrome (FBSS)
f. back syndrome with documented
  pseudarthrosis
f. suicide attempt
failure
chronic acquired hepatic f.
congestive heart f.
f. of conservative management
f. to develop
f. to develop empathy
f. to develop relatedness
f. of drug trial
fatigue f.
fear of f. (FF)
f. to fulfill
f. to gain weight
Harrington rod instrumentation f.
hepatic f.
instrumentation f.
isolated gait ignition f.
f. of lateralization
metal f.
multiple organ f.

F

failure *(continued)*
  myoglobinuric renal f.
  poliomyelitis-induced respiratory f.
  f. of problem solving
  renal f.
  reproductive f.
  f. in social adaptation
  spinal implant load to f.
  f. to sustain consistent work
    behavior
  f. to sustain a monogamous
    relationship
  therapeutic f.
  f. to thrive (FTT)
  f. through success
  f. to warn
failure-to-grow syndrome
failure-to-thrive syndrome
fair shake
Fairbanks change
faire
  savoir f.
fair sex
Fairview Language Evaluation Test
  (FLET)
fair-weather friend
Fairweather Lodge
fait accompli
faith
  blind f.
  f. conversion problem
  f. cure
  good f.
  f. healing
  keeping f.
  religious f.
fake cocaine
falces (*pl. of* falx)
falcial
falciform
  f. crest
  f. lobe
falcine
falciparum
  Plasmodium f.
Falconer lobectomy
Falcon plastic flask
falcotentorial meningioma
falcula
falcular
fallacy
  pathologic f.
falling
  f. attack
  f. out
  f. sickness
fallopian neuritis
FALS
  familial forms of amyotrophic lateral
    sclerosis
false
  f. accusation
  f. arrest
  f. association

  f. attribution
  f. belief
  f. conditioning
  f. euphoria
  f. evaluation
  f. fluency
  f. friend
  f. hermaphroditism
  f. image
  f. localizing sign
  f. masturbation
  f. memory
  f. memory syndrome
  f. negative
  f. neuroma
  f. paracusis
  f. perceptions of movement
  f. positive
  f. pregnancy
  f. role disorder
  f. sensory experience
  f. threshold
false-negative
  f.-n. diagnosis
  f.-n. response
false-positive
  f.-p. diagnosis
  f.-p. response
falsetto voice
falsifiable hypothesis
falsification
  memory f.
  retrospective f.
falx, pl. falces
  f. cerebelli
  f. cerebri
  f. meningioma
  parasagittal f.
familial
  f. aggregation
  f. aggregation problem
  f. Alzheimer disease (FAD)
  f. amyloidosis
  f. amyloidotic polyneuropathy
  f. amyotrophic lateral sclerosis
  f. arteriovenous malformation
  f. cervicocephalic arterial dissection
  f. deficiency
  f. dementia
  f. disorder
  f. dysautonomia
  f. encephalopathy
  f. factor
  f. forms of amyotrophic lateral
    sclerosis (FALS)
  f. glioma
  f. gliomatosis cerebri
  f. hemiplegic migraine (FHM)
  f. hypercholesterolemia
  f. hypokalemic periodic paralysis
  f. Mediterranean fever (FMF)
  f. medulloblastoma
  f. melanoma
  f. migraine headache
  f. neuropathy

f. paroxysmal choreoathetosis
f. paroxysmal choreoathetosis disease
f. paroxysmal kinesigenic ataxia
f. pattern
f. periodic paralysis
f. progressive myoclonic epilepsy
f. psychosis
f. pure depressive disease (FPDD)
f. retardation
f. schizophrenia
f. spastic ataxia
f. spastic paraplegia
f. spinal muscular atrophy
f. splenic anemia
f. tendency
f. transmission of schizophrenia
f. tremor
f. unconscious

familial/genetic
familiar surroundings
famille névropathique
family
F. Adaptability and Cohesion Evaluation Scale III (FACES III)
adoptive f.
alcoholic f.
F. Apperception Test (FAT)
F. Aptitudes Questionnaire (FAQ)
f. assessment
F. Attitudes Questionnaire (FAQ)
F. Attitudes Test (FAT)
bilineal f.
blended f.
f. care
f. caregiver
Coalition for the F. (CF)
cohesive f.
f. conflict
f. connectedness
f. constellation
Council on Children, Adolescents, and Their F.'s
f. counseling
f. counselor
f. disruption
F. Drawing Depression Scale (FDDS)
f. dynamics
dysfunctional f.
empowered f.
F. Environment Scale (FES)
f. evaluation
F. Evaluation Form (FEF)
f. evaluation scale
extended f.
f. group intake
f. history (FH)
F. History Assessment Module
F. History Research Diagnostic Criteria
F. History Research Diagnostic Criteria Schedule
f. identity
f. idiocy

f. incubus
f. interaction
f. intervention
F. Inventory of Life Events and Changes (FILE)
Irish Study of High-Density Schizophrenia F.'s
Jukes f.
Kallikak f.
leucine zipper f.
matrilinear f.
matrilocal f.
f. medicine
f. member
f. member therapy
f. method
f. neglect
neolocal f.
f. neurosis
nuclear f.
occupational f.
patriarchal f.
patrilineal f.
patrilocal f.
f. pattern
f. perception
f. physician
f. process
f. psychotherapy
f. pursuit
reconstituted f.
f. relation
f. relationship
F. Relationship Inventory
F. Relations Test (FRT)
F. Relations Test, Children's Version
rigid f.
f. risk study
f. romance
f. routine
runs in f.
F. Satisfaction Scale
f. sculpting
f. separation
single-parent f.
f. situation
f. social work
f. stability
f. stress
f. structural balance
f. studies
f. support
f. support group
f. support system
systemic f.
f. and systemic psychotherapy
f. system interview
f. systems theory
F. Tracking System (FTS)
f. treatment
f. turbulence
f. type
f. unit
f. unit therapy

F

family *(continued)*
  f. violence
  zero f.
  zinc-finger f.
family/system research orientation
Famous Sayings Test
fan
  f. retractor
  f. sign
Fañanás cell
fanatic personality
Fanconi
  F. anemia
  F. syndrome
fancy free
FANPT
  Freeman Anxiety Neurosis and
    Psychosomatic Test
fantasies
  world-destruction f.
fantasized sexual experience
fantasizing
  active f.
fantastica, phantastica
  paraphrenia f.
  pseudologia f.
fantasy, phantasy
  f. absence
  affect f.
  aggressive f.
  anal rape f.
  f. assessment
  autistic f.
  cannibalistic f.
  f. cathexis
  compensatory f.
  erotic f.
  eroticized f.
  fellatio f.
  f. figure
  flight into f.
  forced f.
  grandiosity in f.
  hero f.
  hetaeral f.
  incest f.
  incestuous f.
  intense sexual f.
  internal world of f.
  king-slave f.
  f. life
  magic f.
  masochistic sexual f.
  night f.
  nonpathological sexual f.
  obsessive f.
  paraphiliac f.
  pathognomonic f.
  pathologic sexual f.
  f. period
  f. play
  Pompadour f.
  primal f.
  f. process

  rape f.
  rebirth f.
  rejuvenation f.
  rescue f.
  romance f.
  romantic f.
  schizoid f.
  screen f.
  secondary f.
  sexual f.
  sexually arousing f.
  spider f.
  unconscious f.
  voyeuristic sexually arousing f.
  womb f.
fantod
FAP
  fixed action pattern
FAQ
  Family Aptitudes Questionnaire
  Family Attitudes Questionnaire
FAR
  Flight Aptitude Rating
far
  F. East Russian encephalitis
  f. lateral inferior suboccipital
    approach
Faraday
  F. law of induction
  F. shield
Farber
  F. disease
  F. lipogranulomatosis
far-field
  f.-f. evoked potential
  f.-f. record
Farley retractor
FAS
  fetal alcohol syndrome
fascia, pl. **fasciae**
  f. cinerea
  f. dentata hippocampi
  dentate f.
  infraspinous f.
  f. lata sling
  lumbodorsal f.
  perineal f.
  vertebral f.
fascia-muscle-fascia sandwich
fascicle
  nerve f.
  peripheral nerve f.
fascicular
  f. adaptation
  f. degeneration
  f. graft
  f. ophthalmoplegia
fasciculation
  cramp benign f.
  f. potential
fasciculus, gen. and pl. **fasciculi**
  f. anterior proprius
  arcuate f. (AF)
  Burdach f.
  calcarine f.

central tegmental f.
f. circumolivaris pyramidis
f. corticospinalis anterior
f. corticospinalis lateralis
cuneate f.
f. cuneatus (Fc)
dorsal longitudinal f.
dorsolateral f.
f. dorsolateralis
Flechsig fasciculi
Foville f.
frontooccipital f.
Gowers f.
f. gracilis (Fg)
hooked f.
inferior longitudinal f.
interfascicular f.
f. interfascicularis
intersegmental fasciculi
f. lateralis proprius
f. lenticularis
Lissauer f.
fasciculi longitudinales pontis
f. longitudinalis dorsalis
f. longitudinalis inferior
f. longitudinalis medialis
f. longitudinalis superior
f. macularis
mamillotegmental f.
f. mamillotegmentalis
mamillothalamic f.
f. mamillothalamicus
f. marginalis
medial longitudinal f.
median longitudinal f.
Meynert f.
f. obliquus pontis
occipitofrontal f.
f. occipitofrontalis
oval f.
f. pedunculomamillaris
perpendicular f.
proper fasciculi
fasciculi proprii
f. pyramidalis anterior
f. pyramidalis lateralis
retroflex f.
f. retroflexus
f. rotundus
fasciculi rubroreticulares
semilunar f.
f. semilunaris
septomarginal f.
f. septomarginalis
slender f.
f. solitarius
subcallosal f.
f. subcallosus
superior longitudinal f.
f. thalamicus
f. thalamomamillaris
unciform f.
uncinate f. of Russell
f. uncinatus
wedge-shaped f.

fascinum
fasciola, pl. fasciolae
   f. cinerea
fasciolar gyrus
fascioscapulohumeral dystrophy
fashion
   cookbook f.
   multiaxial f.
   nonaxial f.
   probabilistic f.
   singsong f.
FAST
   Filtered Audiometer Speech Test
   Frenchay Aphasia Screening Test
fast
   f. activity
   anorexic f.
   f. field-potential rhythm
   f. Fourier transformation spectrum
   analyzer
   f. imaging
   f. imaging with steady precession
   (FISP)
   f. low angle shot (FLASH)
   f. saccadic eye movement
   Snooze F.
   f. speech
   F. Track Program
fast-Fourier transform
fast-frequency repetitive transcranial
   magnetic stimulation (FFr-TMS)
fastidium
   f. cibi
   f. potus
fastigial pressor response (FPR)
fastigiobulbar tract
Fastin
fasting
   f. blood glucose (FBS)
   starvation f.
FasTRACKER-18 infusion catheter
fast-scan magnetic resonance
fast-talk
FAT
   Family Apperception Test
   Family Attitudes Test
fat
   f. body
   f. depot
   f. embolism
   f. embolus
   epidural f.
fatal
   f. accident
   f. familial insomnia
   f. overdose
fatale
   femme f.
fatalistic attitude
fata morgana
fate
   f. analysis
   law of common f.
   f. neurosis
fat-free mass (FFM)

F

father
    alleged f. (AF)
    f. complex
    f. confessor
    f. factor
    f. figure
    f. fixation
    foster f.
    f. hypnosis
    f. ideal
    f. image
    primal f.
    f. substitute
    f. surrogate
    surrogate f.
    vaginal f.
father-child bond
father-daughter incest
fatigability
    auditory f.
    battle f.
    chronic f.
    combat f.
    daytime f.
    easy f.
    excessive f.
    nervous f.
    pseudocombat f.
    psychogenic f.
    stimulation f.
    sustained f.
fatigue
    auditory f.
    battle f.
    chronic f.
    combat f.
    f. disease
    ease of f.
    emotional f.
    f. failure
    implant f.
    mental f.
    metal f.
    nervous f.
    f. neurosis
    operational f.
    overwhelming f.
    pseudocombat f.
    psychogenic f.
    F. Questionnaire
    stapedius muscle f.
    f. state
    stimulation f.
    f. strength
    f. stress
    sustained f.
    f. symptom
    f. syndrome
fatiguing vigil
fatness stimulus
fat-patch graft
FATSA
    Flowers Auditory Test of Selective
    Attention

fat-suppression
    f.-s. MR imaging
    f.-s. technique
fatty
    f. acid oxidation
    f. streak
fatuus
    ignis f.
fat/water
    f. chemical shift
    f. signal cancellation
faucial
    f. paralysis
    f. reflex
faulty judgment
faux pas
FAV
    facioauriculovertebral
    FAV syndrome
Favaloro-Morse sternal spreader
Fazekas Scale
Fazio-Londe syndrome
FBS
    fasting blood glucose
FBSS
    failed back surgery syndrome
FC
    formed response of colored area
Fc
    fasciculus cuneatus
    shading response to black areas
    shading response to gray areas
FCP
    Functional Communication Profile
FDA
    Food and Drug Administration
FDCT
    Franck Drawing Completion Test
FDDQ
    Freedom from Distractibility Deviation
    Quotient
FDDS
    Family Drawing Depression Scale
FDG
    [^{18}F]fluoro-2-deoxy-D-glucose
    [^{13}F]fluorodeoxyglucose
    fluorodeoxyglucose
FDTVP
    Frostig Developmental Test of Visual
    Perception
fear
    f. of abandonment
    f. appeal
    bad-people f.
    building f.
    castration f.
    change f.
    childhood f.
    cold f.
    confinement f.
    crowd f.
    f. of death
    f. of disapproval
    f. drive
    eating f.

emptiness f.
epilepsy f.
eternity f.
excrement f.
f. of failure (FF)
free-floating f.
f. of going crazy
f. hypnosis
ictal f.
impregnation f.
impulse f.
incapacitating f.
intense f.
interoceptive f.
irrational f.
lack of f.
life f.
f. of losing control
marriage f.
maturity f.
mirror f.
moisture f.
monster f.
morbid f.
motion f.
mouse f.
obligations f.
obsessive f.
odor f.
overwork f.
paranoid f.
penis f.
performance f.
pleasure f.
point f.
F. Questionnaire
f. reaction
reasonable f.
rejection f.
f. of rejection
f. response
scratch f.
semen f.
sermon f.
sex f.
sexual f.
shock f.
sitting f.
skin disease f.
skin injury f.
skyscraper f.
sleep f.
snow f.
sound f.
sourness f.
star f.
story f.
strangeness f.
stranger f.
street f.
subjective f.
sudden f.
suffocation f.
sunlight f.
sunrise f.

F. Survey Schedule (FSS)
talking f.
tapeworm f.
taste f.
F. Thermometer
thinking f.
thought f.
Three F.'s
time f.
tooth f.
train f.
unreasonable f.
vehicle f.
virgin f.
void f.
vomiting f.
weakness f.
wind f.
writing f.

feared
f. disease
f. object
f. single performance situation
f. situation
f. words

fearfulness
f. disorder of adolescence
f. disorder of childhood

feasible

feature
age-related f.
age-specific f.
agitative f.
f. analysis
associated descriptive f.
atypical f.
catatonic f.
characteristic f.
clinical f.
common shared f.
f. contrasts process
culture-related f.
culture-specific f.
delusional f.
depressive f.
descriptive f.
diagnostic f.
dominant f.
essential f.
gender f.
gender-specific f.
hysteroid f.
insomnia f.
junctural f.
manic f.
melancholic f.
mixed f.
mood-congruent psychotic f.
mood disorder with atypical f.'s
mood disorder with catatonic f.'s
mood disorder with
  melancholic f.'s
mood-incongruent psychotic f.
neurotic f.
nondistinctive f.

F

feature *(continued)*
   obsessive-compulsive f.
   pain disorder associated with
      psychological f.'s
   paralinguistic f.
   paranoid f.
   personality f.
   phenomenological f.
   prosodic f.
   psychotic f.
   schizoid f.
   shared phenomenological f.
   sociodemographic f.
   specific culture f.
   specific culture, age, and gender f.
   specific gender f.
febarbamate
febrifacient
febrile
   f. convulsion
   f. delirium
   f. psychosis
   f. seizure
febriphobia
fecal
   f. continence
   f. incontinence
feces-child-penis concept
fecundatio ab extra
fecundation
   artificial f.
fecundity
**Federal Emergency Management Agency
   (FEMA)**
feeblemindedness
   affective f.
   primary f.
feedback
   acoustic f.
   afferent f.
   alpha f.
   altered auditory f. (AAF)
   auditory f.
   constructive f.
   control f.
   f. control
   corrective f.
   delayed auditory f.
   efferent f.
   electromyographic f.
   haptic f.
   information f.
   f. inhibition factor (FIF)
   inverse f.
   kinesthetic f.
   f. mechanism
   negative f.
   f. noise
   physiological f.
   positive f.
   proprioceptive f.
   f. system
   tactile f.
   video f.

feeding
   f. artery of aneurysm
   f. behavior
   breast f.
   f. center
   f. and eating disorder
   F. and Eating Disorders of Infancy
      or Early Childhood
   fictitious f.
   forced f.
   f. habits
   intravenous f.
   f. mean arterial pressure (FMAP)
   parenteral f.
   f. problem
   f. psychogenic disorder
   sham f.
   f. system
   f. technique
feeling
   absence of f.
   affected by f.
   ambivalent f.
   f.'s analysis
   f.'s of anxiety
   f. apperception
   ataxic f.
   community f.
   compassionate f.
   conflicted f.
   covert f.
   dammed-up f.
   f. of detachment
   f.'s of dirtiness
   f. of disgust
   disturbing f.
   f. of dread
   f. of electricity
   f.'s of estrangement
   exaggerated f.
   expression with f.
   fellow f.
   group f.
   guilt f.
   inferiority f.
   lack of f.
   loving f.
   maladaptive f.
   negative f.
   f. numb
   f. of numbness
   oceanic f.
   positive f.
   premorbid inferiority f. (PIF)
   rageful f.
   range of f.
   reflection of f.
   f.'s of rejection
   repressed f.
   f. sensation
   sinking f.
   subjective f.
   substituting f.
   superiority f.
   f. tone

tone of f.
transference f.
tridimensional theory of f.
unacceptable f.
f.'s of unreality
ventilation of f.
verbalization of f.
Feer disease
FEF
Family Evaluation Form
frontal eye field
Fehling TOP ejector punch
Feighner criteria for alcoholism
feigned
f. bereavement
f. symptom
feigning
death f.
Feingold diet
felbamate
Felbatol
Feldene
felinophobia, galeophobia, gatophobia
fellatio fantasy
fellation
fellator
fellatorism
fellatrice, fellatrix
fellow
f. drug addict
f. feeling
f. man
felo-de-se, pl. **felones-de-se**
felonious
felony behavior
Fels Parent Behavior Rating Scale
felt
f. need
shredded Teflon f.
Teflon f.
Felty syndrome
FEMA
Federal Emergency Management Agency
female
f. biological status
f. castration
f. circumcision
f. climacteric
f. dyspareunia
f. dyspareunia-male dyspareunia
f. ejaculation
f. eunuchoidism
f. fantasy figure
f. genitalia
f. hypoactive sexual desire disorder
f. intersex
marasmic f.
f. menopause
f. orgasm
f. suffrage
female/system research orientation
female-to-male transgender identity
Femcet
feminine
f. attitude

f. identification
f. identity
f. mannerism
f. masochism
f. social role
femininity
f. complex
construction of f.
feminism
feminist
feminization
feminize
feminizing-testes syndrome
femme fatale
femora
coitus inter f.
femoral
f. cutaneous nerve
f. introducer sheath
f. neuropathy
f. reflex
femoroabdominal reflex
fend
fenestra
f. ovalis
f. rotunda
fenestrated
f. aneurysm clip
f. oculomotor nerve
fenestration
bur hole neuroendoscopic f.
cyst f.
fenethylline hydrochloride
fenfluramine hydrochloride
fenmetozole hydrochloride
fenoprofen calcium
Fenoterol
fentanyl
f. citrate
droperidol and f.
F. Oralet
F. patch
Fenton reaction
feral children
Féré
F. effect
F. phenomenon
Féréol-Graux palsy
Ferguson
F. brain suction tip
F. brain suction tube
F. suction
Feridex IV
ferox
delirium f.
ferpentetate
technetium 99m f.
Ferris
F. Smith-Kerrison laminectomy rongeur
F. Smith-Kerrison punch
ferrite
barium f.

F

319

ferritin
serum f.
f. test
ferromagnetic
f. artifact
f. implant
f. intracerebral aneurysm clip
f. monitoring device
ferrugination
fertilization
ferumoxide injectable solution
Fer-Will Object Kit
FES
Family Environment Scale
functional electrical stimulation
FES figure-drawing test
festinans
chorea f.
festinant
festinating gait
festination
fetal
f. adenoma
f. AIDS transmission
f. alcohol effect (FAE)
f. alcohol syndrome (FAS)
f. cell transplantation
f. death
f. development
f. distress
f. hydantoin syndrome
f. infection
f. injury
f. mesencephalic grafting
f. mesencephalic tissue (FMT)
f. movement
f. neural implant
f. neural transplant
f. period
f. planum
f. planum temporal lateralization
f. position
f. position posture
f. response
f. screening
f. substantia nigra
f. tau
f. transfusion
fetalis
erythroblastosis f.
fetalism
fetal-maternal exchange
fetation
fetched
feticide
fetish
f. object
shoe f.
fetishism
beast f.
f. paraphilia
transvestic f. (TF)
fetoprotein
alpha f.

feud
blood f.
Feulgen cytophotometry
fever
Argentinian hemorrhage f.
Bolivian hemorrhagic f.
cabin f.
Central European tick-borne f.
cerebrospinal f.
Colorado tick f. (CTF)
dance f.
dengue f.
diphasic milk f.
drug f.
familial Mediterranean f. (FMF)
hemorrhagic f.
Jarisch-Herxheimer f.
low f.
meningotyphoid f.
Rift Valley f.
Rocky Mountain spotted f.
South African tick-bite f.
spotted f.
stir f.
trypanosome f.
typhus f.
undulant f.
West Nile f.
yellow f.
Zika f.
Feverall
Infants F.
F. Sprinkle Caps
fey
FF
fear of failure
[^{18}F] fluoride solution
[^{18}F]fluoro-2-deoxy-D-glucose (FDG)
[^{13}F]fluorodeoxyglucose (FDG)
FFM
fat-free mass
FFr-TMS
fast-frequency repetitive transcranial
magnetic stimulation
Fg
fasciculus gracilis
FGFR2
fibroblast growth factor receptor 2
FG syndrome
FH
family history
FHM
familial hemiplegic migraine
FI
fixateur interne
fixed interval
Fiamberti hypothesis
fiber
A f.
accelerator f.
A-delta f.
adrenergic f.
afferent f.
alpha f.
amygdalofugal f.

anastomosing f.
anastomotic f.
annulospiral f.
arcuate f.
association f.
augmentor f.
B f.
Bergmann f.
beta f.
C f.
cholinergic f.
circular f.
climbing f.
commissural f.
cone f.
corticobulbar f.
corticonuclear f.
corticopontine f.
corticoreticular f.
corticospinal f.
depressor f.
endogenous f.
exogenous f.
external arcuate f.
gamma f.
Gratiolet f.
gray f.
inhibitory f.
inner cone f.
internal arcuate f.
intrafusal f.
intrinsic f.
lemniscal f.
medullated nerve f.
Micro link f.
micro-thin plastic f.
monoaminergic f.
mossy f.
motor f.
Müller f.
myelinated nerve f.
Myer f.
myoclonus epilepsy with ragged-red f. (MERRF)
nerve f.
nonmedullated f.
outer cone f.
periventricular f.
pilomotor f.
pressor f.
projection f.
pyramidal f.
ragged red f. (RRF)
Reissner f.
Remak f.
Retzius f.
rod f.
Rosenthal f.
striatopetal f.
sudomotor f.
sustentacular f. of retina
tautomeric f.
f. tract transection
transverse f. of pons

ultra high molecular weight polyethylene f. (UHMWPE)
unmyelinated f.
fiberoptics
fiberscope
superfine f.
Fiblast trafermin growth factor
fibra, pl. **fibrae**
fibrae arcuatae cerebri
fibrae arcuatae externae
fibrae arcuatae internae
fibrae circulares
fibrae corticonucleares
fibrae corticopontinae
fibrae corticoreticulares
fibrae corticospinales
fibrae periventriculares
fibrae pontis transversae
fibrae pyramidales
fibrillary
f. astrocyte
f. astrocytoma
f. chorea
f. myoclonia
f. neuroma
f. tremor
fibrillation
atrial f. (AF)
nonrheumatic atrial f.
paroxysmal atrial f.
f. potential
ventricular f.
fibrillinopathy
fibrils
bundles of f.
fibrin
f. film
f. glue
f. glue-soaked Gelfoam
fibrinogen
fibrinoid degeneration
fibrinolysin
fibrinolysis
fibrinolytic agent
fibrin-platelet-fibrin embolus
fibriphobia
fibroblast
f. growth factor receptor 2 (FGFR2)
senescent f.
transfected f.
fibroblastic
f. meningioma
f. proliferation
fibrodysplasia ossificans
fibrogliosis
fibrohistiocytoma
malignant f.
fibrolipoma
fibroma
chondromyxoid f.
ossifying f.
psammomatoid ossifying f.
sinonasal psammomatoid ossifying f.

fibromatosis
    juvenile f.
fibromuscular
    f. dysplasia
    f. hyperplasia
fibromyalgia syndrome
fibronectin synthesis
fibroneuroma
fibropsammoma
fibrosa
    meninx f.
fibrosarcoma
fibrosclerosis
    multifocal f.
    systemic multifocal f.
fibrosing arachnoiditis
fibrosis
    arachnoid f.
    cystic f.
    dural f.
    leptomeningeal f.
    meningeal f.
    muscle f.
    postradiation f.
    progressive leptomeningeal f.
    f. radiation
    retroperitoneal f.
    root sleeve f.
fibrositic headache
fibrositis
    cervical f.
fibrositis/fibromyalgia syndrome
fibrosum
    molluscum f.
fibrosus
    annulus f.
fibrous
    f. astrocyte
    f. dysplasia
    f. mesothelioma
    f. plaque
    f. sarcoma
fibroxanthoma
fibroxanthosarcoma
fibular
    f. allograft
    f. grafting
    f. peg
fictional finalism
fictitious feeding
FID
    free induction decay
    repeated FID
fiddle factor
fide
    bona f.
fidelity
fidgeting behavior
fiducial
    cranium-affixed f.
    inexact f.
    f. marker
    MKM f.
    radiopaque f.

field
    absolute f.
    barrel f.
    behavior f.
    Broca f.
    Brodmann cytoarchitectonic f.
    centrocecal visual f.
    checkerboard f.
    f. of consciousness
    f. contour
    f. data
    f. defect
    f. dependence
    f. dependence-independence
    dipole f.
    electric f.
    electromagnetic focusing f. (EFF)
    excitatory f.
    f. expansion
    f. experiment
    f. of fixation
    f. force
    f.'s of Forel
    fringing f.
    frontal eye f. (FEF)
    f. of gaze
    Goldmann visual f.
    f. gradient
    gradient magnetic f.
    H f.
    harmonic error f.
    f. homogeneity
    Humphrey visual f.
    f. independence
    f. independence-dependence
    f. inhomogeneity
    lattice f.
    f. lock
    f. magnet
    magnetic f.
    main f.
    minimal audible f. (MAF)
    nerve f.
    f. pattern
    perceptual f.
    phenomenal f.
    phenomenological f.
    play the f.
    prerubral f.
    f. property
    psychological f.
    pulsating electromagnetic f. (PEMF)
    radiofrequency electromagnetic f.
    f. of regard
    f. research
    f. shift
    static magnetic f.
    f. strength
    f. structure
    F. suction dissector
    tegmental field of Forel
    terminal neuronal f.
    f. theory
    vector f.
    f. of view

f. of vision
visual f.
Wernicke f.
f. work
z-gradient f.
field-cognition mode
Fielding membrane
FIF
feedback inhibition factor
fifth
f. cranial nerve
f. ventricle
fight
domestic f.
gang f.
physical f.
fight-or-flight reaction
Figueira syndrome
figural
f. aftereffect
f. cohesion
f. memory
figurative
f. blind spot
f. knowledge
F. Language Interpretation Test
(FLIT)
f. meaning
figure
ambiguous f.
attachment f.
authority f.
childhood f.
empiric-risk f.
fantasy f.
father f.
female fantasy f.
fortification f.
f. ground
f. and ground
identification f.
major attachment f.
myelin f.
noise f.
simple f.
f. of speech
figure-drawing test
figure-ground
f.-g. distortion
f.-g. perception
fila (*pl. of* filum)
filament
helical-like f.
paired helical f.
straight f.
FILE
Family Inventory of Life Events and
Changes
filial
f. generation
f. imprinting
f. therapy
filiate
filicide
filioparental

fillet
lateral f.
f. layer
medial f.
triangle of f.
trigone of f.
filling
f. factor
zero f.
film
Accu-Flo dura f.
fibrin f.
Instat fibrin f.
orthogonal f.
filovaricosis
filter
active f.
analog f.
band-pass f.
high-frequency f.
high linear f.
low-frequency f.
low-pass f.
Millipore f.
muscle f.
notch f.
perceptual f.
roll-off f.
shunt f.
Filtered Audiometer Speech Test
(FAST)
filtered-back projection
filtering
antialias f.
perceptual f.
signal f.
Filtzer interbody rasp
filum, pl. **fila**
f. durae matris spinalis
fila olfactoria
fila radicularia
terminal f.
f. terminale
FIM
Functional Independence Measure
fimbria, pl. **fimbriae**
f. hippocampi
fimbria-fornix lesion
fimbriodentate sulcus
final
f. diagnosis
f. tendency
finalism
fictional f.
financial crisis
Finckh Test
finder
hamate f.
finding
angiographic f.
associated laboratory f.
associated physical examination f.
case f.
clinical f.
fact f.

F

finding *(continued)*
  neurophysiological f.
  neuropsychologic f.
  object f.
  Test of Adolescent/Adult Word F.
    (TAWF)
  Test of Word F. (TWF)
fine
  f. electric hair
  f. motor
  f. motor activity
  f. motor coordination
  f. motor movement
  f. motor skill
  f. postural tremor
  f. rapid nystagmus
  f. tactile sensation
fine-cup forceps
**fine-tipped up-and-down-angled bipolar
  forceps**
finger
  f. agnosia
  f. anomia
  f. fracture technique
  f. indicator
  insane f.
  jerk f.
  F. Localization Test
  lock f.
  F. Oscillation Test (FOT)
  f. painting
  f. penetration
  f. phenomenon
  f. pointing
  snap f.
  f. spelling
  spring f.
  stuck f.
  f. sucking
  F. Tapping Test
  trigger f.
finger-biting behavior
finger-nose test
finger-tapping score
finger-thumb reflex
fingertip number writing perception
finger-to-finger test
finish bur
**Finnish Adoptive Family Study of
  Schizophrenia**
Finochietto
  F. retractor
  F. rib spreader
Fiorgen PF
Fioricet
Fiorinal with codeine
FIQ
FIRDA
  frontal intermittent rhythmic delta
  activity
fire
  ball of f.
  baptism by (with) f.
  Saint Anthony f.

  f. setter (FS)
  f. setting
fire-setting
  f.-s. behavior
  deliberate f.-s.
firing
  f. an anchor
  neuronal element f.
firma
  terra f.
firmly held belief
FIRO-B
  Fundamental Interpersonal Relations
    Orientation-Behavior
FIRO-F
  Fundamental Interpersonal Relations
    Orientation-Feelings
FIR.S.T.
  First Seizure Trial Group
first
  f. admission
  f. aid
  f. cranial nerve
  f. rank symptom (FRS)
  f. rank symptoms of delusion
  F. Seizure Trial Group (FIR.S.T.)
  f. stage of anesthesia
  f. temporal convolution
  f. temporal gyrus
first-degree biological relatives
first-episode schizophrenia
first-pass effect
first-signal system
Fisch
  F. drill
  F. dural hook
  F. micro hook
Fischer
  F. grade
  F. stereotaxy system
**Fischer-Leibinger bur hole-mounted
  fixation device**
Fisher
  F. exact test
  F. grading
  F. syndrome
**Fisher-Logemann Test of Articulation
  Competence (FLTAC)**
Fishgold line
fish scales
FISP
  fast imaging with steady precession
FISS
  Flint Infant Security Scale
fissura, pl. **fissurae**
  f. calcarina
  fissurae cerebelli
  f. cerebri lateralis
  f. choroidea
  f. collateralis
  f. dentata
  f. hippocampi
  f. horizontalis cerebelli
  f. longitudinalis cerebri

f. mediana anterior medullae oblongatae
f. mediana anterior medullae spinalis
f. parietooccipitalis
f. petrooccipitalis
f. posterolateralis
f. prima cerebelli
f. secunda cerebelli
f. sphenooccipitalis
f. transversa cerebelli
f. transversa cerebri

fissure
anal f.
f. of annulus
anterior median f. of medulla oblongata
anterior median f. of spinal cord
ape f.
Bichat f.
Broca f.
calcarine f.
callosomarginal f.
central f.
cerebellar f.
cerebellomedullary f.
cerebral f.
choroid f.
Clevenger f.
collateral f.
dentate f.
displacement of interhemispheric f.
great horizontal f.
great longitudinal f.
hippocampal f.
horizontal f. of cerebellum
inferior orbital f.
interhemispheric f.
lateral cerebral f.
longitudinal cerebral f.
longitudinal f. of cerebrum
lunate f.
optic f.
Pansch f.
paracentral f.
parietooccipital f.
postcentral f.
posterior median f. of the medulla oblongata
posterior median f. of spinal cord
posterolateral f.
posthippocampal f.
postlingual f.
postlunate f.
postpyramidal f.
postrhinal f.
prenodular f.
primary f. of the cerebellum
rhinal f.
rolandic f.
f. of Rolando
secondary f. of the cerebellum
simian f.
superior orbital f. (SOF)
superior temporal f.

sylvian f.
f. of Sylvius
transverse f. of cerebellum
transverse f. of cerebrum
vestibular f. of cochlea
zygal f.

fist clenching
fistula, pl. **fistulae, fistulas**
arteriovenous f.
Blom-Singer tracheoesophageal f.
caroticocavernous f.
carotid-cavernous f. (CCF)
carotid-cavernous sinus f.
carotid-dural f.
cavernous sinus f.
cerebrospinal fluid f.
craniosinus f.
dorsal enteric f.
dural arteriovenous f. (DAF)
dural venous f.
durocutaneous f.
iatrogenic carotid-cavernous f.
intradural arteriovenous f.
intradural retromedullary arteriovenous f.
perilymphatic f.
f. perilymphatic
posterior fossa dural arteriovenous f.
radiculomedullary f.
spinal dural arteriovenous f. (SDAVF)
trauma-induced f.
wall f.

fistula-induced sinus thrombosis
fistular
premedullary arteriovenous f.
fistulas (*pl. of* fistula)
FIT
Flanagan Industrial Test
fit
f. of anger
cerebellar f.
goodness of f.
f.'s of horrific temptation
parental f.
poorness of f.
postdormital chalastic f.
psychomotor f.
pupil-teacher f.
running f.
uncinate f.
Fite stain
fitful sleep
fitness
inclusive f.
physical f.
Fitonal
fittest
survival of the f.
five-axis system
Five P's: Parent Professional Preschool Performance Profile
fixateur interne (FI)

F

fixation
- adjunctive screw f.
- affect f.
- f. of affect
- anterior C1-C2 screw f.
- anterior metallic f.
- anterior plate f.
- anterior screw f.
- anterior spinal f.
- anxiety f.
- atlantoaxial f.
- authority figure f.
- cannibalistic f.
- Caspar anterior plate f.
- C1-C2 cable f.
- cervical spine internal f.
- cervical spine screw-plate f.
- child f.
- child-parent f.
- Cotrel-Dubousset f.
- crossed-screw f.
- dens anterior screw f.
- f. device
- Essex-Lopresti axial f.
- external spinal f.
- father f.
- field of f.
- freudian f.
- Galveston f.
- gaze f.
- Halifax clamp posterior cervical f.
- Harrington rod f.
- hook-plate f.
- f. hysteria
- iliac f.
- f. instability
- intermaxillary f. (IMF)
- internal spinal f.
- libido f.
- line of f.
- lumbar pedicle f.
- lumbar spine segmental f.
- lumbar spine transpedicular f.
- Luque-Galveston f.
- Luque loop f.
- Magerl posterior C1-C2 screw f.
- mandibular f.
- Manual of Internal F.
- Modulock posterior spinal f.
- mother f.
- multiple-point sacral f.
- f. neurosis
- f. nystagmus
- occipitocervical f.
- odontoid fracture internal f.
- oral f.
- parent f.
- f. pause
- pedicle screw-rod f.
- pedicular f.
- pelvic f.
- plate f.
- plate-screw f.
- f. point
- posterior cervical f.

- posterior segmental f.
- f. reaction
- reduction f.
- ReFix noninvasive f.
- rigid internal f.
- role f.
- Roy-Camille posterior screw plate f.
- sacral pedicle screw f.
- sacral spine f.
- sacrum fusion screw f.
- scoliotic curve f.
- screw f.
- segmental f.
- SOF'WIRE spinal f.
- spinal f.
- spondylolisthesis reduction f.
- sublaminar f.
- f. technique
- Texas Scottish Rite Hospital rod f.
- transpedicular screw-rod f.
- transverse f.
- visual f.

fixator
- AO internal f.
- DeBastiani external f.
- external spinal skeletal f. (ESSF)
- intermediate head f.
- ReFix stereotactic head f.
- Vermont spinal f.

fixe
- idée f.

fixed
- f. action pattern (FAP)
- f. belief
- f. delusion
- f. delusional system
- f. gaze
- f. idea
- f. internal
- f. interval (FI)
- f. marker
- f. model
- f. pupil
- f. ratio (FR)
- f. reinforcement
- f. torticollis

fixed-ended session

fixed-interval reinforcement schedule

fixedness
- functional f.

fixed-ratio reinforcement schedule

fix and focus attention

Fixity of Beliefs Scale

F-JAS
- Fleishman Job Analysis Survey

FK-506
- F. neurotoxicity

[^{18}F]-labeled fluorodeoxyglucose

flaccid
- f. cerebral palsy
- f. dysarthria
- f. paralysis
- f. speech

flaccidity

flagellation
flagellomania
flagrante delicto
flame-shaped hemorrhage
flame tip bur
Flamm technique
Flanagan
    F. Aptitude Classification Test
     (FACT)
    F. Industrial Test (FIT)
    F. spinal fusion gouge
flank dissection
flap
    axial pattern scalp f.
    bone f.
    craniotomy f.
    C-shaped scalp f.
    Dandy myocutaneous scalp f.
    f. elevation
    free bone f.
    horseshoe-shaped f.
    I-shaped scalp f.
    island pedicle scalp f.
    liver f.
    lumbar periosteal turnover f.
    myocutaneous f.
    neurovascular f.
    osteoplastic bone f.
    pericranial temporalis f.
    scalp f.
    sickle f.
    skin f.
    supraorbital pericranial f.
    trap-door type f.
    U-shaped scalp f.
flappable
flapping
    f. movement
    f. tremor
flare
    axon f.
FLASH
    fast low angle shot
flash
    f.'s of color
    hot f.
    light f.
    f.'s of light
flashback
    acid f.
    combat f.
    f. hallucinosis
    intrusive f.
    marijuana f.
    sodium lactate induced f.
flashbulb memory
flash-frozen tumor specimen
flashing pain syndrome
flask
    Falcon plastic f.
    tissue culture f.
flat
    f. affect
    f. back curette
    f. back deformity

    f. back syndrome
    f. blues
    f. electroencephalogram
    f. top wave
Flatau law
Flatau-Schilder disease
flatness
    emotional f.
flattened
    f. affect
    f. affectivity
flattening
    affective f.
    f. of gyrus
flavin
    f. adenine dinucleotide (FAD)
    f. mononucleotide (FMN)
flavin-containing mono-oxygenase
  metabolic system (FMO)
Flavivirus
flavored cocaine
flavum
    ligamentum f.
Flaxedil
Flechsig
    F. area
    F. bundle in cerebellum
    F. fasciculi
    F. ground bundle
    F. tract
fleeting
    f. delusion
    f. illusion
    f. pain
Fleishman Job Analysis Survey (F-JAS)
Flesch formula
FLET
    Fairview Language Evaluation Test
fletcherism
Flexaphen
FlexDial stimulus control
Flexeril
Flex Foam orthosis
flexibilitas
    cerea f.
    f. cerea
    f. cerea schizophrenia
flexibility
    behavioral f.
    cognitive f.
    Cotrel-Dubousset rod f.
    waxy f.
flexible
    f. arm microretractor
    f. arm retractor
    f. nasopharyngeal examination
    f. wire electrode
Flexicair bed
Flexinet dressing
flexion
    flicker thumb f.
    f. injury posterior atlantoaxial
     arthrodesis
    paraplegia in f.
    f. reflex

F

flexion-compression spine injury stabilization
flexion-distraction injury
flexion-extension injury
flexor
    f. reflex
    f. spasticity
    f. tetanus
flexura, pl. **flexurae**
flexure
    basicranial f.
    cephalic f.
    cerebral f.
    cervical f.
    cranial f.
    mesencephalic f.
    pontine f.
    telencephalic f.
    transverse rhombencephalic f.
F.L. Fischer modular stereotaxy system
figure
    mother f.
flicker
    chromatic f.
    f. frequency
    f. fusion
    f. thumb flexion
flicker-fusion point
Flickinger
    formula of F.
flight
    F. Aptitude Rating (FAR)
    f. of color
    f. or fight response
    f. from reality
    f. of ideas (FOI)
    f. into disease
    f. into fantasy
    f. into health
    f. into illness
    topical f.
Flint Infant Security Scale (FISS)
flip angle
flirtatious behavior
flirting and coquetting
FLIT
    Figurative Language Interpretation Test
flittering scotoma
floating-forehead operation
floating transference
floccillation
floccular
flocculation
floccule
flocculonodular
    f. arteriovenous malformation
    f. lobe
    f. node
flocculus, pl. **flocculi**
    accessory f.
    peduncle of f.
flomoxef
flooding
    emotional f.

    imaginal f.
    implosion f.
floor
    temporal fossa f.
floorstand
    CASS digital read-out f.
    Contraves type f.
flopping tremor
floppy
    f. head syndrome
    f. infant syndrome
Florical
florid
    f. episode
    f. symptoms
Florida Kindergarten Screening Battery
floridly
    f. delusional
    f. paranoid
florimania
Flourens
    F. doctrine
    F. theory
flow
    adventitious motor f.
    axoplasmic f.
    blood f.
    cerebral blood f. (CBF)
    f. chart
    collateral blood f.
    cortical microcirulatory f.
    f. cytometry
    f. detection technique
    f. direction
    f. dynamics
    f. effect
    hypothalamic blood f.
    f. imaging
    intraarterial f.
    local cerebral blood f. (LCBF)
    f. misregistration
    regional cerebral blood f. (rCBF)
    f. regulated suction tube
    retrograde blood f.
    spinal cord blood f. (SCBF)
    spinal cord white matter blood f.
    f. theory
    turbulent f.
    f. velocity (FV)
flow-directed embolization
flower
    f. basket of Bochdalek
    butter f.
    passion f.
Flowers Auditory Test of Selective Attention (FATSA)
flower-spray
    f.-s. ending
    f.-s. organ of Ruffini
flow-induced influx effect
flowmeter
    clinical electromagnetic f.
    electromagnetic f.

flowmetry
Doppler f.
laser Doppler f. (LDF)
flow-related enhancement
flow-sensitive MR imaging
FLP
Functional Limitation Profile
FLS
Functional Life Scale
FLTAC
Fisher-Logemann Test of Articulation
Competence
fluanisone
Fluanxol Depot
flucindole
fluconazole
fluctuant
fluctuating
f. affect
f. ego state
f. level of consciousness
f. mood disturbance
fluctuation
attention f.
fluctuations of mood
5-flucytosine
fludiazepam
fludrocortisone
fluency
association f.
associative f.
basal f.
f. disorder
f. disturbance
false f.
intermodal f.
f. shaping therapy
speech f.
f. of thought
word f.
fluent
f. aphasia
f. aphasic seizure
f. aphasic speech
f. paraphasic speech
FLUFTEX gauze roll
fluid
f. ability
f. balance
body f.
cerebrospinal f. (CSF)
coccidioidal complement fixation of
cerebrospinal f.
f. disturbance
endoneurial f.
hypoglycorrhacia of cerebrospinal f.
f. imbalance
f. intake
lighter f.
limulus lysate assay of
cerebrospinal f.
lymphocyte:PMN ratio in
cerebrospinal f.
lymphocytic pleocytosis-depressed
glucose in cerebrospinal f.

mononuclear pleocytosis of
cerebrospinal f.
f. output
f. overload
f. percussion head injury
pleocytosis of cerebrospinal f.
f. retention
f. retention syndrome (FRS)
Sayk preparation of cerebrospinal f.
subglial cerebrospinal f.
Traube-Hering-Mayer waves in
cerebrospinal f.
Tyndall effect seen in
cerebrospinal f.
ventricular f.
xanthochromia of cerebrospinal f.
fluidity
increased platelet membrane f.
fluke infestation
flu-like syndrome
flumazenil
flunarizine
flunitrazepam
fluorescein
intrathecal f.
fluorescent
f. immunophotography
f. treponemal antibody absorption
test (FTA-ABS)
Fluori-Methane Topical Spray
fluorocytosine
fluorodeoxyglucose (FDG)
$[^{18}F]$-labeled f.
positron emission tomography with
$[^{18}F]$-labeled f. (PET-FDG)
fluorodopa
f. positron emission tomographic
scan
f. positron emission tomography
fluorography
pulsed f.
fluorometer
fluorophores
fluoroptic
f. thermometry probe
f. thermometry system
fluoroquinolone
fluoroscopic
f. control
f. imaging
fluoroscopy
C-arm f.
intraoperative lateral f.
fluorosis
5-fluorouracil
fluoxetine hydrochloride
fluoxymesterone
flupentixol
fluphenazine
f. decanoate
f. enanthate
f. hydrochloride
flurazepam hydrochloride
flurbiprofen
Fluro-Ethyl Aerosol

F

flurothyl
fluroxamine maleate
flurry of myoclonic jerks
flush chamber
flushing
    hemifacial f.
Flushmesh
    F. panel
    F. strap
fluspiperone
fluspirilene
flutamide
flutazolam
flutoprazepam
flutter
    alar f.
    ocular f.
fluvoxamine maleate
flux
    microcirculatory red cell f.
fly agaric
Flynn-Aird syndrome
FMAP
    feeding mean arterial pressure
FMD
    foramen magnum decompression
FMF
    familial Mediterranean fever
FMN
    flavin mononucleotide
FMO
    flavin-containing mono-oxygenase
    metabolic system
fMRI, FMRI
    functional magnetic resonance imaging
FMSTB
    Frostig Movement Skills Test Battery
FMT
    fetal mesencephalic tissue
FNA
    Functional Needs Assessment
foam
    f. cell
    gelatin f.
    Ivalon f.
    polyvinyl alcohol f.
FOC
    frequency of contact
focal
    f. ability
    f. brain syndrome
    f. cerebral head injury
    f. conflict theory
    f. contralateral routing of signals
    (FOCALCROS)
    f. cortical dysplasia
    f. degeneration
    f. delta slow wave activity
    f. dysfunction
    f. epilepsy
    f. epileptiform activity
    f. epileptiform discharge
    f. infection
    f. lesion
    f. muscular atrophy

    f. neurological impairment
    f. neurologic deficit
    f. neurologic disturbance
    f. neurologic sign
    f. neuropathy
    f. nonextrapyramidal neurologic
    sign
    f. organic psychosyndrome
    f. pathology
    f. plaquelike defect
    f. psychotherapy
    f. sclerosis
    f. seizure
    f. slowing of background rhythm
    f. status epilepticus
    f. stereotactic injection
    f. suicide
    f. twitch
FOCALCROS
    focal contralateral routing of signals
focality
focalize
focal/lateralized dysfunction
foci
    epileptogenic f.
focus, pl. foci
    anaplastic f.
    f. of anticipated danger
    f. of anxiety
    attention f.
    centrotemporal paroxysmal f.
    characteristic paraphiliac f.
    f. of clinical attention
    f. of delusional system
    densate f.
    epileptic f.
    epileptogenic f.
    f. group
    f. of hemorrhage
    Loyola Sensate F.
    mirror f.
    multiple f.
    paraphiliac f.
    principal f.
    rolandic paroxysmal f.
    sensate f.
    somatic f.
    f. of thought
    unilateral f.
focused
    f. analysis
    f. delirium
    f. expressive therapy
    f. radiation therapy
focus-execute component of attention
focusing mechanism
fodrin
fog
    brain f.
    mental f.
Fogarty embolectomy catheter
fogy, fogey
FOI
    flight of ideas

foible
    human f.
Foix-Alajouanine
    F.-A. disease
    F.-A. myelitis
    F.-A. syndrome
Foix syndrome
folate
    f. deficiency
    serum f.
fold
    nasolabial f.
    neural f.
    polypoid degeneration of true f.
    postsynaptic f.
    f. of Veraguth
foldover
    image f.
Folex PFS
Foley catheter
folia
    cerebellar f.
folia (*pl. of* folium)
folic acid
folie
    f. démonomaniaque
    f. à deux
    f. à double forme
    f. morale
    f. à pleusirs
    f. à trois
folium, pl. **folia**
    folia cerebelli
    f. vermis
folk
    f. illness
    f. medicine
    f. psychiatry
    f. psychology
    soul f.
    f. soul
follicle
    hair f.
follicle-stimulating hormone (FSH)
follicle-stimulating/luteinizing hormone adenoma
follicularis
    alopecia f.
follicular phase
Folling disease
Fölling test
follower
    camp f.
    f. role
following
    f. behavior
    f. gaze
    f. movement
followup
    f. counseling
    f. examination
    f. study
Follow-up Drinker Profile

Folstein
    F. Mini-Mental Scale
    F. Mini-Mental Status Examination
Folz catheter
fomentation
fomepizole
fomes ventriculi
fondle
fondling
fontanel, fontanelle
fonticulus nasofrontalis
food
    f. addict
    f. additive
    f. craving
    f. deprivation
    F. and Drug Administration (FDA)
    f. faddism
    f. habit
    f. intake
    f. intake abnormality
    f. intake disorder
    junk f.
    f. poisoning
    f. preference
    f. satiation
    f. therapy
    tyramine-rich f.
foot
    drop f.
    dropped foot
    f. of hippocampus
foot-drop
footing
    war f.
footplate of the stapes
for
    criteria are not met f.
    criteria have never been met f.
    shoot f.
    vehicle f.
foramen, pl. **foramina**
    arachnoid f.
    Bichat f.
    f. cecum medullae oblongatae
    f. cecum posterius
    cervical neural foramina
    f. of Froesch
    great f.
    greater sciatic f.
    interventricular f.
    f. interventriculare
    jugular f.
    f. of Key-Retzius
    f. lacerum
    f. lateralis ventriculi quarti
    f. of Luschka
    Magendie f.
    f. of Magendie
    f. magnum
    f. magnum cyst
    f. magnum decompression (FMD)
    f. magnum line
    Monro f.
    f. of Monro

F

foramen *(continued)*
    foramina nervosa
    neural f.
    open exit f.
    f. ovale
    parietal f.
    Retzius f.
    f. rotundum
    f. spinosum
    stylomastoid f.
    f. of Vesalius
    Vicq d'Azyr f.
foramina
    emissary f.
foraminal
    f. approach
    f. decompression
    f. encroachment
    f. extraforaminal
    f. herniation
    f. stenosis
foraminotomy
foraminulum, pl. **foraminula**
Forbes-Cori disease
Forbes disease
forbidden impulse
force
    anti-instinctual f.
    f. application
    catabolic f.
    F. 2 CEM generator
    central f.
    deflection f.
    distraction f.
    electromotive f.
    exchange f.
    external f.
    field f.
    fraction maximal voluntary
      contraction f.
    f. of habit
    labor f.
    National Gay Task F. (NGTF)
    nerve f.
    f. nucleus
    outside f.
    psychic f.
    f. transducer
    work f.
forced
    f. alimentation
    f. attitude
    f. choice
    f. choice of recognition test
    f. cross-dressing
    f. cross-gender
    f. fantasy
    f. feeding
    f. grasping reflex
    f. hyperventilation
    f. impulse
    f. laughter
    f. movement
    f. sex

    f. sleep
    f. smile
    f. treatment
    f. vibration
    f. vital capacity (FVC)
    f. whisper
forced-choice span of apprehension task
forceps
    Adson bipolar f.
    Adson-Brown f.
    Adson clip-introducing f.
    Adson cup f.
    Adson dressing f.
    Adson hemostatic f.
    Adson hypophyseal f.
    Adson-Mixter neurosurgical f.
    Adson tissue f.
    alligator cup f.
    f. anterior
    Babcock f.
    bayonet f.
    bipolar bayonet f.
    bipolar coagulating f.
    bipolar electrocautery f.
    bipolar long-shaft f.
    brain clip f.
    brain spatula f.
    brain tumor f.
    Brown-Adson f.
    Cairs hemostatic f.
    Castroviejo eye suture f.
    Cherry-Kerrison laminectomy f.
    Cone skull punch f.
    Cone wire-twisting f.
    contact compressive f.
    cranial rongeur f.
    Crile artery f.
    cup f.
    curved knot-tying f.
    Cushing bayonet f.
    Cushing bipolar f.
    Cushing brain f.
    Cushing dressing f.
    Cushing monopolar f.
    Cushing tissue f.
    Dandy scalp hemostatic f.
    Davis coagulating f.
    Davis monopolar f.
    DeBakey f.
    Decker alligator f.
    Decker microsurgical f.
    DeMartel scalp flap f.
    D'Errico bayonet pituitary f.
    D'Errico hypophyseal f.
    D'Errico pituitary f.
    D'Errico tissue f.
    DeTakats-McKenzie brain clip f.
    DeVilbiss rongeur f.
    dissecting f.
    dressing f.
    dura protecting f.
    ear f.
    Ewald-Hudson f.
    fine-cup f.

fine-tipped up-and-down-angled bipolar f.
Fox bipolar electrocautery f.
Gerald f.
Greenwood bipolar and suction f.
Gruenwald ear f.
Hajek-Koffler bone punch f.
Halsted artery f.
Halsted mosquito f.
Hardy bayonet dressing f.
Hardy microsurgical bayonet bipolar f.
Hardy sella punch f.
Heifetz cup serrated ring f.
hemostatic f.
Hirsch hypophysis punch f.
Housepian f.
Howmedica Microfixation System plate-holding f.
Hudson f.
Hunt angled serrated ring f.
Hunt angled tip f.
Hunt grasping f.
Hunt-Yasargil pituitary f.
Hurd bone-cutting f.
hypophysectomy f.
hypophysial f.
hypophysis punch f.
Ingraham skull punch f.
Jacobson mosquito f.
Jannetta alligator f.
Jannetta bayonet f.
Jansen-Middleton f.
Jansen monopolar f.
Jarell f.
Jarit brain f.
Jarit tendon-pulling f.
Jerald f.
jeweler's bipolar f.
Johnson brain tumor f.
Knight f.
laminectomy punch f.
Leibinger Micro System plate-holding f.
LeRoy scalp clip-applying f.
Love-Gruenwald intervertebral disk f.
Love-Gruenwald pituitary f.
Love-Kerrison rongeur f.
Luc ethmoid f.
MacCarty f.
f. major
Malis angled bayonet f.
Malis irrigation f.
Malis-Jensen micro bipolar f.
Malis jeweler's bipolar f.
McGill f.
McKenzie brain clip f.
McKenzie clip-applying f.
McKenzie clip-bending f.
McKenzie clip-introducing f.
microartery f.
microbipolar f.
microcup f.
microsurgery f.

Micro-Two f.
microvascular f.
Miles punch biopsy f.
f. minor
monopolar tissue f.
mosquito f.
Moynihan f.
Nicola f.
Oldberg pituitary f.
Olivecrona-Toennis clip-applying f.
Péan f.
peapod intervertebral disk f.
pituitary f.
plain f.
f. posterior
Preston ligamentum flavum f.
Raimondi infant scalp hemostatic f.
Raney coagulating f.
Raney rongeur f.
Raney scalp clip-applying f.
Rhoton f.
Rhoton-Cushing f.
Rhoton dissecting f.
Rhoton-Tew bipolar f.
Richter laminectomy punch f.
ringed formed f.
round-handled f.
scalp clip f.
scalp flap f.
Scharff microbipolar and suction f.
Scheicker laminectomy punch f.
Scoville brain clip-applying f.
Scoville brain spatula f.
Scoville clip-applying f.
Scoville spatula f.
sella punch f.
Spencer biopsy f.
spinal perforating f.
sponge-holding f.
straight knot-tying f.
straight line bayonet f.
f. tip
tissue f.
Toennis tumor f.
transsphenoidal bipolar f.
tying f.
Yasargil artery f.
Yasargil bayonet f.
Yasargil clip-applying f.
Yasargil flat serrated ring f.
Yasargil hypophyseal f.
Yasargil knotting f.
Yasargil micro f.
Yasargil tumor f.

forebrain
limbic f.
f. vesicle

foreconscious

forehead
remodeled f.

foreign
f. body
f. body granuloma
f. custom
f. language

foreign *(continued)*
    f. standard
    f. value
Forel
    F. decussation
    fields of F.
    tegmental field of F.
forensic
    f. determination
    f. medicine
    f. pathology
    f. proof
    f. psychiatrist
    f. psychiatry
    f. psychology
    f. setting
forensics
Forer Structured Sentence Completion Test
foresight
Forestier disease
forgetfulness
    benign senescent f.
    senescent f.
forgetting
    intentional f.
    motivated f.
fork
    Hardy 3-prong f.
    f. head gene
    f. head response factor
    Jannetta f.
    Sugita f.
forked tongue
forking of sylvian aqueduct
form
    Adjective Rating F. (ARF)
    California Test of Mental Maturity-Short F. (CTMM-SF)
    Clinical Analysis Questionnaire (Short F.)
    Conners Hyperkinesis Index, Parent F.
    Conners Hyperkinesis Index, Teacher F.
    consent f.'s
    Cornell Word F. (CWF)
    Curtis Completion F.
    f. discrimination
    equivalent f.
    Family Evaluation F. (FEF)
    free f.
    Gifted and Talented Screening F.
    Hamburg Obsessional-Compulsion Inventory-Short F.
    ICP wave f.
    Medical Outcomes Study Short F.-36
    Multiaxial Evaluation Report F.
    f. perception
    Personality Research F. (PRF)
    Policy and Program Information F.
    Premenstrual Assessment F. (PAF)
    Psychiatric Evaluation F. (PEF)

    f.'s of psychodrama
    Readiness Scale - Self Rating and Manager Rating F.'s
    Resident and Staff Information F.
    f. response (F)
    f.'s of satisfactory relating
    thought f.
    trimeric f.
formal
    f. contract
    f. discipline
    f. logic
    f. method
    f. operation
    f. operations period
    f. operations stage
    f. thought disorder
    f. universals
formalized contract
format
    nonaxial f.
    f. treatment
formate
    butyl f.
formatio, pl. **formationes**
    f. hippocampalis
    f. reticularis
formation
    brainstem reticular f.
    Chiari f.
    compromise f.
    concept f.
    ego f.
    gender identity f.
    habit f.
    hemostatic plug f.
    hippocampal f.
    identity f.
    inhibition f.
    leukodystrophy with diffuse Rosenthal fiber f.
    mesencephalic reticular f.
    midbrain reticular f. (MRF)
    mucocele f.
    omen f.
    pathologic character f.
    personality f.
    pontine paramedian reticular f. (PPRF)
    pontine parareticular f. (PPRF)
    reaction f.
    replacement f.
    reticular f.
    reversal f.
    Rosenthal fiber f.
    rouleaux f.
    substitute f.
    symptom f.
    syrinx f.
formboard
forme
    folie à double f.
    f. tardive
formed
    f. image

f. response of colored area (FC)
f. visual hallucination
former identity
formes frustes
formication
formula
Abercrombie neuronal cell count f.
Arthritis Pain F.
Bayer Select Pain Relief F.
empirical f.
Flesch f.
f. of Flickinger
Penn cube function f.
formulary
formulation
American Law Institute F.
cultural f.
psychodynamic f.
fornicate
fornication
forniceal column
fornix, gen. **fornicis**, pl. **fornices**
body of f.
transverse f.
for-profit hospital
Fortaz
forte
Aristocort F.
Citanest F.
Enduronyl F.
Norgesic F.
Parafon F.
Phrenilin F.
Serenid F.
fortification
f. figure
f. scotoma
f. spectrum
Fortis
Mepergan F.
Fortovase
fortune
soldier of f.
forward masking
Fosamax
fosphenytoin
fossa, gen. and pl. **fossae**
f. incudis
infratemporal f.
interpeduncular f.
f. interpeduncularis
lateral f. of brain
lateral cerebral f.
f. lateralis cerebri
middle cranial f.
f. ovalis
posterior f.
posterior pituitary f.
pterygopalatine f.
rhomboid f.
f. rhomboidea
f. of Rosenmüller
sphenoidal f.

f. of Sylvius
temporal f.
fossula, pl. **fossulae**
foster
f. care
f. father
F. Kennedy syndrome
F. Mazes
f. mother
f. parenting
f. placement
fostering
cross f.
FOT
Finger Oscillation Test
Fothergill
F. disease
F. neuralgia
Foundation for Accountability (FaAct)
fountain
f. decussation
F. House
four
F. Factor Index
oriented and alert times f.
F. Picture Test
f. times a day
four-channel Aesculap ventriculoscope
Four-Factor Theory of Etiology
Fourier
F. analysis
F. law
F. pulsatility index
F. spectroscopy
F. synthesis
F. transform
F. transform algorithm
F. transformation zeugmatography
F. transform technique
Fournier test
four-point restraint
four-poster frame
four-repeat isoform
fourth
f. cranial nerve
f. nerve palsy
f. ventricle
four-vessel cerebral angiogram
four-way session
fovea, pl. **foveae**
f. anterior
f. centralis retinae
f. inferior
f. superior
foveal vision
Foville
F. fasciculus
F. syndrome
fowleri
Naegleria f.
Fox bipolar electrocautery forceps
FPA
frontopolar artery
FPDD
familial pure depressive disease

F

FPI
Freiburger Personality Inventory
FPR
fastigial pressor response
Functional Performance Record
FR
fixed ratio
fraction
ejection f.
f. maximal voluntary contraction force
regional oxygen extraction f.
S-phase f.
fractional analysis
fractionated
f. radiotherapy
f. StaRT
fractionation
f. protocol
fractious
fracture
acute f.
articular mass separation f.
atlantal f.
atlas-axis combination f.
atlas burst f.
axial loading f.
axis-atlas combination f.
basal skull f.
basilar skull f.
blow-out f.
burst f.
capillary f.
Chance f.
clay-shoveler f.
closed skull f.
combined flexion-distraction injury and burst f.
comminuted skull f.
complicated f.
compound skull f.
compression f.
f. by contrecoup
cranial f.
depressed skull f.
derby hat f.
diastatic skull f.
direct f.
dishpan f.
f. dislocation
expressed skull f.
facial f.
f. fixation device
growing f.
gutter f.
hairline f.
hangman's f.
indirect f.
Jefferson f.
linear skull f.
low lumbar spine f.
lumbar spine burst f.
lumbosacral junction f.
maxillofacial f.
neurogenic f.

odontoid f.
open skull f.
orbital floor f.
ping-pong f.
pond f.
f. reduction
rib f.
sagittal slice f.
seatbelt f.
sentinel spinous process f.
simple skull f.
skull f.
slice f.
slot f.
spinous process f.
f. stabilization
stellate skull f.
teardrop f.
thoracic spine f.
thoracolumbar burst f.
T8-L3 thoracolumbar burst f.
T11-L5 thoracolumbar burst f.
translational f.
vertebral f.
wedge-compression f.
f. with scoliosis
zygomatic f.
fracture-dislocation
f.-d. reduction
thoracolumbar spine f.-d.
f.-d. with anterior ligament
fragesucht
fragile
f. X chromosome
f. X syndrome
fragility
vascular f.
fragilize
fragment
free f.
proteolytic f.
tangle f.
fragmentary
f. delusion
f. dream image
f. hallucination
f. hallucinations in schizophrenia
f. seizure
fragmentation
f. of ego
f. of nocturnal sleep
f. of thinking
fragmented
f. communication
f. nighttime sleep
f. social network
frailty
frame
analytic f.
Andrews f.
Brown-Roberts-Wells head f.
Budde-Greenberg-Sugita stereotactic head f.
CHOP f.

Cor-Tech guidance to stereotatic
head f.
Cosman-Roberts-Wells stereotactic f.
couch-mounted head f.
CRW base f.
CRW head f.
DeBastiani f.
designs for vision f.
Elekta stereotactic head f.
f. fixation-scanner assisted target
localization
four-poster f.
gNomos head f.
Greenberg retractor f.
head f.
Horsley-Clarke stereotactic f. (HCF)
Komai stereotactic head f.
Laitinen stereoguide 2000 arc-
centered stereotactic f.
Laitinen stereotactic head f.
Leksell-Elekta stereotactic f.
Leksell Model G stereotactic f.
Leksell stereotactic f.
Lex-Ton spinal f.
Mayfield fixation f.
Mussen f.
OBT stereotactic f.
Olivier-Bertrand-Talairach stereotactic
head f.
Olivier-Bertrand-Tipal f.
operative wedge f.
Patil stereotactic head f.
Pelorus stereotactic f.
Radionics CRW stereotactic head f.
f. of reference
Reichert-Mundinger-Fischer
stereotactic head f.
Reichert-Mundinger stereotactic
head f.
Relton-Hall f.
self-retaining brain retractor f.
stereotactic f.
f. stereotaxy
Stryker f.
Sugita multipurpose head f.
Talairach stereotactic f.
Todd-Wells stereotactic f.
Wilson f.
ZD f.
frameless
f. and armless stereotactic
neuronavigation
f. stereotactic technique
Framingham Heart Study
franca
lingua f.
Franceschetti syndrome
**Franck Drawing Completion Test
(FDCT)**
francomania
francophile
francophobia
frank
f. delirium
f. disk herniation
f. lesion
f. psychotic symptoms
**Fränkel classification of spinal cord
injury**
Frankel scale
Frankenhäuser ganglion
Frankenstein factor
Frankfurt Questionnaire of Complaints
frataxin gene PCR
fraternal twin
fraternize
fratricide
frayed disk
Frazier
F. brain-exploring cannula
F. brain trocar
F. cordotomy knife
F. dural elevator
F. dural guide
F. dural hook
F. dural scissors
F. dural separator
F. laminectomy retractor
F. lighted brain retractor
F. nerve hook
F. pituitary knife
F. stylet
F. suction tip
F. suction tube
F. ventricular cannula
F. ventricular needle
Frazier-Spiller
F.-S. operation
F.-S. rhizotomy
FRC
functional residual capacity
freaked out
freckling
inguinal f.
free
f. access to process
f. association
f. bone flap
F. and Cued Selective Reminding
Task
fancy f.
f. field room
f. form
f. fragment
f. fragment disk
f. induction decay (FID)
f. induction signal
f. living
f. nerve ending
f. play
f. radical
f. radical homeostasis
f. radical scavenger
f. radical scavenging mechanism
f. recall
f. recall bias
f. rein
f. response
symptom f.
f. will

F

free-access environment
freebase
    cocaine f.
freeborn
freedom
    f. to choose
    degree of f.
    escape from f.
    F. from Distractibility Deviation
      Quotient (FDDQ)
    loss of f.
free-floating
    f.-f. anxiety
    f.-f. attention
    f.-f. fear
Freehand neuroprosthetic system
Freeman Anxiety Neurosis and
  Psychosomatic Test (FANPT)
Freer
    F. chisel
    F. dissector
    F. septal elevator
Freer-Swanson ganglion knife
freeze-dried cadaveric dura
freezing
    f. behavior
    f. of movement
    f. phenomenon
Fregoli
    F. phenomenon
    F. syndrome
Freiberg
    F. craniotome
    F. so-called infarction
Freiberg-Kohler disease
Freiburger Personality Inventory (FPI)
Frenactil
French
    F. blue
    F. brain retractor
    F. catheter
    F. leave
    F. polio
    F. rod bender
Frenchay
    F. Activities Index
    F. Aphasia Screening Test (FAST)
    F. Dysarthria Assessment
freneticism
Frenkel
    F. movement
    F. symptom
frenula
    buccal f.
    multiple buccal f.
frenulum, pl. frenula
    f. cerebelli
    f. of Giacomini
    f. of superior medullary velum
    f. veli medullaris superius
Frenzel glasses
frequency (f)
    f. aliasing
    alpha f.

angular f.
f. of anxiety
band f.
f. combination
f. of contact (FOC)
critical flicker f.
disease f.
f. dispersion curve
f. distribution
f. disturbance
dominant waking f.
f. encoding
f. encountered association
f. error
expected f.
flicker f.
gene f.
high-filter f. (HFF)
f. jitter
Larmor f.
law of f.
low-filter f. (LFF)
low linear f.
f. masking
Nyquist f.
offset f.
f. offset
precessional f.
f. range
relative f.
resonant f.
f. response
seizure f. (SF)
f. shift
spatial f.
f. of treatment
f. of violent act
waking f.
frequency-encoding gradient
frequent derailment
Fresnel
    F. paste-on prism
    F. prism
Freud
    F. cathartic method
    F. syndrome
    F. theory
    F. view of depressive disorder
freudian
    f. approach
    f. censor
    f. fixation
    f. psychoanalysis
    f. psychotherapy
    f. slip
    f. theory
    f. theory of personality
freudian-free association
Freund adjuvant
Frey
    F. irritation hair
    F. syndrome
friable artery
fricative

Friedmann
    F. complex
    F. disease
Friedreich
    F. ataxia
    F. disease
friend
    fair-weather f.
    false f.
friendliness
    active f.
    attitude of active f.
friendship
    f. model
    platonic f.
frightening stimulus
frigidity
    sexual f.
frigophobia
fringe
    f. of consciousness
    subliminal f.
fringing field
frippery
frise
    chevaux de f.
Frisin
Frisium
Froesch
    foramen of F.
Fröhlich syndrome
Frohman factor
Frohse
    arcade of F.
Froin syndrome
Froment sign
frontal
    f. abasia
    f. abscess
    anterior f. (AF)
    f. area
    f. artery
    f. convexity meningioma
    f. cortex
    f. corticectomy
    f. craniotomy
    f. dysequilibrium
    f. eye field (FEF)
    f. gait disorder
    f. groove
    f. gyrectomy
    f. gyrus
    f. headache
    f. horn
    f. interhemispheric space
    f. intermittent rhythmic delta
      activity (FIRDA)
    f. intermittent rhythmic delta
      activity on EEG
    f. lobe
    f. lobe dementia
    f. lobe dysfunction
    f. lobe epilepsy
    f. lobe infarction

    f. lobe interstitial neuron
    f. lobe lesion
    f. lobe neuronal density
    f. lobe syndrome
    f. lobotomy
    f. neoplasm
    f. operculum
    f. perceptual disorder
    f. phosphocreatinine
    f. plane
    f. plane growth abnormality
    f. polar branch
    f. pole
    f. release sign
    f. sulcus
    f. upswap
frontalis
    alopecia liminaris f.
frontal-lobe abstraction/problem solving
frontocortical aphasia
frontoethmoidal encephalocele
frontolenticular aphasia
frontonasomaxillary osteotomy
frontooccipital fasciculus
frontoorbital
    f. advancement
    f. area
    f. osteotomy
frontoparietal
    ascending f. (ASFP)
    f. convexity cyst
    f. operculum
frontopolar
    f. artery (FPA)
    f. lead
frontopontine tract
frontopontocerebellar pathway
frontosphenoidal encephalocele
frontostriatal-pallidalo-thalamic circuit
frontosubcortical dementia
frontotemporal
    f. approach
    f. brain atrophy
    f. craniotomy
    f. hypometabolism
    f. tract
frontotemporoparietal craniotomy
frontothalamic circuit
front-tap reflex
Froriep ganglion
frost anesthesia
Frostig
    F. Developmental Test of Visual
      Perception (FDTVP)
    F. Movement Skills Test Battery
      (FMSTB)
Frostig-Horne training program
Frost Self-Description Questionnaire
  (FSDQ)
frotteurism paraphilia
frovatriptan
frozen
    f. section
    f. watchfulness

F

FRS
first rank symptom
fluid retention syndrome
FRT
Family Relations Test
frucosidosis
fruition
frustes
formes f.
frustration
control f.
f. dream
level of f.
f. response
f. tolerance
frustration-aggression hypothesis
FS
fire setter
FSDQ
Frost Self-Description Questionnaire
FSH
facioscapulohumeral
follicle-stimulating hormone
FSH dystrophy
FSI
Functional Status Index
FSIQ
Full-Scale Intelligence Quotient
Full Scale IQ
FSQ
Functional Status Questionnaire
FSS
Fear Survey Schedule
Functional Systems Scale
FSST
Full-Scale Score Total
FTA-ABS
fluorescent treponemal antibody
absorption test
FTEQ
Functional Time Estimation
Questionnaire
FTS
Family Tracking System
FTT
failure to thrive
fucosidosis
fuddle
Fuerstner disease
fugax
amaurosis f.
amaurosis partialis f.
proctalgia f.
fugitive
fugue
dissociative f.
epileptic f.
hysterical f.
poriomanic f.
psychogenic f.
psychotic f.
f. state
Fujita suction cannula

Fukushima
F. cavernous bypass
F. monopolar malleable coagulator
Fukuyama
F. congenital muscular dystrophy
F. disease
Fuld
F. Object-Memory Evaluation
F. Object Memory Test
fulfill
failure to f.
fulfillment
asymptotic wish f.
wish f.
fulgurating migraine
full
f. blood
f. interepisode recovery
f. relapse
F. Scale Broad Cognitive Ability
F. Scale IQ (FSIQ)
F. Scale IQ score
f. symptom criterion
f. wakefulness
full-blown
f.-b. delirium
f.-b. panic attack
Fullerton Language Test for Adolescents
Full-Scale
F.-S. Intelligence Quotient (FSIQ)
F.-S. Score Total (FSST)
fully organized belief
fulminant
f. hepatic encephalopathy
f. hydrocephalus
f. necrotizing encephalitis
fulminating anoxia
Fulton laminectomy rongeur
fulvius
antivenin (*Micrur f.*)
fumarate
quetiapine f.
fumigatus
Aspergillus f.
function
affective f.
allomeric f.
arousal f.
autonomous ego f.
bowel f.
brainstem f.
caloric stimulation test for
vestibular f.
cerebral cortical f.
cognitive f.
communicative f.
f. complex
compromised f.
concept of brain f.
conflict-free f.
cortical mapping of memory f.
day-to-day f.
deteriorating f.
differential f.

diffuse f.
discrepant intellectual f.
dream f.
ego f.
f. engram
executant ego f.
executive ego f.
existential ego f.
expressive f.
gnostic f.
granulopoietic f.
harmonic f.
hepatic f.
higher cortical f.
higher intellectual f. (HIF)
higher level cognitive f.
immune f.
impaired f.
impairment of cognitive f.
inability to f.
indolamine f.
integrated f.
integrity of brain f.
intellectual f.
intrapsychical f.
inverted-U f.
isomeric f.
language f.
Legendre f.
localization of f.
localized f.
LSUMC classification of motor
  and sensory f.
maintenance f.
mapping of cortical f.
marginal f.
mediated f.
mental f.
motor f.
neurobehavioral f.
neuroendocrine f.
occupational f.
parathyroid f.
performance-intensity f.
personal f.
phasic f.
f. pleasure
premorbid intellectual f.
primary autonomous f.
psychophysical f.
psychosocial f.
receptive f.
recovery of f.
referential f.
role f.
secretory f.
semi-autonomous systems concept
  of brain f.
semiotic f.
sensory f.
seriatim f.
social f.
spectral density f.
spiritual f.
splinter f.

subaverage academic f.
symbolic f.
synthetic f.
vestibular f.
vicarious f.
f. word
functional
f. activation PET scanning
f. activity
f. age
f. aid
f. ailment
F. Ambulation Categories (FAC)
f. anosmia
f. aphasia
f. aphonia
f. apoplexy
f. assessment
F. Assessment Inventory
f. assessment stage
f. asymmetry
f. autonomy
f. blindness
f. bradykinesia
f. brain imaging
f. budgeting
F. Communication Profile (FCP)
f. conformance
f. contracture
f. deafness
f. death
f. disability
f. disease
f. disorder
f. distance
f. dysfunction
f. dyspareunia
f. dyspareunia psychosexual
  dysfunction
f. dyspnea
f. electrical stimulation (FES)
f. encopresis
f. enuresis
F. Ergonomic Prolo Scale
f. fixedness
f. gain testing
f. headache
f. illiteracy
f. illiterate
f. illness
f. impairment
f. impotence
f. incapacity
F. Independence Measure (FIM)
f. invariant
f. irritation
f. leadership
F. Life Scale (FLS)
f. limitation
F. Limitation Profile (FLP)
f. loss
f. magnetic resonance imaging
  (fMRI, FMRI)
f. movement
F. Needs Assessment (FNA)

F

functional *(continued)*
 f. neuroimaging
 f. neurosis
 f. neurosurgery
 f. pain
 f. pathology
 F. Performance Record (FPR)
 f. plasticity
 F. Pragmatic Procedure
 f. psychology
 f. psychosis
 f. relatedness
 f. residual capacity (FRC)
 f. shift
 f. skill
 f. spasm
 F. Status Index (FSI)
 F. Status Questionnaire (FSQ)
 f. stereotaxy
 f. superego structure
 f. symbolism
 F. Systems Scale (FSS)
 f. terminal innervation ratio
 F. Time Estimation Questionnaire
  (FTEQ)
 f. type
 f. unity
 f. vaginismus
 f. vaginismus psychosexual
  dysfunction
functionally impaired
functioning
 anxiety-induced impaired social f.
 body f.
 borderline intellectual f.
 competent, optimal relational f.
 competent relational f.
 Comprehensive Test of Visual F.
  (CTVF)
 decline in academic f.
 f. deterioration
 disrupted, dysfunctional relational f.
 disruptive family f.
 f. disturbance
 dysfunctional relational f.
 educational f.
 executive f.
 general intellectual f.
 Global Assessment of F. (GAF)
 Global Assessment of Relational F.
  (GARF)
 good f.
 grossly impaired f.
 hierarchical f.
 impaired cognitive f.
 impaired social f.
 impairment in cognitive f.
 independent f.
 intellectual subaverage f.
 interepisode f.
 interpersonal f.
 f. level
 level of intellectual f.
 major impairment of f.

 marked decline in academic f.
 McMaster Structured Interview of
  Family F.
 neurological f.
 normal neurological f.
 optimal relational f.
 personality f.
 premorbid level of f.
 Process for the Assessment of
  Effective Student F.
 psychosocial f.
 quality of sexual f.
 receptor f.
 school f.
 sensory f.
 sexual f.
 social f.
 social-emotional f.
 subaverage academic f.
 subaverage intellectual f.
 superior f.
 unequivocal change in f.
 vasculogenic loss of erectile f.
 vocational f.
 voluntary motor f.
 voluntary sensory f.
fund
 f. of information
 f. of information test
 f. of intelligence
 f. of knowledge
fundamental
 f. approach
 f. attribution error
 F. Interpersonal Relations
  Orientation-Behavior (FIRO-B)
 F. Interpersonal Relations
  Orientation-Feelings (FIRO-F)
 f. response process
 f. rule of psychoanalysis
 f. social impulse
 f. symptom
 f. tone
 f. wish
fundamentals
 Clinical Evaluation of
  Language F.-Revised
fundus of aneurysm
fungal infection
fungus, pl. fungi
 f. cerebri
funicular
 f. graft
 f. myelitis
 f. myelosis
funiculitis
funiculus, pl. funiculi
 anterior f.
 f. anterior
 cuneate f.
 dorsal f.
 f. dorsalis
 f. gracilis
 f. lateralis
 lateral f. of spinal cord

funiculi medullae spinalis
f. posterior
posterior f.
f. separans
f. solitarius
f. teres
Funkenstein test
funnel
pial f.
furifosmin
technetium 99m f.
furlough psychosis
furor
epileptic f.
f. epilepticus
furosemide
furthest-neighbor analysis
Fused Rhymed Dichotic Words Test
fusiform
f. aneurysm
f. cell of cerebral cortex
f. gyrus
f. layer
fusimotor
fusion
Adkins spinal f.
Albee lumbar spinal f.
anterior cervical f. (ACF)
anterior cervical discectomy and f.
anterior interbody f.
anterior lumbar spine interbody f.
atlantoaxial f.
Bailey-Badgley cervical spine f.
Bosworth spinal f.
Brooks cervical f.
Brooks-Jenkins atlantoaxial f.
cervical spine posterior f.
cervicooccipital f.
Cloward back f.
degenerative lumbar spine f.
degenerative spondylosis
  decompression and f.
faculty f.
f. faculty
flicker f.
Gallie cervical f.
Gallie spinal f.
Goldstein spinal f.
Harris-Smith cervical f.
Henry-Geist spinal f.
Hibbs-Jones spinal f.
instinctual f.
interbody f.

interfacet wiring and f.
f. limit determination
long segment spinal f.
lower cervical spine f.
lumbar interbody f.
lumbar spinal f.
lumbosacral f.
f. nonunion rate
occipitoatlantoaxial f.
occipitocervical f.
posterior-interbody lumbar spinal f.
posterior-lateral lumbar spinal f.
posterior lumbar interbody f.
  (PLIF)
posterior spinal f.
posterolateral lumbosacral f.
Robinson anterior cervical f.
sacral spine f.
selective thoracic spine f.
short segment spinal f.
Simmons cervical spine f.
single-level spinal f.
in situ spinal f.
spinal f.
f. state
f. stiffness
f. technique
telencephalic f.
thoracic spinal f.
unity and f.
upper cervical spine f.
variable stereotactic image f.
vertebral f.
Wiltberger f.
fustigate
futile cycling
futility
medical f.
futural outlook
future
f. danger
f. misfortune
f. pace
f. shock
futuristic thinking
futurology
FV
flow velocity
FVC
forced vital capacity
F-wave test
F-zero

F

γ (*var. of* gamma)
G
   G factor
   G protein
   G protein abnormality
   G response including entire inkblot
G5
   G5 Fleximatic massage/percussion
      unit
   G5 Vibramatic massage/percussion
      unit
GA
   Gamblers Anonymous
Gaab endoscope
GABA
   gamma aminobutyric acid
      hydroxyl derivative of GABA
         (Gabob)
      GABA receptor complex
      GABA transaminase (GABA-T)
gabapentin
   g. capsule
GABA-T
   GABA transaminase
GABHS
   group A β-hemolytic streptococcus
Gabitril
Gabob
   hydroxyl derivative of GABA
GAD
   generalized anxiety disorder
   glutamate decarboxylase
gadodiamide
gadolinium
   g. contrast
   g. diethylenetriamine-penta-acetate
   g. diethylenetriamine penta-acetic
      acid (Gd-DTPA)
   g. DTPA
   g. enhancement
gadolinium-diethylenetriamine penta-
   acetic acid-enhanced MR
gadolinium-enhanced
   g.-e. MRI
   g.-e. MR imaging
gadopentetate dimeglumine
gadoteridol
GAF
   Global Assessment of Functioning
   GAF scale
   GAF scale
gag
   Dingman mouth g.
   g. reflex
   g. reflex loss
Gagel granuloma
GAI
   guided affective imagery
gain
   desire for personal g.
   epinosic g.
   expected weight g.

material g.
paranosic g.
peak acoustic g.
primary g.
secondary g.
tertiary g.
weight g.
gainfully employed
gain-loss theory of attraction
gain-of-function abnormality
Gairdner disease
gait
   abnormal g.
   g. abnormality
   G. Abnormality Rating Scale
      (GARS)
   g. analysis
   antalgic g.
   g. apraxia
   ataxic g.
   cerebellar g.
   cerebral g.
   Charcot g.
   g. disorder
   g. disorder, autoantibody, late-age
      onset, polyneuropathy (GALOP)
   g. disturbance
   dromedary g.
   equine g.
   festinating g.
   halting g.
   helicopod g.
   hemiplegic g.
   high steppage g.
   hysterical g.
   narrow-based g.
   parkinsonian g.
   g. problem
   retropulsion of g.
   scissor g.
   shuffling g.
   slowed g.
   spastic g.
   staggering g.
   steady g.
   steppage g.
   stuttering g.
   g. stuttering
   swaying g.
   uncoordinated g.
   unsteady g.
   waddling g.
   wide-based g.
galactorrhea
galactose
galactosemia
galactosidase defect
galactosylceramide lipidosis
galanin
galanthamine
Galant reflex

G

Galassi
  G. classification system
  G. pupillary phenomenon
galea
  g. aponeurotica
  closed g.
galeanthropy
galeatomy
Galen
  G. anastomosis
  G. nerve
  vein of G.
galenic medicine
Galen-vein malformation
galeophobia (*var. of* felinophobia)
Galgenhumor
gallamine triethiodide
Gall craniology
galli
  crista g.
Gallie
  G. cervical fusion
  G. spinal fusion
  G. wiring technique
Gallie-Rodgers technique
gallium
  g. nitrate
  g. scan
gallium-67
gallivant
gallomania
gallophobia
gallows humor
GALOP
  gait disorder, autoantibody, late-age
    onset, polyneuropathy
Galtac device
Galton law of regression
Galt skull trephine
galvanic
  g. skin reaction
  g. skin reflex
  g. skin resistance
  g. skin response (GSR)
  g. skin response biofeedback
  g. vertigo
galvanometer
galvanotropism
Galveston
  G. fixation
  G. fixation with TSRH crosslink
  G. Orientation and Awareness Test
    (GOAT)
GAMA
  General Ability Measure for Adults
Gambian trypanosomiasis
Gambierdiscus toxicus
Gamblers Anonymous (GA)
gambling
  g. addict
  g. behavior
  binge g.
  compulsive g.
  pathologic g.
  professional g.

  social g.
  g. strategy
game
  experimental g.
  hallucinatory g.
  language g.
  middle g.
  mixed motive g.
  model g.
  g. plan
  play the g.
  g. playing
  psychological g.
  g. theory
games people play
gamete
gametophobia
gamine
gamma, γ
  g. alcoholism
  g. aminobutyric acid (GABA)
  g. carboxylated protein
  g. efferent
  g. efferent system
  g. fiber
  g. globulin
  g. glutamyl transpeptidase (GGT)
  g. hydroxybutyrate (GHB)
  g. hydroxybutyrate and
    amphetamines
  g. hypothesis
  g. irradiation
  g. knife
  G. knife instrument
  g. knife radiosurgery
  g. linolenic acid
  g. loop
  G. Maxicamera
  g. motor neuron
  g. motor system
  g. movement
  g. ray
  g. thalamotomy
  g. wave
gamma-acetylenic-GABA
gammacism
gamma-glutamyltransferase (GGT)
gamma-hydroxybutyrate
gamma-interferon treatment
gamma-vinyl-GABA
gammopathy
  monoclonal g.
gamomania
gamophobia
ganaxolone
ganciclovir
gang
  g. behavior
  g. fight
  g. rape
  street g.
  g. war
  g. warfare
ganglia (*pl. of* ganglion)
gangliectomy

gangliitis
gangliocyte
gangliocytoma
    dysplastic g.
    sellar g.
ganglioglioma
    desmoplastic infantile g.
    infantile g.
ganglioglioneurocytoma
gangliolysis
    percutaneous radiofrequency g.
ganglioma
    intracerebral g.
ganglion, pl. ganglia, ganglions
    aberrant g.
    acousticofacial g.
    Andersch g.
    aorticorenal ganglia
    ganglia aorticorenalia
    Arnold g.
    auditory g.
    Auerbach ganglia
    auricular g.
    autonomic g.
    ganglia of autonomic plexuses
    basal ganglia
    Bezold g.
    Bochdalek g.
    Bock g.
    Böttcher g.
    calcification of the basal g.
    cardiac ganglia
    ganglia cardiaca
    carotid g.
    celiac ganglia
    ganglia celiaca
    g. cell
    g. cervicale inferius
    g. cervicale medium
    g. cervicale superius
    cervicothoracic g.
    g. cervicothoracicum
    g. ciliare
    ciliary g.
    coccygeal g.
    Corti g.
    dorsal root g. (DRG)
    Ehrenritter g.
    g. extracraniale
    g. of facial nerve
    Frankenhäuser g.
    Froriep g.
    gasserian g.
    geniculate g.
    g. geniculi
    Gudden g.
    g. habenulae
    g. hook
    hypogastric ganglia
    g. impar
    inferior cervical g.
    inferior g. of glossopharyngeal
      nerve
    inferior mesenteric g.
    inferior g. of vagus

    g. inferius nervi glossopharyngei
    g. inferius nervi vagi
    intercrural g.
    ganglia intermedia
    intermediate ganglia
    g. of intermediate nerve
    interpeduncular g.
    intervertebral g.
    intracranial g.
    g. isthmi
    jugular g.
    Laumonier g.
    Lee g.
    lenticular g.
    Lobstein g.
    Ludwig g.
    ganglia lumbalia
    lumbar ganglia
    marbled appearance of basal g.
    Meckel g.
    g. mesentericum inferius
    g. mesentericum superius
    middle cervical g.
    nasal g.
    nerve g.
    neural g.
    nodose g.
    otic g.
    g. oticum
    parasympathetic ganglia
    paravertebral ganglia
    pelvic ganglia
    ganglia pelvina
    petrosal g.
    petrous g.
    phrenic ganglia
    ganglia phrenica
    ganglia plexuum autonomicorum
    posterior root g.
    prevertebral ganglia
    pterygopalatine g.
    g. pterygopalatinum
    radiocapitellar joint g.
    Remak ganglia
    renal ganglia
    ganglia renalia
    Ribes g.
    sacral ganglia
    ganglia sacralia
    Scarpa g.
    Schacher g.
    semilunar g.
    sensory g.
    Soemmering g.
    solar ganglia
    sphenopalatine g.
    spinal g.
    g. spinale
    spiral g. of cochlea
    g. spirale cochleae
    splanchnic g.
    g. splanchnicum
    stellate g.
    g. stellatum
    sublingual g.

G

ganglion (*continued*)
    g. sublinguale
    submandibular g.
    g. submandibulare
    submaxillary g.
    superior cervical g.
    superior g. of glossopharyngeal
     nerve
    superior mesenteric g.
    superior g. of the vagus nerve
    g. superius nervi glossopharyngei
    g. superius nervi vagi
    sympathetic ganglia
    ganglia of sympathetic trunk
    terminal g.
    g. terminale
    thoracic ganglia
    ganglia thoracica
    trigeminal g.
    g. trigeminale
    ganglia trunci sympathici
    g. of trunk of vagus
    tympanic g.
    g. tympanicum
    Valentin g.
    vertebral g.
    g. vertebrale
    vestibular g.
    g. vestibulare
    Vieussens g.
    Walther g.
    Wrisberg ganglia
ganglionectomy
    Meckel sphenopalatine g.
    sphenopalatine g.
    superior cervical g.
ganglioneuritis
ganglioneuroblastoma
ganglioneurocytoma
ganglioneuroma
    central g.
    dumbbell g.
ganglioneuromatosis
ganglionic
    g. blocking agent
    g. crest
    g. cyst in synovial tendon sheath
    g. layer of cerebellar cortex
    g. layer of cerebral cortex
    g. layer of optic nerve
    g. layer of retina
    g. motor neuron
ganglionitis
ganglionostomy
ganglions (*pl. of* ganglion)
ganglioplegic
ganglioradiculitis
ganglioside
    disialyl g.
    GM-1 g.
    g. lipidosis
    g. monosialic acid
gangliosidosis
    G_{M1} g., GM_1 g.

    G_{M2} g., GM_2 g.
    generalized g.
gangrene
    trophic g.
Gann Act
GANS
    granulomatous angiitis of the central
     nervous system
Ganser
    G. commissure
    nucleus basalis of G.
    G. syndrome
gantry rotation
GAP
    Gardner Analysis of Personality Survey
    growth-associated protein
gap
    air-bone g.
    generation g.
    g. junction
    memory g.
GAPS
    Guidelines for Adolescent Preventive
    Services
Garamycin
Garcin syndrome
Gardner
    G. Analysis of Personality Survey
     (GAP)
    G. headholder
    G. meningocele repair
    G. neurosurgical skull clamp
    G. operation
    G. and Robertson classification
     system
    G. syndrome
Gardner-Wells
    G.-W. headrest
    G.-W. tongs
GARF
    Global Assessment of Relational
    Functioning
    GARF scale
gargoylism
Garrett orientation line
garrulous affect
GARS
    Gait Abnormality Rating Scale
GAS
    general adaptation syndrome
    Global Assessment Scale
    Goal Attainment Scale
gas
    g. chamber
    g. chromatography mass
     spectrometry
    nerve g.
    g. poisoning
    tear g.
    war g.
Ga scintigraphy
Gaskell nerve
gasoline intoxication
gasper

gasserian
    g. ganglion
    g. ganglion area
    g. ganglion neuroma
gastric
    g. bypass
    g. crisis
    g. lavage
    g. neurasthenia
    g. psychogenic disorder
    g. tetany
    g. vertigo
gastrica
    tetania g.
gastrin
gastrin-inhibiting peptide
gastritis
    alcoholic g.
    nervous g.
gastrocolic reflex
gastroenteritis
Gastrografin
gastroileac reflex
gastrointestinal
    g. disorder
    g. functional psychogenic
    g. symptom grouping
    G. Symptom Rating Scale
gastroparalysis
gastroparesis
gastropath
gastroplasty
gastrostomy
gastrostomy/jejunostomy
Gastrozepine
GAT
    Gerontological Apperception Test
    group adjustment therapy
GATB
    General Aptitude Test Battery
gate
    g. theory
    g. theory of pain
gate-control
    g.-c. hypothesis
    g.-c. theory
Gates-MacGinitie Reading Test
Gates-McKillop-Horowitz Reading Diagnostic Test
gateway drug
gathering
    injustice g.
gating
    cardiac g.
    g. mechanism
    g. theory
gatophobia (*var. of* felinophobia)
Gaucher disease
gauge
    20-g. catheter
    Durkan CTS g.
    Padgett baseline pinch g.
    pressure g.
    strain g.
Gault decision

gauntlet anesthesia
gauss
gaussian
    g. curve
    g. distribution
    g. noise
gavage
gay
    g. liberation
    g. rights
gayness
gaze
    cardinal directions of g.
    conjugate fixed g.
    conjugate horizontal g.
    consensual g.
    g. coordinating aggregate
    g. deficit
    down g.
    dysconjugate g.
    dysjunctive g.
    field of g.
    g. fixation
    fixed g.
    following g.
    horizontal g.
    g. impairment
    ipsilateral tonic conjugate g.
    lateral g.
    g. mechanism in brain stem
    g. palsy
    g. paralysis
    g. paresis
    ping-pong g.
    g. pontine center
    g. preference
    g. refixational shift
    restriction of inward g.
    spasticity of conjugate g.
    tense g.
    vertical g.
gaze-evoked
    g.-e. nystagmus
    g.-e. visual loss
gaze-paretic nystagmus
gazing
    crystal g.
GBCE
    Grassi Basic Cognitive Evaluation
GBM
    glioblastoma multiforme
GBS
    group B streptococcus
    Guillain-Barré syndrome
GC
    gonococcus
GCDAS
    Gesell Child Development Age Scale
GCI
    General Cognitive Index
GCS
    Generalized Contentment Scale
    Glasgow Coma Scale
GCT
    General Clerical Test

G

GCTSPS
germ-cell tumor with synchronous lesions in pineal and suprasellar region
GDC
Guglielmi detachable coil
Gd-DTPA
gadolinium diethylenetriamine penta-acetic acid
Gd-DTPA-enhanced cranial MR imaging
GDNF
glial-cell-line derived neurotrophic factor
GDP
guanosine diphosphate
GDS
Global Deterioration Scale
G-D syndrome
gearshift probe
GE 9800 CT system
GEFT
Group Embedded Figures Test
gegenhalten
GEI
Grief Experience Inventory
Geigel reflex
gel
Dermaflex G.
diazepam rectal g.
H.P. Acthar G.
Tac g. for EMS unit
Tac g. for TENS unit
gelasmus
gelastic epilepsy
gelatin
g. foam
g. phantom
g. sponge
gelatinous
g. hematoma
g. substance
Gelfoam
fibrin glue-soaked G.
G. pad
papaverine-soaked G.
G. pledget
G. powder emboli
thrombin-soaked G.
Gélineau syndrome
Gellman instrumentation
gelotripsy
Gelpi retractor
Gelpirin
Gelusil
gemästete cell
gemistocyte
gemistocytic
g. astrocyte
g. astrocytoma
g. cell
g. reaction
gemistocytoma
gemmule
Gemnisyn
Gemonil
Genahist Oral
Genapap

Gencalc 600
gender
g. ambiguity psychosis
appropriate in g.
boundaries and g.
g. confusion
g. difference
g. difference psychiatric syndrome
g. differences in anxiety
g. discrimination
g. dysphoria
g. dysphoria syndrome
g. feature
g. identification
g. identity
g. identity board
g. identity confusion
g. identity disorder (GID)
g. identity disorder in adolescence
g. identity disorder of adulthood
g. identity disorder in adults
g. identity disorder of childhood
g. identity disorder in children
g. identity formation
g. identity psychosexual development
multiple personality and g.
g. orientation
personality and g.
g. reassignment
g. role
g. role persistent discomfort
gender-based attitude
gender-sensitive psychopharmacology
gender-specific feature
gene
aberrant g.
amyloid precursor protein g.
autosomal dominant g.
c-fos g.
c-jun g.
DMD g.
dominant g.
elastin g.
enzyme g.
fork head g.
g. frequency
growth arrest-specific g.
hedgehog g.
homeodomain g.
homeotic g.
housekeeping g.
Hox g.
immediate early g.
inverse polymerase chain reaction-based detection of frataxin g.
leucine zipper g.
LIM-kinase g.
low penetrance-high frequency g.
g. marker
g. mutation
myotonic dystrophy g.
p53 g.
persenilin g.
polypeptide hormone g.

g. pool
potassium channel g.
g. product
recessive g.
retinoblastoma g.
g. splicing
g. therapy
g. therapy immunoconjugate
tumor suppressor g.
zinc-finger g.

genealogy
genera (*pl. of* genus)
general
G. Ability Measure for Adults (GAMA)
g. adaptation reaction
g. adaptation syndrome (GAS)
G. Aptitude Test Battery (GATB)
G. Clerical Test (GCT)
G. Cognitive Index (GCI)
G. Electric CT 9800 scanner
G. Electric Hispeed Advantage helical scanner
G. Electric signa 1.5-Tesla magnetic resonance scanner
g. endotracheal anesthesia
g. factor
G. Health Questionnaire (GHQ)
G. High Altitude Questionnaire (GHAG, GHAQ)
g. image
G. Inquiry (GI)
g. intellectual functioning
g. language disability
g. learning ability
g. medical condition (GMC)
g. medical etiology
g. medical/surgical population
g. orotracheal anesthesia
g. paralysis
g. paralysis of the insane (GPI)
g. paresis
g. paresis of the insane
g. personality assessment
g. population
g. relaxation training
g. semantics
g. somatic afferent column
g. somatic efferent column
g. stress sensitivity
g. systems theory
g. transfer
g. will
generalist
generalities
glittering g.
generalization
g. gradient
g. response
stimulus g.
transfer by g.
verbal g.
generalized
g. amnesia
g. anxiety

g. anxiety disorder (GAD)
g. anxiety neurosis
g. auditory agnosia
G. Contentment Scale (GCS)
g. flexion epilepsy
g. gangliosidosis
g. headache
g. hyperreflexia
g. intellectual impairment
g. neurotic anxiety state
g. periodic sharp wave
g. polyneuropathy
g. pruritus
g. sexual dysfunction
g. tetanus
g. tonic clonic (GTC)
g. tonic-clonic epilepsy
g. tonic-clonic seizure
generalized-type dyspareunia
generandi
impotentia g.
generation
filial g.
g. gap
hypothesis g.
lesion g.
me g.
mitochondrial free radical g.
pericyte edema g. (PEG)
sandwich g.
generational responsibility
generative
g. empathy
g. intervention
g. semantics
generativity versus stagnation
generator
distal stimulation g.
Force 2 CEM g.
high-frequency g.
Itrel pulse g.
Neuro N-50 lesion g.
programmable pulse g.
pulse g.
radiofrequency g.
Radionics RF lesion g.
generic skill
genesial cycle
genesis
genetic
behavior g.'s
behavioral g.'s
biochemical g.'s
g. block
g. code
g. counseling
g. counselor
g. defect
g. directive
g. disease
g. disorder
g. drift
g. endowment
g. engineering
g. epistemology

G

genetic *(continued)*
  g. equilibrium
  g. error
  g. heterogenicity
  g. linkage study
  g. loading
  g. map
  g. marker
  g. material
  g. memory
  g. method
  molecular g.'s
  political g.'s
  population g.'s
  g. predisposition
  psychiatric g.'s
  g. psychology
  g. redundancy
  g. research
  g. screening
  g. sequence
  g. technology
  g. theory
  g. vulnerability
genetic-epidemiologic
geneticism
geneticist
genetotrophic disease
genetous idiocy
genic
  g. balance
  g. drift
genicula (*pl. of* geniculum)
geniculate
  g. body
  g. ganglion
  g. herpes
  g. neuralgia
  g. nucleus
  g. otalgia
geniculocalcarine
  g. radiation
  g. tract
geniculocalvarium
geniculocortical pathway
geniculum, pl. **genicula**
  g. of facial nerve
  g. nervi facialis
genidentic
geniophobia
genital
  g. character
  g. corpuscle
  g. erotism
  g. herpes
  g. intercourse
  g. love
  g. maturity
  g. mutilation
  g. organ
  g. pain
  g. phase
  g. primacy
  g. sexual contact

  g. stage
  g. stimulation
  g. ulceration
  g. zone
genitalia
  ambiguous g.
  external g.
  female g.
  male g.
genitalis
  herpes g.
genitality
genitalization
genitofemoral nerve
genitourinary
  g. psychogenic disorder
  g. tract
Gen-K
Gennari
  G. band
  G. stria
  stripe of G.
genocide
genocopy
genogram
genome
genomic
  g. alteration
  g. imprinting
genophobia
genotropism
genotype
  dominant g.
  schizophrenic g.
  tryptophan hydroxylase allelic g.
genotypical
genotypic programming
Genpril
gentamicin
  g. sulfate
genu, gen. **genus**, pl. **genua**
  g. capsulae internae
  g. corporis callosi
  g. of corpus callosum
  facial g.
  g. of facial nerve
  g. of the facial nerve
  g. of internal capsule
  g. nervi faciallis
genuine epilepsy
genus, pl. **genera**
Gen-Xene
geographic
  g. displacement
  g. mobility
GeoMedica
geometric
  g. design
  g. hallucination
  g. mean
Geopen
geophagia
geophagy
geophasia
gephyromania

gephyrophobia
gepirone
Gerald forceps
gerascophobia
Gerbode-Burford rib spreader
Gerhardt disease
Gerhardt-Semon law
geriatric
- g. abuse
- g. delinquency
- G. Depression Scale
- g. depressive disorder
- g. diagnosis
- g. factor
- g. medicine
- g. neuropsychiatry
- g. patient
- g. psychiatry
- g. psychology
- g. psychopharmacology
- g. rehabilitation

geriatrics
geri-chair
geriopsychosis
Gerlier disease
germanomania
germanophile
germanophobia
germ cell tumor
germ-cell tumor with synchronous lesions in pineal and suprasellar region (GCTSPS)
germinal
- g. matrix
- g. matrix hemorrhage

germinally affected
germinoma
gerocomia
gerocomy
geromorphism
gerontological
- G. Apperception Test (GAT)
- g. psychiatry

gerontologic psychiatry
gerontology
gerontophilia
gerontophobia
gerophilia
geropsychiatry
geropsychology
Gerson therapy
Gerstmann-Straussler-Scheinker disease
Gerstmann-Sträussler syndrome (GSS)
Gerstmann syndrome
GES
- Gifted Evaluation Scale
- Group Encounter Scale
- Group Encounter Survey
- Group Environment Scale

Gesell
- G. Child Development Age Scale (GCDAS)
- G. developmental model
- G. Developmental Scale
- G. Developmental Schedules

- G. Infant Scale
- G. Preschool Test
- G. School Readiness Test

gesellschaft
gestalt
- autochthonous g.
- Bender G. (BG)
- g. factor
- g. phenomenon
- g. psychology
- g. psychotherapy
- g. theory
- g. therapy
- G. therapy marathon

gestalten
gestaltism
gestaltist
gestate
gestational
- g. diabetes
- g. diestrus
- g. epilepsy
- g. polyneuropathy
- g. psychosis

gesticulate
gesticulation
gestural
- g. automatism
- g. communication

gestural-postural language
gesture
- bizarre g.
- body g.
- clumsy g.
- g. of good will
- g. of goodwill
- kinesic g.
- g. language
- obscene g.
- overt g.
- paucity of expressive g.'s
- subtle g.
- suicidal g.

gesturing communication pattern
getting along
GFAP
- glial fibrillary acidic protein

G-F-W
- Goldman-Fristoe-Woodcock
- G-F-W Battery

G_{M1} gangliosidosis
G_{M2} gangliosidosis
GGT
- gamma-glutamyltransferase
- gamma glutamyl transpeptidase

GH
- growth hormone

GHAG
- General High Altitude Questionnaire

Ghajar guide
GHAQ
- General High Altitude Questionnaire

GHB
- gamma hydroxybutyrate

Gheel colony

G

ghetto
    psychiatric g.
ghost
    Bidwell g.
    g. image
    I/Q imbalance g.
    g. sickness
    white g.
GHQ
    General Health Questionnaire
GHRH
    growth hormone-releasing hormone
GHRIF
    growth hormone-release inhibiting factor
GI
    General Inquiry
    Imagent GI
Giacomini
    band of G.
    frenulum of G.
    uncus band of G.
Giannetti On-Line Psychosocial History (GOLPH)
giant
    g. axonal neuropathy
    g. cell arteritis
    g. cell astrocytoma
    g. cell glioblastoma
    g. cell tumor
    g. cervical carotid artery aneurysm
    g. glomus tumor
    g. hive
    g. motor unit action potential
    g. neuron
    g. petroclival hemangiopericytoma
    g. pyramidal Betz cell
    g. sacral perineural cyst
    g. tortuous basilar artery
    g. urticaria
giant-cell
    g.-c. granuloma
    g.-c. granulomatous hypophysitis
giantism
gibberish aphasia
Gibbs
    G. artifact
    G. phenomenon
    G. ring
GID
    gender identity disorder
    GID of adolescence
    GID of adulthood
GIDAANT
giddy headache
Gierke respiratory bundle
Giessing syndrome
Gifford reflex
gifted
    g. child
    G. Evaluation Scale (GES)
    G. Program Evaluation Survey
    SOI-Learning Abilities Test: Screening Form for G.
    G. and Talented Screening Form

gigans
    urticaria g.
gigantea
    urticaria g.
gigantism
    cerebral g.
gigantocellular glioma
giggling
    nervous g.
Gigli
    G. guide
    G. saw
Gill
    G. laminectomy
    G. procedure
    G. Thomas locator
Gilles
    G. de la Tourette
    G. de la Tourette disease
    G. de la Tourette syndrome
Gilliat-Summer nerve-damaged hand
ginger paralysis
gingival hyperplasia
ginkgo
Ginkgo biloba
girdle
    Ace halo pelvic g.
    g. anesthesia
    Hitzig g.
    g. pain
    g. sensation
Girdlestone laminectomy
githagism
gitter cell
gitterzelle
giver
    fact g.
giving
    transgenerational role of g.
Gjessing syndrome
glabella-inion
    g.-i. line
    g.-i. line landmark
glabellar exposure osteotomy
glabella tap reflex
glancines
gland
    adrenal g.
    apocrine g.
    Bartholin g.
    eccrine g.
    endocrine g.
    lacrimal g.
    master g.
    pacchionian g.
    parathyroid g.
    pineal g.
    pituitary g.
    salivary g.
    thyroid g.
    von Ebner g.
glandula, pl. glandulae
    g. basilaris
    g. pituitaria

glans
    g. clitoridis
    g. penis
Glanzmann disease
Gla-protein
Glaser automatic laminectomy retractor
Glasflex material
Glasgow
    G. Assessment Schedule
    G. Coma Scale (GCS)
    G. Outcome Scale (GOS)
glass
    optical g.
    g. syringe
    window g.
Glasscock triangle
glasses
    Frenzel g.
    protective g.
    rose-colored g.
glassy eye
glatirama copolymer-1
glatiramer acetate
glaucoma
    angle-closure g.
    chronic angle-closure g.
    low tension g.
glazed look
Glees
    method of G.
glia
    g. limitans
    g. limitons externa
    radial g.
gliacyte
Gliadel
    G. implant
    G. wafer
    G. wafer treatment protocol
gliae
    membrana limitans g.
glial
    g. cell
    g. disease
    g. fibrillary acidic protein (GFAP)
    g. neuronal interaction
    g. nodule
    g. parenchymal cyst
    g. reaction
    g. scarring
    g. tumor
    g. tumorigenesis
glial-cell-line derived neurotrophic factor (GDNF)
glib
Glick effect
glide
    after g.
    off g.
glioblastoma
    cerebral g.
    giant cell g.
    g. multiforme (GBM)
    occipital g.
    g. xenograft

glioblastosis cerebri
gliocytoma
glioma
    anaplastic g.
    36B10 g. cell
    brainstem g.
    butterfly-type g.
    cerebral g.
    childhood optic g.
    diffuse pontine g.
    familial g.
    gigantocellular g.
    high-grade g.
    hypothalamic/chiasmatic g.
    intracranial g.
    low-grade g. (LGG)
    malignant g.
    medullary g.
    mixed g.
    multifocal g.
    nasal g.
    non-aplastic g.
    optic g.
    g. of optic chiasm
    optic nerve g.
    optic pathway g.
    pediatric brain stem g.
    pontine g.
    radiation-induced g.
    rolandoparietal g.
    g. of the spinal cord
    subependymal mixed g.
    supratentorial g.
    tectal g.
    telangiectatic g.
    g. telangiectodes
    thalamic g.
gliomatosis
    arachnoidal g.
    g. cerebri
    leptomeningeal g.
gliomatous
gliomyxoma
glioneuroma
glioneuronal element
gliosarcoma
    cerebellar g.
gliosis
    g. of aqueduct
    astrocytic g.
    Chaslin g.
    isomorphous g.
    piloid g.
    progressive subcortical g.
    reactive g.
glissando technique
glittering generalities
global
    g. amnesia
    g. aphasia
    G. Assessment of Functioning (GAF)
    G. Assessment of Functioning Scale

G

global *(continued)*
    G. Assessment of Relational Functioning (GARF)
    G. Assessment of Relational Functioning Scale
    G. Assessment Scale (GAS)
    g. assessment of sensory disturbance
    g. attractor state
    G. Burden of Disease Study
    g. cerebral ischemia
    G. Clinical Judgments Scale
    g. cognitive deficit
    g. course
    g. delay
    g. dementia
    g. deterioration
    G. Deterioration Scale (GDS)
    g. gene replacement therapy
    g. ischemic neuronal injury
    g. loss of language
    G. Obsessive Compulsive Scale
    g. paralysis
    g. rating
    G. Severity Index (GSI)
    G. Sexual Satisfaction Index (GSSI)
    G. Utilization of Streptokinase and Tissue Plasminogen Activator for Occluded Coronary (GUSTO-1)
    g. ward behavior scale (GWBS)
globe
    pale g.
globi (*pl. of* globus)
globoid
    g. cell
    g. cell leukodystrophy
globosa
    dysphagia g.
globose cell
globulin
    gamma g.
    human tetanus immune g. (HTIG)
    intravenous gamma g.
    intravenous immune g. (IVIG)
    testosterone-estradiol-binding g.
globus, pl. **globi**
    g. epilepticus
    g. hystericus
    g. pallidus (GP)
    g. pallidus externa
glomectomy
glomera (*pl. of* glomus)
glomerule
glomeruli
glomerulonephritis
    crescentic g.
    hypocomplementemic g.
    poststreptococcal g.
glomerulus, pl. **glomeruli**
    olfactory g.
glomus, pl. **glomera**
    g. aorticum
    g. arteriovenous malformation

    g. body
    choroid g.
    g. choroideum
    g. intravagale
    g. jugulare
    g. jugulare tumor
    g. jugulotympanicum
    g. pulmonale
    g. vagale
glorified self
glossocinesthetic (*var. of* glossokinesthetic)
glossodontotropism
glossodyniotropism
glossokinesthetic, glossocinesthetic
glossokinetic
    g. artifact
    g. potential
glossolabiolaryngeal paralysis
glossolabiopharyngeal
    g. paralysis
glossolalia
glossolysis
glossopharyngeal
    g. nerve
    g. neuralgia (GPN)
    g. neuropathy
    g. tic
glossopharyngeus
    nervus g.
glossophobia
glossoplegia
glossoptosis
glossospasm
glossosteresis
glossosynthesis
glossotomy
    labiomandibular g.
gloss over
glossy skin
glottal attack
glottidospasm
glove
    g. anesthesia
    Biogel Sensor surgical g.
glubionate
    calcium g.
glucagon
glucepate
    technetium 99m g.
gluceptate
    calcium g.
glucocerebrosidase
glucocorticoid
    hypothalamic g.
glucocorticoid-induced
    g.-i. bone loss
    g.-i. osteoporosis
glucogenesis
glucomineralocorticoid
gluconate
    calcium g.
    clorhexidine g.
    magnesium g.
    potassium g.

potassium chloride and
  potassium g.
potassium citrate and potassium g.

glucose
  fasting blood g. (FBS)
  g. metabolism in the brain
  g. transporter molecule
glucosephosphate isomerase (GPI)
glucuroconjugation
glucuronidase
  beta g.
  g. deficiency
glucuronide
glue
  acrylic g.
  autologous fibrin sealant g.
  cyanoacrylate g.
  g. ear
  fibrin g.
  g. sniffer's rash
  g. sniffing
GluR1
  glutamide receptor subunit
glutamate
  g. decarboxylase (GAD)
  g. excitotoxicity
  g. metabolism
  monosodium g.
  g. neurotoxicity
  g. toxicity
  g. transport velocity
glutamatergic
  g. excitotoxicity
  g. neurotransmission
glutamic
  g. acid
  g. acid decarboxylase
glutamide receptor subunit (GluR1)
glutamyl transaminase
glutaraldehyde
glutaric
  g. acid
  g. aciduria type I
glutathione synthetase deficiency
gluteal
  g. nerve
  g. reflex
glutethimide
  g. and codeine cough syrup
  g. group
  g. intoxication
  g. with codeine
gluttonous
glyburide
glycerin
glycerol
  g. chemoneurolysis
  g. rhizotomy
  g. test
glyceryl trinitrate
glycinate
  aluminum g.
glycine
glycogenosis (type I–VII)
glycogen storage disease

glycogeusia
glycolipid
glycoprotein
  integral membrane g.
  myelin-associated g. (MAG)
  myelin/oligodendrocyte g. (MOG)
  g. storage disorder
glycoprotein-secreting adenoma
glycopyrrolate
glycorrhachia
glycosaminoglycan
glycoside
  cardiac g.
glycosphingolipid metabolic defect
glycosylase
glycyl
GM-1 ganglioside
GMA
  gross motor activity
GMC
  general medical condition
GMFM
  gross motor function measure
GM$_2$ gangliosidosis
GM$_1$ gangliosidosis
gnathic
Gnathostoma
gNomos
  g. head frame
  g. stereotactic system
gnosia
gnostic function
gnosticism
GnRH, GRH
  gonadotropin-releasing hormone
goal
  Assessment of Core G.'s (ACG)
  g. attainment
  G. Attainment Scale (GAS)
  g. gradient
  gradient g.
  latent g.
  life g.
  manifest g.
  g. orientation
  Planning Career G.'s (PCG)
  g. setting
  short-term g. (STG)
goal-directed
  g.-d. activity
  g.-d. behavior
goal-limited adjustment therapy
goal-oriented process
goal-setting
  vocational g.-s.
GOAT
  Galveston Orientation and Awareness
  Test
GOCL-II
  Gordon Occupational Checklist-II
God
  act of G.
  G. complex
  G. drug
godless

G

godlike
godly
godsend
Golay gradient coil
gold
　　g. peripheral neuropathy
Golda reflex
Goldberg Index
golden-ager
Goldenhar syndrome
Goldflam disease
Goldman-Fristoe Test of Articulation
Goldman-Fristoe-Woodcock (G-F-W)
　　G.-F.-W. Auditory Skills Test
　　Battery
　　G.-F.-W. Test
Goldmann-Offner reference of electrode
Goldmann visual field
Goldman perimetry
Goldscheider test
Goldstein
　　G. spinal fusion
　　G. toe sign
Goldstein-Scheerer Tests of Abstract
　　and Concrete thinking
golf-stick dissector
Golgi
　　G. epithelial cell
　　G. reflex
　　G. staining
　　G. system
　　G. tendon organ
　　G. type II neuron
　　G. type I neuron
　　vesiculation of the G.
Golgi-Mazzoni corpuscle
Goll column
Golombok-Rust Inventory of Marital
　　State (GRIMS)
golpe
GOLPH
　　Giannetti On-Line Psychosocial History
goma
Gombault
　　G. degeneration
　　G. triangle
Gomori
　　G. trichome stain
　　G. trichrome
gonad
gonadal
　　g. agenesis
　　g. cycle
　　g. dysgenesis
　　g. hormone
gonadocentric
gonadotroph cell
gonadotropin, gonadotrophin
　　beta-human chorionic g.
　　chorionic g.
　　human chorionic g.
gonadotropin-producing adenoma
gonadotropin-releasing hormone (GnRH,
　　GRH)

gondii
　　Toxoplasma g.
gondola
gong
gonococcal
gonococcus (GC)
gonorrhea
good
　　g. and evil test
　　g. faith
　　g. form response (F+)
　　g. functioning
　　g. object
　　g. shape
　　g. sleep efficiency
Goodenough
　　G. Animal Test
　　G. Draw-A-Man Test
　　G. Draw-A-Person Test
good-enough
　　g.-e. mother
　　g.-e. mothering
Goodenough-Harris Drawings Test
good H
Goodman Lock Box
goodness of fit
goods
　　bill of g.
goodwill
　　gesture of g.
Goody's Headache Powders
gooseneck rongeur
Gordon
　　G. Diagnostic System Test
　　G. Occupational Checklist-II
　　　(GOCL-II)
　　G. Personal Inventory (GPI)
　　G. Personal Profile Inventory
　　　(GPPI)
　　G. reflex
　　G. sign
　　G. symptom
Gore-Tex
gorger-vomiter
Gorlin
　　G. sign
　　G. syndrome
gormandize
gormiess
GORT-3
　　Gray Oral Reading Test, Third Edition
GOS
　　Glasgow Outcome Scale
Gosling
　　G. pulsatility
　　G. pulsatility index
gouge
　　AO g.
　　Flanagan spinal fusion g.
　　Hibbs spinal fusion g.
　　Hoen lamina g.
　　Killian g.
　　spinal fusion g.
gouging
　　eye g.

Goulet retractor
gouty arthritis
governess psychosis
government
 patient g.
 PSI Basic Skills Test for Business,
 Industry and G.
Gowers
 G. bundle
 G. bundle in cerebellum
 G. column
 G. disease
 G. fasciculus
 G. maneuver
 G. muscular dystrophy
 G. sign
 G. syndrome
 G. tract
 vasovagal attack of G.
gown restriction
GP
 globus pallidus
GPI
 general paralysis of the insane
 glucosephosphate isomerase
 Gordon Personal Inventory
GPN
 glossopharyngeal neuralgia
GPPI
 Gordon Personal Profile Inventory
GPR
 Grenoble-Paris-Rennes
 GPR robot neurosurgical
 microscope
G-protein coupling
gracile
 g. nucleus
 g. tubercle
gracilis
 fasciculus g. (Fg)
gradation method
grade
 g. equivalent
 Fischer g.
 Hunt and Hess g.
 Hunt and Hess G.'s I-III
 g. I astrocytoma
 g. II astrocytoma
 g. III astrocytoma
 g. IV astrocytoma
 g. IV spondylolisthesis
 g. norm
 g. rating
 g. scale
 Simpson G.
 g. skipping
 Spetzler-Martin g.
graded
 g. activity
 g. exposure
 G. Naming Test
 g. potential
 G. Word Spelling Test
Gradenigo syndrome

gradient
 g. amplifier
 approach g.
 avoidance g.
 axial g.
 bipolar g.
 g. coil
 g. compensation
 g. echo
 effect g.
 excitation g.
 field g.
 frequency-encoding g.
 generalization g.
 g. goal
 goal g.
 magnetic g.
 g. magnetic field
 g. moment
 g. moment nulling
 phase-encoding g.
 pulsed g.
 readout g.
 g. recalled echo technique (GRE)
 rephasing g.
 rewinder g.
 slice-select encoding g.
 steep-dose g.
 x g.
 y g.
gradient-echo
 g.-e. MR image
 g.-e. MR imaging
gradient-recalled
 g.-r. acquisition in the steady state
 (GRASS)
 g.-r. echo image
gradient-refocused
 g.-r. imaging
 g.-r. sequence
grading
 De Monte g.
 Fisher g.
 Hirsch g.
 Kernohan g.
 Simpson g.
gradiometer
 axial g.
gradual topic shift
graduate
 college g.
 Committee of International
 Medical G.'s
 international medical g. (IMG)
 G. and Managerial Assessment
 G. Record Examination (GRE)
 G. Record Examination Aptitude
 Test (GREAT)
Graefe
 G. disease
 G. sign
 G. spot
graft
 adipose g.
 adrenal medulla g.

G

graft *(continued)*
    aortobifemoral bypass g.
    autochthonous g.
    autogenous bone g.
    autologous fat g.
    barrel staved g.
    bone g.
    bovine percardium dural g.
    bypass g.
    cable g.
    carotid-vertebral vein bypass g.
    circumferentially aortofemoral g.
    clip g.
    cranial bone g.
    dural g.
    fascicular g.
    fat-patch g.
    funicular g.
    greater auricular nerve g.
    Hemashield enhanced g.
    human dural substitute g.
    hydroxyapatite g.
    interbody g.
    interfascicular g.
    intracranial-extracranial nerve g.
    intracranial-intratemporal nerve g.
    Keystone g.
    g. material alternative
    g. migration
    nerve g.
    petrous carotid-to-intradural carotid saphenous vein g.
    posterior bone g.
    posterolateral bone g.
    radial artery g.
    rib g.
    roof-patch g.
    saphenous vein bypass g.
    saphenous vein patch g.
    g. site
    in situ tricortical iliac-crest block bone g.
    skull bone g.
    sleeve g.
    split calvarial g.
    split-thickness calvarial g.
    strut g.
    sural nerve bridge g.
    sural nerve cable g.
    Teflon tube g.
    temporosuboccipital bone g.
    tricortical iliac crest bone g.
    Unilab Surgibone bovine bone g.
    vascular patch g.
    xenogeneic g.

grafting
    allograft bone g.
    g. anastomosis
    autograft bone g.
    bone g.
    fetal mesencephalic g.
    fibular g.
    hypophysial g.

    posterolateral bone g.
    strut g.
graft-versus-host disease (GVHD)
grammar
    g. development stage
    g. formation stage
    g. language quotient
grammatical
    g. analysis
    g. equivalent
gramophone symptom
grand
    g. mal
    g. mal epilepsy
    g. mal seizure
    g. mal status
grande attaque hysterique
grandeur
    delusion of g.
    g. delusion
grandfather complex
grandiloquence
grandiose
    g. concept
    g. content
    g. delirium
    g. delusion
    g. expansiveness
    g. ideation
    g. theme
    g. type
grandiose-type schizophrenia
grandiosity in fantasy
Grandma rule
Granit loop
Grantham lobotomy
granular
    g. cell
    g. cell myoblastoma
    g. cell tumor
    g. cortex
    g. ependymitis
    g. layers of cerebral cortex
    g. layers of retina
    g. neuron
granularis
    ependymitis g.
granulated opium
granulatio, pl. granulationes
    granulationes arachnoideales
granulation
    arachnoid g.
    pacchionian g.
granulatum
    opium g.
granule
    azurophilic g.
    Birbeck g.
    g. cell
    chromatic g.
    chromophil g.
    Crooke g.
    Nissl g.
granulocyte

granulocytic
  g. brain edema
  g. sarcoma
granulocytopenia
granuloma
  cholesterol g.
  g. cryptococcal
  eosinophilic g.
  foreign body g.
  Gagel g.
  giant-cell g.
  intrasellar g.
  lethal midline g.
  parenchymal g.
  petroclival cholesterol g.
granulomatosis
  eosinophilic g.
  Langerhans cell g.
  lymphomatoid g.
  Wegener g. (WG)
granulomatous
  g. angiitis
  g. angiitis of the central nervous
    system (GANS)
  g. angiitis of the CNS
  g. arteritis
  g. colitis
  g. encephalomyelitis
  g. hypophysitis
  g. ileocolitis
granulopoietic function
granulovacuolar degeneration
grape ending
graph
  bar g.
graphanesthesia
graphesthesia
graphic
  g. aphasia
  g. description
  g. disorientation
  g. impairment
  g. rating scale
graphica
  asemasia g.
graphic-arts therapy
graphology
graphomania
graphometry
graphomotor
  g. aphasia
  g. technique
graphopathology
graphophobia
graphorrhea
graphospasm
Grashey aphasia
grasper
  lion's claw g.
  lion's paw g.
grasping
  g. and groping reflex
  g. reflex
grasp and reach

GRASS
  gradient-recalled acquisition in the steady
    state
    2DFT GRASS
    3DFT GRASS
    interleaved GRASS
    sequential GRASS
Grasset
  G. law
  G. phenomenon
  G. sign
Grasset-Gaussel phenomenon
Grassi
  G. Basic Cognitive Evaluation
    (GBCE)
  G. Block Substitution Test
Grass stimulator S-44
grata
  non g.
  persona g.
  persona non g.
grate on the nerves
gratification
  delayed g.
  g. of dependent wishes
  immediate g.
  inability to delay g.
  material g.
  oral g.
  sexual g.
Gratiolet
  G. fiber
  G. radiation
grave
  delirium g.
  g. delirium
gravel voice
graven image
Graves
  G. disease
  G. ophthalmopathy
gravidarum
  chorea g.
  tetania g.
gravior
  epilepsia g.
gravireceptor
gravis
  congenital myasthenia g.
  dementia paranoides g.
  myasthenia g. (MG)
  neonatal myasthenia g.
  neurasthenia g.
  oneirodynia g.
  paranoia dementia g.
gravity perception
Gravol
gray (Gy)
  central g.
  g. column
  g. degeneration
  g. fiber
  g. layer of superior colliculus
  g. matter
  G. Oral Reading Test

G

gray *(continued)*
    G. Oral Reading Test, Third
      Edition (GORT-3)
    periaqueductal central g. (PAG)
    periventricular g.
    g. shield
    g. substance
    g. tuber
    g. tubercle
    g. wing
gray-out
    g.-o. episode
    g.-o. syndrome
gray-white matter junction
GRE
    gradient recalled echo technique
    Graduate Record Examination
GREAT
    Graduate Record Examination Aptitude
      Test
great
    g. anterior medullary artery
    g. cerebral vein
    g. cerebral vein of Galen
      aneurysm
    g. foramen
    g. horizontal fissure
    g. longitudinal fissure
    g. toe reflex
    g. vein of Galen
greater
    g. auricular nerve graft
    g. occipital nerve
    g. rhomboid muscle
    g. sciatic foramen
    g. superficial petrosal nerve
grecomania
Greenberg
    G. retracting system
    G. retractor
    G. retractor frame
    G. retractor set
Greenberg-Sugita retractor
Greenberg-type bar
Greenfield
    G. classification of spinocerebellar
      ataxia
    G. disease
Greenwood bipolar and suction forceps
Gregorc Style Delineator
Greig
    G. cephalopolysyndactyly
    G. cephalopolysyndactyly syndrome
Grenoble-Paris-Rennes (GPR)
Grenoble stereotactic robot
GRH *(var. of* GnRH)
grid
    subdural g.
**Grid Test of Schizophrenic Thought
Disorder (GTSTD)**
grief
    anticipatory g.
    g. counselor
    delayed g.

    denied g.
    distorted g.
    G. Experience Inventory (GEI)
    impacted g.
    inhibited g.
    Inventory of Complicated G.
    g. management
    G. Measurement Scale
    mutual g.
    prolonged g.
    g. reaction
    Texas Revised Inventory of G.
    g. therapy
    traumatic g.
    unresolved g.
    g. work
Griesinger sign
grievance-seeker
grieving
    inhibited g.
grievous bodily harm
grimace
    facial g.
    tic-like facial g.
grimacing
    prominent g.
grimly adhered-to routine
GRIMS
    Golombok-Rust Inventory of Marital
      State
grin
    sardonic g.
grinding
    jaw g.
    teeth g.
    tooth g.
gringophobia
grip
    pencil g.
    pincer g.
    pistol g.
    g. strength test
    syringe g.
Griselda complex
griseofulvin peripheral neuropathy
grisi siknis
grobelsucht
Grocott stain
groomed
    neatly g.
    poorly g.
grooming deterioration
groove
    anterior intermediate g.
    anterolateral g.
    anteromedian g.
    frontal g.
    meningioma of the olfactory g.
    neural g.
    olfactory g.
    parasagittal g.
    pontomedullary g.
    posterior intermediate g.
    posterolateral g.

sagittal g.
vascular g.
grooved
g. pegboard
G. Pegboard Test
gross
g. impairment
g. impairment of reality testing
g. motor
g. motor activity (GMA)
g. motor deficit
g. motor function measure
  (GMFM)
g. motor skill
g. neurologic deficit
g. sensory deficit
g. stress reaction
grossly
g. disorganized behavior
g. impaired functioning
g. pathogenic care
ground
g. bundle
g. electrode
figure and g.
figure g.
middle g.
g. rule
group
g. acceptance
G. Achievement Identification
  Measure
action g.
g. activity
g. adjustment therapy (GAT)
adolescent support g.
aftercare g.
age g.
g. A β-hemolytic streptococcus
  (GABHS)
g. analytic psychotherapy
AO g.
aspirational g.
attitudinal g.
g. behavior
blood g.
g. boundary
g. B streptococcus (GBS)
g. centered
g. climate
closed g.
CNS disease g.
g. cohesion
community-action g.
g. consciousness
continuous g.
g. contract
control g.
g. counseling
crisis g.
criterion g.
cultural reference g.
g. delinquency
g. delinquent reaction
diagnosis-related g. (DRG)

diagnostic related g. (DRG)
g. difference
g. dimension
diverse g.
g. diversity
g. dynamics
G. Embedded Figures Test (GEFT)
encounter g.
G. Encounter Scale (GES)
G. Encounter Survey (GES)
G. Environment Scale (GES)
equivalent g.
ethnic reference g.
g. experience
experiential g.
experimental g.
family support g.
g. feeling
First Seizure Trial G. (FIR.S.T.)
focus g.
glutethimide g.
g. harmony
heterogeneous g.
high-risk g.
g. home
horizontal g.
human relations g.
g. identification
intake-orientation g.
integrity g.
interact g.
interest g.
International Medical News G.
g. interview
G. Inventory for Finding Creative
  Talent
laissez-faire g.
leaderless g.
g. living
g. marriage
matched g.
g. medicine
g. mind
minority g.
g. morale
mutual aid g.
natural g.
g. norm
nurse support g.
open g.
g. participation
pedunculopontine cholinergic g.
peer g.
personal growth g.
g. phase
Pittsburgh gamma knife g.
g. play
g. pressure
primary support g.
g. problem-solving
g. process
psychoanalytic g.
g. psychosis
rap g.
G. Reading Test (GRT)

G

group *(continued)*
    reference g.
    regressive-inspirational g.
    g. relations theory
    g. rule
    self-help g.
    sensitivity g.
    sensitivity-training g.
    g. session
    g. setting
    social reference g.
    socioeconomic g.
    Spinal Fixation Study G.
    splinter g.
    g. stage
    g. stress reaction
    g. structure
    structured interactional g.
    study g.
    G. Styles Inventory (GSI)
    substance g.
    g. superego
    support g.
    Swedish gamma knife g.
    symptom g.
    T g.
    task-oriented g.
    G. Tests of Musical Ability
    thematically related g.'s
    therapeutic play g. (TPG)
    training g. (T-group)
    transient g.
    work g.
    g. work
grouping
    clavus clinical g.
    gastrointestinal symptom g.
    heterogenous g.
    homogeneous g.
    homogenous g.
    pain symptom g.
    pseudoneurological symptom g.
    sexual symptom g.
    symptom g.
group-type conduct disorder
growing
    g. fracture
    g. pain
growth
    g. arrest-specific gene
    cognitive g.
    g. cone
    continuous g.
    g. factor
    g. hormone (GH)
    g. hormone-producing adenoma
    g. hormone-release inhibiting factor
      (GHRIF)
    g. hormone-releasing factor
    g. hormone-releasing hormone
      (GHRH)
    g. hormone-secreting adenoma
    mental g.
    neurite g.

    g. period
    personal g.
    surgent g.
    tumultuous g.
    zero population g. (ZPG)
growth-associated protein (GAP)
GRT
    Group Reading Test
Gruca-Weiss spring
grudge bearing
Gruenwald
    G. ear forceps
    G. neurosurgical rongeur
grumbling mania
gryochrome
GSI
    Global Severity Index
    Group Styles Inventory
GSR
    galvanic skin response
GSS
    Gerstmann-Sträussler syndrome
GSSI
    Global Sexual Satisfaction Index
GSWH
    gunshot wound to head
GTC
    generalized tonic clonic
    GTC convulsion
GTP
    guanosine triphosphate
GTSTD
    Grid Test of Schizophrenic Thought
      Disorder
guaiac
    g. negative
    g. positive
guaifenesin
Guam
    parkinsonism-dementia complex
      of G.
    G. parkinsonism-dementia complex
guanethidine sulfate
guanfacine
guanidine
guanine/cytosine ratio
guanine nucleotide
guanosine
    g. diphosphate (GDP)
    g. monophosphate
    g. triphosphate (GTP)
guanylate cyclase
guanylyl cyclase
guard
    depth g.
    Midas Rex bur g.
    old g.
    UltraPower bur g.
guarded
    g. manner
    g. tripole
guardedness
    adolescent g.
Gubler
    G. hemiplegia

G. line
G. paralysis
G. syndrome
Gudden
G. atrophy
G. commissure
G. ganglion
G. tegmental nuclei
guerrilla warfare
Guglielmi detachable coil (GDC)
guidance
anticipatory g.
axon g.
Brown-Roberts-Wells computerized
tomography stereotaxic g.
child g.
g. counselor
electrophysiological g.
image g.
real-time g.
StealthStation system real-time g.
stereotactic g.
ultrasonographic g.
vocational g.
guidance-cooperation model
guide
action g.
Adson dural protector g.
AdTech electrode g.
AO stopped-drill g.
Bristol Social Adjustment G.'s
Cognitive Observation G. (COG)
contoured anterior spinal plate
drill g.
Cook stereotaxic g.
Cushing saw g.
Davis saw g.
drill g.
Frazier dural g.
Ghajar g.
Gigli g.
Hall-Dundar drill g.
nut alignment g.
Prevocational Assessment and
Curriculum G. (PACG)
stereotactic g.
Yasargil ligature g.
guided affective imagery (GAI)
guideline
G.'s for Adolescent Preventive
Services (GAPS)
Steering Committee on
Practice G.'s
guidepin
AO g.
guidewire
delivery g.
J-tipped g.
guileless
Guilford-Zimmerman
G.-Z. Aptitude Survey (GZAS)
G.-Z. Interest Inventory (GZII)
G.-Z. Personality Test (GZPT)
G.-Z. Temperament Survey (GZTS)

Guillain-Barré
G.-B. postinfection peripheral
neuropathy
G.-B. reflex
G.-B. syndrome (GBS)
Guillain-Barré-Strohl syndrome
Guillain-Garcin syndrome
Guillain-Mollaret triangle
guilt
g. displacement
g. feeling
initiative versus g.
misattribution of g.
g. obsession
pathologic g.
pervasive proneness to g.
self-attribution of g.
survival g.
survivor g.
g. theme
unconscious g.
guinea worm infestation
Guinon
G. disease
tic de G.
Guiot-Talairach construct
gullwing pattern
gum
brick g.
bubble g.
dream g.
Nicorette G.
Nicorette DS G.
gumma
cerebral g.
gumption
gun
Omni clip g.
riot g.
smoking g.
stun g.
submachine g.
tommy g.
top g.
Gunn
Marcus G.
G. phenomenon
G. syndrome
gunshot
g. wound
g. wound to head (GSWH)
gustation
gustatism
gustatory
g. anesthesia
g. audition
g. aura
g. cell
g. hallucination
g. hyperesthesia
g. lemniscus
g. nerve
g. nucleus
g. organ
g. seizure

G

gustatory (continued)
　　g. sensory modality
　　g. sweating syndrome
gustatory-sudorific reflex
GUSTO-1
　　Global Utilization of Streptokinase and
　　　Tissue Plasminogen Activator for
　　　Occluded Coronary
gusto
gustometry
Guthrie test
gutless
gutsy
gutter fracture
guttering
gutturotetany
Guyon canal
GVHD
　　graft-versus-host disease
gwa sha
Gwathmey anesthesia
GWBS
　　global ward behavior scale
Gy
　　gray
gymnomania
gymnophobia
gynander
gynandrism
gynandroid
gynandromorph
gynatresia
gynecic
gynecogenic
gynecomania
gynecomastia
gynecopathy
gynecophonous
gynephobia, gynophobia
gynergon
gynesic
gyniatrics
gynomonoecism
gynopathic
gynophobia (var. of gynephobia)
gyral infarction
gyrate
gyration
gyrectomy
　　frontal g.
gyrencephalic
gyri (gen. and pl. of gyrus)
gyriform calcification
gyrochrome
　　g. cell
gyromagnetic ratio
gyrosa
Gyroscan
　　Philips G. S5
　　Philips G. S15
gyrose
gyrospasm
gyrus, gen. and pl. **gyri**
　　angular g. (AG)

　　g. angularis
annectent g.
anterior central g.
anterior cingulate g.
anterior piriform g.
ascending frontal g.
ascending parietal g.
gyri breves insulae
Broca g.
callosal g.
central gyri
gyri cerebri
gyri of cerebrum
cingulate g.
g. cinguli
contiguous supramarginal g.
deep transitional g.
dentate g.
g. dentatus
fasciolar g.
g. fasciolaris
first temporal g.
flattening of g.
g. fornicatus
frontal g.
g. frontalis inferior
g. frontalis medius
g. frontalis superior
fusiform g.
g. fusiformis
Heschl g.
hippocampal dentate g.
inferior frontal g.
inferior occipital g.
inferior parietal g.
inferior temporal g.
infracalcarine g.
gyri insulae
insular g.
interlocking gyri
lamination of g.
lateral occipitotemporal g.
lingual g.
g. lingualis
long g. of insula
g. longus insulae
marginal g.
medial frontal g.
medial occipitotemporal g.
middle frontal g.
middle temporal g.
occipital gyri
g. occipitotemporalis lateralis
g. occipitotemporalis medialis
olfactory g.
orbital gyri
gyri orbitales
paracentral g.
parahippocampal g.
g. parahippocampalis
paraterminal g.
g. paraterminalis
parietal g.
postcentral g.
g. postcentralis

posterior central g.
posterior cingulate g.
precentral g.
g. precentralis
preinsular g.
prepiriform g.
quadrate g.
g. rectus
Retzius g.
short gyri of the insula
short insular g.
splenial g.
straight g.
subcallosal g.
g. subcallosus
subcollateral g.
superior frontal g.
superior occipital g.
superior parietal g.
superior temporal g.
supracallosal g.
supramarginal g.

g. supramarginalis
tail of dentate g.
temporal g.
gyri temporales transversi
g. temporalis inferior
g. temporalis medius
g. temporalis superior
transitional g.
transverse temporal g.
Turner marginal g.
uncal g.
uncinate g.

GZAS
Guilford-Zimmerman Aptitude Survey
GZII
Guilford-Zimmerman Interest Inventory
GZPT
Guilford-Zimmerman Personality Test
GZTS
Guilford-Zimmerman Temperament
Survey

G

H
- H field
- H reflex

h
- human response

HA
- high anxiety

HAART
- highly active antiretroviral therapy

habeas corpus

habena, pl. **habenae**

habenula, pl. **habenulae**
- habenulae perforata
- pineal h.
- trigone of h.

habenular
- h. commissure
- h. nucleus

habenulointerpeduncular tract

habilitation

habit
- acculturation problem with expression of h.'s
- alcohol h.
- baby h.
- benign h.
- h. chorea
- chronic h.
- h. complaint
- h. deterioration
- h. disorder
- h. disturbance
- drug h.
- eating h.
- feeding h.'s
- food h.
- force of h.
- h. formation
- h. hierarchy
- h. interference
- king's h.
- laxative h.
- motor h.
- narcotic h.
- nicotine h.
- opium h.
- h. pattern
- h. reversal
- h. spasm
- steal to support a h.
- h. strength
- temporary h.
- h. tic
- h. training
- h. treatment

habitability

habit-forming

Habitrol Patch

habit-training

habitual
- h. act
- h. criminal

- h. offender
- h. runaway

habituate

habituation
- cocaine h.
- electrical h.

habitude

habitue

habitus
- h. apoplecticus
- marfanoid h.
- h. phthisicus

habromania

hache

Hachinski
- H. Ischemia Scale
- H. ischemic score

Hacker procedure

HACS
- hyperactive child syndrome

Haddad syndrome

hadephobia

HADS
- Hospital Anxiety and Depression Scale

Haeckel biogenic law

Haemophilus
- *H. aerophilus*
- *H. influenzae*
- *H. influenzae b*
- *H. influenzae* meningitis
- *H. parainfluenzae*

Haenel symptom

Hageman factor

Hagen-Poiseuille law

haggard appearance

hagiophobia

hagiotherapy

Haglund disease

Hahn echo

Hahnemann
- H. Elementary School Behavior Rating Scale
- H. High School Behavior Rating Scale

Haid universal bone plate system

Haight-Finochietto rib spreader

Haight rib spreader

hair
- h. cell
- h. denuding
- eating h.
- fine electric h.
- h. follicle
- Frey irritation h.
- h. pulling
- spiked h.

hairline fracture

hairpiece

hair-pulling behavior

Hajdu-Cheney syndrome

Hajek
- H. chisel

H

Hajek *(continued)*
   H. laminectomy punch
   H. mallet
Hajek-Ballenger
   H.-B. dissector
   H.-B. septal elevator
Hajek-Koffler
   H.-K. bone punch forceps
   H.-K. laminectomy rongeur
   H.-K. punch
Håkanson technique
Hakim
   H. high-pressure valve
   H. precision valve
   H. syndrome
Hakin-Cortis ventriculoperitoneal shunt
Hakuba
   medial triangle of H.
halazepam
Halcion
Haldol Decanoate
Haldrone
half-and-half exposure
half-Fourier imaging
half-hearted attempt at suicide
half-Nex imaging
Halfprin 81
half track
halfway
   h. children
   h. house
Halifax
   H. clamp posterior cervical fixation
   H. interlaminar clamp
   H. interlaminar clamp system
halitosis
Hall
   H. neurosurgical craniotome
   H. Occupational Orientation
     Inventory (HOOI)
   H. Osteon drill system kit
   H. Osteon irrigation kit
   H. Surgairtome II drill
   H. UltraPower drill
   H. Versipower drill
Hall-Dundar drill guide
Halle
   H. bone curette
   H. dura knife
   H. nasal speculum
   H. speculum
Haller
   H. ansa
   H. circle
   H. unguis
Hallervorden-Spatz
   H.-S. disease
   H.-S. syndrome
Hallervorden syndrome
Halloween effect
Hallpike
   H. maneuver
   H. test
hallucal abnormality
hallucinate

hallucination
   accusatory h.
   affective h.
   alcoholic h.
   alcohol-induced psychotic disorder
     with h.'s
   amphetamine-induced psychotic
     disorder with h.'s
   anxiolytic-induced psychotic disorder
     with h.'s
   auditory h.
   blank h.
   body-image h.
   cannabis-induced psychotic disorder
     with h.'s
   cenesthesic h.
   cocaine-induced psychotic disorder
     with h.'s
   command h.
   command auditory h.'s
   complex h.
   h. of conception
   content of h.
   depressive h.
   dreamlike h.
   drug-induced h.
   elementary h.
   formed visual h.
   fragmentary h.
   geometric h.
   gustatory h.
   hallucinogen-induced psychotic
     disorder with h.'s
   haptic h.
   hypnagogic h.
   hypnopompic h.
   hypnotic-induced psychotic disorder
     with h.'s
   induced h.
   inhalant-induced psychotic disorder
     with h.'s
   kinesthetic h.
   lilliputian h.
   memory h.
   microptic h.
   mood-congruent h.
   mood-incongruent h.
   nocturnal h.
   nonaffective h.
   olfactory h.
   opioid-induced psychotic disorder
     with h.'s
   organic h.
   palinoptic h.
   h. of perception
   phencyclidine-induced psychotic
     disorder with h.'s
   posttraumatic h.
   prominent h.
   psychotic disorder with h.'s
   reflex h.
   sedative-induced psychotic disorder
     with h.'s
   self-destructive h.
   simple h.

sleep-related h.
somatic h.
structured h.
stump h.
tactile h.
tactual h.
teleologic h.
temporal h.
threatening h.
transient auditory h.
transient tactile h.
transient visual h.
unformed visual h.
unpleasant h.
vestibular h.
visual h.
vivid h.
hallucinative
hallucinatoria
paranoia h.
hallucinatory
h. behavior
h. dementia
h. drug
h. epilepsy
h. game
h. image
h. mania
h. neuralgia
h. paranoia
h. state
h. state drug psychosis
h. transient organic
h. transient organic psychosis
h. verbigeration
hallucinatory-type psychoorganic syndrome
hallucinogen
h. abuse
h. dependence
h. hallucinosis
h. intoxication delirium
h. persisting perception disorder
h. toxic effect
h. use disorder
hallucinogen-affective disorder
hallucinogen-delusional disorder
hallucinogenesis
hallucinogenic
h. drug
h. intoxication
hallucinogen-induced
h.-i. delirium and anxiety disorder
h.-i. psychotic disorder with delusions
h.-i. psychotic disorder with hallucinations
hallucinogen-related disorder, not otherwise specified
hallucinosis
acute h.
h. alcoholic psychosis
alcohol withdrawal h.
bromide h.
drug-induced h.

flashback h.
hallucinogen h.
organic h.
peduncular h.
h. peduncular
psychoactive substance h.
withdrawal h.
hallucinotic
halo
Ace low profile MR h.
Ace Mark III h.
h. apparatus
h. brace
Bremer h.
Brown-Roberts-Wells head ring h.
h. effect
Houston h.
hypoechogenic peritumoral h.
h. of light
object h.'s
h. phenomenon
Philadelphia h.
pulsating visual h.
h. retractor system
h. ring
h. vest
halogenated inhalational anesthesia
haloperidol decanoate
halo-ring adapter
Halotestin
halothane anesthesia
halo-vest immobilization
haloxazolam
Halperon
Halstead
H. Aphasia Test (HAT)
H. Category Test
H. Impairment Index
H. modified technique
H. Russell Neuropsychological Evaluation System (HRNES)
Halstead-Reitan
H.-R. Battery (HRB)
H.-R. category subtest
H.-R. Neurological Battery and Allied Procedures
H.-R. Neuropsychological Test Battery (HRNTB)
Halstead-Wepman Aphasia Screening Test
Halsted
H. artery forceps
H. mosquito forceps
HALT
heroin antagonist and learning therapy
halting
h. gait
h. manner
h. movement
h. speech
haltlose-type personality
Haltran
HAM
HTLV-I associated myelopathy

H

HAMA
    Hamilton Anxiety Scale
hamartoma
    cortical h.
    eccrine angiomatous h.
    hypothalamic h.
    subependymal h.
    vascular h.
    ventromedial hypothalamic h.
hamartomania
hamartomatous lipoma
hamartophobia
hamate finder
hamaxophobia (*var. of* amaxophobia)
Hamburg
    H. Obsessional-Compulsion
        Inventory-Short Form
    H. Obsession/Compulsion Inventory
Hamburg-Wechsler Intelligence Test for Children (HAWIC)
HAMD
    Hamilton Depression Scale
Hamilton
    H. Anxiety Rating Scale (HARS)
    H. Anxiety Scale (HAMA)
    H. Depression Rating Scale (HDRS)
    H. Depression Scale (HAMD)
    H. Depression Score
    H. Rating Scale for Anxiety
hammer
    Babinski percussion h.
    Berliner percussion h.
    Buck neurological h.
    Buck percussion h.
    Davis percussion h.
    Dejerine-Davis percussion h.
    Dejerine percussion h.
    Epstein neurological h.
    Küntscher h.
    Monreal reflex h.
    neurological h.
    percussion h.
    Rabiner neurological h.
    slotted h.
    Taube neurological percussion h.
    Taylor percussion h.
    Trömner percussion h.
hammock bandage
Hammond disease
HAM/TSP
    HTLV-associated myelopathy/tropical spastic paraparesis
hand
    accoucheur's h.
    all-median nerve h.
    all-ulnar nerve h.
    ape h.
    h. ataxia
    black h.
    h. deformity
    h. dominant
    dominant h.
    drop h.
    H. Dynamometer Test (HDT)

    Gilliat-Summer nerve-damaged h.
    laying on of h.'s
    Marinesco succulent h.
    mechanic's h.'s
    nondominant h.
    h. nondominant handedness
    obstetrical h.
    h. preference
    h. shaking
    striatal h.
    h. test (HT)
    h. tremor
    h. waving
    h. wringing
    wringing of h.'s
    writing h.
handcuff neuropathy
handedness
    hand nondominant h.
    left h.
hand-foot-and-mouth disease
handicap
    emotional h. (EH)
    International Classification of Impairments, Disabilities, H.'s (ICIDH)
    severe emotional h. (SEH)
handicapped
    educationally mentally h. (EMH)
    h. emotionally
    mentally h.
    perceptually h.
    Questionnaire on Resources and Stress for Families with Chronically Ill or H.
    trainable mentally h. (TMH)
handle
    bayonet h.
    Cloward double hinge cervical retractor h.
    Hardy lateral knife h.
    h. of the malleus
handpiece
    CUSA system 200 straight autoclavable h.
Hand-Schüller-Christian disease
hand-to-mouth
    h.-t.-m. reaction
    h.-t.-m. reflex
hand-washing obsession
handwashing ritual
handwriting analysis
HANE
    hereditary angioneurotic edema
Hanfmann-Kasanin Concept Formation Test
hang
hanging
    accidental h.
    erotized h.
hanging-drop equilibration
hangman's fracture
hangover
    h. effect
    h. headache

hanky panky
Hannover
   H. classification
   H. system
Hansen disease
hapax legomenon
haphalgesia
haphazard
haphephobia (var. of haptephobia)
haploid
haplology
haplotype analysis
happy puppet syndrome
haptephobia, haphephobia
haptic
   h. feedback
   h. hallucination
   H. Intelligence Scale
   h. perception
   h. system
haptodysphoria
haptometer
haptophobia
haptophonia
HAQ
   Health Assessment Questionnaire
harassment
   sexual h. (SH)
hard
   h. chancre
   h. disk herniation
   h. of hearing
   h. line
   h. palate dissection
   h. tissue replacement (HTR)
   h. tissue replacement-malleable
     facial implant (HTR-MFI)
Harding W87 Test
hardware
   TiMesh h.
Hardy
   H. approach
   H. attachment
   H. bayonet dressing forceps
   H. bivalve speculum
   H. curette
   H. dissector
   H. lateral knife handle
   H. lip retractor
   H. microsurgical bayonet bipolar
     forceps
   H. microsurgical enucleator
   H. 5 mm mirror
   H. pituitary spoon
   H. 3-prong fork
   H. sella punch forceps
   H. sellar punch
   H. suction tube
Hardy-Rand-Rittler plate
Hardy-Weinberg equilibrium
Harken rib spreader
harm
   h. avoidance
   grievous bodily h.

   physical h.
   H. posterior cervical plate
harmaline
harm-avoidance need
harmine
harming
   h. others
   h. self
harmless wit
Harmon cervical approach
harmonic
   h. analysis
   h. error field
   h. function
   h. mean
harmony
   group h.
   h. process
harpaxophobia
Harriluque
   H. sublaminar wiring modification
   H. technique
Harrington
   H. distraction
   H. pedicle hook
   H. rod
   H. rod fixation
   H. rod and hook system
   H. rod instrumentation
   H. rod instrumentation compression
   H. rod instrumentation distraction
     outrigger device
   H. rod instrumentation failure
   H. rod instrumentation force
     application
   H. scissors
   H. spreader
Harris
   H. migraine
   H. syndrome
   H. Tests of Lateral Dominance
Harris-Lingoes Subscales - MMPI
Harrison Antinarcotic Act
Harris-Smith cervical fusion
HARS
   Hamilton Anxiety Rating Scale
harsh discipline
Hartel technique
Harter Self-Perception Profile for
  Children
Hartnup
   H. disease
   H. disorder
Hartshill
   H. Ransford loop
   H. rectangle
   H. rectangle rod
Harvard Group Scale of Hypnotic
  Susceptibility (HGSHS)
Hasegawa Dementia Scale
Hashimoto disease
HAT
   Halstead Aphasia Test

H

hatchet
    h. facies
    h. job
hate
HATH
    Heterosexual Attitudes Toward
    Homosexuality
Hatha yoga
haughty behavior
Hauser ambulation index
haut
    h. mal
    h. mal epilepsy
Haverfield-Scoville hemilaminectomy
retractor
haversian canal
Havlane
Hawaii Early Learning Profile
HAWIC
    Hamburg-Wechsler Intelligence Test for
    Children
Haws Screening Test for Functional
Articulation Disorders
Hay Aptitude Test Battery
Hayem encephalitis
Haynes brain cannula
hazard
    environmental h.
    moral h.
    occupational h.
hazardous treatment
Hb
    hemoglobin
HBI
    Hutchins Behavior Inventory
HBr
    citalopram HBr
HC
    Huntington chorea
HCA
    heterocyclic antidepressant
HCD
    higher cerebral dysfunction
HCF
    Horsley-Clarke stereotactic frame
HcG-secreting suprasellar immature
teratoma
HCHWA-D
    hereditary cerebral hemorrhage with
    amyloidosis, Dutch type
HCl
    hydrochloride
        donepezil HCl
        Isocaine HCl
        naratriptan HCl
        nefazodone HCl
        paroxetine HCl
        sertraline HCl
        tacrine HCl
        ticlopidine HCl
        venlafaxine HCl
HCR
    hysterical conversion reaction
HCT
    Lotensin HCT

Hct
    hematocrit
HD
    Huntington disease
Hd
    human figure parts response
hdDXM
    high-dose dexamethasone
HDH
    Hostility and Direction of Hostility
HDHQ
    Hostility and Direction of Hostility
    Questionnaire
HDRS
    Hamilton Depression Rating Scale
HDSA
HDT
    Hand Dynamometer Test
HE
    hepatic encephalopathy
head
    h. banging
    base h.
    h. clamp
    h. coil
    h. consciousness
    h. fixation device
    h. frame
    gunshot wound to h. (GSWH)
    h. injury
    h. jerking
    h. knocking
    H. line
    h. movement
    h. and neck tremor
    perception of sound inside the h.
    perception of sound outside the h.
    h. ring
    h. rolling
    h. shadow effect
    sound inside the h.
    sound outside the h.
    H. Start program
    swelled h.
    swimming in the h.
    swimming h.
    h. tetanus
    h. tilt
    h. trauma
    h. turn technique
    voices inside h.
    voices outside h.
    h. weaving
    whole h. (WH)
    H. zone
headache
    acute confusional migraine h.
    alarm clock h.
    aphasic migraine h.
    band-like h.
    basilar artery migraine h.
    benign exertional h.
    Bickerstaff migraine h.
    bifrontal h.
    bilious h.

bioccipital h.
blind h.
cataclysmic h.
catamenial migraine h.
cervicogenic h. (CH)
cheese reaction h.
chronic h.
ciliary migraine h.
circumstantial migraine h.
classical migraine h.
cluster h.
coital h.
combination h.
common migraine h.
complicated migraine h.
confusional migraine h.
cough h.
cyclic h.
disabling h.
dull h.
episodic tension-type h. (ETTH)
essential h.
evening h.
exertional h.
facioplegic migraine h.
familial migraine h.
fibrositic h.
frontal h.
functional h.
generalized h.
giddy h.
hangover h.
hemiparesthetic migraine h.
hemiplegic migraine h.
histaminic h.
Horton h.
hot dog h.
ice cream h.
ice pick h.
ipsilateral h.
late-life migraine h.
leakage h.
matutinal h.
migraine h.
mixed h.
Monday morning h.
morning h.
muscle contraction h.
nitrite h.
nodular h.
nonpulsating h.
ocular migraine h.
organic h.
paroxysmal migraine h.
pectoralgic migraine h.
peri-ictal h.
postcoital h.
postconcussion h.
postictal migrainous h.
post-LP h.
post-lumbar puncture h.
posttraumatic h.
preictal h.
psychogenic h.
pulsating h.

radiation-injury h.
recurrent migraine h.
recurring h.
reflex h.
retinal migraine h.
seasonal migraine h.
sex h.
sick h.
sinus h.
sleep-related cluster h.
spinal puncture h.
suboccipital h.
sudden-onset h.
Symonds h.
symptomatic h.
syncopal migraine h.
h. syndrome
temporal h.
tension migraine h.
tension-vascular h.
throbbing h.
thunderclap h.
traumatic h.
unilateral migraine h.
vacuum h.
vascular h.
vasodilator h.
vasomotor h.
vestibular migraine h.
weekend h.
whole cranial h.
Willis h.
Wolff h.
head-banging behavior
head-bobbing doll syndrome
head-dropping test
headframe
    Kannon h.
    Sugita h.
    thousand-hands Kannon universal h.
headholder
    Gardner h.
    integrated h.
    Malcolm-Rand carbon-composite h.
    Mayfield-Kees h.
    Mayfield radiolucent h.
    Mayfield skull-pin h.
    pin h.
    pinion h.
    radiolucent cranial pin h.
    Sugita h.
headlamp
    Keeler video h.
headlight
    high beam fiberoptic h.
    LightWear h.
    Orascoptic fiberoptic h.
    Quadrilite 6000 fiberoptic h.
    QuietLite Quadrilite 6000
        fiberoptic h.
headrest
    Brown-Roberts-Wells h.
    Gardner-Wells h.
    horseshoe h.
    Light-Veley h.

H

headrest *(continued)*
    Mayfield h.
    Mayfield horseshoe h.
    Mayfield-Kees h.
    Mayfield radiolucent h.
    multipurpose h.
    pediatric h.
    pin fixation h.
    3-point h.
    Reston foam-padded h.
    Veley h.
headset
    Instatrak h.
heads-up
    h.-u. adjunctive endoscopy
    h.-u. imaging system
healing
    faith h.
    holistic h.
    mental h.
    h. ritual
health
    H. Assessment Questionnaire (HAQ)
    h. behavior
    H. Care Questionnaire
    community mental h.
    Department of Mental H. (DMH)
    emotional h.
    flight into h.
    H. and Human Services
    h. law
    h. maintenance organization (HMO)
    mental h.
    H. Plan Employer Data and Information Set (HEDIS)
    H. Problems Checklist
    h. risk
    h. systems agency (HSA)
health-related
    h.-r. consequence
    h.-r. facility
    h.-r. psychology
    h.-r. quality of life (HRQL)
healthy
    h. aggression
    h. identification
Healy Pictorial Completion Test
hearing
    audiometric h.
    color h.
    h. deficit
    h. disorder
    hard of h.
    h. impairment
    h. loss
    organ of h.
    pure tone h.
    Riese h.
    speech and h. (S&H)
    h. theory
    thought h.
    visual h.
    h. voices

heart
    change of h.
    h. disease
    h. disorder
    irritable h.
    h. murmur
    pounding h.
    purple h.
    h. reflex
    soldier's h.
heat
    h. effect
    h. exhaustion
    h. loss
    h. shock protein
    h. stress
heat-induced asthenia
heating
    eddy current h.
    radiofrequency h.
heavy
    h. metal intoxication
    h. metal neuropathy
    h. metal screen
    h. particle radiotherapy
heavy-duty straight clip
heavy-metal neuritis
hebbian
    h. modification
    h. potentiation of synapse
    h. property
Hebb rule
hebephilia
hebephrenia
    manic h.
hebephrenic
    h. dementia
    h. schizophrenia
hebetic
hebetis
    cynobex h.
hebetude
heboid
    h. paranoia
    h. praecox
heboidophrenia
hecateromeric, hecatomeral, hecatomeric
hederiform ending
hedgehog gene
HEDIS
    Health Plan Employer Data and Information Set
hedonia
hedonic
    h. capacity
    h. drive
    h. level
    h. response
    h. volition
hedonic-tone factor
hedonism
hedonistic
    h. activity
    h. orientation
    h. utilitarianism

hedonomania
hedonophobia
heel
    Achilles h.
    h. jar
    h. tap
heel-tap
    h.-t. reaction
    h.-t. test
heel-to-knee test
Heidelberg concept
Heidenhain
    H. disease
    H. type of spongiform
      encephalopathy
Heifetz
    H. carotid occluder
    H. clip
    H. cranial perforator
    H. cup serrated ring forceps
    H. procedure
    H. skull perforator
Heifetz-Weck clip
height
    h. phobia
    h. vertigo
heightened
    h. attention
    h. attention state
    h. awareness
    h. awareness state
Heilbronner thigh
Heinis constant
heinous crime
heir of the Oedipus complex
held
    H. bundle
    H. decussation
Helfergin
helical CT angiography
helical-like filament
helicat
helices
helicopod gait
helicopodia
heliencephalitis
helienologomania
heliomania
heliophobia
heliotrope rash
helix-loop-helix (HLH)
    h.-l.-h. response factor
hellenologophobia
hellenophobia
Heller
    H. dementia
    H. disease
    H. syndrome
helmet
    collimator h.
    cooling h.
    neurasthenic h.
    Sheffield collimator h.
Helmholtz coil
helminthic infection

helminthophobia
help
helper
    h. role
    h. therapy
helping
    h. behavior
    h. model
    h. relationship
helplessness
    learned h.
    psychic h.
help-rejecting complaining
help-seeking behavior
Helweg bundle
hemangioblastoma
    benign capillary h.
    third ventricular h.
hemangioendothelioma
    epithelial h. (EH)
    epithelioid h. (EH)
    kaposiform h.
    Masson vegetant intravascular h.
hemangioma
    h. of the brain
    calvarial h.
    cavernous h.
    dumbbell-shaped spinal
      cavernous h.
    epidural cavernous h.
    extraaxial cavernous h.
    extramedullary h.
    histiocytoid h.
    infantile hemangioblastic h.
    pontomesencephalic cavernous h.
    sacral h.
    vertebral h.
hemangiomatosis
hemangiopericytoma
    giant petroclival h.
    meningeal h.
Hemashield enhanced graft
hematemesis
hematencephalon
hematin
hematocephaly
hematocrit (Hct)
hematogenous cell infiltration
hematoma
    acute subdural h.
    balancing subdural h.
    carotid plaque h.
    cerebellar h.
    dural h.
    epidural h.
    h. evacuation
    evolving h.
    extracerebral h.
    extradural h.
    facial h.
    gelatinous h.
    hemispheral h.
    hypertensive h.
    iatrogenic h.
    infratemporal h.

H

hematoma *(continued)*
  interhemispheric h.
  intracerebral h.
  intracranial h.
  intramural h.
  intraparenchymal h.
  intraventricular h.
  isodense subdural h.
  nasal septum h.
  posterior fossa h.
  retromembranous h.
  retropharyngeal h.
  scalp h.
  spinal epidural h.
  spontaneous spinal epidural h.
    (SSEH)
  subdural h.
  subgaleal h.
  subperiosteal h.
  sylvian h.
  traumatic h.
Hematome system
hematomyelia
hematomyelopore
hematophobia
hematopoietic
hematoporphyrin derivative
hematorrhachis, hemorrhachis
  h. externa
  extradural h.
  h. interna
  subdural h.
hematoxylin
  Mayer h.
hematoxylin-eosin stain
hematuria
heme biosynthesis
hemeralopia
hemeraphonia
hemiacrosomia
hemialgia
hemiamyosthenia
hemianalgesia
hemianesthesia
  alternate h.
  crossed h.
hemianopia, hemianopsia
  altitudinal h.
  bilateral homonymous h.
  bitemporal h.
  congruous h.
  contralateral h.
  dense h.
  heteronymous h.
  homonymous h.
  ipsilateral h.
  macular h.
  paracentral h.
  partial h.
  quandrantic h.
hemianopic scotoma
hemianopsia
  bitemporal h.
  homonymous h.

hemiapraxia
hemiasynergia
hemiataxia
hemiathetosis
hemiatrophy
  facial h.
  progressive lingual h.
hemiballismic movement
hemiballismus, hemiballism
hemibasal syndrome
hemicephalalgia
hemicerebrum
hemichorea
hemichorea-hemiballism syndrome
**hemiconvulsions, hemiplegia, and
  epilepsy (HHE)**
hemicord
hemicorporectomy
hemicorticectomy
  cerebral h.
hemicrania
  chronic paroxysmal h.
  episodic paroxysmal h.
hemicranial pain
hemicranicus
  status h.
hemicraniectomy
hemicraniosis
hemicraniotomy
hemidecortication
  cerebral h.
hemideficit
  motor h.
  sensible h.
hemidepersonalization
hemidysesthesia
hemiepilepsy
hemifacial
  h. flushing
  h. microsomia
  h. spasm (HFS)
  h. weakness
hemifield
  contralesional h.
  ipsilesional h.
  h. loss
  h. of vision
hemihydranencephaly
hemihypalgesia
hemihyperesthesia
hemihyperkinesis
hemihypertonia
hemihypertrophy
hemihypesthesia, hemihypoesthesia
hemihypotonia
hemilaminectomy
  complete lateral h.
  lumbar h.
  partial h.
  unilateral h.
hemilateral chorea
hemimegalencephaly
hemimyelomeningocele
hemineglect syndrome
hemiopalgia

hemiopia
hemiparaplegia
hemiparesis
    ataxic h. (AH)
    contralateral h.
    dense h.
    hemiparetic h.
    herald h.
    hypesthetic ataxic h.
    ipsilateral h.
    paradoxical ipsilateral h.
    pure motor h. (PMH)
    residual h.
    spastic h.
hemiparesthesia
hemiparesthetic
    h. migraine
    h. migraine headache
hemiparetic hemiparesis
hemiparkinsonian stiffness
hemiplegia
    acute acquired h.
    acutely acquired h.
    h. alternans
    alternating hypoglossal h.
    contralateral h.
    crossed h.
    h. cruciata
    dense h.
    double h.
    facial h.
    Gubler h.
    hysterical h.
    infantile h.
    left h.
    motor h.
    nocturnal h.
    pure motor h.
    right h.
    spastic h.
    spinal h.
    superior alternating h.
    Wernicke-Mann spastic h.
hemiplegic
    h. amyotrophy
    h. gait
    h. idiocy
    h. migraine
    h. migraine headache
hemisensory
    h. loss
    h. syndrome
hemisoma
hemisomatognosia
hemispasm
    facial h.
hemispatial arousal neglect
hemispheral
    h. dysfunction
    h. hematoma
    h. mass
hemisphere
    cerebellar h.
    cerebral h.
    h. competition

    dominant h.
    language-dominant h.
    left h.
    mesial h.
    nondominant h.
    right h.
    h. sequence
    h. stroke
    ventricle of cerebral h.
hemispherectomy
hemispheric
    h. collapse
    h. disconnection syndrome
    h. infarction
    h. lateralization
    h. reliance
hemispherical
    h. contact probe
    h. deafferentation
    h. dysfunction
hemispherium
    h. cerebelli
    h. cerebri
hemithermoanesthesia
hemitonia
hemitransfixion incision
hemitremor
hemivertebra
hemizygosity
hemizygous
hemlock
    poison h.
    H. Society
hemochromatosis
Hemoclip
    Samuels-Weck H.
hemodialysis
hemodilution
    isovolemic h.
    prophylactic hypertensive
     hypervolemic h.
hemodynamic
hemoglobin (Hb)
hemoglobinopathy
hemoglobinuria
    nocturnal h.
hemolysis
    sleep-related h.
hemolytic anemia
hemophilia
hemophobia
hemorrhachis (*var. of* hematorrhachis)
hemorrhage
    aneurysmal h.
    aneurysmal subarachnoid h.
     (ASAH)
    apoplectic h.
    arterial h.
    artery of cerebral hemorrhage
    brainstem h.
    central nervous system h.
    cerebellar h.
    cerebral h.
    delayed traumatic intracerebral h.
     (DTICH)

H

hemorrhage *(continued)*
Duret h.
eight-ball h.
epidural h.
extradural h.
flame-shaped h.
focus of h.
germinal matrix h.
hypertensive basal ganglia h.
hypotensive h.
Icelandic form of intracranial h.
internal h.
intertrabecular h.
intracapsular h.
intracerebral h.
intracranial h. (ICrH)
intraocular h.
intraparenchymal h.
intratumor h.
intraventricular h. (IVH)
Kistler classification of
  subarachnoid h.
lobar h.
mesencephalic h.
neonatal intraventricular h.
nonaneurysmal perimesencephalic
  subarachnoid h.
nondominant putaminal h.
parenchymal cerebral h.
parenchymatous h.
perianeurysmal h.
periaqueductal h.
perimesencephalic nonaneurysmal
  subarachnoid h. (PNSH)
periventricular-intraventricular h.
petechial h.
pontine h.
primary subarachnoid
  supratentorial h.
putaminal h.
retrobulbar h.
slit h.
spinal cord h.
spinal epidural h. (SHE)
spinal subarachnoid h.
spinal subdural h. (SSH)
splinter h.
striate h.
subacute h.
subarachnoid h. (SAH)
subconjunctival h.
subcortical h.
subdural h.
subependymal h.
subgaleal h.
subhyaloid h.
subintimal h.
supratentorial subdural h.
syringomyelic h.
thalamic h.
thalamic-subthalamic h.
traumatic meningeal h.

traumatic subarachnoid h. (TSAH,
  tSAH)
vitreous h.
hemorrhagic
h. dysangiogenesis
h. fever
h. infarct
h. infarction
h. lesion
h. metastasis
h. necrosis
h. pachymeningitis
h. shearing injury
hemorrhagica
encephalitis h.
hemorrheology
hemosiderin
h. deposition
h. scar
hemosiderin-laden cell
hemosiderosis
cerebral h.
hemostasis
chemical h.
hemostasis-related protein
hemostat
Avitene microfibrillator collagen h.
Crile h.
Surgicel fibrillator absorbable h.
hemostatic
h. forceps
h. plug formation
hemothymia
hemotympanum
Hemovac Hydrocoat drain
henbane
**Henderson-Moriarty ESL/Literacy
  Placement Test**
Hendler
H. test
H. Test for Chronic Pain (HTCP)
Henle
H. fiber layer
ligament of H.
H. nervous layer
H. sheath
H. spine
Henmon-Nelson
H.-N. Ability Test, Canadian
  Edition
The H.-N. Tests of Mental Ability
Henoch chorea
Henoch-Schönlein purpura
Henry-Geist spinal fusion
henselae
Rochalimaea h.
Hensen
H. canal
H. cell
H. duct
H. node
heparin
low-molecular weight h. (LMWH)
h. sulfate
heparinization

heparinized
hepatic
    h. coma
    h. disease-associated neuropathy
    h. encephalopathy (HE)
    h. encephalopathy tremor
    h. failure
    h. function
    h. porphyria
    h. steatosis
hepatitis
    alcoholic h. (AH)
    h. A virus
    h. B virus
    h. B virus infection
    h. C virus
    h. D virus
    h. E virus
    h. F virus
    h. G virus
    infectious h.
    toxic h.
hepatobiliary system
hepatocellular
hepatocerebral
    h. degeneration
    h. disease
hepatocyte
hepatolenticular
    h. degeneration
    h. disease
hepatorenal syndrome
hepatosplenomegaly
hepatotoxicity
hepatropic virus
Heplock catheter
heptachlor
Heptalac
herald hemiparesis
Herbal Ecstasy
herbivorous
herd instinct
here-and-now approach
hereditaria
    adynamia episodica h.
    alopecia h.
hereditarian
hereditary
    h. angioneurotic edema (HANE)
    h. areflexic dystasia
    h. branchial myoclonus
    h. cerebellar ataxia of Marie
    h. cerebral hemorrhage with
      amyloidosis, Dutch type
      (HCHWA-D)
    h. deficiency
    h. dementia
    h. disorder
    h. hemorrhagic telangiectasia
    h. motor and sensory neuropathy
      (HMSN)
    h. myokymia
    h. neuropathy with susceptibility to
      pressure palsy (HNPP)
    h. nonprogressive chorea

    h. photomyoclonus
    h. posterior column ataxia
    h. sensorimotor neuropathy (HSMN)
    h. sensory neuropathy (HSN)
    h. spastic paraplegia
    h. spinal ataxia
    h. spinocerebellar ataxia syndrome
    h. striatopallidal disease
heredity
    environment and h. (E&H)
heredoataxia
heredofamilial
    h. psychosis
    h. tremor
heredo-familial essential microsomia
heredopathia atactica polyneuritiformis
Hereford Parental Attitude survey
    (HPA)
heregulin
heresiarch
heretic
Hering-Breuer reflex
Hering sinus nerve
Hering-Traube wave
heritability
    broad h.
heritable
heritage
hermaphrodism
hermaphrodite
hermaphroditism
    bilateral h.
    false h.
    transverse h.
    true h.
    unilateral h.
Hermetian symmetry
hermetic
    H. external ventricular drainage
      system
    H. II drainage management system
    H. lumbar drainage system
    h. medicine
hermsii
    Borrelia h.
hernia
    cerebral h.
    meningeal h.
herniated
    h. cervical disk
    h. intervertebral disk (HID)
    h. nucleus pulposus
herniation
    brain h.
    caudal transtentorial h.
    central transtentorial h.
    cerebellar tonsillar h.
    cerebral h.
    cervical disk h.
    cingulate h.
    concentric h.
    disk h.
    extraforaminal lumbar disc h.
      (ELDH)
    foraminal h.

H

herniation *(continued)*
 frank disk h.
 hard disk h.
 hippocampal h.
 impending h.
 incipient downward central brain h.
 internal disk h.
 intervertebral disk h.
 intraspongy nuclear disk h.
 lumbar disk h.
 rostral transtentorial h.
 soft disk h.
 sphenoidal h.
 subfalcial h.
 subfalcine h.
 subligamentous disk h.
 temporal lobe h.
 tentorial h.
 thoracic disk h.
 tonsillar h.
 transtentorial uncal h.
 traumatic cervical disk h.
 uncal h.
hero
 h. daydream
 h. fantasy
 h. worship
heroin
 h. addiction
 h. antagonist and learning therapy (HALT)
 black tar h.
 cannabis and h.
 cannabis, cocaine and h.
 h. and cocaine
 h. and crack use
 h. injection
 intranasal h.
 liquefied h.
 h. mixed with powdered milk
 h. and morphine
 h. overdose
 phencyclidine and h.
 h. withdrawal
heroinomania
herone
herophili
 torcular h.
herpes
 geniculate h.
 genital h.
 h. genitalis
 h. simplex
 h. simplex virus (HSV)
 h. simplex virus encephalitis (HSVE)
 h. zoster
 h. zoster meningitis
 h. zoster neuritis
 h. zoster ophthalmicus
 h. zoster oticus
herpesvirus
 h. encephalitis
 human h. 6 (HHV-6)

Herpesvirus simiae
herpetic
 h. encephalitis
 h. meningoencephalitis
 h. neuritis
herpetophobia
Herring body
Herrmann syndrome
hersage
Hertel
 H. exophthalmometer
 H. exophthalmometry examination
hertz (Hz)
Heschl
 H. convolution
 H. gyrus
hesitant speech
hesitation phenomenon
Hess
 H. School Readiness Scale (HSRS)
 trophotropic zone of H.
Heston Personality Index (HPI)
hetacillin
hetaeral fantasy
heteresthesia
heterocentric
heteroclite
heterocyclic
 h. agent
 h. antidepressant (HCA)
 h. antidepressant drug
heterodimer
heterodimeric receptor
heteroeroticism
heteroerotism
heterogeneity
 allelic h.
 neurophysiological h.
heterogeneous
 h. clinical presentation
 h. group
 h. nuclear RNA (hnRNA)
 h. system disease
heterogenicity
 genetic h.
 locus h.
heterogenous grouping
heterogeny
heterohypnosis
heterokinesia
heterokinesis
heterolalia
heteroliteral
heterologous stimulus
heteromeral
heteromeric cell
heteromerous
heteromorphic
heteronomous
 h. psychotherapy
 h. stage
 h. superego
heteronomy
heteronymous hemianopia
heteropathy

heterophasia
heterophemia, heterophemy
heterophonia
heterophoria
heteroplasm
heteropsychologic
heterorexia
heterosexual
    h. anxiety
    H. Attitudes Toward Homosexuality
      (HATH)
    h. behavior
    h. lover
    h. marriage
    h. orientation
    h. pedophile
    h. pedophilia
heterosociality
heterosome
heterosuggestion
heterotopia
    band h.
    incomplete band h.
heterotopic
    h. ossification
    h. pain
heterotopy
heterotrimeric
    h. G protein
    h. postreceptor
heterotypic cortex
heterozygosity
heterozygous
Heubner
    artery of H.
    recurrent artery of H.
heuristic
heuroscopy
hex, pl. hexes
    h. doctor
Hexabrix
Hexadrol Phosphate
hexafluorodiethyl ether
hexagon
    Bender-Gestalt h.
hexamethylpropyleneamineoxime
hexamethyl-propyleneamine oxime
    (HMPAO)
hexapropymate
hexenbesen
hexes (pl. of hex)
hexing
    illness ascribed to h.
hexobarbital
hexosaminidase deficiency
hexose
Heyer-Pudenz valve
Heyer-Schulte
    H.-S. antisiphon device
    H.-S. bur hole valve
    H.-S. neurosurgical shunt
    H.-S. wound drain
HFD
    Human Figure Drawing

HFF
    high-filter frequency
      HFF on electroencephalogram
HFPV
    high-frequency percussive ventilation
HFS
    hemifacial spasm
HGF
    human growth factor
HGSHS
    Harvard Group Scale of Hypnotic
      Susceptibility
HHE
    hemiconvulsions, hemiplegia, and
      epilepsy
      HHE syndrome
HHF35 muscle-specific actin tumor
  marker
HHS
HHV-6
    human herpesvirus 6
HI
    hypoglycemic index
5-HIAA
    5-hydroxyindoleacetic acid
hiatus
    tentorial h.
Hibbs
    H. spinal curette
    H. spinal fusion gouge
Hibbs-Jones spinal fusion
Hibbs-Spratt spinal fusion curette
hiccup, hiccough
    psychogenic h.
Hickman catheter
HID
    herniated intervertebral disk
HIDA
    technetium 99m HIDA
hidden
    h. clue test
    h. figures test
    h. meaning
    h. message
    h. observer
    h. self
hiding behavior
hidradenoma
hidrocystoma
hidrosis
HIE
    hypoxic-ischemic encephalopathy
hierarchial structure
hierarchical
    h. functioning
    h. organization
    h. regression analysis
    h. structure
    h. theory of instinct
hierarchy
    anxiety h.
    h. construction
    dominance h.
    exposure h.
    habit h.

H

hierarchy *(continued)*
    lifetime h.
    Maslow h.
    motivational h.
    motives h.
    h. of motives
    h. of need
    occupational h.
    response h.
    social h.
hieromania
hierophobia
hierotherapy
HIF
    higher intellectual function
high
    h. adaptive level
    h. affectivity ratio
    h. anxiety (HA)
    h. beam fiberoptic headlight
    h. cervical spinal cord lesion
    h. density area
    h. energy level
    h. energy X-ray beam
    h. frequency deafness
    h. impulsiveness high anxiety
      (HIHA)
    h. impulsiveness low anxiety
      (HILA)
    h. linear filter
    h. muscular resistance bed
    h. pontine lesion
    h. risk
    H. School Career-Course Planner
      (HSCCP)
    H. School Personality Questionnaire
      (HSPQ)
    h. steppage gait
    h. tolerance potential
    h. voltage slow and sharp activity
high-affinity binding site
high-air-loss bed
high-alcoholic elixir
high-altitude illness
highbrow
    ethical h.
high-calorie diet
high-density transient signals (HITS)
high-dose
    h.-d. dexamethasone (hdDXM)
    h.-d. drug
high-energy
    h.-e. bond
    h.-e. brachytherapy
higher
    h. brain center
    h. cerebral dysfunction (HCD)
    h. cortical dysfunction
    h. cortical function
    h. dementia
    h. echelon
    h. integrative language processing
    h. intellectual function (HIF)
    h. level cognitive function

    h. level of consciousness
    h. level skill
    h. mental process
    h. order conditioning
    h. order interaction
    h. order motion
    h. state of consciousness
    h. status
high-fat diet
high-fiber diet
high-filter frequency (HFF)
high-force Sundt clip system
high-frequency
    h.-f. activity
    h.-f. filter
    h.-f. generator
    h.-f. percussive ventilation (HFPV)
high-grade
    h.-g. defect
    h.-g. glioma
    h.-g. spondylolisthesis
    h.-g. stenosis
high-intensity
    h.-i. click stimulation
    h.-i. lesion
    h.-i. signal
    h.-i. transition
high-lesion load
high-level perceptual disturbance
highly active antiretroviral therapy
    (HAART)
high-molecular weight cytokeratin tumor
    marker
high-osmolar contrast medium
high-pitched voice
high-protein diet
high-resolution
    h.-r. brain SPECT system
    h.-r. CCT
    h.-r. 3DFT MR imaging
high-risk
    h.-r. activity
    h.-r. approach
    h.-r. behavior
    h.-r. group
    h.-r. patient
    h.-r. study
high-signal lesion
high-speed
    h.-s. air drill
    h.-s. microdrill
high-torque bur
High-Vision surgical telescope
high-voltage deflection
high-volume hospital
highway hypnosis
HIHA
    high impulsiveness high anxiety
HILA
    high impulsiveness low anxiety
hila (*pl. of* hilum)
Hilal
    H. coil
    H. microcoil
hilar

Hilger facial nerve stimulator
Hill Interaction Matrix (HIM)
hillock
    axon h.
    facial h.
Hillside Akathisia Scale
Hilson
    H. Adolescent Profile
    H. Personnel Profile/Success
    Quotient (HPP/SQ)
Hilton
    H. law
    H. method
hilum, pl. **hila**
    h. of dentate nucleus
    h. nuclei dentati
    h. nuclei olivaris
    h. of olivary nucleus
    h. ovarii
    h. of ovary
hilus
HIM
    Hill Interaction Matrix
H-imipramine binding
hindbrain
    h. decompression
    h. deformity
    h. ischemia
    h. vesicle
Hind III enzyme
Hinduism
hinged cast
Hinman syndrome
HIP
    Hypnotic Induction Profile
hip-flexion phenomenon
hippanthropy
Hippel disease
Hippel-Lindau
    H.-L. disease
    von H.-L.
hip phenomenon
hippocampal
    h. amnesia
    h. commissure
    h. convolution
    h. damage
    h. dentate gyrus
    h. epilepsy
    h. fissure
    h. formation
    h. formation atrophy
    h. herniation
    h. infarction
    h. monoamine concentration
    h. neuron
    h. sclerosis
    h. seizure
    h. synaptic plasticity
    h. volume loss
hippocampal-amygdala complex
hippocampectomy
hippocampus
    h. major

    mammalian h.
    h. minor
Hippocratic
    H. aphorism
    H. oath
hippomania
hippophobia
hippotherapy
Hirano body
Hirsch
    H. endonasal technique
    H. grading
    H. hypophysis punch forceps
Hirschberg test
Hirschsprung disease
hirsutism
hirundinis
    nidus h.
**Hiskey-Nebraska Test of Learning
Aptitude (HNTLA)**
HISMS
    How-I-See-Myself Scale
His perivascular space
Histacryl Blue
histamine
    h. cephalalgia
histaminic
    h. cephalalgia
    h. headache
histidinemia aminoaciduria
histidyl
histiocyte
    epithelioid h.
histiocytoid hemangioma
histiocytoma
histiocytosis
    diffuse cerebral h.
    kerasin h.
    h. X
histoacryl embolization
histocompatability
histogram
histolytica
    Entamoeba h.
histomorphometric
histonectomy
histoneurology
histopathologic
histopathology
Histoplasma
    H. capsulatum
    H. infection
histoplasmosis
    disseminated CNS h.
historical
    h. data
    h. method
    h. presentation
history
    alcohol-positive h. (APH)
    Automated Child/Adolescent
    Social H. (ACASH)
    biopsychosocial h.
    case h.

H

history *(continued)*
    Comprehensive Assessment of Symptoms and H. (CASH)
    cyclic h.
    depression h.
    detailed h.
    drinking h.
    educational h.
    family h. (FH)
    Giannetti On-Line Psychosocial H. (GOLPH)
    life h.
    lifetime h.
    marijuana h.
    marital h. (MH)
    medical h.
    military h.
    neurologic-ophthalmologic h.
    occupational h. (OH)
    oral h.
    pain h.
    past h. (PH)
    past personal h.
    perinatal h.
    personal h. (PH)
    personal and social h. (P&SH)
    h. and physical (H&P)
    premorbid h.
    prenatal h.
    h. of present illness (HPI)
    previous h.
    psychiatric h.
    psychosexual h.
    psychosocial h.
    relationship h.
    reliable h.
    school h.
    seizure h.
    sexual h.
    social h. (SH)
    suicide attempt h.
    h. of suicide attempt
histotoxic hypoxia
histrionic
    h. character
    h. neurotic personality disorder
    h. paralysis
    h. personality
    h. personality disorder
    h. presentation
    h. scale
    h. situation
    h. spasm
histrionism
HIT
    Holtzman Inkblot Technique
Hitachi scanning electron microscope
HITS
    high-density transient signals
hitting own body
Hitzig girdle
HIV
    human immunodeficiency virus

HIV disease
    HIV illness stage
HIV-based dementia
hive
    giant h.
Hivid
HIV-related
    H.-r. neuropathy
    H.-r. seizure
HLA DR15 (DR2) typing
HLH
    helix-loop-helix
    HLH factor
HMO
    health maintenance organization
HMPAO
    hexamethyl-propyleneamine oxime
H/M ratio
HMSN
    hereditary motor and sensory neuropathy
HMT
    Hodkinson Mental Test
HNB angiographic catheter
HNK
    human natural killer
    HNK cell
HNPP
    hereditary neuropathy with susceptibility to pressure palsy
hnRNA
    heterogeneous nuclear RNA
HNTLA
    Hiskey-Nebraska Test of Learning Aptitude
HO
    holmium
hoarding
    h. character
    h. orientation
    h. personality
hoarseness
    rough h.
Hoche
    H. bundle
    H. tract
hockey-stick
    h.-s. dissector
    h.-s. strategy
Hodgkin disease
Hodgkin-Huxley assumption
Hodkinson Mental Test (HMT)
hodomania
hodophobia
Hoehn and Yahr scale
Hoen
    H. dural separator
    H. intervertebral disk rongeur
    H. lamina gouge
    H. nerve hook
    H. pituitary rongeur
    H. ventricular needle
Hoffman and Mohr procedure
Hoffmann
    H. muscular atrophy
    H. phenomenon

H. reflex
H. sign

Hogan
H. Personality Inventory
H. Personnel Selection Series

Hoge 10-Item Intrinsic Religiosity Scale

holder
Adson dural needle h.
Ayers needle h.
CBI stereotactic head h.
cordotomy hook h.
Crile needle h.
curved micro-needle h.
Donaghy angled suture needle h.
Holinger endarterectomy
  dissector h.
Jacobson needle h.
Malis needle h.
Micro-One needle h.
microsurgery needle h.
Micro-Two needle h.
needle h.
neurosurgical needle h.
Patil stereotactic head h.
ReFix stereotactic head h.
Sugita head h.
Texas Scottish Rite Hospital
  hook h.
three-point head h.
Vari-Angle clip h.
Wangensteen needle h.
Webster needle h.
Yasargil needle h.

holding exercise

hole
bur h.
precoronal bur h.
h. preparation method

holergasia

holiday
h. depression
drug h.
Roman h.
h. syndrome
therapeutic drug h.

holier-than-thou attitude

**Holinger endarterectomy dissector
  holder**

holism

holistic
h. analysis
h. healing
h. medicine
h. psychology
h. treatment

Hollander test

Hollenhorst plaque

Hollingshead Index

Holmes
H. cerebellar degeneration
H. cerebellar degeneration disease
H. cortical cerebellar degeneration

Holmes-Adie
H.-A. pupil
H.-A. syndrome

Holmes-Rahe questionnaire

holmium (HO)
h. YAG laser

Holocaust

holocoenosis

holocord hydromyelia

holocrania

holography
volumetric multiple exposure
  transmission h. (VMETH)

holohemispheric vasogenic edema

holophrases

holophrastic

holoprosencephaly

holorachischisis

holotelencephaly

Holscher nerve root retractor

Holter
H. high-pressure valve
H. medium-pressure valve
H. monitor test
H. valve

Holter-Hausner valve

Holtzman Inkblot Technique (HIT)

Homans sign

homatropine

home
adult h.
adult foster h.
h. assessment
board-and-care h.
h. care
detention h.
domiciliary care h.
h. environment
H. Environment Questionnaire
h. evaluation
group h.
h. language
H. Observation for Measurement of
  the Environment
personal care h.
H. School Situations Questionnaire-
  Revised
H. Screening Questionnaire
h. setting
sheltered h.
single-parent h.
h. visit

home-based family management

homebody

homebound

home-health aide

homemaking responsibility

homeodomain
h. gene
h. protein

homeopathic principle

homeopathy

homeostasis
cellular ion h.
free radical h.

homeostatic
h. balance
h. equilibrium

H

homeostatic *(continued)*
    h. model
    h. principle
homeostenosis
homeotic gene
home-service agency
HomeTrac
    Saunders cervical H.
homichlophobia
homicidal
    h. behavior
    h. ideation
    h. intent
    h. plan
    h. preoccupation
    h. rumination
homicidomania
homilopathy
homilophobia
hominem
    ad h.
homoclite
homocysteine acid
homocystinuria
homoerotic
    subject h.
homoeroticism, homoerotism
homofenazine
homogamy
homogeneity
    Black Intelligence Test of
      Culture H. (BITCH)
    field h.
    spatial h.
homogeneous
    h. grouping
    h. lesion
    h. reinforcement
homogenic love
homogenitality
homogenous
    h. grouping
    h. scintillating scotoma
homogeny
homograph
homolateral
homologous stimulus
homonomy
    analysis of h.
    h. drive
homonymous
    h. hemianopia
    h. hemianopsia
    h. scintillating scotoma
homophile
homophobe
homophobia
homophone
homoplasmy
homorganic
homosexual
    h. behavior
    closet h.
    h. community

    h. complex
    h. conflict disorder
    h. incest
    h. lover
    h. marriage
    h. neurosis
    h. orientation
    h. panic
    h. pedophile
    h. pedophilia
    h. rape
homosexuality
    accidental h.
    adolescent h.
    effeminate h.
    ego dystonic h.
    Heterosexual Attitudes Toward H.
      (HATH)
    iatrogenic h.
    latent h.
    masked h.
    overt h.
    pedophilic h.
    situational h.
    unconscious h.
homosocial
homosociality
homotopic pain
homotypic cortex
homovanillic acid (HVA)
homozygosity
homozygote
homozygous
homuncular organization phase reversal
homunculus
honorable discharge
honor financial obligation
hood
    clitoral h.
    dorsal aponeurotic expansion h.
    H. masking technique
hoodwink
HOOI
    Hall Occupational Orientation Inventory
hook
    Adson dissecting h.
    Adson dural h.
    Adson nerve h.
    anatomic h.
    André anatomical h.
    ball tip nerve h.
    bifid h.
    blunt nerve h.
    Bobechko sliding barrel h.
    calvarial h.
    caudal h.
    cautery h.
    circular laminar h. with offset top
    clawed pedicle h.
    closed Cotrel-Dubousset h.
    closed transverse process TSRH h.
    Cloward cautery h.
    Cloward dural h.
    corkscrew dural h.
    cranial Jacobs h.

Crile nerve h.
Culler h.
Cushing dural h.
Cushing gasserian ganglion h.
Cushing nerve h.
Dandy nerve h.
DePuy nerve h.
h. dislodgement
dissecting h.
downsized circular laminar h.
drop-entry (closed body) h.
dura h.
Fisch dural h.
Fisch micro h.
Frazier dural h.
Frazier nerve h.
ganglion h.
Harrington pedicle h.
Hoen nerve h.
h. hollow-ground connection design
intermediate C-D h.
Isola spinal implant system h.
Jannetta h.
Kennerdell-Maroon h.
Kilner h.
Krayenbuehl nerve h.
Lahey Clinic dural h.
Lahey Clinic nerve h.
laminar C-D h.
large ball nerve h.
Leatherman h.
Love nerve root h.
Lucae nerve h.
Malis nerve h.
Marino transsphenoidal h.
microball h.
Moe alar h.
Moe spinal h.
Moe square-ended h.
multispan fracture h.
Murphy ball h.
nerve h.
open C-D h.
pear-shaped nerve h.
pediatric C-D h.
pediatric TSRH h.
pedicle C-D h.
ribbed h.
Rosser crypt h.
Sachs dural h.
Scoville nerve root h.
Selverstone cordotomy h.
side-opening laminar h.
h. site
Smithwick button h.
Smithwick ganglion h.
Smithwick sympathectomy h.
Speare dural h.
square-ended h.
straight nerve h.
Strully dural h.
Texas Scottish Rite Hospital
   trial h.
Toennis dural h.
top-entry (open body) h.

transsphenoidal h.
TSRH buttressed laminar h.
TSRH circular laminar h.
TSRH pedicle h.
h. V-groove connection design
von Graefe strabismus h.
Weary nerve h.
Yasargil spring h.
Zielke bifid h.
Zimmer caudal h.
hookean body
hooked
   h. bundle of Russell
   h. fasciculus
hook-plate fixation
hook-to-screw L4-S1 compression
   construct
Hooper Visual Organization Test
Hoover sign
Hopkins
   H. Symptom Checklist (HSCL)
   H. Symptom Checklist-90 (HSCL-
      90)
   H. Symptom Checklist-90 Total
      Score (HSCL-90 T)
   H. syndrome
Hoppe-Goldflam disease
horizon
   closed h.
   open h.
   white h.
horizontal
   h. cell of Cajal
   h. fissure of cerebellum
   h. gaze
   h. gaze palsy
   h. gaze paresis
   h. group
   h. inhibition
   h. mobility
   h. nystagmus
   h. pedicle diameter
   h. vertigo
hormephobia
hormism
hormonal
   h. level
   h. self-treatment
   h. sex-reassignment
   h. sexual reassignment
hormone
   adrenocorticotropic h. (ACTH)
   antidiuretic h. (ADH)
   corticotropin-releasing h. (CRH)
   ectopic h.
   follicle-stimulating h. (FSH)
   gonadal h.
   gonadotropin-releasing h. (GnRH,
      GRH)
   growth h. (GH)
   growth hormone-releasing h.
      (GHRH)
   hypothalamic regulating h.
   h. ingestion
   luteinizing h. (LH)

H

hormone *(continued)*
    luteinizing hormone-releasing h.
      (LHRH)
    natriuretic h.
    parathyroid h. (PTH)
    polypeptide h.
    resistance to thyroid h. (RTH)
    syndrome of inappropriate secretion
      of antidiuretic h. (SIADH)
    thyroid stimulating h. (TSH)
    thyrotropin-releasing h. (TRH)
    thyrotropin-stimulating h. (TSH)
horn
    Ammon h.
    anterior h.
    cutaneous h.
    dorsal h.
    frontal h.
    inferior h. of lateral ventricle
    lateral h.
    occipital h.
    posterior h.
    temporal h.
    ventral h.
Horner syndrome
Horn-Hellersberg
    H.-H. Drawing Completion
    H.-H. Drawing Completion Test
Horrax
horrific
    h. impulse
    h. temptation
hors de combat
horseback riding accident
horseshoe
    h. headrest
    h. incision
horseshoe-shaped flap
Horsley
    H. bone wax
    H. dural separator
    H. rongeur
Horsley-Clarke
    H.-C. stereotactic frame (HCF)
    H.-C. stereotaxic apparatus
Hortega cell
Horton
    H. disease
    H. giant cell arteritis
    H. headache
    H. histamine cephalalgia
hospice
    h. care
    h. movement
hospital
    h. addiction syndrome
    H. Anxiety and Depression Scale
      (HADS)
    h. and community psychiatry
    day h.
    for-profit h.
    high-volume h.
    mental h.
    night h.

    not-for-profit h.
    open h.
    open-door h.
    private psychiatric h.
    psychiatric h.
    state h. (SH)
    state mental h. (SMH)
    Texas Scottish Rite H. (TSRH)
    VA H. (VA)
    Veterans Administration H.
    weekend h.
hospital-based psychiatry
hospitalism
hospitalitis
hospitalization
    involuntary h.
    long-term h.
    partial h.
    short-term h.
    voluntary h.
host
    h. culture
    h. mother
hostile
    h. aggression
    h. aggressiveness
    h. behavior
    h. identity
    h. response
    h. transference
hostility
    covert h.
    H. and Direction of Hostility
      (HDH)
    H. and Direction of Hostility
      Questionnaire (HDHQ)
    open h.
    paranoid h.
    penalty, frustration, anxiety,
      guilt, h. (PFAGH)
hot
    h. dog headache
    h. flash
    h. knife
    h. line
hotline
    abused-child h.
    abused-wife h.
    crisis h.
    runaway h.
    suicide h.
hot-seat technique
hot-spot phantom
Hounsfield unit (HU)
hour
    twenty-minute h.
hour-glass dressing
hourglass tumor
house
    h. arrest
    cooperative urban h.
    Fountain H.
    halfway h.
    National Mental Health Consumers
      Self-Help Clearing H.

Phoenix H.
h. physician
quarter-way h.
h. rule
Soteira H.
transitional halfway h.
House-Brackmann
H.-B. facial nerve function grading scale
H.-B. Grading Scale
H.-B. Scale
H.-B. Score
House-Fisch
H.-F. dural retractor
H.-F. dural spatula
household
h. product inhalant
h. responsibility
housekeeping gene
Housepian
H. aneurysm clip
H. forceps
House-Tree (HT)
H.-T. Test (HT)
House-Tree-Person (HTP)
H.-T.-P. Technique
H.-T.-P. Test
housewife
h. neurosis
h. psychosis
h. syndrome
housing
satellite h.
Houston
H. halo
H. Test for Language Development
Howard spinal curette
Howell Prekindergarten Screening Test
How-I-See-Myself Scale (HISMS)
Howmedica
H. Microfixation cranial plate
H. Microfixation System drill bit
H. Microfixation System plate cutter
H. Microfixation System plate-holding forceps
H. Microfixation System pliers
H. VSF fixation system
Hox gene
Ho:YAG laser
HP
hyperphoria
Nicoderm HP
Vicodin HP
H&P
history and physical
HPA
Hereford Parental Attitude survey
hypothalamic-pituitary-adrenal
hypothalamic-pituitary-adrenocortical
H.P. Acthar Gel
HPI
Heston Personality Index
history of present illness

HPNT
Hundred Pictures Naming Test
HPP/SQ
Hilson Personnel Profile/Success Quotient
HRB
Halstead-Reitan Battery
H-reflex
HRNES
Halstead Russell Neuropsychological Evaluation System
HRNTB
Halstead-Reitan Neuropsychological Test Battery
HRQL
health-related quality of life
Hs
hypochondriasis scale
HSA
health systems agency
HSCCP
High School Career-Course Planner
HSCL
Hopkins Symptom Checklist
HSCL-90
Hopkins Symptom Checklist-90
HSCL-90 T
Hopkins Symptom Checklist-90 Total Score
H-shaped microplate
HSMN
hereditary sensorimotor neuropathy
HSN
hereditary sensory neuropathy
HSPQ
High School Personality Questionnaire
HSRS
Hess School Readiness Scale
HSV
herpes simplex virus
HSV encephalitis
HSVE
herpes simplex virus encephalitis
HT
hand test
House-Tree
House-Tree Test
hypertension
5-HT
5-hydroxytryptamine
5-HT receptor assay
HTCP
Hendler Test for Chronic Pain
5-HT$_2$-D$_2$-antagonist
HTIG
human tetanus immune globulin
HTLV
human T-cell leukemia virus
human T-cell lymphoma virus
human T-cell lymphotropic virus
HTLV-associated myelopathy/tropical spastic paraparesis (HAM/TSP)
HTLV-I associated myelopathy (HAM)

H

HTP
  House-Tree-Person
  HTP test
HTR
  hard tissue replacement
  HTR polymer
HTR-MFI
  hard tissue replacement-malleable facial
  implant
    HTR-MFI chin implant
    HTR-MFI curved implant
    HTR-MFI malar implant
    HTR-MFI paranasal implant
    HTR-MFI premaxillary implant
    HTR-MFI ramus implant
    HTR-MFI straight implant
HTR-PMI implant
HU
  Hounsfield unit
huang
    ma h.
Hudson
    H. brace
    H. brace bur
    H. cerebellar attachment
    H. cranial drill set
    H. cranial rongeur
    H. drill
    H. forceps
    H. perforator
hue
    blue de h.
    h. and cry
    primary h.
Hulka instrument
human
    h. botulism
    Children's Apperception Test-H.
    (CAT-H)
    h. chorionic gonadotropin
    h. dural substitute
    h. dural substitute graft
    h. ecology
    h. engineering
    h. factor psychology
    H. Figure Drawing (HFD)
    h. figure parts response (Hd)
    h. foible
    H. Genome Project
    h. growth factor (HGF)
    h. herpesvirus 6 (HHV-6)
    h. immunodeficiency virus (HIV)
    H. Information Processing Survey
    h. movement response
    h. natural killer (HNK)
    h. nature
    h. neurofilament light chain
    h. potential
    h. prion disease
    h. relation
    h. relations group
    h. resources
    h. response (h)
    h. surrogate
    h. T-cell leukemia virus (HTLV)

    h. T-cell lymphoma virus (HTLV)
    h. T-cell lymphotropic virus
    (HTLV)
    h. tetanus immune globulin (HTIG)
    h. therapeutic experience
humane
humanism
humanistic
    h. conscience
    h. perspective
    h. psychology
    h. school
    h. theory
    h. therapy
humanitarian
human-motivation theory
human-pet bonding
human-potential
    h.-p. model
    h.-p. movement
human-relations training
humanus
    morsus h.
humeroperoneal muscular dystrophy
humidity effect
humor
    anal h.
    gallows h.
    sense of h.
humoral
    h. immune response
    h. immune system
    h. immunity
    h. phototransduction
    h. synapse
    h. theory
Humphrey visual field
Hundred Pictures Naming Test (HPNT)
hunger
    affect h.
    air h.
    h. drive
    h. edema
    narcotic h.
    h. pain
    psychogenic air h.
    social h.
Hunstad infusion needle
Hunt
    H. angled serrated ring forceps
    H. angled tip forceps
    H. atrophy
    H. disease
    H. grasping forceps
    H. and Hess criteria
    H. and Hess grade
    H. and Hess Grades I-III
    H. and Kosnik classification
    H. neuralgia
    H. paradoxical phenomenon
    H. syndrome
    H. tremor
Hunt-Early technique
Hunter
    H. canal

H. disease
H. dural separator
H. open cord tendon implant
H. operation
H. syndrome
hunterian
h. ligation
h. ligation of aneurysm
Hunt-Hess
H.-H. aneurysm classification
H.-H. aneurysm grading system
H.-H. neurological classification
H.-H. subarachnoid hemorrhage
scale
hunting behavior
huntingtin protein
Huntington
H. chorea (HC)
H. chorea organic psychosis
H. disease (HD)
Hunt-Kosnik classification of aneurysm
**Hunt-Minnesota Test for Organic Brain
Damage**
Hunt-Yasargil pituitary forceps
Hurd bone-cutting forceps
Hurler
H. disease
H. syndrome
Hurler-Scheie disease
Hurst disease
Hurteau skull plate anvil
husband-to-wife aggression
Husk bone rongeur
Hutchins Behavior Inventory (HBI)
Hutchinson
H. facies
H. mask
H. pupil
H. type neuroblastoma
HVA
homovanillic acid
HVS
hyperventilation syndrome
hwa-byung
wool h.-b.
H-wave test
hyaline
h. arteriosclerosis
h. body of pituitary
h. thickening
hyalinization
Crooke h.
hyalophobia, hyelophobia
hyaluron-binding region
hyaluronidase
hyatari
hybridization
Northern h.
in situ h.
hybridoma
Hydantoin
hydatid
cerebral h.
h. cyst
h. disease

Hydergine LC
hydralazine
h. hydrochloride
h. and hydrochlorothiazide
**hydralazine, hydrochlorothiazide, and
reserpine**
hydranencephaly
Hydrap-ES
hydrargyromania
hydrate
chloral h.
H. Injection
hydrencephalocele
hydrencephalomeningocele
hydrencephalus
hydride
butyl h.
hydrobulbia
hydrocarbons
aromatic h.
volatile h.
hydrocele spinalis
hydrocephalic
h. dementia
h. idiocy
h. periventricular radiolucency
hydrocephalocele
hydrocephaloid
hydrocephalus
acquired h.
acute h.
asymptomatic h.
bilateral h.
chronic communicating h.
communicating h.
congenital h.
delayed h.
double compartment h.
external h.
h. ex vacuo
fulminant h.
idiopathic normal pressure h.
infantile h.
internal h.
kaolin-induced h.
meningitic h.
multiloculated h.
noncommunicating h.
normal pressure h. (NPH)
normotensive h.
obstructive h.
occult h.
otitic h.
h. oversecretion
posthemorrhagic h.
postinfectious h.
postmeningitic h.
posttraumatic h.
primary h.
secondary h.
shunted h.
subdural effusion with h. (SEH)
symptomatic h.
thrombotic h.
toxic h.

H

hydrocephalus *(continued)*
   triventricular h.
   unilateral h.
   unshunted h.
hydrocephaly
Hydrocet
hydrochloride (HCl)
   alphaprodine h.
   amantadine h.
   amitriptyline h.
   amphetamine h.
   apomorphine h.
   aptiganel h.
   Aventyl H.
   benactyzine h.
   benzphetamine h.
   bromodiphenhydramine h.
   bupropion h.
   buspirone h.
   butaciamol h.
   butamoxane h.
   butethamine h.
   butoxamine h.
   butriptyline h.
   chlordiazepoxide h.
   chlorphentermine h.
   chlorpromazine h.
   cinnamedrine h.
   clonidine h.
   cocaine h.
   cyclobenzaprine h.
   cycrimine h.
   cyproheptadine h.
   desipramine h.
   dexciamol h.
   dexfenfluramine h.
   diacetylmorphine h.
   dibenzepin h.
   dibucaine h.
   diethylpropion h.
   dihydromorphinone h.
   diphenhydramine h.
   dipipanone h.
   donepezil h.
   dopamine h.
   doxepin h.
   doxorubicin h.
   etazolate h.
   ethaverine h.
   ethomoxane h.
   ethopropazine h.
   etoxadrol h.
   fenethylline h.
   fenfluramine h.
   fenmetozole h.
   fluoxetine h.
   fluphenazine h.
   flurazepam h.
   hydralazine h.
   hydromorphone h.
   hydroxyzine h.
   imipramine h.
   isoetharine h.
   levomethadyl acetate h.

levoxadrol h.
mebeverine h.
medazepam h.
meperidine h.
methadone h.
methamphetamine h.
methaqualone h.
methylphenidate h.
metopon h.
molindone h.
morphine h.
nalbuphine h.
nalmefene h.
nalorphine h.
naloxone h.
naratriptan h.
nefazodone h.
nitrosourea h.
opipramol h.
oxycodone h.
oxymorphone h.
oxyphencyclimine h.
papaverine h.
perphenazine and amitriptyline h.
phenadoxone h.
phencyclidine h.
phentermine h.
phenylpropanolamine h.
procarbazine h.
promethazine h.
proparacaine h.
propoxyphene h.
propranolol h.
ropinirole h.
sertraline h.
thiothixene h.
tiagabine h.
ticlopidine h.
tizanidine h.
trazodone h.
trifluoperazine h.
trifluperidol h.
triflupromazine h.
trihexyphenidyl h.
trimethobenzamide h.
tryptizol h.
venlafaxine h.
ziprasidone h.
hydrochlorothiazide
   amiloride and h.
   benazepril and h.
   bupropion h.
   captopril and h.
   enalapril and h.
   hydralazine and h.
   lisinopril and h.
   losartan and h.
   methyldopa and h.
   propranolol and h.
   h. and reserpine
   h. and spironolactone
   h. and triamterene
hydrocodone
   h. and acetaminophen
   h. and aspirin

h. bitartrate
h. and ibuprofen
hydrocortisone
Hydrocortone
H. Acetate
H. Phosphate
hydrodipsomania
HydroDIURIL
hydroencephalocele
hydroencephaly
Hydro-Ergoloid
hydroflumethiazide and reserpine
hydrogel
copper sulfate h.
hydrogen ion concentration
Hydrogesic
Hydrolene polymer
Hydroloid-G
hydroma
cystic h.
hydromania
hydromeningocele
hydromeningoencephalocele
hydromicrocephaly
hydromorphine
hydromorphone hydrochloride
Hydromox
hydromyelia
holocord h.
hydromyelocele
Hydro-Par
hydroperoxide
phospholipid h.
4-hydroperoxycyclophosphamide
hydrophilicity
hydrophobia
hydrophobica
agriothymia h.
hydrophobicity algorithm
hydrophobic tetanus
hydrophobophobia
hydrophorograph
hydropneumatic massage
hydropneumogony
Hydropres
hydrops
endolymphatic h.
labyrinthine h.
vestibular h.
Hydro-Serp
Hydroserpine
HydroStat IR
hydrosyringomyelia
hydrotherapy
5-hydrotryptophan
hydroxide
aluminum h.
magnesium aluminum h.
hydroxyapatite
APS h.
h. graft
hydroxybutyrate
beta h.
gamma h. (GHB)
hydroxychloroquine

17-hydroxycorticosteroid
6-hydroxydopamine (OHDA)
hydroxyethylmethacrylate
2-hydroxyethylmethacrylate
hydroxyethyl methacrylate polymerizing solution
5-hydroxyindoleacetic acid (5-HIAA)
hydroxyisovaleric aminoaciduria
hydroxyl
h. derivative of GABA (Gabob)
h. radical
hydroxylase
dopamine-beta h. (DBH)
h. immunohistochemical
tyrosine h.
hydroxylase-positive
tyrosine h.-p.
hydroxylation
5-hydroxytryptamine (5-HT)
5-h. receptor assay
hydroxyurea
hydroxyzine
h. hydrochloride
h. pamoate
hyelophobia (*var. of* hyalophobia)
hygieiolatry
hygiene
criminal h.
h. deterioration
inadequate sleep h.
industrial h.
mental h.
minimal personal h.
personal h.
sleep h.
hygienic inducement
hygroma
subdural h.
hygrophobia
Hygroton
hyla
hylomania
hylophobia, hylephobia
hymen
imperforate h.
hymenal membrane
hymenectomy
Hymovich Chronicity Impact and Coping Instrument (CICI)
hyoid bone
hyoscyamine sulfate
hypacusic
hypacusis, hypoacusis
hypalgesia, hypoalgesia
h. dolorosa
hypalgesic, hypalgetic
hypalgia
Hy-Pam
hypapoplexia
Hypaque
hypaxial
hypegiaphobia
hypengyophobia
hyperabduction syndrome

H

hyperactive
- h. behavior
- h. child syndrome (HACS)
- h. disorder
- h. sexual arousal
- h. sexual desire

hyperactive-impulse attention-deficit/hyperactivity disorder
hyperactive-impulsive combined behavior
hyperactivity
- attention deficit disorder with h. (ADD-HA)
- autonomic h.
- developmental h.
- h. disorder
- dopaminergic h.
- h. index
- motoric h.
- prefrontal h.
- spontaneous neuronal h.

hyperactivity-impulsivity dimension
hyperacusis, hyperacusia
hyperadrenal constitution
hyperadrenalism
hyperadrenergic response
hyperadrenocorticism
hyperaesthetic personality
hyperaggressivity
hyper-β-alaninemia aminoaciduria
hyperaldosteronism
hyperalert
hyperalgesia
- auditory h.

hyperalgesic, hyperalgetic
hyperalgia
hyperalimentation
hyperammonemia
- cerebroatrophic h.

hyperamnesia
hyperamylasemia
hyperaphia
hyperarousal
- autonomic h.

hyperbaric
- h. medicine
- h. oxygen

hyperbeta-alaninemia
hyperbilirubinemia
- nonhemolytic h.

hyperbulimia
hypercalcemia
hypercalciuria
hypercapnia
hypercarbia
- depressed ventilatory response to h.

hypercatabolism
hypercathexis
hypercenesthesia, hypercoenesthesia
hypercholesterolemia
- familial h.

hypercinesis, hypercinesia
hyper-CKemia
- idiopathic h.

hypercoagulability
hypercoagulable state

hypercoagulation
hypercoenesthesia (*var. of* hypercenesthesia)
hypercompensatory type
hypercortisolemia
hypercortisolism
hypercritical
hypercryalgesia
hypercryesthesia
hyperdefensive attitude
hyperdopaminergic state
hyperdynamia
hyperechema
hyperemia
- occlusive h.
- relative h.

hyperemic response
hyperemotional
hypereosinophilic syndrome
hyperepithymia
hyperergasia
hyperergia, hypergia
hyperergic encephalitis
hypereridic state
hyperesthenia
hyperesthesia
- auditory h.
- cerebral h.
- gustatory h.
- muscular h.
- h. olfactoria
- olfactory h.
- h. optica
- tactile h.

hyperesthetic
- h. memory
- h. zone

hyperexcitability
- neuronal h.

hyperexplexia
hyperextension
- intraoperative neck h.

hyperextension-hyperflexion injury
hyperflexion
hyperfractionated
- h. irradiation
- h. radiotherapy

hyperfractionation
hyperfrontality
hyperfunction
- adrenal cortical h.

hyperfusion
hypergammaglobulinemia
hypergamy
hypergargalesthesia
hypergasia
hypergenitalism
hypergeusia
hypergia (*var. of* hyperergia)
hyperglycemia
- nonketotic h.

hyperglycorrhachia
hypergnosis
hypergraphia

hyperhidrosis
  palmar h.
hyperindependence
hyperingestion
hyperinsulinism
hyperintense
  h. hyperosmolality
  h. lesion
hyperintensity
  incidental punctate white matter h.
  punctate white matter h.
  white matter h.
hyperirritability
hyperkalemia
hyperkalemic periodic paralysis
hyperkeratosis
hyperkeratotic plantar lesion
hyperkinesis, hyperkinesia
  axial h.
  developmental disorder associated
    with h.
  h. index
hyperkinetic
  h. conversion reaction
  h. disorder
  h. disturbance
  h. dysarthria
  h. dysphonia
  h. encephalopathy
  h. reaction of childhood
  h. speech
  h. syndrome
  h. syndrome of childhood
hyperkyphoscoliosis
  neuropathic h.
hyperlexia
hyperlipidemia
hyperlogia
hyperlysinemia aminoaciduria
hypermagnesemia
hypermania
hypermetabolic tumor component
hypermetabolism
  prefrontal h.
hypermetamorphosis
hypermethylation
hypermetria
hypermimia
hypermnesia
hypermyelination
hypermyesthesia
hypermyotonia
hypernatremia
hypernatremic encephalopathy
hypernephroma
hypernoia
hypernomia
hyperobesity
hyperontomorph
hyperorality
hyperorexia
hyperosmia
hyperosmolality
  hyperintense h.

**hyperosmolar (hyperglycemic) nonketotic
  coma**
hyperosmolarity
hyperosmotic agent
hyperosphresia, hyperosphresis
hyperostosis
  Caffey h.
  diffuse idiopathic skeletal h.
  h. frontalis interna
hyperostotic
  h. lesion
  h. spondylosis
hyperoxia
hyperparathyroidism
hyperpathia
hyperperfusion
  h. syndrome
  tissue h.
hyperphagia
hyperphagic obesity
hyperphoria (HP)
hyperphrasia
hyperphrenia
hyperpipecolatemia
hyperpituitarism
hyperplasia
  adrenal h.
  arachnoidal h.
  cerebral h.
  congenital adrenal h.
  congenital virilizing adrenal h.
  fibromuscular h.
  gingival h.
  multiglandular h.
  papillary mucosal h.
  somatotroph h.
  vessel h.
hyperplastic
hyperplastic-hypertrophic obesity
hyperpolarization
hyperponesis
hyperpragia
hyperpraxia
hyperprolactinemia
hyperprolinemia aminoaciduria
hyperprosexia
hyperprosody
hyperpselaphesia
hyperpsychosis
hyperpyrexia
hyperquantivalent idea
hyperreflexia
  asymmetric h.
  autonomic h.
  bilateral h.
  generalized h.
  pathologic h.
  spastic h.
  unilateral h.
hyperreligiosity
hyperresponsible worry
hypersalivation
hypersarcosinemia
hypersecretion
hypersecretory adenoma

H

hypersensibility
hypersensitive
hypersensitivity
    h. syndrome
    h. vasculitis
hypersensitization
hyperserotonemia
hypersexual complex
hypersomnia
    h. associated with depression
    h. disorder
    idiopathic h.
    persistent h.
    primary h.
    transient h.
hypersomnia-type sleep disorder
hypersomnolence
    central nervous system h.
    h. disorder
    idiopathic CNS h.
hypersomnolent
hyperstimulation
    adrenergic h.
hypertelorism
    orbital h.
hypertension (HT)
    benign intracranial h. (BIH)
    cerebral h.
    essential h.
    idiopathic intracranial h. (IIH)
    intracranial h.
    orthostatic h.
    venous h.
hypertensive
    h. basal ganglia hemorrhage
    h. crisis
    h. encephalopathy
    h. hematoma
hypertensive, hypervolemic,
  hemodilutional therapy
hypertensor
hyperthermalgesia
hyperthermia
    malignant h.
hyperthermoesthesia
hyperthymia
hyperthymic
    h. personality disorder
    h. temperament
hyperthyroidism
    apathetic h.
hyperthyroid neuropathy
hypertonia
    sympathetic h.
hypertonic absence
hypertrichosis
hypertriglyceridemia
hypertrophic
    h. arthritis
    h. cervical pachymeningitis
    h. cranial pachymeningitis
    h. interstitial neuropathy
    h. obesity
    h. olivary degeneration
    h. pachymeningitis dorsalis

hypertrophica
    pachymeningitis cranialis h.
hypertrophied frenula syndrome
hypertrophy
    facet h.
    pseudomuscular h.
    uncovertebral joint h.
hypertropia
    over-right h.
hypertychia
hyperuricemia
hypervalinemia
hypervascularity
    intratumoral h.
hyperventilation
    h. activating technique
    autonomic h.
    central neurogenic h.
    forced h.
    neurogenic h.
    psychogenic h.
    h. syndrome (HVS)
    h. test
    h. tetany
hyperverbal
hypervigilant
hyperviscosity syndrome
hypervolemia
hypervolemic treatment
hypesthesia, hypoesthesia
    brachiofacial cortical h.
    olfactory h.
    trigeminal h.
    vaginal h.
hypesthetic ataxic hemiparesis
hyphedonia
hyphema
Hy-Phen
hypnagogic
    h. hallucination
    h. hallucination image
    h. hallucination imagery
    h. intoxication
    h. perception
    h. reverie
    h. state
    h. vision
hypnagogue
hypnalgia
hypnesthesia
hypnic jerk
hypnoanalysis
hypnoanesthesia
hypnocarthosis
hypnocatharsis
hypnodrama
hypnogenesis
hypnogenic
    h. spot
    h. zone
hypnogenous
hypnogogic
hypnograph
hypnoid state
hypnolepsy

hypnologist
hypnology
hypnomania
Hypnomidate
hypnonarcosis
hypnopathy
hypnopedia
hypnophobia
hypnophrenosis
hypnopompic
    h. hallucination
    h. image
    h. perception
    h. state
hypnosis
    diagnostic use of h.
    direct suggestion under h. (DSUH)
    father h.
    fear h.
    highway h.
    lethargic h.
    major h.
    minor h.
    mother h.
    suggestion h.
    suggestion under h.
    symptom relief through h.
    waking h.
hypnosophy
hypnotherapy
hypnotic
    h. abreaction
    h. abuse
    h. amnesia
    h. anesthesia
    h. capacity
    h. delirium
    h. dependence
    h. dependency
    h. drug
    h. induction
    H. Induction Profile (HIP)
    h. interview
    h. intoxication
    h. patient
    h. psychotherapy
    h. relationship
    h. relaxation technique training
    h. response
    h. sedative
    h. sleep
    h. state
    h. suggestion
    h. trance
    h. use disorder
    h. withdrawal
    h. withdrawal symptom
hypnotic-dependent patient
hypnotic-induced
    h.-i. anxiety
    h.-i. disorder
    h.-i. persisting dementia
    h.-i. psychotic disorder with delusions

    h.-i. psychotic disorder with hallucinations
    h.-i. sexual dysfunction
hypnotic-sedative drug
hypnoticus
    status h.
hypnotism
hypnotizability
hypnotization
    collective h.
hypnotize
hypnotoid
hypoactive
    h. sexual arousal
    h. sexual desire
    h. sexual desire disorder
hypoacusis (*var. of* hypacusis)
hypoadrenalism
hypoaffective
hypoalgesia (*var. of* hypalgesia)
hypoboulia, hypobulia
hypocalcemia
hypocapnia
hypocathexis
hypochondriaca
    melancholia h.
hypochondriacal
    h. melancholia
    monosymptomatic h.
    h. neurosis
    h. paranoia
    h. preoccupation
    h. psychogenic disorder
    h. psychoneurosis
    h. psychoneurotic reaction
    h. psychosis
    h. symptom
hypochondriac language
hypochondrial reflex
hypochondriasis
    monosymptomatic h.
    h. neurotic disorder
    h. scale (Hs)
Hypochondriasis With Poor Insight Type
hypochondroplasia
hypochoresis
hypocomplementemic glomerulonephritis
hypocortisolemia
hypodensity
    white matter h.
hypodepression
hypodermatic medication
hypodermic
    h. injection
    intracutaneous h.
    intramuscular h.
    intravenous h.
    h. needle
hypodopaminergic state
hypoechogenic peritumoral halo
hypoesthesia (*var. of* hypesthesia)
hypoesthetic
hypoevolutism
hypofibrinogenemia

H

hypofolatemia
hypofrontality phenomenon
hypofunction
    prefrontal h.
    testicular h.
hypoganglionosis
hypogastric
    h. ganglia
    h. reflex
hypogenetic corpus callosum
hypogeusia
    idiopathic h.
hypoglossal
    h. eminence
    h. nerve
    h. nerve paresis
    h. neuralgia
    h. neuropathy
    h. nucleus
    h. triangle
hypoglossal-facial nerve anastomosis
hypoglossi
    nucleus prepositus h. (NPH)
hypoglossus
    nervus h.
hypoglycemia
hypoglycemic
    h. delirium
    h. encephalopathy
    h. index (HI)
    h. peripheral neuropathy
hypoglycorrhachia
hypoglycorrhacia of cerebrospinal fluid
hypogonadal
hypogonadism
    h. with anosmia
hypogonadism with anosmia
hypohypnotic
hypointensity
hypokalemia
    thiazide-induced h.
hypokalemic
    h. metabolic acidosis
    h. periodic paralysis
hypokinesia, hypokinesis
    cardiac wall h.
hypokinetic
    h. anoxia
    h. dysarthria
    h. speech
    h. syndrome
hypokrisia
hypokyphosis
    right thoracic curve with h.
    thoracic h.
hypolepsiomnia
hypologia
hypomagnesemia
hypomania scale
hypomanic
    bipolar I disorder, most recent
     episode h.
    h. disorder
    h. episode
    h. manic-depressive reaction

    h. mood episode
    h. personality
    h. psychosis
    h. reaction
    h. scale
    h. tendency
hypomanic-depressive reaction
hypomelancholia
hypomelanosis of Ito
hypometabolism
    frontotemporal h.
    striatal h.
hypometamorphosis
hypometria
hypomimia
hypomnesia
hypomotility
hypomyelinating condition
hypomyelination, hypomyelinogenesis
hyponatremia
hyponatremic encephalopathy
hyponoia
hyponomic
hypoparathyroid
    h. encephalopathy
    h. tetany
hypoparathyroidism
hypoperfusion
    cerebral h.
    delayed postischemic h.
hypophonia
hypophonic aphasia
hypophoria
hypophosphatemia
hypophrasia
hypophrenic
hypophrenosis
hypophyseal (*var. of* hypophysial)
hypophysectomize
hypophysectomy
    h. forceps
    partial central h.
    total h.
    transethmosphenoidal h.
    transsphenoidal h.
    unilateral h.
hypophyseopriva, hypophysiopriva
    cachexia h.
hypophysial, hypophyseal
    h. aneurysm
    h. cachexia
    h. forceps
    h. grafting
    h. syndrome
hypophysiosphenoidal syndrome
hypophysis
    catecholamine h.
    h. cerebri
    pharyngeal h.
    h. punch forceps
hypophysitis
    giant-cell granulomatous h.
    granulomatous h.
    lymphocytic h.

lymphoid h.
pseudotumoral lymphocytic h.
hypopituitarism
hypopituitary coma
hypoplasia
cerebral h.
condylar h.
optic nerve h.
hypoplasticus
status h.
hypopraxia
hypoprosessis
hypoprosody
hypopsychosis
hyporeflexia
multisegmental h.
radicular h.
hyposensitive
hyposexuality
hyposmia
hyposomnia
h. associated with anxiety
h. associated with depression
h. associated with psychosis
hyposphresia
hyposthenia
hypostheniant
hypotaxia
hypotelorism
hypotension
acute severe h.
idiopathic orthostatic h.
intracranial h.
neurogenic orthostatic h.
orthostatic h.
postural h.
spontaneous intracranial h.
sympathotonic orthostatic h.
hypotensive
h. hemorrhage
h. retinopathy
h. surgery
hypothalamic
h. acromegaly
h. astrocytoma
h. blood flow
h. glucocorticoid
h. hamartoma
h. hypophyseal gonadal axis
h. infundibulum
h. lesion
h. obesity
h. regulating hormone
h. sulcus
hypothalamic/chiasmatic glioma
hypothalamic-pituitary
h.-p. axis
h.-p. axis dysfunction
h.-p. dysfunction
hypothalamic-pituitary-adrenal (HPA)
h.-p.-a. axis
hypothalamic-pituitary-adrenocortical
(HPA)

hypothalamohypophysial
h. portal system
h. tract
hypothalamus
ventromedial h.
Hypotherm Gel Kap
hypothermia
accidental h.
regional h.
hypothermic
h. disorder
h. metabolic index
hypothesis
adaptive h.
anniversary h.
apertural h.
as-if h.
beta h.
biogenic amine h.
congenital h.
degenerative h.
disconnection h.
dopamine h.
drift h.
ethical risk h.
experimental h.
falsifiable h.
Fiamberti h.
frustration-aggression h.
gamma h.
gate-control h.
h. generation
intergroup-contact h.
lipid h.
matching h.
maturation h.
mediumistic h.
mnemenic h.
monoamine h.
neurohumoral h.
null h.
Penfield h.
quantal h.
segregation h.
serotonergic deficiency h.
specificity h.
h. testing
topographic h.
viral h.
hypothesize
hypothetical
h. continuum
h. deductive thinking
hypothetical-deductive reasoning
hypothymia
hypothymic personality disorder
hypothymism
hypothyroidism
congenital h.
hypothyroid neuropathy
hypotonia
essential h.
neonatal h.
hypotonic cerebral palsy
hypotonicity

H

hypotonus, hypotony
hypotropia
hypoventilation
hypovigility
hypovolemia
hypovolemic shock
hypoxemia
hypoxia
 anemic h.
 anoxic h.
 cerebral h.
 histotoxic h.
 hypoxic h.
 ischemic h.
 stagnant h.
 toxic h.
hypoxic
 h. brain damage
 h. encephalopathy
 h. hypoxia
 h. ventilatory response
hypoxic-ischemic
 h.-i. brain damage
 h.-i. encephalopathy (HIE)
hypoxyphilia
hypoxyphilia-caused death
hypsarhythmia, hypsarrhythmia
hypsicephalic
hypsicephaly
hypsiphobia, hypsophobia
hypsokinesis
Hyrexin-50 Injection
hysteresis
hysteria
 anxiety h.
 Arctic h.
 canine h.
 Charcot grand h.
 collective h.
 combat h.
 communicable h.
 conversion h.
 defense h.
 dissociative h.
 epidemic h.
 fixation h.
 major h.
 mass h.
 minor h.
 h. neurotic disorder
 h. psychoneurosis
 h. psychosis
 h. scale
 studies on h.
 h. study
hysteric
 h. amaurosis
 h. amblyopia
 aura h.'s
 h. coma-like state
 h. lethargy
 megalopia h.'s
 h. paralysis
 suffocation h.'s

hysterica
 aura h.
hysterical
 h. abasia
 h. amnesia
 h. anesthesia
 h. aphonia
 h. astasia-abasia
 h. ataxia
 h. aura
 h. blindness
 h. character
 h. character defense
 h. chorea
 h. conversion reaction (HCR)
 conversion-type neurotic h.
 h. convulsion
 h. deafness
 h. delirium
 h. delirium hysterical depression
 dissociative-type neurotic h.
 h. dysphoria hysterophilia
 h. epilepsy
 h. fugue
 h. fugue state
 h. gait
 h. gait disorder
 h. hemiplegia
 h. insanity
 h. joint
 h. laughter
 h. lithiasis
 h. mania
 h. mutism
 h. myodynia
 h. neurosis
 h. personality
 h. polydipsia
 h. pregnancy
 h. pseudodementia
 h. psychoneurotic reaction
 h. psychosis
 h. puerilism
 h. seizure
 h. stuttering
 h. syncope
 h. trance
 h. tremor
 h. vertigo
 h. visual loss
hystericism
hystericoneuralgic
hystericum
 delirium h.
hystericus
 globus h.
hysteriform
hysterique
 grande attaque h.
hysterocatalepsy
hysteroepilepsy
hysterofrenatory
hysterofrenic
hysterogenic, hysterogenous
 h. zone

hysteroid
    h. convulsion
    h. defense
    h. dysphoria
    h. feature
    h. personality
hysteromania
hysteronarcolepsy
hysterophilia
    hysterical dysphoria h.

hysteropia
hysterosyntonic
hysterotrismus
Hytakerol
Hytrast
Hyzaar
Hyzine-50
Hz
    hertz

H

I
I marker
I tracing
IA
inactive alcoholic
IAA
inhibitory amino acid
IAAT
Iowa Algebra Aptitude Test
IABP
intraaortic balloon pump
intra-ortic balloon pump
IAC
Inventory of Anger Communication
isolated angiitis of the CNS
IADL
instrumental activities of daily living
IADSA
intraarterial digital subtraction angiogram
iamatology
iambic stress
IAP
intermittent acute porphyria
IAS
Integrated Assessment System
iatric
iatrogenesis
iatrogenic
i. addiction
i. carotid-cavernous fistula
i. discitis
i. disease
i. disorder
i. elevatus
i. hematoma
i. homosexuality
i. illness
i. induction
i. lumbar kyphosis
i. psychosis
i. schizophrenia
i. seizure
iatrogeny
iatrology
iatrophobia
iatrophysics
IB
index of body build
Dynafed IB
Excedrin IB
Midol IB
Motrin IB
Sine-Aid IB
IBBB
intra-blood-brain barrier
IBC
Illness Behavior Checklist
ibogaine
I-bolt
Texas Scottish Rite Hospital I-b.
IBQ
Illness Behavior Questionnaire

IBS
Interpersonal Behavior Study
Interpersonal Behavior Survey
IBT
inkblot test
Ibuprin
ibuprofen
hydrocodone and i.
pseudoephedrine and i.
Ibuprohm
Ibu-Tab
IBW
ideal body weight
ICA
internal carotid artery
ICA-occluded stable Xe/CT CBF study
ICD
impulse control disorder
International Classification of Diseases
Inventory for Counseling and
Development
ICD-9
International Classification of Diseases,
9th Edition
International Classification of Diseases,
9th edition
ICD-9-CM
International Classification of Diseases,
9th Edition, Clinical Modification
ICD-10
International Classification of Diseases
and Related Health Problems, 10th
Edition
ICDS
Integrated Child Development Scheme
ICE
Individual Career Exploration
ice
i. cream headache
i. pick headache
i. pick-like pain
iceblock theory
ICEDP
intracranial epidural pressure
ICEEG
intracranial electroencephalography
Iceland disease
**Icelandic form of intracranial
hemorrhage**
ICET
48-Item Counseling Evaluation Test
ichnogram
ichthyoacanthotoxin
ichthyohemotoxin
ichthyohemotoxism
ichthyomania
ichthyophagia
ichthyophobia
ichthyosarcotoxin
ichthyosarcotoxism
ichthyotoxin
ichthyotoxism

ICI
Interpersonal Communication Inventory
IC-IC
intracranial to intracranial
IC-IC bypass
ICIDH
International Classification of
Impairments, Disabilities, Handicaps
iconic
i. memory
i. sign
i. storage
iconoclast
iconolatry
iconomania
iconophobia
ICP
intracranial pressure
ICP Camino bolt
ICP catheter
ICP monitor
ICP wave form
ICPS
interpersonal cognitive problem solving
ICP-T
I.-T. fiberoptic ICP intracranial
temperature catheter
I.-T. fiberoptic ICP monitoring
catheter
ICrH
intracranial hemorrhage
ICRT
Individualized Criterion Referenced
Testing
ICRTM
Individualized Criterion Reference
Testing Mathematics
ICRTR
Individualized Criterion Reference
Testing Reading
ICS
intracranial stimulation
ICSD
International Classification of Sleep
Disorders: Diagnostic and Coding
Manual
ICT
insulin coma therapy
ictal
i. amnesia
i. automatism
i. confusional seizure
i. depression
i. depression phase of seizure
i. emotion
i. epileptiform activity
i. epileptiform pattern
i. fear
i. focal epileptiform discharge
i. pattern on EEG
i. period
icteric
icterogenic
icterohepatitis
icteroid

icterus
icthyomania
ictus
i. epilepticus
i. paralyticus
ICU
intensive care unit
ICU psychosis
ICVM
intracerebroventricular administration of
morphine
ID
identification
id
i. anxiety
i. ego
i. interpretation
i. psychology
i. resistance
i. sadism
i. wish
ida
tripa i.
idazoxan
IDEA
Individuals with Disabilities Education
Act
IDEA Oral Language Proficiency
Test II
idea
abstract i.
associated i.
association of i.'s
i. association
autochthonous i.
bizarre i.
complex of i.'s
compulsive i.
disconnected i.
dominant i.
expansive i.
fixed i.
flight of i.'s (FOI)
hyperquantivalent i.
imperative i.
inappropriate i.
i. of influence
intruding i.
intrusive distressing i.
morbid i.
obliquely related i.
obsessional i.
obtrusive i.
overcharged i.
overvalued i.
permanent dominant i.
persecutory i.
persistent inappropriate i.
persistent intrusive i.
poverty of i.
pressure of i.'s
recurring i.
i. of reference
referential i.
repetitive i.

ruminative i.
strongly held i.
i. of unreality
unreasonable i.
unwarranted i.

ideal
body i.
i. body weight (IBW)
ego i.
i. ego
father i.
i. masochism
narcissistic ego i.
i. personality
i. spinal implant
transient ego i.

idealism

idealist

idealization
i. defense mechanism
primitive i.

idealized
i. image
i. self
i. value

IDEAS
Interest Determination, Exploration and
Assessment System
Interest Determination, Exploration and
Assessment System, Enhanced Version

ideation
adolescent sexual i.
AWOL i.
elopement i.
grandiose i.
homicidal i.
incoherent i.
paranoid i.
persecution i.
recurrent suicidal i.
stress-related paranoid i.
suicidal i.
suspicious i.
transient i.
transient stress-related paranoid i.

ideational
i. agnosia
i. apraxia
i. shield
i. style of coping

ideatory apraxia

idebenone

idée fixe

id-ego

idem

idenenone

identical
i. element
i. twin

identifiable
i. stress
i. stressor

identification (ID)
anthropometric i.
cosmic i.

cross-gender i.
deep trance i.
i. defense mechanism
empathic i.
facial i.
feminine i.
i. figure
gender i.
group i.
healthy i.
letter-word i.
multiple i.
object i.
i. phenomenon
phenomenon i.
primary i.
projective i.
secondary i.
social i.
i. test
i. transference
trial i.
i. with the aggressor
Word Intelligibility by Picture I.
(WIPI)

identifying
i. data
i. with aggression

identity
adolescent personal i.
adolescent sexual i.
alteration in i.
alternate i.
assumption of new i.
body i.
i. confusion
controlling i.
core gender i.
core sense of i.
i. crisis
cultural i.
i. disorder
i. disorder of adolescence
i. disorder of childhood
i. disturbance
ego i.
family i.
female-to-male transgender i.
feminine i.
i. formation
former i.
gender i.
hostile i.
inflated i.
loss of personal i.
male-to-female transgender i.
masculine i.
multiple distinct i.'s
i. need
personal i.
place i.
primary i.
i. problem
protector i.
psychosexual i.

identity *(continued)*
    sense of i.
    sexual i.
    i. state
    i. theme
    i. versus role diffusion
    vocational i.
    i. vs. role confusion
ideodynamism
ideogenetic
ideogenic
ideogenous
ideoglandular
ideogram
ideographic
ideokinetic
    i. apraxia
    i. praxis
ideological commitment
ideology
ideometabolic
ideometabolism
ideomotion
ideomotor
    i. aphasia
    i. apraxia
    i. dyspraxia
    i. signal
ideomuscular
ideo-obsessional constitution
ideophobia
ideophrenia
ideoplastia
ideoplastic stage
ideosynchysia
ideovascular
idiochromosome
idiocrasy
idiocy
    amaurotic axonal i.
    amaurotic familial i. (AFI)
    athetosic i.
    axonal i.
    Aztec i.
    Bielschowsky i.
    cretinoid i.
    developmental i.
    diplegic i.
    eclamptic i.
    epileptic i.
    erethismic i.
    family i.
    genetous i.
    hemiplegic i.
    hydrocephalic i.
    infantile i.
    intrasocial i.
    juvenile i.
    Kalmuk i.
    microcephalic i.
    mongolian i.
    moral i.
    paralytic i.
    paraplegic i.

    plagiocephalic i.
    profound i.
    scaphocephalic i.
    sensorial i.
    spastic amaurotic axonal i.
    torpid i.
    traumatic i.
    Vogt-Spielmeyer i.
    xerodermic i.
idiodynamic control
idiogamist
idiogenesis
idiogenic osmoles
idioglossia
idiogram
idiographic approach
idiohypnotism
idioimbecile
idiolalia
idiolect
idiolog
idiologism
idiom
    personal i.
idiomatic usage
idiomuscular
idioneurosis
idiopathic
    i. CNS hypersomnolence
    i. dystonia
    i. encephalopathy
    i. facial nerve palsy
    i. generalized epilepsy
    i. growth hormone deficiency
    i. hyper-CKemia
    i. hypersomnia
    i. hypogeusia
    i. inflammatory myopathy (IIM)
    i. insomnia
    i. intracranial hypertension (IIH)
    i. intracranial pachymeningitis
    i. language retardation
    i. meningitis
    i. muscular atrophy
    i. neuralgia
    i. neuropathy
    i. normal pressure hydrocephalus
    i. orbital pseudotumor
    i. orthostatic hypotension
    i. Parkinson disease
    i. Parsonage-Turner syndrome
    i. plexus neuritis
    i. polyneuropathy
    primary thrombocytopenia i.
    i. psychosis
    i. recurring stupor (IRS)
    i. scoliosis
    i. seizure
idiophonia
idiophrenic
    i. insanity
    i. psychosis
idiopsychologic
idioreflex
idiospasm

idiosyncrasia olfactoria
idiosyncrasy
idiosyncratic
    i. alcohol intoxication
    i. behavior
    evidence of intrusion of i.
    i. material
    i. meaning
    i. process
    i. reaction
    i. reasoning
    i. side effect
    i. thinking
    i. topic shifting
idiot
    erethismic i.
    mongolian i.
    oxycephalic i.
    pithecoid i.
    profound i.
    i. savant
    superficial i.
    torpid i.
idiotism
idiotrophic
idiotropic type
idiovariation
idolatrous
idolomania
IDT
    interdisciplinary team
I-E
    internal versus external
    I-E Scale
    I-E Scale of Rotter
IER
    IER test
IES
    introversion-extroversion scale
IFI
    Institutional Functioning Inventory
ifiasochism
    verbal i.
IFN
    interferon
IFN-γ
    interferon-γ
IFN-B1a
    interferon-β 1a
IFN-B1b
    interferon-β 1b
IFROS
    ipsilateral frontal routing of signals
IGF
    insulin-like growth factor
IgG
    immunoglobulin G
IGI
    Institutional Goals Inventory
IgM
    immunoglobulin M
    IgM antibody capture (MAC EIA)
ignipedites
ignis fatuus

IHD
    ischemic heart disease
iich'aa
IIH
    idiopathic intracranial hypertension
IIM
    idiopathic inflammatory myopathy
I-it relationship
ikota
IL
    interleukin
ILD
    interstitial lung disease
ILDCSI
    Individual Learning Disabilities
    Classroom Screening Instrument
ILEAD
    Instructional Leadership Evaluation and
    Development Program
ileitis
    regional i.
ileocolitis
    granulomatous i.
Iletin
    Semilente I. I
    Protamine Zinc and I. I
    Regular I. I
    Ultralente I. I
ileus
    adynamic i.
    paralytic i.
Ilhéus encephalitis
iliac
    i. artery injury
    i. crest bone graft stabilization
    i. crest resection
    i. crest syndrome
    i. fixation
    i. post
    i. screw
iliocostal muscle
iliofemoral thrombosis
iliohypogastric nerve
ilioinguinal nerve
iliopsoas muscle
iliosacral
    i. and iliac fixation construct
    i. screw
Ilizarov corticotomy
ill
    chronically mentally i. (CMI)
    mentally i.
    object i.
    terminally i.
    i. will
    i. wisher
illegal drug
illegitimate
illicit
    i. drug
    i. lover
    i. psychoactive substance
Illinois
    I. Children's language Assessment
    Test

Illinois *(continued)*
    I. Test of Psycholinguistic Ability
      (ITPA)
illiteracy
    functional i.
    technological i.
illiterate
    functional i.
illness
    advantage by i.
    i. ascribed to hexing
    i. as self-punishment
    i. behavior
    I. Behavior Checklist (IBC)
    I. Behavior Questionnaire (IBQ)
    bipolar i. (BPI)
    catastrophic i.
    chronic factitious i.
    course of i.
    cyclic i.
    dysautonomic i.
    emotional i.
    escape into i.
    factitious i.
    flight into i.
    folk i.
    functional i.
    high-altitude i.
    history of present i. (HPI)
    iatrogenic i.
    length of i.
    life-threatening i.
    manic-depressive i.
    models of i.
    monophasic i.
    no mental i. (NMI)
    petition of mental i. (PMI)
    i. phase
    i. phobia
    preexisting i.
    present i. (PI)
    progressive dementing i.
    psychiatric i.
    psychogenic i.
    psychosomatic i.
    psychotic i.
    social class and mental i.
    I. and Symptom History Schedule
    usual childhood i. (UCI)
illogical
    i. attitude
    i. communication
    i. reasoning
    i. thinking
illogicality
illumination
    i. condition
    Luxtec coaxial i.
illuminator
    XL i.
illusion
    bodily i.
    i. of doubles
    dream i.

fleeting i.
memory i.
movement i.
optic i.
optical i.
i. of orientation
Poggendorf i.
recurrent i.
tactile i.
temporal lobe i.
transient auditory i.
transient tactile i.
transient visual i.
visual i.
windmill i.
Zollner i.
illusionary misconception
illusory memory
ILSA
    Interpersonal Language Skills and
      Assessment
IM
    intramuscular
    Loxitane IM
image
    accidental i.
    i. acquisition time
    i. agglutination
    angio i.
    autoradiographic i.
    axial spin-echo i.
    B-mode i.
    body i.
    changed body i.
    cohesive i.
    concrete i.
    contrast-enhanced MR i.
    i. control
    i. correlation
    cross-sectional i.
    direct i.
    distorted body i.
    disturbed body i.
    eidetic i.
    false i.
    father i.
    i. foldover
    i. formation principle
    formed i.
    fragmentary dream i.
    general i.
    ghost i.
    gradient-echo MR i.
    gradient-recalled echo i.
    graven i.
    i. guidance
    i. guided solution
    hallucinatory i.
    hypnagogic hallucination i.
    hypnopompic i.
    idealized i.
    inappropriate i.
    incidental i.
    in-phase i.

i. integrated surgery treatment
    planning
i. intensification
i. intensifier
intrusive obsessional i.
inverted i.
long pulse repetition time/echo
    time i.
memory i.
mental i.
midsagittal i.
mirror i.
mother i.
motor i.
negative body i.
obsessional mental i.
out-of-phase i.
parent i.
percept i.
peripheral field i.
persistent inappropriate i.
persistent intrusive i.
personal i.
PET i.
phantom i.
primary mental i.
proton-weighted i.
i. quality
real i.
reformatted i.
sagittal spin-echo i.
sagittal T1-weighted SE i.
sensory i.
short pulse repetition time/echo
    time i.
source i.
SPECT i.
stereotactic PET i.
tactile i.
thin-section i.
tilting of visual i.'s
trailing i.
transient i.
T1-weighted MR i.
T2-weighted MR i.
T1-weighted spin-echo i.
T2-weighted spin-echo i.
unformed i.
visual i.
vivid dream i.
image-distorting level
imaged pseudohallucination
image-guided stereotactic brain biopsy
imageless thought
Imagent
    I. BP
    I. GI
    I. LN
    I. US
imager
    Magnes 2500 WH i.
    1.5-T i.
imagery
    affective i.
    auditory i.

i. code
eidetic i.
emotive i.
guided affective i. (GAI)
hypnagogic hallucination i.
mental i.
paraphiliac i.
pictorial i.
smell i.
tactile i.
taste i.
i. therapy
visual i. (VI)
imaginal
    i. desensitization
    i. exposure
    i. flooding
    i. process
imaginary
    i. companion
    i. language
imaginative play
imagined
    i. abandonment
    i. defect
    i. loss
    I. Process Inventory (IPI)
imaging
    blood pool i.
    brain i.
    i. brain
    cerebral dynamic i.
    chemical-shift i.
    Chopper-Dixon hybrid i.
    color-flow i.
    computerized infrared
        telethermographic i.
    continuous-wave Doppler i.
    contrast-enhanced MR i.
    2DFT gradient-echo i.
    3DFT gradient-echo i.
    3DFT gradient-echo MR i.
    Diasonics magnetic resonance i.
    diffusion i.
    digital vascular i. (DVI)
    direct multiplanar i.
    Dixon method opposed i.
    Doppler i.
    echo planar i.
    fast i.
    fat-suppression MR i.
    flow i.
    flow-sensitive MR i.
    fluoroscopic i.
    functional brain i.
    functional magnetic resonance i.
        (fMRI, FMRI)
    gadolinium-enhanced MR i.
    Gd-DTPA-enhanced cranial MR i.
    gradient-echo MR i.
    gradient-refocused i.
    half-Fourier i.
    half-NEX i.
    high-resolution 3DFT MR i.
    line i.

imaging *(continued)*
    MAGNES magnetic source i.
    magnetic resonance i. (MRI)
    magnetic source i. (MSI)
    i. multiplanar
    multiple line-scan i. (MLSI)
    multiple plane i.
    neurodiagnostic i.
    neurovascular i.
    nonproton magnetic resonance i.
    nuclear i.
    oblique sagittal gradient-echo
      MR i.
    partial flip angle i.
    partial Fourier i.
    phase-sensitive gradient-echo MR i.
    planar spin i.
    point i.
    proton i.
    pulsed Doppler i.
    quantitative i.
    radionuclide i.
    rapid acquisition radiofrequency-
      echo steady state i.
    real-time color Doppler i.
    reproducible target i.
    sequential plane i.
    sequential point i.
    short inversion recovery i. (STIR)
    simultaneous volume i.
    spin-echo i.
    spin-warp i.
    structural brain i.
    subtraction i.
    surface coil spectroscopic i.
    ^{99m}Tc-HMPAO SPECT i.
    Tc-99m HMPAO cerebral perfusion
      SPECT i.
    three-dimensional fast low-angle
      shot i.
    three-dimensional Fourier
      transform i.
    three-dimensional Fourier transform
      gradient-echo i.
    transcranial real-time color
      Doppler i.
    two-dimensional i.
    two-dimensional Fourier
      transform i.
    two-dimensional Fourier transform
      gradient-echo i.
imago, pl. **imagines**
imbalance
    acid-base i.
    autonomic i.
    biochemical i.
    central language i.
    developmental i.
    effort-reward i.
    electrolyte i.
    fluid i.
    intellectual i.
    language i.

    sympathetic i.
    vasomotor i.
imbecility
    moral i.
    old age i.
    old-age i.
    phenylpyruvic i.
    senile i.
IMC
    information memory concentration
IMF
    intermaxillary fixation
IMG
    international medical graduate
IMI
    Impact Message Inventory
imipenem-cilastatin
    i.-c. injection
imipramine
    i. hydrochloride
    i. pamoate
imitation
    elicited i.
    interiorized i.
    morbid i.
    repetition by i.
    spontaneous i.
imitative
    i. behavior
    i. speech
    i. tetanus
Imitrex
immanence theory
immature
    i. personality
    i. personality disorder
immaturity
    emotional i.
    emotionally unstable i.
    perceptual i.
    i. reaction
    social i.
immediacy behavior
immediate
    i. anxiety
    i. early gene
    i. early gene induction
    i. echolalia
    i. ejaculation
    i. environment
    i. experience
    i. gratification
    i. memory
    i. memory test
    i. posttraumatic automatism
    i. posttraumatic convulsion
immediate-early gene cascade
immediately
immigrant status
immigration
    macrophage i.
imminent justice
immissio penis
immitis
    Coccidioides i.

immix
immobile state
immobility
    motor i.
    motoric i.
immobilization
    halo-vest i.
    i. method
    i. paralysis
    postoperative i.
    sternal occipital mandibular i.
      (SOMI)
    Treponema pallidum i. (TPI)
immobilizer
    sternooccipitomanubrial i.
immoral imperative
immune
    i. body
    chorea i.
    i. complex
    i. deficiency
    i. deficiency syndrome
    i. disorder
    i. function
    i. mediated mechanism
    i. response
    i. system
    i. system regulation
immunity
    active i.
    humoral i.
    passive i.
    stress i.
immunoblot analysis
immunocompetent macrophage
immunocompromised
immunoconjugate
    gene therapy i.
immunocytochemistry
immunocytology
immunodeficiency
    sexually acquired i. (SAID)
immunodiagnosis
immunoelectrophoresis
    countercurrent i. (CIE)
immunoelectrotransfer blot technique
immunofluorescence test
immunogen
    behavioral i.
immunoglobulin
    i. G (IgG)
    intravenous i. (IVIG)
    i. M (IgM)
    oligoclonal i. (OI)
    plasmapheresis and intravenous i.
immunohistochemical
    hydroxylase i.
immunologic
    cellular i.
    i. nitric oxide synthase (iNOS)
immunological paralysis
immunology
    clinical i.
immunomodulatory

immunoperoxidase
    i. method
    i. staining
immunophotography
    fluorescent i.
immunoreaction
immunoreactivity
    c-fos protein i.
    metenkephalin-like i.
immunosorbent assay
immunostain
    cytokeratin i.
immunostaining
immunosuppression
immunosuppressive therapy
immunotherapy
    adoptive i.
immunotoxin
immunoturbidimetry analyzer
Imovane
IMPA cephalometric measurement
impact
    i. analysis
    developmental i.
    I. of Events Scale
    I. Message Inventory (IMI)
    potential i.
impacted grief
impactor
    Cloward bone graft i.
    vertebral body i.
impaired
    i. affect
    i. affect modulation
    i. arousal
    i. balance
    i. cognition
    i. cognitive functioning
    communicatively i.
    i. concentration
    i. concentration ability
    i. connectedness
    consciousness i.
    i. consciousness
    i. development
    i. effective communication
    emotionally i.
    i. function
    functionally i.
    i. impulse control
    i. insight
    i. language
    learning i.
    i. memory
    mentally i.
    i. orientation
    i. performance
    i. relationship
    severely mentally i. (SMI)
    i. sexual desire
    i. social functioning
    i. social interaction
    i. social judgment
    speech and language i. (SLI)

impaired *(continued)*
   i. thinking ability
   i. vision
impairment
   age-associated memory i. (AAMI)
   anterior horn cell motor i.
   aphasic i.
   aphasic phonological i.
   attentional i.
   category specific semantic i.
   cerebral i.
   clinically significant i.
   cognitive i.
   i. of cognitive function
   i. in cognitive functioning
   i. of consciousness
   constructional i.
   i. criterion
   degree of i.
   i. of dementia
   disproportionate i.
   emotional i.
   focal neurological i.
   functional i.
   gaze i.
   generalized intellectual i.
   graphic i.
   gross i.
   hearing i.
   i. index
   intellectual i.
   interpersonal i.
   language i.
   major i.
   marked i.
   measurable i.
   memory i.
   mental i.
   motor i.
   neurologic i.
   neuropsychologic i.
   no more than slight i.
   occupational i.
   organic i.
   Patient Rated Overall Life I.
   perceptual-motor i.
   perceptual-motor abilities i.
   peripheral nerve level motor i.
   permanent residual i.
   physical i.
   Rated Overall Life I.
   reading comprehension i.
   residual i.
   reversible memory i.
   root level motor i.
   saccade i.
   school functioning i.
   sensory i.
   serious i.
   significant i.
   sleep-induced respiratory i.
   social functioning i.
   spinal nerve level motor i.
   supranuclear vertical gaze i.

   i. symptom
   upper motor neuron i.
   visual i.
   visual-motor i.
impar
   nervus i.
imparity
impasse
   therapeutic i.
impedance
   i. artifact
   i. audiometry
   electrode i.
   i. matching
   i. method
   middle ear i.
   static acoustic i.
impending
   i. death
   i. decompensation
   i. doom
   i. herniation
   i. relapse
imperative
   categorical i.
   i. conception
   ethical i.
   i. idea
   immoral i.
   i. mood
imperfecta
   dentinogenesis i.
imperforate hymen
imperious act
impersistence
   motor i.
impersonal
   i. projection
   i. relationship
   i. unconscious
impingement
   anterior cord i.
   corpus callosal i.
implant
   Activa Tremor Control System i.
   Arenberg-Denver inner-ear valve i.
   breast i.
   broken existing i.
   Christoferson disk bony i.
   cochlear i.
   custom i.
   DTT i.
   embryonic i.
   epidural i.
   epilepsy i.
   i. fatigue
   ferromagnetic i.
   fetal neural i.
   Gliadel i.
   hard tissue replacement-malleable
     facial i. (HTR-MFI)
   HTR-MFI chin i.
   HTR-MFI curved i.
   HTR-MFI malar i.
   HTR-MFI paranasal i.

HTR-MFI premaxillary i.
HTR-MFI ramus i.
HTR-MFI straight i.
HTR-PMI i.
Hunter open cord tendon i.
ideal spinal i.
iodine-125 i.
KLS-Martin i.
lumbar anterior-root stimulator i.
   (LARSI)
malleable facial i. (MFI)
metallic otologic i.
NeuroControl Freehand i.
otologic i.
patient-matched i.
Polaris adjustable spinal cage i.
i. removal
Schwann-cell i.
silicone i.
i. survival rate
tissue i.
TSRH i.
vagal nerve i.
vagus stimulator i.
Zielke VDS i.

implantation
brachytherapy seed i.
i. cone
DBS electrode i.
nerve i.
screw i.
subdural grid i.

implanted infusion pump
implausible phenomenon
implicit
i. behavior
i. language
i. memory
i. personality theory
i. response
i. role

implied criticism
implosion flooding
implosive therapy
impossible
impostor
juvenile i.
i. psychotic manifestation
i. syndrome

impotence, impotency
anal i.
anatomic i.
atonic i.
ejaculatory i.
erectile i.
erective i.
functional i.
muscular and anal i.
organic i.
orgastic i.
paretic i.
penile i.
primary i.
psychic i.
psychogenic i.

relative i.
secondary i.
sexual i.
symptomatic i.

impotentia
i. coeundi
i. erigendi
i. generandi

impoverished
i. early environment
i. fantasy life
i. speech
i. thought

impoverishment
intellectual i.
personality i.
i. in thinking

impregnation
Bodian silver i.
i. fear

impressio, pl. **impressiones**
i. petrosa pallii

impression
absolute i.
basilar i.
clinical i.
Clinical Global I.'s (CGI)
erroneous i.
i. management
mental i.
i. method
Nurse's Global I.'s (NGI)
petrosal i. of the pallium
sensory i.

impressive aphasia
imprinting
filial i.
genomic i.

improper diet
improved
Isollyl I.

improvement
Battery of Health I. (BHI)
Clinical Global I. (CGI)
Committee on Quality Assurance
   and I.
plateau in i.
teacher's reading global i. (TRGI)
i. training
transference i.

**Improving Writing, Thinking and
Reading Skills test**
IMPS
Inpatient Multidimensional Psychiatric
   Scale

impulse
aggressive i.
i. asynchrony
base i.
i. control
i. control conduct disorder
i. control disorder (ICD)
excitatory i.
i. fear
forbidden i.

impulse *(continued)*
    forced i.
    fundamental social i.
    horrific i.
    inappropriate i.
    inhibitory i.
    intrusive i.
    irresistible i.
    libidinal i.
    i. life
    maladaptive i.
    morbid i.
    nerve i.
    nervous i.
    nociceptive i.
    obsessional i.
    obsessive i.
    oral i.
    persistent inappropriate i.
    persistent intrusive i.
    i. regulation
    repressed i.
    stealing i.
    unacceptable i.
    unconscious i.
    voluntary i.
    wandering i.
impulse-control
    i.-c. disorder NOS
    i.-c. problem
impulsive
    i. act
    i. activity
    i. behavior
    i. character
    i. dyscontrol
    i. insanity
    i. madness
    i. neurosis
    I. Nonconformity Scale
    i. obsession
    i. petit mal epilepsy
    i. raptus
    i. tendency
impulsive/compulsive psychopathology
impulsiveness
    low i.
impulsivity
    self-damaging i.
impunitive response
imu
Imura
in
    i. absentia
    acting i.
    i. articulo mortis
    i. control
    i. extremis
    i. loco parentis
    i. propria persona
    run i.
    shut i.
    sit i.
    i. situ hybridization

    i. situ photocoagulation
    i. situ spinal fusion
    i. situ tricortical iliac-crest block
      bone graft
    i. toto
    turn i.
    i. utero
    i. utero teratologic agent
    i. vitro
    i. vitro spectra
    i. vivo
    i. vivo benzodiazepine receptor
      binding
    i. vivo ^{1}H magnetic resonance
      spectroscopy
    i. vivo optical spectroscopy
      (INVOS)
    i. vivo situational exposure
    i. vivo stereological assessment
inability
    i. to delay gratification
    i. to function
inactive alcoholic (IA)
inactivity
    alert i.
    electrocerebral i. (ECI)
inadequacy
    intellectual i.
    personal i.
inadequate
    i. discipline
    i. information
    i. personality
    i. personality disorder
    i. rapport
    i. response
    i. school environment
    i. sleep hygiene
    i. stimulus
inappropriate
    i. affect
    i. attitude
    i. behavior
    i. circumstance
    i. dependent care
    i. idea
    i. image
    i. impulse
    i. laughter
    i. posture
    i. quality of obsession
    i. response
    i. social relatedness
    i. thought
    i. urge
    i. voiding
inappropriateness
    sexual i.
    social i.
Inapsine
inattention
    i. dimension
    selective i.
    sensory i.
    visual i.

inattentive behavior
inattentive-type attention-
   deficit/hyperactivity disorder
inaudible
inborn error of metabolism
inbreeding
   coefficient of i.
incapacitating fear
incapacity
   functional i.
incendiare
   monomania i.
incentive
   aversive i.
   i. motivation
   positive i.
   i. system
   i. theory
inception
incertitude
incessant speech
incest
   i. barrier
   i. fantasy
   father-daughter i.
   homosexual i.
   mother-daughter i.
   mother-son i.
   i. taboo
incestual relationship
incestuous
   i. desire
   i. fantasy
   i. ties
incidence
   myelopathy i.
   nonunion i.
   i. rate
   suicide i.
incidental
   i. aneurysm
   i. image
   i. learning
   i. learning language
   i. learning language retardation
   i. memory
   i. punctate white matter
     hyperintensity
   i. stimulus
incipient
   i. downward central brain
     herniation
   i. schizophrenia
   i. schizophrenic psychosis
incision
   anteromedial i.
   battledore i.
   bifrontal i.
   Brunner modified i.
   Caldwell-Luc i.
   circumscribing i.
   coronal scalp i.
   C-shaped i.
   curved i.
   deltoid-splitting i.

   dural i.
   elliptical i.
   exploratory i.
   hemitransfixion i.
   horseshoe i.
   Kocher collar i.
   laterally convex dural i.
   lateral rhinotomy i.
   Lynch i.
   Mayfield i.
   midline i.
   muscle-splitting i.
   Naffzinger straight midline i.
   palatal mucosal i.
   posterolateral costotransversectomy i.
   right-sided submandibular
     transverse i.
   S i.
   scalp i.
   skin i.
   standard retroperitoneal flank i.
   straight i.
   tangential i.
   transcortical i.
   transverse i.
   T-shaped i.
   vertical midline i.
   V-shaped i.
   Weber-Fergusson i.
   webspace i.
   Y i.
incisional neuroma
incisura, pl. **incisurae**
   i. cerebelli anterior
   i. cerebelli posterior
   i. preoccipitalis
   tentorial i.
   i. tentorii
incisural
   i. dissection
   i. space
incisure
   Lanterman i.
   Schmidt-Lanterman i.
incitement premium
inclusion
   i. body encephalitis
   class i.
   i. lipoma
   i. tumor
inclusion-body myositis
inclusive fitness
incoherent
   i. behavior
   i. ideation
   i. patient
   i. speech
income
   Supplemental Security I. (SSI)
incompatibility
   Rh i.
incompatible
   i. behavior
   i. response

incompetence
    ejaculatory i.
    level of i. (LOI)
incompetency
    certificate of i.
    i. proceeding
incompetent
    mentally i.
incomplete
    i. alexia
    i. band heterotopia
    i. neurofibromatosis
    i. sentence blank test
    I. Sentences Survey
    I. Sentences Task
incomplete-pictures test
incomplete-sentence test
incomprehensible
    i. speech
    i. thinking
    i. thought
incongruity
    insensitivity to i.
incongruous affect
inconsistent
    i. manner
    i. parental discipline
    i. recall
incontestable
incontinence
    active i.
    affective i.
    bowel i.
    emotional i.
    encopresis, with constipation and
        overflow i.
    encopresis, without constipation and
        overflow i.
    fecal i.
    overflow i.
    paradoxical i.
    passive i.
    reflex i.
    urge i.
    urgency i.
    urinary i.
incontinent
incontinentia
    i. pigmenti
    i. pigmenti achromians
incontrovertible
    i. evidence
    i. proof
incoordination
incorporation defense mechanism
incorrect inference
increased
    i. arousal
    i. energy
    i. interpersonal conflict
    i. platelet membrane fluidity
    i. responsibility
    i. speed of thought
incredible
incredulous

increment
    sensation i.
incubation of avoidance
incubus
    family i.
incudis
    fossa i.
incudostapedial joint
incurable problem drinker (IPD)
incus
IND
    internodal distance
indapamide
indecent
    i. assault
    i. exposure
indecisiveness
    parental i.
indefinable
indefinite
indeloxazine
independence
    Balthazar Scales for Adaptive
        Behavior I: Scales of
        Functional I.
    field i.
    moral i.
    physical i.
independence-dependence
    field i.-d.
independent
    i. action
    i. event
    i. functioning
    i. living
    I. Living Behavior Checklist
    i. physical reality
    i. play
    i. variable
in-depth
Inderal LA
Inderide
indeterminant
indeterminate
    i. sex
    i. sleep
indeterminism
index, gen. **indicis**, pl. **indices, indexes**
    active hostility i. (AHI)
    Addiction Severity I. (ASI)
    ADL i.
    Adolescent Alienation I. (AAI)
    Adolescent Drinking I. (ADI)
    Adolescent Problem Severity I.
        (ASPI)
    Affective Style I.
    air pollution i.
    allergy i. (AI)
    alpha i.
    ambulation i.
    American Psychiatric Association I.
    ankle-brachial i. (ABI)
    anterior horn i. (AHI)
    anxiety i. (AI)
    Anxiety Sensitivity I. (ASI)

anxiety status i. (ASI)
APA I.
articulation i.
Barthel Activities of Daily Living I.
Barthel ADL I.
beta i.
i. of body build (IB)
body mass i. (BMI)
Campbell Leadership I. (CLI)
cardiac risk i.
Caregiver Strain I. (CSI)
i. case
case i.
cephalic i.
cephalorrhachidian i.
cerebrospinal i.
Chippaux-Smirak arch i.
Classroom Environment I.
College Characteristics I. (CCI)
Composite Risk I. (CRI)
Computer Anxiety I.
Convery polyarticular disability i.
Cornell Medical I.
delta i.
deterioration i. (DI)
i. of discrimination
Doppler pulsatility i.
Drug Use I.
Duke Religion I.
Egocentricity I.
Emotions Profile I.
empathic i.
Evans i.
Four Factor I.
Fourier pulsatility i.
Frenchay Activities I.
Functional Status I. (FSI)
General Cognitive I. (GCI)
Global Severity I. (GSI)
Global Sexual Satisfaction I. (GSSI)
Goldberg I.
Gosling pulsatility i.
Halstead Impairment I.
Hauser ambulation i.
Heston Personality I. (HPI)
Hollingshead I.
hyperactivity i.
hyperkinesis i.
hypoglycemic i. (HI)
hypothermic metabolic i.
impairment i.
Jansky Screening I. (JSI)
Jette Functional Status I.
Job Description I. (JDI)
K i.
Katz ADL I.
Keitel i.
Kenny ADL i.
Klaus height i.
Kolbe Conative I. (KCI)
labeling i. (LI)
Life Satisfaction I. (LSI)
Lucas and Drucker Motor I.

maturation i.
McDowell Impairment I. (MII)
Motricity I.
multi-item i.
New Haven Schizophrenia I.
Northwick Park Index of Independence in ADL i.
Nottingham Extended ADL I.
organism-specific antibody i. (OSAI)
Organizational Climate I.
Parenting Stress I.
perceptual organizational i.
Peritraumatic Dissociation I.
Personality I. (PI)
physiological sleepiness i.
PICA i.
Picture Identification for Children-Standardized I. (PICSI)
pipe stemming of ankle-brachial i.
Pittsburgh Sleep Quality I.
poststress ankle/arm Doppler i.
Potential for Addiction I.
I. of Potential Suicide
pressure-volume i.
I. of Primitive Thought
pulsatility i. (PI)
putative i.
radiological pressure-volume i.
referential i.
Reintegration to Normal Living I.
i. of reliability
response i.
resting ankle/arm Doppler i.
Retirement Descriptive I. (RDI)
Ritchie i.
Rivermead ADL i.
Rivermead Mobility I. (RMI)
schizophrenia i.
Self-Esteem I. (SEI)
Sexual Functioning I. (SFI)
i. of sexuality (IS)
sexuality i.
shift referential i.
Short Increment Sensitivity I. (SISI)
Social Adequacy I. (SAI)
Social Function I. (SFI)
Speech with Alternating Masking I. (SWAMI)
Spinal Cord Motor Index and Sensory Indices
I. of Spouse Abuse
spouse abuse i.
State-Trait Anxiety I.
status i.
steal i.
stimulation i. (SI)
switch referential i.
tabular i.
TCD pulsatility i.
Teen Addiction Severity I. (T-ASI)
therapeutic i.
theta i.
Thought Disorder I.

index *(continued)*
    total response i. (TRI)
    Trait Evaluation I.
    i. variable
    verbal comprehension i.
    Vocational Opinion I. (VOI)
    I. of Well-Being (IWB)
    Work Interest I.
    I. of Work Satisfaction (IWS)
indexical
    i. communication
    i. sign
Indiana tome carpal tunnel release system
Indian medicine
Indica
indicatio
    i. causalis
    i. curativa
    i. symptomatica
indication
    causal i.
    symptomatic i.
indicative mood
indicator
    Activity Pattern I. (API)
    finger i.
    Keegan Type I.
    Myers-Briggs Type I. (MBTI)
    Occupational Stress I. (OSI)
    Rehabilitation I. (RIs)
    risk i.
    sensor position i. (SPI)
    Skill I.'s (SKI)
    Status I.'s
    type i.
indices *(pl. of* index)
indicis *(gen. of* index)
indifference
    i. to pain syndrome
    i. point
    sexual i.
indifferent
    i. euphoria
    i. to surroundings
indigenous
    i. family culture
    i. worker
indigestion
    nervous i.
indigotin disulfonate sodium
indinavir
indirect
    i. aggression
    i. association
    i. evidence
    i. fracture
    i. method of therapy
    i. motor system
    i. object
    i. self-destructive behavior (ISDB)
    i. survey
    i. wit

indiscretion
    sexual i.
indiscriminate
    i. lesion
    i. sexual encounter
indium cisternogram
indium-111 octreotide scintigraphy
individual
    age-matched i.
    i. analysis
    androgynous i.
    i. care
    I. Career Exploration (ICE)
    i. counseling
    i. counselor
    i. difference
    insightless i.
    I. Learning Disabilities Classroom Screening Instrument (ILDCSI)
    i. psychology
    i. psychotherapy
    i. response
    i. response-specificity
    i. responsibility
    i.'s subsystem
    i. test
    i. therapy (IT)
    I.'s with Disabilities Education Act (IDEA)
    i. with Schizophrenia
individualistic
    i. motive
    i. reward structure
individualized
    I. Criterion Referenced Testing (ICRT)
    I. Criterion Reference Testing Mathematics (ICRTM)
    I. Criterion Reference Testing Reading (ICRTR)
    i. education program
    i. instruction
individual's
    i. age
    i. culture
individuation stage
Indochron E-R capsule
Indocin
    I. IV
    I. SR
indoctrination while captive
Indoklon therapy
indolamine function
indole derivative
indolence
indolent
indomethacin
indomitable
indubitable
induced
    i. abortion
    i. association
    i. hallucination
    i. insanity
    i. lethargy

i. paranoid disorder
i. psychosis
i. psychotic disorder
i. schizophrenia
i. trance
inducement
hygienic i.
inducer
angiogenic i.
inductance
induction
i. coil
dream i.
enzyme i.
Faraday law of i.
hypnotic i.
iatrogenic i.
immediate early gene i.
i. loop
magnetic i.
mood i.
negative mood i.
perceptual i.
positive i.
inductive
i. problem solving
i. reactance
i. reasoning
inductor
indulgence
plenary i.
indulgent
indurate
indusium, pl. **indusia**
i. griseum
industrial
i. hygiene
i. psychiatry
i. psychology
i. rehabilitation counselor
i. sociology
i. therapy
industrialized culture
industry
Attitude Survey Program for
Business and I.
Personnel Tests for I. (PTI)
i. versus inferiority
inebriant
ineffective
i. anger
i. decision making
i. stimulus
i. treatment
ineffectual parent
inelasticity of thought
ineptness
social i.
Inerpan flexible burn dressing
inertia
motor i.
principle of i.
psychic i.
i. time

inevitability
sensation of ejaculatory i.
inexact fiducial
In-Exsufflator respiratory device
infamy
infancy
adjustment reaction of i.
attachment in i.
attachment disorder of i.
bonding in i.
i. developmental stage
diencephalic syndrome of i.
i. and early childhood disturbance
melanotic neuroectodermal tumor
of i.
reactive attachment disorder of i.
i. research
rumination disorder of i.
infant
i. at risk
i. behavior record
I.'s Feverall
i. mortality
Mother's Assessment of the
Behavior of Her I. (MABI)
i. narcotic withdrawal
i. and preschool test
i. psychiatry
I. Reading Test
i. stimulation program
infanticide
infantile
i. acid maltase deficiency
i. affect
i. amnesia
i. aphasia
i. articulation
i. autism
i. behavior
i. botulism
i. convulsion
i. dementia
i. diplegia
i. dynamics
i. encephalopathy
i. ganglioglioma
i. hemangioblastic hemangioma
i. hemiplegia
i. hydrocephalus
i. idiocy
i. masturbation
i. muscular atrophy
i. myofibromatosis
i. neuroaxonal dystrophy
i. neuronal degeneration
i. neuropathy
i. paresis
i. perseveration
i. progressive spinal muscular
atrophy
i. psychosis
i. sadism
i. seduction
i. seizure
i. sexuality

infantile *(continued)*
    i. spasm
    i. spastic paraplegia
    i. speech
    i. tetany
    i. X-linked ataxia
    i. X-linked deafness
infantilis
    dementia i.
    mania phantastica i.
infantilism
    Brissaud i.
    cachectic i.
    regressive i.
    sex i.
    sexual i.
    static i.
infantilization
Infants' Silapap
Infant/Toddler Environment Rating Scale (ITERS)
infantum
    autismus i.
infarct
    bilateral occipital i.'s
    cerebral i.
    cystic lacunar i.
    i. dementia
    hemorrhagic i.
    lacunar i.
    large-artery i.
    multiple cortical i.
    right frontoparietal i.
    watershed i.
infarction
    anterior communicating artery distribution i.
    atherosclerotic i.
    bicerebral i.
    bilateral upper brain stem i.
    borderzone i.
    brain i.
    brainstem i.
    calcarine cortex i.
    capsular i.
    capsulocaudate i.
    capsuloputaminal i.
    capsuloputaminocaudate i.
    cerebellar i.
    cerebral artery i.
    cortical i.
    cryptogenic i.
    dominant hemisphere i.
    embolic i.
    Freiberg so-called i.
    frontal lobe i.
    gyral i.
    hemispheric i.
    hemorrhagic i.
    hippocampal i.
    inferolateral i.
    ischemic brainstem i.
    ischemic cerebral i.
    lacunar brain i.

    medullary i.
    mesencephalic i.
    midbrain i.
    migraine-induced i.
    migrainous i.
    multiple cortical i.
    myocardial i.
    nonembolic i.
    nonhemorrhagic cerebral i.
    nonseptic embolic brain i.
    occipital lobe i.
    optic nerve i.
    paramedian i.
    parietooccipital i.
    photochemically-induced graded spinal cord i.
    photothrombotic i.
    pontine i.
    posterior cerebral territory i.
    retinal i.
    silent cerebral i.
    small, deep, recent i. (SDRI)
    spinal cord i.
    striatocapsular i.
    subendocardial myocardial i.
    temporal lobe i.
    thalamic i.
    thalamopeduncular i.
    tuberothalamic i.
    ventral pontine i.
    vertebrobasilar i.
    watershed i.
    white matter i.
Infatab
    Dilantin I.
infatuation
infection
    Absidia i.
    Acanthamoeba i.
    arenavirus i.
    bacterial i.
    Candida i.
    central nervous system i.
    cerebral i.
    chronic spinal epidural i.
    chronic spinal intradural i.
    closed disk space i.
    Coccidioides i.
    Cryptococcus i.
    cryptogenic i.
    cysticercal i.
    dental i.
    disk space i.
    enteric virus i.
    enterovirus i.
    epidural i.
    extradural i.
    fetal i.
    focal i.
    fungal i.
    helminthic i.
    hepatitis B virus i.
    Histoplasma i.
    Legionella pneumophila i.
    lytic i.

Mucor i.
Mycoplasma i.
myxovirus i.
Naegleria i.
neonatal i.
nervous system i.
odontogenic i.
opportunistic i.
i. organic psychosis
parasitic i.
paraspinal i.
perinatal i.
postoperative i.
i. prevention
protozoan i.
rhabdovirus i.
Rhizopus i.
rickettsial i.
scalp i.
slow-virus i.
spinal i.
spinal cord i.
viral i.

infection-exhaustion psychosis
infection-related neuropathy
infectious
i. aneurysm
i. disease
i. hepatitis
i. hepatitis peripheral neuropathy
i. insanity
i. ophthalmoplegia
i. polyneuritis
i. polyneuritis syndrome
i. retinopathy

infectious-exhaustive
i.-e. psychosis
i.-e. syndrome

infectiva
polioencephalitis i.

infective
i. endocarditis
i. psychosis

inference
incorrect i.
logical i.
statistical i.
i. strategy
Test of Social I.'s (TSI)

inferential
i. behavioral monitoring
i. behavioral monitoring distortion
i. perception
i. perception distortion
i. statistics
i. thinking

inferior
i. anastomotic vein
area vestibularis i.
i. cerebellar artery
i. cerebellar peduncle
i. cervical ganglion
i. colliculus
constitutional psychopathia i. (CPI)
i. dental nerve

i. extradural approach
i. frontal convolution
i. frontal gyrus
i. frontal sulcus
i. ganglion of glossopharyngeal nerve
i. ganglion of vagus
i. horn of lateral ventricle
i. laryngeal nerve
i. longitudinal fasciculus
macula cribrosa i.
i. medullary velum
i. mesenteric ganglion
i. occipital gyrus
oliva i.
i. olivary nucleus
i. olive
i. orbital fissure
i. parietal gyrus
i. parietal lobule
i. part of vestibulocochlear nerve
i. polioencephalitis
i. pontine syndrome
i. quadrigeminal brachium
i. rectus muscle
i. root of cervical loop
i. root of vestibulocochlear nerve
i. salivary nucleus
i. semilunar lobule
i. sibling lifestyle
i. surface of cerebellar hemisphere
i. temporal convolution
i. temporal cortex (ITC)
i. temporal gyrus
i. temporal sulcus
i. thalamic peduncle
i. transvermian approach
i. veins of cerebellar hemisphere
i. vena cava
i. vertebra
i. vestibular area
i. vestibular nucleus

inferiority
i. complex
constitutional psychopathic i. (CPI)
i. feeling
industry versus i.
organ i.
psychopathic i.

inferior-lateral endonasal transsphenoidal approach
inferolateral
i. infarction
i. pontine artery

inferred
i. conflict
i. delusional conviction
i. Self-Concept Scale

infestation
i. delusion
fluke i.
guinea worm i.

infibulation
infidelity
delusion of i.

infidelity *(continued)*
    i. delusion
    marital i.
infiltrate
    lymphocytic i.
infiltrating tumor
infiltration
    i. anesthesia
    hematogenous cell i.
    paraneural i.
    perineural i.
infiltrative
infinity neurosis
inflammation
    i. bowel disease
    cartilage i.
    ear cartilage i.
    ischemic ocular i.
inflammatory
    i. demyelinating disease
    i. demyelinating neuropathy
    i. demyelinating
      polyradiculoneuropathy
    i. lesion
inflated
    i. appraisal
    i. identity
    i. knowledge
    i. power
    i. worth
    i. worth theme
inflexibility
    enduring pattern of i.
inflexible
    i. attitude
    i. pattern
    i. personality trait
inflow effect
influence
    cocaine i.
    contextual i.
    i. delusion
    delusion of i.
    driving under the i. (DUI)
    drug i.
    evil i.
    idea of i.
    passive i.
    prenatal i.
influenced psychosis
influenzae
    Haemophilus i.
informal
    i. admission
    i. contract
    i. method
    I. Reading Comprehension
      Placement Test
    i. retention
information
    assimilating i.
    i. assimilation
    autobiographical i.
    contradictory i.

drug i. (DI)
educational i.
i. feedback
fund of i.
inadequate i.
i. input process
kinetic i.
learning i.
i. memory concentration (IMC)
neurocognitive i.
nonverbal i.
i. optimization position
i. overload
i. processing
i. processing deficit
rapidity of analyzing i.
rapidity of assimilating i.
i. retrieval
i. subtest
System for Interactive Guidance I.
    (SIGI)
i. test
i. theory
thirdhand i.
unbiased i.
informational support
informed consent
infracalcarine gyrus
infraclinoid aneurysm
infradian rhythm
infragranular layer
infranuclear
    i. lesion
    i. paralysis
    i. weakness
infraorbital
    i. injection
    i. nerve
infrapsychic
infraspinous fascia
infrastriate layer
infratemporal
    i. fossa
    i. hematoma
infratentorial
    i. arteriovenous malformation
    i. compartment
    i. lateral supracellular approach
    i. lesion
    i. neoplastic syndrome
    i. neurological tumor
    i. structural syndrome
    i. supracerebellar
infratentorial-Lindau tumor
infrequency scale
infrequent interpersonal conflict
Infumorph Injection
infundibula (*pl. of* infundibulum)
infundibular
    i. part of anterior lobe of
      hypophysis
    i. recess
    i. stalk
    i. stem

infundibulo-hypophysitis
  necrotizing i.-h.
infundibuloma
infundibulum, pl. **infundibula**
  i. hypothalami
  hypothalamic i.
Infusaid M400 constant flow pump
infusion
  i. computed tomography
  continuous intrathecal baclofen i.
  (CIBI)
  diastole-phased pulsatile i.
  etomidate-propylene glycol i.
  lactate i.
  propofol i.
  i. pump
Inge
  I. cervical lamina spreader
  I. laminectomy retractor
  I. laminectomy spreader
ingestion
  caustic i.
  drug i.
  hormone i.
Ingraham-Fowler tantalum clip
Ingraham skull punch forceps
ingratiating behavior
ingravascent
ingravescent apoplexy
ingredient
  toxic i.
ingrowth
  neuronal i.
inguinal freckling
inhabit
inhalant
  absorption of i.
  i. abuse
  aerosol i.
  amyl nitrate i.
  i. dependence
  household product i.
  i. intoxication
  i. intoxication delirium
  nitrate i.
  nitrite i.
  i. sniffing
  i. use
  i. use disorder
inhalant-induced
  i.-i. delirium
  i.-i. disorder
  i.-i. persisting dementia
  i.-i. psychotic disorder with
    delusions
  i.-i. psychotic disorder with
    hallucinations
inhalant-related disorder
inhalation
  i. convulsive treatment
  i. of drug
inhaled
  i. anesthesia
  i. octane booster

inhaler
  amphetamine i.
  nasal i.
  Nicorette I.
  Nicotrol i.
inharmonious
inherent contrast
inheritable
inheritance
  archaic i.
  autosomal dominant i.
  autosomal recessive i.
  mendelian rules of i.
  mode of i.
  multifactorial i.
  polygenic i.
inherited
  i. abnormality
  i. ataxia
  i. global neurodegenerative disorder
  i. progressive degenerative disease
  i. releasing mechanism (IRM)
inhibin
inhibited
  i. communication
  emotionally i.
  i. female orgasm psychosexual
  i. grief
  i. grieving
  i. male orgasm psychosexual
  i. mania
  i. orgasm
  i. sexual arousal
  i. sexual desire
  i. sexual desire psychosexual
  i. sexual excitement (ISE)
  i. sexual response
inhibited-type
  i.-t. reactive attachment disorder
  i.-t. reactive attachment disorder of
    infancy or early
inhibition
  academic i.
  aim i.
  associative i.
  central i.
  collagenase i.
  conditioned i.
  i. of delay
  emotional i.
  i. epilepsy
  external i.
  i. formation
  horizontal i.
  internal i.
  i. mechanism
  motor i.
  occupational i.
  proactive i. (PI)
  i. profile
  reactive i.
  reciprocal i.
  retroactive i. (RI)
  sexual i.
  social i.

inhibition *(continued)*
    specific academic or work i.
    work i.
inhibition-action balance
inhibitor
    calpain i.
    carbonic anhydrase i.
    cholinesterase i.
    cyclooxygenase i.
    cytokine i.
    leukocyte adhesion i. (LAI)
    MAO i.
    monoamine oxidase i. (MAOI)
    nonselective phosphodiesterase i.
    physiological hyaluronidase i. (PHI)
    polyamine biosynthesis i.
    reuptake i.
    reversible cholinesterase i.
    selective phosphodiesterase i.
    selective serotonin reuptake i.
     (SSRI)
    serotonin reuptake i. (SRI)
    xanthine oxidase i.
inhibitory
    i. amino acid (IAA)
    i. epilepsy
    i. fiber
    i. impulse
    i. obsession
    i. postsynaptic current
    i. postsynaptic potential (IPSP)
    i. protein
    i. tone
    i. virus
inhomogeneity
    field i.
in-house evaluation
iniencephaly
inion
initial
    bystander dominates i.
    i. insomnia
    i. interview
    i. lag
    i. masking
    i. phase of insomnia
    i. spurt
    I. Teaching Alphabet
    i. upward deflection
initiating
    i. insomnia
    i. structure
initiation
    i. of goal-directed behavior
    i. of treatment
initiative
    lack of i.
    i. versus guilt
initio
    ab i.
injectable cocaine
Inject-Ease
injection
    Adlone I.

Alfenta I.
A-methaPred I.
AquaMEPHYTON I.
Astramorph PF I.
Benadryl I.
Ben-Allergin-50 I.
Calciferol I.
Calcimar I.
Carnitor I.
cerebral i.
Cibacalcin I.
Cytoxan I.
death by lethal i.
depMedalone I.
Depoject I.
Depo-Medrol I.
Depopred I.
depot medication i.
D.H.E. 45 I.
Diazemuls I.
Dinate I.
D-Med I.
Dopascan i.
drug i.
Duralone I.
Duramorph I.
Dymenate I.
Enlon I.
epidural steroid i.
etomidate i.
extradural i.
focal stereotactic i.
heroin i.
Hydrate I.
hypodermic i.
Hyrexin-50 I.
imipenem-cilastatin i.
infraorbital i.
Infumorph I.
i. injury
intracutaneous i.
intradermal i.
intramuscular i.
intraneural phenol i.
intrathecal i.
intravascular i.
intravenous i.
intraventricular i.
Key-Pred I.
Key-Pred-SP I.
Konakion I.
Largon I.
lethal i.
Medralone I.
Mestinon I.
Metastron I.
Miacalcin I.
M-Prednisol I.
Narcan I.
Neosar I.
Novocain I.
Octocaine I.
Osmitrol I.
Osteocalcin I.
paramagnetic contrast i.

Pontocaine With Dextrose I.
Predcor-TBA I.
Prednisol TBA I.
Prolixin Decanoate I.
Prolixin Enanthate I.
Regonol I.
Relefact TRH i.
retrobulbar i.
retrogasserian i.
Reversol I.
saline i.
Salmonine I.
Seconal I.
Solu-Medrol I.
stereotactic intracystic i.
subcutaneous i.
Sublimaze I.
Sufenta I.
sumatriptan succinate i.
Tensilon I.
THAM I.
THAM-E I.
Toradol I.
Ureaphil I.
Valium I.
injector
injunction
paradoxical i.
injury
acceleration extension i.
acute burst i.
acute central cervical spinal cord i.
(ACCSCI)
acute lung i. (ALI)
avulsion i.
axonal i.
axonotmetic i.
birth i.
brachial plexus avulsion i.
brain i.
burst i.
cervical nerve root i.
cervical spine i.
chemical i.
closed head i. (CHI)
common iliac artery i.
contrecoup i.
contrecoup i. of brain
coup i. of brain
crush i.
current of i.
deceleration i.
dementia due to traumatic brain i.
diffuse axonal i. (DAI)
diffuse brain i. (DBI)
diffuse white matter shearing i.
discoligamentous i.
electrical i.
endothelial i.
Erb i.
Erb-Duchenne-Klumpke i.
extension i.
extension-type cervical spine i.
fetal i.
flexion-distraction i.

flexion-extension i.
fluid percussion head i.
focal cerebral head i.
Fränkel classification of spinal
cord i.
global ischemic neuronal i.
head i.
hemorrhagic shearing i.
hyperextension-hyperflexion i.
iliac artery i.
injection i.
i. of intervertebral disk
laryngeal nerve i.
LSUMC classification of nerve i.
middle column i.
mild head i. (MHI)
Mini Inventory of Right Brain I.
(MIRBI)
missile i.
multiple impact i.
neural i.
neuronal i.
non-missile head i.
old nerve i. (ONI)
open head i.
operative i.
optic nerve i.
oxygen radical-induced cellular i.
parasympathetic nerve i.
penetrating i.
peripheral nerve i.
i. potential
radiation i.
retraction i.
rotational i.
rotationally induced shear-strain i.
Seddon classification of nerve i.'s
self-induced i.
self-inflicted bodily i.
severe head i. (SHI)
I. Severity Scale (ISS)
I. Severity Score (ISS)
shearing i.
soft tissue i.
spinal cord i.
spleen i.
stable cervical spine i.
suction i.
thoracic duct i.
thoracolumbar spine flexion-
distraction i.
three-column cervical spine i.
toxic i.
tracheal i.
transient plexus i.
traumatic brain i. (TBI)
two-column cervical spine i.
unstable cervical spine i.
ureter i.
vascular i.
vena cava i.
vertebral artery i.
whiplash i.
Wilbrandt knee i.
injury-healing theory

injustice gathering
inkblot
    G response including entire i.
    i. test (IBT)
in-line telesensor
inmate personality
innate
    i. behavior
    i. drive
    i. reflex
    i. releasing mechanism
    i. response system
innateness theory
inner
    i. barrenness
    i. battery cluster
    i. child issue
    i. cone fiber
    i. conflict
    i. control
    i. directed
    i. estrangement
    i. experience
    i. language
    i. life
    i. need
    i. self-helper
    i. slight
    i. space
    i. tension
    i. vision
inner-directed person
innervate
innervation
    adrenergic i.
    i. apraxia
    motor i.
innervatory
    i. apraxia
    i. dyspraxia
innominata
    substantia i.
innominate
    i. angiogram
    i. artery
    i. substance
    i. vein
Innovar
INO
    internuclear ophthalmoplegia
inoculation
    emotional i.
    stress i.
inoperable
iNOS
    immunologic nitric oxide synthase
inositol triphosphate (IP$_3$)
inpatient
    I. Multidimensional Psychiatric
      Scale (IMPS)
    i. psychiatric setting
    i. treatment
in-phase image
input
    acoustic i.

    cerebral sensory i.
    positivity of i. 1
    positivity of i. 2
input-output mechanism
INQ
    Inquiry Mode Questionnaire: A Measure
      of How You Think and Make Decisions
inquiry
    General I. (GI)
    I. Mode Questionnaire: A
      Measure of How You Think and
      Make Decisions (INQ)
    Systematic I. (SI)
inquisition
inquisitor
INR
    International Normalized Ratio
insane
    criminally i.
    i. finger
    general paralysis of the i. (GPI)
    general paresis of the i.
    paralysis of the i.
insania lupina
insaniens
    chorea i.
insanity
    acute confusional i.
    adolescent i.
    affective i.
    alcoholic i.
    alternating i.
    American Law Institute formulation
      of i.
    basedowian i.
    choreic i.
    circular i.
    climacteric i.
    communicated i.
    compulsive i.
    confusional i.
    consecutive i.
    constitutional i.
    criminal i.
    cyclic i.
    i. defense
    degenerative i.
    delusional i.
    double i.
    doubting i.
    dread of i.
    drug i.
    emotional i.
    hysterical i.
    idiophrenic i.
    impulsive i.
    induced i.
    infectious i.
    intermittent i.
    interpretational i.
    manic-depressive i.
    moral i.
    i. of negation
    not guilty by reason of i. (NGI,
      NGRI)

partial i.
periodic i.
plea of i.
religious i.
senile i.
simultaneous i.
subacute confusional i.
toxic i.
triple i.
insanoid
insatiable appetite
insecticide
cannabis mixed with i.'s
organophosphate i.
i. peripheral neuropathy
insecurity
social i.
insemination
insenescence
insensate
insensible thirst
insensitivity to incongruity
insentient
inseparability
linear i.
inserter
Texas Scottish Rite Hospital
hook i.
insertion
C-D rod i.
i. equipment
oblique screw i.
pedicle screw i.
screw i.
sphenoidal electrode i.
Syracuse anterior I-plate i.
thought i.
inside density
inside-out signaling
insidious onset
insight
absence of i.
analytic i.
emotional i.
impaired i.
intellectual i.
judgment and i.
lack of i.
myopic i.
poor i.
Schedule for Assessment of I.
(SAI)
sudden i.
i. therapy
I. and Treatment Attitudes
Questionnaire (ITAQ)
I. to Treatment Questionnaire
true i.
insightless
i. individual
i. tendency
insight-oriented
exploratory i.-o.
i.-o. psychotherapy
i.-o. treatment

insipidus
diabetes i.
insomnia
alcohol-related i.
i. associated with anxiety
i. associated with depression
i. associated with psychosis
bout of i.
childhood-onset i.
chronic i.
i. disorder
drug-dependent i.
drug-related i.
i. due to nonorganic origin
fatal familial i.
i. feature
idiopathic i.
initial i.
initial phase of i.
initiating i.
intermittent i.
maintenance i.
middle i.
midwinter i.
nonorganic origin i.
persistent i.
i. phase
primary i.
psychophysiological i.
rebound i.
i. related to another mental
disorder
situational i.
sleep disorder i.
sleep-onset i.
stimulant-induced i.
i. symptom
terminal i.
transient i.
withdrawal i.
insomniac patient
insomnia-type
i.-t. sleep disorder due to general
medical condition
i.-t. substance-induced sleep
disorder
insomnium dream
inspirational group therapy
inspiratory center
instability
affective i.
atlantoaxial i.
fixation i.
i. in interpersonal relationship
lumbar spine i.
marital i.
occipitoatlantoaxial i.
phase i.
postural i.
sagittal plane i.
vasomotor i.
vertebral cervical i.
Insta-Char

instantaneous
  i. axotomy
  i. power
instant scan
Instat fibrin film
Instatrak
  I. guidance system
  I. headset
instigation therapy
instill
instillation procedure
instinct
  acquisitive i.
  aggressive i.
  complementary i.
  death i.
  destructive i.
  ego i.
  erotic i.
  herd i.
  hierarchical theory of i.
  life i.
  mother i.
  i. need
  part i.
  partial i.
  i. ridden
  sexual i.
  social i.
instinctive behavior
instinctoid need
instinct-training interlocking
instinctual
  i. aim
  i. anxiety
  i. dyscontrol
  i. fusion
  i. renunciation
  i. tension
  i. vicissitude
institute
  I. of Educational Research Test
  I. for Personality and Ability Test
  I. of Personality and Ability
    Testing (IPAT)
institution
  mental i.
  religious i.
institutional
  i. care
  i. commitment
  i. environment
  I. Functioning Inventory (IFI)
  I. Goals Inventory (IGI)
  i. peonage
  I. Review Board
  i. transference
institutionalize
instruction
  competency-based i.
  individualized i.
instructional
  I. Leadership Evaluation and
    Development Program (ILEAD)
  I. Leadership Inventory

  i. objective
  The I. Environment Scale (TIES)
instrument
  action i.
  assessment i.
  Backlund stereotactic i.
  20-channel Beckman EEG i.
  Clarke stereotactic i.
  Cloward i.
  Craig vertebral body biopsy i.
  Dartmouth Assessment of
    Lifestyle I. (DALI)
  digitized i.
  Dwyer i.
  Eby Elementary identification I.
  Evershears surgical i.
  Gamma knife i.
  Hulka i.
  Hymovich Chronicity Impact and
    Coping I. (CICI)
  Individual Learning Disabilities
    Classroom Screening I. (ILDCSI)
  interspinous segmental spinal i.
    (ISSI)
  Kinetix i.
  Kloehn craniofacial i.
  Malis bipolar i.
  Micro-Three microsurgery i.
  i. migration
  Millet neurological test i.
  Model TC2-64B pulsed-range gated
    Doppler i.
  Nicolet Compass EMG i.
  Nucleotome Endoflex i.
  Nucleotome Flex II cannula i.
  Parental Bonding I.
  pencil-grip i.
  Philadelphia Multilevel
    Assessment I.
  pistol-grip i.
  pulsed-range gated Doppler i.
  Radionics bipolar i.
  Richmond subarachnoid screw i.
  Ruggles Surgical I.'s
  solid-state i.
  spark-gap i.
  SpeedReducer i.
  stereotactic i.
  I. Timbre Preference Test
  Ware i.
  Yasargil i.
  Yasargil-Aesculap i.
  Zielke i.
instrumental
  i. activities of daily living (IADL)
  i. ADL
  i. ADL measurement
  i. affair
  i. aggression
  i. avoidance act
  i. conditioning
  i. dependence
  i. need
  i. response

i. support
i. task
instrumental-relativist orientation
instrumentation
anterior distraction i.
AO fixateur interne i.
AO notched i.
C-D i.
compression U-rod i.
Cotrel-Dubousset pedicle screw i.
Cotrel-Dubousset pedicular i.
Cotrel-Dubousset spinal i.
distraction i.
double Zielke i.
dynamic compression plate i.
Edwards i.
i. failure
Gellman i.
Harrington rod i.
interspinous segmental spinal i.
(ISSI)
Jacobs locking hook spinal rod i.
Jacobs locking spinal rod i.
Kambin i.
Kaneda anterior spinal i.
Louis i.
lumbar spine i.
lumbosacral spine transpedicular i.
Luque II segmental spinal i.
Luque segmental spinal i.
Luque semirigid segmental spinal i.
modular i.
Moss-Miami spinal i.
multiple hook assembly C-D i.
posterior cervical spinal i.
posterior distraction i.
posterior hook-rod spinal i.
sacral spine modular i.
sacral spine universal i.
segmental spinal i. (SSI)
spinal i.
Steffee i.
stereotactic i.
transpedicular spinal i.
TSRH i.
universal i.
variable screw placement system i.
VSP plate i.
Zielke i.
Z-plate anterior thoracolumbar i.
insufficiency
adrenal cortical i.
adrenocortical i.
anterior pituitary i.
aortic i.
basilar i.
cerebrovascular i.
corticoadrenal i.
i. of eyelid
mechanical i.
mental i.
muscular i.
role i.
testicular i.
vertebrobasilar i.

insufficient
i. nocturnal sleep
i. stimulation
insufflation anesthesia
insula, gen. and pl. **insulae**
long gyrus of the i.
i. operculum
insular
i. area
i. cistern
i. cortex
i. epilepsy
i. gyrus
i. lobe
i. sclerosis
insularity
insular-opercular syndrome
insulate
insulated electrode needle
insulation
i. anesthesia
emotional i.
insulator
insulin
i. abnormality
i. coma therapy (ICT)
i. coma treatment
i. growth factor
i. hypoglycemia test
Protamine Zinc I.
i. shock
insulin-like growth factor (IGF)
insult
bihemispheral i.
CNS i.
nutritional i.
insuperable
insupportable
insurable
insurance carrier
insurgent
insurmountable
insusceptibility
intact
judgment, orientation, memory,
abstraction and calculation i.
(JOMACI)
naming i.
i. spinous lamina
i. spinous process
intake
caloric i.
family group i.
fluid i.
food i.
i. worker
intake-orientation group
integral membrane glycoprotein
integrated
I. Assessment System (IAS)
I. Child Development Scheme
(ICDS)
i. function
i. headholder

integrated *(continued)*
    i. psychological therapy
    i. sideport access portal
integrating anchors/responses
integration
    Beery-Buktinica Developmental Test of Visual Motor I.
    Beery Test of Visual Motor I.
    cerebral i.
    Developmental Test of Visual Motor I. (DVMI)
    Developmental Test of Visual-Motor I., Third Edition
    ego i.
    message i.
    personality i.
    primary i.
    secondary i.
    sensory i.
    social i.
    structural i.
    I. Test
    Test of Visual Motor I.
    visual motor i. (VMI)
integration-disintegration
    social i.-d.
integrative
    i. aspect
    i. learning
    i. problem
integrity
    i. of brain function
    ego i.
    electrophysiologic i.
    i. group
    i. versus despair
intellect
    ambivalence of the i.
    structure of i. (SI)
intellectual
    i. ability
    i. aphasia
    i. aura
    i. capacity
    i. deterioration
    i. development
    i. faculty
    i. function
    i. functioning level
    i. imbalance
    i. impairment
    i. impoverishment
    i. inadequacy
    i. insight
    i. maturity
    i. monomania
    i. resource
    i. rigidity
    i. skill
    i. subaverage functioning
intellectualization communication pattern
intelligence
    above-average i.
    abstract i.

    AH5 Group Test of High Grade I.
    AH6 Group Test of High Level I.
    artificial i. (AI)
    aura i.
    biologic i.
    Cattell Infant Scale for I. (CISI)
    coefficient of i. (CI)
    concrete i.
    crystallized i.
    i. disorder
    fund of i.
    low i.
    marginal i.
    measured i.
    mechanical i.
    Pictorial Test of I. (PTI)
    psychomotor i.
    i. quotient (IQ)
    I. Quotient test
    representative i.
    i. scale
    i. score
    social i.
    superior i.
    Test of Nonverbal I. (TONI)
    verbal i.
    Wechsler Preschool and Primary Scale of I. (WPPSI)
intelligibility
    i. test
    i. threshold
intense
    i. affect
    i. anger
    i. anxiety
    i. apprehension
    i. autonomic arousal
    i. desire
    i. episodic dysphoria
    i. fear
    i. intoxication
    i. psychological distress
    i. relationship
    i. sexual behavior
    i. sexual fantasy
    i. sexual urge
    i. wish
intensification
    image i.
intensified action
intensifier
    image i.
    OEC-Diasonics mobile C-arm image i.
intensity
    delusional i.
    i. modulated radiation therapy
    i. of mood
    i. of reaction
    signal i.
Intensity, Severity, and Discharge (ISD)
intensive
    i. care syndrome
    i. care unit (ICU)
    i. habit pattern

I

i. psychotherapy
i. treatment unit (ITU)
intensive-care community residence
Intensol
Diazepam I.
intent
homicidal i.
suicidal i.
intention
i. to deceive
motor i.
i. myoclonus
paradoxical i. (PI)
i. spasm
i. tremor
intentional
i. death
i. fire setting
i. forgetting
i. involuntary behavior
i. production of symptoms
i. stereotyped movement
i. tremor
intentionally produced symptom
interact group
interacting cytokine
interaction
accelerated i.
affective i.
afferent stimulus i.
alcohol-methadone i.
communicative i.
complementarity of i.
dipole-dipole i.
drug i. (DI)
i. effect
electron-coupled nuclear spin-spin i.
family i.
glial neuronal i.
higher order i.
impaired social i.
interpersonal i.
occupational i.
peer i.
person-environment i.
physicochemical i.
proton-electron dipole-dipole i.
reciprocal social i.
sexual i.
social i.
i. territory
interactional
i. childhood psychosis
i. contract
i. group psychotherapy
i. theory of personality
interaction-oriented group therapy
interaction-process analysis
interactive
i. measurement
i. phenomenon
interannular segment
interarticularis
pars i.
interbehavioral psychology

interbody
i. fusion
i. graft
intercalary neuron
intercalated nucleus
intercavernous sinus
intercellular
i. collagen
i. matrix
intercerebral
interclinoid ligament
intercostal
i. artery angiogram
i. neuralgia
intercostohumeralis
intercourse
anal i.
i. anxiety
buccal i.
extramarital i.
genital i.
painful i.
sexual i.
unprotected i.
intercrural ganglion
interculture
intercurrent anxiety
interdigital neuritis
interdigitate
interdisciplinary
i. approach
i. environmental
i. environmental design
i. team (IDT)
interdural tumor
interear difference
interego
interelectrode
interenvironmental
interepisode
i. functioning
i. recovery
interest
i. blank
I. Check List
conflict of i.
cross-gender i.
decreased i.
I. Determination, Exploration and
Assessment System (IDEAS)
I. Determination, Exploration and
Assessment System, Enhanced
Version (IDEAS)
diminished sexual i.
i. factor
i. group
i. inventory
lack of i.
loss of i.
low sexual i.
range of i.'s
region of i. (ROI)
i. scale
i. schedule
sex i.

interest *(continued)*
    sexual i.
    social i.
    stereotyped i.
    i. survey
    i. test
    What I Like to Do: An Inventory
      of Students' I.'s (WILD)
interface
    acoustic i.
    air-brain i.
    emotion-cognition i.
    long-term bone-instrumentation i.
interfaceable minds
interfacet wiring and fusion
interfamily
interfascial approach
interfascicular
    i. fasciculus
    i. graft
interference
    anterograde memory i.
    background i.
    habit i.
    i. modification
    i. pattern of discharge
    retrograde memory i.
    sleep i.
    theme i.
    i. theory
    treatment i.
interferon-β
    i. 1a (IFN-B1a)
    i. 1b (IFN-B1b)
interferon (IFN)
    alpha i.
    i.-γ (IFN-γ)
interfibrillary migration
interforniceal approach
interganglionic
intergemmal
intergenerational
    i. relation
    i. transmission
intergradation
intergroup-contact hypothesis
intergroup exercise
intergyral
interhemicerebral
interhemispheric
    i. approach
    i. asymmetry
    i. cyst
    i. fissure
    i. hematoma
    i. propagation time
    i. synchrony
    transcallosal i.
    i. transfer
interictal
    i. behavior
    i. epileptic personality
    i. epileptiform abnormality
    i. epileptiform activity
    i. epileptiform spike
    i. focal epileptiform discharge
    i. generalized spike-and-wave
      discharge
    i. period
    i. phenomenon
    i. psychosis
    i. spike discharge
interindividual differences
interinstitutional relation
interior band of Baillarger
interiorized imitation
interjudge reliability
interlaminar
    i. clamp
    i. decompression
interleaved
    i. GRASS
    i. learning
interleukin (IL)
    i. 4
    i. 5
    i. 6
    i. 7
    i. 8
    i. 9
    i. 10
    i. 11
    i. 12
interlocking
    i. gyri
    instinct-training i.
interloctus
intermale
intermanual conflict
intermarriage
intermasculine
intermaxillary fixation (IMF)
intermedia
    massa i.
intermediate
    I. Booklet Category Test
    i. brain syndrome
    i. C-D hook
    i. ganglia
    i. head fixator
    i. layer
    i. nerve
    obligatory i.
    i. part
    I. Personality Questionnaire (IPQ)
    i. sex
    i. structure
intermediate-acting insulin preparation
intermediate-care facility
intermediolateral
    i. cell column of spinal cord
    i. mesencephalic syndrome
    i. nucleus
intermediomedial nucleus
intermedius
    ventralis i. (VIM)
intermeningeal
intermenstrual
intermenstruum

intermetamorphosis
intermittent
    i. acute porphyria (IAP)
    i. aphonia
    i. cramp
    i. emotional conflicts or reaction
    i. explosive behavior
    i. explosive disorder
    i. explosive disturbance
    i. insanity
    i. insomnia
    i. melancholia
    i. pain
    i. psychosis
    i. reinforcement
    i. reinforcement schedule
    i. rhythmic delta activity (IRDA)
    i. tetanus
    i. torticollis
    i. wakefulness
intermodal
    i. competition
    i. fluency
intermorbid
interna
    hematorrhachis i.
    hyperostosis frontalis i.
    mediodorsal globus pallidus i.
    ophthalmoplegia i.
    pachymeningitis i.
    protuberantia occipitalis i.
    tabula i.
internal
    i. acoustic meatus
    i. arcuate fiber
    i. auditory canal
    i. capsule
    i. capsule syndrome
    i. carotid angiogram
    i. carotid artery (ICA)
    i. carotid artery aneurysm
    i. carotid artery balloon test
      occlusion
    i. carotid balloon test
    i. conflict
    i. cue
    i. decompression
    i. disk herniation
    i. drive
    i. fixation plate-screw system
    i. fixation of spine
    i. fixation spring
    fixed i.
    i. hemorrhage
    i. hydrocephalus
    i. inhibition
    i. locus of control
    i. meningitis
    i. neurolysis
    i. ophthalmoplegia
    i. pillar cell
    i. popliteal nerve
    i. pulse generating unit
    i. pyocephalus
    i. respiration

    i. second messenger system
    i. spinal fixation
    i. state
    i. stimulus
    i. stressor
    i. value
    i. versus external (I-E)
    i. versus external scale
    i. world of belief
    i. world of expectation
    i. world of fantasy
    i. world of perception
internal-external control
internalization
internalize
internalized
    i. sense
    i. speech
    i. validity
internalized-state rating
international
    I. Classification of Diseases (ICD)
    I. Classification of Diseases and
      Related Health Problems, 10th
      Edition (ICD-10)
    I. Classification of Diseases, 9th
      Edition (ICD-9)
    I. Classification of Diseases, 9th
      Edition, Clinical Modification
      (ICD-9-CM)
    I. Classification of Impairments,
      Disabilities, Handicaps (ICIDH)
    I. Classification of Sleep Disorders
    I. Classification of Sleep Disorders:
      Diagnostic and Coding Manual
      (ICSD)
    I. Cooperative Study on the
      Timing of Aneurysm Surgery
    I. Headache Society
    i. medical graduate (IMG)
    I. Medical News Group
    I. Normalized Ratio (INR)
    I. Pilot Study of Schizophrenia
      (IPSS)
    I. Primary Factors (IPF)
    I. Primary Factors test battery
    I. Society for Traumatic Stress
      Studies
    I. Statistical Classification of
      Diseases and Related Health
      Problems
    I. 10–20 system of electrode
      placement
    I. Test for Aphasia
    I. Version of the Mental Status
      Questionnaire
    I. Working Formulation
      classification
interne
    AO/ASIF fixateur i.
    AO fixateur i.
    Dick AO fixateur i.
    fixateur i. (FI)
Internet
    I. addiction

Internet *(continued)*
   I. psychotherapy
   I. sex
interneuron
interneuronal
   i. calcium modulation
   i. connection
internodal
   i. distance (IND)
   i. segment
internode
internship
internuclear
   i. ophthalmoplegia (INO)
internuclearis
   ophthalmoplegia i.
internuncial neuron
interobserver reliability
interoceptive
   i. awareness
   i. exposure
   i. fear
interofective system
interolivary
interoreceptive
interparietal sulcus
interpeak latency
interpedicular distance
interpeduncular
   i. cistern
   i. fossa
   i. fossa lesion
   i. ganglion
   i. nucleus
interpenetration
interpersonal
   i. accommodation
   i. behavior
   I. Behavior Study (IBS)
   I. Behavior Survey (IBS)
   i. cognitive problem solving (ICPS)
   I. Communication Inventory (ICI)
   i. conflict
   i. control
   i. dependency
   i. difficulty
   i. distrust
   i. dysfunction
   i. effectiveness skill
   i. exploitation
   i. functioning
   i. impairment
   i. interaction
   I. Language Skills and Assessment (ILSA)
   i. loss
   i. morality
   i. network
   I. Perception Scale (IPS)
   i. personality trait
   i. process
   i. psychiatry
   i. psychotherapy (IPT)
   i. rapport

   I. Reaction Test (IPRT)
   i. rejection
   i. relation
   i. relationship
   i. relationship deficit
   i. research orientation
   i. responsibility
   i. role
   i. spacing communication pattern
   i. strain
   i. style
   I. Style Inventory
   i. theory
   i. therapy (IPT)
   i. trust
   i. withdrawal
Inter-Person Perception Test (IPPT)
interpolation algorithm
interpose
interpositi
   cavum veli i. (CVI)
interpositum
   velum i.
interpositus nuclei
interpretation
   abstract i.
   action i.
   anagogic i.
   analytic i.
   aura i.
   defense i.
   i. delusion
   distortion of i.
   dream i.
   id i.
   mutative i.
   personalized i.
   psychoanalytic i.
   psychodynamic i.
   test i.
   i. test
interpretational insanity
interpreter role
interpretive therapy
interprofessional relation
interpsychic
   i. relationship
interpsychology
interpulse time
InterQual Intensity, Severity, and Discharge
interrater reliability
interrelate
interrupted tracing
interrupter device
interruption
   evidence of i.
   repeated REM sleep i.'s
   i. of thought
interruptus
   coitus i.
interscapular reflex
intersegmental
   i. aberration

I

i. fasciculi
i. reflex
intersensory
    i. disorder
    i. transfer
intersex
    i. condition
    female i.
    male i.
    true i.
intersexual disorder
intersociety
interspace
    ballooning of vertebral i.
    cervical i.
    lumbar i.
    thoracic i.
interspike interval
interspinous
    i. segmental spinal instrument (ISSI)
    i. segmental spinal instrumentation (ISSI)
    i. segmental spinal instrumentation technique
interstitial
    i. brachytherapy
    i. hydrocephalic edema
    i. lung disease (ILD)
    i. neuritis
    i. neurosyphilis
    i. nucleus of Cajal
    i. radiation source
    i. radiation therapy (IRT)
    i. radiotherapy
interstriate layer
interthalamic adhesion
intertrabecular hemorrhage
interuncal distance
interval
    atlantoaxial i.
    class i.
    confidence i.
    fixed i. (FI)
    interspike i.
    lucid i.
    mean interpotential i. (MIPI)
    i. psychosis
    i. reinforcement
    i. scale
    variable i. (VI)
intervening
    i. validity
    i. variable
intervention
    active i.
    associated i.
    barrier to i.
    clinical-facilitated i.
    cognitive-behavioral i.
    community i.
    crisis i.
    educative i.
    emergency i.
    evolutionary i.

family i.
generative i.
opportunities from i.
optimal therapeutic i.
outpatient i.
paradoxical i.
pharmacotherapeutic i.
postdisaster psychosocial i.
preventive i.
psychological i.
psychopharmaceutical i.
psychosocial i.
remedial i.
i. research
selective preventive i.
static i.
stop, look and listen i.
strategic i.
therapeutic i.
interventional
    i. material
    i. neuroradiology
    i. radiology
interventricular foramen
intervertebral
    i. discitis
    i. disk
    i. disk herniation
    i. disk rupture
    i. ganglion
    i. osteochondrosis
    i. punch
intervertebralis
    annulus fibrous disci i.
interview
    Adolescent Diagnostic I. (ADI)
    adolescent-parent i.
    amobarbital i.
    Amytal i.
    Autism Diagnostic I.
    barbiturate-facilitated i.
    Camberwell Family I.
    clinical i.
    Composite International Diagnostic I.
    Compulsive Sexual Disorders I.
    conjoint i.
    counseling i.
    diagnostic i.
    direct i.
    employment i.
    evaluation i.
    exit i.
    family system i.
    group i.
    i. group psychotherapy
    hypnotic i.
    initial i.
    Iowa Structured Psychiatric I. (IPSI)
    job i.
    Lehman Quality of Life I.
    Mini International Neuropsychiatric I.
    Minnesota Impulsive Disorders I.

interview *(continued)*
  open-ended i.
  Parent Attachment Structured I.
  patterned i.
  psychiatric i.
  Psychiatric Diagnostic I.
  Psychiatric Epidemiology
    Research I. (PERI)
  psychological i.
  Quality of Life I. (QOLI)
  Rutler-Graham Psychiatric I.
  semistructured diagnostic i.
  Sexual Abuse I.
  stress i.
  structured i.
  i. technique
  i. therapy
  unstructured i.
interviewer
  i. effect
  i. training
intestinal
  i. polyposis
  i. trauma
intimacy
  I. Potential Quotient (IPQ)
  i. principle
  sexual i.
  i. versus isolation
  i. versus self-absorption
intimate zone
intimidating
  i. behavior
  i. others
intolerance
  alcohol i.
  caffeine i.
  drug i.
intonation
intoxicated
  driving while i. (DWI)
  legally i.
intoxication
  acute i.
  acute alcohol i.
  alcohol acute i.
  alcoholic i.
  alcohol idiosyncratic i.
  alcohol pathological i.
  aluminum i.
  ammonia i.
  amphetamine i.
  anticonvulsant i.
  anxiolytic i.
  anylcyclohexylamine i.
  barbiturate i.
  bromide i.
  Burundanga i.
  caffeine i.
  cannabis i.
  carbon dioxide i.
  carbon disulfide i.
  carbon monoxide i.
  chronic i.

  cocaine i.
  i. delirium
  drug pathological i.
  i. episode
  ethanol i.
  gasoline i.
  glutethimide i.
  hallucinogenic i.
  heavy metal i.
  hypnagogic i.
  hypnotic i.
  idiosyncratic alcohol i.
  inhalant i.
  intense i.
  i. level
  manganese i.
  marijuana i.
  mercury i.
  metal i.
  narcotic chemical i.
  nicotine i.
  opioid i.
  i. organic psychosis
  organic psychosis drug i.
  pathologic i.
  pathologic alcohol i.
  pathologic drug i.
  PCP i.
  phencyclidine i.
  physiological i.
  psychoactive substance i.
  sedative i.
  serum heavy metal i.
  severe i.
  signs of alcohol i.
  substance i.
  substance-induced i.
  sympathomimetic i.
  i. syndrome
  water i.
intoxication-type organic psychosis
intra
  i. vitam
intraabdominal neuroblastoma
intraaortic balloon pump (IABP)
intraarachnoid
  i. leptomeningeal malformation
  i. neurovascular structure
intraarterial
  i. Amytal testing
  i. digital subtraction angiogram
    (IADSA)
  i. drug delivery
  i. flow
intraaural attenuation
intraaxial brain lesion
intra-blood-brain barrier (IBBB)
intracapsular hemorrhage
**intracarotid sodium Amytal memory
  testing**
intracavernous
  i. carotid aneurysm
  i. tumor
intracavitary irradiation
intracelial

intracellular
- i. calcium block
- i. deoxyhemoglobin
- i. ion
- i. metabolic pathway
- i. second messenger system
- i. signal

intraception
intraceptive signaling
intracerebellar
intracerebral
- i. aneurysm
- i. arteriovenous malformation
- i. depth electrode
- i. depth electrode monitoring
- i. ganglioma
- i. hematoma
- i. hemorrhage
- i. Hodgkin lymphoma
- i. hydatid cyst
- i. lesion
- i. steal

intracerebroventricular administration of morphine (ICVM)
intracisternal
intraconal mass
intraconscious personality
intracorporeal pharmacological testing
intracranial
- i. aneurysm
- i. arachnoid cyst
- i. arterial dolichoectasia
- i. astrocytoma
- i. cavernous angioma
- i. compliance
- i. cryptococcosis
- i. disorder
- i. electroencephalography (ICEEG)
- i. epidural abscess
- i. epidural pressure (ICEDP)
- i. ganglion
- i. glioma
- i. hematoma
- i. hemorrhage (ICrH)
- i. Hodgkin lymphoma
- i. hypertension
- i. hypotension
- i. infection organic psychosis
  intracranial to i. (IC-IC)
- i. mass lesion
- i. meningioma
- i. meningioma resection
- i. MR angiography
- i. neoplasm
- i. neuroblastoma
- i. occlusion
- i. pachymeningitis
- i. pneumatocele
- i. pneumocele
- i. pressure (ICP)
- i. pressure Express digital monitor
- i. rhizotomy
- i. sarcoidosis
- i. seminoma
- i. steal phenomenon

- i. steal syndrome
- i. stimulation (ICS)
- i. tumor
- i. vascular malformation
- i. venous malformation (IVM)
- i. venous sinus

intracranial-extracranial
- i.-e. nerve graft
- i.-e. transplantation

intracranial-intratemporal nerve graft
intractable
- i. epilepsy
- i. pain

intractive pain
intracutaneous
- i. hypodermic
- i. injection

intracytoplasmic
intradermal
- i. angioma
- i. injection

intradiploic epidermoid cyst
intradural
- i. abscess
- i. anastomosis
- i. approach
- i. arteriovenous fistula
- i. dissection
- i. draining vein
- i. extramedullary mass lesion
- i. inflammatory disease
- i. lipoma
- i. phase
- i. retractor
- i. retromedullary arteriovenous fistula
- i. segment
- i. tumor
- i. tumor surgery

intradural-extradural meningioma
intrafamilial
- i. conflict
- i. relationship

intrafascicular migration
intraforaminal approach
intrafusal fiber
intragemmal
intragyral
intrahippocampal microdialysis
Intra- and Interpersonal Relations Scale
intralaminar
- i. nuclei
- i. nuclei of thalamus

intraloctus
intraluminal thrombolysis
intrameatal
- i. earphone
- i. electrode

Intramedic PE-50 polyethylene tubing
intramedullary
- i. canal
  ependymoma i.
- i. ependymoma
- i. epidermoid cyst
- i. lymphoma

intramedullary *(continued)*
    i. nail
    i. spinal cord tumor
    i. spinal lesion
    i. toxoplasmosis
    i. tractotomy
intrameningeal
intramolecular
    i. dipole-dipole mechanism
    i. relaxation
intramucosal
intramural hematoma
intramuscular (IM)
    i. hypodermic
    i. injection
intranasal heroin
intraneural
    i. edema
    i. ganglion cyst
    i. neurofibrillary tangle
    i. phenol injection
intraneuronal
    i. argentophilic Pick inclusion body
    i. fibrillary tangles
    i. inclusion disease
intranidal aneurysm
intranuclear ophthalmoplegia
intraocular
    i. hemorrhage
    i. neuritis
    i. pressure
intraoperative
    i. angiography
    i. balloon occlusion
    i. B-mode ultrasound
    i. cell saver
    i. dural tear
    i. electrical cortical stimulation
    (IOECS)
    i. electrical stimulation
    i. facial nerve monitoring
    i. lateral fluoroscopy
    i. microendoscopy
    i. neck hyperextension
    i. neurophysiological monitoring
    i. rupture
    i. stereotactic spatial localization
    i. stress-relaxation
    i. ultrasonic probe
    i. ultrasound
    i. x-ray
intraorbital
    i. arteriovenous malformation
    i. granular cell tumor
    i. lesion
    i. meningioma
    i. surgery
intraosseous schwannoma
intraparenchymal
    i. cyst
    i. hematoma
    i. hemorrhage
    i. meningioma
    i. periventricular echodensity

intraparietal
    i. sulcus
    i. sulcus of Turner
intrapersonal
    i. conflict
    i. space
intrapontine
intrapsychic
    i. ataxia
    i. conflict
    i. distortion
    i. distress
    i. personality trait
intrapsychical function
Intrascan ultrasound
intrasegmental reflex
intrasellar
    i. extension
    i. granuloma
    i. lesion
    i. neuroadenohyphophyseal
    choristoma
    i. paraganglioma
    i. Rathke cleft cyst
intrasocial idiocy
intraspinal
    i. adenoma
    i. drug infusion system
    i. epidural pressure (ISEDP)
    i. herniated disk
    i. lesion
    i. meningioma
    i. vascular malformation
intraspinous muscle
intraspongy nuclear disk herniation
intrasynaptic
intratentorial
    i. malformation
    i. supracerebellar approach
intraterritorial anastomoses
intratest scatter
intrathecal
    i. antibiotic
    i. fluorescein
    i. IgG synthetic rate
    i. injection
    i. morphine analgesia
    i. morphinotherapy
    i. octreotide
    i. pain management
intratumoral hypervascularity
intratumor hemorrhage
intrauterine sonographic diagnosis
intravagal paraganglioma
intravaginal
intravascular
    i. balloon occlusion
    i. device
    i. injection
    i. ligature
    i. lymphoma
    i. streaming
intravenous (IV)
    i. drug user (IVDU)
    i. feeding

i. gamma globulin
i. hypodermic
i. immune globulin (IVIG)
i. immune globulin humoral
therapy
i. immunoglobulin (IVIG)
i. injection
i. medication
i. oxygen-15 water bolus technique
i. regional anesthesia (IVRA)
i. regional sympathetic blockade
i. treatment

intraventricular (I-V)
i. catheter
i. endoscopy
i. hematoma
i. hemorrhage (IVH)
i. injection
i. meningioma
i. septation
i. tumor

intravoxel phase dispersion
Intrex Questionnaire
intrinsic
i. asthma
i. behavior
i. brainstem tumor
i. cell suicide mechanism
i. constancy
i. disease
i. fiber
i. motivation
i. reflex
i. reward
i. transverse connector
i. transverse connector role

intrinsic-negative runners
intrinsic-positive runners
introintensive personality style
introject
introjection defense mechanism
intromission
intromit
intromittent organ
intron
Intropaque
Intropin
intropunitiveness
anxious i.

intropunitive response
introspection
phenomenalistic i.

introspective method
introtensive problem-solving style
introversion
passive i.
social i. (SI)

introversion-extroversion
i.-e. continuum
i.-e. scale (IES)

introversive
i. tendency
i. trait

introvert
introverted
i. disorder of adolescence
i. disorder of childhood
i. personality disorder
i. schizoid personality
i. schizothymia
i. type

Introvertive Anhedonia Scale
intruding idea
intrusion
ego-dystonic i.

intrusive
i. distressing idea
i. flashback
i. impulse
i. obsessional image
i. recollection
i. sexual disorder
i. thought
i. treatment
i. urge

intubation
aqueductal i.
nasogastric i.
oral i.

intuitive
i. stage
i. type

intumescence
tympanic i.

intumescentia
i. cervicalis
i. ganglioformis
i. lumbalis
i. tympanica

invagination
basilar i.

invalidating environment
invariable behavior
invariance
factorial i.

invariant
functional i.

invasion
aggressive i.
personal space i.

invasive
i. operation
i. pituitary adenoma
i. treatment
i. tumor

inventory
ABC I. - Extended
academic i.
Acute Panic I.
adaptive behavior i.
Addiction Research Center I.
i. adjustment
adjustment i.
adolescent i.

inventory *(continued)*
    Adolescent Multiphasic
      Personality I.
    Adult Career Concerns I. (ACCI)
    Adult Personal Data I. (APDI)
    Adult Personality I. (API)
    Alcohol Use I. (AUI)
    Analytical Reading I.
    I. of Anger Communication (IAC)
    anxiety i.
    Anxiety States I.
    anxiety status i. (ASI)
    aptitude i.
    assessment i.
    Assessment of Chemical Health I.
    Association Adjustment I.
    Athletic Motivation I. (AMI)
    attitude i.
    Barclay Classroom Climate I.
      (BCCI)
    Barclay Learning Needs
      Assessment I. (BLNAI)
    Basic Concept I.
    Basic Personality I. (BPI)
    Basic Reading I. (BRI)
    Basic School Skills I. (BSSI)
    Batelle Developmental I.
    Batelle Developmental I.
    Beck Depression I. (BDI)
    behavior i.
    Behavior Status I. (BSI)
    Bell Object Relations-Reality
      Testing I.
    Bem Sex-Role I.
    Bernreuter Personality I.
    Bipolar Psychological I. (BPI)
    Botel Reading I.
    Brief Life History I. (BLHI)
    Brief Symptom I. (BSI)
    Burns/Roe Informal Reading I.
    Buss-Durkee Hostility I.
    California Critical Thinking
      Dispositions I. (CCTDI)
    California Personality I. (CPI)
    California Psychological I. (CPI)
    Canfield Instructional Styles I.
    career i.
    Career Assessment I. (CAI)
    Career Beliefs I. (CBI)
    Career Development I.
    Career Maturity I. (CMI)
    Caregiver's School Readiness I.
      (CSRI)
    Caring Relationship I. (CRI)
    Carnegie Interest I. (CII)
    Carrow Elicited Language I.
      (CELI)
    Cattell Infant Scale I. (CISI)
    child abuse i.
    Child Abuse Potential I.
    Child Care I.
    child depression i.
    child development i.

Children's Academic Intrinsic
      Motivation I.
    Children's Depression I. (CDI)
    Children's Diagnostic I. (CDI)
    Children's Perception of Support I.
      (CPSI)
    clinical i.
    College Major Interest I. (CMII)
    Communication Sensitivity I.
    I. of Complicated Grief
    coping i.
    Coping Resources I. (CRI)
    COPSystem Interest I.
    Cornell Learning and Study
      Skills I. (CLASSI)
    counseling i.
    I. for Counseling and Development
      (ICD)
    Couples Pre-Counseling I.
    Cross-Cultural Adaptability I.
      (CCAI)
    Crown-Crisp Experiential I.
    cultural i.
    Cultural Attitude I. (CAI)
    Culture-Free Self-Esteem I.'s,
      Second Edition (CFSEI-2)
    Culture Shock I.
    Decision Making I.
    Defense Mechanism I. (DMI)
    depression i.
    Depression Status I. (DSI)
    development i.
    Developmental Activities
      Screening I. (DASI)
    Devine I.
    I. to Diagnose Depression
    diagnostic i.
    Diagnostic Mathematics I. (DMI)
    Driver Risk I. (DRI)
    Dynamic Personality I. (DPI)
    Early Child Development I.
    Early Coping I.
    Early Screening I.
    Eating I.
    Eating Disorder I. (EDI)
    Eating Disorder I., 2nd edition
      (EDI-2)
    Edinburgh Handedness I.
    Ego State I. (ESI)
    El Senoussi Multiphasic Marital I.
    Employability I.
    Employee Attitude I.
    Employee Reliability I. (ERI)
    employment i.
    environmental i.
    Environmental Language I. (ELI)
    Environmental Response I. (ERI)
    Experiential World I. (EWI)
    Eysenck Personality I. (EPI)
    Family Relationship I.
    Freiburger Personality I. (FPI)
    Functional Assessment I.
    Gordon Personal I. (GPI)
    Gordon Personal Profile I. (GPPI)
    Grief Experience I. (GEI)

Group Styles I. (GSI)
Guilford-Zimmerman Interest I. (GZII)
Hall Occupational Orientation I. (HOOI)
Hamburg Obsession/Compulsion I.
Hogan Personality I.
Hutchins Behavior I. (HBI)
Imagined Process I. (IPI)
Impact Message I. (IMI)
I. of Individually Perceived Group Cohesiveness
Institutional Functioning I. (IFI)
Institutional Goals I. (IGI)
Instructional Leadership I.
interest i.
Interpersonal Communication I. (ICI)
Interpersonal Style I.
Inwald Personality I. (IPI)
Jackson Personality I. (JPI)
Jesness I. (JI)
Johnston Informal Reading I. (JIRI)
Junior Eysenck Personality I. (JEPI)
Khatena-Torrance Creative Perception I.
leadership i.
Leadership Practices I. (LPI)
Leadership Skills I.
learning i.
Learning and Study Strategies I. (LASSI)
Learning and Study Strategies I.-High School Version (LASSI-HS)
Learning Styles I.
Leisure Interest I. (LII)
Leyton Obsessional I.
Leyton Obsessive I. (LOI)
i. of loss
management i.
Management Styles I.
Mandsley Personality I. (MPI)
Marital Satisfaction I.
Marriage Adjustment I. (MAI)
Martin Suicide-Depression I. (MSDI)
Maslach Burnout I. (MBI)
Maudsley Obsessional-Compulsive I.
Maudsley Obsessional Compulsive I. (MOCI)
Maudsley Personality I. (MPI)
Michigan Picture I.
Military Environment I.
Millon Adolescent Clinical I. (MACI)
Millon Adolescent Personality I. (MAPI)
Millon Behavioral Health I. (MBHI)
Millon Clinical Multiaxial I. (MCMI)
Millon Clinical Multiaxial i. II (MCMI-II)

Millon Clinical Multiaxial I. III (MCMI-III)
Milwaukee Academic Interest I. (MAII)
Minnesota Child Development I. (MCDI)
Minnesota Infant Development I.
Minnesota Multiphasic Personality I. (MMPI)
Minnesota Multiphasic Personality I., Second Edition (MMPI-2)
Minnesota Teacher Attitude I. (MTAI)
Minnesota Vocational Interest I. (MVII)
Morbid Anxiety I. (MAI)
motivational i.
Motivational Patterns I.
Multidimensional Pain I. (MPI)
Multilevel Informal Language I.
Multiphasic Personality I. (MPI)
Multiscore Depression I. (MDI)
Multivariate Personality I. (MPI)
NEO Five Factor I.
Neuroticism-Extroversion-Openness Personality I.
New Sucher-Allred Reading Placement I.
obsessive-compulsive i. (OCI)
occupational i.
Ohio Work Values I. (OWVI)
Omnibus Personality I. (OPI)
Oral Language Sentence Imitation Diagnostic I. (OLSIDI)
Organizational Culture I. (OCI)
Orientation I.
orientation i. (OI)
PACG I.
Pair Attraction I. (PAI)
parent i.
Parent as a Teacher I. (PAAT)
Parent Opinion I.
Partner Relationship I. (PRI)
PDI Employment I.
I. of Peer Influence on Eating Concern
perception i.
I. of Perceptual Skills (IPS)
Personal I.
personal data i.
Personality I. (PI)
Personality Assessment I. (PAI)
Personal Orientation I. (POI)
Personal Relationship I. (PRI)
Personal Style I. (PSI)
Personal Values I. (PVI)
Personnel Selection I.
picture i.
Premarital Communication I. (PCI)
Preschool Development I.
Prescriptive Reading I. (PRI)
Primary Self-Concept I. (PSCI)
Problem Solving I.
Professional Sexual Role I. (PSRI)

inventory *(continued)*
psychological i.
Psychological Distress I.
Psychological Screening I. (PSI)
I. of Psychosocial Development (IPD)
psychosomatic i. (PSI)
Psychotherapy Supervisory I.
Quality of Life I. (QOLI)
Racial Perceptions I. (RPI)
Reaction to Loss I.
readiness i.
Reading Comprehension I.
Reading-Free Vocational Interest I. (RFVII)
Reading Miscue I. (RMI)
Reasons for Living I. (RLI)
relationship i.
Revised NEO Personality I.
Riley Motor Problems I.
Riley Preschool Developmental Screening I. (RPDSI)
risk i.
Risk-Taking, Attitude, Values I. (RTAVI)
Safran Student's Interest I. (SSII)
Salience I. (SI)
satisfaction i.
School Climate I.
School Interest I.
School Problem Screening I. (SPSI)
screening i.
Self-Concept and Motivation I. (SCAMI, SCAMIN)
Self-Control I.
Self-Description I. (SDI)
Self-Esteem I. (SEI)
Self-Perception I. (SPI)
self-report personalities i.
self-report psychological i.
Senoussi Multiphasic Marital I. (SMMI)
Separation Anxiety Symptom I. (SASI)
Sequential Assessment of Mathematics Inventories: Standardized I.
sex i. (SI)
Shipley Personal I. (SPI)
Short Imaginal Processes I. (SIPI)
skill i.
Social Behavior Assessment I. (SBAI)
social stress and functionability i. (SSFI)
Spielberger Anxiety I.
Spielberger State-Trait Anger Expression I.
Spielberger State-Trait Anxiety I.
State-Trait Anger Expression I. (STAXI)
State-Trait Anxiety I. (STAI)
State-Trait Personality I. (STPI)

stress i.
Stress Evaluation I.
stress and functionability i.
Strong-Campbell Interest I. (SCII)
Student Adjustment I. (SAI)
Student Opinion I. (SOI)
Style of Management I.
Style of Mind I. (SMI)
Substance Abuse Subtle Screening I. (SASSI)
suicide i.
Suicide Intervention Response I.
I. of Suicide Orientation-30 (ISO-30)
Supervisory Practices I.
task i.
teacher i.
teacher attitude i.
Teacher Opinion I.
Teacher School Readiness I. (TSRI)
Teacher Stress I.
Teaching Style I.
Temperament and Values I. (TVI)
i. test
test anxiety i.
Time Perception I.
Time Problems I.
TLC-Learning Preference I.
values i.
Vocational Interest I.
Vocational Planning I. (VPI)
Vocational Preference I. (VPI)
Wahler Physical Symptoms I.
Wahler Self-Description I. (WSDI)
Wakefield Self-Assessment Depression I.
Western Personality I.
What I Like to Do: An I. of Students' Interests (WILD)
Wilson-Patterson Attitude I. (WPAI)
Wisconsin Psychosocial Pain I.
Word and Number Assessment I. (WNAI)
Work Information I. (WII)
Work Motivation I. (WMI)
Work Values I. (WVI)
World of Work I. (WWI)
inversal
language i.
inverse
i. agonist
i. Anton syndrome
i. Argyll Robertson pupil
i. feedback
i. ocular bobbing
i. polymerase chain reaction-based detection of frataxin gene
i. relationship
i. square rule
i. treatment planning (ITP)
inversion
absolute i.
affect i.
amphigenic i.

I

inversion recovery imaging with
short-time i.
occasional i.
i. recovery
i. relationship
sex role i.
sexual i.
sleep i.
i. time (TI)
visual image i.
inverted
i. image
i. Oedipus
i. radial reflex
inverted-U function
investigation
Luria's Neuropsychological I.
principal i.
investigatory reflex
investment
emotional i.
inveterate drinking
inviolacy motive
Invirase
invisible college
invocational psychosis
involuntary
i. admission
i. behavior
i. civil commitment
i. discharge
i. hospitalization
i. manslaughter
i. motion
i. motor movement
i. nervous system
i. pauses in speech
i. premonitory urge
i. repetitive movement disorder
antineuronal antibody assay
i. response
i. retention
i. state of trance
i. treatment
i. twitch
i. vocalization
i. whispering
involuntomotor
involuntomotory
involution
senile i.
involutional
i. depression
i. melancholia
i. paranoia
i. paranoid state
i. paraphrenia
i. period
i. psychosis
i. reaction
involvement
ego i.
extraocular muscle i.
extrapyramidal i. (EPI)
lack of i.

subcortical brain i.
tumorous i.
INVOS
in vivo optical spectroscopy
INVOS 3100 cerebral oximeter
monitoring system
INVOS transcranial cerebral
oximeter
Inwald Personality Inventory (IPI)
inward
i. aggression
i. picture
iobenzamic acid
iobutoic acid
iocarmate meglumine
iocarmic acid
iocetamate
iodamic acid
iodamide
Iodamoeba buetschlii **cerebral amebiasis**
iodatol
iodide
metocurine i.
radioactive i.
iodinated
iodine
isotopic i.
i. 131 MIBG
protein-bound i. (PBI)
iodine-125 implant
iodipamide
i. meglumine
i. methylglucamine
iodized oil
iodoalphionic acid
iodohippurate
iodomethamate
iodophendylate
iodophthalein
iodopyracet
iodoxamate
iodoxamic acid
iodoxyl
IOECS
intraoperative electrical cortical
stimulation
ioglicate
ioglicic acid
ioglucol
ioglucomide
ioglunide
ioglycamic acid
ioglycamide
iogulamide
iohexol
i. CT ventriculogram
i. myelography
iomide
ion
argon i.
calcium i.
intracellular i.
positive i.
Ionamin

iopamidol
 i. contrast medium
iopanoate
iopanoic acid
iophendylate
iophenoxic acid
iophobia
ioprocemic acid
iopromide
iopronic acid
iopydol
iopydone
iosefamate
iosefamic acid
ioseric acid
iosulamide
iosumetic acid
iotacism
iotasul
ioteric acid
iothalamate
 meglumine i.
iothalamic acid
iotrol
iotroxamide
iotroxic acid
ioversol
Iowa
 I. Algebra Aptitude Test (IAAT)
 I. Conners Rating Scale
 I. Pressure Articulation Test
  (IPAT)
 I. Structured Psychiatric Interview
  (IPSI)
 I. Stuttering Scale
 I. Tests of Basic Skills
 I. Tests of Educational
  Development, Forms X-8 and Y-
  8
ioxaglate
 i. meglumine
 i. sodium
ioxaglic acid
ioxithalamate
ioxithalamic acid
iozomic acid
IP₃
 inositol triphosphate
IPAR
I-Paracaine
IPAT
 Institute of Personality and Ability
  Testing
 Iowa Pressure Articulation Test
 IPAT Anxiety Scale
 IPAT Depression Scale
IPD
 incurable problem drinker
 Inventory of Psychosocial Development
ipecac
I-persona
IPF
 International Primary Factors
 IPF test battery

IPI
 Imagined Process Inventory
 Inwald Personality Inventory
I.P.I Aptitude-Intelligence Test Series
I-plate
 Syracuse anterior I-p.
ipodate acid
IPPT
 Inter-Person Perception Test
IPQ
 Intermediate Personality Questionnaire
 Intimacy Potential Quotient
iprindole
iproclozide
iproniazid
IPRT
 Interpersonal Reaction Test
IPS
 Interpersonal Perception Scale
 Inventory of Perceptual Skills
ipsapirone
ipsation
ipsative score
IPSI
 Iowa Structured Psychiatric Interview
ipsilateral
 i. approach
 i. cerebellar ataxia
 i. cerebellar sign
 i. corticospinal tract sign
 i. deficit
 i. facial palsy
 i. facial paralysis
 i. facial paresis
 i. frontal routing of signals
  (IFROS)
 i. gaze palsy
 i. headache
 i. hemianopia
 i. hemiparesis
 i. loss
 i. mesial temporal sclerosis
 i. middle cerebral artery
 i. monocular blindness
 i. reflex
 i. stroke
 i. tonic conjugate gaze
 i. tonic deviation
 i. tragus
 i. transcallosal technique
 i. vasogenic edema
ipsilesional hemifield
IPSP
 inhibitory postsynaptic potential
IPSS
 International Pilot Study of
  Schizophrenia
IPT
 interpersonal psychotherapy
 interpersonal therapy
IQ
 intelligence quotient
 Full Scale IQ (FSIQ)
 IQ Test
I/Q imbalance ghost

IR
   HydroStat IR
IRDA
   intermittent rhythmic delta activity
   IRDA on electroencephalogram
iridis
   rubeosis i.
Iriditope
iridium
iridium-192
iridocyclitis
iridoparalysis
iridoplegia
   complete i.
   reflex i.
   sympathetic i.
Irish Study of High-Density Schizophrenia Families
iris neovascularization
iritis
   white i.
irkunii
IRM
   inherited releasing mechanism
iron
   i. deficiency
   i. deficiency anemia
   i. lung
   i. poisoning
   serum i.
iron-ascorbate-DTPA
   technetium 99m i.-a.-D.
ironic aspect
irradiation
   conventional fractionated i.
   convergent beam i. (CBI)
   excitatory i.
   gamma i.
   hyperfractionated i.
   intracavitary i.
   selective i.
   stereotactic i.
irradiation-induced mental deterioration
irrational
   i. action
   i. anger
   i. behavior
   i. desire
   i. fear
   i. type
irrationality
irreal
irreality level
irregular
   i. movement
   i. nystagmus
   i. sleep pattern
   i. sleep-wake pattern
irrelevant
   i. answer
   i. external stimuli
   i. language
irresistible
   i. apprehension
   i. impulse

   I. Impulse Test
   i. sleep
irresponsibility
   consistent i.
   criminal i.
irresponsible
   i. parenting
   i. work behavior
irreverent communication
irreversibility
irreversible
   i. coma
   i. shock
irrigant
   Neosporin GU I.
irrigation bipolar system
irritability
   acoustic i.
   electric i.
   marked i.
   myotatic i.
Irritability/Depression and Anxiety Scale
irritable
   i. bowel syndrome
   i. heart
   i. mood
   i. testis
irritate
irritation
   cerebral i.
   functional i.
   i. therapy
irritative lesion
irrumation
irruption
IRS
   idiopathic recurring stupor
I-R specificity
IRT
   interstitial radiation therapy
   item response theory
IS
   index of sexuality
Isaacs syndrome
Isakower phenomenon
ischemia
   anoxic i.
   brain i.
   brainstem i.
   cerebral i.
   cortical transient i.
   global cerebral i.
   hindbrain i.
   ischemic i.
   myoneural i.
   i. organic psychosis
   rostral brain stem i.
   tourniquet i.
   transient brain stem i.
   vasomotor i.
   vertebrobasilar i.
ischemic
   i. brain damage
   i. brain edema
   i. brainstem infarction

ischemic *(continued)*
    i. cerebral infarction
    i. disease
    i. forearm exercise test
    i. heart disease (IHD)
    i. hypoxia
    i. ischemia
    i. lesion
    i. lumbago
    i. muscular atrophy
    i. neuritis
    i. neuropathy
    i. ocular inflammation
    i. penumbra
    i. stroke
    i. vascular dementia
ischemic-hypoxic encephalopathy
ischialgia
ischiodynia
ischioneuralgia
ischonophonia
ischophonia
ISD
    Intensity, Severity, and Discharge
ISDB
    indirect self-destructive behavior
ISE
    inhibited sexual excitement
ISEDP
    intraspinal epidural pressure
^{125}**I seed**
ISG viewing wand
I-shaped scalp flap
Ishihara plate
island
    i. of Calleja
    i. of control
    i. pedicle scalp flap
    i. of Reil
    social i.
    syncytial i.
    Three Mile I.
islet
    i. cell adenoma
    i. of precocity
ISO-30
    Inventory of Suicide Orientation-30
isobutyl
    i. nitrate
    i. nitrite
isobutyl-2 cyanoacrylate
isobutyl-2-cyanoacrylate
Isocaine HCl
Isocal
isocaloric
isocarboxazid
isocentric
    i. linear accelerator
    i. linear accelerator x-ray
Isocet
isochromosome
isochronal
isochronism
    law of i.

Isocom
isocoric pupil
isocortex
isodense
    i. mass
    i. subdural hematoma
isodose
    i. curve
    i. line
isodynamic
isoeffect
isoelectric
    i. electroencephalogram
    i. encephalogram
isoenergetic
isoenzyme
isoetharine hydrochloride
isoflavone
isoflurane anesthesia
isoform
    brain i.
    embryonic i.
    four-repeat i.
    recombinant tau i.
    three-repeat i.
isogamous
isogenic
isointense lesion
Isola
    I. spinal implant system
    I. spinal implant system accessory
    I. spinal implant system anchor
    I. spinal implant system application
    I. spinal implant system complication
    I. spinal implant system component
    I. spinal implant system design
    I. spinal implant system dimension
    I. spinal implant system eye rod
    I. spinal implant system hook
    I. spinal implant system iliac post
    I. spinal implant system iliac screw
    I. spinal implant system longitudinal member contouring
    I. spinal implant system plate-rod combination
isolate
    social i.
isolated
    i. angiitis
    i. angiitis of the central nervous system
    i. angiitis of the CNS (IAC)
    i. delusion
    emotionally i.
    i. explosive disorder
    i. explosive disturbance
    i. gait ignition failure
    i. phobia
    i. radial nerve palsy
isolation
    i. of affect
    i. amentia
    i. aphasia

autistic i.
i. effect
intimacy versus i.
mononuclear leukocyte i.
social i.
i. syndrome
isolative behavior
isolé
cerveau i.
encephale i.
isoleucyl
Isollyl Improved
isolophobia
isomerase
glucosephosphate i. (GPI)
isomeric function
isometheptene mucate
isomorphism
isomorphous gliosis
Isonate
isoniazid neuropathy
isonicotinic acid peripheral neuropathy
Isopap
Isopaque
isopathic principle
isophane
isophilia
isopotential
isopropyl alcohol
isopropylparaiodoamphetamine
isoproterenol
electroblotting i.
Mucomyst with I.
i. tilt table test
isopterophobia
Isoptin
Isordil
isosexual
isosorbide dinitrate
isotope
i. cisternogram
i. cisternography
isotopic
i. cisternography
i. iodine
isotropic
i. 3DFT
i. three-dimensional Fourier
transform
isotypical
isovaleric acidemia aminoaciduria
isovolemic hemodilution
Isovue M
isozyme
ISS
Injury Severity Scale
Injury Severity Score
ISSI
interspinous segmental spinal instrument
interspinous segmental spinal
instrumentation
issue
extratransference i.
inner child i.

legal i.
nature-nurture i.
preexisting underlying emotional i.
process i.
reality i.
skirt the i.
take i.
termination i.
underlying emotional i.
"I" statement
isthmi (*pl. of* isthmus)
isthmoparalysis
isthmoplegia
isthumus, pl. **isthmi, isthmuses**
i. of cingular gyrus
i. gyri cinguli
i. of gyrus fornicatus
i. of His
i. of limbic lobe
i. rhombencephali
rhombencephalic i.
Isuprel
IT
individual therapy
italomania
ITAQ
Insight and Treatment Attitudes
Questionnaire
ITC
inferior temporal cortex
ITC radiopaque balloon catheter
item
i. analysis
I. Counseling Evaluation Test
48-I. Counseling Evaluation Test
(ICET)
cultural i.
i. difficulty
i. discrimination parameter
15-I. Memorization Test
i. response theory (IRT)
i. scaling
i. selection
i. validity
i. weighting
iterate
ITERS
Infant/Toddler Environment Rating Scale
iter a tertio ad quartum ventriculum
I-Thou
I-thou relationship
ithykyphosis, ithycyphosis
itylordosis
IT-MS infusion therapy
Ito
hypomelanosis of I.
ITP
inverse treatment planning
ITPA
Illinois Test of Psycholinguistic Ability
Itrel
I. pulse generator
I. II spinal cord stimulation system
I. II spinal cord stimulator
I. 3 spinal cord stimulation system

ITSC
  It Scale for Children
It Scale for Children (ITSC)
ITU
  intensive treatment unit
IV
  intravenous
    IV drug abuse
    Feridex IV
    Indocin IV
    mucolipidosis, type IV (ML4)
I-V
  intraventricular
Ivalon
  I. embolic sponge
  I. foam
  I. particle
  I. wire coil

IVDU
  intravenous drug user
IVEC-10 neurotransmitter analyzer
IVH
  intraventricular hemorrhage
IVIG
  intravenous immune globulin
  intravenous immunoglobulin
IVM
  intracranial venous malformation
IVRA
  intravenous regional anesthesia
Iwabuchi clip
IWB
  Index of Well-Being
IWS
  Index of Work Satisfaction
ixomyelitis

JACE-STIM electrotherapy stimulation device
jack
    j. box
    turnbuckle j.
jacket
    Minerva j.
    strait j.
    yellow j.
jackknife
    j. attack
    j. seizure
Jackson
    J. epilepsy
    J. Evaluation System
    J. law
    J. Personality Inventory (JPI)
    J. rule
    J. sign
    J. syndrome
    J. vagoaccessory hypoglossal paralysis
    J. Vocational Interest Survey (JVIS)
jacksonian
    j. convulsion
    j. epilepsy
    j. march
    j. seizure
Jackson-Pratt drain
Jackson-Weiss syndrome
Jacobs
    J. locking hook spinal rod
    J. locking hook spinal rod instrumentation
    J. locking hook spinal rod instrumentation modification
    J. locking hook spinal rod technique
    J. locking spinal rod instrumentation
Jacobson
    J. endarterectomy spatula
    J. microneurosurgical scissors
    J. microprobe
    J. microvascular knife
    J. mosquito forceps
    J. needle holder
    J. nerve
    J. probe
    J. reflex
    J. suture pusher
    J. vessel knife
    J. view of depressive disorder
Jacobson-Potts vascular clamp
Jacod syndrome
jactatio
    j. capitis nocturna
    j. capitis nocturnus
jactitation, jactation
    periodic j.
Jadassohn nevus

jade
jaded
Jaeger-Hamby procedure
jag
    arousal j.
    crying j.
    j. drinker
    j. drinking
Jahnke syndrome
jail sentence
Jak
    Janus kinase
jake paralysis
Jakob-Creutzfeldt
    J.-C. disease
    J.-C. disease organic psychosis
Jak-STAT mechanism
Jamaica
    J. ginger paralysis
    J. ginger poisoning
Jamaican
    J. neuropathy
    J. vomiting sickness
jamais
    j. phenomenon
    j. vu
    j. vu aura
James-Lange
    J.-L. theory
    J.-L. theory of emotion
James-Lange-Sutherland theory
James Language Dominance Test
Jamestown Canyon virus
Janet
    J. disease
    J. test
Janimine Oral
Jannetta
    J. alligator forceps
    J. aneurysm neck dissector
    J. bayonet forceps
    J. duckbill elevator
    J. fork
    J. hook
    J. knife
    J. microvascular decompression procedure
    J. posterior fossa retractor
    J. probe
Jannetta-Kurze dissecting scissors
Jansen
    J. bone curette
    J. mastoid retractor
    J. monopolar forceps
    J. rasp
    J. rongeur
    J. scalp retractor
Jansen-Middleton
    J.-M. forceps
    J.-M. rongeur
    J.-M. scissors
Jansen-Wagner retractor

J

Jansky-Bielschowsky disease
Jansky Screening Index (JSI)
Janus-faced
janusian thinking
Janus kinase (Jak)
Janz
    J. juvenile myoclonic seizure
    J. response
    J. response on electroencephalogram
Japanese
    J. B encephalitis
    J. encephalitis (JE)
    J. encephalitis virus
    J. suction tip
japanophobia
japonica
    encephalitis j.
jar
    heel j.
Jarcho-Levin syndrome
Jarell forceps
jargon
    j. agraphia
    j. aphasia
    organic j.
    j. paraphasia
    semantic j.
jargonistic
Jarisch-Herxheimer
    J.-H. fever
    J.-H. fever reaction
Jarit
    J. brain forceps
    J. periosteal elevator
    J. rotator
    J. tendon-pulling forceps
Jarit-Kerrison laminectomy rongeur
Jarit-Liston bone rongeur
Jarit-Ruskin bone rongeur
JAS
    Jenkins Activity Survey
    Job Attitude Scale
jaundice
    allergic j.
    nuclear j.
Javid
    J. carotid clamp
    J. shunt
jaw
    j. claudication
    j. grinding
    j. jerk
    j. reflex
    j. winking reflex
jaw-closing muscle reflex
jaw-winking
    j.-w. phenomenon
    j.-w. syndrome
jaw-working reflex
JBC
    Jesness Behavior Checklist
JCMHC
    Joint Commission on Mental Health of
    Children

JCV
    JC virus
JC virus (JCV)
JDI
    Job Description Index
JE
    Japanese encephalitis
jealous
    j. rage
    j. type
jealous-type
    j.-t. delusion
    j.-t. schizophrenia
jealousy
    alcoholic j.
    delusional j.
    morbid j.
    projected j.
    sibling j.
JedMed TRI-GEM microscope
Jeep driver's disease
Jefferson fracture
jejunal bypass operation
jejuni
    Campylobacter j.
jejunostomy
Jekyll and Hyde personality
jelly nystagmus
Jendrassik maneuver
Jenkins
    J. Activity Survey (JAS)
    J. Non-Verbal Test
Jenny Craig diet
JEPI
    Junior Eysenck Personality Inventory
Jerald forceps
jerk
    Achilles j.
    ankle j.
    chin j.
    crossed adductor j.
    crossed knee j.
    elbow j.
    j. finger
    flurry of myoclonic j.'s
    hypnic j.
    jaw j.
    knee j.
    myoclonic j.
    nystagmoid j.
    j. nystagmus
    paretic j.
    photomyoclonic j.
    square-wave j.
    supinator j.
jerking
    head j.
    j. movement
Jesness
    J. Behavior Checklist (JBC)
    J. Inventory (JI)
jet
    j. lag phenomenon
    j. lag syndrome

j. lag-type dyssomnia
j. set
Jette Functional Status Index
Jevs Work Sample Battery
jeweler's bipolar forceps
Jewett wave
JI
Jesness Inventory
jig
Ace Hershey halo j.
jinjinia bemar
JIRI
Johnston Informal Reading Inventory
jiryan
jitter
frequency j.
JKST
Johnson-Kenney Screening Test
JLO
Judgment of Line orientation
JND
just noticeable difference
job
j. analysis
J. Attitude Scale (JAS)
j. change
j. characteristics model
j. component method
J. Description Index (JDI)
j. design
j. dimensions
j. enlargement
j. enrichment
j. evaluation
hatchet j.
j. interview
j. placement
j. requirement
j. satisfaction
J. Seeking Skills Assessment
snow j.
j. stress
job-sample experience
job-specific test
Jocasta complex
Joffroy
J. reflex
J. sign
Johnson
J. brain tumor forceps
Masters and J.
Johnson-Kenney Screening Test (JKST)
Johnston
J. alopecia
J. Informal Reading Inventory
(JIRI)
joint
amp j.
apophysial j.
atlantoaxial j.
atlantooccipital j.
Charcot j.
J. Commission on Mental Health
of Children (JCMHC)
j. custody

j. disorder
facet j.
hysterical j.
incudostapedial j.
neuropathic j.
j. play
radiohumeral j.
sacroiliac j.
j. sense
super j.
temporomandibular j. (TMJ)
zygapophyseal j.
joker dissector
joking mania
Jolly
J. reaction
J. test
JOMACI
judgment, orientation, memory,
abstraction and calculation intact
Jonah words
Jordan Left-Right Reversal Test
Joseph
J. disease
J. Pre-School and Primary Self-
Concept Screening Test
Joubert syndrome
joule
journaling exercise
JPI
Jackson Personality Inventory
Jr.
Caltrate, J.
J-sella deformity
JSI
Jansky Screening Index
J-tipped guidewire
Juan
Don J.
Juana
Dona J.
Juanita
Dona J.
jubilation
judeophobia
judgment
automatic j.
clinical j.
comparative j.
critical j.
diagnostic j.
faulty j.
impaired social j.
j. and insight
J. of Line orientation (JLO)
moral j.
negative j.
J. of Occupational Behavior-
Orientation
j., orientation, memory, abstraction,
and calculation
j., orientation, memory, abstraction
and calculation intact (JOMACI)
personal j.
poor j.

J

judgment *(continued)*
    qualitative j.
    quantitative j.
    social j.
    value j.
judgment,
judicial process
jugular
    j. bulb
    j. bulb venous oxygen saturation
    j. foramen
    j. foramen muscle
    j. foramen syndrome
    j. ganglion
    j. vein
    j. vein dissection
    j. venous oxygen saturation (SjO_2)
jugulation
jugulocephalic vein
jugulosubclavian junction
jugulotympanicum
    glomus j.
Jukes family
jumper disease of Maine
jumping
    j. Frenchmen of Maine
    j. Frenchmen of Maine syndrome
jumpy stump
junction
    anterior cervical approach to
      cervicothoracic j.
    cervical medullary j.
    cervicothoracic j.
    craniocervical j.
    craniovertebral j.
    electrotonic j.
    gap j.
    gray-white matter j.
    jugulosubclavian j.
    liponeural j.
    lumbosacral j.
    myoneural j.
    neuromuscular j.
    pontomedullary j.
    pontomesencephalic j.
    posterior craniocervical j.
    sylvian/rolandic j.
    temporal-occipital j.
    thoracolumbar j.
junctional
    j. dilation
    j. kyphosis
junctural feature
juncture
    closed j.
    open j.
Jung
    J. association test
    J. method
    J. theory
jungian
    j. psychoanalysis
    j. psychology
    j. theory

Junin virus
Junior
    J. Eysenck Personality Inventory
      (JEPI)
    J. Strength Motrin
    J. Strength Panadol
junk food
jurisprudence
    dental j.
    medical j.
jurisprudential teaching model
jury
    special j.
    traverse j.
    trial j.
jus primae noctis
justice
    imminent j.
justifiable reaction
just noticeable difference (JND)
juvantibus
    diagnosis ex j.
juvenescence
juvenile
    j. amyotrophy
    j. angiofibroma
    j. arteriovenous malformation
    j. cerebellar astrocytoma
    j. chorea
    j. court
    j. delinquent
    dementia paralytica j.'s (DPJ)
    j. dermatomyositis
    j. era
    j. fibromatosis
    j. fire setting
    j. idiocy
    j. impostor
    j. muscular atrophy
    j. myoclonic epilepsy
    j. myxedema
    j. neurotic delinquency
    j. nonneuropathic Niemann-Pick
      disease
    j. officer
    j. papillomatosis
    j. paralytic dementia
    j. paresis
    j. parkinsonism
    j. pilocytic astrocytoma
    j. psychosis
    j. rheumatoid arthritis
    j. tabes
juxtacortical
    j. chondroma
    j. sarcoma
juxtallocortex
juxtapapillary uveitis
juxtarestiform body
JVIS
    Jackson Vocational Interest Survey

K
K complex
K index
K index value

K+
K. Care
K. Care Effervescent

KAB
knowledge, attitude, behavior

KABC
Kaufman Assessment Battery for Children

Kadian sustained-release morphine capsule

Kahn
K. Intelligence Test (KIT)
K. syndrome
K. Test of Symbol Arrangement (KTSA)

kainomania

kainotophobia, kainophobia

KAIT
Kaufman Adolescent and Adult Intelligence Test

kakergasia

kakké

kakorrhaphiophobia

kakosmia

kakotrophy

Kaksonjae

Kales
criteria of Rechtschaffen and K.

Kallikak family

Kallmann syndrome

Kalmuk idiocy

Kaltostat dressing

Kambin instrumentation

kanamycin

Kanavel approach

Kandel stereotactic apparatus

Kaneda
K. anterior spinal instrumentation
K. anterior spinal/scoliosis system (KASS)
K. anterior spine stabilizing device

kangaroo

Kanner
K. disease
K. syndrome

Kannon headframe

Kaochlor
K.-Eff
K. SF

kaolin clotting time

kaolin-induced hydrocephalus

Kaon
K.-Cl
K.-Cl-10

kap
Hypotherm Gel K.

Kaplan agnesis

Kaplan-Meier
K.-M. survival analysis
K.-M. survival curve

kaposiform hemangioendothelioma

Kaposi sarcoma

kappa
k. coefficient
k. light chain
k. opiate receptor
k. wave

kapseals
Dilantin K.

Karlin microknife

Karma yoga

Karnofsky
K. Performance Scale
K. performance score (KPS)
K. Performance Status
K. Rating Scale

Karolinska Scales of Personality

Karpman triangle

Kartchner carotid artery clamp

karyochrome cell

karyotyping
spectral k. (SKY)

KAS
Katz Adjustment Scale

Kasabach-Merritt syndrome

Kasanin-Hanfmann Concept Formation Test

KASS
Kaneda anterior spinal/scoliosis system

KAST
Kindergarten Auditory Screening Test

katagelophobia (*var. of* catagelophobia)

katagogic tendency

katasexuality

kathisomania

kathisophobia (*var. of* cathisophobia)

Kato
technique of Miyazaki and K.

Katz
K. Adjustment Scale (KAS)
K. ADL Index

Katzman test

Kaufman
K. Adolescent and Adult Intelligence Test (KAIT)
K. Assessment Battery for Children (KABC)
K. Brief Intelligence Test (K-BIT)
K. Development Scale
K. Infant and Preschool Scale
K. Survey of Early Academic and Language Skills (K-SEALS)
K. Test of Educational Achievement (K-TEA)

Kayexalate

Kayser-Fleischer ring

K-BIT
Kaufman Brief Intelligence Test

K

kc
  kilocycle
KCI
  Kolbe Conative Index
K-complex
K-corrected raw score
56kD protein
K-Dur
  K-D. 10
  K-D. 20
Keane Mobility bed
Kearns-Sayre
  K.-S. disease
  K.-S. syndrome (KSS)
Keegan Type Indicator
Keeler
  K. Galilean loupe
  K. panoramic loupe
  K. polygraph
  K. video headlamp
Keen
  K. operation
  K. point
keep
  recognize, empathize, think, hear,
    integrate, notice, k. (RETHINK)
keeping faith
keirospasm
Keirsey Temperament sorter
Keitel index
K-Electrolyte Effervescent
Kelly-Goerss COMPASS stereotactic
  system
Kelly stereotactic system
Kelvin body
Kemadrin
Kempf disease
Kenacort
Kenaject-40
Kenalog
  K.-10
  K.-40
Kendrick Cognitive Tests for the
  Elderly
Kennedy-Fischbeck disease
Kennedy syndrome
Kennerdell-Maroon
  K.-M. dissector
  K.-M. elevator
  K.-M. hook
  K.-M. orbital retractor
  K.-M. technique
Kenney Self-Care Questionnaire
Kenny
  K. ADL index
  K. Self-Care Evaluation
kenophobia, cenophobia
Kent
  K. EGY Test
  K. Infant Development Scale
  K. Series of Emergency Skills
Kent-Rosanoff Test
Kerandel symptom
kerasin histiocytosis
keratan sulfate

keratitis
  neuroparalytic k.
  neurotrophic k.
keratoacanthoma
keratoconjunctivitis
  k. sicca
keratoderma blennorrhagicum
keratopathy
  band k.
  exposure k.
keratosis
  actinic k.
  k. obturans
  seborrheic k.
keratotic lesion
keraunoneurosis
keraunophobia (*var. of* ceraunophobia)
Kerlix dressing
kernel complex
kernicterus
Kernig
  K. sign
  K. test
Kernohan
  K. classification of brain tumor
  K. grading
  K. notch
  K. notch phenomenon
  K. notch syndrome
  K. system
  K. system of glioma classification
Kerr clip
Kerrison
  K. bone punch
  K. microronguer
  K. rongeur
Ketalar
ketamine
ketazolam
ketoacidosis
  alcoholic k. (AKA)
  diabetic k.
ketoaciduria
  branched-chain k.
ketoconazole
ketogenic diet
ketoprofen
ketorolac tromethamine
ketosis
ketosteroid
key
  k. concept
  K. elevator
  k. question
keyhole surgery
keying
  empirical-criterion k.
KeyMath Revised: A Diagnostic
  Inventory of Essential Mathematics
Key-Pred Injection
Key-Pred-SP Injection
Key-Retzius
  foramen of Key-Retzius
Keystone graft

KFD
Kinetic Family Drawings
K-Gen Effervescent
Khatena-Torrance Creative Perception Inventory
kHz
kilohertz
KIDDIE-SADS
Schedule for Affective Disorders and Schizophrenia for School-Age Children
K-Ide
Kiel classification
killer
k. cult
human natural k. (HNK)
serial sexual k.
time k.
Killian
K. gouge
K. operation
K. septum speculum
killing
mercy k.
Kilner hook
kilobytophobia
kilocycle (kc)
kilogram
kilohertz (kHz)
Kiloh-Nevin
K.-N. ocular form or progressive muscular dystrophy
K.-N. ocular myopathy
K.-N. syndrome
kilounit
kilovolt (kV)
kilovoltage peak (kVp)
KinAir bed
kinanesthesia
kinase
calcium-calmodulin k. II (CaMKII)
Janus k. (Jak)
protein k.
protein k. C (PKC)
kindergarten
K. Auditory Screening Test (KAST)
K. Language Screening Test (KLST)
K. Readiness Test (KRT)
Kindergartners
Rating Inventory for Screening K.
kindling
k. effect
Kindling pattern
Kindt carotid clamp
kinematograph
kinephantom
kinergety
kinesalgia
kinesia paradoxica
kinesiatrics
kinesic
k. behavior
k. gesture
kinesics

kinesigenic
k. ataxia
k. attack
k. chorea
k. choreoathetosis
kinesiology
kinesioneurosis
kinesiotherapy
kinesipathy
kinesis
kinesomania
kinesophobia
kinesthesia
kinesthesiometer
kinesthetic
k. analysis
k. apraxia
k. aura
k. cue
k. feedback
k. hallucination
k. method
k. perception
k. sensation
k. sense
k. technique
kinetic
k. analysis
k. ataxia
k. cervical spine
k. drive
k. energy
K. Family Drawings (KFD)
k. information
k. strabismus
k. tremor
kinetics
cellular k.
chemical k.
kinetism
Kinetix instrument
kinetogenic
kinetosis
kinetotherapy
King
K. type I curve
K. type II curve
K. type III curve
K. type II scoliosis
K. type IV curve
K. type IV curve posterior correction
K. type V curve
K. type V scoliosis
king's habit
king-slave fantasy
kink
cervicomedullary k.
kinky-hair disease
Kinnier-Wilson disease
kinohapt
kinship
k. network
k. system

K

KIPS
knowledge information processing system
Kirby-Bauer disk diffusion method
Kirschner
   K. pin
   K. wire
   K. wire placement
Kisch reflex
kissing
   k. behavior
   k. disease
Kistler
   K. classification of subarachnoid
     hemorrhage
   K. subarachnoid hemorrhage
     classification
KIT
Kahn Intelligence Test
kit
   Ceretec imaging k.
   cyanide antidote k.
   Fer-Will Object K.
   Hall Osteon drill system k.
   Hall Osteon irrigation k.
   KLS-Martin modular neuro k.
   KTP dual disk k.
   Laitinen high precision stereotactic-
     assisted radiation therapy k.
   Laitinen percutaneous tumor
     biopsy k.
   Laserscope discography k.
   MICRO E irrigation k.
   MICRO 100 irrigation k.
   Ototome irrigation k.
   PainBuster infusion pump
     management k.
   Radiofocus introducer B k.
   Shiley distention k.
   START k.
   stereotactic-assisted radiation
     therapy k.
Kiver-Bucy syndrome
Klaus height index
klazomania
K-Lease
Klebedenken
Klebenbleiben
kleeblattschädel
Klein
   K. death wish
   K. suffocation alarm theory
   K. view of depressive disorder
Kleine-Levin syndrome
Klemme laminectomy retractor
kleptolagnia
kleptomania
kleptophobia
Klinefelter syndrome
Klippel disease
Klippel-Feil syndrome
Klippel-Trenaunay syndrome
Klippel-Trenaunay-Weber syndrome
klismaphilia
Kloehn craniofacial instrument
Klonopin

K-Lor
Klor-Con
   K.-C. 8
   K.-C. 10
Klor-Con/25
Klor-con/EF
Klorvess Effervescent
Klotrix
Klover-Bucy syndrome
KLS-Martin
   K.-M. center-drive screw
   K.-M. implant
   K.-M. modular neuro kit
KLST
Kindergarten Language Screening Test
Klumpke
   K. palsy
   K. paralysis
Klumpke-Dejerine syndrome
Klüver
   method of K.
Klüver-Bucy syndrome
K-Lyte/Cl
K-Lyte Effervescent
knee
   k. jerk
   k. phenomenon
knee-chest position
knee-jerk reflex
Kneerdell-Maroon dissector
kneippism
knife
   Adson dural k.
   Adson right-angle k.
   angular k.
   arachnoid k.
   Bucy cordotomy k.
   canal k.
   clasp k.
   Cottle k.
   Crile gasserian ganglion k.
   Cushing dural hook k.
   DeMarneffe meniscotomy k.
   diamond k.
   discission k.
   electric k.
   Frazier cordotomy k.
   Frazier pituitary k.
   Freer-Swanson ganglion k.
   gamma k.
   Halle dura k.
   hot k.
   Jacobson microvascular k.
   Jacobson vessel k.
   Jannetta k.
   Koos microvascular k.
   Leksell gamma k.
   Olivecrona trigeminal k.
   platelet-shaped k.
   Rayport dural dissector and k.
   roentgen k.
   201-source cobalt-60 gamma k.
   Stecher arachnoid k.
   Toennis dura k.
   Weary cordotomy k.

Yasargil arachnoid k.
Yasargil microvascular k.
knight
K. forceps
k. move
Knighton hemilaminectomy retractor
knismogenic
knismolagnia
knob
synaptic k.
knochenschädel
knocking
head k.
knock over
Knodt rod
K-Norm
knot
lover's k.
primitive k.
vital k.
knowledge
acquired k.
k., attitude, behavior (KAB)
carnal k.
competence k.
figurative k.
fund of k.
inflated k.
k. information processing system (KIPS)
lack of k.
K. of Occupations Test (KOT)
k. test
k. theme
known organic factor
Knox Cube Test
knuckle
cervical aortic k.
Koala Pad graphics tablet
Kobayashi retractor
Kocher
K. clamp
K. collar incision
K. dissector
K. point
Kocher-Debré-Semelaigne syndrome
Kocher-Lovelace clamp
Koerber-Salus-Elschnig syndrome
Koerte-Ballance operation
Koerte procedure
Kohlberg developmental model
Kohnstamm
K. phenomenon
K. Test
Kohs
K. Block Design
K. Block-Design Test
K. Block Test
koinotropy
KOIS
Kuder Occupational Interest Survey
Kojewnikoff epilepsy
Kolbe Conative Index (KCI)
Kölliker reticulum
kolyphrenia

kolytic
Kolyum
Komai stereotactic head frame
Konakion Injection
koniocortex
auditory k.
koniophobia
koniphobia
Kontrast U
Kool-Aid
Koos microvascular knife
kopophobia
Koppitz Scoring System for Organicity
koro
k. psychosis
k. syndrome
Korsakoff
K. alcoholic psychosis
K. amnesia
K. disease
K. nonalcoholic psychosis
K. psychosis
K. syndrome
korsakoffian amnesia
Koshevnikoff epilepsy
Kostuik
K. rod
K. screw
Kostuik-Harrington
K.-H. device
K.-H. distraction system
KOT
Knowledge of Occupations Test
Kozhevnikov spring-summer encephalitis
K-Phos Neutral
KPR-V
Kuder Preference Record-Vocational
KPS
Karnofsky performance score
Krabbe
K. Arnold-Chiari malformation
K. diffuse sclerosis
K. disease
K. leukodystrophy
K. syndrome
Krabbe-Weber-Dimitri disease
Kraepelin
K. diagnostic system
K. disease
Kraepelina paranoia
kraepelinian
k. subtype
k. view of psychosis
krauomania
Krause
K. denervation
K. end bulb
K. respiratory bundle
Krayenbuehl nerve hook
Kretschmer type
Krimsky test
Kronecker aneurysm needle
KRT
Kindergarten Readiness Test
Kryptonite

K

K's
  K's disease
  K's psychosis
  K's syndrome
K-SADS
  Schedule for Affective Disorders and
  Schizophrenia for School-Age Children
K-SADS-E
  Schedule for Affective Disorders and
  Schizophrenia for School-Age Children-
  Epidemiologic Version
K-SADS-P
  Schedule for Affective Disorders and
  Schizophrenia for School-Age Children-
  Present Episode
K-SEALS
  Kaufman Survey of Early Academic and
  Language Skills
KSS
  Kearns-Sayre syndrome
KT
  Orudis KT
K-Tab
K-TEA
  Kaufman Test of Educational
  Achievement
KTP/532 surgical laser
KTP dual disk kit
KTSA
  Kahn Test of Symbol Arrangement
kubisagari, kubisaguru
Kuder
  K. General Interest Survey, Form
  E
  K. Occupational Interest Survey
  (KOIS)
  K. Preference Record
  K. Preference Record-Vocational
  (KPR-V)
Kufs disease
Kugelberg-Welander
  K.-W. disease
  K.-W. juvenile spinal muscle
  atrophy
  K.-W. syndrome
Kühne
  K. phenomenon
  K. spindle
kulangeta
Kümmell spondylitis
Kundalini yoga
Küntscher
  K. hammer
  K. nail

Kurtzke Expanded Disability Status
  Scale
kuru
Kurze
  K. dissection scissors
  K. suction-irrigator
Kussmaul
  K. aphasia
  K. coma
Kussmaul-Landry paralysis
kV
  kilovolt
Kveim test
K-Vescent
kVp
  kilovoltage peak
K-wire placement
Kwoh-Young stereotactic robot
kymatism
kymogram
kymograph
kynophobia
kynurenic acid
kyofusho
  taijin k.
kyphoscoliosis
  neurofibromatosis k.
  k. secondary to neurofibromatosis
  severe k.
  thoracolumbar k.
kyphosis
  acute angular k.
  k. brace
  Cobb method of measuring k.
  congenital k.
  k. correction
  k. creation
  iatrogenic lumbar k.
  junctional k.
  lumbar k.
  postlaminectomy k.
  posttraumatic k.
  right thoracic curve with
  junctional k.
  Scheuermann k.
  thoracic k.
  thoracolumbar k.
kyphotic
  k. deformity
  k. deformity pathomechanics

L4-5 disk disease
LA
    low anxiety
    lupus anticoagulant
      Dexone LA
      Inderal LA
L.A.
      Dexasone L.A.
      Solurex L.A.
L-a-acetylmethadol (LAMM)
L-AAM
    L-alpha-acetylmethadiol 3
LAB
    Leisure Activities Blank
Labbé
    L. neurocirculatory syndrome
    vein of L.
    L. vein
labeling
    l. index (LI)
    l. theory
labetalol
labial
    l. dysarthria
    l. paralysis
labialism
labile
    l. emotionality
    l. mood
    l. personality disorder
    l. range of affect
lability
    affective l.
    emotional l.
    mood l.
labiochorea
labiochoreic stuttering
labioglossolaryngeal
    l. palsy
    l. paralysis
labioglossomandibular approach
labioglossopharyngeal paralysis
labiomandibular
    l. approach
    l. glossotomy
labiorum
    morsicatio l.
laboratory
    l. abnormality
    Automated Multitest L. (AML)
    clinical l.
    l. data
    l. diagnosis
    diagnostic l.
    National Training L.'s (NTL)
    NIDA-certified forensic
      toxicology l.
    personal growth l.
    l. test
    l. training
    Venereal Disease Research L.
      (VDRL)

laboratory-method model
laborer
    manual l.
labor force
labyrinth
    vestibular l.
labyrinthectomy
labyrinthine
    l. aplasia
    l. concussion syndrome
    l. disease
    l. disorder
    l. fistula test
    l. hydrops
    l. righting reflex
    l. sense
    l. speech
    l. torticollis
    l. vertigo
labyrinthitis
laceration
    brain l.
    cerebral l.
    scalp l.
lacerum
    foramen l.
lachrymose
lacing agent
lack
    l. of boundary
    l. of clear-cut cerebral dominance
    l. of control
    l. of energy
    l. of fear
    l. of feeling
    l. of initiative
    l. of insight
    l. of interest
    l. of interoceptive awareness
    l. of involvement
    l. of knowledge
    l. of memory
    l. of motivation
    l. of penetrance
    l. of reactivity
    l. of remorse
    l. of restraint
    l. of self-confidence
    l. of speech
    l. of structure
    l. of will
laconic speech
laconism
Lacri-Lube
lacrimal
    l. duct
    l. gland
    l. gland dysfunction
    l. nerve
    l. reflex
lacrimation
lacrimogustatory reflex

L

La Crosse encephalitis
LACT
    Lindamood Auditory Conceptualization
    Test
lactate
    calcium l.
    l. dehydrogenase (LHD)
    l. dehydrogenase phenomenon
    l. dehydrogenase test
    l. infusion
    Ringer l.
    sodium l.
lactational diestrus
lactic acidosis
lactoferrin
lactoovovegetarian diet
lactotroph cell
lactotrophic
lactovegetarian diet
Lactrodectus mactans
lactulose
Lactulose PSE
lacuna, pl. **lacunae, lacunas**
    l. cerebri
    lacunae laterales
    superego l.
lacunaire
    état l.
lacunar
    l. amnesia
    l. brain infarction
    l. dementia
    l. infarct
    l. state
    l. stroke
    l. syndrome
lacunaris
    status l.
lacunas (*pl. of* lacuna)
LAD
    language acquisition device
ladder
    abstraction l.
    counseling l.
Ladd fiberoptic system
Laennec cirrhosis
Lafayette pegboard
Lafora
    L. body
    L. disease
    L. familial myoclonic epilepsy
lag
    circadian rhythm sleep disorder,
      jet l.
    cultural l.
    initial l.
    maturational l.
    terminal l.
lagophthalmos
Lahey
    L. Clinic dural hook
    L. Clinic nerve hook
    L. score
LAI
    leukocyte adhesion inhibitor

laissez-faire
    l.-f. group
    l.-f. leader
    l.-f. leadership pattern
Laitinen
    L. high precision stereotactic-
      assisted radiation therapy kit
    L. percutaneous tumor biopsy kit
    L. stereoadapter
    L. stereoguide 2000 arc-centered
      stereotactic frame
    L. stereotactic head frame
    L. stereotactic system
lake
    lateral l.'s
    venous l.
laliatry
laliophobia, lalophobia
lalochezia
lalognosis
lalomania
laloneurosis
lalopathology
lalopathy
lalophobia (*var. of* laliophobia)
laloplegia
lalorrhea
L-alpha-acetylmethadiol
L-alpha-acetylmethadiol 3 (L-AAM)
lamarckian theory
Lamaze technique
lambdacism
lambda light chain
lambdoid
    l. activity
    l. craniosynostosis
    l. plagiocephaly
    l. synostosis
lambdoidal suture
**Lambert-Eaton myasthenic syndrome
(LEMS)**
**Lambeth Disability Screening
Questionnaire**
lambitus
lamella, pl. **lamellae**
    triangular l.
lamellated corpuscle
Lamictal
lamina, pl. **laminae**
    l. affixa
    l. alaris
    alar l. of neural tube
    laminae albae cerebelli
    l. arcus vertebrae
    basal l.
    l. basalis
    basal l. of neural tube
    basilar l.
    l. basilaris cochleae
    l. choroidea
    l. choroidea epithelialis
    l. cinerea
    l. cribrosa
    l. dorsalis
    epithelial l.

l. epithelialis
intact spinous l.
lateral medullary l. of corpus
   striatum
medial medullary l. of corpus
   striatum
laminae medullares cerebelli
laminae medullares thalami
l. medullaris lateralis corporis
   striati
l. medullaris medialis corporis
   striati
periclaustral l.
l. quadrigemina
Rexed l.
rostral l.
l. rostralis
l. septi pellucidi
l. of septum pellucidum
l. spreader
l. supraneuroporica
l. tecti mesencephali
l. terminalis
l. terminalis cerebri
l. ventralis
l. of vertebral arch
laminaplasty
Tsuji l.
laminar
l. C-D hook
l. cortex posterior aspect
l. cortical necrosis
l. cortical sclerosis
laminated cortex
lamination of gyrus
laminectomized spine
laminectomy
Beckman-Eaton l.
Beckman-Weitlaner l.
cervical l.
cervical spine l.
decompressive l.
Gill l.
Girdlestone l.
multilevel l.
osteoplastic l.
4-place l.
l. punch forceps
l. roll
single-level decompressive l.
laminin
laminoplasty
Domen l.
open door l.
spinous process-splitting l.
l. with extended foraminoplasty for
   cervical myelopathy
laminotomy
unilateral l.
Lamitrode lead
lamivudine
zidovudine and l.
LAMM
L-a-acetylmethadol
levo-α-acetylmethadol

lamotrigine
Lancaster red-green screen
Lance-Adams syndrome
lancinating
Landau
L. reflex
L. syndrome
Landau-Kleffner syndrome
landmark
Copying Drawings with L.'s (CDL)
developmental l.
glabella-inion line l.
pedicle l.
surface l.
Landolt
L. pituitary speculum
L. spreader
Landouzy-Dejerine
L.-D. disease
L.-D. dystrophy
Landouzy-Grasset law
Landry
L. paralysis
L. syndrome
Landry-Guillain-Barré-Strohl syndrome
Landry-Guillain-Barré syndrome
lane of childhood
Langat viral encephalitis
Langenbach elevator
Langenbeck periosteal elevator
Langerhans
L. cell
L. cell granulomatosis
language
l. ability
l. acquisition device (LAD)
l. area
artificial l.
l. assessment
l. associated cortex
automatic l.
l. barrier
Basic Inventory of Natural L.
l. behavior
behavior l.
l. boundary
l. center
l. change
l. and communication
l. and communication distortion
l. comprehension
l. comprehension and production
l. content
daughter l.
l. deficit
delayed l.
l. development
l. developmental delay disorder
deviant l.
l. difficulty
l. disability
l. disorder in dementia
l. disturbance
dominant l.
l. dysfunction

L

language *(continued)*
    egocentric l.
    emotive l.
    English as a second l. (ESL)
    l. enrichment therapy (LET)
    executive l.
    l. experience approach (LEA)
    expressive l.
    l. faculty
    foreign l.
    l. function
    l. function deterioration
    l. game
    gestural-postural l.
    gesture l.
    global loss of l.
    home l.
    hypochondriac l.
    imaginary l.
    l. imbalance
    impaired l.
    l. impairment
    implicit l.
    incidental learning l.
    inner l.
    l. inversal
    irrelevant l.
    l. lateralization
    l. localization
    loss of l.
    metaphoric l.
    mixed receptive-expressive l.
    L. Modalities Test for Aphasia
        (LMTA)
    negotiating l.
    nonspecific l.
    nonverbal l.
    obscene l.
    oral l.
    organic l.
    l. origin
    l. pathology
    primitive psychosomatic l.
    l. problem
    l. processing
    L. Processing Test
    l. purist
    l. quotient
    Receptive-Expressive Emergent L.
        (REEL)
    l. recovery
    l. retardation
    L. Sampling, Analysis and Training
    l. scale
    scatological l.
    school l.
    l. screening
    L. Screening Test
    Screening Test of Adolescent L.
    Screening Test for Auditory
        Comprehension of L. (STACL)
    sign l.
    l. skills learning retardation
    l. and speech disorder

spoken l.
subcultural l.
syntaxic l.
target l.
Test of Adolescent L. (TOAL)
Test for Auditory Comprehension
    of L. (TACL)
Test of Pragmatic L. (TOPL)
Tests for Auditory Comprehension
    of L.-Revised (TACL-R)
Test of Written L. (TOWL)
l. theory
l. therapist
twin l.
unknown l.
vulgar l.
written l.
l. zone
language-dominant hemisphere
language-processing
    receptive l.-p.
**Language-Structured Auditory Retention
    Span (LARS)**
Lanorinal
Lanoxin
Lanterman
    L. incisure
    L. segment
lanthanide
lanugo
laparotomaphilia
Lapidus bed
**Laplacian montage on
    electroencephalogram**
Lapras catheter
lapse
    l. of awareness
    memory l.
lapsus
    l. calami
    l. lingua
    l. memoriae
large-artery infarct
large ball nerve hook
large-egress cannula
Largon Injection
Larmor
    L. equation
    L. frequency
    L. precession
Larodopa
laroxyl
LARS
    Language-Structured Auditory Retention
        Span
LARSI
    lumbar anterior-root stimulator implant
larval
    l. epilepsy
    l. sadism
    l. schizophrenia
larvated epilepsy
laryngeal
    l. anesthesia
    l. anomaly

l. atresia
l. chorea
l. crisis
l. dysarthria
l. epilepsy
l. nerve injury
l. paresthesia
l. psychophysiologic reaction
l. syncope
l. vertigo
laryngectomy
anterior partial l.
laryngoparalysis
laryngoplegia
laryngospasm
laryngospastic reflex
LAS
laxative abuse syndrome
lascivia
lasciviency forced laughter
lascivious hysterical laughter
LASE
laser-assisted spinal endoscopy
Lasègue
L. disease
L. sign
L. syndrome II
L. test
laser
argon l.
l. beam
carbon dioxide l.
Cavitron l.
l. Doppler flowmetry (LDF)
holmium YAG l.
Ho:YAG l.
KTP/532 surgical l.
Nd:YAG l.
l. nucleotomy
orthogonal l.
Sharplan l.
l. surgery
Surgica K6 l.
VersaPulse holmium l.
laser-assisted spinal endoscopy (LASE)
laser-Doppler
l.-D. spectroscopy
l.-D. velocimetry
Laserflo Doppler probe
Laserflow
L. blood perfusion monitor
L. BPM² real time cerebral
perfusion monitor
Laserscope discography kit
Lasix
LASS
Linguistic Analysis of Speech Samples
Lassa fever virus
LASSI
Learning and Study Strategies Inventory
LASSI-HS
Learning and Study Strategies Inventory-
High School Version
lassitude
last word

lata
Tutoplast fascia l.
latah, lata, lattah
l. syndrome
latchkey children
late
l. adolescence
l. adulthood
l. epilepsy
l. life
l. life developmental stage
l. luteal phase
l. luteal phase dysphoric disorder
(LLPDD)
l. luteal phase of menstrual cycle
l. Lyme neuroborreliosis
l. paraphrenia
l. reaction
l. speech development
l. traumatic epilepsy
l. whiplash syndrome
late-age trauma
late-life
l.-l. migraine
l.-l. migraine headache
latency
blink reflex l.
distal motor l.
l. distal motor
Erickson theory of l.
interpeak l.
mean sleep l.
l. period (LP)
l. period psychosexual development
l. phase
prolonged sleep l.
l. proximal
rapid eye movement l.
reduced rapid eye movement l.
reflex l.
REM l.
l. of reply
l. of response
short REM l.
short sleep l.
sleep l.
l. stage
latency-age children
latency-evoked potential
latent
l. class analysis
l. content
l. epilepsy
l. goal
l. homosexuality
l. learning
l. meaning
l. period
l. psychosis
l. reflex
l. response
l. schizophrenia
l. schizophrenic reaction
l. tetany

L

465

latent *(continued)*
    l. thought
    l. zone
late-onset
    l.-o. ataxia
    l.-o. schizophrenia
lateral
    l. aperture of the fourth ventricle
    l. cerebral fissure
    l. cerebral fossa
    l. cerebral sulcus
    l. column of spinal cord
    l. cuneate nucleus
    l. dominance
    L. Dominance Examination (LDE)
    l. dorsal tegmentum
    l. extracavitary approach
    l. femoral cutaneous nerve
    l. fillet
    l. fossa of brain
    l. funiculus of spinal cord
    l. gaze
    l. gaze nystagmus
    l. gaze palsy
    l. geniculate body
    l. geniculate nucleus (LGN)
    l. ground bundle
    l. horn
    l. intradural approach
    l. lakes
    l. listhesis
    l. longitudinal stria
    l. medullary lamina of corpus striatum
    l. neocortex
    l. nucleus of medulla oblongata
    l. nucleus of thalamus
    l. occipital sulcus
    l. occipitotemporal gyrus
    l. orbitofrontal circuit
    l. posterior choroidal (LPCh)
    l. preoptic nucleus
    l. projection
    l. recess of fourth ventricle
    l. recess stenosis
    l. rectus muscle
    l. rectus palsy
    l. reticular nucleus
    l. rhinotomy
    l. rhinotomy incision
    l. roentgenogram
    l. root of median nerve
    l. root of optic tract
    l. sellar compartment
    l. sinus
    l. spinal sclerosis
    l. sulcus
    l. tarsorrhaphy
    l. temporal epileptogenic lesion
    l. temporal resection
    l. thalamic peduncle
    l. thoracic meningocele
    l. tuberal nuclei
    l. ventricle

    l. vertigo
    l. vestibular nucleus
lateralis
    cisterna sulci l.
    ventralis l. (VL)
    ventralis posterior l.
laterality
    crossed l.
    dominant l.
    mixed l.
    L. Preference Schedule
lateralization
    cortical l.
    failure of l.
    fetal planum temporal l.
    hemispheric l.
    language l.
lateralized
    l. activity
    l. artifact
    l. brain language system
    l. dysfunction
    l. rapid activating task
lateralizing abnormality
laterally convex dural incision
lateropolaris
lateropulsion
    l. of body movement
    l. of eye movement
latex
    l. balloon
    l. covered pledget
lathyrism
latissimus dorsi muscle
lattah *(var. of* latah)
lattice
    l. degeneration
    l. field
latticed layer
laudanum
laugh
    nervous l.
    sardonic l.
laughing
    l. disease
    l. sickness
laughter
    compulsive l.
    drawn l.
    forced l.
    hysterical l.
    inappropriate l.
    lasciviency forced l.
    lascivious hysterical l.
    obsessive l.
    l. reflex
    spasmodic l.
    spontaneous l.
    uncontrolled l.
Laumonier ganglion
Laurence-Biedl syndrome
Laurence-Moon-Bardet-Biedl syndrome
Laurence-Moon-Biedl syndrome
Laurence-Moon syndrome
Lausanne stereotactic robot

lavage
  gastric l.
law
  l. of advantage
  American Academy of Psychiatry
    and L.
  l. of assimilation
  assimilation l.
  l. of association
  autonomic-affective l.
  l. of avalanche
  l. of average localization
  Baruch l.
  Bell l.
  Bell-Magendie l.
  Bernoulli l.
  biogenetic mental l.
  Boltzmann distribution l.
  Briggs l.
  Broadbent l.
  Charpentier l.
  l. of closure
  l. of coercion to the biosocial
    mean
  l. of cohesion
  l. of combination
  command l.
  l.'s of commitment
  common l.
  l. of common fate
  l. of constancy
  l. of contiguity
  l. of contrast
  court of l.
  Dale l.
  l. of denervation
  l. of diminishing return
  effect l.
  l. of effect
  empirical l.
  l. of equality
  equality l.
  equipotentiality l.
  eugenic sterilization l.
  l. of exercise
  exercise l.
  Flatau l.
  Fourier l.
  l. of frequency
  Gerhardt-Semon l.
  Grasset l.
  Haeckel biogenic l.
  Hagen-Poiseuille l.
  health l.
  Hilton l.
  l. of initial value
  l. of isochronism
  Jackson l.
  Landouzy-Grasset l.
  Leyden l.
  Magendie l.
  Mendel l.
  mendelian l.
  Merkel l.
  Müller l.

  Murphy's l.
  natural l.
  Ohm l.
  parallel l.
  Pitres l.
  Poiseuille l.
  poor l.
  l. of precision
  l. of referred pain
  l. of relativity
  l. of retrogenesis
  Ritter l.
  Rosenbach l.
  Semon l.
  Semon-Rosenbach l.
  Sherrington l.
  Stokes l.
  talion l.
  van der Kolk l.
  wallerian l.
  Weber-Fechner l.
  Wilder l. of initial value
  Yerkes-Dodson l.
law-and-order orientation
Lawford syndrome
lawful behavior
laxative
  l. abuse
  l. abuse syndrome (LAS)
  l. addiction
  l. of choice (LOC)
  l. dependence
  l. habit
lay analysis
layer
  arachnoid l.
  bacillary l.
  l. of Bechterew
  l. of cerebellar cortex
  l. of cerebral cortex
  cerebral l. of retina
  claustral l.
  dysfibrous l.
  ependymal l.
  epithelial choroid l.
  fillet l.
  fusiform l.
  ganglionic l. of cerebellar cortex
  ganglionic l. of cerebral cortex
  ganglionic l. of optic nerve
  ganglionic l. of retina
  granular l.'s of cerebral cortex
  granular l.'s of retina
  gray l. of superior colliculus
  Henle fiber l.
  Henle nervous l.
  infragranular l.
  infrastriate l.
  intermediate l.
  interstriate l.
  latticed l.
  magnocellular l.
  mantle l.
  marginal l.
  medullary l.'s of thalamus

L

layer *(continued)*
    Meynert l.
    molecular l. of cerebellar cortex
    molecular l. of cerebral cortex
    molecular l.'s of olfactory bulb
    molecular l. of retina
    multiform l.
    neural l. of retina
    neuroepithelial l. of retina
    nuclear l.'s of retina
    olfactory nerve l. (ONL)
    optic l.
    pigmented l. of retina
    l. of piriform neurons
    plexiform l. of cerebral cortex
    plexiform l.'s of retina
    polymorphous l.
    Purkinje l.
    pyramidal cell l.
    l. of rods and cones
    rostral l.
    spindle-celled l.
    suprastriate l.
    tangential l.
    ventricular l.
    Waldeyer zonal l.
    zonular l.
laying on of hands
lazabemide
lazaroid
LBAII
    Leader Behavior Analysis II
LBDQ
    Leader Behavior Description
      Questionnaire
LBE
    line bisection error
LBS
    low back syndrome
LC
    Hydergine LC
LCBF
    local cerebral blood flow
LCMV
    lymphocytic choriomeningitis virus
LCT
    Listening Comprehension Test
LCU
    life change unit
LD
    learning disability
    lethal dose
LDA
    low-density area
LDD
    LDD delivery system
    LDD procedure
LDE
    Lateral Dominance Examination
LDES
    Learning Disability Evaluation Scale
LDF
    laser Doppler flowmetry

L-dopa
    on-off effect of L.-d.
    L.-d. stimulation test
L-dopa/benserazide
LE
    lupus erythematosus
LEA
    language experience approach
lead
    colic l.
    l. colic
    deep brain l.
    dual octapolar l.
    dual quadrapolar l.
    EEG with NP l.
    l. encephalitis
    l. encephalopathy
    frontopolar l.
    Lamitrode l.
    NCP l.
    l. neuropathy
    octapolar l.
    l. palsy
    l. paralysis
    l. pipe contraction
    l. poisoning
leaden paralysis
leader
    authoritarian l.
    L. Behavior Analysis II (LBAII)
    L. Behavior Description
      Questionnaire (LBDQ)
    laissez-faire l.
    l. match
    l. role
    team l. (TL)
leaderless
    l. group
    l. group discussion (LGD)
    l. group therapy
leadership
    L. Ability Evaluation
    l. behavior
    dual l.
    L. Evaluation and Department
      Scale
    functional l.
    l. inventory
    L. Opinion Questionnaire (LOQ)
    l. potential
    l. power struggle
    L. Practices Inventory (LPI)
    l. role
    L. Skills Inventory
    l. theory
    l. training
lead-pipe rigidity
leaf, pl. **leaves**
    cassina l.
    mint l.
    mugwort leaves
leak
    leaky l.
    sentinel l.

leakage
- cerebrospinal fluid l.
- chylous l.
- l. headache
- verbal l.

leaky leak

Lear complex

learned
- l. autonomic control
- l. drive
- l. dysfunctional behavior
- l. helplessness

learner
- auditory l.
- Self-Concept as a L. (SCAL)
- slow l.

learning
- l. ability
- L. Accomplishment Profile
- l. aptitude
- associate l.
- association l.
- associative l.
- attachment l.
- avoidance and escape l.
- cognitive theory of l.
- conceptual l.
- l. cue
- l. curve
- l. defect
- l. development
- l. developmental disorder
- Developmental Indicators for Assessment of L. (DIAL)
- Developmental Indicators for Assessment of L., Revised/AGS Edition (DIAL-R)
- l. difficulty
- l. disability (LD)
- L. Disability Evaluation Scale (LDES)
- L. Disability Rating Procedure
- l. disabled
- discrimination l.
- dissociated l.
- dissociation of l.
- l. by doing
- L. Efficiency Test-II (LET-II)
- escape l.
- l. impaired
- incidental l.
- l. information
- integrative l.
- interleaved l.
- l. inventory
- L. Inventory of Kindergarten Experiences (LIKE)
- latent l.
- maze l.
- l. mechanism
- l. model
- Mullen Scales of Early L.
- l. new information disturbance
- observational l.
- operant l.
- paired-associates l.
- l. paradigm
- passive-avoidance l.
- perceptual-motor l.
- probability l.
- l. problem
- problem-based l.
- l. retardation
- reversal l.
- rote l.
- self-directed l. (SDL)
- sensate focus l.
- serial list l.
- l. session
- l. set
- sexual l.
- state-dependent l.
- l. strategy
- stress effect on l.
- L. and Study Strategies Inventory (LASSI)
- L. and Study Strategies Inventory-High School Version (LASSI-HS)
- L. Style Profile (LSP)
- L. Styles Inventory
- subliminal l.
- l. test
- l. theory
- Thorndike trial-and-error l.
- transfer of l.
- trial-and-error l.
- verbal l.
- vicarious l.
- visceral l.
- Wide Range Assessment of Memory and L. (WRAML)

learning-disabilities specialist

least
- L. Preferred Coworker Score
- l. resistance
- l. restrictive alternative

least-effort principle

least-square residual

Leatherman
- L. hook
- L. Leadership Questionnaire (LLQ)

leather restraint

leave
- l. of absence (LOA)
- absent without l. (AWOL)
- authorized l.
- extended sick l.
- French l.
- l. on pass (LOP)
- sick l.
- unauthorized l. (UL)

leaves (*pl. of* leaf)

Leber
- L. congenital amaurosis
- L. disease
- L. hereditary optic atrophy
- L. optic atrophy

Leboyer method

LEC
- Life Experiences Checklist

L

lecanomancy
lechery
LED
    light-emitting diode
    LED probe
Leeds Scales for the Self-Assessment of Anxiety and Depression
Lee ganglion
LeFort
    L. classification
    L. osteotomy
left
    l. bundle branch block
    l. common carotid artery
    l. frontal lobe
    l. handedness
    l. hemiplegia
    l. hemisphere
    l. hemisphere dominance
    l. parietal association metabolism
    l. thoracolumbar major curve pattern
    l. ventricle
left-bearing nystagmus
left-hand dominant
left-out sibling profile
left-right asymmetry
left/right hemisphere dominance
left-sided
    l.-s. apraxia
    l.-s. thoracotomy
leftward asymmetry
leg
    champagne-bottle l.
    cold mottled insensate l.
    l. pain
    l. phenomenon
    restless l.
    stork l.
legal
    l. age
    l. blindness
    l. capacity
    l. contract
    l. counselor
    l. determination
    l. divorce
    l. issue
    l. medicine
    l. psychiatry
    l. psychology
    l. responsibility
    l. sanction
    l. standard
legally
    l. committed
    l. drunk
    l. intoxicated
    l. separated (LS)
Legendre
    L. function
    L. sign
Legg disease
Legionella pneumophila **infection**

legomenon
    hapax l.
leg-raising test
Lehman Quality of Life Interview
Leibinger
    L. 3-D plate
    L. microplate
    L. Micro Plus plate
    L. Micro Plus screw
    L. Micro System cranial fixation plate
    L. Micro System drill bit
    L. Micro System plate cutter
    L. Micro System plate-holding forceps
    L. Micro System pliers
    L. titanium mini-Würzburg implant system
Leica vibrating knife microtome
Leichtenstern
    L. encephalitis
    L. phenomenon
    L. sign
Leigh
    L. disease
    L. necrotizing encephalopathy
    L. subacute necrotizing encephalomyelitis
    L. syndrome
leiomyoma
    extraspinal l.
leiomyosarcoma
    disseminated l.
leipolalia
Leisure
leisure
    L. Activities Blank (LAB)
    l. activity
    l. awareness
    L. Diagnostic Battery
    L. Interest Inventory (LII)
    l. skill
    l. time
Leiter
    L. Adult Intelligence Scale
    L. International Performance Scale (LIPS)
    L. Recidivism Scale
Leksell
    L. adapter to Mayfield device
    L. arc
    L. gamma knife
    L. gamma knife target series
    L. GammaPlan computerized program
    L. Micro-Stereotactic system
    L. Model G stereotactic frame
    L. posteroventral pallidotomy
    L. rongeur
    L. selector
    L. stereotactic frame
    L. stereotactic gamma unit
    L. SurgiPlan computerized program
    L. technique
Leksell-Elekta stereotactic frame

Lembrol
Lemmon sternal spreader
lemniscal
    l. fiber
    l. pathway
lemniscus, pl. lemnisci
    acoustic l.
    auditory l.
    gustatory l.
    l. lateralis
    medial l.
    l. medialis
    l. spinalis
    trigeminal l.
    l. trigeminalis
LEMS
    Lambert-Eaton myasthenic syndrome
length
    chord l.
    crown-rump l.
    cycle l.
    l. of episode
    l. of illness
    l. of patient stay (LOPS)
    pedicle screw chord l.
    pedicle screw path l.
    pulse l.
    l. of stay (LOS)
Lengthened-Off-Time (LOT)
lengthening
    distal catheter l.
    l. reaction
Lenhossék process
Lennert lymphoma
Lennon-Gastaut seizure
Lennox-Gastaut
    L.-G. pattern
    L.-G. syndrome
Lennox syndrome
lens
    275mm objective l.
    nucleus of l.
Lente
    L. Iletin I
    L. Iletin II
lenticula
lenticular
    l. ansa
    l. aphasia
    l. ganglion
    l. loop
    l. nucleus
    l. progressive degeneration
lenticularis
    dystonia l.
lenticulooptic
lenticulostriate
    l. arteries
lenticulothalamic
lentiform nucleus
lentis
    ectopia l.
leontiasis ossea
Leponex

leprae
    Mycobacterium l.
lepraphobia, leprophobia
leprosy
    anesthetic l.
    articular l.
    dry l.
    mutilating l.
    l. peripheral neuropathy
    trophoneurotic l.
leprotica
    alopecia l.
leprous neuropathy
leptin
leptomeningeal (LM)
    l. anastomosis
    l. angiomatosis
    l. carcinoma
    l. carcinomatosis
    l. cyst
    l. disease
    l. fibrosis
    l. gliomatosis
    l. metastasis
    l. tumor
leptomeningeal/wedge cortical biopsy
leptomeninges
leptomeningitis
    basilar l.
leptomeninx
leptomyelolipoma
Leptomyxid
leptophonia, leptophonic
leptospirosis
    l. lymphocytic meningitis
Leriche
    L. operation
    L. sympathectomy
    L. syndrome
Leri sign
Leroy-Raney scalp clip
LeRoy scalp clip-applying forceps
LES
    Life Experience Survey
    Liquid Embolic System
lesbianism
Lesch-Nyhan
    L.-N. disease
    L.-N. syndrome
Leser-Trélat sign
lesion
    acute cerebellar hemispheric l.
    afferent digital l.
    afferent nerve l.
    angiocentric immunoproliferative l.
    anterior parietal l.
    anterochiasmatic l.
    atrophic l.
    auricular l.
    basal ganglionic l.
    biparietal l.
    brachial plexus l.
    brain l.
    brainstem l.
    callosal l.

L

lesion *(continued)*
cavernous sinus l.
central l.
cerebral l.
cerebrovascular l.
cervical cord l.
chiasmal l.
chiasmatic l.
circumscribed l.
conus medullaris l.
cortical l.
corticospinal pathway l.
cyclops l.
deep white matter l. (DWML)
demyelinating l.
diffuse pontine l.
discharging l.
discoid skin l.
dominant hemisphere l.
dorsal root entry zone l.
Duret l.
entry zone l.
epicortical l.
epileptogenic temporal l.
excitatory l.
extraaxial l.
extracranial mass l.
fimbria-fornix l.
focal l.
frank l.
frontal lobe l.
l. generation
hemorrhagic l.
high cervical spinal cord l.
high-intensity l.
high pontine l.
high-signal l.
homogeneous l.
hyperintense l.
hyperkeratotic plantar l.
hyperostotic l.
hypothalamic l.
indiscriminate l.
inflammatory l.
infranuclear l.
infratentorial l.
interpeduncular fossa l.
intraaxial brain l.
intracerebral l.
intracranial mass l.
intradural extramedullary mass l.
intramedullary spinal l.
intraorbital l.
intrasellar l.
intraspinal l.
irritative l.
ischemic l.
isointense l.
keratotic l.
lateral temporal epileptogenic l.
l. load
low-density l.
lower motor neuron l.
mass l.

Meckel cave l.
median nerve l.
mesial temporal epileptogenic l.
metabolic l.
midbrain l.
midline l.
mucous membrane l.
multiple focal l.
nail l.
neoplastic l.
neurofibrillary l.
neurogenic l.
nondominant hemisphere l.
nonmeningiomatous malignant l.
nucleus basalis l.
occipital l.
ocular l.
optic nerve l.
orbitomedial/cingulate l.
paraorbital l.
parasagittal l.
parasellar l.
parietal cortex l.
parietal lobe l.
parietooccipital l.
peripheral nerve l.
periventricular hyperintense l.
periventricular white matter l.
Perthes-Bankart l.
petroclival l.
pigment epithelial l.
pituitary stalk l.
pontine l.
posterior column l.
posterior compartment l.
posterior fossa l.
posterior language area l.
pretectal l.
pseudocystic hypodense l.
pseudomedial longitudinal
  fasciculus l.
radiofrequency l.
regurgitant l.
retrochiasmal l.
retrochiasmatic l.
retrocochlear l.
ring-wall l.
root entry-zone l.
rotationally induced shear-strain l.
sciatic nerve l.
single enhancing CT l. (SECTL)
skin l.
space-occupying brain l.
spinal l.
striatal l.
subcortical l.
subtentorial l.
supranuclear l.
suprasellar l.
supratentorial structural l.
synchronous l.
tectal l.
thalamic l.
transverse cord l.
ulnar nerve l.

upper motor neuron l.
white matter l. (WML)
lesionectomy
lesioning
dorsal root entry zone l.
DREZ l.
nucleus caudalis-nucleus solitarius
DREZ l.
radiofrequency l.
trigeminal nucleus caudalis l.
less
l. pervasive disorder
l. than maximal effect
lesson
object l.
trial l.
LET
language enrichment therapy
linear energy transfer
lethal
l. blow
l. catatonia
l. dose (LD)
l. factor
l. injection
l. midline granuloma
l. overdose
l. weapon
lethality scale
lethargic
l. hypnosis
l. patient
l. stupor
lethargica
encephalitis l.
lethargy
hysteric l.
induced l.
lucid l.
letheomania
lethica
aphasia l.
l. aphasia
lethologica
LET-II
Learning Efficiency Test-II
"Let's Talk" Inventory for Adolescents
letter
l. blindness
Dear John l.
scarlet l.
Snellen l.
Letterer-Siwe disease
letter-word identification
lettuce opium
leucine
l. zipper family
l. zipper gene
leucotomy
leucovorin
leukemia inhibitory factor (LIF)
Leukeran
leukocyte
l. adhesion inhibitor (LAI)

eosinophilic l.
l. scintigraphy
leukocytoclastic vasculitides
leukocytosis
emotional l.
leukodystrophia cerebri progressiva
leukodystrophy
Canavan l.
globoid cell l.
Krabbe l.
metachromatic l. (MLD)
Pelizaeus-Merzbacher l.
spongy degeneration l.
sudanophilic l.
l. with diffuse Rosenthal fiber
formation
leukoencephalitis
acute epidemic l.
acute hemorrhagic l.
acute necrotizing hemorrhagic l.
necrotizing hemorrhagic l.
postinfectious l.
postvaccinial l.
subacute sclerosing l.
van Bogaert sclerosing l.
viral l.
leukoencephalopathy
cerebral autosomal dominant
arteriopathy with subcortical
infarcts and l. (CADASIL)
diffuse necrotizing l.
multifocal l.
progressive multifocal l. (PML)
l. radiation
subacute sclerosing l.
leukokoria
leukomalacia
cystic periventricular l.
leukomyelopathy
leukopenia
leukopoiesis
leukotome
leukotomy
bimedial l.
bimedial frontal l.
prefrontal l.
transorbital l.
ventromedial frontal l.
leukotriene
leukotrienes B4 and C4
leuprolide
levacecarnine
levallorphan tartrate
levamphetamine
levator
l. palpebrae muscle
l. scapulae
level
action l.
l. of activity
activity l.
alertness l.
l. of alertness
alpha l.
androgen l.

L

level (*continued*)
   annoyance l. (AL)
   l. of anxiety
   anxiety l.
   aspiration l.
   l. of aspiration
   Assessment Program of Early
    Learning L.'s (APELL)
   automatic phrase l.
   basal resistance l.
   below detectable l.'s (BDL)
   beta l.
   blood l.
   blood alcohol l. (BAL)
   l. of care
   cognitive-awareness l.
   cognitive impairment l.
   l. of cohesiveness
   cohesiveness l.
   confidence l.
   l. of confidence
   conflict l.
   l. of conflict
   l. of consciousness (LOC)
   current defense l.
   defense l.
   l. of defensive dysregulation
   defensive dysregulation l.
   delta l.
   denervation l.
   desire l.
   l. of development
   developmental l.
   difficulty l.
   disability l.
   disavowal l.
   discomfort l.
   drug l.
   educational l.
   effort l.
   endurance l.
   energy l.
   engagement l.
   l. of frustration
   functioning l.
   hedonic l.
   high adaptive l.
   high energy l.
   hormonal l.
   image-distorting l.
   l. of incompetence (LOI)
   l. of intellectual functioning
   intellectual functioning l.
   intoxication l.
   irreality l.
   lithium l.
   low educational l.
   maintenance l.
   major image-distorting l.
   meningioma prostaglandin l.
   mental inhibition l.
   microscopic l.
   minor image-distorting l.
   neural noise l.

   occupational functioning l.
   operant l.
   l. of pain tolerance
   peak and trough l.
   phallic l.
   plasma homocysteine l.
   pragmatic l.
   predominant current defense l.
   pre-oedipal l.
   psychopathology l.
   L. of Psychosocial Stress
   reference zero l.
   l. of resistance
   resistance l.
   l. of response
   risk l.
   l. of risk
   sensory l.
   serotonin l.
   serum caffeine l.
   significance l.
   social functioning l.
   society l.
   spinal l.
   therapeutic blood l.
   theta l.
   tolerance l. (TL)
   toxic l.
   uncertainty l.
   vegetative l.
   vertebral l.
Levine-Critchley syndrome
Levine-Pilowsky Depression
   Questionnaire
Levin thermocouple cordotomy electrode
levirate
levitation
levo-α-acetylmethadol (LAMM)
levoamphetamine
levobupivacaine
levocarnitine
levodopa and carbidopa
levodopa/carbidopa
levodopa-induced dyskinesia
Levo-Dromoran
Levolist
levomepromazine
levomethadyl
   l. acetate
   l. acetate hydrochloride
levophobia
levopromazine
Levoprome
levorphanol tartrate
Levothroid
levothyroxine (T_4)
   l. sodium
levoxadrol hydrochloride
Levoxine
Levy Draw-and-Tell-a-Story Technique
Lewy
   L. body dementia
   L. body variant of Alzheimer
   disease
   L. inclusion body

lexica concept
lexical
    l. access
    l. agraphia
    l. ambiguity
    l. process
    l. processing
lexipafant
lex talionis
Lex-Ton spinal frame
Leyden
    L. ataxia
    L. law
    L. neuritis
Leyden-Möbius muscular dystrophy
Leyla
    L. brain retractor
    L. self-retaining tractor bar
Leyton
    L. Obsessional Inventory
    L. Obsessive Inventory (LOI)
LFF
    low-filter frequency
    LFF on electroencephalogram
LGD
    leaderless group discussion
LGG
    low-grade glioma
LGN
    lateral geniculate nucleus
LH
    luteinizing hormone
LHD
    lactate dehydrogenase
Lhermitte
    L. phenomenon
    L. sign
Lhermitte-Duclos disease
LHRH
    luteinizing hormone-releasing hormone
LI
    labeling index
liability abuse
liaison
    l. nursing
    l. psychiatry
liar
    pathologic l.
lib
    ad l.
liberation
    gay l.
liberomotor
libidinal
    l. development
    l. energy
    l. impulse
    l. object constancy
    l. phase
    l. transference
    l. type
libidinal-cathexis
libidinization
libidinous

libido
    l. analog
    l. binding
    bisexual l.
    dammed-up l.
    diminished l.
    displaceability of l.
    ego l.
    l. fixation
    mobility of l.
    normal l. (NL)
    object l.
    organ l.
    l. organization
    plasticity of l.
    primal l.
    l. quantum
    sexual l.
    l. stasis
    l. theory
    traumatization of the l.
    viscosity of l.
    l. wish
library
    Committee on History and L.
Librax
Libritabs
Librium
licensed
    L. Marriage Family and Child Counselor (LMFCC)
    L. Marriage and Family Therapist (LMFT)
    l. professional counselor (LPC)
    l. psychologist
    l. vocational nurse (LVN)
Lichtheim
    L. aphasia
    L. disease
    L. sign
licostinel
lid
    l. nystagmus
    l. tic
Liddell-Sherrington reflex
lidocaine
    crack cut with l.
    l. and epinephrine
    l. and prilocaine
    l. test
LidodexNS
lidofenin
    technetium 99m l.
lie
    l. detection
    l. detector
    l. scale
liebestod
Liepmann apraxia
lieutenant
LIF
    leukemia inhibitory factor
life
    adjustment reaction of later l.
    change of l.

L

life (continued)
l. change rating scale
l. change unit (LCU)
l. circumstance problem
l. course
l. crisis
l. cycle
l. cycle change
l. cycle theory
l. difficulty
l. energy
l. event
L. Event Scale Adolescents
L. Event Scale Children
l. expectancy
expectation of l.
l. experience
L. Experiences Checklist (LEC)
L. Experience Survey (LES)
fact of l.
fantasy l.
l. fear
l. goal
health-related quality of l. (HRQL)
l. history
L. History of Aggression
  Assessment
impoverished fantasy l.
impulse l.
inner l.
l. instinct
L. Interpersonal History Enquiry
  (LIPHE)
late l.
mental l.
noon of l.
l. organization
phase of l.
l. plan
prime of l.
Profile of Adaptation to L. (PAL)
purpose in l. (PIL)
quality of l. (QOL)
reading/everyday activities in l.
real l.
L. Satisfaction Index (LSI)
l. script
l. sentence
sexual l.
sheltered l.
L. Skills, Forms 1 & 2
L. Skills Program
l. space
spastic paraparesis of middle l.
l. stage
l. stress
L. Study Sample (LSS)
l. support system
l. table
vegetative l.
vicissitudes of l.
life-cycle
l.-c. adjustment
l.-c. transition

life-event stress theory
lifelikelihood
vegetative l.
lifelong obesity
life-long sexual dysfunction
lifelong-type
l.-t. disorder
l.-t. dyspareunia
l.-t. vaginismus
life-span development
life's stressor
lifestyle
alternative l.
inferior sibling l.
nomadic l.
sedentary l.
life-threatening
l.-t. behavior (LTB)
l.-t. disease
l.-t. illness
lifetime
l. expectancy
l. hierarchy
l. history
l. personality
l. prevalence
l. risk
life-years
quality adjusted l.-y. (QUALY)
Li-Fraumeni syndrome
Lifril
lift
pneumatic chair l.
lifter
weight l.
Yasargil tissue l.
Ligaclip
L. applier
L. clip
Ethicon L.
ligament
alar l.
anterior longitudinal l.
atlantoepistrophic l.
axial-occipital l.
costotransverse l.
costovertebral l.
cruciate l.
dentate l.
denticulate l.
fracture-dislocation with anterior l.
l. of Henle
interclinoid l.
longitudinal l.
occipital-atlas-axis l.
ossification of the posterior
  longitudinal l. (OPLL)
petrosphenoidal l.
posterior longitudinal l.
Struthers l.
transverse atlantal l.
yellow l.
ligamentectomy
bilateral l.
ligamentum, pl. **ligamenta**

l. denticulatum
l. flavum

ligand
l. occupation
putative endogenous l.
receptor l.

ligand-gated ion channel

ligation
hunterian l.
sigmoid sinus l.

ligature
intravascular l.

light
l. chain paraprotein
l. diet
l. drinking
l. flash
flashes of l.
halo of l.
l. sleep (LS)
l. therapy
l. touch sensation
l. trance
l. treatment
l. treatment for winter depression

light-emitting diode (LED)

lighter
l. fluid
l. fluid dependence

light-prompted button task
light-therapy-induced mood disorder
Light-Veley headrest
LightWare micro retractor
LightWear headlight
LII
Leisure Interest Inventory

likability
peer l.

likable
LIKE
Learning Inventory of Kindergarten
Experiences

Likert scale
Lilienthal rib spreader
Liliequist
membrane of L.

lilliputian hallucination
limb
abnormal position of distal l.'s
ampullary l.'s of semicircular ducts
anterior l. of internal capsule
l.'s of bony semicircular canals
common l. of membranous
semicircular ducts
l. movement disorder
phantom l.
posterior l. of internal capsule
retrolenticular l. of internal capsule
simple membranous l. of
semicircular duct
sublenticular l. of internal capsule
l. weakness

limb-girdle muscular dystrophy
limb-girdle-trunk paresis

limbic
l. circuit
l. cortex
l. dysregulation
l. encephalitis
l. epilepsy
l. forebrain
l. lobe
l. neuronal firing rate
l. system
l. system disorder
l. system pathway
l. zone

Limbitrol
L. DS
L. DS 10-25

limb-kinetic
l.-k. apraxia
l.-k. dyspraxia

limbus vertebra
limen, pl. **limina**
difference l.
l. insulae

liminal stimulus
liminometer
limit
class l.
extreme narrowing l.
method of l.'s
normal l.'s
off l.'s
physiological l.
l. setting
within normal l.'s (WNL)

limitans
glia l.
sulcus l.

limitation
functional l.
l. of movement (LOM)
receiver l.
sex l.

limited
l. activity
l. diet
l. responsibility
l. support
l. war

limited-capacity retrieval
limited-symptom attack
limiting
l. sulcus of Reil
l. sulcus of rhomboid fossa

limit-setting for adolescent
limit-testing behavior
LIM-kinase gene
limnophobia
Limon Self-Image Assessment
limophoitas
limophthisis
limosis
limotherapy
limp
antalgic l.

L

limulus lysate assay of cerebrospinal fluid
LINAC
    linear accelerator
        Boston LINAC
        LINAC system
LINAC-based radiosurgical system
LINAC radiosurgery
Linac radiosurgery system
Lincoln-Oseretsky
        L.-O. Motor Development Scale
        L.-O. Motor Performance Test
        (LOMPT)
Lindamood
        L. Auditory Conceptualization
        L. Auditory Conceptualization Test
        (LACT)
Lindau
        L. disease
        L. tumor
Lindermann bur
Linde XeScan
line
        AC-PC l.
        anterior commissure-posterior
        commissure l.
        l. artifact
        Baillarger l.
        basal l.
        l. of Bechterew
        bimastoid l.
        l. bisection error (LBE)
        central sacral l. (CSL)
        Chamberlain palatooccipital l.
        Chaussier l.
        clivus canal l.
        digastric l.
        l. of duty
        l.'s of expression
        Fishgold l.
        l. of fixation
        foramen magnum l.
        l. frequency noise dot
        Garrett orientation l.
        l. of Gennari
        glabella-inion l.
        Gubler l.
        hard l.
        Head l.
        hot l.
        l. imaging
        isodose l.
        l. of Kaes
        Lorentzian l.
        McGregor basal l.
        McRae foramen magnum l.
        Mees l.
        midpoint to meatal l.
        Obersteiner-Redlich l.
        palatooccipital l.
        posterior canal l.
        pure l.
        radiosignal l.
        recruitment l.
        Reid base l.

        rolandic l.
        l. scanning
        simian l.
        spinolamellar l.
        spinous interlaminar l.
        Sydney l.
        sylvian l.
        tender l.
        Ullmann l.
        Voigt l.
        Wackenheim clivus canal l.
        l. width
linear
        l. accelerator (LINAC)
        l. accelerator radiosurgery
        l. accelerator system
        l. chromosome
        l. craniectomy
        l. energy transfer (LET)
        l. inseparability
        l. nevus sebaceous syndrome
        l. regression analysis
        l. skull fracture
        l. thought process
        l. type
line-of-sight link
liner
        Teflon l.
lingua, gen. and pl. **linguae,** pl. **linguae**
        l. cerebelli
        l. franca
        lapsus l.
linguadental
lingual
        l. airway dysfunction
        l. delirium
        l. gyrus
        l. muscle
        l. paralysis
        l. trophoneurosis
        l. vein
linguistic
        L. Analysis and Remediation
        Procedure
        L. Analysis of Speech Samples
        (LASS)
        l. approach
        l. content of task
        l. determinism
        l. disorganization
        l. disturbance
        l. savant
linguistic-kinesic method
linguistics
        anthropological l.
lingula, pl. **lingulae**
        l. cerebelli
lingular
linguofacial vein
link
        causal l.
        line-of-sight l.
linkage
        l. analysis
        associative l.

l. object
rod l.
sex l.
l. worker
linonophobia
lion's
l. claw grasper
l. paw grasper
Lioresal
liothyronine (L-T$_3$)
l. sodium
lip
l. biting
l. erotism
l. pursing
l. reading
l. reflex
l. smacking
l. smacking automatism
lipase
acid l.
lipectomy
lipedematous alopecia
LIPHE
Life Interpersonal History Enquiry
lipid
l. bilayer
cell membrane l.
l. hypothesis
l. metabolism disorder
l. peroxidation
l. recycling
lipid-laden stromal cell
lipidosis, pl. lipidoses
cerebral l.
cerebroside l.
galactosylceramide l.
ganglioside l.
neuronal l.
sphingomyelin l.
sulfatide l.
Lipiodol
lipodermatosis
lipofuscinosis
ceroid l.
neuronal ceroid l.
lipogranulomatosis
Farber l.
lipohyalinosis
lipoid metabolism
lipoidosis
lipolysis
membrane l.
lipoma
dorsal brain stem l. (DBSL)
epidermoid l.
hamartomatous l.
inclusion l.
intradural l.
quadrigeminal cistern l. (QCL)
spinal l.
subarachnoid l.
tectal l.
lipomatosis

lipomeningocele
lipomyelocele
lipomyelomeningocele
lipomyeloschisis
liponeural junction
lipophilic
l. chloroethylnitrosourea
l. compound
l. morpholino anthracycline
lipoprotein
low-density l.
liposarcoma
Lipoxide
lipoxygenase pathway
LIPS
Leiter International Performance Scale
liquefied heroin
Liqui-Char
liquid
l. diet
L. Ecstasy
L. Embolic System (LES)
ethylene vinyl alcohol copolymer l.
L. Pred
Tums Extra Strength L.
liquidation of attachment
Liquipake
Liquiprin
liquor, gen. liquoris, pl. liquores
l. cerebrospinalis
Lisch nodule
lisinopril and hydrochlorothiazide
Lissauer
L. bundle
L. dementia paralytica
L. fasciculus
L. marginal zone
L. paralysis
L. tract
L. tracts of spinal cord
Lissauer-type paresis
lissencephalia, lissencephaly
lissencephalic syndrome
list
Career Problem Check L.
Interest Check L.
Occupational Check L.
Personality Adjective Check L.
(PACL)
l.'s preoccupation
Sales Attitude Check L. (SACL)
Tourette Syndrome Symptom L.
listening
l. attitude
L. Comprehension Test (LCT)
diotic l.
l. language quotient
passive l.
l. with the third ear
Listeria monocytogenes
listhesis
lateral l.
Listomin
lisuride

L

literacy
  Standardized Test of Computer L.
    (STCL)
  l. test
  Test of Economic L. (TEL)
  visual l.
literal
  l. agraphia
  l. alexia
  l. meaning
  l. paraphasia
  l. paraphrasia
literalis
  anarithmia l.
  anarthria l.
  dysarthria l.
  paralalia l.
lithiasis
  hysterical l.
lithium
  l. action on first messenger
  l. action on membranes
  l. action on second messenger
  l. carbonate
  l. level
  l. monotherapy
  l. therapy
  l. toxicity
  l. tremor
lithium-induced postural tremor
Lithobid
Lithonate
Lithotabs
litigious
  l. delusional state
  l. paranoia
Litmosoides carinii
Little disease
live
  l. birth
  l. one
  will to l.
livedo reticularis (LR)
liver
  l. cirrhosis
  cirrhotic l.
  l. disease
  l. disease organic psychosis
  l. flap
  l. function test
  l. transplantation
living
  activities of daily l. (ADL)
  capacity for independent l.
  Communicative Abilities in
    Daily L. (CADL)
  daily l.
  l. death
  existential l.
  free l.
  group l.
  independent l.
  instrumental activities of daily l.
    (IADL)

  simulated activities of daily l.
    (SADL, SADLs)
  standard of l.
  l. standard
  vicarious l.
  l. will
LLPDD
  late luteal phase dysphoric disorder
LLQ
  Leatherman Leadership Questionnaire
LM
  leptomeningeal
LMFCC
  Licensed Marriage Family and Child
    Counselor
LMFT
  Licensed Marriage and Family Therapist
LMN
  lower motor neuron
LMR
  localized magnetic resonance
LMTA
  Language Modalities Test for Aphasia
LMWH
  low-molecular weight heparin
LN
  Imagent LN
LNB
  Lyme neuroborreliosis
LNNB
  Luria-Nebraska Neuropsychological
    Battery
LOA
  leave of absence
  loosening of associations
load
  axial l.
  high-lesion l.
  lesion l.
loading
  axial l.
  Edwards modular system
    dynamic l.
  factor l.
  genetic l.
loaner
  psychological l.
lobar
  l. atrophy
  l. division
  l. hemorrhage
  l. sclerosis
lobe
  anterior l. of hypophysis
  l. of cerebrum
  contralateral parietal l.
  cuneiform l.
  l. dysfunction
  falciform l.
  flocculonodular l.
  frontal l.
  insular l.
  left frontal l.
  limbic l.
  medial temporal l.

mesial aspect of temporal l.
mesial part of frontal l.
mesiobasal temporal l.
mesiotemporal l.
occipital l.
parietal l.
posterior l. of hypophysis
posterodorsal temporal l.
quadrate l.
right frontal l.
temporal l.
uncus of temporal l.

lobectomy
anterior l.
anterior temporal l. (ATL)
anteromesial temporal l.
Falconer l.
temporal l.
transorbital l.

lobi (*gen. and pl. of* lobus)
lobotomy
frontal l.
Grantham l.
prefrontal l.
radical prefrontal l.
l. syndrome
transorbital l.

Lobstein ganglion
lobule
ansiform l.
anterior lunate l.
biventral l.
central l.
crescentic l.'s of the cerebellum
inferior parietal l.
inferior semilunar l.
myxoid l.
paracentral l.
posterior lunate l.
quadrangular l.
quadrate l.
simple l.
slender l.
superior parietal l.
superior semilunar l.

lobulet, lobulette
lobulus, gen. and pl. **lobuli**
l. biventer
l. biventralis
l. centralis cerebelli
l. clivi
l. culminis
l. cuneiformis
l. folii
l. fusiformis
l. gracilis
l. paracentralis
l. parietalis inferior
l. parietalis superior
l. quadrangularis
l. quadratus
l. semilunaris inferior
l. semilunaris superior
l. simplex

lobus, gen. and pl. **lobi**

l. anterior hypophyseos
lobi cerebri
l. clivi
l. falciformis
l. frontalis cerebri
l. glandularis hypophyseos
l. nervosus
l. occipitalis cerebri
l. parietalis cerebri
l. posterior hypophyseos
l. temporalis

LOC
laxative of choice
level of consciousness
locus of control
loss of consciousness

local
l. anesthesia
l. cerebral blood flow (LCBF)
l. convulsion
l. epilepsy
l. excitatory state
l. field distortion
l. potential
l. reduction in amplitude
l. response
l. sign
l. syncope
l. tetanus
l. tic

localis paracusis
locality attachment
locality-specific pattern of aberrant
  behavior
localization
l. agnosia
auditory l.
autoradiographic l.
l. of behavior
cerebral l.
2D graphic l.
dipole l.
frame fixation-scanner assisted
  target l.
l. of function
intraoperative stereotactic spatial l.
language l.
law of average l.
manual target l.
pedicle l.
pneumotaxic l.
point l.
scanner assisted target l.
spatial l.
stereotactic l.
stereotactic anatomic target l.
subcellular l.
l. of symptoms
target l.
ultrasonographic l.
X-ray l.

localized
l. amnesia
l. epilepsy
l. evoked potential

L

localized *(continued)*
    l. function
    l. magnetic resonance (LMR)
    l. pruritus
    l. restorative central nervous
        system gene therapy
    l. weakness
localizer
    Mayfield fiducial l.
    Risser l.
    Suetens-Gybels-Vandermeulen
        angiographic l.
    ultrasonic l.
location
    action l.
    cerebral l.
    cervical sympathetic chain l.
    l. constancy
    pedicle l.
locative
locator
    Gill Thomas l.
LOC-C
    locus of control-chance
LOC-E
    locus of control-external
LOC-I
    locus of control-internal
loci (*pl. of* locus)
LOCI score
lock
    field l.
    l. finger
    l. nut
    scalp l.
locked
    l. cell
    l. facet
    l. hospital unit
    l. room
    l. seclusion
    l. in state
    l. ward
locked-in syndrome
locking
    phase l.
lockjaw, lock-jaw
**Lock Wallace Short Marital
Adjustment Scale**
locomotor
    l. activity
    l. arrest
    l. ataxia
    l. maze
locomotor-genital stage
locomotorium
LOC-PO
    locus of control-powerful others
loculation
    l. syndrome
locum tenens
locura
locus, pl. loci
    l. ceruleus

    l. ceruleus neuron
    chromosomal loci
    l. cinereus
    l. of control (LOC)
    L. of Control of Behavior Scale
    l. of control-chance (LOC-C)
    l. of control-external (LOC-E)
    l. of control-internal (LOC-I)
    l. of control-powerful others (LOC-
        PO)
    l. ferrugineus
    l. heterogenicity
    l. minoris resistentiae
    l. niger
    l. perforatus anticus
    l. perforatus posticus
locution
LOD
    logarithm of odds
    LOD score
Lodge
    Fairweather L.
Lodine XL
Lodosyn
**Loevinger's Washington University
Sentence Completion Test**
Loewenthal
    L. bundle
    L. tract
lofepramine
loflazepate
    ethyl l.
log
    activity l.
    drug information l. (DIL)
logagnosia
logagraphia
logamnesia
logaphasia
logarithm of odds (LOD)
logasthenia
logic
    formal l.
    perverted l.
    trance l.
logical
    l. inference
    l. memory
    l. memory test
    L. Memory and Visual
        Reproduction subtest Russell's
        revised
    l. operation
    l. positivism
logicogrammatical disorder
logistic
    l. curve
    l. regression
logoclonia
logographic
logokophosis
logomania
logoneurosis
logopathy
logophobia

logoplegia
Logor
logorrhea
logospasm
logotherapy
LOI
    level of incompetence
    Leyton Obsessive Inventory
Lollipop Test: A Diagnostic Screening Test of School Readiness
LOM
    limitation of movement
    loss of movement
Lombard Test
LOMPT
    Lincoln-Oseretsky Motor Performance Test
lomustine
London Psychogeriatric Scale (LPS)
loner
    psychological l.
long
    L. Beach stereotactic robot
    l. gyrus of insula
    l. gyrus of the insula
    l. latency response
    l. pulse repetition time/echo time image
    l. pulse repetition time/long echo time
    l. pulse repetition time/long echo time spin-echo
    l. root of ciliary ganglion
    l. segment spinal fusion
    l. spinal white matter
    l. thoracic nerve
    l. thoracic palsy
long-acting
    l.-a. barbiturate
    l.-a. insulin preparation
long-chain fatty acid
longevity
    marital l.
long-half-life anxiolytic substance
long-hot-summer effect
longing
    passive-receptive l.
longitudinal
    l. cerebral fissure
    l. course
    l. course specifier
    l. fissure of cerebrum
    L. Interval Follow-up Evaluation
    l. ligament
    l. ligament rupture
    l. magnetization
    l. member to anchor connector
    l. mental status examination
    l. method
    l. observation
    l. pontine bundle
    l. relaxation
    l. spinal bar
    l. study

long-term
    l.-t. bone-instrumentation interface
    l.-t. care
    l.-t. care facility
    l.-t. commitment
    l.-t. course of abuse
    l.-t. data
    l.-t. dependency
    l.-t. disability (LTD)
    l.-t. effect
    l.-t. heavy use
    l.-t. hospitalization
    l.-t. memory (LTM)
    l.-t. mortality rate
    l.-t. outcome
    l.-t. pattern
    l.-t. potentiation (LTP)
    l.-t. psychotherapy
    l.-t. therapy
    l.-t. treatment
longus
    l. capitis muscle
    l. cervicis colli muscle
    l. colli muscle
look
    glazed l.
    paranoid l.
look-alike
    amphetamine l.-a.
looking-glass self
loop
    basal ganglia-cingulate gyrus-frontal lobe l.
    Blair-Ivy l.
    calibrated l.
    l. diuretic
    gamma l.
    Granit l.
    Hartshill Ransford l.
    induction l.
    lenticular l.
    Meyer l.
    Meyer-Archambault l.
    peduncular l.
    Ransford l.
    l.'s of spinal nerves
    subclavian l.
    unipolar cutting l.
    Vieussens l.
loose
    l. association
    l. boundary
loosening
    l. of associations (LOA)
    screw l.
LOP
    leave on pass
Lophophora williamsii
loprazolam
Lopressor
LOPS
    length of patient stay
LOQ
    Leadership Opinion Questionnaire
loquacious

L

lorazepam
Lorcet-HD
Lorcet Plus
lordosis
    l. creation
    lumbar spine l.
    l. preservation
    thoracic spine l.
Lorentzian line
Lorenz
    L. cranial plate
    L. cranial screw
    L. Neuro/skull base titanium
       osteosynthesis system
    L. titanium screws and plate
Lorenzo oil
Lorfan
Lorge-Thorndike
    L.-T. Cognitive Abilities Test
    L.-T. Intelligence Test
lormetazepam
Lorr Scale
Lortab ASA
LOS
    length of stay
losartan and hydrochlorothiazide
losing
    l. control
    l. time
loss
    age-related hearing l.
    allelic l.
    appetite l.
    l. of appetite
    approval l.
    l. of autonomy
    autonomy l.
    axonal l.
    l. of belief
    l. of biographical memory
    blood l.
    l. of boundaries of ego
    l. of breadwinner
    central sensory l.
    cognitive l.
    color vision l.
    complete visual l.
    l. of consciousness (LOC)
    contralateral l.
    l. of control
    cortical sensory l.
    Dejerine onion peel sensory l.
    dense sensory l.
    l. discrimination
    dissociated sensory l.
    l. of effect
    l. of ego boundary
    ego boundary l.
    l. of energy
    l. experience
    l. of freedom
    functional l.
    gag reflex l.
    gaze-evoked visual l.
    glucocorticoid-induced bone l.
    hearing l.
    heat l.
    hemifield l.
    hemisensory l.
    hippocampal volume l.
    hysterical visual l.
    imagined l.
    l. of interest
    interpersonal l.
    inventory of l.
    ipsilateral l.
    l. of language
    l. of loved one
    lumbar lordosis iatrogenic l.
    major l.
    mechanical functional l.
    mechanical visual l.
    memory l.
    monocular visual l.
    l. of motivation
    motor l.
    l. of movement (LOM)
    multiple l.
    natural hearing l.
    nerve l.
    neuronal l.
    nonnormative hair l.
    object l.
    l. of orientation
    parental l.
    partial visual l.
    perceived l.
    peripheral sensory l.
    personal l.
    l. of personal identity
    l. of pleasure
    pregnancy l.
    psychogenic hearing l.
    real l.
    saddle-area sensory l.
    self-induced hair l.
    l. of semen
    semen l.
    l. of sensation
    sensory l.
    signal l.
    significant l.
    sleep l.
    soul l.
    stocking-glove sensory l.
    surgical hearing l.
    symbolic l.
    threat of job l.
    transient monocular visual l.
    unresolved l.
    visual acuity l.
    weight l.
    l. of zest
loss-of-resistance technique
lost privileges (LP)
LOT
    Lengthened-Off-Time
Lotensin HCT
LOTE Reading and Listening Test
loud speech

Lou Gehrig disease
Louis-Bar syndrome
Louisiana State University Medical
    College (LSUMC)
Louis instrumentation
Louisville Behavior Checklist
lounging position
loupe
    Keeler Galilean l.
    Keeler panoramic l.
    l. magnification
lovastatin
love
    anal-sadistic l.
    l. child
    deficiency l.
    Dorian l.
    genital l.
    homogenic l.
    mother l.
    l. need
    L. nerve root hook
    L. nerve root retractor
    l. object
    object l.
    passive object l.
    phallic l.
    L. pituitary rongeur
    platonic l.
    Polybus l.
    pregenital l.
    primary object l.
    productive l.
    puppy l.
    sexual l.
    smother l.
    tough l.
    transference l.
Love-Adson wire tightener
Love-Gruenwald
    L.-G. cranial rongeur
    L.-G. disk rongeur
    L.-G. intervertebral disk forceps
    L.-G. pituitary forceps
    L.-G. pituitary rongeur
Love-Kerrison
    L.-K. laminectomy rongeur
    L.-K. rongeur forceps
Lovén reflex
lover
    heterosexual l.
    homosexual l.
    illicit l.
lover's knot
loving
    delusional l.
    l. feeling
low
    l. anxiety (LA)
    l. back syndrome (LBS)
    l. cervical approach
    l. current monopolar coagulation
    l. delirium
    l. dose
    l. educational level

    l. energy
    l. fever
    l. impulsiveness
    l. intelligence
    l. linear frequency
    l. lumbar spine fracture
    l. molecular weight cytokeratin
    l. penetrance-high frequency gene
    l. profile
    L. Profile valve
    l. self-confidence
    l. sensory environment
    l. sexual desire
    l. sexual interest
    l. single thoracic curve
    l. stimulation environment
    l. tension glaucoma
    l. tolerance potential
low-activity situation
low-air-loss bed
low-amplitude activity
low-calorie diet
low-complexity movement
low-degree astrocytoma
low-density
    l.-d. area (LDA)
    l.-d. lesion
    l.-d. lipoprotein
Löwenberg
    L. canal
    L. scala
low-energy gamma radiation
lower
    l. abdominal periosteal reflex
    l. basilar aneurysm
    l. cervical spine
    l. cervical spine fusion
    l. cervical spine posterior
      stabilization
    l. cervical spine procedure
    l. clivus
    l. hook trial
    l. limb dysmetria
    l. lumbar spine
    l. motor neuron (LMN)
    l. motor neuron lesion
    l. motor neuron paralysis
    l. motor neuron syndrome
    l. pons
    l. posterior lumbar spine and
      sacrum surgery
    l. thoracic pedicle
    l. thoracic spine
lowered mood
Lowe syndrome
low-fat diet
low-filter frequency (LFF)
low-frequency
    l.-f. activity
    l.-f. filter
low-grade
    l.-g. astrocytoma
    l.-g. glioma (LGG)
low-magnitude stressor subscale

L

low-melt temperature agarose
low-molecular weight heparin (LMWH)
low-pass filter
low-quality drug
low-salt diet
low-stimulation situation
low-tyramine diet
low-voltage
   l.-v. activity
   l.-v. calibration
loxapine succinate
loxazolam
loxia
Loxitane
   L. C
   L. IM
loyalty
   doubts of l.
   unjustified doubt of l.
Loyola Sensate Focus
Lozol
LP
   latency period
   lost privileges
   lumbar puncture
LPC
   licensed professional counselor
LPCh
   lateral posterior choroidal
   LPCh artery
LPI
   Leadership Practices Inventory
LPS
   London Psychogeriatric Scale
LR
   livedo reticularis
LS
   legally separated
   light sleep
   Micro-K LS
L5-S1
   L5-S1 disk disease
   L5-S1 disk space
LSD
   lysergic acid diethylamide
   LSD abuse
   LSD dependence
   LSD reaction
LSD-type perception
LSES
   Salamon-Conte Life Satisfaction in the
   Elderly Scale
L-shaped
   L.-s. aneurysm clip
   L.-s. microplate
LSI
   Life Satisfaction Index
LSM-GB200 confocal laser scanning
   microscope
LSP
   Learning Style Profile
LSS
   Life Study Sample

LSUMC
   Louisiana State University Medical
   College
   LSUMC classification of motor
      and sensory function
   LSUMC classification of nerve
      injury
LSV2
   Vocational Learning Styles
L-T$_3$
   liothyronine
LTB
   life-threatening behavior
LTD
   long-term disability
LTM
   long-term memory
LTP
   long-term potentiation
L-triiodothyronine
L-tryptophan
lubeluzole
Luborsky Health-Sickness Rating Scale
Lucae
   L. bone mallet
   L. nerve hook
Lucas and Drucker Motor Index
Luc ethmoid forceps
lucid
   l. interval
   l. lethargy
lucidity
luding out
Ludiomil
ludotherapy
Ludwig
   L. ganglion
   L. nerve
Luer-Lok stopcock
lues
luetic
   l. aneurysm
   l. curve
   l. meningitis
Luft disease
lugubrious
Luhr
   L. Microfixation cranial plate
   L. Microfixation System drill bit
   L. Microfixation System pliers
   L. micro plate
   L. microplate
   L. mini plate
   L. pan plate
lumbago
   ischemic l.
lumbar
   l. anterior-root stimulator implant
      (LARSI)
   l. arachnoid peritoneal shunt
   l. catheter
   cisterna l.
   l. curve
   l. discectomy
   l. disk disease

l. disk herniation
l. drainage
l. enlargement of spinal cord
l. epidural steroid
l. facet disease
l. flat back syndrome
l. ganglia
l. hemilaminectomy
l. interbody fusion
l. interspace
l. kyphosis
l. lordosis iatrogenic loss
l. lordosis preservation
l. meningocele
l. pedicle
l. pedicle fixation
l. pedicle marker
l. pedicle screw
l. periosteal turnover flap
l. plexus
l. port
l. puncture (LP)
l. puncture needle
l. puncture pain
l. rheumatism
l. scoliosis
l. spinal fusion
l. spinal stenosis
l. spine
l. spine biopsy
l. spine burst fracture
l. spine decompression
l. spine instability
l. spine instrumentation
l. spine kyphotic deformity
l. spine lordosis
l. spine model
l. spine pedicle diameter
l. spine rotational stability
l. spine segmental fixation
l. spine stabilization
l. spine transpedicular fixation
l. spine trauma
l. spine vertebral osteosynthesis
l. spondylosis
l. sympathectomy
l. synovial cyst
l. theco-peritoneal shunt syndrome
l. tumor
l. vertebra
lumbarization
lumbar-peritoneal
l.-p. shunt
l.-p. shunting
lumbodorsal fascia
lumboperitoneal shunt
lumbosacral
l. corset
l. fusion
l. junction
l. junction bone density
l. junction cortical thickness
l. junction fracture
l. myelomeningocele
l. plexus

l. plexus neuritis
l. radiculopathy
l. spine
l. spine transpedicular
instrumentation
l. vertebra
luminal occlusion
luminescence of object
Lumsden
pneumotaxic center of L.
lunate
l. fissure
l. sulcus
Lundborg myoclonic epilepsy
lung
l. disorder
iron l.
trench l.
lupina
insania l.
Lupron
lupus
l. anticoagulant (LA)
l. cerebritis
l. erythematosus (LE)
l. erythematosus peripheral
neuropathy
Luque
L. II segmental spinal
instrumentation
L. instrumentation concave
technique
L. instrumentation convex technique
L. loop fixation
L. rectangle
L. ring
L. rod
L. rod migration
L. segmental spinal instrumentation
L. semirigid segmental spinal
instrumentation
L. sublaminar wiring technique
L. wire
Luque-Galveston
L.-G. fixation
L.-G. post
lura
lural
Luria
L. technique
L. Test
**Luria-Nebraska Neuropsychological
Battery (LNNB)**
Luria's Neuropsychological Investigation
Luschka
foramen of L.
lust
l. dynamism
l. murder
lusterless eye
lutea
macula l.
luteal
l. phase
l. phase assessment

L

luteinizing
l. hormone (LH)
l. hormone-releasing hormone (LHRH)
Luvox
luxation
rotatory l.
Luxtec
L. coaxial illumination
L. illuminated surgical telescope
luxury
l. perfusion
l. perfusion syndrome
Luys body
luysii
corpus l.
LVN
licensed vocational nurse
lycanthropy
lycomania
lycorexia
lygophilia
lying
pathologic l.
repetitive l.
Lyme
L. borreliosis
L. disease
L. neuroborreliosis (LNB)
L. neuropathy
lymphadenopathy
lymphangioma
lymphoblastoid
lymphocyte
CD4 l.
tumor-infiltrating l. (TIL)
lymphocyte:PMN ratio in cerebrospinal fluid
lymphocytic
l. adenohypophysitis
l. choriomeningitis
l. choriomeningitis virus (LCMV)
l. hypophysitis
l. infiltrate
l. pleocytosis-depressed glucose in cerebrospinal fluid
lymphocytopenia
lymphocytosis
atypical l.
lymphoepithelial parotid tumor
lymphoepithelioma
lymphogranuloma venereum encephalitis
lymphoid hypophysitis
lymphokine
lymphokine-activated killer cell

lymphoma
angiotropic l.
Burkitt l.
central nervous system l.
centroblastic B-cell l.
cerebral l.
CNS l.
intracerebral Hodgkin l.
intracranial Hodgkin l.
intramedullary l.
intravascular l.
Lennert l.
malignant l.
primary brain l.
primary CNS l.
primary intramedullary l.
primary leptomeningeal l.
solitary extranodal l.
lymphomagenesis
lymphomatoid granulomatosis
lymphomatous
l. meningitis
l. tumor
lymphoproliferative disorder
lymphotoxin
Lynch incision
Lyodura
Lyodura-associated Creutzfeldt-Jakob disease
lyophilized
l. cadaveric dura
l. dura
lypressin
lyra davidis
lysatotherapy
lysergic
l. acid
l. acid amide
l. acid diethylamide (LSD)
l. acid diethylamide and strychnine
l. acid diethylamide use
l. acid monoethylamide
lysolecithin patching
lysosomal
l. enzymatic activity
l. storage disease
lyssa
lyssophobia
lytic
l. cocktail
l. infection
Lytico-Bodig disease
lz R
total response

M
M segment
M vector
M wave

M1
M1 agonist
M1 segment aneurysm

99m
CEA-Tc 99m
Pertscan 99m

MA
mental age
migraine with aura

M/A
mood and/or affect

MAACL
Multiple Affect Adjective Checklist

Maalox

MAAS-R
Maastricht History and Advice Checklist-Revised

Maastricht
M. History and Advice Checklist-Revised (MAAS-R)
M. Interview for Vital Exhaustion

MAB
management of assaultive behavior

MABI
Mother's Assessment of the Behavior of Her Infant

MABP
mean arterial blood pressure

MAC
maximum allowable cost
McAndrews Alcoholism Scale
membrane attack complex
MAC EIA

MacAndrew Addiction Scale (MAS)
MacCarty forceps
MacDonaldd dissector
MacDougall diet for multiple sclerosis
macerate
maceration
Macewen
M. sign
M. symptom

Machado-Joseph
Machado-Joseph disease

machiavellianism
machine
Accuray Neurotron 1000 m.
m. artifact
Burdick Eclipse ECG m.
slot m.
TECA-TD20 EMG m.

macho manner
Machover Draw-A-Person Test (MDAP)
Mach Scale
Machupo virus
MACI
Millon Adolescent Clinical Inventory

MacKenzie syndrome

Macmillan Graded Word Reading Test
MacQuarrie Test for Mechanical Ability
macrencephaly, macrencephalia
macroadenoma
enclosed m.

macroaneurysm
macrobiotic diet
macrocephalic, macrocephalous
macrocephaly, macrocephalia
m. with somatic and genital growth delay

macrocheilia
macrocranium
macrocryoglobulinemia peripheral neuropathy
macrocytic megaloblastic anemia
macro-eCVR-FV circulation
macroelectrode technique
macroencephalon
macroesthesia
macroglia cell
macroglobulinemia
m. peripheral neuropathy
Waldenstrom m.
m. of Waldenstrom

macrognathia
macrographia, macrography
macrogyria
macroinstrument
macromania
macromaniacal delirium
macromolecule
myelin m.

macrophage
m. immigration
immunocompetent m.

macrophthalmos
macropsia
macroscopic
m. magnetization moment
m. magnetization vector

macrostereognosis
macro stimulation
macrostomia
Macrotec
mactans
Lactrodectus m.

macula, pl. maculae
m. communicans
m. cribrosa
maculae cribrosae
m. cribrosa inferior
m. cribrosa media
m. cribrosa quarta
m. cribrosa superior
m. densa
m. lutea
neuroepithelium of m.
neuroepithelium maculae
m. retinae

macula *(continued)*
    m. sacculi
    m. utriculi
macular
    m. hemianopia
    m. sparing
maculocerebral
maculoneural bundle
Madame Butterfly syndrome
madazolam
MADD
    mixed anxiety depression disorder
    Mothers Against Drunk Driving
made-to-order dream
Mad Hatter syndrome
madness
    impulsive m.
    myxedema m.
    raving m.
Madonna complex
Madonna-prostitute complex
madreporic coral
MADRS
    Montgomery-Åsberg Depression Rating Scale
madurae
    Actinomadura m.
MAE
    Multilingual Aphasia Examination
MAF
    minimal audible field
Maferr Inventory of Masculine Values (MIMV)
Maffucci syndrome
MAG
    myelin-associated glycoprotein
MAG3
    Technescan MAG3
magaldrate
magdalen
Magenblase syndrome
Magendie
    foramen of M.
    M. foramen
    M. law
Magendie-Hertwig
    M.-H. sign
    M.-H. syndrome
Magerl
    M. hook-plate system
    method of M.
    M. plate-screw system
    M. posterior C1-C2 screw fixation
magic
    black m.
    communication m.
    compulsive m.
    cursing m.
    m. fantasy
    M. microcatheter
    new m.
    m. omnipotence
    m. phase
magical thinking

magicked
MAGIC syndrome
magna
    chorda m.
    cisterna m.
    M. Mater
    mega cisterna m.
Magnacal
magnae
    cisterna venae m.
Magnan
    M. sign
    M. trombone movement
magnanimity
MAGNES
    M. magnetic source imaging
    M. MEG system
magnesia
    milk of m.
    Phillips' Milk of M.
magnesium
    m. aluminum hydroxide
    m. carbonate
    m. chloride
    m. gluconate
    m. hydroxide suspension
    m. oxide
    m. pemoline
    m. salicylate
    serum m.
    m. sulfate
Magnes 2500 WH imager
magnet
    Alnico Magneprobe m.
    cobalt samarium m.
    C-shaped resistive m.
    field m.
    main field m.
    permanent m.
    m. quench
    m. reaction
    m. reflex
    resistive m.
    m. shielding
    superconducting m.
    0.5-T superconducting m.
magnetic
    m. apraxia
    m. attraction
    m. crisis
    m. dipole
    m. disk
    m. field
    m. field vector
    m. gradient
    m. induction
    m. moment
    m. personality
    m. resonance (MR)
    m. resonance angiogram
    m. resonance angiography (MRA)
    m. resonance imaging (MRI)
    m. resonance neurography (MRN)
    m. resonance signal
    m. resonance spectroscopy (MRS)

m. shielded cabin
m. source imaging (MSI)
m. stimulator
m. susceptibility
m. susceptibility artifact
magnetism
    animal m.
magnetization
    longitudinal m.
    spatial modulation of m. (SPAMM)
    spin m.
    transverse m.
magnetoelectric stimulation
magnetoelectrophysiology
magnetoencephalogram (M-EEG, MEG)
magnetoencephalograph (MEG)
magnetoencephalography (MEG)
magnetohydrodynamic effect
magnetometer
Magnetom SP 4000 1.5-Tesla system
magnetophosphene
Magnevist
magnification
    loupe m.
magniloquence
magnitude
magnocellular
    m. layer
    m. visual system
magnocellularis
magnum
    M. 800 bed
    foramen m.
magnus
    nucleus raphe m.
Magonate
MAGS
    Multidimensional Assessment of Gains in School
Magstim 200
magusucht
ma huang
MAI
    Marriage Adjustment Inventory
    Morbid Anxiety Inventory
maidica
    psychoneurosis m.
maieusiophobia
MAII
    Milwaukee Academic Interest Inventory
main
    m. d'accoucheur
    m. en crochet
    m. field
    m. field magnet
    m. sensory nucleus of the trigeminus
    M. syndrome
Maine
    jumper disease of M.
    jumping Frenchmen of M.
mainlining
maintenance
    m. dose
    m. drug

drug m.
m. drug therapy
m. function
m. insomnia
m. level
methadone m.
minimum m.
perceptual m.
physiological m.
m. striving
m. treatment
major
    m. attachment figure
    chorea m.
    m. depression
    m. depressive affective psychosis
    m. depressive disorder (MDD)
    m. depressive disorder, recurrent
    m. depressive disorder, single episode
    m. depressive episode (MDE)
    epilepsia m.
    m. epilepsy
    m. histocompatibility complex (MHC)
    m. hypnosis
    m. hysteria
    m. image-distorting level
    m. impairment
    m. impairment of functioning
    m. life activity
    m. life change
    m. loss
    m. motor aphasia
    m. motor seizure
    M. Role Adjustment Scale II
    m. role obligation
    m. role therapy (MRT)
    M. Symptoms of Schizophrenia Scale
    m. tranquilizer
majority society
make believe
make-believe play
makeup
    mental m.
making
    Assessment of Career Decision M. (ACDM)
    m. change test
    competent decision m.
    decision m.
    ineffective decision m.
    tyrannical decision m.
makros
mal
    cerebral m.
    comitial m.
    m. de la rosa
    m. de ojo
    m. de pelea
    grand m.
    haut m.
    petit m.

M

mal *(continued)*
    m. puesto
    m. rosso
malabsorption
    disaccharide m.
    m. syndrome peripheral neuropathy
Malacarne
    M. pyramid
    M. space
maladaptation
maladaption
maladaptive
    m. behavior
    m. behavioral change
    m. defense mechanism
    m. feeling
    m. impulse
    m. pattern of substance abuse
    m. personality
    m. personality pattern
    m. personality trait
    m. psychological change
    m. reaction
    m. reaction to a stressor
    m. response
    m. thought
    m. way
maladjustment
    sexual m.
    social m.
    Structured and Scaled Interview to Assess M. (SSIAM)
    vocational m.
malaise
    postexertional m.
malapert
malar eminence
malaria
    cerebellar m.
    cerebral m.
    therapeutic m.
Malcolm-Rand carbon-composite headholder
maldevelopment
male
    m. alcoholism subtype
    m. biological status
    m. bond
    m. castration
    m. climacteric
    m. climacteric syndrome
    m. dyspareunia
    m. dyspareunia male erectile disorder
    m. erectile dysfunction
    m. genitalia
    m. hypoactive sexual desire disorder
    M. Impotence Test (MIT)
    m. intersex
    m. menopause
    m. orgasm
    m. pattern alopecia
    m. rape

maleate
    chlorpheniramine m.
    clothixamide m.
    dazadrol m.
    fluroxamine m.
    fluvoxamine m.
    methyergol carbamide m.
    methysergide m.
    prochlorperazine m.
    pyrilamine m.
    timolol m.
    velnacrine m.
male-to-female transgender identity
malevolent
    m. behavior
    m. distrust
malformation
    angiographically occult intracranial vascular m. (AOIVM)
    angiographically occult vascular m. (AOVM)
    angiographically visualized vascular m. (AVVM)
    Arnold-Chiari m.
    arteriovenous m. (AVM)
    bone occipital m.
    brain arteriovenous m.
    cavernous m.
    cerebral venous m. (CVM)
    cerebrovascular m.
    Chiari I m.
    Chiari II m.
    Chiari III m.
    congenital m.
    craniofacial m.
    cryptic arteriovenous m.
    cryptic vascular m. (CVM)
    Dandy-Walker m.
    developmental m.
    dural arteriovenous m.
    familial arteriovenous m.
    flocculonodular arteriovenous m.
    Galen-vein m.
    glomus arteriovenous m.
    infratentorial arteriovenous m.
    intraarachnoid leptomeningeal m.
    intracerebral arteriovenous m.
    intracranial vascular m.
    intracranial venous m. (IVM)
    intraorbital arteriovenous m.
    intraspinal vascular m.
    intratentorial m.
    juvenile arteriovenous m.
    Krabbe Arnold-Chiari m.
    medial hemispheric arteriovenous m.
    occipital m.
    occult cerebrovascular m. (OCVM)
    Osler-Weber-Rendu arteriovenous m.
    radiculomeningeal spinal vascular m.
    Spetzler-Martin classification of arteriovenous m.
    split-cord m. (SCM)
    structural m.

supratentorial arteriovenous m.
thalamocaudate arteriovenous m.
vascular m.
vein of Galen m.
Wyburn-Mason arteriovenous m.

Malibu orthosis
malicious mischief
malignancy
   nasopharyngeal m.
malignant
   m. astrocytoma
   m. atrophic papulosis
   m. brain neoplasm
   m. endovascular papillary
     angioendothelioma
   m. external otitis
   m. fibrohistiocytoma
   m. germ cell tumor
   m. glioma
   m. hyperthermia
   m. lymphoma
   m. melanoma
   m. neuroleptic syndrome
   m. neurosis
   m. psychosis
   m. stupor
   m. teratoma
   m. trend
mali-mali
malinger
malingerer
malingering disorder
Malin syndrome
Malis
   M. angled bayonet forceps
   M. bipolar cautery scissors
   M. bipolar instrument
   M. bipolar microcoagulator
   M. brain retractor
   M. CMC-II bipolar coagulator
   M. CMC-III electrosurgical system
   M. curette
   M. dissector
   M. electrocoagulation unit
   M. elevator
   M. irrigating bipolar CMC III
   M. irrigation forceps
   M. jeweler's bipolar forceps
   M. ligature passer
   M. needle holder
   M. nerve hook
   M. neurological scissors
   M. solid state coagulator
   M. vessel supporter
Malis-Jensen micro bipolar forceps
Mallamint
malleability
malleable
   m. endoscope
   m. facial implant (MFI)
   m. microsurgical suction device
   m. multipore suction tube
   m. sucker
malleatory chorea

mallet
   anger m.
   Hajek m.
   Lucae bone m.
malleus
   handle of the m.
malnourished
malnutrition
malocclusion
malodorous
maltreatment
   child m.
   elder m.
malum vertebrale suboccipitale
mama coca
mamillary
   m. body (MB)
   m. body volume
   m. tubercle of hypothalamus
mamillotegmental fasciculus
mamillothalamic
   m. fasciculus
   m. tract
mammalian
   m. hippocampus
   m. teratology
   m. tissue
mammalingus
mammary
   m. body
   m. neuralgia
mammas
   coitus intra m.
MaMT
   Maudsley Mentation Test
man
   effeminate m.
   eight stages of m.
   enlisted m.
   Erikson eight stages of m.
   fellow m.
   personal m.
   wise old m.
managed
   m. care
   M. Care Appropriateness Protocol
management
   M. Appraisal Survey (MAS)
   m. of assaultive behavior (MAB)
   behavioral m.
   clinical m.
   conflict m.
   contingency m.
   crisis m.
   M. Development Profile
   diet m.
   drug m.
   exhaustion m.
   failure of conservative m.
   grief m.
   home-based family m.
   impression m.
   intrathecal pain m.
   m. inventory

M

management *(continued)*
    M. Inventory on Leadership, Motivation and Decision-Making (MILMD)
    multidimensional pain m.
    participative m.
    pharmacological m.
    M. Philosophies Scale (I-V) (MPS)
    M. Position Analysis Test
    psychological m.
    M. Readiness Profile
    reflux m.
    Style of Leadership and M.
    M. Styles Inventory
    M. Transactions Audit (MTA)
manager
    M. Profile Record
    M. Style Appraisal
Managerial Style Questionnaire (MSQ)
MANCOVA
    multivariate analysis of covariance
Mandel Social Adjustment Scale (MSAS)
mandible
    osteotomy of m.
mandibular
    m. condylectomy
    m. fixation
    m. nerve
    m. osteotomy
    m. reflex
    m. retraction
    m. swing technique
mandibulofacial dysostosis
mandibulotomy
mandrel, mandril
    steam-shaping m.
Mandsley Personality Inventory (MPI)
Manegan
Maneon
maneuver
    Adson modified m.
    Bielschowsky m.
    body concept-exploration m.
    body contact-exploration m.
    Buzzard m.
    Dandy m.
    Dix-Hallpike m.
    doll's eye m.
    Gowers m.
    Hallpike m.
    Jendrassik m.
    Phalen m.
    Spurling m.
    tactical m.
    Valsalva m.
manganese
    m. chloride
    m. intoxication
    m. mask
    m. toxicity
    m. toxin
mania
    absorbed m.

    acute alcoholic m.
    acute hallucinatory m.
    adolescent m.
    akinetic m.
    alcoholic m.
    atypical m.
    Bell m.
    biting m.
    chronic alcoholic m.
    collecting m.
    compulsive m.
    copying m.
    dancing m.
    delirious m.
    doubting m.
    ephemeral m.
    epileptic m.
    grumbling m.
    hallucinatory m.
    hysterical m.
    inhibited m.
    joking m.
    m. mitis
    peracute m.
    periodic m.
    m. phantastica infantilis
    postpartum m.
    m. á potu
    primary m.
    puerperal m.
    pure m.
    M. Rating Scale (MRS)
    Ray m.
    reactive m.
    reasoning m.
    m. of recommencement
    recommencement m.
    recurrent m.
    recurrent episode chronic m.
    religious m.
    M. "9" Scale
    seaman m.
    m. secandi
    secondary m.
    senile m.
    single episode chronic m.
    stage 3 m.
    stupor m.
    transitory m.
    unipolar m.
    unproductive m.
maniacal grief reaction
maniac catatonia
mania/hypomania
manic
    m. bipolar disorder
    m. delirium
    m. depression
    m. depressive
    m. episode
    m. excitement
    m. feature
    m. hebephrenia
    m. mood
    m. mood episode

m. mood theme
m. phase
m. psychosis
m. reaction
m. speech
m. state
m. stupor
m. symptom
m. temperament

manic-depressive
m.-d. affective psychosis
m.-d. disorder
m.-d. illness
m.-d. insanity
perplexed-type m.-d.
m.-d. reaction
m.-d. syndrome

manicky
manic-like episode
Manic-State Rating Scale
manifest
m. anxiety
M. Anxiety Scale (MAS)
m. content
m. destiny
m. dream
m. goal
m. tetany

manifesta
spina bifida m.

manifestation
behavioral m.
impostor psychotic m.
neurotic m.
objective m.
physiological m.
psychiatric m.
psychogenic physiological m.
psychophysiologic m.
psychotic m.
subjective m.

manifested disability
manipulability
manipulation
m. communication pattern
cranial nerve m.
emotional m.
environmental m.

manipulative
M. Aptitude Test (MAT)
m. behavior
m. device
m. drive
m. pseudohallucination
m. technique

manipulatory task
man-machine system
manner
bedside m.
detached m.
m.'s deterioration
devious m.
elementary m.
guarded m.
halting m.

inconsistent m.
macho m.
part-object m.
patronizing m.
psychical m.
secretive m.
superior m.
sustained m.
unkempt m.
unusual m.

mannerism
feminine m.
speech m.

mannitol
mannitol-induced cerebral vasodilatation
Mannkopf sign
mannose-terminated-glucocerebrosidase
mannosidase
mannosidosis
alpha m.
beta m.

Mann-Whitney
M.-W. test
M.-W. U Test

manometry
anal sphincter m.

MANOVA
multivariate analysis of variance

manslaughter
involuntary m.

mansoni
Schistosoma m.

Mantel-Haenszel
M.-H. Test
M.-H. Test for Linear Trend

mantle
brain m.
cerebral m.
m. layer
m. sclerosis

mantra
manual
m. communication
Crime Classification M. (CCM)
m. dexterity
m. dominance
M. of Internal Fixation
International Classification of Sleep
  Disorders: Diagnostic and
  Coding M. (ICSD)
m. laborer
m. sadism
m. stimulation
m. target localization
m. vernier scale

manubrium
MAO
monoamine oxidase
MAO inhibitor
MAO spectrophotometric assay

MAOI
monoamine oxidase inhibitor

MAOI-serotonergic agent
Maolate
Maox

M

MAP
　Musical Aptitude Profile
map
　　brain electrical activity m.
　　cognitive m.
　　genetic m.
　　Personal Skills M.
　　phase-contrast m.
Mapap
MAPI
　Millon Adolescent Personality Inventory
maple syrup urine disease (MSUD)
maplike skull
mapping
　　behavioral m.
　　brain electrical activity m. (BEAM)
　　brainstem diencephalic m.
　　cognitive m.
　　cortical m.
　　m. of cortical function
　　electrical stimulation m.
　　electrophysiological m.
　　phase m.
　　radiotherapy brain m.
　　somatosensory m.
　　speech and motor m.
　　stimulation m.
　　Talairach whole-brain m.
　　topographic m.
　　two-dimensional m.
maprotiline
MAPS
　Make-A-Picture-Story
Maranox
marantic endocarditis
marasmic
　　m. female
　　m. state
marasmus
Marateaux-Lamy disease
marathon
　　Gestalt therapy m.
　　m. group psychotherapy
　　m. session
marbled appearance of basal ganglion
Marcaine
march
　　jacksonian m.
Marchac forehead template
Marchant zone
marche a petits plantar aspect
Marchi
　　M. degeneration
　　M. tract
Marchiafava-Bignami
　　M.-B. aminoaciduria
　　M.-B. disease
Marcus
　　M. grading scale for avascular
　　　necrosis
　　M. Gunn
　　M. Gunn phenomenon
　　M. Gunn pupil
　　M. Gunn sign
　　M. Gunn syndrome

mareos
Marezine
marfanoid habitus
Marfan syndrome
Margesic H
margin
　　dural m.
marginal
　　m. consciousness
　　m. function
　　m. gyrus
　　m. intelligence
　　m. layer
　　m. sinus
　　m. thinking
　　m. transvestite
marginalis
　　alopecia m.
marginalization
Marie
　　M. ataxia
　　hereditary cerebellar ataxia of M.
Marie-Foix-Alajouanine
　　M.-F.-A. cerebellar atrophy
　　M.-F.-A. disease
Marie-Robinson syndrome
Marie-Strümpell disease
marijuana, marihuana
　　m. abuse
　　m. delirium
　　m. delusional disorder
　　m. dependence
　　m. flashback
　　m. history
　　m. intoxication
　　m. preparation
　　m. psychosis
　　sinsemillan m.
Marin Amat syndrome
Marinesco-Garland syndrome
Marinesco-Sjögren syndrome
Marinesco succulent hand
Marino
　　M. transsphenoidal curette
　　M. transsphenoidal dissector
　　M. transsphenoidal enucleator
　　M. transsphenoidal hook
Marinol
marital
　　m. adjustment
　　M. Attitudes Evaluation (MATE)
　　M. Communication Scale
　　m. conflict
　　m. counseling
　　m. counselor
　　m. couples group therapy
　　m. discord
　　m. disruption
　　m. dissatisfaction
　　m. history (MH)
　　m. infidelity
　　m. instability
　　m. longevity
　　m. problem
　　M. Satisfaction Inventory

m. schism
m. skew
m. stability
marked
m. anger
m. anxiety
m. decline in academic functioning
m. depression
m. impairment
m. irritability
m. tension
marker
biochemical tumor m.
biologic m.
circadian m.
desmin tumor m.
discoid m.
DNA m.
epithelial membrane antigen
   tumor m.
Factor VIII antigen tumor m.
fiducial m.
fixed m.
gene m.
genetic m.
HHF35 muscle-specific actin
   tumor m.
high-molecular weight cytokeratin
   tumor m.
I m.
lumbar pedicle m.
metallic skin m.
pedicle m.
psychological m.
roentgenographic opaque m.
Schwann cell m.
S-100 tumor m.
surface fiducial m.
thoracic pedicle m.
tumor m.
vimentin tumor m.
marketing personality
Markham-Meyerding hemilaminectomy
   retractor
marking
analog m.
Markov decision analysis model
Marks-Sheehan Phobia Scale
Marlex
Marlow-Crowne Scale (MCS)
Marlowe-Crowne Scale of Social
   Desirability
marmoratus
status m.
Marnal
Maroon-Jannetta dissector
Maroteaux-Lamy
M.-L. disease
M.-L. syndrome
Marplan
Marpres
marriage
M. Adjustment Inventory (MAI)
civil m.
cluster m.

compassionate m.
consanguineous m.
m. contract
m. of convenience
m. counseling
m. counselor
m. encounter
experimental m.
M. and Family Attitude Survey
m. fear
group m.
heterosexual m.
homosexual m.
nonconsanguineous m.
open-end m. (OEM)
pluralism m.
m. response
m. ritual
same-sex m.
sandbox m.
shotgun m.
M. Skills Analysis (MSA)
symbiotic m.
synergic m.
m. therapy
trial m.
unconsummated m.
m. vows
MARS
Mathematics Anxiety Rating Scale
MARS-A
Mathematics Anxiety Rating Scale-
   Adolescents
marsupial notch
Marthritic
martialis
psychopathia m.
Martin
M. nerve root retractor
M. Suicide-Depression Inventory
   (MSDI)
Martin-Bell syndrome
Martinez Assessment of the Basic Skills
Martin-Gruber anastomosis
Martinotti cell
martyr complex
marxist
Maryland Parent Attitude Survey
MAS
MacAndrew Addiction Scale
Management Appraisal Survey
Manifest Anxiety Scale
Maternal Attitude Scale
Memory Assessment Scales
masculation
masculine
m. attitude
m. attitude in female neurotic
m. identity
m. protest
m. social role
masculinity
masculinity-femininity scale
masculinization
Masini sign

M

mask
    death m.
    Hutchinson m.
    manganese m.
masked
    m. affection
    m. anxiety
    m. depression
    m. deprivation
    m. epilepsy
    m. facies
    m. homosexuality
    m. obsession
masking
    background m.
    backward visual m.
    central m.
    effective m.
    m. efficiency
    forward m.
    frequency m.
    initial m.
    maximum m.
    perceptual m.
    peripheral m.
    m. stimulus
    upward m.
    white noise m.
masklike facies
Maslach Burnout Inventory (MBI)
Maslow hierarchy
masochism
    erotogenic m.
    feminine m.
    ideal m.
    mental m.
    moral m.
    sadism and m.
    sexual m.
    social m.
masochist
masochistic
    m. character
    m. character defense
    m. component
    m. personality
    m. personality disorder
    m. ritual
    m. sabotage
    m. sexual activity
    m. sexual behavior
    m. sexual fantasy
    m. sexual urge
    m. wish
    m. wish dream
mass
    m. action theory
    apperceptive m.
    m. behavior
    cerebellar m.
    congenital nasal m.
    m. doubling time
    fat-free m. (FFM)
    hemispheral m.
    m. hysteria

    intraconal m.
    isodense m.
    m. lesion
    m. method
    m. movement
    m. murderer
    parasagittal intracranial m.
    parasellar m.
    m. polarization
    m. psychology
    m. reflex
    serpiginous m.
    m. spectrometer
    suprasellar m.
    supratentorial m.
    m. therapy
massa, gen. and pl. massae
    m. intermedia
massage
    carotid sinus m.
    digital temple m.
    electrovibratory m.
    hydropneumatic m.
    nerve-point m.
    tremolo m.
    vibratory m.
massager
    Cryocup ice m.
masse
    en m.
massed negative practice
masseter
    m. reflex
    m. strength
massive
    m. parallel processing system
      (MPPS)
    m. seizure
Masson
    M. trichrome stain
    M. vegetant intravascular
      hemangioendothelioma
Masson-Fontana stain
massotherapy
MAST
    Michigan Alcoholism Screening Test
master
    m. gland
    M. of Science in Nursing (MSN)
    M. of Social Work (MSW)
Masters and Johnson
mastery
    motive m.
    m. motive
mastication disorder
masticatoria
    monoplegia m.
masticatory
    m. attack
    m. diplegia
    m. nucleus
    m. spasm
mastigophobia
mastocytosis
    systemic m.

mastoid
    m. air cell
    m. antrum
    m. complex
    m. process
    m. retractor
mastoidectomy
    cosmetic m.
mastoiditis
Mast syndrome
masturbation
    anal m.
    compulsive m.
    m. equivalent
    false m.
    infantile m.
    mutual m.
    psychic m.
    symbolic m.
masturbator
masturbatory
    m. activity
    m. pain
MAT
    Manipulative Aptitude Test
    Metropolitan Achievement Test
    Miller Analogies Test
    Motivation Analysis Test
    Music Achievement Test (1-4)
MAT7
    Metropolitan Achievement Test, Seventh
    Edition
Matas
    M. operation
    M. test
match
    leader m.
    perceptual-motor m.
matched group
matching
    M. Familiar Figures Test (MFFT)
    m. hypothesis
    impedance m.
    m. test
    m. and tuning network
MATE
    Marital Attitudes Evaluation
mater
    arachnoid m.
    dura m.
    Magna M.
    pia m.
material
    alloplastic m.
    American Society for Testing
      and M.'s
    ballistic m.
    Elgiloy clip m.
    evidence of intrusion of
      idiosyncratic m.
    evidence of intrusion of private m.
    m. gain
    genetic m.
    Glasflex m.
    m. gratification

    idiosyncratic m.
    interventional m.
    MP-35 clip m.
    nonferrous m.
    Phynox cobalt alloy clip m.
    precollagenous filamentous m.
    m. symbolism
materialization
maternal
    m. attachment
    m. attitude
    M. Attitude Scale (MAS)
    m. behavior
    m. depression
    m. deprivation
    m. desertion
    m. drive
    m. neglect
    m. overprotection
    m. rejection
    m. role
    m. stress
    M. Trait Anxiety Score (MTAS)
maternity blues
math achievement
mathematical
    m. ability
    m. optimization and logical
      dimensioning for radiotherapy
      (MOLDR)
    m. skill
    m. symbol
mathematics
    M. Anxiety Rating Scale (MARS)
    M. Anxiety Rating Scale-
      Adolescents (MARS-A)
    Assessment in M.
    m. disorder
    Individualized Criterion Reference
      Testing M. (ICRTM)
    KeyMath Revised: A Diagnostic
      Inventory of Essential M.
    Test of Cognitive Style in M.
      (TCSM)
mating
    assortive m.
    m. behavior
    nonrandom m.
    random m.
matriarchy
matrices (*pl. of* matrix)
matricide
matrilineal
matrilinear family
matrilocal family
matrix, pl. **matrices**
    Advanced Progressive Matrices
    M. Analogies Test
    Coloured Progressive Matrices
    dural graft m.
    extracellular m. (ECM)
    factor m.
    germinal m.
    Hill Interaction M. (HIM)
    intercellular m.

M

matrix *(continued)*
    m. metalloproteinase (MMP)
    parenchymal m.
    Raven Standard Progressive
      Matrices (RSPM)
    rigid body transformation m.
    Standard Progressive Matrices
    therapeutic m.
matroclinous
matrocliny
matronism
matter
    anisotropy of white m.
    central gray m. (CGM)
    cortical gray m.
    dorsal gray m.
    m. of fact
    gray m.
    long spinal white m.
    midbrain m.
    periaqueductal gray m.
    periventricular gray m. (PVG)
    periventricular white m.
    pontine gray m.
    sclerosis of white m.
    subcortical white m.
    white m.
Mattis Dementia Rating Scale
Mattis-Kovner Scale
mattoid
mattress
    Akros extended care m.
    Akros pressure m.
    eggcrate m.
Matulane
maturate
maturation
    cognitive m.
    m. hypothesis
    m. index
    mitosis, migration and m.
    neurological m.
    pandys m.
    principle of anticipatory m.
    m. rate
    retarded m.
maturational
    m. crisis
    m. lag
mature
    m. defense
    m. minor rule
maturity
    biologic m.
    California Short-Form Test of
      Mental M. (CTMM-SF)
    California Test of Mental M.
      (CTMM)
    emotional m.
    m. fear
    genital m.
    intellectual m.
    mental m.

    m. rating
    m. scale
matutinal
    m. epilepsy
    m. headache
maudlin drunkenness
Maudsley
    M. Mentation Test (MaMT)
    M. Obsessional Compulsive
      Inventory (MOCI)
    M. Obsessional-Compulsive
      Inventory
    M. Personality Inventory (MPI)
Mauthner
    M. cell
    M. sheath
mauve factor
Maxalt-MLT
Maxenon 300 watt xenon light source
Maxfield-Buchholz Social Maturity Scale
   for Blind Preschool Children
maxibolin
Maxicamera
    Gamma M.
maxilla
maxillary
    m. antrum
    m. artery
    m. osteotomy
    m. sinus
    m. vein
maxillectomy
maxillofacial
    m. fracture
    m. plating system
    m. trauma
maxillomandibular artery
maxillotomy
Maxillume 250 watt quartz halogen
   light source
Maxima II TENS unit
maximal
    m. contrast
    m. effect
    m. electroshock (MES)
    m. electroshock seizure (MES)
    m. stimulus
    m. voluntary contraction (MVC)
maximation
    ego m.
maximum
    m. acoustic output
    m. allowable cost (MAC)
    m. intensity pixel reconstruction
    m. masking
    m. permissible dose
    m. recommended human dose
      (MRHD)
    m. security unit
    M. Strength Nytol
    m. tolerated dose (MTD)
Maxwell pair
Maxzide

Mayer
    M. hematoxylin
    M. reflex
Mayerson sign
Mayfield
    M. aneurysm clip
    M. brain spatula
    M. disposable skull pin
    M. fiducial localizer
    M. fixation frame
    M. head clamp
    M. headrest
    M. headrest system
    M. horseshoe headrest
    M. incision
    M. miniature clip applier
    M. neurosurgical skill clamp
    M. pinion
    M. radiolucent base unit
    M. radiolucent headholder
    M. radiolucent headrest
    M. rongeur
    M. skull cap pin
    M. skull-pin headholder
    M. spinal curette
    M. surgical system
    M. temporary aneurysm clip applier
    M. tongs
Mayfield/ACCISS stereotactic device
Mayfield-Kees
    M.-K. headholder
    M.-K. headrest
    M.-K. skull fixation apparatus
    M.-K. table attachment
Mayo
    M. Alzheimer Disease Center/Alzheimer Disease Patient Registry
    M. Asymptomatic Carotid Endarterectomy Study
    M. block anesthesia
    M. Clinic stereotactic robot
    M. scissors
May-White syndrome
Mazanor
maze
    m. behavior
    Elithorn m.
    Foster M.'s
    m. learning
    locomotor m.
    m. test
Mazicon
mazindol
Mazzoni corpuscle
MB
    mamillary body
MBD
    minimal brain dysfunction
MBHI
    Millon Behavioral Health Inventory
MBI
    Maslach Burnout Inventory

MBP
    myelin basic protein
MBSP
    Monitoring Basic Skills Progress
MBTI
    Myers-Briggs Type Indicator
MCA
    middle cerebral artery
    motorcycle accident
    multiple congenital anomaly
MCAB
    Minnesota Clerical Assessment Battery
McAndrews
    M. Alcoholism
    M. Alcoholism Scale (MAC)
MCAT
    Medical College Admission Test
    Minnesota Clerical Aptitude Test
McCain
    M. TMJ cannula
    M. TMJ trocar
McCarthy
    M. reflex
    M. Scales of Children's Ability (MCSA, MSCA)
    M. Screening Test
MCCS
    Minnesota Cocaine Craving Scale
McCullough-Pitts
    M.-P. model
    M.-P. neuron
MCD
    mean consecutive difference
MCDI
    Minnesota Child Development Inventory
McDowell Impairment Index (MII)
MCE
    medical care evaluation
McFadden clip
McFadden-Kees clip
McGill
    M. forceps
    M. Pain Questionnaire (MPQ)
McGregor basal line
m-chlorophenylpiperazine
McKenzie
    M. brain clip forceps
    M. clip-applying forceps
    M. clip-bending forceps
    M. clip-introducing forceps
    M. enlarging bur
    M. hemostasis clip
    M. perforating twist drill
    M. reservoir
    M. silver clip
McLain-Weinstein classification of spinal tumors
McLeod syndrome
McLone and Knepper etiological theory
McMaster
    M. Health Index Questionnaire
    M. Structured Interview of Family Functioning
MCMI
    Millon Clinical Multiaxial Inventory

M

MCMI-II
Millon Clinical Multiaxial Inventory II
MCMI-III
Millon Clinical Multiaxial Inventory III
MCPS
Missouri Children's Picture Series
MCR
mother-child relationship
McRae foramen magnum line
MCRE
Mother-Child Relationship Evaluation
MCS
Marlow-Crowne Scale
MCSA
McCarthy Scales of Children's Ability
MCT
Minnesota Clerical Test
MCTD
mixed connective tissue disease
MCV
mean corpuscular volume
MD
mentally deficient
MDAP
Machover Draw-A-Person Test
MDB
Mental Deterioration Battery
MDD
major depressive disorder
MDDA
Minnesota Differential Diagnosis of
Aphasia
MDE
major depressive episode
MDEA
N-ethyl-3,4-methylenedioxyamphetamine
MDI
Multiscore Depression Inventory
MDQ
Menstrual Distress Questionnaire
MDSO
mentally disordered sex offender
meals
after m. (p.c.)
before m. (a.c.)
skip m.
mean
arithmetic m.
m. arterial blood pressure (MABP)
assumed m.
m. consecutive difference (MCD)
m. corpuscular volume (MCV)
m. deviation
geometric m.
harmonic m.
m. interpotential interval (MIPI)
law of coercion to the
biosocial m.
m. sleep latency
m. sorted difference (MSD)
standard error of the m. (SEM)
statistical m.
meaning
double m.
figurative m.

hidden m.
idiosyncratic m.
latent m.
literal m.
m. reframing
sliding of m.'s
subtle m.
symbolic m.
transferred m.
unknown m.
will to m.
meaningful interpersonal relationship
MEAP
Multiphasic Environmental Assessment
Procedure
measles
m. encephalitis
m. peripheral neuropathy
measles, rubella and zoster (MRZ)
measurable impairment
measure
adjustment m.
Affect Intensity M.
avoidance m.
biologic m.
central tendency m.
m. of central tendency
Functional Independence M. (FIM)
gross motor function m. (GMFM)
Group Achievement
Identification M.
M.'s of Musical Ability
M.'s of Psychosocial Development
(MPD)
psychotherapeutic m.
reactive m.
Schütz M.'s
social adjustment m.
unobtrusive m.
measured
m. capacity
m. dose
m. intelligence
m. stress
measurement
absolute m.
ANB cephalometric m.
Aptitude Interest M.
blood flow m.
educational m.
EEG activity m.
error of m.
IMPA cephalometric m.
instrumental ADL m.
interactive m.
M. of Language Development
mental m.
M-mode electrocardiographic m.
psychomotor m.
reference m.
vasodilator-stimulated rCBF single
photon emission computed
tomographic m.
xenon CT m.

MEAT
Minnesota Engineering Analogies Test
meatus
acoustic m.
external acoustic m.
internal acoustic m.
mebanazine
Mebaral
mebendazole
mebeverine hydrochloride
MECA
Methodology for Epidemiology in
Children and Adolescents
mecamylamine
mechanical
m. anosmia
m. aptitude
m. articulated arm
m. functional loss
m. insufficiency
m. intelligence
m. plate design
m. ventilation
m. vertigo
m. visual loss
mechanicoreceptor
mechanics
body m.
quantum m.
spinal m.
mechanic's hands
mechanism
abnormalities in sleep-wake
timing m.
acting out defense m.
adaptation m.
adaptive defense m.
adjustment m.
airstream m.
alerting m.
arousal boost m.
arousal reduction m.
association m.
balance m.
clamping m.
compensation defense m.
compensatory m.
conversion defense m.
coping m.
m. of correction
cross-correlation m.
defense m.
denial defense m.
direct causative
pathophysiological m.
disengagement m.
displacement defense m.
dissociation defense m.
ego defense m.
escape m.
feedback m.
focusing m.
free radical scavenging m.
gating m.
idealization defense m.

identification defense m.
immune mediated m.
incorporation defense m.
inherited releasing m. (IRM)
inhibition m.
innate releasing m.
input-output m.
intramolecular dipole-dipole m.
intrinsic cell suicide m.
introjection defense m.
Jak-STAT m.
learning m.
maladaptive defense m.
mediating m.
mental m.
mote-beam m.
neutralizing m.
one-way flow m.
outgoing m.
pain m.
paracrine m.
pathophysiological m.
physiological m.
Pollyanna m.
projection defense m.
rationalization defense m.
reaction formation defense m.
regression defense m.
rotating m.
sex arousal m. (SAM)
shared m.
sleep m.
sour-grapes m.
specific pathophysiological m.
spring m.
sublimation defense m.
substitution defense m.
sunburst m.
sweet-lemon m.
symbolization defense m.
triggering m.
undoing defense m.
mechanistic approach
mechanology
mechanophobia
mechanoporation
mechanoreceptor
pacinian m.
Ruffini m.
mechanoreflex
mechanotherapy
mechanothermy
Meckel
M. cave
M. cave lesion
M. ganglion
M. sphenopalatine ganglionectomy
Meckel-Gruber syndrome
meckelii
cavum m.
meclizine, meclozine
meclobemide
meclofenamate sodium
meclofenoxate
Meclomen

M

mecloqualone
meclozine (*var. of* meclizine)
meconism
medazepam hydrochloride
MEDnext **bone dissecting system**
Medea complex
Medelec five-channel neurophysiological
    device
media
    adhesive otitis m.
    contrast m.
    macula cribrosa m.
    otitis m.
    scala m.
medial
    m. accessory olivary nucleus
    m. central nucleus of thalamus
    m. eminence
    m. epicondylectomy
    m. extradural approach
    m. fillet
    m. forebrain bundle
    m. frontal gyrus
    m. geniculate body
    m. geniculate nucleus (MGN)
    m. hemispheric arteriovenous
        malformation
    m. lemniscus
    m. longitudinal bundle
    m. longitudinal fasciculus
    m. longitudinal stria
    m. medullary lamina of corpus
        striatum
    m. nucleus of thalamus
    m. occipitotemporal gyrus
    m. operculum
    m. plantar nerve
    m. posterior choroidal (MPCh)
    m. preoptic nucleus
    m. rectus muscle
    m. root of median nerve
    m. root of optic tract
    m. striate artery
    m. superior temporal (MST)
    m. surface of cerebral hemisphere
    m. temporal lobe
    m. triangle of Hakuba
    m. vestibular nucleus
median
    m. aperture of the fourth ventricle
    center m.
    m. corpectomy
    m. eminence
    m. frontal sulcus
    m. longitudinal fasciculus
    m. mixed nerve action potential
    m. nerve
    m. nerve entrapment
    m. nerve lesion
    m. sagittal plane
    statistical m.
    m. sulcus of fourth ventricle
mediated
    m. function
    m. response

mediating mechanism
mediation
    cognitive m.
    verbal m.
Medica
    Excerpta M.
medicable
Medicaid
medical
    m. advice
    m. anthropology
    m. audit
    m. care
    m. care evaluation (MCE)
    M. College Admission Test
        (MCAT)
    m. condition
    m. discharge
    m. ethics
    m. etiology
    m. examiner
    m. futility
    m. history
    m. jurisprudence
    m. model
    M. Outcomes Study
    M. Outcomes Study Short Form-36
    M. Outcomes Study Short-Form
        General Health Survey Physical
        Functioning Scale
    m. psychology
    m. psychotherapy
    m. record
    M. Research Council (MRC)
    m. review
    m. sociology
    m. stress
    m. syndrome
    m. taper schedule
    m. treatment
medicalization
medical/neurological disorder
medical/psychiatric sleep disorder
medicament
medicamentosa
    alopecia m.
Medicare
medicaster
medication
    m. abuse
    adverse effects of m.
    agonist m.
    agonist/antagonist m.
    antagonist m.
    antianxiety m.
    antidepressant m.
    antiepileptic m.
    antihypertensive m.
    antiparkinsonian m.
    antipsychotic m.
    anxiolytic m.
    beta adrenergic m.
    black-market m.
    m. Cardex
    cheeking m.

conservative m.
cyclic m.
depot m.
experimental m.
hypodermatic m.
intravenous m.
prescription m.
psychoactive m.
sublingual m.
substitutive m.
targeted m.
m. trial
medication-induced
    m.-i. movement
    m.-i. movement disorder, not
      otherwise specified
    m.-i. parkinsonism
    m.-i. postural tremor
    m.-i. tardive dyskinesia
medicinal
    abuse of patent m.'s
    patent m.'s
medicine
    Artificial Intelligence in M. (AIM)
    aviation m.
    behavioral m.
    clinical m.
    comparative m.
    compound m.
    m. concept
    Diploma in Psychological M.
      (DPM)
    domestic m.
    dosimetric m.
    emergency m.
    environmental m.
    experimental m.
    family m.
    folk m.
    forensic m.
    galenic m.
    geriatric m.
    group m.
    hermetic m.
    holistic m.
    hyperbaric m.
    Indian m.
    legal m.
    mental m.
    neo-Hippocratic m.
    Office of Alternative M. (OAM)
    patent m.
    physical m.
    preclinical m.
    prescription-only m. (POM)
    preventive m.
    psychologic m.
    psychosomatic m. (PSMed)
    rational m.
    social m.
    socialized m.
    suggestive m.
medicolegal
medicomechanical
medicopsychological

medicopsychology
medicosocial
Medicus bed
Mediflow pillow
medifoxamine
Medigesic
Medihaler ergotamine
mediodorsal
    m. globus pallidus interna
    m. nucleus
mediopubic reflex
Medipain 5
Medipren
Medisorb drug delivery system
MediSpacer
    Airlife M.
meditatio mortis
meditation
    Transcendental M. (TM)
medium
    culture m.
    Eagle minimum essential m.
    high-osmolar contrast m.
    iopamidol contrast m.
    spiritual m.
    m. trance
    ^{133}XeSPECT contrast m.
mediumistic hypothesis
mediumship
medley
    chance m.
Medos-Hakim valve
Medos valve
Medpacific LD 5000 Laser-Doppler
   perfusion monitor
Medralone Injection
Medrol Oral
medronate
    technetium 99m m.
medroxyprogesterone acetate
MED system
Medtronic SynchroMed implantable
   pump
medulla, pl. medullae
    adrenal m.
    m. oblongata
    m. spinalis
    ventrolateral m. (VLM)
medullar
medullaris
    conus m.
medullary
    m. artery
    m. canal
    m. center
    m. chemoreceptor
    m. cone
    m. glioma
    m. infarction
    m. layers of thalamus
    m. narcosis
    m. plate
    m. protrusion
    m. pyramidotomy
    m. raphe

M

medullary *(continued)*
    m. raphe nucleus
    m. sheath
    m. sign
    m. solitary tract
    m. striae of the fourth ventricle
    m. stria of the thalamus
    m. substance
    m. syndrome
    m. teniae
    m. tube
    m. tumor
medullated nerve fiber
medullation
medullectomy
medulloblastoma
    desmoplastic m.
    familial m.
    vermian m.
medullocell
medulloepithelioma
medullomyoblastoma
medullovasculosa
    zona m.
M-EEG
    magnetoencephalogram
Mees line
Meeting Street School Screening Test (MSSST)
mefenamic acid
mefexamide
Meffill-Palmer Scale
Mefoxin
MEG
    magnetoencephalogram
    magnetoencephalograph
    magnetoencephalography
    MEG head-based coordinate system
    MEG sensor
    MEG sensorimotor mapping coordinate
mega
    m. cisterna magna
    The M. Test
    M. Tilt and Turn bed
Mega-Air bed
megacephalic
megacephalous
megacolon
    psychogenic m.
megadolichobasilar anomaly
megadolichovertebrobasilar anomaly
megalencephaly
    unilateral m.
megalgia
megaloblastic anemia
megalocephaly, megalocephalia
megaloencephalic
megaloencephalon
megaloencephaly
megalographia, megalography
megalomania
megalomanic, megalomaniac
megalopapilla

megalophobia
megalopia, megalopsia
    m. hysterics
Megasedan
megavitamin therapy
me generation
meglumine
    diatrizoate m.
    m. diatrizoate
    iocarmate m.
    iodipamide m.
    m. iothalamate
    ioxaglate m.
    m. metrizoate
megohm
megrim
Meige
    M. disease
    M. syndrome
meiosis
Meissner
    M. corpuscle
    M. plexus
melancholia
    acute m.
    affective m.
    m. affective psychosis
    m. agitata
    agitated m.
    m. attonita
    chronic m.
    climacteric m.
    convulsive m.
    m. hypochondriaca
    hypochondriacal m.
    intermittent m.
    involutional m.
    menopausal m.
    panphobic m.
    paranoid m.
    paretic m.
    puberty m.
    puerperal m.
    reactive m.
    recurrent m.
    m. religiosa
    senile m.
    sexual m.
    m. simplex
    m. stuporosa
    stuporous m.
    suicidal m.
    m. vera
    m. with delirium
    m. zoanthropy
melancholic, melancholiac
    m. constitutional type
    m. depression
    m. feature
    m. involutional reaction
    m. mood
    m. personality
melancholicus
    raptus m.
melancholium

melanin pigment
melanocyte
melanocyte-inhibiting factor
melanocytoma
 meningeal m.
melanoma
 familial m.
 malignant m.
 ocular m.
melanosis
 neurocutaneous m.
melanotic
 m. neuroectodermal tumor
 m. neuroectodermal tumor of
 infancy
melarsoprol
MELAS
 mitochondrial encephalomyopathy with
 lactic acidosis and strokelike episode
 MELAS syndrome
melatonin test
meliorism
melioristic
melissophobia
melitensis
 Brucella m.
melitracen
Melkersson-Rosenthal syndrome
Mellanby effect
Mellaril-S
mellitus
 diabetes m.
Melmon and Rosen classification
melomania
melperone
melphalan
Melzack and Wall gate theory
member
 couple m.
 family m.
 team m. (TM)
membrana, gen. and pl. **membranae**
 m. basilaris
 m. cerebri
 m. limitans gliae
 m. versicolor
membrane
 arachnoid m.
 m. attack complex (MAC)
 basement m. (BM)
 basilar m.
 brain synaptic m.
 caroticooculomotor m.
 diencephalic m.
 Fielding m.
 hymenal m.
 m. ion channel
 m. of Liliequist
 m. lipolysis
 lithium action on m.'s
 mesencephalic m.
 neuronal m.
 pial-glial m.
 postsynaptic m.
 m. potential

Preclude spinal m.
presynaptic m.
Reissner m.
sarcolemma m.
spiral m.
vestibular m.
membranectomy
membranous cochlea
memoriae
 lapsus m.
memory
 m. ability
 affect m.
 m. afterimage
 amnesia loss of m.
 m. amplification
 anterograde m.
 anterograde loss of m.
 M. Assessment Scales (MAS)
 associative m.
 auditory m.
 autobiographical m.
 automatic m.
 behavioral m.
 m. bias
 biographical m.
 body m.
 m. buffer
 buffer m.
 childhood trauma m.
 coast m.
 conscious m.
 constructive m.
 decreased m.
 m. defect
 m. deficit
 delayed m.
 m. for design (MFD)
 m. difficulty
 Digit-Symbol and Incidental M.
 m. disability
 m. disorder
 m. distortion
 distributed m.
 disturbance of m.
 m. disturbance
 echoic m.
 m. encoding
 episodic m.
 explicit m.
 eye m.
 false m.
 m. falsification
 figural m.
 flashbulb m.
 m. gap
 genetic m.
 m. hallucination
 hyperesthetic m.
 iconic m.
 m. illusion
 illusory m.
 m. image
 immediate m.
 impaired m.

M

memory *(continued)*
    m. impairment
    implicit m.
    incidental m.
    lack of m.
    m. lapse
    logical m.
    long-term m. (LTM)
    m. loss
    loss of biographical m.
    minute m.
    non-autobiographical m.
    overconsolidation of m.
    painful m.
    panoramic m.
    m. passage
    permanent m.
    photographic m.
    physiological m.
    primary m.
    priming m.
    m. questionnaire
    m. quotient (MQ)
    racial m.
    recall m.
    m. recall
    recent past m.
    recognition m.
    recursive autoassociative m.
    m. reference
    remote m.
    replacement m.
    m. retention
    retrograde m.
    retrograde loss of m.
    retrospective gaps in m.
    m. romance
    rote m.
    m. scale
    m. score
    screen m.
    m. screen
    selective m.
    semantic m.
    senile m.
    sequence m.
    sequential m.
    short-term m. (STM)
    short-term visual m.
    m. skill
    somatic m.
    m. span
    state-dependent m.
    m. storage
    stress effect on m.
    subconscious m.
    m. symbol
    m. for symbolic unit (MSU)
    m. test
    m. theory
    m. trace
    m. training
    m. transfer
    traumatic m.

    unconscious m.
    verbal working m.
    veridical m.
    visual spatial m.
    working m.
Memory-for-Designs Test
MEMPHIS
    Memphis Educational Model Providing
        Handicapped Infant Services
Memphis Educational Model Providing
  Handicapped Infant Services
  (MEMPHIS)
MEN
    multiple endocrine neoplasia
        MEN I
        MEN II
        MEN III
menace
Menadol
menage à trois
mendacious
mendacity
Mendel
    M. instep reflex
    M. law
Mendel-Bechterew reflex
mendelian
    m. law
    m. rules of inheritance
mendelism
mendicancy
    pathologic m.
menerik
Menezes
    method of M.
Mengo encephalitis
Meni-D
Ménière
    M. disease
    M. syndrome
meningeal
    m. angiomatosis
    m. artery
    m. biopsy
    m. carcinoma
    m. carcinomatosis
    m. diverticula
    m. fibrosis
    m. hemangiopericytoma
    m. hernia
    m. melanocytoma
    m. neurosarcoidosis
    m. neurosyphilis
    m. pachymeningitis
    m. plexus
    m. sign
    m. tumor
    m. vein
meningeocortical
meningeorrhaphy
meninges (*pl. of* meninx)
meningioangiomatosis
meningioma
    angioblastic m.
    angioplastic m.

angle m.
bifrontal malignant m.
cavernous sinus m.
clinoidal m.
clival m.
clivus m.
complex m.
convexity m.
craniospinal m.
cutaneous m.
cystic intraparenchymal m.
dermal m.
endotheliomatous m.
en plaque m.
epidural m.
extracranial m.
extradural m.
falcotentorial m.
falx m.
fibroblastic m.
frontal convexity m.
intracranial m.
intradural-extradural m.
intraorbital m.
intraparenchymal m.
intraspinal m.
intraventricular m.
meningothelial m.
metastasizing m.
olfactory groove m.
m. of the olfactory groove
parasagittal m.
parasellar tentorial m.
parietal m.
perioptic m.
peritorcular m.
petroclinoclival m.
petroclival m.
petroclivotentorial m.
pineal m.
posterior fossa m.
m. prostaglandin level
psammomatous m.
sphenoid ridge m.
sphenoid wing m.
sphenoorbital m.
spinocranial m.
subdural m.
subfrontal m.
suprasellar m.
tentorial apex m.
tentorial leaf m.
thoracic m.
torcular m.
transitional m.
tuberculum sellae m.
meningioma-associated cerebral edema
meningiomatosis
meningis (*gen. of* meninx)
meningism
meningismus psychosis
meningitic
m. hydrocephalus
m. neurosyphilis
m. streak

meningitidis
Neisseria m.
meningitis, pl. **meningitides**
Acanthamoeba m.
actinomycosis lymphocytic m.
acute purulent m.
aseptic uremic m.
bacterial m.
basilar m.
benign lymphocytic m.
beta hemolytic streptococcus m.
blastomyocotic m.
candidal m.
cerebrospinal m.
CMV m.
coccidioidal m.
coxsackievirus m.
cryptococcal m.
echinomycosis lymphocytic m.
echovirus m.
enterovirus m.
eosinophilic m.
epidemic cerebrospinal m.
epidural m.
external m.
Haemophilus influenzae m.
herpes zoster m.
idiopathic m.
internal m.
leptospirosis lymphocytic m.
luetic m.
lymphomatous m.
meningococcal m.
Mollaret m.
mumps m.
Naegleria m.
neoplastic m.
occlusive m.
ornithosis lymphocytic m.
otitic m.
paragonimiasis lymphocytic m.
pneumococcal m.
serosa m.
serous m.
m. serous spinalis
sinogenic m.
staphylococcal m.
streptococcal m.
subacute m.
sympathetic m.
syphilitic m.
tubercular m.
tuberculous m.
viral m.
meningitophobia
meningocele
lateral thoracic m.
lumbar m.
sacral m.
spurious m.
traumatic m.
meningocerebral cicatrix
meningococcal meningitis
meningocortical
meningocyte

M

meningoencephalitis
    acute primary hemorrhagic m.
    amebic m.
    arbovirus m.
    bacterial m.
    biundulant m.
    eosinophilic m.
    herpetic m.
    mumps m.
    murine typhus m.
    nonvasculitic autoimmune
      inflammatory m. (NAIM)
    primary amebic m. (PAM)
    Rocky Mountain spotted fever m.
    sterile m.
    syphilitic m.
meningoencephalocele
    basal m.
    ethmoidal m.
    sphenoethmoidal m.
    sphenoorbital m.
    sphenopharyngeal m.
    transsphenoidal m.
meningoencephalomyelitis
meningoencephalopathy
meningohypophyseal
    m. branch
    m. trunk (MHT)
meningomyelitis
meningomyelocele
meningopolyneuritis
    tick-borne m.
meningorachidian vein
meningoradicular
meningoradiculitis
meningorhachidian, meningorrhachidian
meningorrhagia
meningothelial
    m. appearance
    m. meningioma
meningothelioma
meningotyphoid fever
meningovascular
    m. neurosyphilis
    m. syphilis
meninx, gen. **meningis,** pl. **meninges**
    m. fibrosa
    m. primitiva
    m. serosa
    m. tenuis
    m. vasculosa
meniscus, pl. **menisci**
    tactile m.
    m. tactus
menkeiti
Menkes
    M. disease
    M. kinky hair syndrome
Menninger Clinic Treatment
  Intervention Project
menopausal
    m. depression
    m. distress
    m. melancholia
    m. paranoid psychosis

    m. paranoid reaction
    m. paranoid state
    m. paraphrenia
menopause
    adjustment reaction of m.
    female m.
    male m.
    m. neurosis
menses
mens rea
menstrual
    m. cycle
    m. disorder
    M. Distress Questionnaire (MDQ)
    m. migraine
    m. molimen
    m. period
menstrual-associated syndrome
menstruation
    psychogenic painful m.
mensuration
mental
    m. aberration
    m. ability
    m. abuse
    m. act
    m. activity
    m. age (MA)
    m. agitation
    m. agraphia
    m. anesthesia
    m. apparatus
    m. asthenia
    m. asymmetry
    m. ataxia
    m. audition
    m. blind spot
    m. block
    m. capacity
    m. capacity evaluation
    m. chemistry
    m. chronometry
    m. claudication
    m. competence
    m. competency
    m. concept
    m. confusion
    m. control
    m. defect
    m. deficiency
    m. deficit
    m. depression
    m. derangement
    m. deterioration
    M. Deterioration Battery (MDB)
    m. development
    m. disability
    m. discipline
    m. disease
    m. disorder due to alcoholism
    m. disorder due to a general
      medical condition
    M. Disorders Due to a General
      Medical Condition Not Elsewhere
      Classified

m. disorganization
m. disturbance
m. dynamism
m. dysfunction
m. eclipse
m. ego
m. energy
m. evolution
m. excitement
m. exhaustion
m. faculty
m. fatigue
m. fog
m. function
m. growth
m. healing
m. health
m. health clinic (MHC)
m. health counselor
m. health resource
m. health worker
m. hospital
m. hygiene
m. image
m. imagery
m. impairment
m. impression
m. inhibition level
m. institution
m. insufficiency
m. life
m. makeup
m. masochism
m. maturity
m. measurement
M. Measurements Yearbook
  (MMY)
m. mechanism
m. medicine
m. metabolism
m. obtundation
m. pain
m. process
m. psychoneurotic disorder
m. retardation (MR)
m. retardation, severity unspecified
m. scale
m. scotoma
m. set
m. shock
m. stability
m. state
m. status
m. status change
m. status cognitive task
m. status examination (MSE)
m. status examination report
  (MSER)
M. Status Questionnaire (MSQ)
m. status schedule (MSS)
m. status test
m. stress
m. structure
m. subnormality
m. subnormality disorder

m. tension
m. testing
m. topography
trichorrhexis nodosa with m.
m. upset
mental-hygiene clinic
mentalis
mentalism
mentality
dominant m.
mentally
m. deficient (MD)
m. deranged
disordered m.
m. disordered offender
m. disordered sex offender
  (MDSO)
m. handicapped
m. ill
m. impaired
m. incompetent
m. obtunded
m. retarded
m. retarded child
m. retarded persons' rights
mental-patient organization
Mentane
mentation
altered m.
change in m.
normal m.
m. rate
subjective m.
menticide
mentis
abalienatio m.
alienatio m.
compos m.
non compos m.
mentulomania
menu
registration m.
Menzel
M. olivopontocerebellar atrophy
M. olivopontocerebellar degeneration
MEP
motor evoked potential
multimodality evoked potential
meparfynol
mepazine acetate
Mepergan Fortis
meperidine
analog of m. (PEPAP)
m. hydrochloride
m. and promethazine
mephenesin
mephenoxalone
mephenytoin
mephobarbital
Mephyton Oral
mepivacaine
MEPOP
mitochondrial encephalomyopathy with
  sensorimotor polyneuropathy,
  ophthalmoplegia, and paralysis

M

meprobamate
    aspirin and m.
meralgia paresthetica
mercurial
    m. behavior
    m. tremor
mercurialis
    erethism m.
mercury
    m. encephalopathy
    m. intoxication
    m. peripheral neuropathy
    m. poisoning
    m. toxicity
    m. toxin
mercy killing
mere-exposure effect
merergasia
merergastic
meretricious
mergent
    partial m.
    total m.
merger state
merinthophobia
merit
    m. ranking
    m. rating
Merkel
    M. corpuscle
    M. law
    M. tactile cell
    M. tactile disk
Merocel tampon
merorachischisis, merorrhachischisis
merosmia
MERRF
    myoclonus epilepsy with ragged-red fiber
    MERRF syndrome
Merrill-Palmer
    M.-P. Scale
    M.-P. Scale of Mental Tests
MERRLA syndrome
Mersiline tape
mertazepine
Mertens Visual Perception Test (MVPT)
mertiatide
    technetium 99m m.
Merzbacher-Pelizaeus disease
MES
    maximal electroshock
    maximal electroshock seizure
Mesantoin
mesaxon
mescaline
    methylenedioxymethamphetamine and m.
mescalism
mesem
    per m.
mesencephalic
    m. cistern
    m. flexure
    m. hemorrhage

    m. infarction
    m. membrane
    m. nucleus of the trigeminus
    m. premotor structure
    m. reticular formation
    m. sign
    m. tegmentum
    m. tractotomy
    m. tract of trigeminal nerve
    m. transition area
    m. vein
mesencephalitis
mesencephalon
    m. aqueduct
    ventral m.
mesencephalooculofacial angiomatosis
mesencephalotomy
mesenchymal drift
mesenchyme
    paraxial m.
mesenteric vasculitis
mesh
    Dumbach cranial titanium m.
    tantalum m.
    Teflon m.
mesial
    m. aspect of temporal lobe
    m. cerebral structure
    m. cortex
    m. hemisphere
    m. part of frontal lobe
    m. prefrontal cortex
    m. temporal epileptogenic lesion
    m. temporal sclerosis (MTS)
mesial-frontal cortex
mesiobasal
    m. limbic epilepsy
    m. temporal lobe
mesiotemporal lobe
mesmeric crisis
mesmerism
mesmerize
mesmeromania
mesoblastic sensibility
mesocortical dopaminergic system deficit
mesocorticolimbic
mesoderm
mesoglia
mesoglial cell
mesolimbic
    m. dopamine
    m. dopamine system
mesolimbic-mesocortical tract
mesolobus
mesomorph
mesomorphic constitutional type
mesoneuritis
    nodular m.
mesontomorph
mesopsychic
mesorhachischisis
mesoridazine besylate
mesothelioma
    fibrous m.

message
- conflicting m.
- covert m.
- dichotic m.
- diotic m.
- hidden m.
- m. integration
- mixed m.
- overt m.
- subliminal m.
- two-sided m.

messenger
- chemical m.
- eukaryotic m.
- external chemical m. (ECM)
- lithium action on first m.
- lithium action on second m.
- m. ribonucleic acid (mRNA)
- m. RNA
- second m.

messiah complex
messianic
messorole
Mestinon
- M. Injection
- M. Oral

mesulergin
mesylate
- benztropine m.
- bromocriptine m.
- Desferal M.
- dihydroergotamine m.
- ergoloid m.
- ergot m.
- pergolide m.
- reboxetine m.
- tirilazed m. (TM)

MET
- Minimum Essentials Test

meta-analysis
metabolic
- m. abnormality
- m. acidosis
- m. alkalosis
- m. amyloidosis
- m. anomaly
- m. anoxia
- m. asymmetry
- m. coma
- m. defect
- m. derangement
- m. disease organic psychosis
- m. disorder
- m. disturbance
- m. dysperception
- m. encephalitis
- m. encephalopathy
- m. energy
- m. flow uncoupling
- m. lesion
- m. nutritional model
- m. tolerance
- m. tremor
- m. volume depletion

metabolism
- arachidonic acid m.
- basal m.
- brain m.
- carbohydrate m.
- cerebral glucose m.
- glutamate m.
- inborn error of m.
- left parietal association m.
- lipoid m.
- mental m.
- metal m.
- mineral m.
- myelin m.
- neuronal m.
- nitrogen m.
- nucleic acid m.
- phosphate m.
- porphyrin m.
- purine m.
- pyrimidine m.

metabolite
- dopamine m.
- neurotransmitter m.
- phosphoinositol m.

metacarpohypothenar reflex
metacarpothenar reflex
metachlorophenylpiperazine
metachromatic
- m. leukodystrophy (MLD)
- m. leukodystrophy neuropathy

metaclazepam
metacommunication
metaerotism
metaethics
metaevaluation
metagenesis
metagnosis
Metahydrin
metaiodobenzyl-guanidine (MIBG)
metakinesis
metal
- m. electrode
- m. failure
- m. fatigue
- m. intoxication
- m. metabolism
- m. neuropathy
- m. plate

metalanguage
metalinguistic
metallic
- m. cranioplasty
- m. foreign body
- m. otologic implant
- m. skin marker
- m. tremor

metalloendoprotease
metallophobia
metalloproteinase
- matrix m. (MMP)

metal-produced neuropathy
metameric nervous system
metamorphic paralogia
metamorphopsia

M

metamorphosis
   behavioral m.
   m. sexualis paranoica
metamotivation
Metamucil
metapathology
metapelet
metaphase
metaphoric
   m. language
   m. paralogia
   m. symbolism
metaphrenia
metaphysics
metaplexus
metapore
metapramine
Metaprel
metaproterenol sulfate
metapsyche
metapsychiatry
metapsychics
metapsychological profile
metapsychology
metaraminol bitartrate
metastasis, pl. metastases
   brain m.
   cerebral m.
   choroidal m.
   distant m.
   drop m.
   dural m.
   extradural spinal m.
   hemorrhagic m.
   leptomeningeal m.
   miliary brain m.
   ocular m.
   retrobulbar orbital m.
   spinal m.
metastasizing meningioma
metastatic
   m. breast cancer
   m. disease
   m. tumor
   m. tumor removal
Metastron Injection
metasyncrisis
metatabi
metatarsalgia
metatarsal reflex
metathalamus
metatrophia
metatrophy
metatropism
metaxalone
metempirical
metempsychosis
metencephalic
metencephalon
metenkephalin
metenkephalin-like immunoreactivity
meteorophobia
meter
   biofeedback m.

BioTrainer exercise m.
   clip force m.
methacrylate
   dimethylaminoethyl m.
methadone
   m. addiction
   m. block
   m. center
   m. dependence
   m. hydrochloride
   m. maintenance
   m. maintenance treatment
Methadose
methamphetamine
   m. abuse
   m. addiction
   m. dependence
   m. hydrochloride
methamphetamine-like substance
methandrostenolone
methanol poisoning
methantheline
methapyrilene
methaqualone hydrochloride
metharbital
methazolamide
methcathinone and cocaine
Methedrine
methemoglobin
methenolone
methicillin sodium
methilepsia
methiodal
methocarbamol and aspirin
method
   adjustment m.
   m. of administration
   adoptee family m.
   analytic m.
   anecdotal m.
   Anel m.
   Antyllus m.
   approximation m.
   aristotelian m.
   m. of ascertainment
   avidin-biotin-complex-peroxidase m.
   behavior m.
   biofeedback m.
   biographical m.
   bisensory m.
   Brasdor m.
   bundle-nailing m.
   case m.
   cathartic m.
   Cavalieri direct estimator m.
   chewing m.
   classification m.
   complete-learning m.
   confluence m.
   m. of constant stimuli
   correlational m.
   cross-sectional m.
   m. of defining criterion
   m. of delivery
   m. of Dickman

Dubois m.
equal-and-unequal-cases m.
equal-appearing-intervals m.
equivalent m.
exosomatic m.
experimental m.
expression m.
m. factor
factor comparison m.
family m.
formal m.
Freud cathartic m.
genetic m.
m. of Glees
gradation m.
Hilton m.
historical m.
hole preparation m.
immobilization m.
immunoperoxidase m.
impedance m.
impression m.
informal m.
introspective m.
job component m.
Jung m.
kinesthetic m.
Kirby-Bauer disk diffusion m.
m. of Klüver
Leboyer m.
m. of limits
linguistic-kinesic m.
longitudinal m.
m. of Magerl
mass m.
m. of Menezes
metric m.
Milligan annihilation m.
minimal-change m.
minimum separable m.
Montessori m.
Moore m.
need-press m.
nonpurging m.
numerical cipher m.
observational m.
obstruction m.
operant m.
optimal m.
part-learning m.
Pavlov m.
pedigree m.
phase-contrast m.
plateau m.
preferred m.
proband m.
Projective Assessment of Aging M.
purging m.
Purmann m.
Q m.
recall m.
reconstruction m.
reduction m.
relearning m.
review m.

rhythm m.
Rochester m.
Scarpa m.
School Apperception M.
scientific m.
Seldinger m.
sibship m.
m. of successive approximation
suicide m.
swallow-belch m.
synthetic m.
systematic m.
Tadoma m.
Thane m.
Trager m.
Turnbull m.
Wardrop m.
Westergren m.
Winston-Lutz m.
Wintrobe m.
xenon m.
zeta m.
methodical chorea
methodologic
methodology
    M. for Epidemiology in Children
      and Adolescents (MECA)
    Q m.
methods analysis
methohexital sodium
methomania
methotrexate
    m. poisoning
    m. sodium
methotrimeprazine
methoxamine
3-methoxy-4-hydroxyphenylglycol
  (MHPG)
5-methoxy-3,4-
  methylenedioxyamphetamine (MMDA)
methprylon
methsuximide
methyclothiazide
    m. and deserpidine
    m. and pargyline
methyergol carbamide maleate
methyl
    m. alcohol
    m. alcohol addiction
    m. alcohol peripheral neuropathy
    m. alcohol poisoning
    m. alcohol toxicity
    m. alcohol toxin
    m. dopa
methylal
methylated spirit addiction
methylcobalamin
β-methylcrotonylglycinuria
methyldichlorarsin
methyldimethoxyamphetamine
methyldopa
    alpha m.
    chlorothiazide and m.
    m. and hydrochlorothiazide

M

methylene
  m. blue
  m. chloride
  m. dioxyamphetamine
methylenedioxymethamphetamine
  m. and mescaline
  m. and phencyclidine
3,4-methylenedioxymethamphetamine
methylenedioxy-5-
  methoxyphenylisopropylamine
methylglucamine
  iodipamide m.
methylglyoxal *bis*-**guanylhydrazone**
  (MGBG)
methylmalonic
  m. acidemia
  m. aciduria
  m. aminoaciduria
methylmethacrylate
  m. block
  m. cranioplastic plug
  m. cranioplasty
  m. spacer
methylmorphine
methylphenidate
  m. challenge test
  m. hydrochloride
methylphenobarbital
methylphenyltetrahydropyridine
methylprednisolone
  m. acetate
  m. and sodium succinate
methyltestosterone
5-methyltetrahydrofolate
methylxanthine
methylxanthine-induced postural tremor
methyprylon
5-methy-S-adenosylmethionine
methysergide maleate
metiapine
Meticorten
metoclopramide
metocurine iodide
metolazone
metonymic distortion
metonymy
metopic
  m. craniectomy
  m. suture
  m. synostosis
metopon hydrochloride
metopoplasty
metoprolol tartrate
Metrazol
  M. shock therapy
  M. shock treatment
metric method
Metrifonate
metrizamide
  m. contrast study
  m. myelography
metrizamide-enhanced CT
metrizamide-filled balloon
metrizoate
  meglumine m.

metrizoic acid
metromania
metronidazole
metronoscope
Metropolitan
  M. Achievement Test (MAT)
  M. Achievement Test, Seventh
    Edition (MAT7)
  M. Language Instructional Test
  M. Readiness Test (MRT)
metyrapone test
Metz
  Bad Wildungen M. (BWM)
Metzenbaum scissors
mevinolin
Mexate-AQ
mexazolam
mexiletine
Meyer
  M. loop
  M. sublaminar wiring technique
  M. theory
Meyer-Archambault loop
Meyerding
  M. laminectomy blade
  M. laminectomy retractor
Meyerding-Scoville blade
Meyer-Kendall Assessment Survey
  (MKAS)
Meynert
  M. cell
  M. commissure
  M. decussation
  M. fasciculus
  M. layer
  nucleus basalis of M.
  M. retroflex bundle
MF
  multifactorial model
MFD
  memory for design
  monorhythmic frontal delta
  MFD activity
  MFD Test
  MFD waves on
    electroencephalogram
MFFT
  Matching Familiar Figures Test
MFI
  malleable facial implant
MFMN
  multifocal motor neuropathy
MG
  myasthenia gravis
MGBG
  methylglyoxal *bis*-guanylhydrazone
MGN
  medial geniculate nucleus
MGUS
  monoclonal gammopathies of
    undetermined significance
MH
  marital history

MHAQ
Modified Health Assessment
Questionnaire
MHC
major histocompatibility complex
mental health clinic
MHI
mild head injury
MHPA
Minnesota-Hartford Personality Assay
MHPG
3-methoxy-4-hydroxyphenylglycol
MHT
meningohypophyseal trunk
MHT artery
MIA
missing in action
multiple intracranial aneurysms
Miacalcin
M. Injection
M. Nasal Spray
Miami
M. Acute Care collar
M. J collar
mianserin
miasma theory
MIBG
metaiodobenzyl-guanidine
iodine 131 MIBG
Michele vertebral body trephine
Michel scalp clip
Michigan
M. Alcoholism Screening Test
(MAST)
M. English Language Assessment
Battery
M. Picture Inventory
M. Picture Stories
M. Screening Profile of Parenting
micosis
paralytic m.
spastic m.
Micrainin
micrencephalia, micrencephaly
micrencephalous
MICRO
M. E irrigation kit
M. 100 irrigation kit
Micro
M. link fiber
M. Plus screw
microabscess
candidal m.
microadenoma
cystic m.
pituitary m.
microadenomectomy
selective m.
Micro-Aire blade
microalbuminuria
microaneurysm
microangiopathy
mineralizing m.
microartery forceps
microball hook

microbiophobia
microbipolar forceps
microbore Tygon tube
microcatheter
Magic m.
m. system
Tracker m.
variable stiffness m.
microcephalic idiocy
microcephalus
microcephaly
encephaloclastic m.
schizencephalic m.
microcheilia
MicroChoice electric powered surgical system
microcirculation
nerve root m.
microcirculatory
m. perfusion
m. red cell flux
microclip
Yasargil m.
microcoagulator
Malis bipolar m.
microcoil
endothelin-1 platinum-Dacron m.
Hilal m.
platinum m.
platinum-Dacron m.
microconnector
titanium m.
microcosm of words
microcrania
microcup forceps
microcurette, microcuret
Yasargil m.
microcyst
microdactyly
microdialysis
intrahippocampal m.
micro-dipole
microdiscectomy, microdiskectomy
microdissector
Rhoton m.
Yasargil m.
microdrill
high-speed m.
microdysgenesia
micro-eCVR-FV circulation
microelectrode
m. recording
m. technique
microembolism
cerebral m.
silent m.
microencephaly
microendoscopic discectomy system
microendoscopy
intraoperative m.
MicroFet 2 muscle test
microfibrillar collagen
microforceps
Yasargil m.
microgeny

M

microglia cell
microgliacyte
microglioma
microgliomatosis
microgliosis
microglobulin
micrognathia
micrograph
    electron m.
micrographia
micrography
microguidewire
microgyria
microinfarction
Micro-K
    M.-K. 10
    M.-K. 10 Extencaps
    M.-K. LS
microknife
    Karlin m.
microlumbar discectomy
micromania
micromaniacal delirium
microMax drill system
micromelia
micromesh
    titanium m.
microneurovascular anastomosis
Micro-One needle holder
micro-operative
    m.-o. procedure
    m.-o. treatment
microorchidism
    primary m.
microorganism
Micropaque
microphobia
microphonia
microphthalmos
microphthalmos-corneal opacity-spasticity
    syndrome
micropituitary rongeur
microplate
    C-shaped m.
    H-shaped m.
    Leibinger m.
    L-shaped m.
    Luhr m.
    Storz Microsystem m.
    Synthes Microsystem m.
Micro-Plus titanium plating system
microporosity
microprobe
    Jacobson m.
micropsia
micropsy
micropsychophysiology
micropsychosis
micropsychotic episode
microptic
    m. delirium
    m. hallucination
microrasp
    Yasargil m.

microretractor
    flexible arm m.
microronguer
    Kerrison m.
microsaw
    oscillating m.
    Zimmer m.
microscissors
    curved conventional m.
    straight m.
    Yasargil m.
microscope
    GPR robot neurosurgical m.
    Hitachi scanning electron m.
    JedMed TRI-GEM m.
    LSM-GB200 confocal laser
        scanning m.
    MKM m.
    Moller m.
    Omni 2 m.
    operating m.
    operating m. VM 900
    operative m.
    Philips 400 transmission
        electron m.
    pneumatic m.
    surgical m.
    VARIMIC 900 m.
    Zeiss-Contraves operating m.
    Zeiss MKM m.
    Zeiss OpMi CS-NC2 surgical m.
    zoom m.
microscopic level
microscopy
    electron m.
    scanning electron m. (SEM)
microseme
microsleep
microsmatic
microsmic
microsocial engineering
Micro-Softplate
micro-Soft Stream sidehole infusion
    catheter
microsomal isoenzyme metabolism
    profile
microsomia
    hemifacial m.
    heredo-familial essential m.
MicroSpan Capnometer 8800
microstaple
    Barouk m.
microstomia
Microsulfon
microsurgery
    m. discectomy
    endoscope-controlled m. (ECM)
    m. forceps
    m. needle holder
microsurgical
    m. DREZotomy
    m. neck clipping
    m. procedure
    m. thoracoscopic vertebrectomy
microsuture

microsystem
    Sun m.
micro-thin plastic fiber
Micro-Three microsurgery instrument
microtia
microtome
    Leica vibrating knife m.
Microtrast
microtubule
    cytoplasmic m.
microtubule-associated protein
microtubule-binding
    m.-b. domain
    m.-b. repeat
Micro-Two
    M.-T. forceps
    M.-T. needle holder
    M.-T. scissors
Micro-Vac suction catheter
microvascular
    m. anastomosis
    m. clip
    m. decompression (MVD)
    m. forceps
microvesicular steatosis
microvolt
Microzide
Micro-Z neuromuscular stimulator
MICS
    Mother/Infant Communication Screening
micturate
micturition
    m. disorder
    m. reflex
    m. syncope
Midamor
Midas
    M. punishment
    M. Rex bur guard
    M. Rex craniotome
    M. Rex craniotomy saw
    M. Rex drill
    M. Rex power system
midazolam
midbrain
    m. deafness
    m. dysfunction
    m. infarction
    m. lesion
    m. matter
    m. reticular formation (MRF)
    rostral m.
    m. tegmentum
    m. vesicle
midcervical flexion myelopathy
midchildhood
Midchlor
middle
    m. adolescence
    m. adulthood
    m. age
    m. age pedophilia
    m. cerebellar peduncle
    m. cerebral artery (MCA)
    m. cervical ganglion

    m. column injury
    m. cranial fossa
    m. cranial fossa approach
    m. cranial fossa cyst
    m. ear impedance
    m. fossa craniotomy approach
    m. fossa exposure
    m. fossa floor/petrous dissection
    m. fossa transtentorial
      translabyrinthine approach
    m. frontal convolution
    m. frontal gyrus
    m. frontal sulcus
    m. game
    m. ground
    m. insomnia
    m. radicular syndrome
    m. temporal convolution
    m. temporal gyrus
    m. temporal sulcus
midface
    m. degloving
    m. degloving technique
    m. retrusion
midfrontal
midget bipolar cell
midgracile
midlife crisis
midline
    anatomical m.
    m. exposure
    m. fusion defect
    m. incision
    m. lesion
    m. myelotomy
    m. nuclei
    m. shift
    m. spinal approach
    m. syndrome
midnight oil
Midol
    M. 200
    M. IB
    M. PM
    M. PMS
midpoint to meatal line
midpontine
    m. syndrome
    m. wakefulness
Midrin
midsagittal image
Midtown Manhattan Study
midwinter insomnia
mifepristone
Mignon delusion
migraine
    abdominal m.
    acephalgic m.
    acute confusional m. (ACM)
    affective prodrome of m.
    aphasic m.
    autosomal dominant m.
    basilar artery m.
    Bickerstaff m.

M

migraine *(continued)*
    Brobdingnagian disorder of visual perception in m.
    catamenial m.
    catastrophic m.
    ciliary m.
    circumstantial m.
    classic m.
    cluster m.
    common m.
    complicated m.
    confusional m.
    m. equivalent
    Miller-Fisher syndrome
    facial m.
    facioplegic m.
    familial hemiplegic m. (FHM)
    fulgurating m.
    Harris m.
    m. headache
    hemiparesthetic m.
    hemiplegic m.
    late-life m.
    menstrual m.
    ocular m.
    ophthalmic m.
    ophthalmoplegic m.
    paroxysmal m.
    pectoralgic m.
    m. personality
    retinal m.
    seasonal m.
    syncopal m.
    tension m.
    unilateral m.
    vestibular m.
    m. with aura (MA)
    m. without aura (MwoA)
migraine-induced
    m.-i. infarction
    m.-i. stroke
migraine-neuralgia analgesic
migraineur
migrainoid
migrainous
    m. aura
    m. cranial neuralgia
    m. infarction
    m. syndrome
Migralam
Migranal Nasal Spray
migrans
    erythema chronicum m. (ECM)
    visceral larva m.
migrate
migrateur
Migratine
migration
    m. abnormality
    m. adaptation
    adjustment following m.
    cultural adjustment following m.
    electrode m.
    graft m.

    instrument m.
    interfibrillary m.
    intrafascicular m.
    Luque rod m.
    neuronal m.
    perifascicular m.
    m. psychosis
    rod m.
    transendothelial m.
    vertical m.
migratory arthralgia
MII
    McDowell Impairment Index
Mikulicz operation
mild
    anxiety reaction, m. (ARM)
    m. ataxia
    m. depression
    m. disability
    m. head injury (MHI)
    m. mental retardation
    m. mental subnormality
    m. neurocognitive disorder
mildly ungrammatical construction
milenperone
Miles
    M. ABC Test of Ocular Dominance
    M. Nervine Caplets
    M. punch biopsy forceps
milestone
    developmental m.
    m. event
miliary
    m. aneurysm
    m. brain metastasis
milieu
    sociocultural m.
    structured m.
    therapeutic m.
    m. therapy
milipertine
militaristic
military
    M. Environment Inventory
    m. forensic psychiatry
    m. history
    m. neurosis
    m. psychology
militate
milk
    heroin mixed with powdered m.
    m. of magnesia
milk-ejection reflex
Millard-Gubler syndrome
mille
    m. pattes screw
    m. pattes technique
Miller
    M. Analogies Test (MAT)
    M. Assessment for Preschoolers
Miller-Dieker syndrome
Miller-Fisher
    M.-F. test

M.-F. variant of Guillain-Barré syndrome

Miller-Yoder Language Comprehension Test

Milles syndrome

Millet neurological test instrument

Mill Hill Vocabulary Scale

Milligan
M. annihilation method
M. dissector

Millipore
M. filter
M. suture

millivolt

Millon
M. Adolescent Clinical Inventory (MACI)
M. Adolescent Personality Inventory (MAPI)
M. Behavioral Health Inventory (MBHI)
M. Clinical Multiaxial Inventory (MCMI)
M. Clinical Multiaxial Inventory II (MCMI-II)
M. Clinical Multiaxial Inventory III (MCMI-III)

Mills dressing

MILMD
Management Inventory on Leadership, Motivation and Decision-Making

Milontin

Milpath

milrinone

Miltex rib spreader

Milton
M. disease
M. model

Miltown-600

Milwaukee
M. Academic Interest Inventory (MAII)
M. brace

mimesis

mimetic
m. chorea
m. convulsion
m. paralysis
m. seizure

mimic
m. convulsion
m. seizure
m. spasm
m. speech
m. tic

mimica
asemasia m.

mimicry
molecular m.

mimmation

MIMV
Maferr Inventory of Masculine Values

Minamata disease

minaprine

minatory

Mincep
Minnesota Comprehensive Epilepsy Program

mind
m. blindness
m. control
group m.
interfaceable m.'s
miniature m.
mortal m.
open m.
m. pain
prelogical m.
m. reading
state of m.
subconscious m.
wandering m.

mind-altering drug

mind/body dualism

mind-body problem

minded
social m.

mindedness
psychological m.
small m.
weak m.

mind's eye

mine postural tremor

mineralizing microangiopathy

mineral metabolism

Minerin

miner's
m. cramp
m. nystagmus

Minerva
M. jacket
M. vest

mini
m. applier
M. International Neuropsychiatric Interview
M. Inventory of Right Brain Injury (MIRBI)
M. Orbita plate
M. Würzburg implant system
M. Würzburg screw

miniaccomplishment

miniature
m. mind
m. system

minilaparotomy

minimal
m. audible field (MAF)
m. audible pressure
m. brain damage
m. brain dysfunction (MBD)
m. cue
m. personal hygiene
m. provocation
m. residual symptom
m. risk

minimal-change method

Minimax 200 watt light source

Mini-Mental State Examination (MMSE)

minimization of emotional detail

M

minimum
m. dose
M. Essentials Test (MET)
m. incision surgery (MIS)
m. maintenance
m. separable method
minimum-change therapy
miniplate
m. strut
titanium m.
mini-Sugita clip
Minizide
Minnesota
M. Child Development Inventory (MCDI)
M. Clerical Aptitude Test (MCAT)
M. Clerical Assessment Battery (MCAB)
M. Clerical Test (MCT)
M. Cocaine Craving Scale (MCCS)
M. Comprehensive Epilepsy Program (Mincep)
M. Differential Diagnosis of Aphasia (MDDA)
M. Engineering Analogies Test (MEAT)
M. Importance Questionnaire (MIQ)
M. Impulsive Disorder Interview Model for Compulsive Buying
M. Impulsive Disorders Interview
M. Infant Development Inventory
M. Job Description Questionnaire (MJDQ)
M. Mechanical Assembly Test (MMAT)
M. Multiphasic Personality Inventory (MMPI)
M. Multiphasic Personality Inventory, Adolescent (MMPI-A)
M. Multiphasic Personality Inventory, Second Edition (MMPI-2)
M. Occupational Classification System (MOCS-III)
M. Paper Form Board Test (MPFBT)
M. Percepto-Diagnostic (MPD)
M. Percepto-Diagnostic Test (MPDT)
M. Preschool Scale
M. Rate of Manipulation Test
M. Satisfaction Questionnaire (MSQ)
M. Satisfaction Scale (MSS)
M. Scholastic Aptitude Test (MSAT)
M. Spatial Relations Test (MSRT)
M. Teacher Attitude Inventory (MTAI)
M. Test for the Differential Diagnosis of Aphasia (MTDDA)
M. Twin Family Study

M. Vocational Interest Inventory (MVII)
Minnesota-Hartford Personality Assay (MHPA)
minocycline
minor
m. analysis
chorea m.
m. depressive disorder
emancipated m.
epilepsia m.
m. epilepsy
forceps m.
m. hypnosis
m. hysteria
m. image-distorting level
m. penalty
m. stimulus
m. tranquilizer
minority
m. group
m. group psychiatry
minoxidil
mint leaf
minute memory
miosis
paralytic m.
spastic m.
MIPI
mean interpotential interval
MIQ
Minnesota Importance Questionnaire
Mira
M. cautery
M. Mark III cranial drill
M. Mark III cranial drill set
M. Mark V craniotome
M. Mark V craniotome set
mira
mirabile
rete m.
MIRAGE
Multi-Institutional Research in Alzheimer Genetic Epidemiology
MIRAGE study
Mirapex
MIRBI
Mini Inventory of Right Brain Injury
mirror
m. drawing
m. exercise
m. fear
m. focus
Hardy 5 mm m.
m. image
one-way m.
m. sign
m. speech
m. technique
m. transference
m. of Wernicke
m. writing
mirroring
crossover m.
m. the transference

mirror-writing
mirtazapine tablet
miryachit, myriachit
MIS
    minimum incision surgery
misala
misandry
misanthropia
misanthropy
misattribution of guilt
misbisection
mischief
    malicious m.
mischievous behavior
misconception
    illusionary m.
misdirection phenomenon
miserotia
misery perfusion
misfortune
    future m.
Mishler valve
misinformation effect
Miskimins Self-Goal-Other Discrepancy Scale
Miskimon cerebellar retractor
misocainia
misogamy
misogynist
misogyny
misologia
misology
misoneism
misonidazole
misopedia, misopedy
misophobia
misperception
    sleep state m.
misplaced objects test
misprision
misregistration
    flow m.
    oblique flow m.
missed abortion
missense mutation
missile
    m. basing
    m. effect
    m. injury
missing in action (MIA)
missing-parts test
Mississippi Scale for Combat-Related Posttraumatic Stress Disorder
Missouri
    M. Auditory Learning Test
    M. Children's Picture Series (MCPS)
    M. Kindergarten Inventory of Developmental Skills
    M. Occupational Card Sort
mistake
    basic m.
    category m.
mistrust
    basic m.

    trust vs. m.
    m. versus trust
MIT
    Male Impotence Test
    Motor Impersistence Test
Mitchell
    M. disease
    M. treatment
mite
    delirium m.
Mithracin
mitigated echolalia
mitior
    epilepsia m.
mitis
    catatonia m.
    dementia paranoides m.
    epilepsia m.
    mania m.
mitissima
mitochondria
mitochondrial
    m. condensation
    m. cytopathy
    m. deoxyribonucleic acid analysis
    m. DNA
    m. encephalomyelopathy
    m. encephalomyopathy
    m. encephalomyopathy with lactic acidosis and strokelike episode (MELAS)
    m. encephalomyopathy with sensorimotor polyneuropathy, ophthalmoplegia, and paralysis (MEPOP)
    m. encephalopathy
    m. free radical generation
    m. myopathy
    m. neurogastrointestinal encephalomyopathy (MNGIE)
    m. neuropathy
mitogen
    pokeweed m.
mitosis
mitosis, migration and maturation
mitotane
mitotic
    m. segregation
    m. spindle apparatus (MSA)
mitral
    m. annulus calcification
    m. cell
    m. valve disorder
    m. valve prolapse (MVP)
Mitran Oral
mitten pattern
Mivacron
mivacurium
mix
    case m.
mixed
    m. anxiety depression disorder (MADD)
    m. aphasia
    m. bipolar affective psychosis

M

mixed *(continued)*
    m. bipolar disorder
    bipolar I disorder, most recent episode m.
    m. cerebral dominance
    m. compulsive psychasthenia
    m. compulsive states psychasthenia
    m. conduct/emotional disturbance
    m. conduct/emotional disturbance adjustment disorder
    m. conduct/emotional disturbance adjustment reaction
    m. conduct/emotions conduct disorder
    m. connective tissue disease (MCTD)
    m. design
    m. development developmental delay disorder
    m. disturbance stress reaction
    m. emotions/conduct adjustment reaction
    m. feature
    m. foot dominant
    m. germ cell tumor
    m. glioma
    m. growth hormone-prolactin cell adenoma
    m. headache
    m. laterality
    m. manic-depressive psychosis
    m. message
    m. model
    m. mood episode
    m. motive game
    m. nerve
    m. neurosis
    m. paralysis
    m. paralytic conversion reaction
    paranoid-affective organic psychosis, m.
    m. paranoid/affective organic psychotic state
    m. phobic
    m. presentation
    m. psychoneurosis
    m. psychopathic personality
    m. receptive-expressive language
    m. receptive-expressive language disorder
    m. reinforcement
    m. schizophrenia
    m. sleep apnea
    m. specific developmental disorder
    m. stress reaction
    m. symptom picture with perceptual disturbance
    m. type
    m. type epilepsy
mixed-mood state
mixed-type
    m.-t. delusion
    m.-t. psychopathic
    m.-t. schizophrenia

mixoscopia bestialis
mixoscopy
Mixter ventricular needle
mixture
    m. approach
    color m.
    epinephrine-anesthetic m.
    m. theory
    thrombogenic ferrous m.
Mizuho surgical Doppler
MJDQ
    Minnesota Job Description Questionnaire
MKAS
    Meyer-Kendall Assessment Survey
MKM
    MKM fiducial
    MKM microscope
    MKM stereotactic image-guided system
    MKM workstation
ML4
    mucolipidosis, type IV
MLD
    metachromatic leukodystrophy
MLQ
    Multifactor Leadership Questionnaire
MLSI
    multiple line-scan imaging
MMAT
    Minnesota Mechanical Assembly Test
MMDA
    5-methoxy-3,4-methylenedioxyamphetamine
MMECT
    multimonitored electroconvulsive treatment
M-mode electrocardiographic measurement
MMP
    matrix metalloproteinase
MMPI
    Minnesota Multiphasic Personality Inventory
    MMPI Code Type
    Harris-Lingoes Subscales - MMPI
MMPI-2
    Minnesota Multiphasic Personality Inventory, Second Edition
MMPI-A
    Minnesota Multiphasic Personality Inventory, Adolescent
    MMPI-Adolescent
MMPI-Adolescent (MMPI-A)
MMSE
    Mini-Mental State Examination
MMTIC
    Murphy-Meisgeier Type Indicator for Children
MMY
    Mental Measurements Yearbook
M'Naghten
    M. rule
    M. test
MNC
    mononuclear cell

mneme
    phylogenetic m.
mnemenic, mnemic
    m. hypothesis
    m. theory
mnemism
mnemonic
    m. strategy
    m. system
    m. trace
MNGIE
    mitochondrial neurogastrointestinal
      encephalomyopathy
    myo-neuro-gastrointestinal
      encephalopathy
mobbing behavior
Mobidin
mobile spasm
mobility
    m. disability
    geographic m.
    horizontal m.
    M. Inventory for Agoraphobia
    m. of libido
    upward m.
    vertical m.
mobilization reaction
Möbius
    M. disease
    M. syndrome
mobocracy
mob psychology
MOCI
    Maudsley Obsessional Compulsive
      Inventory
moclobemide
MOCS-III
    Minnesota Occupational Classification
      System
modafinil
modal adaptive task
modality
    gustatory sensory m.
    sensory m.
    tactile sensory m.
    therapeutic m.
    treatment m.
    visual sensory m.
modality-specific
modams
mode
    enactive m.
    field-cognition m.
    m. of inheritance
    parataxic m.
    protaxic m.
    prototaxic m.
    quiet wakefulness m.
model
    active-passive m.
    adversary m.
    awareness training m.
    behavioral m.
    biopsychosocial m.
    Blos developmental m.

Bowen m.
Bowlby developmental m.
brain m.
categorical m.
cognitive m.
contingency m.
corpectomy m.
cost-reward m.
dimensional m.
dual-arousal m.
ecological systems m.
educational-socialization m.
ego m.
Erickson developmental m.
fixed m.
friendship m.
m. game
Gesell developmental m.
guidance-cooperation m.
helping m.
homeostatic m.
human-potential m.
m.'s of illness
job characteristics m.
jurisprudential teaching m.
Kohlberg developmental m.
laboratory-method m.
learning m.
lumbar spine m.
Markov decision analysis m.
McCullough-Pitts m.
medical m.
metabolic nutritional m.
Milton m.
mixed m.
multifactorial m. (MF)
Munich cooperative m.
mutual participation m.
parent-child m.
M. Penal Code
PLISSIT M.
psychodynamic-experiential m.
psychological m.
m. psychosis
public health m.
random m.
role m.
single-major-locus m.
SML m.
social integration-disintegration m.
socially intimate m.
stress-diathesis m.
M. TC2-64B pulsed-range gated
    Doppler instrument
teacher-student m.
vitro matrigel m.
modeled behavior
modeling
    abstract m.
    behavioral m.
    covert m.
    m. exercise
    participant m.
moderate
    m. ataxia

M

moderate *(continued)*
    m. depression
    m. difficulty
    m. mental retardation
    m. mental subnormality
moderator variable
Modern Occupational Skills Test (MOST)
modification
    active m.
    behavior m. (B-mod)
    carbonyl m.
    C-D screw m.
    environment m.
    environmental m.
    Harriluque sublaminar wiring m.
    hebbian m.
    interference m.
    Jacobs locking hook spinal rod
       instrumentation m.
    posttranslational m.
modified
    m. ECT therapy
    m. Fischer classification
    m. Gilsbach technique
    m. Harrington rod
    M. Health Assessment
       Questionnaire (MHAQ)
    m. McGill Pain Questionnaire
    M. Rankin Scale
    m. Robert Jones dressing
    M. Simpson Dyskinesia Scale
    M. Vygotsky Concept Formation
       Test
    M. Word Learning Test (MWLT)
modifier
    biologic response m.
Modirax
Modiur
modular instrumentation
modulated affect
modulation
    affect m.
    amplitude m. (AM)
    emotional m.
    impaired affect m.
    interneuronal calcium m.
    pain m.
module
    CUSA electrosurgical m. (CEM)
    Family History Assessment M.
    Nd:YAG m.
Modulock posterior spinal fixation
Moduretic
modus operandi
Moe
    M. alar hook
    M. rod
    M. spinal hook
    M. square-ended hook
    M. system
MOG
    myelin/oligodendrocyte glycoprotein
Mogadon

mogiarthria
mogigraphia
mogilalia
mogiphonia
moieties
Moire topographic scoliosis assessment
moisture
    m. fear
    m. fear-molar approach
MOJAC
    mood, orientation, judgment, affect,
    content
molar
    m. approach
    m. behavior
MOLDR
    mathematical optimization and logical
    dimensioning for radiotherapy
molecular
    m. approach
    m. behavior
    m. genetics
    m. layer of cerebellar cortex
    m. layer of cerebral cortex
    m. layer of retina
    m. layers of olfactory bulb
    m. mimicry
    m. neuropathology
    m. neurosurgery
    m. psychiatry
molecule
    adenine m.
    cell adhesion m. (CAM)
    glucose transporter m.
    nerve-cell adhesion m. (NCAM)
    neural cell adhesion m. (NCAM)
    second-messenger m.
molestation
    child m.
molester
    child m.
molesting
    child m.
molilalia
molimen, pl. **molimina**
    menstrual m.
molindone hydrochloride
Mollaret meningitis
Moller microscope
mollis
    chorea m.
molluscum, pl. **mollusca**
    m. fibrosum
molysmophobia
moment
    gradient m.
    macroscopic magnetization m.
    magnetic m.
    three-point bending m.
momentum
    angular m.
momism
Monakos tract
Monakow
    M. bundle

M. nucleus
M. syndrome
monandry
monarchical
monastic
monathetosis
monaxonic
Monday morning headache
monde
beau m.
Mondonesi reflex
MO needle
monesthetic
monestrous
mongolian
m. idiocy
m. idiot
mongolism
translocation m.
mongoloid
monism
monistic
monitor
body m.
Camino fiberoptic ICP m.
Camino OLM ICP m.
Cortexplorer cerebral blood
flow m.
Datex infrared CO_2 m.
Doppler ultrasound m.
ICP m.
intracranial pressure Express
digital m.
Laserflow blood perfusion m.
Laserflow BPM^2 real time cerebral
perfusion m.
Medpacific LD 5000 Laser-Doppler
perfusion m.
Moor MBF3D m.
Nerve Integrity M. 2
PAM2 m.
PAM3 m.
SentiLite EEG m.
SentiLite neurological m.
Sentinel-4 neurological m.
Steritek ICP mini m.
Xomed nerve integrity m.-2
Xomed-Treace nerve integrity m.-2
monitoring
anesthetic m.
baseline m.
M. Basic Skills Progress (MBSP)
bedside multimodality m.
behavioral m.
cranial nerve m.
distortion of inferential
behavioral m.
Doppler m.
Doppler precordial end-tidal carbon
dioxide m.
ECoG m.
end-tidal nitrogen m.
exaggeration of inferential
behavioral m.
inferential behavioral m.

intracerebral depth electrode m.
intraoperative facial nerve m.
intraoperative neurophysiological m.
neurophysiological m.
m. probe
real-time m.
scalp EEG m.
screw position perioperative m.
somatosensory evoked potential m.
spinal cord function
intraoperative m.
subdural ICP m.
video/EEG m.
monkey therapist
monoamine
m. hypothesis
m. oxidase (MAO)
m. oxidase inhibitor (MAOI)
m. oxidase inhibitor agent
m. oxidase inhibitor-serotonergic
agent
m. oxidase inhibitor-tricyclic agent
monoaminergic fiber
monobactam
monobloc advancement
monochorea
monoclonal
m. gammopathies of undetermined
significance (MGUS)
m. gammopathy
m. gammopathy of unknown
significance (MUGUS)
monocular
blindness m.
m. blindness
m. heads-up display imaging
system
m. visual loss
monocyclic antidepressant
monocystic craniopharyngioma
monocyte
monocytogenes
Listeria m.
monoecious
monoecism
monoethylamide
lysergic acid m.
monogamous relationship
monogenetic disorder
Mono-Gesic
monogyny
monoideic somnambulism
monoideism
monologue
collective m.
monomania
affective m.
emotional m.
m. incendiare
intellectual m.
monomaniac
monomelic
m. amyotrophy
m. muscular atrophy
m. paresis

M

monomer
    acrylamide m.
monomoria
monomorphic activity
monomyoplegia
mononeural, mononeuric
mononeuralgia
mononeuritis multiplex
mononeuropathy
    entrapment m.
    m. multiplex
    phrenic m.
mononoea
mononuclear
    m. cell (MNC)
    m. leukocyte isolation
    m. pleocytosis
    m. pleocytosis of cerebrospinal
      fluid
mononucleosis peripheral neuropathy
mononucleotide
    flavin m. (FMN)
monoparesis
monoparesthesia
monopathophobia
monophagia
monophagism
monophasia
monophasic
    m. action potential
    m. illness
Monophen
monophobia
monophosphate
    adenosine m.
    cyclic adenosine m. (cAMP)
    cyclic guanosine m. (cGMP)
    guanosine m.
monoplegia
    crural m.
    m. masticatoria
monoplegic disorder
monopolar
    m. cautery
    m. coagulation
    m. depression
    m. electrocautery
    m. electrode
    m. tissue forceps
monopolization communication pattern
monoportal ventriculoscopy
monopsychosis
monorhythmic
    m. frontal delta (MFD)
    m. frontal delta activity
    m. sinusoidal delta activity
monos
monoscenism
monosexual
monosodium glutamate
monosomy
    chromosome (9_p) m.
monospasm
monosyllabic speech
monosymptom

monosymptomatic
    m. circumscription
    m. hypochondriacal
    m. hypochondriacal psychosis
    m. hypochondriasis
    m. neurosis
monosynaptic
    m. reflex arc
    m. segmental reflex response
monotheism
monotherapy
    lithium m.
Monotic Word Memory Test (MWMT)
monotone speech
monotonic
monotonous speech
monotreme
monotropic
monoxide
    carbon m. (CO)
monozygotic
    m. twin (MZ)
Monreal reflex hammer
Monro
    M. aqueduct
    foramen of M.
    M. foramen
    M. sulcus
monster fear
montage
    bipolar m.
    reference m.
Montessori method
**Montgomery-Åsberg Depression Rating
  Scale (MADRS)**
monticulus, pl. **monticuli**
mood
    abnormal m.
    absence of depressed m.
    absence of elevated m.
    adjustment disorder with
      depressed m.
    adjustment disorder with mixed
      anxiety and depressed m.
    m. and/or affect (M/A)
    anxious m.
    change in m.
    m. change
    m. congruent
    dejected m.
    depressed m.
    depth of m.
    m. deterioration
    m. disorder
    m. disorder due to a general
      medical condition
    m. disorder with atypical features
    m. disorder with catatonic features
    m. disorder with melancholic
      features
    m. disorder with postpartum onset
    m. disorder with rapid cycling
    m. disorder with seasonal pattern
    m. disturbance
    duration of m.

dysphoric m.
elevated m.
m. elevator
m. episode
erratic m.
euphoric m.
euthymic m.
expansive m.
fluctuations of m.
imperative m.
indicative m.
m. induction
intensity of m.
irritable m.
labile m.
m. lability
lowered m.
manic m.
melancholic m.
nondepressed m.
normal range of m.
M. and Physical Symptoms Scale
  (MPSS)
m. profile
prominent irritable m.
pure m.
quality of m.
m. reactivity
m. shift
somber m.
m. stabilizer
subjunctive m.
m. swing
m. swings affective psychosis
m. swing syndrome
m. symptom
m. symptomatology
unpleasant m.
usual nondepressed m.
vascular dementia with
  depressed m.
mood-altering
  m.-a. drug
  m.-a. substance
mood-balance
mood-congruent
  m.-c. delusion
  m.-c. hallucination
  m.-c. psychotic feature
mood-cyclic disorder
mood-elevating drug
mood-incongruent
  m.-i. delusion
  m.-i. hallucination
  m.-i. psychotic feature
**mood, orientation, judgment, affect,
  content (MOJAC)**
mood-stabilizing agent
moon
  m. facies
  m. phase
Mooney
  M. Faces Closure Test

M. Problem Checklist (MPC,
  MPCL)
M. Test
Moonies
moon-phase study
Moonwalker
Moore
  M. method
  M. syndrome
Moor MBF3D monitor
mooseri
  Rochalimaea m.
Moos Family Environment Scale
moperone
moral
  m. anxiety
  m. ataxia
  m. behavior
  m. code
  m. conduct
  m. consistency
  m. deficiency
  m. deficiency personality disorder
  m. development
  m. hazard
  m. idiocy
  m. imbecility
  m. independence
  m. insanity
  m. judgment
  m. masochism
  m. oligophrenia
  m. outrage
  m. philosophy
  m. pride
  m. principle
  m. realism
  m. relativism
  m. right
  m. treatment
  m. turpitude
  m. value
morale
  acquired folie m.
  folie m.
  group m.
moralism
morality
  m. of constraint
  m. of conventional role conformity
  m. of cooperation
  interpersonal m.
  m. of self-accepted moral principle
  sphincter m.
Morand spur
moratorium
  psychosexual m.
  psychosocial m.
morbid
  m. anxiety
  M. Anxiety Inventory (MAI)
  m. dependency
  m. desire
  m. doubt
  m. fear

M

morbid *(continued)*
    m. idea
    m. imitation
    m. impulse
    m. jealousy
    m. obesity
    m. perplexity
    m. response
    m. risk
    m. rumination
    m. thirst
morbidity
    perinatal m.
morbidostatic
morcellation
morcellement
morcellize
mordancy
mordant
Morel-Kraepelin disease
mores
    sexual m.
    social m.
Morgagni
    M. disease
    M. syndrome
Morgagni-Adams-Stokes syndrome
morgana
    fata m.
Morganella morganii
morganii
    Morganella m.
moria
moribund state
Morita
    M. psychotherapy
    M. therapy
morning
    m. bright light therapy
    m. drinking
    m. glory seeds dependence
    m. glory syndrome
    m. headache
morning-after pill
moronity
Moro reflex
morose
morosis
morpheme
    bound m.
    circumfix m.
morphine
    m. abuse
    m. addiction
    cocaine, heroin and m.
    m. dependence
    heroin and m.
    m. hydrochloride
    intracerebroventricular administration
      of m. (ICVM)
    m. sulfate
    m. withdrawal
morphine-like action
morphine-naloxone test

morphinic
morphinism
morphinium sulfate
morphinomania
morphinotherapy
    intrathecal m.
morphiomania
morphogenetic
morphological rule
morphology
    planum temporale m.
    Test for Examining Expressive M.
      (TEEM)
morphometric analysis
morphometry
    brain m.
    pedicle m.
morphosynthesis
Morquio
    M. disease
    M. syndrome
Morscher
    M. anterior cervical plate
    M. titanium cervical plate
Morse sternal spreader
morsicatio
    m. buccarum
    m. labiorum
morsus humanus
mortal
    m. combat
    m. mind
    m. sin
mortality
    actual m.
    infant m.
    prediction of m.
    m. rate
    reproductive m.
    m. trend
mortido
mortis
    in articulo m.
    meditatio m.
mortisemblant
Morton
    M. neuralgia
    M. neuroma
Morvan
    M. chorea
    M. disease
mosaicism
Mosaic Test
MOSP
    myelin/oligodendrocyte-specific protein
mosquito
    m. clamp
    m. forceps
Moss-Harms basket
Moss-Miami spinal instrumentation
mossy
    m. cell
    m. fiber
MOST
    Modern Occupational Skills Test

mota/moto
mote-beam mechanism
moth-eaten alopecia
mother
>M.'s Against Drunk Driving (MADD)
>M. Card
>complete m.
>m. complex
>m. confessor
>m. fixation
>m. flgure
>foster m.
>good-enough m.
>host m.
>m. hypnosis
>m. image
>m. instinct
>M. Jones dressing
>m. love
>phallic m.
>schizophrenogenic m.
>m. substitute
>M. Superior complex
>m. surrogate
>surrogate m.
>working m.

mother-child
>m.-c. attachment
>m.-c. bond
>m.-c. relationship (MCR)
>M.-c. Relationship Evaluation (MCRE)

mother-daughter incest
mother-infant
>m.-i. attachment
>m.-i. bonding
>m.-i. proximity
>m.-i. relationship

Mother/Infant Communication Screening (MICS)
mothering
>good-enough m.
>multiple m.

Mother's Assessment of the Behavior of Her Infant (MABI)
mother-son incest
motilin
motility
>m. disorder
>ocular m.
>m. ocular
>m. psychosis

motion
>active integral range of m. (AIROM)
>m. artifact
>brownian m.
>m. concentration
>m. fear
>higher order m.
>involuntary m.
>m. perception
>phenomenal m.
>m. segment

>set in m.
>m. sickness
>spinal range of m. (SROM)
>Thinking Creatively in Action and M.
>voluntary m.

motivated
>m. error
>m. forgetting

motivating operation
motivation
>achievement m.
>adult m.
>m. analysis
>M. Analysis Test (MAT)
>m. analysis testing
>being m.
>childhood m.
>competence m.
>competing theories of m.
>m. for cross-dressing
>decreased m.
>deficiency m.
>m. deterioration
>expressed m.
>external incentive m.
>extrinsic m.
>incentive m.
>intrinsic m.
>lack of m.
>loss of m.
>personal m.
>positive m.
>primary m.
>psychological m.
>m. research
>secondary m.
>m. for self-injury
>sexual m.
>SPECTRUM-I: A Test of Adult Work M.
>suicide m.
>true m.
>unconscious m.
>work m.

motivational
>m. factor
>m. hierarchy
>m. inventory
>M. Patterns Inventory
>m. selectivity

motivational/behavioral factor
motive
>abundancy m.
>achievement m.
>m. achievement
>aroused m.
>autonomy of m.'s
>competitive m.
>conflicting m.
>cooperative m.
>deficiency m.
>effectance m.
>m.'s hierarchy
>hierarchy of m.'s

M

motive *(continued)*
    individualistic m.
    inviolacy m.
    mastery m.
    m. mastery
    personal social m.
    physiological m.
    safety m.
motiveless resistance
motoneuron
motor
    m. ability
    m. abreaction
    m. activity
    m. agraphia
    m. alexia
    m. amusia
    m. aphasia
    m. apraxia
    m. area
    m. ataxia
    m. aura
    m. behavior
    m. cell
    m. center
    m. compliance
    m. conduction block
    m. control
    m. control of the ego
    m. conversion symptom
    m. coordination
    m. cortex
    m. cortical center
    m. dapsone neuropathy
    m. decussation
    m. deficit
    m. depressant
    m. development
    m. disability
    m. disinhibition
    m. end plate
    m. endplate
    m. evoked potential (MEP)
    m. fiber
    fine m.
    m. function
    gross m.
    m. habit
    m. hemideficit
    m. hemiplegia
    m. image
    m. immobility
    m. impairment
    m. impersistence
    M. Impersistence Test (MIT)
    m. inertia
    m. inhibition
    m. innervation
    m. intention
    m. jacksonian attack
    latency distal m.
    m. learning theory
    m. loss
    m. movement

    m. nerve
    m. nerve conduction
    m. neuron
    m. neuron disease
    m. neuron paralysis
    m. neurosis
    m. nucleus of facial nerve
    m. nucleus of trigeminus
    m. paradigm
    m. passivity
    m. pathways disease
    m. performance
    m. performance test
    m. perseveration
    m. persistence
    m. planning
    m. point
    m. psychosis
    m. restlessness
    m. retardation developmental delay disorder
    m. root of ciliary ganglion
    m. root of trigeminal nerve
    m. skill
    m. skill disturbance
    m. skills disorder
    m. speech center
    m. speed
    M. Steadiness Battery
    m. strength
    m. strip
    m. system
    m. thalamus
    m. theory of thought
    m. tic
    m. tic disorder
    transcortical m.
    m. unit
    m. unit action potential (MUAP)
    m. unit potential (MUP)
    vane-type m.
    m. vocalization
    m. zone
motorcycle accident (MCA)
Motor-Free Visual Perception Test (MVPT)
motori
motoric
    m. hyperactivity
    m. immobility
    m. phenomenon
    m. region
    m. reproduction process
    m. slowing
motorically
motoricity
motorium
motorneuronal pool
    inhibitory neuron
motorphobia
motor-verbal
    m.-v. tic
    m.-v. tic disorder
motor-vocal tic disorder
Motricity Index

Motrin
- Children's M.
- M. IB
- M. IB Sinus
- Junior Strength M.

moulage

Mount laminectomy rongeur

mourn

mourning work

mouse fear

mouth
- m. disorder
- dry m.
- nothing by m. (NPO)
- poor m.
- tapir m.
- twisted m.

MouthGuard oral protector

mouthing
- object m.

movable, moveable

move
- knight m.
- opening m.

movement
- abnormal involuntary m.
- m. abnormality
- active m.
- adventitious m.
- alpha m.
- anomalous m.
- arcuate m.
- m. artifact
- associated m.
- athetoid m.
- automatic m.
- ballistic m.
- beta m.
- bodily m.
- body m.
- brownian m.
- cardinal ocular m.
- choreic m.
- choreiform m.
- choreoathetoid m.
- choreoathetotic m.
- clonic m.
- cocaine-induced choreoathetoid m.'s
- compensatory m.
- complex whole body m.
- conjugate contraversive eye m.
- conjugated eye m.
- constraint of m.
- coreoathetoid m.
- decomposition of m.
- m. disorder
- m. disorder effect
- M. Disorder Questionnaire
- dysconjugate m.
- dyskinetic m.
- dysmetric hand m.
- dyspractic m.
- dysrhythmic m.
- dystonic m.
- encounter m.

- epsilon m.
- expressive m.
- extraneous m.
- eye m.
- false perceptions of m.
- fast saccadic eye m.
- fetal m.
- fine motor m.
- flapping m.
- following m.
- forced m.
- freezing of m.
- Frenkel m.
- functional m.
- gamma m.
- halting m.
- head m.
- hemiballismic m.
- hospice m.
- human-potential m.
- m. illusion
- intentional stereotyped m.
- involuntary motor m.
- irregular m.
- jerking m.
- lateropulsion of body m.
- lateropulsion of eye m.
- limitation of m. (LOM)
- loss of m. (LOM)
- low-complexity m.
- Magnan trombone m.
- mass m.
- medication-induced m.
- motor m.
- myoclonic m.
- neurobiotactic m.
- nonrapid eye m. (non-REM, NREM)
- nonrhythmic stereotyped motor m.
- orofacial m. (OFM)
- paradoxical abdominal m.
- passive m.
- paucity of m.
- perseverative m.
- poverty of m.
- purposeful m.
- purposeless m.
- purposive m.
- pursuit eye m.
- quasi-purposive m.
- random m.
- rapid alternating m. (RAM)
- rapid eye m. (REM)
- rapid fine m.
- rapid motor m.
- rapid repetitive m.
- recurrent motor m.
- reflex eye m.
- reflexive m.
- repetitive imitative m.
- rhythmic slow eye m.
- roving eye m.
- roving ocular m.
- saccadic eye m.
- m. scale

movement *(continued)*
    sleep m.
    slow lateral eye m. (SLEM)
    smooth pursuit eye m. (SPEM)
    spontaneous m.
    stereotyped body m.
    stereotyped motor m.
    stereotypic motor m.
    sudden motor m.
    m. symptom
    synkinetic motor m.
    m. therapy
    tonic-clonic m.
    tremulous m.
    vergence m.
    vermicular m.
    vestibular m.
    visual pursuit m.
    volitional m.
    voluntary muscle m.
    withdrawal m.
    women's liberation m.
movie star drug
moving object
moxa
Moxadil
moxalactam disodium
Moxam
moxibustion
moxie
moyamoya
    m. collateral enlargement
    m. disease
    m. syndrome
Moynahan syndrome
Moynihan forceps
MP-35 clip material
MPC, MPCL
    Mooney Problem Checklist
MPCh
    medial posterior choroidal
        MPCh artery
MPD
    Measures of Psychosocial Development
    Minnesota Percepto-Diagnostic
    multiple personality disorder
MPDT
    Minnesota Percepto-Diagnostic Test
MPFBT
    Minnesota Paper Form Board Test
MPI
    Mandsley Personality Inventory
    Maudsley Personality Inventory
    Multidimensional Pain Inventory
    Multiphasic Personality Inventory
    Multivariate Personality Inventory
MPM I multi-parameter monitoring system
MPO
    myeloperoxidase
MPPS
    massive parallel processing system
MPQ
    McGill Pain Questionnaire

M-Prednisol Injection
MPS
    Management Philosophies Scale (I-V)
    mucopolysaccharidoses
    mucopolysaccharidosis
MPSS
    Mood and Physical Symptoms Scale
MPTP-induced parkinsonism
MQ
    memory quotient
MR
    magnetic resonance
    mental retardation
        MR angiogram
        gadolinium-diethylenetriamine penta-acetic acid-enhanced MR
        MR imaging with gadolinium enhancement
        MR spectroscopy
        surface coil MR
MRA
    magnetic resonance angiography
MRC
    Medical Research Council
MRF
    midbrain reticular formation
MRHD
    maximum recommended human dose
MRI
    magnetic resonance imaging
        MRI compatibility
        contrast-enhanced MRI
        gadolinium-enhanced MRI
        nonproton MRI
        MRI scan
        whole-spine MRI
MRN
    magnetic resonance neurography
mRNA
    messenger ribonucleic acid
MRS
    magnetic resonance spectroscopy
    Mania Rating Scale
MRT
    major role therapy
    Metropolitan Readiness Test
MRZ
    measles, rubella and zoster
        MRZ reaction
MS
    multiple sclerosis
        MS Contin
        MS Contin Oral
        Rebif MS
MSA
    Marriage Skills Analysis
    mitotic spindle apparatus
MSAS
    Mandel Social Adjustment Scale
MSAT
    Minnesota Scholastic Aptitude Test
MSCA
    McCarthy Scales of Children's Ability
MSCS
    Multidimensional Self Concept Scale

MSD
    mean sorted difference
MSDI
    Martin Suicide-Depression Inventory
MSE
    mental status examination
MSER
    mental status examination report
MSI
    magnetic source imaging
MSIR Oral
MSIS
    multistate information system
MS/L
MSLT
    Multiple Sleep Latency Test
      MSLT with electroencephalogram
MSN
    Master of Science in Nursing
MSQ
    Managerial Style Questionnaire
    Mental Status Questionnaire
    Minnesota Satisfaction Questionnaire
MSRPP
    multidimensional scale for rating
      psychiatric patients
MSRT
    Minnesota Spatial Relations Test
MSS
    mental status schedule
    Minnesota Satisfaction Scale
MSSST
    Meeting Street School Screening Test
MST
    medial superior temporal
MSU
    memory for symbolic unit
MSUD
    maple syrup urine disease
MSW
    Master of Social Work
    multiple stab wounds
MT
    music therapy
MTA
    Management Transactions Audit
MTAI
    Minnesota Teacher Attitude Inventory
MTAS
    Maternal Trait Anxiety Score
99mTc
    technetium 99m, or 99mTc
99mTc-HMPAO
MTC Ventcontrol ventricular catheter
MTD
    maximum tolerated dose
MTDDA
    Minnesota Test for the Differential
      Diagnosis of Aphasia
mtDNA depletion syndrome
MTM 2 bur
MTP
    multidisciplinary treatment plan
MTR
    Music Therapist, Registered

MTS
    mesial temporal sclerosis
      MTS electrohydraulic piston
mu
    m. opiate receptor
    m. rhythm
    m. wave
MUAP
    motor unit action potential
      MUAP on electromyogram
mucate
    isometheptene m.
Much-Holzmann reaction
mucinosa
    alopecia m.
mucin-secreting adenocarcinoma
mucocele
    clival m.
    erosive sphenoid m.
    m. formation
    paranasal m.
    sphenoid m.
mucolipidosis
mucolipidosis, type IV (ML4)
Mucomyst with Isoproterenol
mucopolysaccharide
mucopolysaccharidoses (MPS)
mucopolysaccharidosis (MPS)
    m. I
    m. II
    m. III
    m. IV
    m. V
    m. VI
mucopyocele
    m. of the clivus
    nasal sinus m.
Mucoraceae
Mucor infection
mucormycosis
mucosal
Mucosil
mucous membrane lesion
Muenzer-Rosenthal syndrome
MUGUS
    monoclonal gammopathy of unknown
      significance
mugwort leaves
mulato
mulberry-like nodule
Mulholland and Gunn criteria
muliebrity
Mullan
    M. percutaneous trigeminal ganglion
      microcompression set
    M. triangle
    M. wire
Mullen Scales of Early Learning
Müller
    M. fiber
    M. law
    M. muscle
    M. radial cell
    M. trigone

M

mullerian duct aplasia, renal aplasia, cervicothoracic somite dysplasia (MURCS)
Müller-König
   M.-K. procedure
   M.-K. transposition
multiapproach
multiarc LINAC radiosurgery
multiaxial
   m. classification
   m. classification system
   m. evaluation
   M. Evaluation Report Form
   m. fashion
   Obsessive-Compulsive Personality Disorder Subscale from Millon Clinical M.
multicausal
multicomponent
multicore disease
multicultural environment
multicystic encephalomalacia
multidetermination
multidetermined behavior
multidimensional
   M. Aptitude Battery
   M. Assessment of Gains in School (MAGS)
   m. construct
   m. Fourier transform
   M. Pain Inventory (MPI)
   m. pain management
   m. scale for rating psychiatric patients (MSRPP)
   M. Self Concept Scale (MSCS)
multidirectional
multidisciplinary
   m. group psychiatry
   m. treatment plan (MTP)
MultiDop XS system
multidrug
multifactorial
   m. inheritance
   m. model (MF)
Multifactor Leadership Questionnaire (MLQ)
multifamilial
multifamily
multifocal
   m. fibrosclerosis
   m. glioma
   m. leukoencephalopathy
   m. motor neuropathy (MFMN)
   m. myoclonus
   m. placoid pigment epitheliopathy
   m. subcortical demyelination
   m. thought
multiforme
   erythema m.
   glioblastoma m. (GBM)
multiforme-like
   erythema m.-l.
multiform layer
multifunctional
multiglandular hyperplasia

multihandicapped
multi-impulsivity syndrome
multi-infarct
   m.-i. dementia
   m.-i. progressive supranuclear palsy
   m.-i. psychosis
Multi-Institutional Research in Alzheimer Genetic Epidemiology (MIRAGE)
multi-item
   m.-i. index
   m.-i. test
multilayered
multilevel
   M. Informal Language Inventory
   m. laminectomy
Multilingual Aphasia Examination (MAE)
multiloculated hydrocephalus
multimodal behavior therapy
multimodality evoked potential (MEP)
multimonitored electroconvulsive treatment (MMECT)
multiorgasmic
multiphase
Multiphasic
   M. Environmental Assessment Procedure (MEAP)
   M. Personality Inventory (MPI)
multiplanar
   imaging m.
multiple
   M. Affect Adjective Checklist (MAACL)
   m. analysis
   M. Aptitude Test
   m. baseline design
   m. birth
   m. buccal frenula
   m. cognitive deficits
   m. congenital anomaly (MCA)
   m. correlation
   m. cortical infarct
   m. cortical infarction
   m. delusions
   m. distinct identities
   m. ego state
   m. endocrine neoplasia (MEN)
   m. endocrine neoplasia, type 1
   m. endocrine neoplasia, type 2
   m. endocrine neoplasia, type 3
   m. family therapy
   m. focal lesion
   m. focus
   m. hook assembly
   m. hook assembly C-D instrumentation
   m. identification
   m. impact injury
   m. intracranial aneurysms (MIA)
   m. life difficulty
   m. line-scan imaging (MLSI)
   m. loss
   m. mothering
   m. mucosal neuroma syndrome

m. myeloma
m. myeloma peripheral neuropathy
m. neuritis
m. operations syndrome
m. organ failure
m. personality
m. personality crime
m. personality disorder (MPD)
m. personality and gender
m. plane imaging
m. psychotherapy
m. regression
m. regression technique
m. reinforcement
m. role playing
m. sclerosis (MS)
m. sclerosis dementia
m. sclerosis organic psychosis
m. sclerosis-type organic
m. sensitive point
M. Sleep Latency Test (MSLT)
m. spontaneous orgasms
m. stab wounds (MSW)
m. subpial transection
m. system atrophy
m. targeting
m. therapy
m. tics with coprolalia

multiple-point sacral fixation
multiplex
arthrogryposis congenita m.
dysostosis m.
mononeuritis m.
mononeuropathy m.
myoclonus m.
multiplication
m. of personality
m. table test
multiplicity
target m.
multipolar
m. cell
m. neuron
multipore suction tip
multipotential cell
multipurpose headrest
Multiscore Depression Inventory (MDI)
multisegmental hyporeflexia
multisensory
multispan fracture hook
multistate information system (MSIS)
multistep task
multisynaptic
multitalented
multitudinous
multivalence
multivariable
multivariate
m. analysis
m. analysis of covariance
(MANCOVA)
m. analysis of variance
(MANOVA)
M. Personality Inventory (MPI)
m. study

multiversity
mumbling automatism
mummy attitude
mumps
m. encephalitis
m. meningitis
m. meningoencephalitis
m. peripheral neuropathy
Munchausen
M. disease by proxy
M. by proxy syndrome
M. syndrome
mundane realism
Munich cooperative model
MUP
motor unit potential
mural thrombus
MURCS
mullerian duct aplasia, renal aplasia,
cervicothoracic somite dysplasia
murder
lust m.
m. one
murderer
mass m.
serial m.
murderous predation behavior
murine typhus meningoencephalitis
murmur
brain m.
heart m.
Murphy
M. ball hook
M. rake retractor
**Murphy-Meisgeier Type Indicator for
Children (MMTIC)**
MurphyScope neurologic device
Murphy's law
Murray Valley encephalitis
muscaria
Amanita m.
muscarine
m. blockade
m. poisoning
muscarine-agonist-induced
muscarinic
m. cholinergic receptor
m. receptor blockade
m. side effect
muscimol
muscle
anterior digastric m.
anterior scalene m.
anterior serratus m.
m. biopsy
buccinator m.
cervicis m.
m. contraction headache
m. cramp
cranial m.
digastric m.
m. disorder
m. dissection
m. erotism
external intercostal m.

M

muscle *(continued)*
  m. fibrosis
  m. filter
  greater rhomboid m.
  iliocostal m.
  iliopsoas m.
  inferior rectus m.
  intraspinous m.
  jugular foramen m.
  lateral rectus m.
  latissimus dorsi m.
  levator palpebrae m.
  lingual m.
  longus capitis m.
  longus cervicis colli m.
  longus colli m.
  medial rectus m.
  Müller m.
  nuchal m.
  ocular m.
  omohyoid m.
  orbicularis orbis m.
  orbicularis oris m.
  orbicular oculi m.
  m. pain
  paraspinal m.
  pectoralis major m.
  platysma m.
  m. pleasure
  psoas m.
  m. relaxant
  m. rigidity
  Rouget m.
  scalenus anticus m.
  m. spasm
  m. spindle
  sternocleidomastoid m.
  sternohyoid m.
  sternomastoid m.
  sternothyroid m.
  strap m.
  m. stretch reflex
  striated m. (StrAbs)
  superior rectus m.
  temporalis m.
  teres major m.
  m. tone
  trapezius m.
  m. twitch
muscle-fascia-Gelfoam combination
muscle-paretic nystagmus
muscle-splitting incision
muscular
  m. and anal impotence
  m. anesthesia
  m. atrophy
  m. body
  m. dystrophy
  m. hyperesthesia
  m. insufficiency
  m. reflex
  m. sense
  m. tension
  m. trophoneurosis

muscular-anal stage
muscularis
  ataxia m.
musculature
  axial m.
musculocutaneous nerve
musculoskeletal disorder
musculospiral paralysis
music
  m. ability sparing
  M. Achievement Test (1-4) (MAT)
  m. blindness
  m. deafness
  M. Therapist, Registered (MTR)
  m. therapy (MT)
Musical
  M. Aptitude Profile (MAP)
musical
  m. agraphia
  m. alexia
  m. stimulus
  m. therapy
musician's cramp
musicogenic epilepsy
musicomania
musicophobia
musicotherapy
musomania
musophobia
Mussen frame
mussitans
  delirium m.
mussitation
mustard
  nitrogen m.
Mustargen
mutable
mutacism
mutagenicity
mutation
  deletion m.
  gene m.
  missense m.
  point m.
  m. rate
  single point m.
  tandem double m.
  testicular feminization m. (TFM)
mutative interpretation
muteness
mute state
mutilating
  m. acropathy
  m. leprosy
mutilation
  genital m.
  sadistic m.
mutism
  akinetic m.
  apathetic akinetic m.
  catatonic m.
  elective m.
  hysterical m.
  pure word m.
  relative elective m.

selective m.
traumatic m.
voluntary m.
muttering delirium
Mutt and Jeff approach
mutual
m. affective responsiveness
m. aid group
m. grief
m. masturbation
m. participation model
m. pretense awareness
m. regard
m. respect
mutual-help services
mutualism
mutuality
mutually exclusive
MVC
maximal voluntary contraction
MVD
microvascular decompression
MVII
Minnesota Vocational Interest Inventory
MVP
mitral valve prolapse
MVPT
Mertens Visual Perception Test
Motor-Free Visual Perception Test
MWLT
Modified Word Learning Test
MWMT
Monotic Word Memory Test
MwoA
migraine without aura
MX2
3'-deamino-3'-morpholino-13-deoxo-10-
hydroxycarminomycin
myalgia
myasthenia
m. gravis (MG)
m. gravis evaluation
myasthenic
m. crisis
m. facies
m. reaction
m. syndrome
myatonia, myatony
m. congenita
mycetism, mycetismus
m. cerebralis
Mycobacterium
M. leprae
M. tuberculosis
mycophagy
Mycoplasma
M. arthritidis
M. infection
M. pneumoniae encephalitis
mycosis
mycotic
m. aneurysm
m. intracranial aneurysm
mydriasis
alternating m.

paralytic m.
spasmodic m.
spastic m.
springing m.
mydriatic rigidity
myelapoplexy
myelatelia
myelauxe
myelencephalic vein
myelencephalon
myelic
myelin
m. basic protein (MBP)
m. body
m. breakdown
m. degradation
m. figure
m. macromolecule
m. metabolism
oral bovine m.
peripheral nerve m. (PNM)
m. sheath
myelin-associated glycoprotein (MAG)
myelinated
m. axonal tract
m. nerve fiber
myelinating phenotype
myelination of axon
myelinic
myelinization
myelinoclasis
myelinoclastic disease
myelinogenesis
myelin/oligodendrocyte glycoprotein (MOG)
myelin/oligodendrocyte-specific protein (MOSP)
myelinolysis
central pontine m.
myelitic
myelitis
acute transverse m.
ascending m.
bulbar m.
complete transverse m.
concussion m.
Foix-Alajouanine m.
funicular m.
subacute necrotizing m.
systemic m.
transverse m.
myeloarchitectonics
myelocele
myelocyst
myelocystocele
terminal m.
myelocystomeningocele
myelocyte
myelodiastasis
myelodysplasia
myelofibrosis
myelogram
myelography
computed tomographic m. (CTM)

M

myelography *(continued)*
  computed tomographic
    metrizamide m. (CTMM)
  delayed computed tomographic m.
  iohexol m.
  metrizamide m.
  water-soluble contrast m.
myeloid elastase
myelolysis
myeloma
  multiple m.
myeloma-associated neuropathy
myelomalacia
  angiodysgenetic m.
  cystic m.
myelomeningocele
  lumbosacral m.
  spina bifida m.
myeloneuritis
myeloneuropathy
  cassava plant tropical m.
  tropical m.
myeloparalysis
myelopathic
myelopathy
  acute partial m.
  acute transverse m. (ATM)
  AIDS-related m.
  carcinomatous m.
  cervical spondylosis without m.
  cervical spondylotic m. (CSM)
  chronic progressive m.
  compressive m.
  diabetic m.
  HTLV-I associated m. (HAM)
  m. incidence
  laminoplasty with extended
    foraminoplasty for cervical m.
  midcervical flexion m.
  necrotizing m.
  paracarcinomatous m.
  paraneoplastic m.
  radiation m.
  spondylotic m.
  subacute necrotic m.
  subacute necrotizing m.
  m. syndrome
  tropical spastic paraparesis/HTLV-I
    associated m. (TSP/HAM)
myeloperoxidase (MPO)
myelopetal
myelophthisic
myelophthisis
myeloplegia
myeloproliferative disorder
myeloradiculitis
myeloradiculodysplasia
myeloradiculopathy
myeloradiculopolyneuronitis
myelorrhagia
myelorrhaphy
myeloschisis
myelosis
  funicular m.

myelosyphilis
myelosyringosis
myelotome
myelotomography
myelotomy
  Bischof m.
  commissural m.
  extralemniscal m.
  midline m.
  T m.
myenteric plexus
Myer fiber
Myers-Briggs
  M.-B. psychological test
  M.-B. Type Indicator (MBTI)
Myerson
  M. reflex
  M. sign
myesthesia
Mykrox
Mylanta
Myloral
myoblastoma
  granular cell m.
myobradia
myocardial infarction
myocardiopathy
  alcoholic m.
myocarditis
  toxic m.
myocelialgia
myoclonia
  fibrillary m.
myoclonic
  m. absence
  m. astatic epilepsy
  m. convulsion
  m. encephalitis
  m. encephalopathy
  m. jerk
  m. movement
  m. seizure
myoclonica
  dementia m.
  dyssynergia cerebellaris m.
myoclonus
  cortical m.
  m. epilepsy
  m. epilepsy with ragged-red fiber
    (MERRF)
  hereditary branchial m.
  intention m.
  multifocal m.
  m. multiplex
  nocturnal m.
  ocular m.
  oculopalatal m.
  palatal m.
  palatoocular m.
  propriospinal m.
  spinal segmental m.
  stimulus sensitive m.
  tardive m.
  m. tardive
myocutaneous flap

Myodil
myodynia
> hysterical m.

myodystony
myodystrophy, myodystrophia
myoedema
myoepithelium
myoesthesis, myoesthesia
myofascial
> m. pain
> m. pain syndrome

myofibrillary disarray
myofibromatosis
> infantile m.

Myoflex
myofunctional therapy
myogenic
> m. motor evoked potential
> m. paralysis

myoglobin
myoglobinuria
myoglobinuric renal failure
myogram
myography
myoinositol
Myokinetic Psychodiagnosis Test
myokymia
> facial m.
> hereditary m.

myokymic discharge
myomedulloblastoma
myoneural
> m. ischemia
> m. junction

myoneuralgia
> postural m.

myoneurasthenia
myo-neuro-gastrointestinal
encephalopathy (MNGIE)
myoneuroma
myopalmus
myoparalysis
myoparesis
myopathic
> m. atrophy
> m. carnitine deficiency
> m. facies
> m. paralysis

myopathy
> acute alcoholic m.
> acute steroid quadriplegic m.
> alcoholic m.
> centronuclear m.
> critical illness m.
> distal m.
> idiopathic inflammatory m. (IIM)
> Kiloh-Nevin ocular m.
> mitochondrial m.
> nondystrophin m.
> proximal m.
> quadriceps m.
> thyrotoxic m.
> Xp21 m.

myophosphorylase deficiency

myopia
> axial m.

myopic insight
myopsychic
myopsychopathy
myopsychosis
myorhythmia
> oculomasticatory m.

myosalgia
Myoscint
myoseism
myositis
> cancer-associated m.
> cervical m.
> cervical tension m. (CTM)
> childhood m.
> eosinophilic m.
> inclusion-body m.
> orbital m.
> m. ossificans

myospasm, myospasmus
> cervical m.

myotatic
> m. contracture
> m. irritability
> m. reflex

myotone
myotonia
> m. acquisita
> m. atrophica
> chondrodystrophic m.
> m. chondrodystrophic
> m. congenita
> m. dystrophica
> m. neonatorum

myotonic
> m. discharge
> m. dystrophy gene
> m. dystropy
> m. facies
> m. muscular dystrophy
> m. pupil

myotonica
> dystrophia m.

myotonoid
myotonus
myotony
myriachit (*var. of* miryachit)
myristic acid
Mysoline
mysophilia
mysophobia
mysophobic
mystic
> m. paranoia
> m. union

mystical experience
mytacism
Mytelase Caplets
myth
> personal m.
> sexual m. (SM)

mythological theme
mythomania
mythophobia

M

myxedema
    m. coma
    juvenile m.
    m. madness
    m. peripheral neuropathy
    m. reflex
myxedematous
myxoid lobule
myxoma
    atrial m.

myxomatous
    m. cell
    m. thickening
myxoneuroma
myxopapillary ependymoma
myxophobia
myxovirus infection
MZ
    monozygotic twin

N
numerical aptitude
N protein
NA
Narcotics Anonymous
nonadherent
NAA
N-acetylaspartate
NAAG
N-acetylaspartylglutamate
nabumetone
N-acetylaspartylglutamate (NAAG)
n-Ach
achievement need
NAD
no acute distress
nadolol
Naegleria
N. fowleri
N. infection
N. meningitis
nafate
cefamandole n.
Nafcil
nafcillin sodium
Naffziger
N. syndrome
N. test
Naffzinger straight midline incision
Naftidrofuryl
Nageotte cell
Nager Miller syndrome
nail
n. biting
intramedullary n.
Küntscher n.
n. lesion
NAIM
nonvasculitic autoimmune inflammatory
meningoencephalitis
naive wit
nalbuphine hydrochloride
Nalfon
Nalline test
nalmefene hydrochloride
nalorphine hydrochloride
naloxone hydrochloride
naltrexone
name
n. the date test
N.'s Learning Test (NLT)
naming
category-specific n.
n. common objects test
n. intact
nandrolone decanoate
NAP
nerve action potential
napalm burn
naphtha
napping phenomenon
Naprelan

Naprosyn
naproxen
napsylate
Naqua
Nar-Anon
naratriptan
n. HCl
n. hydrochloride
Narcan Injection
Narcanon
narcissism
body n.
ego n.
primary n.
primitive n.
secondary n.
narcissistic
n. character
n. ego ideal
n. equilibrium
n. neurotic personality disorder
n. object choice
n. personality
n. rage
n. scale
n. self-peeping
n. tendency
n. transference
n. vulnerability
n. wounding
narcoanalysis
narcoanesthesia
narcocatharsis
narcohypnia
narcohypnosis
narcolepsy
n. cataplexy syndrome
n. experience
narcoleptic tetrad
narcoma
narcomania
narcomatous
narcoplexy
narcose
narcosis
basal n.
continuous n.
medullary n.
nitrogen n.
narcosomania
narcostimulant
narcosuggestion
narcosynthesis
narcotherapy
narcotic
n. abuse
n. addict
n. addiction
n. agent
n. agonist drug
N.'s Anonymous (NA)
n. antagonist

N

narcotic *(continued)*
- n. antagonist drug
- n. blockade
- n. blocking drug
- n. chemical intoxication
- n. dependence
- n. detoxification
- n. habit
- n. hunger
- n. poisoning
- n. withdrawal

narcotism
narcotize
Nardil
Naropin
narrative therapy
narrow
- n. AO dynamic compression plate
- n. bipole
- n. tripole

narrow-based gait
narrow-bite bone rongeur
narrowing
- degenerative n.

NART
- National Adult Reading Test

nasal
- n. ala
- n. cavity
- n. chondritis
- n. dermoid
- n. dissection
- n. ganglion
- n. glioma
- n. inhaler
- n. mucosal sac
- n. septum hematoma
- n. sinus
- n. sinus mucopyocele
- n. surgery

nasality
- assimilated n.

nascentium
- trismus n.

nascent motor unit potential
NASCET
Nashold
- N. biopsy needle
- N. TC electrode

nasion
nasociliaris nerve
nasociliary
- n. nerve
- n. neuralgia
- n. root

nasoethmoidal encephalocele
nasofrontal encephalocele
nasofrontalis
- fonticulus n.

nasogastric
- n. intubation
- n. tube

nasolabial fold
nasomental reflex

nasoorbital encephalocele
nasopharyngeal
- n. angiofibroma
- n. blastomycosis
- n. cooling
- n. malignancy
- n. mucus retention cyst

nasopharynx
NAT
- National Attention Test
- Nonverbal Ability Test
- Numerical Attention Test

NATB
- Non-Reading Aptitude Test Battery

Natecor
national
- N. Adult Reading Test (NART)
- N. Attention Test (NAT)
- N. Board of Medical Examiners
- N. Center for Health Statistics
- n. character
- N. Comorbidity Survey
- N. Educational Development Test
- n. epithet
- N. Gay Task Force (NGTF)
- n. Information Center for Children & Youth with Disabilities
- N. Institute of Allergy and Infectious Disease (NIAID)
- N. Institute of Mental Health-Epidemiologic Catchment Area Program
- N. Institute of Mental Health-Global Obsessive Compulsive Scale (NIMH-OC)
- N. Institute on Deafness & Other Communication Disorders
- N. Institute on Drug Abuse (NIDA)
- N. Institutes of Health Stroke Scale
- N. Mental Health Consumers Self-Help Clearing House
- N. Occupation Competency Testing (NOCT)
- N. Police Officer Selection Test (POST)
- N. Training Laboratories (NTL)

nativism
nativist theory
natriuresis
natriuretic hormone
natural
- n. environment
- n. group
- n. hearing loss
- n. law
- N. Process Analysis
- n. selection
- n. theology

naturalism
nature
- dilatory n.
- human n.
- negative n.

pathologic n.
pejorative n.
n. versus nurture
nature-nurture issue
Naturetin
naturopath
naturopathy
nauseam
ad n.
nauseant
nausea and vomiting (N&V)
nautomania
Navane
navigator
Operating Arm stereotactic n.
Naylor-Harwood
N.-H. Adult Intelligence Scale
(NHAIS)
N.-H. Intelligence Scale (NHIS)
nazism, naziism
NBAS
Neonatal Behavioral Assessment Scale
NBAS-K
Neonatal Behavioral Assessment Scale
with Kansas Supplements
N-butyl cyanoacrylate
NCAM
nerve-cell adhesion molecule
neural cell adhesion molecule
NCC
neurocysticercosis
NCO
noncommissioned officer
NCP
NeuroCybernetic prosthesis
NCP lead
NCP System
NCS
nerve conduction study
NCV
nerve conduction velocity
N-desmethylclozapine
1505 NDSB occlusion balloon catheter
Nd:YAG
neodymium:yttrium-aluminum-garnet
Nd:YAG laser
Nd:YAG module
NE
norepinephrine
near
n. reflex spasm
n. syncope
near-field record
NEAT
Norris Educational Achievement Test
neatly groomed
Nebcin
nebulaphobia
nebulous
necessary
as n. (PRN)
n. condition
n. task
Nec-Hugger cervical support pillow

neck
n. of aneurysm
bent-over n.
buffalo n.
n. dissection
n. pain
potato tumor of n.
n. reflex
n. sign
stiff n.
n. weakness
wry n.
necrolysis
epidermal n.
toxic epidermal n.
necromancy
necromania
necromimesis
necrophagous
necrophilia, necrophilism, necrophily
necrophilous
necrophobia
necrosadism
necrosis
acute tubular n.
aseptic n.
avascular n.
caseous n.
cell n.
cerebral radiation n. (CRN)
coagulative n.
cystic medial n.
hemorrhagic n.
laminar cortical n.
Marcus grading scale for
avascular n.
n. negation
neuronal n.
postpartum n.
pressure n.
radiation n.
tubular n.
tumor n.
necrotizing
n. angiitis
n. encephalitis
n. encephalomyelitis
n. encephalomyelopathy
n. hemorrhagic leukoencephalitis
n. infundibulo-hypophysitis
n. myelopathy
n. vasculitis
NECYSYS home neck care system
need
achievement n. (n-Ach)
n. for admiration
affective n.
affiliative n.
blithely ignored n.
n. for care
certificate of n.
N. for Cognition Scale
cognitive n.
community n.
n. for constant attention

N

need *(continued)*
    n. to control
    dependency n.
    emotional n.
    esteem n.
    excessive n.
    exhibitionist n.
    existence n.
    felt n.
    harm-avoidance n.
    hierarchy of n.
    identity n.
    inner n.
    instinct n.
    instinctoid n.
    instrumental n.
    love n.
    oral n.
    personal n.
    Personal Inventory of N.'s
    physiological n.
    primary n.
    psychological n.
    n. for punishment
    repressed n.
    rootedness n.
    Screening Children for Related
      Early Educational N.'s (SCREEN)
    seclusion n.
    n. a sentence test
    submerged individual n.
    succorance n.
    n. tension
    togetherness n.
    transcendence n.
    unmet dependency n.
need-fear dilemma
needle
    Adson n.
    aneurysm n.
    angled n.
    n. aspiration
    Backlund biopsy n.
    Bier lumbar puncture n.
    brain biopsy n.
    butterfly n.
    Colorado MicroDissection n.
    Cone ventricular n.
    Cournand arteriogram n.
    Cournand-Grino arteriogram n.
    Cushing ventricular n.
    Dandy ventricular n.
    D'Errico ventricular n.
    dirty n.
    n. dissector
    n. electrode
    n. electromyographic
    n. electromyography
    epidural n.
    Espocan combined spinal/epidural n.
    Estridge biopsy n.
    Frazier ventricular n.
    Hoen ventricular n.
    n. holder

    Hunstad infusion n.
    hypodermic n.
    insulated electrode n.
    Kronecker aneurysm n.
    lumbar puncture n.
    Mixter ventricular n.
    MO n.
    Nashold biopsy n.
    neurography n.
    Pace ventricular n.
    Parhad-Poppen arteriogram n.
    Poppen ventricular n.
    Quincke spinal n.
    Retter aneurysm n.
    Scoville ventricular n.
    Sedan-Nashold n.
    Shaw aneurysm n.
    Sheldon-Spatz vertebral
      arteriogram n.
    Smiley-Williams arteriogram n.
    spinal n.
    Sprotte epidural n.
    Sprotte spinal n.
    n. stick
    straight n.
    Thermistor n.
    titanium alloy n.
    n. track
    n. trephination system
    Tuohy n.
    ventricular n.
    ventriculostomy n.
    Whitacre spinal n.
needle-nose rongeur
needless repetition
need-press method
needs-assessment survey
NEEG
    neoelectroencephalography
nefazodone
    n. HCl
    n. hydrochloride
Neftel disease
neg
    negative
negate
negation
    delirium of n.
    delusion of n.
    n. delusion
    n. of the ego
    insanity of n.
    necrosis n.
negative (neg)
    n. affect
    n. aspiration
    n. attitude
    n. behavior
    n. body image
    n. command
    n. conditioning
    n. conditioning for sleep
    n. correlation
    n. delusion
    n. diagnosis

n. emotion
n. emotionality
n. eugenics
n. evaluation
n. factor
false n.
n. feedback
n. feeling
guaiac n.
n. judgment
n. life event
n. mood induction
n. mood state
n. nature
n. Oedipus
n. practice
n. predictive power
n. quality
n. reinforcement
n. reinforcer
n. relationship
n. response
n. ruler of the soul
n. scotoma
n. self-comparison
n. self-image
n. symptom
n. transference
true n.
n. utilitarianism
n. variation
n. voice

negative-affect alcoholism
negatively bathmotropic
negative-symptom schizophrenia
negativism
active n.
adolescent n.
catatonic n.
command n.
extreme n.
sexual n.
toddler n.
negativistic
n. behavior
n. personality disorder
n. response
negativity
endogenous n.
n. of Input 1
n. of Input 2
negi
negi n.
neglect
adult survivor of n.
child n.
n. of child
n. of duty
elder adult n.
family n.
hemispatial arousal n.
maternal n.
organic n.
parent n.
paternal n.

perceived n.
problems related to abuse or n.
sensory n.
spatial n.
survivor of n.
n. syndrome
thalamic n.
unilateral organic n.
unilateral spatial n.
unilateral visual n.
visual n.
neglected child
negligence
contributory n.
professional n.
negligible routine
negotiating
n. goals skills
n. language
n. routines skills
n. rules skills
negotiation
problem-solving n.
Negro phenomenon
negrophile
negrophobia
Neisseria meningitidis
nelfinavir
Nelson
N. rib spreader
N. syndrome
N. tumor
Nembutal
nemonapride
NEO
neuroticism/extroversion/openness
NEO Five Factor Inventory
NEO personality questionnaire
neoassociationism
neoatavism
Neo-Calglucon
neocerebellum
neoconnectionism
neocortex
lateral n.
NeoDerm dressing
neodymium
neodymium:yttrium-aluminum-garnet
(Nd:YAG)
neoelectroencephalography (NEEG)
neoencephalon
neoformans
Cryptococcus n.
neofreudian
neographism
neography
neo-Hippocratic medicine
Neo-Iopax
neokinetic
neo-kraepelian classification
neolallism
neolocal family
neologism
neomimism
neomnesis

N

neomycin
neo-myerian era
neonatacide
neonatal
- n. apoplexy
- N. Behavioral Assessment Scale (NBAS)
- N. Behavioral Assessment Scale with Kansas Supplements (NBAS-K)
- n. familial seizure
- n. hypotonia
- n. infection
- n. intraventricular hemorrhage
- n. myasthenia gravis
- n. opiate withdrawal
- n. poliomyelitis
- n. tetany
- n. tyrosinemia aminoaciduria

neonate asphyxia
neonatorum
- encephalitis n.
- myotonia n.
- tetanus n.
- trismus n.

neo-Nazi
neopallium
Neopap
neophasia
- polyglot n.

neophilia
neophilism
neophobia
neophrenia
neoplasia
- adenohypophyseal n.
- multiple endocrine n. (MEN)
- multiple endocrine n., type 1
- multiple endocrine n., type 2
- multiple endocrine n., type 3

neoplasm
- benign brain n.
- cranial nerve n.
- extensive n.
- frontal n.
- intracranial n.
- malignant brain n.
- pearly n.
- pineal parenchymal n.
- spinal cord n.
- temporal horn n.
- trochlear nerve n.

neoplastic
- n. aneurysm
- n. angioendotheliomatosis
- n. arachnoiditis
- n. disease
- n. disorder
- n. encephalopathy
- n. lesion
- n. meningitis

neopsychic
neopterin
- serum n.

Neosar Injection

neosleep
Neosporin GU Irrigant
neostigmine test
neostriatum
neoteny
neothalamus
neovascularization
- iris n.

nepenthe
nephophobia
nephritis
- shunt n.

Nephro-Calci
nephrosis
nephrotopic
Néri sign
nerve
- abducens n.
- accelerator n.'s
- accessory n.
- accommodation of n.
- acoustic n.
- n. action potential (NAP)
- afferent digital n.
- anomalous nonrecurrent right inferior laryngeal n.
- antebrachial cutaneous n.
- anterior interosseous n.
- aortic n.
- auditory n.
- augmentor n.
- autonomic n.
- axillary n.
- baroreceptor n.
- brachial cutaneous n.
- carotid sinus n.
- n. cell
- n. cell body
- n. cell death
- n. cell destruction
- n. cell survival
- centrifugal n.
- centripetal n.
- cervical n.
- cluneal n.
- cochlear n.
- common peroneal n.
- n. conduction
- n. conduction study (NCS)
- n. conduction velocity (NCV)
- cranial n.
- cutaneous n.
- Cyon n.
- n. deafness
- n. decompression
- dental n.
- depressor n. of Ludwig
- digital n.
- n. discontinuity
- dorsal scapular n.
- efferent n.
- eighth cranial n.
- eleventh cranial n.
- n. ending
- n. entrapment

n. entrapment neuralgia
esodic n.
excitor n.
excitoreflex n.
exodic n.
external popliteal n.
facial n.
n. fascicle
femoral cutaneous n.
fenestrated oculomotor n.
n. fiber
n. field
fifth cranial n.
first cranial n.
n. force
fourth cranial n.
Galen n.
n. ganglion
n. gas
Gaskell n.
genitofemoral n.
genu of the facial n.
glossopharyngeal n.
gluteal n.
n. graft
grate on the n.'s
greater occipital n.
greater superficial petrosal n.
n. growth factor (NGF)
gustatory n.
Hering sinus n.
n. hook
hypoglossal n.
iliohypogastric n.
ilioinguinal n.
n. implantation
n. impulse
inferior dental n.
inferior laryngeal n.
infraorbital n.
N. Integrity Monitor 2
intermediate n.
internal popliteal n.
Jacobson n.
lacrimal n.
lateral femoral cutaneous n.
long thoracic n.
n. loss
Ludwig n.
mandibular n.
medial plantar n.
median n.
mixed n.
motor n.
musculocutaneous n.
nasociliaris n.
nasociliary n.
ninth cranial n.
nuclei of cranial n.'s
nucleus of abducent n.
nucleus of hypoglossal n.
nucleus of trochlear n.
obturator n.
occipital n.
oculomotor n.

olfactory n.
optic n.
n. pain
n. palsy
n. papilla
pathetic n.
peripheral n.
petrosal n.
plantar n.
n. plexus
plexus of spinal n.'s
pneumogastric n.
popliteal n.
posterior communicating n.
posterior interosseous n. (PIN)
posterior tibial n.
pressor n.
pressoreceptor n.
pudendal n.
radial n.
recurrent laryngeal n.
n. root
n. root avulsion
n. root block
n. root edema
n. root embarrassment
root of facial n.
n. root microcirculation
n. root retractor
n. root sheath effacement
roots of trigeminal n.
sacral n.
scapular n.
sciatic n.
second cervical n.
second cranial n.
secretory n.
sensory n.
seventh cranial n.
n. sheath tumor
sinus n. of Hering
sinuvertebral n.
sixth cranial n.
n. of smell
spinal accessory n.
n. stimulator
n. stump
superficial petrosal n.
superior laryngeal n.
supraorbital n.
suprascapular n.
sural n.
n. suture
sympathetic n.
tenth cranial n.
third cranial n.
thoracic n.
tibial n.
n. tract
trifacial n.
trigeminal n.
trigone of auditory n.
trigone of hypoglossal n.
trigone of vagus n.
trochlear n.

N

nerve *(continued)*
    twelfth cranial n.
    ulnar n.
    vagus n.
    vestibular n.
    vestibulocochlear n.
    war of n.'s
    Wrisberg n.
    n. of Wrisberg
nerve-cell adhesion molecule (NCAM)
nerve-point massage
nervi (*gen. and pl. of* nervus)
nervimotility
nervimotion
nervimotor
nervine
nervios, nevra
    ataque de n.
Nervocaine
nervosa
    anorexia n. (AN)
    bulimia n.
    chronic anorexia n.
    dysphagia n.
    dysphoria n.
nervosus
    status n.
nervous
    n. asthma
    n. bladder
    n. breakdown
    n. debility
    n. depression
    n. disease
    n. distribution
    n. exhaustion
    n. fatigability
    n. fatigue
    n. gastritis
    n. giggling
    n. impulse
    n. indigestion
    n. laugh
    n. system
    n. system infection
    n. tension
    n. vomiting
nervus, gen. and pl. nervi
    n. abducens
    n. accessorius
    n. acusticus
    n. cochlearis
    nervi craniales
    n. facialis
    n. glossopharyngeus
    n. hypoglossus
    n. impar
    n. intermedius neuralgia
    n. octavus
    n. oculomotorius
    nervi olfactorii
    n. opticus
    n. statoacusticus
    n. trigeminus

    n. trochlearis
    n. vagus
    n. vestibularis
    n. vestibulocochlearis
NES
    norepinephrine-selective
Nesacaine
Nesacaine-MPF
nest
    bees' n.
    choristoma n.
    empty n.
    n. syndrome
net
    Neuro n.
N-ethyl-3,4-methylenedioxyamphetamine (MDEA)
netilmicin
network
    artificial neural n.
    Body Awareness Resource N. (BARNY)
    communication n.
    cortical n.
    delusional n.
    Drug Abuse Warning N. (DAWN)
    fragmented social n.
    interpersonal n.
    kinship n.
    matching and tuning n.
    Practice Research N.
    n. therapy
    wide area n.
Neucalm
Neumann syndrome
neuradynamia
neuragmia
neural
    n. arch resection
    n. axis
    n. canal
    n. cell adhesion molecule (NCAM)
    n. crest
    n. crest precursor
    n. crest syndrome
    n. crest tumor localization study
    n. cyst
    n. cytoarchitecture
    n. deafness
    n. deficit
    n. dissector
    n. ectoderm
    n. efficiency
    n. fold
    n. foramen
    n. foramen remodeling
    n. ganglion
    n. groove
    n. growth factor
    n. imaging study
    n. injury
    n. layer of retina
    n. noise level
    n. placode
    n. plasticity

n. plate
n. progenitor cell
n. prosthesis
n. regeneration
n. segment
n. tube
n. tube closure
n. tube defect (NTD)
n. tube floor plate cell

neuralgia
abdominal n.
atypical n.
chronic migrainous n.
ciliary n.
cranial n.
delayed-onset postherpetic n.
epileptiform n.
facial n.
n. facialis vera
Fothergill n.
geniculate n.
glossopharyngeal n. (GPN)
hallucinatory n.
Hunt n.
hypoglossal n.
idiopathic n.
intercostal n.
mammary n.
migrainous cranial n.
Morton n.
nasociliary n.
nerve entrapment n.
nervus intermedius n.
occipital n.
paratrigeminal n.
periodic migrainous n.
petrosal n.
postherpetic n.
posttraumatic n.
pterygopalatine n.
Raeder paratrigeminal n.
red n.
reminiscent n.
sciatic n.
Sluder n.
sphenopalatine n.
stump n.
suboccipital n.
supraorbital n.
symptomatic n.
Trélate-Charlin n.
trifacial n.
trigeminal n. (TN)
trigger point n.
vagoglossopharyngeal n.

neuralgic
n. amyotrophy
n. pain

neuralgiform
Neuramate
neuramebimeter
neuranagenesis
neurapophysis
neurapraxia

neurasthenia
acoustic n.
angioparalytic n.
angiopathic n.
aviator's n.
experimental n.
gastric n.
n. gravis
n. neurotic disorder
n. praecox
primary n.
professional n.
pulsating n.
sexual n.
traumatic n.

neurasthenic
n. helmet
n. neurosis
n. psychoneurosis
n. psychoneurotic reaction

neuraxis staging
neuraxon, neuraxone
neurectasis, neurectasia, neurectasy
neurectomy, neuroectomy
Cotte presacral n.
obturator n.
presacral n.
retrogasserian n.
Sonneberg n.
vestibular n.

neurectopia, neurectopy
Neurelan
neuremia
neurepithelium
neurergic
neurexeresis
neurexin
neuriatria, neuriatry
neurilemma, neurolemma
n. cell

neurilemoma
acoustic n.
Antoni type A n.
Antoni type B n.

neurility
neurimotility
neurimotor
neurinoma
acoustic n.
dumbbell-shaped n.
trigeminal nerve n.

neurite, neurit
dystrophic n.
n. extension
n. growth
n. outgrowth
n. overgrowth

neuritic
n. atrophy
n. plaque

neuriticum
atrophoderma n.

neuritis, pl. neuritides
adventitial n.
ascending n.

N

neuritis *(continued)*
    axial n.
    brachial plexus n.
    central n.
    descending n.
    Eichhorst n.
    eighth nerve herpetic n.
    endemic n.
    fallopian n.
    heavy-metal n.
    herpes zoster n.
    herpetic n.
    idiopathic plexus n.
    interdigital n.
    interstitial n.
    intraocular n.
    ischemic n.
    Leyden n.
    lumbosacral plexus n.
    multiple n.
    occipital n.
    optic n.
    parenchymatous n.
    peripheral n.
    relapsing hypertrophic n.
    retrobulbar n.
    sciatic n.
    segmental n.
    suboccipital n.
    toxic n.
    traction n.
    traumatic n.
    unilateral optic n.
neuro
    n. cognition
    n. convex transducer
    N. net
    N. N-50 lesion generator
    n. trend probe
neuroacanthocytosis
neuroactive
    n. amino acid
    n. peptide
neuroadaptation
neuroadenolysis
neuro-AIDS
neuroallergy
neuroanalysis
neuroanastomosis
    autogenous cable graft interposition
    VII-VII n.
neuroanatomy
    n. of aging
    behavioral n.
neuroanesthesia
neuroarthropathy
    atrophic n.
neuroastrocytoma
neuroaugmentation
neuroaugmentive
NeuroAvitene applicator
neuroaxonal dystrophy
neurobehavioral
    N. Cognitive Status Examination

    n. function
    n. readaptation
    n. syndrome
neuro-Behçet disease
neurobiochemistry
neurobiological factor
neurobiology
    behavioral n.
neurobiotactic movement
neurobiotaxis
neuroblast
neuroblastoma
    cerebral n.
    dumbbell-type n.
    Hutchinson type n.
    intraabdominal n.
    intracranial n.
    occipital n.
    olfactory n.
    Pepper n.
neuroborreliosis
    late Lyme n.
    Lyme n. (LNB)
neurocardiac
neurocardiogenic syncope
neurocele
NeuroCell-HD neural cell transplant
    product
NeuroCell-PD porcine neural cell
    transplant product
neurochemical research
neurochemistry
    behavioral n.
neurochitin
neurochorioretinitis
neurochoroiditis
neurocirculatory
    n. asthenia
    n. psychogenic disorder
neurocladism
neurocognition
neurocognitive
    n. deficit
    n. disorder
    n. information
NeuroCol neurosurgical sponge
NeuroControl Freehand implant
neurocristopathy
neurocutaneous
    n. angiomatosis
    n. melanosis
    n. syndrome
NeuroCybernetic
    N. prosthesis (NCP)
    N. Prosthesis System
neurocysticercosis (NCC)
neurocyte
neurocytolysis
neurocytoma
neurodegeneration
neurodegenerative
    n. disease
    n. process
neurodendrite
neurodendron

neurodevelopmental
  n. disorder
  n. dysfunction
  n. pattern
  n. telencephalic ontogenic process
neurodiagnostic imaging
neurodissector
  Penfield n.
NeuroDrape surgical drape
neurodynia
neuroectodermal tumor
neuroectodermatosis
neuroectomy (*var. of* neurectomy)
neuroencephalomyelopathy
neuroendocrine
  n. challenge
  n. function
  n. system
  n. test
  n. transducer cell
  n. tumor localization study
neuroendocrinology
neuroendoscope
  Neuroview n.
neuroendoscopy
  computer-assisted n. (CANE)
neuroenteric cyst
neuroepithelial
  n. cell
  n. cyst
  n. layer of retina
  n. tumor
neuroepithelium
  n. of ampullary crest
  n. cristae ampullaris
  n. of macula
  n. maculae
neuroethology
neurofeedback training (NT)
neurofibril
neurofibrillar
neurofibrillary
  n. degeneration
  n. lesion
  n. tangle
neurofibrillatory
  n. degeneration (NFD)
  n. tangle (NFT)
neurofibroma
  aryepiglottic fold n.
  dumbbell n.
  nonplexiform cutaneous n.
  orbital n.
  plexiform n.
  solitary n.
  spinal n.
neurofibromatosis
  abortive n.
  central n.
  cutaneous n.
  incomplete n.
  n. kyphoscoliosis
  kyphoscoliosis secondary to n.
  peripheral n.
  segmental n.

  n. type 1 (NF-1)
  n. type 2 (NF-2)
  von Recklinghausen n.
neurofibrosarcoma
neurofilament expression
neuroganglion
neurogenic, neurogenetic
  n. atrophy
  n. bladder
  n. claudication
  n. disorder
  n. dysphagia
  n. fracture
  n. hyperventilation
  n. lesion
  n. orthostatic hypotension
  n. pulmonary edema (NPE)
  n. reaction
  n. shock
  n. shock syndrome
neurogenous
neurogerontology
neuroglia cell
neurogliacyte
neuroglial, neurogliar
neurogliocytoma
neuroglioma
neurogliomatosis
neurogram
neurography
  magnetic resonance n. (MRN)
  n. needle
Neuroguard transcranial Doppler
neurohemal
neurohistology
neurohormone
neurohumor
neurohumoral
  n. hypothesis
  n. transmission
neurohypophyseal peptide
neurohypophysial
neurohypophysis
neuroid
neuroimaging
  functional n.
  n. studies
  three-dimensional n.
neuroimmunology
neuroinduction
neurointerventional
neurokeratin
neurokinin
neurokym
neurolemma (*var. of* neurilemma)
neuroleptanalgesia
neuroleptic
  n. agent
  n. anesthesia
  atypical n.
  n. bioavailability
  n. dose-dependent akathisia
  n. drug
  n. malignant syndrome (NMS)
  n. responsivity

N

neuroleptic *(continued)*
    n. treatment
    n. treatment of childhood conduct disorder
neuroleptic-induced
    n.-i. acute dystonia
    n.-i. acute movement disorder
    n.-i. akathisia
    n.-i. akinesia
    n.-i. dysphoria
    n.-i. parkinsonian tremor
    n.-i. parkinsonism
    n.-i. postural tremor
    n.-i. tardive dyskinesia
neuroleptic-related event
neuroleptic-resistant schizophrenic
neuroleptization
    rapid n.
neurolinguist
neurolinguistic
    n. assessment
    n. deficit
NeuroLink II EEG data acquisition system
Neurolite
neurologic
    n. complication
    n. deterioration
    n. diagnosis
    n. disability
    n. disease
    n. disorder
    n. disturbance
    n. evaluation
    n. impairment
    n. rehabilitation
    n. restitution
neurological
    n. amnesia
    n. condition
    n. control
    n. defect
    n. deficit
    n. disorder
    n. dysfunction
    N. Dysfunctions of Children
    n. evaluation
    n. examination
    n. functioning
    n. hammer
    n. maturation
    n. soft sign
neurologic-ophthalmologic history
neurologic-otology
neurologist
neurology
    behavioral n.
    environmental n.
    psychiatry and n. (P&N)
    restorative n.
neurolymph
neurolymphomatosis
neurolysis
    internal n.

neurolytic
neuroma
    acoustic n.
    amputation n.
    n. cutis
    extracanicular acoustic n.
    facial n.
    false n.
    fibrillary n.
    gasserian ganglion n.
    incisional n.
    Morton n.
    neuromata n.
    peripheral nerve n.
    plexiform n.
    posttraumatic n.
    n. telangiectodes
    traumatic n.
    trigeminal n.
    Verneuil n.
neuromalacia
neuromata neuroma
neuromatosa
neuromatosis
Neuromed Octrode implantable device
Neuromeet nerve approximator
neuromere
neuromessenger
neurometabolic disorder
Neurometer CPT/C for nerve evaluation
neurometric analysis
neurometrics
neuromimesis
neuromodulator
neuromotor
neuromuscular
    n. blockade
    n. blocking agent
    n. condition
    n. disorder
    n. electrical stimulation (NMES)
    n. junction
    n. rehabilitation
    n. scoliosis
    n. scoliosis orthotic treatment
    n. spindle
    n. transmission
neuromusculoskeletal syndrome
neuromyasthenia
    epidemic n.
neuromyelitis optica
neuromyopathy
    carcinomatous n.
neuromyositis
neuromyotonia
neuromyotonic discharge
neuron
    A9 n.
    abnormal epileptic n.
    accumbens n.
    afferent n.
    alpha motor n.
    aspiny n.
    autonomic motor n.
    bipolar n.

cholinergic n.
collateral sprouting n.
cortical n.
corticobulbar motor n.
corticospinal motor n.
n. doctrine
epileptic n.
excitability of n.
excitatory pyramidal n.
frontal lobe interstitial n.
gamma motor n.
ganglionic motor n.
giant n.
Golgi type I n.
Golgi type II n.
granular n.
hippocampal n.
n. II
intercalary n.
internuncial n.
locus ceruleus n.
lower motor n. (LMN)
McCullough-Pitts n.
motor n.
motorneuronal pool
  inhibitory n.
multipolar n.
nonsynaptic n.
noradrenergic n.
pedunculopontine n.
postganglionic motor n.
preganglionic motor n.
presynaptic n.
projection n.
pseudounipolar n.
pyramidal n.
redundant n.
sensory n.
serotonergic n.
somatic motor n.
somesthetic n.
spiny n.
stellate n.
striatal n.
TCR n.
unipolar n.
upper motor n.
visceral motor n.

neuronal
n. activity
n. adhesion
n. aggregate
n. ceroid lipofuscinosis
n. circuit
n. death
n. degeneration
n. differentiation
n. element firing
n. hyperexcitability
n. ingrowth
n. injury
n. lipidosis
n. loss
n. lysosomal storage disorder
n. membrane

n. metabolism
n. migration
n. necrosis
n. nitric oxide synthase (nNOS)
n. plasticity
n. polypeptide
n. pruning
n. regeneration
n. reuptake
n. shrinkage
n. signal
n. spike activity
n. sprouting
n. tumor
n. viability

neuronal/axonal
neuronavigation
frameless and armless
  stereotactic n.
neuronavigator
three-dimensional digitizer n.
neuronavigator-guided brain surgery
neurone
neuronitis
vestibular n.
neuronopathy
sensory n.
neuronophage
neuronophagia, neuronophagy
neuron-specific enolase (NSE)
Neurontin
neuronyxis
neurooncology
neuroophthalmology
neurootology
Neuropak
N. Four EMG/Evoked Response
  Measuring System Model MEM-
  4104K
N. 8 system
neuropapillitis
neuroparalysis
neuroparalytic
n. keratitis
n. ophthalmia
neuropath
neuropathic
n. arthritis
n. arthropathy
n. diathesis
n. hyperkyphoscoliosis
n. joint
neuropathicum
papilloma n.
neuropathogenesis
neuropathology
molecular n.
neuropathy
acquired demyelinative n.
acromegalic n.
acrylamide peripheral n.
acute ischemic brachial n.
AIDS n.
alcoholic peripheral n.
alcohol-induced peripheral n.

N

neuropathy *(continued)*
  alkaloid n.
  amyloid n.
  amyloidosis peripheral n.
  anterior ischemic optic n.
  anterior ischemic otic n.
  anterograde fast component n.
  arsenic peripheral n.
  asymmetric motor n.
  autonomic n.
  autosympathectomy secondary to n.
  avitaminosis B$_{12}$ peripheral n.
  axonal n.
  bacterial peripheral n.
  barbiturate peripheral n.
  Bassen-Kornzweig peripheral n.
  botulism peripheral n.
  brachial plexus n.
  brucellosis peripheral n.
  buffer n.
  B vitamin deficiency n.
  carcinoma peripheral n.
  carcinomatous n.
  chronic hepatic failure peripheral n.
  chronic inflammatory demyelinating
    sensorimotor n.
  chronic inflammatory
    demyelinative n.
  compressive n.
  congenital hypomyelination n.
  cranial n.
  Dejerine-Sottas peripheral n.
  demyelinating n.
  Denis Browne n.
  diabetic n.
  dinitrophenol peripheral n.
  diphtheria peripheral n.
  diphtheritic n.
  distal n.
  dying-back n.
  emetine peripheral n.
  entrapment n.
  ethyl alcohol peripheral n.
  facial n.
  familial n.
  femoral n.
  focal n.
  giant axonal n.
  glossopharyngeal n.
  gold peripheral n.
  griseofulvin peripheral n.
  Guillain-Barré postinfection
    peripheral n.
  handcuff n.
  heavy metal n.
  hepatic disease-associated n.
  hereditary motor and sensory n.
    (HMSN)
  hereditary sensorimotor n. (HSMN)
  hereditary sensory n. (HSN)
  HIV-related n.
  hyperthyroid n.
  hypertrophic interstitial n.
  hypoglossal n.

  hypoglycemic peripheral n.
  hypothyroid n.
  idiopathic n.
  infantile n.
  infection-related n.
  infectious hepatitis peripheral n.
  inflammatory demyelinating n.
  insecticide peripheral n.
  ischemic n.
  isoniazid n.
  isonicotinic acid peripheral n.
  Jamaican n.
  lead n.
  leprosy peripheral n.
  leprous n.
  lupus erythematosus peripheral n.
  Lyme n.
  macrocryoglobulinemia peripheral n.
  macroglobulinemia peripheral n.
  malabsorption syndrome
    peripheral n.
  measles peripheral n.
  mercury peripheral n.
  metachromatic leukodystrophy n.
  metal n.
  metal-produced n.
  methyl alcohol peripheral n.
  mitochondrial n.
  mononucleosis peripheral n.
  motor dapsone n.
  multifocal motor n. (MFMN)
  multiple myeloma peripheral n.
  mumps peripheral n.
  myeloma-associated n.
  myxedema peripheral n.
  nonprogressive n.
  nutritional n.
  occupational n.
  oculomotor n.
  onion bulb n.
  optic n.
  pantothenic acid deficiency
    peripheral n.
  paraneoplastic n.
  paraproteinemic n.
  peripheral autonomic n.
  peroneal entrapment n.
  phrenic n.
  polyarteritis nodosa peripheral n.
  porphyria peripheral n.
  porphyric n.
  progressive hypertrophic n.
  progressive hypertrophic
    interstitial n.
  pure sensory n.
  radiation n.
  radicular n.
  Refsum peripheral n.
  relapsing n.
  retrograde fast component n.
  rheumatoid n.
  sarcoid n.
  sarcoidosis peripheral n.
  segmental n.
  sensorimotor peripheral n.

sensory n.
sensory-motor-autonomic n.
serum sickness peripheral n.
Shy-Drager n.
slow component n.
sprue peripheral n.
steroid-sensitive n.
subacute demyelinating n.
subacute myelo-optic n. (SMON)
subclinical n.
sulfonamide peripheral n.
symmetrical diffuse n.
symmetric distal n.
Tangier peripheral n.
thallium peripheral n.
therapeutic-agent related n.
tomaculous n.
traumatic n.
tricresyl phosphate peripheral n.
trigeminal n.
tropical ataxic n.
tuberculosis peripheral n.
typhoid peripheral n.
ulnar n.
uremia peripheral n.
uremic n.
vaccination peripheral n.
vagus n.
vasculitic n.
vestibulocochlear n.
vincristine peripheral n.
vitamin B12 n.
Wegener granulomatosis-
    associated n.
Whipple disease peripheral n.
neuropeptide
    n. change
    n. oxytocin
    n. Y (NPY)
neuropharmacology
neurophilic
neurophonia
neurophthalmology
neurophysin
neurophysiological
    n. assessment
    n. finding
    n. heterogeneity
    n. monitoring
    n. testing
neurophysiology
neuropil, neuropile
    n. thread
neuroplasm
neuroplastic response
neuroplasty
neuroplegic
neuropodia
neuropore
    caudal n.
    rostral n.
neuroprotective
neuropsychiatric
    n. movement disorder
    N. Rating Schedule

n. systemic lupus erythematosus
    (NP-SLE)
n. test
neuropsychiatrist (NP)
neuropsychiatry (NP)
    geriatric n.
neuropsychic
neuropsychologic, neuropsychological
    n. assessment
    n. deficit
    n. disorder
    n. evaluation
    n. finding
    n. impairment
    n. skill
    n. test
    n. testing
Neuropsychological
    N. Screening Examination
    N. Status Examination
neuropsychology
neuropsychometric test
neuropsychopathic
neuropsychopathy
neuropsychopharmacology
neuropsychophysiological
neuropsychosis
neuroradiology
    interventional n.
    pediatric n.
neuroreceptor
neurorecidive
neurorecurrence
neuroregeneration
neurorelapse
neuroretinal angiomatosis
neuroretinitis
neurorrhaphy
    epineurial n.
neurosarcocleisis
neurosarcoidosis
    meningeal n.
neuroschisis
neuroschwannoma
neuroscience
neurosecretion
neurosecretory
    n. cell
    n. substance
neuroshunting
neurosis, pl. neuroses
    accident n.
    actual n.
    acute conditioned n. (ACN)
    analytic n.
    anancastic n.
    anxiety n.
    artificial n.
    association n.
    asthenic n.
    battle n.
    cardiac n.
    cardiovascular n.
    character n.
    chronic posttraumatic n.

N

neurosis *(continued)*
   climacteric n.
   collective n.
   combat n.
   compensation n.
   compulsion n.
   compulsive n.
   conversion hysteria n.
   countertransference n.
   craft n.
   death n.
   decompensative n.
   depersonalization n.
   depressive n.
   dissociative-type hysterical n.
   ego n.
   environmental n.
   esophageal n.
   existential n.
   expectation n.
   experimental n.
   family n.
   fate n.
   fatigue n.
   fixation n.
   functional n.
   generalized anxiety n.
   homosexual n.
   housewife n.
   hypochondriacal n.
   hysterical n.
   impulsive n.
   infinity n.
   malignant n.
   menopause n.
   military n.
   mixed n.
   monosymptomatic n.
   motor n.
   neurasthenic n.
   noogenic n.
   obsessional n.
   obsessive-compulsive n.
   occlusal n.
   occupational n.
   oedipal n.
   organ n.
   organic n.
   pain-type anxiety n.
   panic-type anxiety n.
   pension n.
   performance n.
   perhaps n.
   phobic n.
   phobic obsessional n.
   postconcussion n.
   posttraumatic n.
   prison n.
   professional n.
   progredient n.
   promotion n.
   psychasthenic n.
   psychoanalytic n.
   railroad n.
   regression n.
   regressive transference n.
   retirement n.
   senile n.
   sexual n.
   situational posttraumatic n.
   success n.
   Sunday n.
   suppression n.
   symptom n.
   n. tarda
   torsion n.
   transference n.
   traumatic n.
   uprooting n.
   vagabond n.
   vegetative n.
   visceral n.
   war n.
   weekend n.
neurosonology
neurospasm
neurosplanchnic
neurospongioma
neurospongium
Neurostation One
neurosthenia
neurostimulation
neurostimulator
neurosurgeon
neurosurgery
   functional n.
   molecular n.
   stereotactic n.
neurosurgical
   N. Cervical Spine Scale
   n. needle holder
   n. stereotactic robot
neurosuture
neurosyphilis
   asymptomatic n.
   cerebral n.
   cerebrovascular n.
   congenital n.
   ectodermogenic n.
   interstitial n.
   meningeal n.
   meningitic n.
   meningovascular n.
   ophthalmic n.
   parenchymatous n.
   paretic n.
   tabetic n.
   vascular n.
neurotabes
   Dejerine peripheral n.
neurotendinous
   n. organ
   n. spindle
neurotensin
neurotension
neurothekeoma
neurothele
neurotherapeutics, neurotherapy
neurothlipsis, neurothlipsia

neurotic
  n. acting out
  alopecia n.
  n. delinquency
  n. depression
  n. direction profile
  n. excoriation
  n. feature
  n. hysteric disorder
  n. manifestation
  masculine attitude in female n.
  n. paradox
  passive-aggressive n.
  n. personality
  N. Personality Factor Test (NPFT)
  n. process
  n. reaction
  n. reaction brain syndrome
  n. resignation
  n. rumination
  n. state
  n. state with depersonalization
  n. state with depersonalization
    episode
neurotica
neurotic-depressive reaction
neuroticism/extroversion/openness (NEO)
**Neuroticism/Extroversion/Openness to
  Experience personality questionnaire**
**Neuroticism-Extroversion-Openness
  Personality Inventory**
Neuroticism Scale Questionnaire (NSQ)
neuroticum
  papilloma n.
neurotization
neurotize
neurotmesis
neurotogenic
neurotology
neurotome
neurotomy
  retrogasserian n.
  Spiller-Frazier n.
neurotonic
neurotony
neurotoxic
neurotoxicity
  FK-506 n.
  glutamate n.
neurotoxin
  therapeutic botulinum n.
neurotransmission
  adrenergic n.
  chemical n.
  glutamatergic n.
  serotonergic n.
neurotransmitter
  acetylcholine as n.
  amino acid n.
  biogenic amine n.
  catecholamine n.
  coexistence of n.
  excitatory n.
  n. metabolite

  peptide n.
  putative n.
  n. receptor
  n. release
  specific n.
  n. synthesizing enzyme
  n. system
neurotrauma
**Neurotrend continuous multiparameter
  system**
neurotripsy
neurotrophasthenia
neurotrophic
  n. atrophy
  brain-derived n.
  n. factor expression
  n. keratitis
neurotrophin
neurotrophy
neurotropic
neurotropy, neurotropism
neurotrosis
neurotubule
neurovaricosis, neurovaricosity
neurovascular
  n. flap
  n. imaging
  n. tree
neurovegetative
  n. sign
  n. symptom
Neuroview
  N. integrated visualization system
  N. neuroendoscope
neurovirology
neurovirulence
neurovisceral
Neurturin
neurula, pl. neurulae
neurulation
neutral
  n. attitude
  K-Phos N.
  n. party
  n. spirit
  n. stimulus
neutrality
  therapeutic n.
neutralization
  anterior n.
  n. rule
neutralize
neutralized anxiety
neutralizing mechanism
Neutra-Phos
Neutra-Phos-K
neutropenia
nevi (*pl. of* nevus)
**Nevin-Jones subacute spongiform
  encephalopathy**
nevios
nevirapine
nevoid amentia
nevra (*var. of* nervios)

N

névropathique
    famille n.
nevus, pl. **nevi**
    basal cell n.
    blue n.
    Jadassohn n.
    Ota n.
    port wine n.
    Spitz n.
new
    n. age
    N. Hampshire rule
    N. Haven Schizophrenia Index
    N. Haven study
    N. Jersey Test of Reasoning Skills
    n. magic
    N. Mexico Attitude Toward Work Test (NMATWT)
    N. Mexico Career Planning Test (NMCPT)
    N. Mexico Job Application Procedures Test (NMJAPT)
    N. Mexico Knowledge of Occupations Test (NMKOT)
    n. responsibility
    N. Sucher-Allred Reading Placement Inventory
    n. wave
    N. York University Parkinson Disease Scale
newer-generation device
newly abstinent alcoholic
Newman-Keuls Test
new-onset seizure
Newport collar
newtonian body
new-work effort
NEX
    number of excitations
nexus, pl. **nexus**
NF-1
    neurofibromatosis type 1
NF-2
    neurofibromatosis type 2
NFD
    neurofibrillatory degeneration
NFT
    neurofibrillatory tangle
NGF
    nerve growth factor
NGI
    not guilty by reason of insanity
    Nurse's Global Impressions
    NGI Scale
NGRI
    not guilty by reason of insanity
NGTF
    National Gay Task Force
NHAIS
    Naylor-Harwood Adult Intelligence Scale
NHIS
    Naylor-Harwood Intelligence Scale
niacin deficiency

NIAID
    National Institute of Allergy and Infectious Disease
nialamide
niaprazine
nicardipine
NicErase-SL
niche
Nichrome cylindrical electrode
nickel deck
Nicoderm
    N. CQ
    N. HP
    N. Patch
Nicola
    N. forceps
    N. pituitary rongeur
    N. rasp
    N. scissors
Nicolet
    N. Compass EMG instrument
    N. Pathfinder I
    N. Pathfinder I recording device
    N. Viking II electrophysiologic system
Nicorette
    N. DS Gum
    N. Gum
    N. Inhaler
nicotine
    n. abstinence
    n. abuse
    n. addiction
    n. dependence
    n. habit
    n. intoxication
    n. organic brain disorder
    n. pharmacology
    n. poisoning
    n. polacrilex
    n. test
    n. use disorder
    n. withdrawal
nicotine-induced disorder
nicotine-related
    n.-r. disorder NOS
    n.-r. disorder, not otherwise specified
nicotinic
    n. acetylcholine receptor
    n. acid deficiency
    n. cholinergic receptor
    n. receptor blockade
Nicotrol
    N. inhaler
    N. NS Nasal Spray
    N. Patch
nictation
nictitans
    spasmus n.
nictitate
nictitating spasm
nictitation
NIDA
    National Institute on Drug Abuse

NIDA-certified forensic toxicology
  laboratory
nidal
nidus, pl. nidi
    n. avis
    n. definition
    n. hirundinis
    n. obliteration
niebla
Nielsen syndrome
Niemann-Pick disease (type A, B, C)
niente
    dolce far n.
nifedipine
nifurtimox
niger
    Aspergillus n.
niggling
night
    every n.
    n. fantasy
    n. hospital
    n. pain
    n. palsy
    n. residue
    slept all n. (SAN)
    n. terror
    wedding n.
night-eating syndrome
nightmare disorder
nightshade poisoning
nighttime
    n. activity
    n. agitation
nigra
    fetal substantia n.
    substantia n.
nigrostriatal
    n. dopaminergic system
    n. pathway
    n. tract
nihilism
    n. theme
    therapeutic n.
nihilistic
    n. delusion
NIH Stroke Scale
Nilain
nimbies
nimetazepam
NIMH
    NIMH data
    NIMH Global Obsessive-Compulsive
      Scale
NIMH-OC
    National Institute of Mental Health-
      Global Obsessive Compulsive Scale
nimodipine
Nimotop
nimustine
nine-digit task
Ninjitsu
Nintendo epilepsy
ninth cranial nerve

niobium-titanium
Niopam
Nipride
Nirvana principle
Nishioka system
Nishizaki-Wakabayashi suction tube
Nissl
    N. body
    N. degeneration
    N. granule
    N. staining
    N. substance
nisus
2-nite
    Sleepwell 2-n.
nitrate
    butyl n.
    gallium n.
    n. inhalant
    isobutyl n.
nitrazepam
nitric
    n. acid (NO)
    n. oxide (NO)
    n. oxide synthase (NOS)
nitrite
    amyl n.
    butyl n.
    ethyl n.
    n. headache
    n. inhalant
    isobutyl n.
Nitro-Bid
nitrocellulose
nitrogen
    blood urea n. (BUN)
    n. metabolism
    n. mustard
    n. narcosis
    n. wasting
nitroglycerin
nitroprusside
    sodium n.
nitrosourea hydrochloride
Nitrostat
nitrous
    n. oxide
    n. oxide dependence
nizofenone
NL
    normal libido
    NL CICI
NLC&C
    normal libido, coitus, and climax
NLT
    Names Learning Test
NMATWT
    New Mexico Attitude Toward Work Test
NMCPT
    New Mexico Career Planning Test
NMDA
    N-methyl-D-aspartate
    NMDA receptor
    NMDA receptor alteration

NMES
    neuromuscular electrical stimulation
N-methyl-D-aspartate (NMDA)
N-methyl-D-aspartate receptor
***N*-methylspiroperidol**
NMI
    no mental illness
NMJAPT
    New Mexico Job Application Procedures
    Test
NMKOT
    New Mexico Knowledge of Occupations
    Test
NMR
    nuclear magnetic resonance
NMS
    neuroleptic malignant syndrome
NNN
    normal neonatal nursery
nNOS
    neuronal nitric oxide synthase
NO
    nitric acid
    nitric oxide
no
    n. acute distress (NAD)
    n. diagnosis or condition on axis
    n. event
    n. fault
    n. mental illness (NMI)
    n. more than slight impairment
    N. Pain-HP
noc
Nocardia asteroides
nocardiosis
    cerebral n.
nocere
    primum non n.
nociassociation
nociceptive
    n. impulse
    n. pain
    n. reflex
nociceptor activation
nocifensor reflex
nociinfluence
nociperception
NOCT
    National Occupation Competency Testing
noctambulation
noctambulism
Noctec
noctimania
noctiphobia
noctis
    jus primae n.
nocturna
    enuresis n.
    jactatio capitis n.
nocturnal
    n. confusion
    n. diarrhea
    n. drinking syndrome
    n. eating syndrome
    n. emission

    n. enuresis
    n. epilepsy
    n. hallucination
    n. hemiplegia
    n. hemoglobinuria
    n. myoclonus
    n. panic attack
    n. paralysis
    n. paroxysmal dystonia
    n. penile tumescence (NPT)
    n. penile tumescence study
    n. penile tumescence test
    n. sleep episode
    n. vertigo
nocturnus
    jactatio capitis n.
    pavor n.
nocuous
nodal behavior
nodding spasm
node
    Dürck n.
    flocculonodular n.
    Hensen n.
    primitive n.
    Ranvier n.
    n. of Ranvier
    Schmorl n.
    vital n.
nodosa
    periarteritis n.
    polyarteritis n. (PAN)
    trichorrhexis n.
nodose ganglion
NoDoz
nodular, nodous
    n. enhancement
    n. headache
    n. induration of temporal artery
    n. mesoneuritis
    n. panencephalitis
nodule
    glial n.
    Lisch n.
    mulberry-like n.
    Schmorl n.
nodulus, pl. noduli
noematachograph
noematachometer
noematic
noesis
noetic anxiety
noeud vital
no-holds-barred
noise
    acoustic n.
    ambient n.
    n. analyzer
    background n.
    complex n.
    extraneous n.
    n. factor
    feedback n.
    n. figure
    gaussian n.

pink n.
random n.
n. reduction device
white n.
noisome
nolo contendere
Noludar
Nolvadex
nomadic lifestyle
nomadism
Nomad-LE EMG
nomatophobia
nomenclature
psychiatric n.
standard psychiatric n.
nomifensine
nominal
n. aphasia
n. standard dose (NSD)
nominalization
nomogram
d'Ocagne n.
nomograph
nomological
nomothetic approach
non
n. compos mentis
n. grata
n. possumus
n. sequitur
non-24-hour sleep-wake syndrome
nonability
cognitive n.
nonabrasive
nonacceptable
nonaddicting
nonadherent (NA)
nonaffective hallucination
nonage
nonaggressive
non-Alzheimer frontal lobe type
dementia
nonamphetamine
central nervous system
stimulant, n.
nonanaplastic oligodendroglioma
nonaneurysmal perimesencephalic
subarachnoid hemorrhage
non-aplastic glioma
nonattentive
nonautistic
non-autobiographical memory
nonaxial
n. fashion
n. format
nonbacterial thrombotic endocarditis
nonbarbiturate
nonbeliever
nonbenzodiazepine
nonbiological artifact
nonbizarre
n. delusion
n. symptoms
noncaloric
noncephalic electrode

noncerebral activity
nonchalance
nonchalant
noncharismatic
nonchromaffin paraganglioma
noncognitive subscale
noncoherent
noncoital stimulation
noncombatant
noncommissioned officer (NCO)
noncommunicating hydrocephalus
noncomparable
noncomplementary role
noncompliance with medical treatment
noncompliant
noncomprehension
nonconclusive
nonconcur
nonconflicting
nonconformance
nonconformist
nonconfrontive therapy
nonconsanguineous marriage
nonconsenting
n. adult
n. partner
noncontrastive distribution
noncontributory
noncontroversial
nonconvulsive status epilepticus
noncooperative
noncued memory pattern
noncustodial parent
nondampened waveform
nondecalcified trabecula
nondefense
nondeficit schizophrenia
nondemented
nondependent adult abuse
nondepolarizing
nondepressed mood
nondescript
nondetachable
n. endovascular balloon
n. occlusive balloon
n. silicone balloon catheter
nondirective
n. approach
n. psychotherapy
n. therapy
nondisclosure
nondiscretionary
nondiscriminatory
nondisease
psychogenic cardiac n.
nondistinctive feature
nondominant
n. hand
n. hemisphere
n. hemisphere lesion
n. putaminal hemorrhage
nondopaminergic
nondouloureux
tic n.
nondystrophin myopathy

N

nonegalitarian
noneloquent area
nonembolic infarction
nonenteric cyst
nonentity
nonepileptic myoclonic contraction
nonepileptiform activity
nonexistent
nonextrapyramidal neurologic sign
nonfatal
nonfattening
nonfeasance
nonferromagnetic clip
nonferrous material
nonfluent
    n. aphasia
    n. aphasic seizure
    n. aphasic speech
nonfunctional and repetitive motor
  behavior
nongeneral phobic
nongeriatric
nonhazardous
nonhemolytic hyperbilirubinemia
nonhemorrhagic cerebral infarction
nonhereditary
nonhero
nonhomonymous field defect
nonictal
nonidentical
noninvasive
    n. diagnosis
    n. operation
noninvolvement
nonionic
nonketotic
    n. hyperglycemia
    n. hyperglycemic hyperosmolar
      coma
non-kraepelinian chronic schizophrenia
nonlacunar syndrome
Non-Language
    N.-L. Learning Test
    N.-L. Multi-Mental Test
nonlesional cortical resection
nonlinear distortion
nonlinguistic
nonmajor depression
nonmedullated fiber
nonmeningiomatous malignant lesion
non-microsurgical procedure
non-missile head injury
nonmoral
nonmyelinated
nonnarcotic analgesic
nonnegative
nonnegotiable
nonneoplastic disease
non-neuroleptic-induced tremor
nonneuronal
nonneuropathic
nonnormative hair loss
nonobjective
no-nonsense
nonoo

nonopioid
nonorganic
    acute paranoid reaction n.
    n. origin
    n. origin insomnia
    psychogenic paranoid n.
    n. psychosis
    n. steep disorder
nonorgasmic
nonorthodox
no-no tremor
nonparametric tests of significance
nonparaphilic compulsive sexual
  behavior
nonparkinsonian tremor
nonparticipant observer
nonparticipatory
nonpartisan
nonpathological
    n. amnesia
    n. anxiety
    n. reaction
    n. sexual fantasy
    n. substance use
nonpenetrating trauma
nonpersistent
nonperson
nonphantom study
nonpharmacologic
nonpharmacologically induced tremor
nonphobic anxiety behavior therapy
nonphysiologic artifact
nonplexiform cutaneous neurofibroma
nonplussed
nonprescription
    n. drug
    n. drug abuse
nonproband
nonproblematic drinking
nonproductive
    n. activity
    n. behavior
nonprogressive neuropathy
nonproton
    n. magnetic resonance imaging
    n. MRI
nonpsychotic
    n. anxiety
    n. mental disorder
    n. onset of symptoms
    n. posttraumatic brain
    n. severity psychoorganic
    n. severity psychoorganic syndrome
    n. unipolar depression
    unspecified mental disorder, n.
nonpsychotropic drug
nonpulsating headache
nonpurging method
nonrandom mating
nonrapid
    n. eye movement (non-REM,
      NREM)
    n. eye movement sleep
nonreactive depression
nonreader

Non-Reading
 N.-R. Aptitude Test Battery
 (NATB)
 N.-R. Intelligence Test, Levels 1-3
 (NRIT)
nonrecognition
 spatial n.
nonrecurrent
non-reduplicated babbling
nonreference recording
nonregressive schizophrenia
non-REM
 nonrapid eye movement
 non-REM sleep
nonreporting
nonresidency
nonresistant
nonrespondent
nonresponsive state
nonrestorative sleep
nonrestraint
nonrestrictive
nonrheumatic atrial fibrillation
nonrhythmic
 n. stereotyped motor movement
 n. vocalization
nonrigid
nonscientific
nonselective
 n. expression of transgene
 n. phosphodiesterase inhibitor
nonsense
 n. syndrome
 n. in wit
nonsensical
 n. speech
 n. statement
nonsensuous
nonseptic embolic brain infarction
nonserotonergic
nonsexist
nonsexual boundary violation
nonsignificant
nonsmoker (NS)
nonsocial
nonspeaking
nonspecific
 n. abnormality
 n. abnormality on EEG
 n. encephalomyeloneuropathy
 n. language
 n. research
 n. stress
 n. syndrome
 n. system
nonstandard
nonstarter
nonstereotactic PET
nonsteroidal anti-inflammatory drug
 (NSAID)
non-substance-induced mental disorder
nonsuffocation panicker
nonsupport
nonsuppression
 dextramethasone n.

nonsymbolic
nonsynaptic
 n. neuron
 n. transmission
nonsystematic schizophrenia
nonsystematized delusion
nontherapeutic
nonthrombogenic
nontoxic
 n. gene expression
 n. lithium tremor
 n. substance
nontranssexual cross-gender disorder
nontraumatic necrosis of bone
nontrivial value
nonturning against self (NTS)
nonunion
 n. incidence
 n. rate
nonunique
nonuser
nonvasculitic autoimmune inflammatory
 meningoencephalitis (NAIM)
nonverbal
 N. Ability Test (NAT)
 n. behavior
 n. communication
 n. expression
 n. information
 n. intellectual capacity
 n. language
 N. Reasoning
 n. task
nonviable
nonviolence
nonviolent behavior
nonvocal communication
noogenic neurosis
nookleptia
noology
Noonan syndrome
noon of life
noopsyche
noothymopsychic ataxia
nootropic
noradrenalin
noradrenaline dementia of Alzheimer
 type
noradrenergic
 n. drug
 n. neuron
 n. receptor
 n. synapse
 n. system
Norcet
Norco
Norcuron
nordazepam
Nordstadt classification
no-reflow phenomenon
norepinephrine (NE)
 n. neurotransmitter systems
norepinephrine-selective (NES)
norfenfluramine
Norflex

norfluoxetine
Norgesic Forte
Norland digital oscilloscope
norm
> age n.
> age-appropriate societal n.
> cultural n.
> deviation from physiological n.
> grade n.
> group n.
> occupational n.
> percentile n.
> physiological n.
> social n.
> societal n.
> subculture n.

normal
> n. affect
> n. anxiety
> n. childhood development
> n. curve
> n. distribution
> n. libido (NL)
> n. libido, coitus, and climax (NL CICI, NLC&C)
> n. limits
> n. mentation
> n. neonatal nursery (NNN)
> n. neurological functioning
> n. perfusion pressure breakthrough (NPPB)
> n. pressure hydrocephalus (NPH)
> n. range of mood
> n. transition
> n. voluntary napping phenomenon

normalcy
normality
normalization
norm-assertive stance
normative
> N. Adaptive Behavior Checklist
> n. aging process
> n. behavior
> n. crisis
> n. data
> n. ethics

normative-referenced
normatologically
normatological research
normatology
normethadone
normokalemic periodic paralysis
normotensive hydrocephalus
normothymatic
normotonic
normotype
normoxic diffusion
Norpace
Norpramin
Norris Educational Achievement Test (NEAT)
North American Depression Inventories for Children and Adults

Northern
> N. hybridization
> N. Manhattan Stroke Study

Northwestern
> N. Syntax Screening Test (NSST)
> N. University Children's Perception of Speech Test

Northwick
> N. Park Index of Independence in ADL
> N. Park Index of Independence in ADL index

nortriptyline
Norvir
NOS
> nitric oxide synthase
> not otherwise specified
> > NOS category
> > impulse-control disorder NOS
> > nicotine-related disorder NOS
> > PDD NOS
> > personality disorder NOS
> > phencyclidine-related disorder NOS

nose-bridge-lid reflex
nosecone
> CEM handswitching n.

nose drops
nose-eye reflex
nosemaphobia
noser
nosey (*var. of* nosy)
nosh
NOSIE
> Nurses' Observation Scale for Inpatient Evaluation

nosocomion, nosocomium
nosogenesis
nosogeny
nosological
nosology
> psychiatric n.

nosomania
nosophilia
nosophobia
nosotropic
> n. drug
> n. drug dementia of Alzheimer type

nostalgist
nostomania
nostophobia
nostrum
nosy, nosey
not
> n. applicable
> n. due to direct physiological effects of a substance or a general medical condition
> n. guilty by reason of insanity (NGI, NGRI)
> n. otherwise specified (NOS)
> n. prisoner of war (NPOW)
> n. significant (NS)

notanencephalia

notch
> anterior n. of cerebellum
> n. filter
> Kernohan n.
> marsupial n.
> posterior n. of cerebellum
> preoccipital n.
> semilunar n.
> n. of tentorium

note blindness
not-for-profit hospital
nothing by mouth (NPO)
Nothnagel syndrome
notification
notochord
Nottingham
> N. Extended ADL Index
> N. Health Profile
> N. Ten-Point ADL Scale

noumenal
noumenon
nourishment
nous
nouveau riche
nouvelle vague
novation
novelistic
novel stimulus
novelty seeking
novelty-seeking trait
novo
> de n.

Novo-10a CBF measuring device
Novocain Injection
Novodorm
Novopaque
Novus
> N. hydrocephalic valve
> N. mini valve

no-win relationship
noxa
noxious
> n. responsibility
> n. stimulus

NP
> neuropsychiatrist
> neuropsychiatry

NPE
> neurogenic pulmonary edema

NPFT
> Neurotic Personality Factor Test

NPH
> normal pressure hydrocephalus
> nucleus prepositus hypoglossi

NPH Iletin I
NPO
> nothing by mouth

NPOW
> not prisoner of war

NPPB
> normal perfusion pressure breakthrough

NP-SLE
> neuropsychiatric systemic lupus
> erythematosus

NPT
> nocturnal penile tumescence

NPY
> neuropeptide Y

NREM
> nonrapid eye movement
> NREM sleep

NRIT
> Non-Reading Intelligence Test, Levels 1-
> 3

NS
> nonsmoker
> not significant
> Stadol NS

NS2000 bipolar generator system
NSAID
> nonsteroidal anti-inflammatory drug

NSD
> nominal standard dose

NSE
> neuron-specific enolase

NSQ
> Neuroticism Scale Questionnaire

NSST
> Northwestern Syntax Screening Test

NT
> neurofeedback training

NTD
> neural tube defect

NTL
> National Training Laboratories

NTS
> nonturning against self

nuance
Nubain
nubility
nubs
nuchal
> n. dystonia
> n. muscle
> n. rigidity

nuchocephalic reflex
nuclear
> n. bag
> n. envelope
> n. family
> n. imaging
> n. jaundice
> n. layers of retina
> n. magnetic relaxation dispersion
> n. magnetic resonance (NMR)
> n. magnetization vector
> n. MR scan
> n. ophthalmoplegia
> n. problem
> n. psuedoinclusion
> n. relaxation
> n. schizophrenia
> n. signal
> n. spin
> n. spin quantum number
> n. transsexual
> n. transvestite
> n. war

nuclei (*pl. of* nucleus)

N

nucleic acid metabolism
nucleofugal
nucleolysis
    percutaneous laser n.
nucleomitaphobia
nucleon
nucleopetal
nucleotide
    guanine n.
nucleotome
    N. aspiration probe
    N. Endoflex instrument
    N. Flex II cannula instrument
    N. Flex II flexible cutting probe
    n. procedure
nucleotomy
    laser n.
nucleus, pl. nuclei
    abducens n.
    n. abducentis
    n. of abducent nerve
    accessory cuneate n.
    accessory oculomotor n.
    accessory olivary nuclei
    n. accumbens septi
    n. acusticus
    n. alae cinereae
    almond n.
    ambiguous n.
    n. ambiguus
    n. amygdalae
    amygdaloid n.
    nuclei anteriores thalami
    n. anterodorsalis
    anterodorsal thalamic n.
    n. anteromedialis
    anteromedial thalamic n.
    n. anteroventralis
    anteroventral thalamic n.
    arcuate n.
    nuclei arcuati
    n. arcuatus
    n. arcuatus thalami
    auditory n.
    n. basalis of Ganser
    n. basalis lesion
    n. basalis of Meynert
    Bechterew n.
    Blumenau n.
    branchiomotor nuclei
    Burdach n.
    n. of Cajal
    n. caudalis
    n. caudalis-nucleus solitarius DREZ
      lesioning
    caudate n.
    n. caudatus
    cell n.
    n. centralis lateralis thalami
    n. centralis tegmenti superior
    central tegmental n.
    centromedian n.
    n. centromedianus
    cerebellar nuclei
    Clarke n.

    cochlear nuclei
    nuclei cochleares
    n. colliculi inferioris
    convergence n. of Perlia
    n. corporis geniculati medialis
    nuclei corporis mamillaris
    cranial motor nuclei (CMN)
    nuclei of cranial nerves
    cuneate n.
    n. cuneatus
    n. cuneatus accessorius
    n. of Darkschewitsch
    deep cerebellar n.
    Deiters n.
    dentate n. of cerebellum
    n. dentatus cerebelli
    descending n. of the trigeminus
    dorsal accessory olivary n.
    dorsal cochlear n.
    n. dorsalis
    n. dorsalis corporis trapezoidei
    n. dorsalis nervi vagi
    dorsal motor n. of vagus
    dorsal raphe nuclei
    dorsal n. of vagus
    dorsomedial hypothalamic n.
    n. dorsomedialis hypothalami
    Edinger-Westphal n.
    ego n.
    emboliform n.
    n. emboliformis
    external cuneate n.
    extrapyramidal n.
    n. facialis
    facial motor n.
    n. fasciculi gracilis
    n. fastigii
    n. fibrosus linguae
    n. filiformis
    force n.
    n. funiculi cuneati
    n. funiculi gracilis
    n. gelatinosus
    geniculate n.
    n. gigantocellularis medullae
      oblongatae
    n. globosus
    n. of Goll
    gracile n.
    n. gracilis
    Gudden tegmental nuclei
    gustatory n.
    n. habenulae
    habenular n.
    hypoglossal n.
    n. of hypoglossal nerve
    inferior olivary n.
    inferior salivary n.
    inferior vestibular n.
    intercalated n.
    n. intercalatus
    intermediolateral n.
    n. intermediolateralis
    intermediomedial n.
    n. intermediomedialis

interpeduncular n.
n. interpeduncularis
n. interpositus
interpositus nuclei
interstitial n. of Cajal
n. interstitialis
intralaminar nuclei
nuclei intralaminares thalami
intralaminar nuclei of thalamus
lateral cuneate n.
lateral geniculate n. (LGN)
n. lateralis medullae oblongatae
n. lateralis thalami
n. of lateral lemniscus
lateral n. of medulla oblongata
lateral preoptic n.
lateral reticular n.
lateral n. of thalamus
lateral tuberal nuclei
lateral vestibular n.
n. lemnisci lateralis
n. of lens
lenticular n.
lentiform n.
n. lentiformis
n. lentis
n. of Luys
main sensory n. of the trigeminus
n. of the mamillary body
n. masticatorius
masticatory n.
medial accessory olivary n.
medial central n. of thalamus
medial geniculate n. (MGN)
n. of medial geniculate body
n. medialis centralis thalami
n. medialis thalami
medial preoptic n.
medial n. of thalamus
medial vestibular n.
mediodorsal n.
medullary raphe n.
mesencephalic n. of the trigeminus
midline nuclei
Monakow n.
motor n. of facial nerve
n. motorius nervi trigemini
motor n. of trigeminus
n. nervi abducentis
nuclei nervi cochlearis
n. nervi facialis
n. nervi hypoglossi
n. nervi oculomotorii
n. nervi trochlearis
nuclei nervi vestibulocochlearis
nuclei nervorum cranialium
n. niger
nucleus ventralis posteromedialis thalami
nucleus ventralis thalami
oculomotor n.
n. of oculomotor nerve
n. olivaris
n. olivaris accessorius dorsalis
n. olivaris accessorius medialis

Onuf n.
nuclei of origin
nuclei originis
oval hyperchromatic n.
parabrachial nuclei
nuclei parabrachiales
n. paracentralis thalami
paracentral n. of thalamus
paraventricular n.
n. paraventricularis
pedunculopontine n.
Perlia n.
phrenic motor n.
pontine nuclei (PN)
nuclei pontis
n. posterior hypothalami
posterior hypothalamic n.
posterior medial n. of thalamus
posterior periventricular n.
n. preopticus lateralis
n. preopticus medialis
n. prepositus hypoglossi (NPH)
prerubral n.
Prosthetic Disc N. (PDN)
n. pulposus
n. pyramidalis
raphe nuclei
n. raphe magnus
nuclei raphes
red n.
reticular nuclei of the brainstem
n. reticularis paragigantocellularis
n. reticularis thalami
reticular thalamic n.
reticular n. of thalamus
n. reuniens
rhombencephalic gustatory n.
Roller n.
roof n.
rostral interstitial n.
n. ruber
n. salivatorius inferior
n. salivatorius superior
Schwalbe n.
secondary sensory nuclei
semilunar n. of Flechsig
n. sensorius principalis nervi trigemini
n. sensorius superior nervi trigemini
sensory n.
serotonergic raphe nuclei
sole nuclei
n. solitarius
n. of solitary tract
somatic motor nuclei
somesthetic relay n.
special visceral efferent nuclei
special visceral motor nuclei
spherical n.
spinal n. of accessory nerve
n. spinalis nervi accessorii
spinal trigeminal n.
spinal n. of the trigeminus
Spitzka n.

N

nucleus *(continued)*
    Staderini n.
    Stilling n.
    subthalamic n. (STN)
    n. subthalamicus
    superior olivary n.
    superior salivary n.
    superior vestibular n.
    suprachiasmatic nuclei
    supraoptic n.
    n. supraopticus hypothalami
    tail of caudate n.
    n. tecti
    nuclei tegmenti
    n. tegmenti pontis caudalis
    n. tegmenti pontis oralis
    terminal nuclei
    nuclei terminales
    nuclei terminationis
    thalamic gustatory n.
    thoracic n.
    n. thoracicus
    n. tractus mesencephali nervi
      trigemini
    n. tractus solitarii
    n. tractus spinalis nervi trigemini
    trochlear n.
    n. of trochlear nerve
    tuberal nuclei
    nuclei tuberales
    ventral anterior n. of thalamus
    ventral intermediate n. of thalamus
    n. ventralis anterior
    n. ventralis anterior thalami
    n. ventralis corporis trapezoidei
    n. ventralis intermedius thalami
    n. ventralis lateralis
    n. ventralis posterior intermedius
      thalami
    n. ventralis posterior thalami
    n. ventralis posterolateralis
    n. ventralis posterolateralis thalami
    n. ventralis posteromedialis
    ventral lateral n. of thalamus
    ventral posterior intermediate n. of
      thalamus
    ventral posterior lateral n. of
      thalamus
    ventral posterior n. of thalamus
    ventral posterolateral n. (VPL)
    ventral posterolateral n. of
      thalamus
    ventral posteromedial n. of
      thalamus
    ventral n. of thalamus
    ventral tier thalamic nuclei
    ventral n. of trapezoid body
    ventrobasal n.
    ventrocaudal n. (Vc)
    n. ventro-intermedius
    ventromedial n. of hypothalamus
    n. ventromedialis hypothalami
    vestibular n.

    vestibular nuclei
    nuclei vestibulares
nudiphobia, nudophobia
nudomania
NuGauze
nugget
nuke
null
    n. hypothesis
    n. position nystagmus
null-cell adenoma
nullify
nulling
    gradient moment n.
numb
    feeling n.
numb-chin syndrome
number
    chromosome n.
    n. dysgnosia
    n. of excitations (NEX)
    nuclear spin quantum n.
    n. one
    quantum n.
    Reynolds n.
    900 n. sex
    n. 3 traced on patient's palm test
numbing
    emotional n.
    psychic n.
    n. sensation
numbness
    feeling of n.
    psychic n.
    sleep n.
    waking n.
numen
numerical
    n. aptitude (N)
    N. Attention Test (NAT)
    n. cipher method
    n. reasoning skills
    n. thinking
numerology
numinous
Numorphan
NUM test
nunnation
Nuprin
nuptial
Nurolon suture
Nurrl protein
nurse
    licensed vocational n. (LVN)
    n. practitioner
    psychiatric n.
    registered n.
    n. support group
    visiting n.
nursery
    normal neonatal n. (NNN)
Nurse's
    N. Global Impressions (NGI)
    N. Global Impressions Scale

Nurses' Observation Scale for Inpatient Evaluation (NOSIE)
nursing
    liaison n.
    Master of Science in N. (MSN)
nurturant
nurture
    nature versus n.
nurturing environment
nut
    n. alignment guide
    betel n.
    lock n.
nutans
    chorea n.
    epilepsia n.
    spasmus n.
nutation
nuthkavihak
nutrient vessel
nutriment
    emotional n.
Nutri/System diet
nutrition
    American Institute of N. (AIN)
    autotrophic n.
    parenteral n.
    total parenteral n. (TPN)
    n. treatment
nutritional
    n. adequacy
    n. amblyopia
    n. amenorrhea
    n. anemia
    n. deficiency
    n. deficiency disorder
    n. edema
    n. insult
    n. neuropathy
    n. polyneuropathy
    n. therapy
    n. type cerebellar atrophy
nutritive
    n. enema
    n. equilibrium
nutriture
N&V
    nausea and vomiting
NX
    Talwin NX
nyctalgia
nyctalopia
nyctaphonia
nyctophilia
nyctophobia
nyctophonia
Nyegaard
nylon
    4-0 n.
    n. suture
Nymox urinary test
nympholepsy
nymphomania
    active n.
    platonic n.

nymphomaniac
Nyquist
    N. frequency
    N. sampling criteria
nystagmoid jerk
nystagmus
    abduction n.
    acquired n.
    alternating n.
    apogeotropic n.
    asymmetric n.
    Bruns n.
    caloric n.
    central n.
    cerebellar n.
    circular n.
    coarse n.
    congenital n.
    conjugate n.
    contralateral monocular n.
    convergence-evoked n.
    convergence-retraction n.
    diagonal n.
    dissociated n.
    downbeat n.
    drug-induced n.
    dysjunctive n.
    elliptical n.
    end-gaze physiologic n.
    fine rapid n.
    fixation n.
    gaze-evoked n.
    gaze-paretic n.
    horizontal n.
    irregular n.
    jelly n.
    jerk n.
    lateral gaze n.
    left-bearing n.
    lid n.
    miner's n.
    muscle-paretic n.
    null position n.
    oblique n.
    ocular n.
    opticokinetic n.
    optokinetic n. (OKN)
    palatal n.
    paroxysmal positional n.
    party n.
    pendular n.
    periodic alternating n.
    phasic n.
    positional n.
    postrotational n.
    railway n.
    rapid n.
    rebound n.
    retraction n.
    retraction-convergence n.
    reversed optokinetic n.
    right-bearing n.
    rotary n.
    rotatory n.
    seesaw n.

N

nystagmus *(continued)*
   sensory-deprivation n.
   third-degree continuous
    spontaneous n.
   torsional n.
   toxic n.
   transient n.
   true n.
   unidirectional n.

   upbeating n.
   vertical n.
   vestibular n.
   vestibular end-organ n.
   voluntary n.

Nytol
   Maximum Strength N.
   N. Oral

O
>opium

O-A
>objective-analytic

OA
>OA subtest
>object assembly
>Overeaters Anonymous
>OA subtest (OA)

OADMT
>Oliphant Auditory Discrimination
>Memory Test

OAM
>Office of Alternative Medicine

OAP
>Occupational Ability Pattern

OARS Multidimensional Functional Assessment Questionnaire (OMFAQ)

OAST
>Oliphant Auditory Synthesizing Test

oasthouse urine disease

oath
>Hippocratic o.

OBD
>organic brain disease
>organic brain disorder

obdormition

obduracy

obdurate

OBE
>out-of-body experience

obedience
>automatic o.
>deferred o.
>destructive o.

obedient behavior

Oberhill laminectomy retractor

Obersteiner-Redlich
>O.-R. line
>O.-R. zone

Oberto mouth prop

obese body

obesity
>adult-onset o.
>alimentary o.
>endocrine o.
>endogenous o.
>exogenous o.
>hyperphagic o.
>hyperplastic-hypertrophic o.
>hypertrophic o.
>hypothalamic o.
>lifelong o.
>morbid o.
>psychogenic o.
>simple o.
>o. treatment

obesogenous

Obetrol

Obex plugging

obfuscate

obfuscation
>terminological o.

object
>o. addict
>o. addiction
>agent, action, and o.
>o. agnosia
>analytic o.
>anxiety o.
>o. assembly (OA)
>o. assembly subtest
>o. attachment
>o. attitude
>bad o.
>o. blindness
>o. cathexis
>o. choice
>O. Classification Test (OCT)
>o. concept
>o. constancy
>o. of a delusion
>feared o.
>fetish o.
>o. finding
>good o.
>o. halos
>o. identification
>o. ill
>indirect o.
>o. lesson
>o. libido
>linkage o.
>o. loss
>o. love
>love o.
>luminescence of o.
>o. mouthing
>moving o.
>paraphiliac o.
>part o.
>o. permanence
>primary transitional o.
>o. relation
>o. relationship
>O. Relations Technique
>o. relations theory
>secondary transitional o.
>sex o.
>o. shadow
>O. Sorting Scale (OSS)
>O. Sorting Test (OST)
>substitute o.
>o. test (OT)
>test o.
>transitional o.
>twirling of o.
>unidentified flying o. (UFO)

objectifying attitude

objectivation

objective
>O. Analytic Battery
>o. anxiety

O

objective *(continued)*
    behavioral o.
    o. correlative
    o. criticism
    o. examination
    instructional o.
    o. manifestation
    275mm o. lens
    operational o.
    O. Opiate Withdrawal Scale
    o. orientation
    o. pain
    performance o.
    principal o.
    o. psychobiology
    o. psychology
    o. psychotherapy
    o. reality
    o. scoring
    o. self-awareness
    o. sensation
    o. sign
    o. sociogram
    o. symptom
    o. test (OT)
    o. type
    o. vertigo
objective-analytic (O-A)
object-love
    primary o.-l.
oblativity
obligation
    honor financial o.
    major role o.
    role o.
    therapist o.
obligations fear
obligatory
    o. intermediate
    o. occurrence
    o. perception
oblique
    o. bundle of pons
    o. flow misregistration
    o. nystagmus
    o. sagittal gradient-echo MR
      imaging
    o. screw insertion
    o. transcorporeal approach
obliquely related idea
obliquity
    pelvic o.
obliterans
    thromboangiitis o.
obliterated basal cistern
obliteration
    nidus o.
    transcatheter o.
obliterative
    o. arachnoiditis
    o. arteritis
oblivious to surroundings
obliviscence

oblongata
    medulla o.
obloquy
obmutescence
obnubilation
O'Brien Vocabulary Placement Test
OBS
    organic brain syndrome
obscene
    o. gesture
    o. language
    o. wit
obscenity-purity complex
obscurantism
observable disability
observation
    around-the-clock o.
    o. commitment
    continuous o.
    delusion of o.
    o. delusion
    direct o.
    evaluation and o. (E&O)
    longitudinal o.
    participant o.
    random o.
    receptive-expressive o. (REO)
    serial o.
    o. technique
    unselective o.
observational
    o. learning
    o. learning theory
    o. method
observer
    o. drift
    hidden o.
    nonparticipant o.
    participant o.
    o. position
obsession
    aggressive o.
    alien o.
    contamination o.
    counting o.
    erotic o.
    guilt o.
    hand-washing o.
    impulsive o.
    inappropriate quality of o.
    inhibitory o.
    masked o.
    o. psychasthenia
    pure o.
    quality of o.
    religious o.
    revenge o.
    rooted o.
    rotted o.
    sexual o.
    somatic o.
    symmetry o.
obsessional
    o. brooding
    o. character

o. disorder
o. idea
o. impulse
o. mental image
o. neurosis
o. personality
o. phobia
o. psychoneurosis
o. psychoneurotic reaction
o. rehearsal
o. rumination
o. slowness
o. state
o. syndrome
o. thought
o. type

obsessive
o. attack
o. behavior
o. disorder
o. doubt
o. fantasy
o. fear
o. impulse
o. laughter
o. personality
o. preoccupation
o. psychogenic disorder
o. psychoneurotic reaction
o. reaction
o. rumination

obsessive-compulsive
o.-c. disorder (OCD)
O.-c. Disorder With Poor Insight Type
O.-c. Drinking Scale (OCDS)
o.-c. feature
o.-c. inventory (OCI)
o.-c. neurosis
o.-c. personality
O.-c. Personality Disorder Subscale from Millon Clinical Multiaxial
o.-c. psychoneurosis
o.-c. reaction
O.-c. Subscale of the Comprehensive Psychopathological Rating Scale

obsessive-ruminative tension state
obsolescence
role o.
obstacle sense
obstetrical, obstetric
o. hand
o. paralysis
obstinate progression
obstipation
obstipatio paradoxa
obstreperous
obstruction
o. box
cranial venous o.
o. drive
o. method

sleep apnea hypersomnolence syndrome associated with upper airway o. (SAHS-UAO)
thought o.
venous outflow o.
venular o.
visual o.
obstructionism
obstructive
o. apnea
o. hydrocephalus
o. sleep apnea
o. sleep apnea syndrome
obstruent
obtrude
obtrusive idea
OBT stereotactic frame
obtundation
mental o.
obtunded
mentally o.
obtundent
obturans
keratosis o.
obturator
o. nerve
o. neurectomy
obtuse
obtusion
obvious proof
Oby-trim
occasional
o. inversion
o. sexual aversion
occipital
o. bone
o. bossing
o. corticectomy
o. dominant intermittent rhythmic delta activity
o. encephalocele
o. glioblastoma
o. gyri
o. horn
o. interhemispheric approach
o. intermittent rhythmic delta activity (OIRDA)
o. lesion
o. lobe
o. lobe infarction
o. lobe tumor
o. malformation
o. nerve
o. neuralgia
o. neuritis
o. neuroblastoma
o. operculum
o. pole
o. sulcus
o. transtentorial
occipital-atlas-axis ligament
occipital-supracerebellar
occipitoatlantoaxial
o. complex

occipitoatlantoaxial *(continued)*
    o. fusion
    o. instability
occipitocervical
    o. arthrodesis
    o. fixation
    o. fusion
    o. stabilization
occipitocollicular tract
occipitofrontal fasciculus
occipitomastoid suture
occipitonuchal region
occipitoparietal artery occlusion
occipitopontine tract
occipitotectal tract
occipitotemporal sulcus
occipitothalamic radiation
occiput
occluded sinus
occluder
    Heifetz carotid o.
occlusal neurosis
occlusion
    aneurysm o.
    aqueductal o.
    artery o.
    o. balloon catheter with silicone
      balloon
    balloon test o.
    branch artery o.
    carotid artery o.
    chronic o.
    o. coil
    distal o.
    dural sinus o.
    endovascular balloon o.
    internal carotid artery balloon
      test o.
    intracranial o.
    intraoperative balloon o.
    intravascular balloon o.
    luminal o.
    occipitoparietal artery o.
    posterotemporal artery o.
    pre-Rolandic artery o.
    proximal balloon o.
    sinovenous o.
    sinus o.
    superior sagittal sinus o.
    transtorcular o.
    vascular o.
    ventricular catheter o.
    vertebral artery o.
occlusive
    o. cerebrovascular disease
    o. hyperemia
    o. meningitis
occulomotor pathway
occult
    o. blood
    o. cerebrovascular malformation
      (OCVM)
    o. head trauma

    o. hydrocephalus
    o. spinal dysraphism
occulta
    amentia o.
    spina bifida o.
occultism
occupation
    British Manual of the Classification
      of O.'s
    ligand o.
    sedative o.
    stimulating o.
occupational
    o. ability
    O. Ability Pattern (OAP)
    o. activity
    o. adjustment
    o. analysis
    O. Check List
    o. checklist (OCL)
    o. choice
    o. cramp
    o. deafness
    o. delirium
    o. disease (OD)
    o. disorder
    o. drinking
    O. Environment Scales, Form E-2
    o. exposure
    o. family
    o. function
    o. functioning level
    o. hazard
    o. hierarchy
    o. history (OH)
    o. impairment
    o. inhibition
    o. interaction
    O. Interests Explorer (OIE)
    O. Interests Surveyor (OIS)
    o. inventory
    o. neuropathy
    o. neurosis
    o. norm
    o. problem
    o. psychiatry
    o. psychoneurosis
    o. rehabilitation
    O. Roles Questionnaire (ORQ)
    o. skill training
    o. spasm
    o. stability
    o. stress
    O. Stress Indicator (OSI)
    o. test
    O. Test Series-Basic Skills Test
    o. therapist (OT)
    o. therapy (OT)
    o. tic
occupationally effective
occurrence
    obligatory o.
OCD
    obsessive-compulsive disorder
    behavioral avoidance test for OCD

OCDS
Obsessive-Compulsive Drinking Scale
oceanic feeling
ochlomania
ochlophobia
ochronosis
OCI
obsessive-compulsive inventory
Organizational Culture Inventory
OCL
occupational checklist
ocnophile
OCS-1 cortical stimulator
OCT
Object Classification Test
octapeptide
cholecystokinin o. (CCK-8)
octapolar lead
octave band analyzer
octavus
nervus o.
Octocaine Injection
OctreoScan scanner
octreotide
intrathecal o.
Ocufen Ophthalmic
ocular
o. apraxia
o. bobbing
o. cup
o. deviation
o. dipping
o. dominance column
o. dyskinesia
o. dysmetria
o. flutter
o. ischemic syndrome
o. lesion
o. melanoma
o. metastasis
o. migraine
o. migraine headache
o. motility
motility o.
o. motility examination
o. motor ataxia
o. motor nerve paresis
o. motor syndrome
o. muscle
o. myoclonus
o. nystagmus
o. pain
o. paralysis
o. photoreceptor
o. pneumoplethysmography
o. pseudomyasthenia
o. pulse
o. tilt reaction
o. torticollis
o. vesicle
ocularis
angor o.
Oculinum
oculocardiac reflex

oculocephalic
o. reflex
o. test
oculocephalogyric
o. crisis
o. reflex
oculocerebrorenal syndrome
oculocerebrovasculometry
oculocraniosomatic disease
oculoencephalic angiomatosis
oculogastrointestinal muscular dystrophy (OGIMD)
oculographic artifact
oculogyric crises
oculomasticatory myorhythmia
oculomotor
o. abnormality
o. apraxia
o. disturbance
o. nerve
o. nerve paralysis
o. nerve paresis
o. neuropathy
o. nucleus
o. response
o. system
oculomotorius
nervus o.
oculopalatal myoclonus
oculopharyngeal muscular dystrophy (OPMD)
oculoplethysmography
oculosympathetic dysfunction
oculovestibular reflex
OCVM
occult cerebrovascular malformation
postirradiation OVM
OD
occupational disease
overdose
od
odaxesmus
odaxetic
ODD
oppositional defiant disorder
odd
o. behavior
o. belief
logarithm of o.'s (LOD)
o. speech
odd-eccentric cluster
odd-even method reliability coefficient
oddities of behavior
Oden syndrome
odious
odium
odogenesis
odonterism
odontogenic infection
odontoid
o. dysplasia
o. fracture
o. fracture internal fixation
o. fracture stabilization
o. process

O

odontoid (*continued*)
  o. process osteosynthesis
  o. process resection
odontoideum
  os o.
odontoneuralgia
odontophobia
odontoprisis
odor
  body o. (BO)
  o. fear
odorant
odoriferous
odorivectory
odorous
ODS
  Operation Desert Storm
odynometer
odynophagia
odynophobia
odynophonia
Odysseus pact
OEC-Diasonics mobile C-arm image intensifier
oecophobia
oedipal
  o. behavior
  o. complex
  o. conflict
  o. neurosis
  o. period
  o. phase
  o. situation
  o. stage
oedipism
Oedipus
  complete O.
  O. complex
  inverted O.
  negative O.
  O. period
OEM
  open-end marriage
oenomania
oenophobia
OFD
  oral-facial-digital syndrome
off
  o. balance
  o. the cuff
  o. effect
  o. glide
  o. limits
offend
offender
  habitual o.
  mentally disordered o.
  mentally disordered sex o. (MDSO)
  repeat o.
  sex o. (SO)
  status o.
  Task Force on Sexually Dangerous O.'s
offending agent

offense
  sex o.
  statutory o.
offensive
Offer
  O. Parent-Adolescent Questionnaire
  O. Self-Image Questionnaire (OSIQ)
  O. Self-Image Questionnaire for Adolescents
office
  O. of Alternative Medicine (OAM)
  o. seclusion
  O. Skills Test
officer
  juvenile o.
  noncommissioned o. (NCO)
officious
offish
offscouring
offset
  frequency o.
  o. frequency
offsetting
OFM
  orofacial movement
OGIMD
  oculogastrointestinal muscular dystrophy
ogoy
Ogura operation
OH
  occupational history
OHDA
  6-hydroxydopamine
Ohio
  O. Vocational Interest Survey (OVIS)
  O. Work Values Inventory (OWVI)
OHIP
ohm
Ohm law
OHS
  Overcontrolled Hostility Scale
OI
  oligoclonal immunoglobulin
  orientation inventory
OIE
  Occupational Interests Explorer
oikiomania
oikiophobia (*var. of* oikophobia)
oikiotropic
oikofugic
oikomania
oikophobia, ecophobia, oikiophobia
oil
  BAL in O.
  brominized o.
  ethiodized o.
  iodized o.
  Lorenzo o.
  midnight o.
  Pitressin Tannate in O.
oilotropic
oinomania
oinophobia

ointment
Polysporin o.
OIRDA
occipital intermittent rhythmic delta
activity
OIRDA on electroencephalogram
OIS
Occupational Interests Surveyor
OISE Picture Reasoning Test (PRT)
OIT
Organic Integrity Test
ojo
mal de o.
okadaic acid
Oklahoma tick fever virus
OKN
optokinetic nystagmus
OKT3 uremic
olan
olanzapine
OLC
ovabain-like compound
Olcadil
old
o. age
o. age imbecility
o. guard
o. nerve injury (ONI)
oldest o.
old o. (over age 75)
old-age
o.-a. dementia
o.-a. imbecility
o.-a. psychiatry
o.-a. therapy
Oldberg
O. brain retractor
O. dissector
O. intervertebral disk rongeur
O. pituitary forceps
O. pituitary rongeur
oldest old
old-old patient
olecranon reflex
olfactie, olfacty
olfaction
olfactism
olfactophobia
olfactoria
hyperesthesia o.
idiosyncrasia o.
olfactorii
nervi o.
olfactory
o. amnesia
o. anesthesia
o. area
o. aura
o. bulb
o. bundle
o. cortex
o. epithelium
o. erotism
o. esthesioneuroblastoma
o. glomerulus

o. groove
o. groove meningioma
o. gyrus
o. hallucination
o. hyperesthesia
o. hypesthesia
o. nerve
o. nerve layer (ONL)
o. neuroblastoma
o. organ
o. pathway
o. peduncle
o. psychomotor seizure
o. pyramid
o. receptor cell
o. reference syndrome
o. root
o. sheathing cell
o. stimulation
o. striae
o. sulcus
o. tract
o. trigone
o. tubercle
olfacty (*var. of* olfactie)
oligemia
oligergasia
oligoastrocytoma
oligoclonal
o. band
o. immunoglobulin (OI)
oligodendria
oligodendrite
oligodendroblast
oligodendroblastoma
oligodendrocyte
oligodendroglia cell
oligodendroglioma
nonanaplastic o.
oligodendrolysis
oligodipsia
oligodontia
oligomania
oligomenorrhea
oligonucleotide
antisense o.
oligophrenia
moral o.
phenylpyruvic o.
o. phenylpyruvica
polydystrophic o.
oligophrenic
oligopsychia
oligoria
oligosthenic
oligosynaptic
oligothymia
oligothymic
oligotrophia
oligotropy
Oliphant
O. Auditory Discrimination Memory
Test (OADMT)
O. Auditory Synthesizing Test
(OAST)

O

olisbos
oliva, pl. olivae
    o. inferior
    o. superior
olivary
    o. body
    o. degeneration
    o. eminence
olive
    inferior o.
    superior o.
Olivecrona
    O. aneurysm clamp
    O. brain spatula
    O. clip
    O. clip applier
    O. dura dissector
    O. dura scissors
    O. rasp
    O. rongeur
    O. trigeminal knife
    O. trigeminal scissors
    O. wire saw
Olivecrona-Gigli saw
Olivecrona-Toennis clip-applying forceps
Olivier-Bertrand-Talairach stereotactic
  head frame
Olivier-Bertrand-Tipal frame
olivifugal
olivipetal
olivocerebellar tract
olivocochlear bundle
olivopontocerebellar
    o. atrophy
    o. degeneration
olivospinal tract
Ollier disease
OLMAT
    Otis-Lennon Mental Ability Test
olonism
OLSIDI
    Oral Language Sentence Imitation
    Diagnostic Inventory
OLSIST
    Oral Language Sentence Imitation
    Screening Test
Olympia VACPAC support
Olympus neonatal cystoscope
ombrophobia
OMC
    short orientation-memory-concentration
    test
OMD
    organic mental disorder
Omega sign
omen formation
Omersch-Woltman syndrome
OMFAQ
    OARS Multidimensional Functional
    Assessment Questionnaire
ominous
omission
    o. of duty
    o. in wit
ommatophobia, ommetaphobia

Ommaya
    O. reservoir
    O. ventriculoperitoneal shunt
Omni
    O. clip gun
    O. 2 microscope
Omnibus Personality Inventory (OPI)
Omnipaque
Omnipen-N
omnipotence
    magic o.
    thought o.
    o. of thought
omnipotent infantile sadism
omnipresent
Omniscan
omniscient
Omni-Vent
omohyoid muscle
omophagia
OMS
    opsoclonus-myoclonus syndrome
    organic mental syndrome
    OMS Oral
on
    o. effect
    o. the skin
    o. top of the world
    o. the wagon
onanism
    buccal o.
onanist
oncocytoma
oncogene
    ras o.
oncoprotein
    c-erbB-2-encoded o.
OncoRad OV103
OncoScint
    O. CR103
    O. CR/OV
    O. OV103
    O. PR
OncoTrac
Oncovin
OND
    other neurological disease
Ondine curse
one
    live o.
    loss of loved o.
    murder o.
    Neurostation O.
    number o.
    o. way
    O. Word Receptive Picture
    Vocabulary Test
one-and-a-half syndrome
one-dimensional
Oneida community
oneiric delirium
oneiric, oniric
oneirism
oneiroanalysis
oneirocritical

oneirodelirium
oneirodynia
    o. activa
    o. gravis
oneirogenic
oneirogmus
oneirogonorrhea
oneirogonos
oneiroid
    o. schizophrenia
    o. state
oneirology
oneiromancy
oneironosus
oneirophobia
oneirophrenia
oneiroscopy
one-on-one supervision
onerous
oneself
    play with o.
    will to be o.
one's own control
ONE TIME sharp debridement tray
one-to-one situation
one-upmanship
one-way
    o.-w. flow mechanism
    o.-w. mirror
ongoing treatment
ONI
    old nerve injury
oniomania
onion
    o. bulb change
    o. bulb neuropathy
oniric
    oneiric, o.
ONL
    olfactory nerve layer
online sex
on-off
    o.-o. effect of L-dopa
    o.-o. flushing reservoir
    o.-o. phenomenon
onology
onomatomania
onomatophobia
onomatopoeia
onomatopoiesis
onotoanalysis
onotogenesis
onset
    abrupt o.
    adolescent o.
    age at o.
    o. of agitation
    childhood o.
    dementia of the Alzheimer type, with early o.
    dementia of the Alzheimer type, with late o.
    insidious o.
    mood disorder with postpartum o.
    o. of sleep
    sudden o.
    o. of symptoms
on-task behavior
ontoanalysis
ontogenesis
ontogenic
ontogeny
    psychic o.
ontology
Onuf nucleus
onus
onychophagia
onychophagy
onychotillomania
OOB
    out of bed
OOC
    out of control
OP
    outpatient
opacity
Opalski cell
open
    o. angiography
    o. awareness
    o. C-D hook
    o. cordotomy
    o. door laminoplasty
    o. exit foramen
    o. group
    o. head injury
    o. horizon
    o. hospital
    o. hostility
    o. juncture
    o. mind
    o. place
    o. posture
    o. quotient
    o. seclusion restriction
    o. skull fracture
    o. stereotactic craniotomy
    o. ward
open-cue situation
open-door hospital
open-ended
    o.-e. interview
    o.-e. question
    o.-e. session
open-end marriage (OEM)
opener
    eye o.
opening
    o. move
    o. sound
open-mouthed anteroposterior tomogram
openness to experience
open-ward status
operandi
    modus o.
operant
    autoclitic o.
    o. behavior
    o. behaviorism
    o. conditioning

O

operant *(continued)*
    o. learning
    o. level
    o. method
    o. reserve
    tact o.
    o. therapy
operating
    O. Arm stereotactic navigator
    o. microscope
    o. microscope VM 900
operation
    Albee-Delbert o.
    aneurysmal clipping o.
    Ball o.
    Brooks-Gallie cervical o.
    Brooks-Jenkins cervical o.
    cingulate o.
    Cloward o.
    concrete o.
    Cotte o.
    Dana o.
    Dandy o.
    decompression o.
    O. Desert Storm (ODS)
    dissectible cognitive o.
    effector o.
    floating-forehead o.
    formal o.
    Frazier-Spiller o.
    Gardner o.
    Hunter o.
    invasive o.
    jejunal bypass o.
    Keen o.
    Killian o.
    Koerte-Ballance o.
    Leriche o.
    logical o.
    Matas o.
    Mikulicz o.
    motivating o.
    noninvasive o.
    Ogura o.
    Schloffer o.
    security o.
    sensor o.
    Smith-Robinson o.
    stereotactic o.
    Stoffel o.
    Stookey-Scarff o.
    synchrocyclotron o.
    tongue-in-groove o.
    O. Versus Aspirin study
operational
    o. definition
    o. evaluation
    o. fatigue
    o. objective
    o. planning
    o. research
    o. sign
    o. thought

operationism
operations research (OR)
operative
    o. approach
    o. behavior
    o. injury
    o. microscope
    o. risk
    o. technique
    o. trajectory
    o. wedge frame
operatoire
    pensee o.
opercular
    o. cortex
    o. epilepsy
operculum, gen. operculi, pl. opercula
    frontal o.
    frontoparietal o.
    insula o.
    medial o.
    occipital o.
    parietal o.
    sylvian o.
    temporal o.
OPG
    ophthalmoplethysmography
ophidiomania
ophidiophilia
ophidiophobia
ophiophobia
ophresiophobia
ophryosis
OphSeg
    ophthalmic segment
Ophthalgan Ophthalmic
ophthalmia
    neuroparalytic o.
ophthalmic
    o. artery
    o. artery aneurysm
    o. migraine
    o. neurosyphilis
    Ocufen O.
    Ophthalgan O.
    o. segment (OphSeg)
    o. segment aneurysm
    o. system
    o. vein
    Voltaren O.
    zoster o.
    o. zoster
ophthalmicus
    herpes zoster o.
ophthalmodynamometer
    Bailliart o.
    compression o.
ophthalmodynamometry
    suction o.
ophthalmoparesis
    progressive external o. (PEO)
ophthalmopathy
    Graves o.
ophthalmoplegia
    o. externa

fascicular o.
infectious o.
o. interna
internal o.
internuclear o. (INO)
o. internuclearis
intranuclear o.
nuclear o.
orbital o.
Parinaud o.
o. partialis
o. progressiva
progressive external o.
pseudo-internuclear o.
supranuclear o.
o. totalis
ophthalmoplegic migraine
ophthalmoplethysmography (OPG)
ophthalmoscopy
Ophthetic
OPI
Omnibus Personality Inventory
opiate
o. abstinence
o. abstinence syndrome
o. addiction
o. antagonist
o. overdose
o. poisoning
o. receptor
opiate-induced emergency
opinionnaire
Purdue Student-Teacher O. (PSTO)
Purdue Teacher O. (PTO)
opinion questionnaire
opinions toward adolescents (OTA)
opioid
o. abuse
o. antagonist
o. dependence
endogenous o.
o. intoxication
o. intoxication delirium
o. intoxication, with perceptual
disturbance
o. overdose
o. peptide
o. poisoning
o. precursor protein
o. receptor
o. substitute
o. tolerance
o. treatment
o. use disorder
o. withdrawal
opioid-induced
o.-i. delirium
o.-i. disorder
o.-i. psychotic disorder with
delusions
o.-i. psychotic disorder with
hallucinations
o.-i. sexual dysfunction
opiomania
opiophagism

opiophagorum
tremor o.
opipramol hydrochloride
opisthoporeia
opisthotonic
opisthotonoid
opisthotonos, opisthotonus
opium (O)
o. addiction
o. alkaloid
belladonna and o. (B&O)
Boston o.
cannabis and o.
crude o.
denarcotized o.
o. deodoratum
deodorized o.
o. dependence
granulated o.
o. granulatum
o. habit
lettuce o.
o. poisoning
powdered o.
pudding o.
o. pulveratum
o. tincture
o. use
o. wine
opiumism
OPLL
ossification of the posterior longitudinal
ligament
OPMD
oculopharyngeal muscular dystrophy
OpMi microscopic drape
opotherapy
Oppenheim
O. disease
O. reflex
O. syndrome
opportunistic infection
opportunity
educational o.
equal employment o.
o.'s from intervention
sexual o.
opposed
diametrically o.
opposite
o. affect state
o. biological sex
o. phase
polar o.
relational o.
o.'s test
opposition
o. breathing
o. respiration
oppositional
o. attitude
o. defiant disorder (ODD)
o. disorder of adolescence
o. disorder of childhood
o. thinking

O

oppression-artifact disorder
opprobrium
OpSite dressing
opsoclonus
opsoclonus-myoclonus syndrome (OMS)
opsomania
optative
optesthesia
optic
- o. agnosia
- o. agraphia
- o. aphasia
- o. ataxia
- o. atrophy
- o. canal
- o. chiasm
- o. chiasmal syndrome
- o. chiasm compression
- o. cup
- o. decussation
- o. disc pallor
- o. disk
- o. fissure
- o. glioma
- o. illusion
- o. layer
- o. nerve
- o. nerve astrocytoma
- o. nerve glioma
- o. nerve hypoplasia
- o. nerve infarction
- o. nerve injury
- o. nerve lesion
- o. neuritis
- o. neuropathy
- o. part of retina
- o. pathway glioma
- o. radiation
- o. recess
- o. tectum
- o. tract
- o. tract compression
- o. tract syndrome
- o. vesicle

optica
- hyperesthesia o.
- neuromyelitis o.

optical
- o. alexia
- American O. (AO)
- o. densitometry
- o. device
- o. glass
- o. illusion
- o. image guided surgery system with dynamic referencing
- o. projection
- o. righting reflex

opticocarotid triangle
opticocerebral syndrome
opticochiasmatic
- o. cistern
- o. depression

opticofacial reflex
opticokinetic nystagmus

opticopyramidal syndrome
opticus
- nervus o.

Optifast diet
optimal
- o. development
- o. diet
- o. interpersonal distance
- o. method
- o. relational functioning
- o. relationship
- o. therapeutic intervention

optimal-stimulation principle
optimism
- oral o.
- therapeutic o.

optimistic atmosphere
optimization
optimum dose
Optiray
optokinetic
- o. disorder
- o. nystagmus (OKN)

optophobia
OR
- operations research

Orabilex
Oragrafin
oral
- Adapin O.
- o. aggressive
- AllerMax O.
- Ansaid O.
- o. anxiety
- o. apraxia
- o. atresia
- Banophen O.
- o. behavior
- Belix O.
- Benadryl O.
- o. biting period
- Blocadren O.
- o. bovine myelin
- Calciferol O.
- Carnitor O.
- Cataflam O.
- Catapres O.
- o. cavity
- o. character
- o. coitus
- o. contraceptive
- o. contraceptive-induced chorea
- o. crisis
- Cytoxan O.
- Delta-Cortef O.
- o. dependence
- Dimetabs O.
- Dormarex O.
- Dormin O.
- Dramamine O.
- Drisdol O.
- o. dyskinesia
- o. ego
- o. erotism
- o. fixation

Genahist O.
o. gratification
o. history
o. impulse
o. intubation
Janimine O.
o. language
O. Language Sentence Imitation Diagnostic Inventory (OLSIDI)
O. Language Sentence Imitation Screening Test (OLSIST)
Medrol O.
Mephyton O.
Mestinon O.
Mitran O.
MS Contin O.
MSIR O.
o. need
Nytol O.
OMS O.
o. optimism
Oramorph SR O.
o. orientation
Pediapred O.
Permitil O.
o. personality
o. pessimism
o. phase
Phendry O.
Prelone O.
o. primacy
Prolixin O.
Reposans-10 O.
o. retraction
Roxanol O.
Roxanol SR O.
o. sadism
o. sensory ability
o. sex
Siladryl O.
Sinequan O.
Sleep-eze 3 O.
Sominex O.
o. stage
o. stage psychosexual development
o. state
o. stereognosis
o. stereotypy
o. stimulation
o. test
Toradol O.
o. triad
Twilite O.
o. ulceration
Valium O.
O. Verbal Intelligence Test (OVIT)
VitaCarn O.
Voltaren O.
Voltaren-XR O.
oralage
oral-aggressive character
oral-buccal-lingual dyskinesia
oral-eroticism phase

Oralet
Fentanyl O.
oral-facial-digital syndrome (OFD)
oral-genital contact
oral-incorporative phase
oralism
orality
Oral-Motor/Feeding Rating Scale
oral-nasal acoustic ratio (TONAR)
oral-passive character
oral-receptive character
oral-sadistic cathexis
oral-sensory stage
Oramorph
O. SR
O. SR Oral
orange
agent o.
Orap
Orascoptic
O. fiberoptic headlight
O. loupe extension
Oravue
Orbeli effect
orbicularis
o. oculi reflex
o. orbis muscle
o. oris muscle
o. pupillary reflex
sign of the o.
tic o.
orbicular oculi muscle
Orbis-Sigma cerebrospinal fluid shunt valve
orbit
orbital
o. apex syndrome
o. chemosis
o. decompression
o. dystopia
o. encephalocele
o. floor fracture
o. granulocytic sarcoma
o. gyri
o. hypertelorism
o. myositis
o. neurofibroma
o. ophthalmoplegia
o. part
o. plate
o. pseudotumor
o. roof
o. solitary fibrous tumor
o. sulci
o. varices
o. vein
o. venous approach
o. zygomatic craniotomy
orbitofrontal
o. cortex
o. epilepsy
o. pathway
o. region
o. syndrome
orbitomedial/cingulate lesion

O

orbitomedial syndrome
orbitopathy
    thyroid o.
orbitotomy
orbitozygomatic
    o. mandibular osteotomy
    o. osteotomy
    o. temporopolar approach
orbivirus
orchidomania
order
    birth o.
    chronological o.
    court o.
    o. of extinction
    pecking o.
    rank o.
ordering and arranging
orderliness
    compulsive o.
    organic o.
    o. preoccupation
ordinal
    o. position
    O. Scales of Psychological
    Development
ordinate
ordure
orectic
Oregon Adolescent Depression Project
Orestes complex
Oretic
orexia
orexigenic
oreximania
orexis
organ
    annulospiral o.
    auxiliary o.
    circumventricular o.
    Corti o.
    o. of Corti
    encapsulated end o.
    end o.
    o. erotic
    o. erotism
    executive o.
    flower-spray o. of Ruffini
    genital o.
    Golgi tendon o.
    gustatory o.
    o. of hearing
    o. inferiority
    o. inferiority complex
    intromittent o.
    o. libido
    o. neurosis
    neurotendinous o.
    olfactory o.
    o. pleasure
    reinnervation of target o.
    sense o.
    o. of smell
    o. speech
    spiral o.

    subcommissural o.
    target o.
    o. of taste
    o. of touch
    o. transplantation
    vestibular o.
    vestibulocochlear o.
    visceral o.
    o. of vision
    o. of Zuckerkandl
organa (*pl. of* organum)
organic
    o. acidemia
    o. aciduria
    o. amnesia
    o. anxiety
    o. approach
    o. brain disease (OBD)
    o. brain disorder (OBD)
    o. brain dysfunction
    o. brain syndrome (OBS)
    o. contracture
    o. deafness
    o. defect
    o. delirium
    delirium transient o.
    delusional transient o.
    o. dementia
    o. disorder
    o. drivenness
    o. dyscontrol
    o. epilepsy
    o. factor
    o. hallucination
    hallucinatory transient o.
    o. hallucinosis
    o. headache
    o. impairment
    o. impotence
    O. Integrity Test (OIT)
    o. jargon
    o. language
    o. mental disorder (OMD)
    o. mental syndrome (OMS)
    multiple sclerosis-type o.
    o. neglect
    o. neurosis
    o. orderliness
    o. pain
    o. persona
    o. pleasure
    o. psychiatry
    psychoactive substance-induced o.
    o. psychosis
    o. psychosis drug intoxication
    o. psychosyndrome
    o. psychotic condition
    o. psychotic state
    o. reaction
    o. repression
    o. solvent
    o. speech
    o. syndrome
    o. therapy

o. variable
o. vertigo
organica
alalia o.
organic-functional dilemma
organicism
organicist
organicity
Koppitz Scoring System for O.
o. screening
organism
o. embolus
empty o.
organismic
o. causation
o. psychology
o. variable
organism-specific antibody index (OSAI)
organization
action o.
Assessment of Conceptual O.
(ACO)
borderline personality o.
care o.
cortical o.
cytoarchitectural o.
defense o.
disrupted sleep o.
health maintenance o. (HMO)
O. Health Survey
hierarchical o.
libido o.
life o.
mental-patient o.
peer review o. (PRO)
perceptual o.
personality o.
pregenital o.
o. preoccupation
Professional Standards Review O.
(PSRO)
psychic o.
sleep o.
social o.
social welfare o.
spatial o.
temporal o.
topographical o.
trait o.
welfare o.
World Health O. (WHO)
organizational
O. Climate Index
O. Culture Inventory (OCI)
o. plan
o. psychology
o. skills
o. structure
O. Value Dimensions Questionnaire
(OVDQ)
organized
o. activity
o. play
organized-care psychiatry

organizer
decision-making o.
organizing principle
organogenesis
organogenetic, organogenic
organoleptic
organophosphate
o. insecticide
o. pesticide poisoning
organophosphorus insecticide poisoning
organotherapy
organum, pl. **organa**
o. auditus
o. gustus
o. olfactus
organa sensuum
o. spirale
o. tactus
o. vestibulocochleare
o. visus
Orgaran
orgasm
alimentary o.
anejaculatory o.
coital o.
dry o.
female o.
inhibited o.
male o.
multiple spontaneous o.'s
paradoxical o.
pharmacogenic o.
premature o.
premature female o.
premature male o.
vaginal o.
orgasmic
o. anhedonia
o. capacity
o. cephalalgia
o. deficiency
o. disorder
o. dysfunction
o. phase
o. phase of sexual response cycle
o. platform
o. problem
o. reconditioning
orgasmus deficiens
orgastic
o. impotence
o. potency
o. release
orgone therapy
oriental nightmare-death syndrome
orientation
academic o. (AO)
autopsychic o.
behavioral research o.
biologic research o.
bisexual o.
cognitive research o.
coronal o.
o. cue
delusion of o.

O

orientation *(continued)*
    o. disorder
    disturbed o.
    double o.
    ego-dystonic o.
    exploitative o.
    family/system research o.
    female/system research o.
    Fundamental Interpersonal
      Relations O.-Behavior (FIRO-B)
    Fundamental Interpersonal
      Relations O.-Feelings (FIRO-F)
    gender o.
    goal o.
    hedonistic o.
    heterosexual o.
    hoarding o.
    homosexual o.
    illusion of o.
    impaired o.
    instrumental-relativist o.
    interpersonal research o.
    O. Inventory
    o. inventory (OI)
    Inventory of Suicide O.-30 (ISO-
      30)
    Judgment of Line o. (JLO)
    law-and-order o.
    loss of o.
    objective o.
    oral o.
    psychodynamic o.
    psychodynamic research o.
    reality o. (RO)
    receptive o.
    reversed o.
    sagittal o.
    same-sex o.
    o. session
    sexual o.
    spatial o.
    subjective o.
    temporal o.
    transverse o.
orientation-memory-concentration test
oriented
    alert and o.
    alert, cooperative, and o. (ACO)
    o. and alert times four
    o. and alert times three
    o. in all sphere
    awake, alert, and o. (AAO)
    past o.
    o. to person, place, and time
    present o.
    reality o. (RO)
    o. to time and place
orienting
    o. reflex
    o. response
orifice
    bodily o.
    body o.
    o. picking

origin
    anomalous o.
    apparent o.
    bleeding of undetermined o. (BUO)
    bruising of undetermined o. (BUO)
    culture of o.
    deep o.
    ectal o.
    ental o.
    insomnia due to nonorganic o.
    language o.
    nonorganic o.
    nuclei of o.
    psychogenic o.
    real o.
    Schwann cell o.
    superficial o.
    tic disorder of organic o.
    undetermined o. (UO)
original
    Doan's, O.
    o. response
originaria
    paranoia o.
Orinase
ORION anterior cervical plate
ORLAAM
Orleans-Hanna Algebra Prognosis Test
orlistat
Ormazine
ornithine
    o. decarboxylase
    o. transcarbamoylase
ornithinemia
ornithomania
ornithophobia
ornithosis lymphocytic meningitis
orobuccal dyskinesia
orofacial
    o. dyskinesia
    o. movement (OFM)
orofaciodigital syndrome
orogenital
    o. activity
    o. sex
orolingual-buccal dyskinesia
oropharyngeal
    o. dystonia
    o. reflex
oropharynx
Orozco cervical plate
orphan
    o. drug
    enteric cytopathic human o.
      (ECHO)
    O. Train Heritage Society
orphenadrine
    o., aspirin, and caffeine
    o. citrate
ORQ
    Occupational Roles Questionnaire
Orthawear antiembolism stockings
orthergasia
orthobiosis
orthochorea

orthodromically
orthogenesis
orthogenetic
orthogenic
orthogonal
 o. angiography
 o. film
 o. laser
 o. x-ray
orthograde degeneration
orthographic
orthography
orthomolecular
 o. psychiatry
 o. therapy
 o. treatment
orthonasia
orthophrenia
orthopnea
orthopsychiatry
orthosis, pl. **orthoses**
 cervicothoracic o.
 Flex Foam o.
 Malibu o.
 postoperative lumbosacral o.
 Pucci pediatrics hand orthoses
 thoracolumbar standing o.
 thoracolumbosacral o. (TLSO)
orthostasis
orthostatic
 o. epileptoid
 o. hypertension
 o. hypotension
 o. tremor
orthosympathetic
orthothaniasia
orthotics
orthotonos, orthotonus
orthriogenesis
ortobiosis
Orudis KT
Oruvail
OS
 overall survival
os
 o. odontoideum
 per o.
OSAI
 organism-specific antibody index
Osaka telesensor
OSBCL
 Ottawa School Behavior Checklist
Osbil
Osborn band
Os-Cal 500
oscillating
 o. microsaw
 o. tremor
oscillation
 behavioral o.
oscillations of attachment
oscillopsia
oscilloscope
 Norland digital o.

OSI
 Occupational Stress Indicator
 OSI modular table system
OSIQ
 Offer Self-Image Questionnaire
Osler-Weber-Rendu arteriovenous
 malformation
osmicate
Osmitrol Injection
osmoceptor
osmodysphoria
Osmoglyn
osmolagnia
osmolality
osmoles
 idiogenic o.
osmophobia
osmoreceptor
osmosis
osmotherapy
osmotic
 o. demyelination syndrome
 o. diuretic
osphresia
osphresiolagnia
osphresiophilia
osphresiophobia
osphresis
OSS
 Object Sorting Scale
ossea
 leontiasis o.
ossicle
 Tutoplast auditory o.
ossificans
 fibrodysplasia o.
 myositis o.
ossification
 heterotopic o.
 o. of the posterior longitudinal
 ligament (OPLL)
ossify
ossifying
 o. arachnoiditis
 o. fibroma
OST
 Object Sorting Test
osteitis deformans
ostentatious
osteoarthritis
osteoarthrosis
osteoblastoma
osteocalcin
Osteocalcin Injection
osteochondroma
osteochondrosis
 intervertebral o.
osteoclastic
osteodiastasis
osteogenic sarcoma
osteoid osteoma
osteolysis
osteoma
 osteoid o.
osteomalacia

O

Osteomed
osteomyelitis
    cranial o.
    pyogenic o.
    spinal o.
osteonecrosis
    syphilitic o.
osteopathic scoliosis
osteopenia
osteopetrosis
    cranial o.
osteophyte
osteoplastic
    o. bone flap
    o. craniotomy
    o. laminectomy
osteoporosis
    o. circumscripta
    o. circumscripta cranii
    disuse o.
    glucocorticoid-induced o.
    posttraumatic o.
    senile o.
    o. with vertebral collapse and
      neurologic deficit
osteoporotic spine
osteoradionecrosis
osteosarcoma
osteosynthesis
    anterior column o.
    cranial o.
    facial o.
    lumbar spine vertebral o.
    odontoid process o.
    plate-screw o.
    posterior column o.
    thoracic spine vertebral o.
    thoracolumbar spine vertebral o.
    vertebral o.
    wire o.
osteotome
    Cherry o.
    Cloward spinal fusion o.
osteotomy
    craniofacial o.
    ethmoidal o.
    frontonasomaxillary o.
    frontoorbital o.
    glabellar exposure o.
    LeFort o.
    o. of mandible
    mandibular o.
    maxillary o.
    orbitozygomatic o.
    orbitozygomatic mandibular o.
    Tessier o.
ostracism
    peer o.
ostracize
OT
    objective test
    object test
    occupational therapist
    occupational therapy

OTA
    opinions toward adolescents
otalgia
    geniculate o.
Ota nevus
OTC
    over the counter
    OTC drug
Othello syndrome
other
    anxiety due to potential evaluation
      by o.'s
    avoidance of o.'s (AO)
    O. Conditions That May Be a
      Focus of Clinical Attention
    dangerous to o.'s
    o. directed
    harming o.'s
    o. interpersonal problem
    intimidating o.'s
    locus of control-powerful o.'s
      (LOC-PO)
    o. neurological disease (OND)
    relating to o.'s
    rights of o.'s
    significant o.
    o. specified family circumstance
    o. type personality disorder
    o. woman
other-directed person
others/self
    danger to o.
otic
    o. abscess
    o. capsule
    o. ganglion
oticus
    herpes zoster o.
otiose
Otis-Lennon
    O.-L. Mental Ability Test
      (OLMAT)
    O.-L. School Ability Test
**Otis Quick Scoring Mental Abilities
  Test**
otitic
    o. hydrocephalus
    o. meningitis
otitis
    malignant external o.
    o. media
otocerebritis
otocyst
otoencephalitis
otoganglion
otohemineurasthenia
Otolaryngology
    American Academy of O.
otologic implant
otoneuralgia
otoneurasthenia
otorhinorrhea
otorrhea
    cerebrospinal fluid o.
otosclerosis

Ototome irrigation kit
Ottawa School Behavior Checklist
 (OSBCL)
Ouchterlony double diffusion technique
Ouija board
ouranophobia, uranophobia
out
 acting o.
 asocial acting o.
 o. of bed (OOB)
 blacking o.
 o. of the blue
 o. of bounds
 o. of control (OOC)
 falling o.
 freaked o.
 luding o.
 neurotic acting o.
 passive-aggressive acting o.
 read o.
 roached o.
 rule o. (R/O)
 sexual acting o.
 shut o.
 sign o.
 sit o.
 skip o.
 speak o.
 spell o.
 stand o.
 take o.
 talk o.
 talking it o.
 throw o.
 o. of touch
 o. of touch with reality
 tripped o.
 wash o.
 washed o.
 o. of wedlock
 wipe o.
 working o.
outburst
 aggressive o.
 o. of anger
 angry o.
 behavioral o.
 explosive o.
 tearful o.
 temper o.
 verbal o.
 violent o.
outcast
 social o.
outcome
 o. domain
 long-term o.
 overall management o.
 o. variable
 well-formed o.
outcome-based therapy
outdoing wit
outer
 o. cone fiber
 o. mesaxon of the myelin sheath

outframing
outgoing mechanism
outgrowth
 neurite o.
outlandish
outlet
 thoracic o.
outlier
outlook
 futural o.
out-of-body
 o.-o.-b. experience (OBE)
 o.-o.-b. sensation
out-of-control behavior
out-of-mind sensation
out-of-phase
 o.-o.-p. image
 o.-o.-p. waveform
outpatient (OP)
 o. intervention
 o. mental health clinic setting
 o. patient population
outpatient-based psychiatry
output
 cardiac o.
 o. disability
 energy o.
 fluid o.
 maximum acoustic o.
 reduced verbal o.
outrage
 moral o.
outre
outreach
 assertive o.
 o. services
outside
 o. control
 o. density
 o. force
 o. the range of normal human
 experience
 o. stimulus
outside-in signaling
OV103
 OncoRad O.
 OncoScint O.
ovabain-like compound (OLC)
oval
 o. area of Flechsig
 o. corpuscle
 o. fasciculus
 o. hyperchromatic nucleus
ovale
 centrum o.
 foramen o.
ovalis
 fenestra o.
 fossa o.
ovarian dysgenesis
ovariectomized
OVDQ
 Organizational Value Dimensions
 Questionnaire

O

over
>bind o.
>o. the counter (OTC)
>gloss o.
>knock o.
>slough o.
>talk o.
>throw o.
>working o.

overabstract speech
overachiever
overactivity
>psychomotor o.

overadequate-inadequate reciprocity
overage
overall
>o. management outcome
>o. survival (OS)

overanxious
>o. disorder
>o. disorder of adolescence
>o. disorder of childhood
>o. reaction

overbearance
>phallic o.

overbearing
overbreathing
>voluntary hysterical o.

overburden
overcharged idea
overcommit
overcompensation
overconcern with sleep
overconcrete speech
overconfident
overconscientious personality disorder
overconsciousness
overconsolidation of memory
Overcontrolled Hostility Scale (OHS)
overcorrection
overdependence
>social o.

overdependency
overdependent attitude
overdetermination
overdistraction
overdominance
overdominant
overdose (OD)
>accidental o.
>amphetamine o.
>barbiturate o.
>benzodiazepine o.
>down from o.
>drug o.
>fatal o.
>heroin o.
>lethal o.
>opiate o.
>opioid o.
>paregoric o.
>talk-down from o.

overdrainage syndrome
Overeaters Anonymous (OA)
over-elaborate speech

overexertion
overextension
overflow
>o. encopresis
>o. incontinence
>receiver o.

overgrowth
>neurite o.

overhang
>bony o.

overidentification
overinclusion
overindependence
overinvolvement
>emotional o.

overlay
>emotional o.
>psychogenic o.
>supratentorial o.

overlearning
overload
>attention o.
>fluid o.
>information o.
>receiver o.
>stimulus o.

overly stimulating treatment
overmanning
overmobilization
overoptimistic
overplay
overpower
overproduction
overprotection
>maternal o.

overreaction
>emotional o.

overreactive disorder
overresponse
over-right hypertropia
oversecretion
>hydrocephalus o.

oversensitive
oversexed
overshadowing
>diagnostic o.

overshooting
>saccadic o.

oversimplify
oversleeping
oversoul
overstatement
overstay
overstep
overstimulation
overstrain
overstress
overt
>O. Aggression Scale
>o. behavior
>o. compliance
>o. compliance masking covert resistance
>o. criticism
>o. gesture

o. homosexuality
o. message
o. response
o. sensitization
overtalkative
over-the-counter
o.-t.-c. drug
o.-t.-c. drug-related disorder
overtone
psychic o.
overture
overvaluation
overvalued idea
overventilation
overweight
overwhelm
overwhelmed subjectivity
overwhelming
o. depression
o. fatigue
overwork fear
overwrought
OVIS
Ohio Vocational Interest Survey
OVIT
Oral Verbal Intelligence Test
ovulation
paracyclic o.
Owen gauze dressing
Owsley's
O. acid
white O.
OWVI
Ohio Work Values Inventory
oxacillin
oxandrolone
oxaprozin
oxazepam
oxazolam
Oxford STA scale
oxidant
oxidase
cytochrome c o. (COX)
monoamine o. (MAO)
platelet monoamine o.
oxidation
fatty acid o.
o. state
oxidative
o. degeneration
o. phosphorylation
o. stress
oxide
magnesium o.
nitric o. (NO)
nitrous o.
superparamagnetic iron o.
oxidized
o. cotton
o. regenerated cellulose
oxidronate
technetium 99m o.
oxime
hexamethyl-propyleneamine o.
(HMPAO)

^{99m}Tc-hexamethylpropyleneamine o.
(^{99m}Tc-HMPAO)
oximeter
INVOS transcranial cerebral o.
pulse o.
Somanetics INVOS 3100
cerebral o.
oximetry
continuous venous o.
pulse o.
oxiracetam
oxitriptan
oxolinic acid
oxtriphylline
oxyacoia, oxyakoia
oxyaphia
oxybarbiturates
oxyblepsia
oxybutynin
Oxycel
oxycellulose
oxycephalia
oxycephalic, oxycephalous
o. idiot
oxycephaly
oxychlorosene
oxycodone
o. and acetaminophen
o. and aspirin
o. hydrochloride
o. terephthalate
oxyesthesia
oxygen
o. deficiency
o. deprivation
hyperbaric o.
partial venous gas tension of o.
(PvO2)
o. radical attack
o. radical-induced cellular injury
regional cerebral metabolic rate
of o.
o. tension
o. therapy
oxygenation
extracorporeal membrane o.
oxygen-carrying capacity
oxygen-deprived sexual arousal
oxygen-depriving activities
oxygeusia
oxyhemoglobin
OxyIR
oxylalia
oxylate
sodium o.
oxymetazoline nasal spray
oxymoron
oxymorphone hydrochloride
oxyopia
oxyosmia
oxyosphresia
oxypathia
oxypertine
oxyphenbutazone
oxyphencyclimine hydrochloride

O

oxyphonia
oxyphresia
oxytetracycline
oxytocin
  neuropeptide o.

Oyst-Cal 500
Oystercal 500
ozoline
  purple o.

P

P segment
P & SH

P-3

Pain Patient Profile

P3 probe

p53 gene

PA

paranoia
passive aggressive
passive-aggressive
physician's assistant
plasminogen activator
psychoanalysis
psychoanalyst
psychogenic aspermia
psychosocial assessment
  subtest PA
  PA subtest
  tissue-type PA (t-PA)
  urokinase-type PA (u-PA)

PAAT

Parent as a Teacher Inventory

PAB

Pabalate-SF

Pabenol

PA-C

physician's assistant, certified

PAC

parent-adult-child
Progress Assessment Chart of Social and
Personal Development

pacchionian

p. body
p. corpuscle
p. gland
p. granulation

PACE

Personal Assessment for Continuing
Education
Professional and Administrative Career
Examination
Psychosocial Assessment of Childhood
Experiences

pace

change of p.
future p.
P. ventricular needle

**Paced Auditory Serial Addition Test
(PASAT)**

pacemaker

cardiac p.
cerebral p.
endogenous circadian p.

PACG

Prevocational Assessment and
Curriculum Guide
PACG Inventory

Pachon test

pachygyria

pachyleptomeningitis

pachymeningitis

chronic hypertrophic p. (CHPM)
p. cranialis hypertrophica
p. externa
hemorrhagic p.
hypertrophic cervical p.
hypertrophic cranial p.
idiopathic intracranial p.
p. interna
intracranial p.
meningeal p.
pyogenic p.
syphilitic cerebral hypertrophic p.

pachymeningopathy

pachymeninx

pacing

p. behavior
ceaseless p.
restless p.

pacinian

p. corpuscle
p. mechanoreceptor

package

California Computerized
Assessment P.

packer

Woodson dura p.

packet

Creativity Assessment P.

packing

Avitene p.
Vaseline gauze p.

packs per day (PPD, Ppd)

PACL

Personality Adjective Check List

PaCO2

partial arterial gas tension of carbon
dioxide

pact

devil's p.
Odysseus p.
suicide p.

PAD

primary affective disorder
psychoaffective disorder
PAD score

pad

Bovie grounding p.
cotton p.
Gelfoam p.
visuospatial scratch p.

padded

p. cell
p. room

paddies

cotton p.

Padgett baseline pinch gauge

PAE

paradoxical air embolism

PAF

Premenstrual Assessment Form

P

PAG
periaqueductal central gray
paganism
paganize
Paget disease
pagoclone
pagophagia
pagophobia, phagophobia
PAI
Pair Attraction Inventory
Personality Assessment Inventory
paidology
pain
abdominal p.
affected p.
anatomical site of p.
P. Apperception Test (PAT)
atypical p.
p. avoidance
back p.
p. behavior
Behavioral Assessment of P. (BAP)
bone p.
burning p.
causalgic p.
central p.
chest p.
chronic intractable p.
p. clinic
p. complaint
p. control
deafferentation p.
degree of p.
diabetic neuropathy neuralgia p.
diminished response to p.
p. disorder, acute
p. disorder associated with both
psychological features and a
general medical condition
p. disorder associated with
psychological features
p. disorder, chronic
p. and distress score
p. drawing
dream p.
p. dysfunction syndrome (PDS)
ecstatic p.
effected p.
ejaculatory p.
endogenous p.
end-zone p.
p. exacerbation
facial p.
faciocephalic p.
fleeting p.
functional p.
gate theory of p.
genital p.
girdle p.
growing p.
hemicranial p.
Hendler Test for Chronic P.
(HTCP)
heterotopic p.
p. history

homotopic p.
hunger p.
ice pick-like p.
intermittent p.
intractable p.
intractive p.
law of referred p.
leg p.
lumbar puncture p.
masturbatory p.
p. mechanism
mental p.
mind p.
p. modulation
muscle p.
myofascial p.
neck p.
nerve p.
neuralgic p.
night p.
nociceptive p.
objective p.
ocular p.
organic p.
pathologic p.
P. Patient Profile (P-3)
pelvic p.
p. perception
P. Perception Profile (PPP)
peripheral deafferentation p.
phantom limb p.
phantom tooth p.
physical manifestation of p.
posttraumatic p.
pounding p.
precordial p.
prepsychotic p.
p. presentation
p. principle
p. prone disorder
psychic p.
psychogenic penis p.
psychogenic testicular p.
psychogenic testis p.
psychogenic uterus p.
psychological p.
psychosocial p.
pulsating p.
p. questionnaire
radicular distribution of p.
p. reaction
recalcitrant p.
p. receptor
recurrent p.
referred p.
p. relief
residual p.
response to p.
rest p.
retroorbital p.
sciatic p.
scrotal p.
searing p.
secondary p.
sexual p.

shooting p.
skin graft harvesting p.
somatic p.
p. somatoform disorder
soul p.
spinal cord p.
stabbing p.
p. state
stinging p.
subjective p.
superficial p.
p. symptom
p. symptom grouping
p. and temperature pathway
temporomandibular joint p.
thalamic p.
p. threshold
p. threshold reduction
throat p.
TMJ p.
p. tolerance
p. transduction
unexplained p.
unrelenting p.
venipuncture p.
vice-like p.
visceral p.
wandering p.

PainBuster infusion pump management kit

Paine retinaculatome

painful
    p. affect
    p. anesthesia
    p. consequence
    p. intercourse
    p. memory
    p. paraplegia
    p. point
    p. rituals
    p. stimulus
    p. symptom

Pain-HP
    No P.-HP

pain-pleasure principle
painter's encephalopathy
painting
    action p.
    finger p.

pain, touch and stroke psychiatric syndrome
pain-type
    p.-t. anxiety
    p.-t. anxiety neurosis

PAIR
    Personal Assessment of Intimacy in Relationships

pair
    P. Attraction Inventory (PAI)
    p. bond
    Maxwell p.

paired
    p. associates
    p. dreams

p. electrode recording
p. helical filament
paired-associates learning
PAIS
    Psychosocial Adjustment to Illness Scale
PAL
    Profile of Adaptation to Life
palatal
    p. mucosal incision
    p. myoclonus
    p. nystagmus
    p. paresis
    p. reflex
    p. split
palatine reflex
palatinum
    velum p.
palatooccipital line
palatoocular myoclonus
palatoplasty
palatoplegia
paleencephalon
pale globe
paleocerebellum
paleocortex
paleokinetic
paleologic thinking
paleomnesis
paleophrenia
paleopsychic
paleopsychology
paleosensation
paleostriatal syndrome
paleostriatum
paleosymbol
paleothalamus
paliacusis
paligraphia
palikinesia, palicinesia
palilalia
palilexia
palilogia
palimony
palindromia
palindromic encephalopathy
palinesthesia
palingnosticum
    delirium p.
palingraphia
palinlexia
palinmnesis
palinopia
palinopsia
palinoptic hallucination
palinphrasia palipraxia
paliopsy
paliphrasia
palipraxia
    palinphrasia p.
pallanesthesia
pallesthesia
pallesthetic sensibility
pallial
palliate
palliative

P

pallid
pallidal
    p. cell
    p. degeneration
    p. syndrome
pallidectomy
pallidoamygdalotomy
pallidoansotomy
pallidotomy
    Leksell posteroventral p.
    posteroventral p. (PVP)
    stereotactic p.
    ventroposterior medial p.
    ventroposterolateral p.
    VPL p.
pallidum
    posteroventral sensorimotor p.
    ventral p.
pallidum
    Treponema p.
pallidus
    globus p. (GP)
    ventral globus p.
pallium
pallolalia
pallor
    optic disc p.
palmar
    p. hyperhidrosis
    p. reflex
palm-chin reflex
palmesthesia
palmi (*pl. of* palmus)
palmic
palmistry
palmitic acid
palmitoylation
palmitoyltransferase
    carnitine p. (CPT)
palmodic
palmomental
    p. reflex
    p. test
palmus, pl. **palmi**
palpebral
palpitant
palpitate
palpitation
PALST
    Picture Articulation and Language
    Screening Test
palsy
    abducens nerve p.
    ataxic cerebral p.
    athetoid cerebral p.
    atonic cerebral p.
    backpack p.
    Bell p.
    bilateral gaze p.
    birth p.
    brachial birth p.
    bridegroom's p.
    bulbar p.
    cerebral p.
    choreoathetoid cerebral p.

clonic cerebral p.
conjugate p.
craft p.
cranial nerve p.
creeping p.
crutch p.
Dejerine-Klumpke p.
diabetic third nerve p.
dyskinetic cerebral p.
dystonic cerebral p.
Erb p.
extraocular muscle p.
extrapyramidal cerebral p.
facial p.
Féréol-Graux p.
flaccid cerebral p.
fourth nerve p.
gaze p.
hereditary neuropathy with
  susceptibility to pressure p.
  (HNPP)
horizontal gaze p.
hypotonic cerebral p.
idiopathic facial nerve p.
ipsilateral facial p.
ipsilateral gaze p.
isolated radial nerve p.
Klumpke p.
labioglossolaryngeal p.
lateral gaze p.
lateral rectus p.
lead p.
long thoracic p.
multi-infarct progressive
  supranuclear p.
nerve p.
night p.
peripheral nerve pressure p.
peroneal nerve p.
persistent facial p.
postganglionic oculosympathetic p.
posticus p.
pressure p.
progressive bulbar p.
progressive supranuclear p. (PSP)
pseudoabducens p.
pseudobulbar p.
pure athetoid p.
pure spastic p.
pyramidal cerebral p.
rigid cerebral p.
saccadic p.
Saturday night p.
scrivener's p.
seventh nerve p.
shaking p.
sixth nerve p.
spastic cerebral p.
spinal accessory p.
supranuclear gaze p.
Tapia vagohypoglossal p.
third nerve p.
trembling p.
tremulous cerebral p.
trochlear nerve p.

vertical gaze p.
wasting p.
PAM
primary amebic meningoencephalitis
PAM2 monitor
PAM3 monitor
pamabrom
Pamelor
pamidronate
pamoate
hydroxyzine p.
imipramine p.
Pamprin
PAN
polyarteritis nodosa
Panadol
Junior Strength P.
Panama cut
pananxiety
Panasal 5/500
panasthenia
panatella
pancakes and syrup
Pancoast
P. syndrome
P. tumor
pancreatic
p. carcinoma
p. encephalopathy
pancreatitis
alcoholic p.
pancuronium bromide
pandemic
pandemonium
pandiculation
pandys maturation
panel
continuous p.
Flushmesh p.
personality p.
panencephalitis
nodular p.
progressive rubella p.
rubella p.
sclerosing p.
subacute sclerosing p. (SSPE)
panendoscopy
panesthesia
panethnic
Panevril
pangenesis
panglossia
Pangonadalot
Pang type agenesis
panhandling
panhypopituitarism
panic
acute homosexual p.
p. agoraphobic
p. attack
p. attack neurotic anxiety
p. attack neurotic anxiety state
p. button
p. delirium
p. diathesis

p. disorder (PD)
P. Disorder Severity Scale
p. disorder with agoraphobia
p. disorder without agoraphobia
homosexual p.
primordial p.
p. state
p. symptomatology
Panic-Agoraphobic
P.-A. Spectrum Questionnaire
panic-agoraphobic
p.-a. spectrum
p.-a. syndrome
panic-disordered patient
panicker
nonsuffocation p.
suffocation p.
panicky
panicogenic effect
panic-related phobia
panic-spectrum phenomenon
panic-type
p.-t. anxiety
p.-t. anxiety neurosis
panky
hanky p.
panneuritis endemica
panneurosis
panodic
panophobia (*var. of* panphobia)
panoply
panoramic memory
panphobia, panophobia, pantophobia
panphobic melancholia
panplegia
panpsychism
Pansch fissure
pansexualism
PANSS
Positive and Negative Stroke Scale
Positive and Negative Syndrome Scale
pansynostosis
pantalgia
pantanencephaly, pantanencephalia
pantaphobia
pantheism
panthodic
pantomime
Pantomime Recognition Test (PRT)
Pantopaque
pantophobia (*var. of* panphobia)
Pantopon
pantothenic acid deficiency peripheral neuropathy
panum phenomenon
PAP
passive-aggressive personality
papaphobia
papaverine hydrochloride
papaverine-soaked Gelfoam
Papaver somniferum
paper
p. pica
p. stop artifact

P

Papez
  P. circuit
  P. theory of emotion
papilla, pl. **papillae**
  acoustic p.
  nerve p.
papillary mucosal hyperplasia
papilledema
  axoplasmic flow and p.
papilliferous cystoma
papillitis
papilloma, pl. **papillomata**
  choroid plexus p.
  p. neuropathicum
  p. neuroticum
papillomatosis
  juvenile p.
papillophlebitis
PAPS
  primary antiphospholipid syndrome
papulosis
  malignant atrophic p.
PAQ
  Personal Attributes Questionnaire
  Position Analysis Questionnaire
PAR
  Proficiency Assessment Report
  PAR Admissions Testing program
paraballism
parablepsia
parabrachial
  p. area
  p. nuclei
parabulia
paracarcinomatous
  p. encephalomyelopathy
  p. myelopathy
paracenesthesia
paracentesis
paracentral
  p. fissure
  p. gray area
  p. gyrus
  p. hemianopia
  p. lobule
  p. nucleus of thalamus
  p. scotoma
paracetamol
parachiasmal epidermoid tumor
parachlorophenylalanine
parachromatopsia
parachromopsia
parachute reflex
paracinesia, paracinesis
paracinesis
paraclinoid
  p. internal carotid artery aneurysm
Paracoccioides brasiliensis
paracrine mechanism
paracusis, paracousia, paracusia
  false p.
  localis p.
  Willis p.
paracyclic ovulation
paradementia

paradigm
  biopsychosocial p.
  p. clash
  cocktail party p.
  diathesis-stress p.
  learning p.
  motor p.
  physiological p.
  p. shift
  transference p.
paradigmatic
  p. response
  p. shift
  p. stress from life experience
Paradione
paradipsia
paradox
  calcium p.
  neurotic p.
paradoxa
  obstipatio p.
paradoxica
  kinesia p.
paradoxical
  p. abdominal movement
  p. air embolism (PAE)
  p. anxiety
  p. cerebral embolism
  p. cold
  p. effect
  p. extensor reflex
  p. incontinence
  p. injunction
  p. intention (PI)
  p. intervention
  p. ipsilateral hemiparesis
  p. orgasm
  p. pupil
  p. pupillary phenomenon
  p. reaction
  p. response
  p. sleep
  p. technique
  p. therapy
  p. undressing
  p. warmth
paraequilibrium
paraeroticism
paraesthetica
  pseudomelia p.
paraffin embedding
Paraflex
Parafon
  P. Forte
  P. Forte DSC
parafunction
paragammacism
paraganglioma
  intrasellar p.
  intravagal p.
  nonchromaffin p.
paragenital
parageusia
paragigantocellularis
  nucleus reticularis p.

paragloboside
  sulfate-3-glucuronyl p. (SGPG)
  sulfate-3-glucuronyllactosaminyl p.
    (SGLPG)
paragnomen
paragonimiasis lymphocytic meningitis
paragrammatism
paragraphia
paragraph-meaning test
paragraph recall test
parahaemolyticus
  Vibrio p.
parahippocampal
  p. activation
  p. gyrus
parahypnosis
parahypophysis
parainfluenzae
  Haemophilus p.
parakinesia, parakinesis
Paral
paralalia literalis
paralambdacism
paralanguage
paraldehyde
paraldehydism
paraleprosis
paralepsy
paralexia
paralgesia
paralgia
paralimbic
paralinguistic feature
paralipophobia
parallax
parallel
  p. dream
  p. law
  p. play
  p. processing
parallelism
  cultural p.
  psychoneural p.
  psychophysical p.
paralog
paralogia
  benign p.
  metamorphic p.
  metaphoric p.
  thematic p.
  themomatic p.
paralogical thinking
paralysis, pl. paralyses
  abducens nerve p.
  acute atrophic p.
  p. agitans
  alcoholic p.
  ascending p.
  backpack p.
  Bell p.
  Benedikt ipsilateral oculomotor p.
  bilateral abductor p.
  bilateral adductor p.
  Brown-Séquard p.
  bulbar p.

catatonic cerebral p.
central p.
chronic basal meningitis with
  cranial nerve p.
compression p.
conjugate p.
contralateral facial p.
conversion p.
cricothyroid p.
crossed p.
crutch p.
decubitus p.
deglutition p.
Dejerine-Klumpke p.
diphtheritic p.
Duchenne p.
Duchenne-Erb p.
Erb spinal p.
exhaustion p.
extraocular p.
facial p.
familial hypokalemic periodic p.
familial periodic p.
faucial p.
flaccid p.
gaze p.
general p.
ginger p.
global p.
glossolabiolaryngeal p.
glossolabiopharyngeal p.
Gubler p.
histrionic p.
hyperkalemic periodic p.
hypokalemic periodic p.
hysteric p.
immobilization p.
immunological p.
infranuclear p.
p. of the insane
ipsilateral facial p.
Jackson vagoaccessory
  hypoglossal p.
jake p.
Jamaica ginger p.
Klumpke p.
Kussmaul-Landry p.
labial p.
labioglossolaryngeal p.
labioglossopharyngeal p.
Landry p.
lead p.
leaden p.
lingual p.
Lissauer p.
lower motor neuron p.
mimetic p.
mitochondrial encephalomyopathy
  with sensorimotor polyneuropathy,
  ophthalmoplegia, and p. (MEPOP)
mixed p.
motor neuron p.
musculospiral p.
myogenic p.
myopathic p.

P

paralysis *(continued)*
    nocturnal p.
    normokalemic periodic p.
    obstetrical p.
    ocular p.
    oculomotor nerve p.
    periodic p.
    postdiphtheritic p.
    postdormital sleep p.
    postepileptic p.
    posticus p.
    Pott p.
    predominantly predormital sleep p.
    predormital sleep p.
    pressure p.
    progressive bulbar p.
    pseudobulbar p.
    pseudohypertrophic muscular p.
    psychogenic p.
    rectus p.
    residual p.
    saccade p.
    sensory p.
    sleep p.
    sodium-responsive periodic p.
    spastic spinal p.
    spinal p.
    supranuclear p.
    thyrotoxic periodic p.
    tick p.
    Todd postepileptic p.
    unilateral abductor p.
    unilateral adductor p.
    upper motor neuron p.
    vasomotor p.
    wasting p.
    work p.
    Zenker p.
paralytic
    p. abasia
    p. chorea
    congenital syphilitic p.
    p. dementia
    p. disorder
    p. idiocy
    p. ileus
    p. micosis
    p. miosis
    p. mydriasis
    p. pontine exotropia
    p. scoliosis
paralytica
    aphonia p.
    p. aphonia
    dementia p.
    Lissauer dementia p.
paralyticus
    ictus p.
paralyzant
paralyze
paralyzing vertigo
paramagnetic
    p. contrast
    p. contrast enhancement

    p. contrast injection
    p. relaxation
paramagnetism
paramania
paramedian
    p. durotomy
    p. infarction
    p. mesencephalic syndrome
    p. region
    p. thalamopeduncular artery
    p. thalamus
    p. triangle
paramedical
parameter
    chance response p.
    item discrimination p.
paramethadione
paramethasone acetate
parametric
    p. study
    p. test of significance
parametrismus
paramilitary
paramimia
paramimism
paramnesia
    reduplicative p.
paramour
paramusia
paramyoclonus
paramyotonia
    atactic p.
    ataxic p.
    p. congenita
    congenital p.
    symptomatic p.
paramyotonus
paranalgesia
paranasal
    p. mucocele
    p. sinus
paraneoplastic
    p. cerebellar degeneration
    p. limbic encephalitis
    p. myelopathy
    p. neuropathy
    p. pain syndrome
paranesthesia
paraneural infiltration
paraneurone
paranodal region
paranoia, pl. **paranoides (PA)**
    acquired p.
    acute hallucinatory p.
    affect-laden p.
    alcoholic p.
    amentia paranoides
    amorous p.
    classical p.
    conjugal p.
    p. and delusions psychiatric syndrome
    dementia paranoides
    p. dementia gravis
    dissociative p.

eccentric p.
erotic p.
exalted p.
p. hallucinatoria
hallucinatory p.
heboid p.
hypochondriacal p.
involutional p.
Kraepelina p.
litigious p.
mystic p.
p. originaria
paranoidal p.
p. paranoid state
persecutory p.
projectional p.
p. querulans
p. querulans paranoid state
querulous p.
reformatory p.
rudimentary p.
P. "6" Scale
senile p.
p. senilis
p. simplex
paranoiac
    p. character
    p. psychosis
paranoica
    aphonia p.
    aphrasia p.
    metamorphosis sexualis p.
paranoic psychosis
paranoid
    p. behavior
    p. belief system
    p. condition
    p. dementia
    p. erotism
    p. fear
    p. feature
    floridly p.
    p. grandiose delusion
    p. hostility
    p. ideation
    p. litigious state
    p. look
    p. melancholia
    p. neurotic personality disorder
    p. personality
    p. psychoneurosis
    p. psychosis
    p. reaction
    p. reaction type
    p. scale
    p. schizophrenia
    schizophrenic reaction, acute, p.
      (SR/AP)
    schizophrenic reaction, chronic, p.
      (SR/CP)
    sensitive Beziehungswahn p.
    P. Sensitivity Profile
    p. tendency
    p. trait
    p. trend

paranoid/affective organic psychosis
paranoid-affective organic psychosis, mixed
paranoidal paranoia
paranoides (*pl. of* paranoia)
paranoidism
paranoid-schizoid position
paranoid-schizotypal personality disorder
paranoid-type arteriosclerotic
paranomasia
paranomia
paranormal
    p. cognition
    p. phenomenon
paranosic gain
paranosis
paraolfactory cortical area
paraorbital lesion
paraparesis
    acute-onset p.
    chronic p.
    HTLV-associated myelopathy/tropical
      spastic p. (HAM/TSP)
    spastic p.
    tropical spastic p. (TSP)
    X-linked spastic p.
paraparetic
parapathetic proviso
parapathy
paraphasia
    extended jargon p.
    jargon p.
    literal p.
    thematic p.
    verbal p.
paraphasic error
paraphasis
paraphemia
paraphenomenon
paraphernalia
    drug p.
    paraphiliac p.
paraphia
paraphilia
    atypical p.
    exhibitionism p.
    fetishism p.
    frotteurism p.
    pedophilia p.
    transvestism p.
    troilism p.
    voyeurism p.
paraphiliac, paraphilic
    p. behavior
    p. coercive disorder
    p. fantasy
    p. focus
    p. imagery
    p. object
    p. paraphernalia
    p. pornography
    p. preference
    p. stimulus
paraphobia
paraphonia

P

paraphonic state
paraphora
paraphrasia
    literal p.
    thematic p.
paraphrenia
    climacteric p.
    p. confabulans
    p. expansiva
    p. fantastica
    involutional p.
    late p.
    menopausal p.
    p. paranoid state
    presenile p.
    p. systematica
paraphrenic
    p. dementia
    p. schizophrenia
paraphysial, paraphyseal
    p. cyst
paraphysis, pl. **paraphyses**
parapineal
parapithymia
paraplectic
paraplegia
    alcoholic p.
    atactic p.
    ataxic p.
    congenital spastic p.
    p. dolorosa
    Erb spastic p.
    p. in extension
    familial spastic p.
    p. in flexion
    hereditary spastic p.
    infantile spastic p.
    painful p.
    postoperative p.
    Pott p.
    senile p.
    spastic p.
    superior p.
    tetanoid p.
paraplegic
    p. idiocy
    p. spasm
parapoplexy
parapraxia
parapraxis, pl. **parapraxes**
paraprofessional
paraprotein
    light chain p.
paraproteinemia
paraproteinemic neuropathy
parapsia
parapsychology
parapsychosis
parareaction
parareflexia
pararhotacism
pararmusia
parasagittal
    p. falx
    p. groove

    p. intracranial mass
    p. lesion
    p. meningioma
parasellar
    p. cistern
    p. dysgerminoma
    p. lesion
    p. mass
    p. tentorial meningioma
    p. tumor
parasexuality
parasigmatism
parasinoidal sinuses
parasite
parasites of the superego
parasitic
    p. brain abscess
    p. infection
    p. superego
    p. vampirism
parasitophobia
parasitosis
parasocial speech
parasomnia
parasomniac
    p. consciousness
    p. conscious state
parasomnia-type
    p.-t. sleep disorder
    p.-t. substance-induced sleep
      disorder
paraspasm
paraspinal
    p. infection
    p. muscle
    p. rod application
Parastep I System
parastriate
    p. area
    p. cortex
parasuicidal behavior
parasympathetic
    p. epilepsy
    p. ganglia
    p. nerve injury
    p. nervous system (PNS)
    p. part
parasympathicotonia
parasympatholytic
parasympathomimetic drug
parasympathotonia
paratactic distortion
parataxic
    p. distortion
    p. mode
parataxis, parataxia
parateresiomania
paraterminal
    p. body
    p. gyrus
parathormone
parathymia
parathyreopriva
    tetania p.

parathyroid
  p. disorder
  p. function
  p. gland
  p. hormone (PTH)
  p. tetany
parathyroprival tetany
paratonia
Paratrend 7 sensor
paratrigeminal neuralgia
paratrophy
paratype
paratypic
paraventricular
  p. cyst
  p. nucleus
paraverbal therapy
paravertebral
  p. ganglia
  p. venous plexus
paraxial mesenchyme
paraxon
parchment crackling
parectropia
paregoric
  p. overdose
  p. poisoning
pareidolia
parencephalia
parencephalitis
parencephalocele
parencephalous
parenchyma
parenchymal
  p. bacillary peliosis
  p. cerebral hemorrhage
  p. granuloma
  p. matrix
parenchymatous
  p. atrophy
  p. cell of corpus pineale
  p. cerebellar degeneration
  p. hemorrhage
  p. neuritis
  p. neurosyphilis
parens patriae
parent
  p. abuse
  p. artery
  P. as a Teacher Inventory (PAAT)
  P. Attachment Structured Interview
  P. Attitude Scale (PAS)
  authoritarian p.
  authoritarian rejecting-neglecting p.
  P. Awareness Skills Survey (PASS)
  battered p.
  p. burnout
  custodial p.
  P. Daily Report
  P. Effectiveness Training (PET)
  p. egostate
  p. fixation
  p. image
  ineffectual p.

  P. Interview for Child Syndrome
    (PICS)
  p. inventory
  p. neglect
  noncustodial p.
  P. Opinion Inventory
  P. Perception of Child Profile
    (PPCP)
  permissive p.
  p. perplexity
  problem p.
  P. Rating of Student Behavior
  rejecting p.
  rejecting-neglecting p.
  Sleep Screening Questionnaire
    for P.'s
  strict p.
  surrogate p.
  p. therapist program
  ungiving p.
  weak p.
  weekend p.
Parent-Adolescent Communication Scale
parent-adult-child (PAC)
parental
  P. Acceptance-Rejection
    Questionnaire
  p. behavior
  P. Bonding Instrument
  p. control
  p. control problem
  p. criticism
  p. custody
  p. fit
  p. indecisiveness
  p. loss
  p. perplexity
  p. rejection
  p. right doctrine
  p. rights
  p. spontaneity
  P. Stressor Scale
  P. Stressor Scale: Neonatal
    Intensive Care Unit (PSS:NICU)
parent-child
  p.-c. conflict
  p.-c. conflict counseling
  p.-c. dyad
  p.-c. model
  p.-c. relational problem
  p.-c. relationship
parenteral
  p. alimentation
  p. drug
  p. drug administration
  p. feeding
  p. nutrition
  p. physostigmine
parenthetical expression
parenthood
  Planned P.
parentified role
parent-infant bonding
parenting
  erratic p.

P

parenting *(continued)*
    foster p.
    irresponsible p.
    Michigan Screening Profile of P.
    positive p.
    reciprocal p.
    refrigerator p.
    p. skill
    P. Stress Index
    p. style
parentis
    in loco p.
parent-offspring bond
parents
    P. Anonymous
    p. subsystem
    P. Without Partners (PWP)
Parent-Teacher Questionnaire (PTQ)
parepithymia
parerethisis
parergasia
paresis
    abducens nerve p.
    accessory nerve p.
    alcoholic p.
    bibrachial p.
    canal p.
    central facial p.
    cerebral gaze p.
    crural p.
    distal motor p.
    downward gaze p.
    elevation p.
    extraocular muscle p.
    facial p.
    gaze p.
    general p.
    horizontal gaze p.
    hypoglossal nerve p.
    infantile p.
    ipsilateral facial p.
    juvenile p.
    limb-girdle-trunk p.
    Lissauer-type p.
    monomelic p.
    ocular motor nerve p.
    oculomotor nerve p.
    palatal p.
    postictal p.
    progressive extraocular p.
    pseudoabducens nerve p.
    trochlear nerve p.
    upward gaze p.
    vertical gaze p.
    watershed area p.
paresthesia
    Berger p.
    laryngeal p.
paresthetica
    digitalgia p.
    meralgia p.
    meralgia p.
paresthetic conversion reaction

paretic
    p. curve
    p. dementia
    p. impotence
    p. jerk
    p. melancholia
    p. neurosyphilis
    p. psychosis
Pargonimus westermani
pargyline
    methyclothiazide and p.
Parhad-Poppen arteriogram needle
Parham decision
Paridol
paries, gen. **parietis**, pl. **parietes**
    p. vestibularis ductus cochlearis
parietal
    p. association area
    p. cortex
    p. cortex lesion
    p. corticectomy
    p. craniotomy
    p. encephalocele
    p. foramen
    p. gyrus
    p. lobe
    p. lobe dysfunction
    p. lobe lesion
    p. lobe syndrome
    p. meningioma
    p. operculum
    p. plane
    p. skull bone
    temporal, occipital, p. (TOP)
parietooccipital
    p. aphasia
    p. craniotomy
    p. fissure
    p. infarction
    p. lesion
    p. sulcus
parietopontine tract
parietosquamous suture
parietotemporal
    p. area
    p. perfusion deficit
parieto-temporo-occipital
Parinaud
    P. ophthalmoplegia
    P. sign
    P. syndrome
park bench position
Parkinson
    P. disease (PD)
    P. facies
    P. triangle
parkinsonian
    p. crisis
    p. dysarthria
    p. facies
    p. gait
    p. muscular rigidity
    p. speech
    p. tremor

parkinsonism
    amyotrophy p.
    drug-induced p.
    juvenile p.
    medication-induced p.
    MPTP-induced p.
    neuroleptic-induced p.
    postencephalitic p.
    primary p.
    vascular p.
parkinsonism-dementia
    p.-d. complex
    p.-d. complex of Guam
parkinsonism-like effect
Parkland Rapid Exam (PRE)
Parlodel
Parmodalin
Parnate
parody in wit
parolfactory area
paroneiria salax
paroniria ambulans
paronomasia
paronymous
parophresis
parorexia
parosmia
parosphresia
parotid
    p. dissection
    p. duct
    p. tumor
parotitis
parousiamania
paroxetine HCl
paroxysmal
    p. activity
    p. alpha activity
    p. atrial fibrillation
    p. cerebral dysrhythmia
    p. convulsion
    p. drinking
    p. dyskinesia
    dyskinesia p.
    p. dystonia
    p. kinesigenic choreoathetosis
    p. migraine
    p. migraine headache
    p. phenomenon
    p. positional nystagmus
    psychogenic p.
    p. psychosis
    p. seizure
    p. sleep
    p. sleep disorder
    p. tachycardia
    p. trepidant abasia
    p. vertigo
parricide
parrotlike speech pattern
Parry-Romberg disease
PARS
    Personal Adjustment and Role Skills
    Personal and Role Skills
    PARS Scale
pars, pl. partes
    p. anterior
    p. anterior commissurae anterioris
    p. anterior commissurae rostralis
    p. anterior facies diaphragmatis
    p. anterior fornix vaginae
    p. autonomica
    p. basilaris pontis
    p. caudalis
    p. centralis ventriculi lateralis
    p. cervicalis arteriae carotis internae
    p. cervicalis esophagi
    p. cervicalis medullae spinalis
    p. coccygea medullae spinalis
    p. cochlearis
    p. compacta
    p. cupularis
    p. distalis
    p. dorsalis pontis
    p. frontalis corporis callosi
    p. infundibularis
    p. insularis
    p. interarticularis
    p. intermedia commissura bulborum
    p. intermedia lobi anterioris hypophyseos
    p. lumbalis diaphragmatis
    p. lumbalis medullae spinalis
    p. nervosa hypophyseos
    p. occipitalis corporis callosi
    p. opercularis
    p. optica retinae
    p. orbitalis glandulae lacrimalis
    p. orbitalis musculi orbicularis oculi
    p. orbitalis nervi optici
    p. orbitalis ossis frontalis
    p. parasympathica
    p. peripherica
    p. pharyngea hypophyseos
    p. plana
    p. plicata
    p. posterior commissurae anterioris
    p. posterior facies diaphragmatis hepatis
    p. posterior fornix vaginae
    p. postlaminalis nervi optici vaginae
    p. pro toto
    p. reticulata
    p. retrolentiformis capsulae internae
    p. sacralis medullae spinalis
    p. sellaris
    p. spinalis
    p. sublentiformis capsulae internae
    p. sympathica
    p. thoracica aortae
    p. thoracica ductus thoracici
    p. thoracica esophagi
    p. thoracica medullae spinalis
    p. triangularis
    p. vagalis

P

pars (*continued*)
    p. ventralis pontis
    p. vertebralis
    p. vestibularis
Parsidol
parsimony
Parsitan
Parsonage-Aldren-Turner syndrome
Parsonage-Turner
    P.-T. disease
    P.-T. syndrome
part
    anterior p. of pons
    autonomic p.
    basilar p. of pons
    coccygeal p. of spinal cord
    cochlear p. of vestibulocochlear
      nerve
    cupular p.
    cupulate p.
    distal p. of anterior lobe of
      hypophysis
    dorsal p. of pons
    inferior p. of vestibulocochlear
      nerve
    infundibular p. of anterior lobe of
      hypophysis
    p. instinct
    intermediate p.
    p. object
    optic p. of retina
    orbital p.
    parasympathetic p.
    superior p. of vestibulocochlear
      nerve
    sympathetic p.
    vagal p. of accessory nerve
    ventral p. of the pons
    vertebral p.
    vestibular p. of vestibulocochlear
      nerve
partes (*pl. of* pars)
parthenium
    Tanacetum p.
parthenophobia
partial
    p. adjustment
    p. agenesis
    p. agonist
    p. aim
    p. amnesia
    p. arterial gas tension of carbon
      dioxide (PaCO2)
    p. central hypophysectomy
    p. complex seizure
    p. correlation
    p. cross-dressing
    p. delirium
    p. delusion
    p. epilepsy
    p. facetectomy
    p. flip angle imaging
    p. Fourier imaging
    p. hemianopia

    p. hemilaminectomy
    p. homonymous field defect
    p. hospitalization
    p. hospital patient population
    p. hospital setting
    p. insanity
    p. instinct
    p. mergent
    p. nominal aphasia
    p. organic psychosyndrome
    p. permanent disability
    p. pressure
    p. recovery
    p. regression
    p. reinforcement
    p. remission
    p. saturation
    p. sensory seizure
    p. thromboplastin time (PTT)
    p. tonic seizure
    p. venous gas tension of oxygen
      (PvO2)
    p. visual loss
partialis
    p. fugax amaurosis
    ophthalmoplegia p.
    psychopathia p.
    rachischisis p.
partialism
    persistent p.
partiality
partially disabled
partial-reinforcement effect (PRE)
partial-thickness craniectomy
participant
    p. modeling
    p. observation
    p. observer
participation
    group p.
participative management
particle
    p. beam
    p. beam radiosurgery
    p. domain
    Ivalon p.
    polyvinyl alcohol p.
    proteinaceous infectious p.
    signal recognition p. (SRP)
particular
    bill of p.'s
    p. complex
    p. task
particularism
particulate embolization
parting of the ways
parti pris
partisan
partitive
part-learning method
partner
    bed p.
    compulsive fixation on an
      unobtainable p.
    consenting p.

nonconsenting p.
Parents Without P.'s (PWP)
phallic p.
p. relational problem
P. Relationship Inventory (PRI)
sleeping p.
surrogate p.
surrogate sexual p.
part-object manner
parturiphobia
parturition
party
drug p.
neutral p.
p. nystagmus
paruresis
parviculata
alopecia p.
PAS
Parent Attitude Scale
periodic acid-Schiff
personality assessment system
Prevocational Assessment Screen
pas
faux p.
petit p.
PASAT
Paced Auditory Serial Addition Test
PASES
Performance Assessment of Syntax
Elicited and Spontaneous
pasmo
PAS-positive circular body
PASS
Parent Awareness Skills Survey
Perception of Ability Scale for Students
pass
leave on p. (LOP)
weekend p.
passage
adiabatic fast p.
bird of p.
p. comprehension
memory p.
rite of p.
wire p.
passer
Malis ligature p.
passing stranger effect
passion
crime of p.
p. flower
passional attitude
passionate attitude
passionelle
attitude p.
psychose p.
passive
p. accommodation
p. aggression
p. aggressive (PA)
p. algolagnia
p. analysis
p. avoidance
p. behavior

p. castration complex
p. dependency
p. euthanasia
p. immunity
p. incontinence
p. influence
p. introversion
p. listening
p. mode of consciousness
p. movement
p. object love
p. parasitic psychopathy
p. personality
p. reaction
p. recreation
p. resistance
p. therapist
p. therapy
p. transport
p. tremor
p. vocabulary
passive-aggressive (PA)
p.-a. acting out
p.-a. behavior
p.-a. neurotic
p.-a. neurotic personality
p.-a. neurotic personality disorder
p.-a. personality (PAP)
p.-a. reaction
p.-a. scale
passive-avoidance learning
passive-dependent
p.-d. personality (PDP)
p.-d. reaction
passive-receptive longing
passivity
active p.
p. in anger expression
delusion of p.
p. delusion
motor p.
past
p. event
p. experience
p. history (PH)
P. History Schedule
p. oriented
p. personal history
p. tic
past-life hypnotic regression
pastoral
p. care
p. counseling
p. counselor
p. psychiatry
PAT
Pain Apperception Test
Photo Articulation Test
Predictive Ability Test
psychoacoustic test
Psychoacoustic Testing
patch
BuSpar p.
Fentanyl p.
Habitrol P.

P

609

patch (*continued*)
  Nicoderm P.
  Nicotrol P.
  ProStep P.
  shagreen p.
  striosome p.
  Tissue-Guard bovine pericardial p.
  Transderm Scop P.
patching
  lysolecithin p.
patchy retrograde amnesia
patellar tendon reflex
patelloadductor reflex
patellometer
patency
  valve p.
patent
  p. medicinal abuse
  p. medicinals
  p. medicine
paterfamilias
paternal
  p. attitude
  p. behavior
  p. deprivation
  p. desertion
  p. drive
  p. neglect
paternalism
paternity
  p. blues
  proof of p.
  p. test
pathematic aphasia
pathemia
pathergasia
pathergy phenomenon
pathetic nerve
pathetism
Pathibamate
pathic
pathoclisis
pathocure
pathodixia
pathoformic
pathogen
  behavioral p.
pathogenesis
pathogenic, pathogenetic
  p. care
  p. dystonia
  p. family pattern
pathogenicity
pathogeny
pathognomic
pathognomonic
  p. fantasy
  p. sign
pathognomy
pathognostic
pathography
  psychoanalytic p.
  psychoanalytical p.
pathohysteria

pathokinesis
patholesia
pathologic, pathological
  p. alcohol intoxication
  p. amenorrhea
  p. behavior
  p. care
  p. character formation
  p. communication
  p. condition
  p. diagnosis
  p. drowsiness
  p. drug intoxication
  p. drug intoxication drug psychosis
  p. drunkenness
  p. emotionality
  p. fallacy
  p. gambling
  p. grief reaction
  p. guilt
  p. hyperreflexia
  p. intoxication
  p. intoxication alcoholic psychosis
  p. liar
  p. lying
  p. mendicancy
  p. nature
  p. pain
  p. personality
  p. preoccupation
  p. process
  p. reaction to alcohol
  p. reflex
  p. sexual fantasy
  p. sexuality
  p. sleepiness
  p. spontaneous activity (PSA)
  p. substance use
  p. swindler
  p. trait
pathology
  association deficit p.
  aural p.
  brain p.
  character p.
  focal p.
  forensic p.
  functional p.
  language p.
  psychosocial p.
  structural p.
pathology-induced memory reconstruction
pathomania
pathomechanics
  kyphotic deformity p.
  spinal fusion p.
pathomimesis
pathomimia
pathomimicry
pathomiosis
pathomorphism
pathoneurosis
pathophilia
pathophobia

pathophrenesis
pathophysiological
    p. mechanism
    p. pattern
    p. process
pathophysiology
pathoplasty
pathopsychology
pathopsychosis
pathos
pathosis
    attitudinal p.
pathway
    abducens p.
    amygdalofugal p.
    anterior cingulate p.
    auditory p.
    biochemical p.
    cerebellar p.
    corticobulbar p.
    corticofugal p.
    corticospinal motor p.
    CSF outflow p.
    dentato-olivary p.
    dopaminergic p.
    dorsolateral p.
    frontopontocerebellar p.
    geniculocortical p.
    intracellular metabolic p.
    lemniscal p.
    limbic system p.
    lipoxygenase p.
    nigrostriatal p.
    occulomotor p.
    olfactory p.
    orbitofrontal p.
    pain and temperature p.
    perforant p.
    pyramidal p.
    ras signaling p.
    reticulocortical p.
    retinal p.
    retrochiasmal visual p.
    signal transduction p.
    spinoreticulothalamic p.
    p. stimulation
    stretch reflex p.
    striatopallidothalamocortical p.
    synaptic p.
    thalamocortical p.
    trigeminovascular p.
    ventral amygdalofugal p.
    visual p.
patico
patient (pt)
    abused p.
    adult scoliosis p.
    agitated p.
    analytic p.
    aphasic p.
    comatose p.
    combative p.
    p. compliance
    p. contract
    dangerous p.

    p. delay
    Diagnostic Interview for
      Borderline P.'s
    disoriented p.
    dual diagnosis p.
    P. and Family Services (PFS)
    geriatric p.
    p. government
    high-risk p.
    hypnotic p.
    hypnotic-dependent p.
    incoherent p.
    insomniac p.
    lethargic p.
    multidimensional scale for rating
      psychiatric p.'s (MSRPP)
    old-old p.
    panic-disordered p.
    peregrinating problem p.
    person in the p.
    p. positioning
    posttraumatic p.
    problem p.
    psychiatric p.
    P. Rated Anxiety Scale (PRAS)
    P. Rated Disability Scale
    P. Rated Impairment Scale
    P. Rated Overall Life Impairment
    p. resistance
    p. responsibility
    p. rights
    p. satisfaction
    P. Satisfaction Questionnaire-III
    self-destructive p.
    stuporous p.
    target p.
    unresponsive p.
    variable screw placement system-
      plated p.
    young-old p.
patient-care audit
patient-centered services
patient-controlled analgesia (PCA)
patient-matched implant
patient-oriented consultation
Patil
    P. stereotactic head frame
    P. stereotactic head holder
    P. stereotactic system II
PATLC
    Progressive Achievement Tests of
    Listening Comprehension
patriae
    parens p.
patriarchal family
patricide
Patrick test
patrilineal family
patrilocal family
patriophobia
patronizing manner
patronymic
pattern
    aberrant p.
    action p.

P

pattern *(continued)*
  activation p.
  advanced sleep-phase p.
  affectomotor p.
  agreed-on p.
  alpha p.
  p. analysis
  p. of antisocial behavior
  Antoni p. (type A & B)
  authoritarian leadership p.
  autosomal dominant p.
  avoidance p.
  beaten copper p.
  behavior p.
  binge eating p.
  blame-placing communication p.
  Boder Test of Reading-
    Spelling P.'s
  changing sleep-wake p.
  characteristic p.
  checkerboard p.
  chronically disabling p.
  communication p.
  p. of conduct
  convergence-divergence p.
  delusional thought p.
  democratic leadership p.
  p. of detachment
  developmental p.
  p. discrimination
  disturbed sleep p.
  double major curve p.
  EEG alpha p.
  electromyographic incomplete
    interference p.
  enduring p.
  erotic-arousal p.
  expressive p.
  extinction-type p.
  familial p.
  family p.
  field p.
  fixed action p. (FAP)
  gesturing communication p.
  gullwing p.
  habit p.
  ictal epileptiform p.
  P.'s of Individual Change Scale
    (PICS)
  inflexible p.
  intellectualization communication p.
  intensive habit p.
  interpersonal spacing
    communication p.
  irregular sleep p.
  irregular sleep-wake p.
  Kindling p.
  laissez-faire leadership p.
  left thoracolumbar major curve p.
  Lennox-Gastaut p.
  long-term p.
  maladaptive personality p.
  manipulation communication p.
  P. Misfit Scale

  mitten p.
  monopolization communication p.
  mood disorder with seasonal p.
  neurodevelopmental p.
  noncued memory p.
  Occupational Ability P. (OAP)
  parrotlike speech p.
  pathogenic family p.
  pathophysiological p.
  persistent p.
  personality p.
  pervasive p.
  p. of pervasive unhappiness
  phenomenal p.
  positive spike p.
  power struggle leadership p.
  prototypical course p.
  radiofrequency homogeneity p.
  rapid-cycling p.
  p. recognition
  recruitment p.
  reflex p.
  repetitive p.
  response p.
  right thoracic left lumbar curve p.
  right thoracic minor curve p.
  role p.
  scapegoating communication p.
  seasonal p.
  semantic argument
    communication p.
  p. sensitive epilepsy
  shared thought p.
  silence communication p.
  sleep p.
  specific dynamic p.
  stable sleep-wake p.
  storiform p.
  symptom response p.
  syndromal p.
  syndrome p.
  thought p.
  touching communication p.
  type II curve p.
  validation communication p.
patterned
  p. alopecia
  p. interview
pattern-induced epilepsy
patterning
  p. exercise
  p. psychotherapy
  p. vision
patting automatism
patty
  polyclot p.
pauci-immune necrotizing vasculitis
paucisynaptic
paucity
  p. of data
  p. of expressive gestures
  p. of movement
  p. of reports
  p. of speech
  p. of speech content

Pauli exclusion principle
Paulus trocar
pauperize
pause
>apneic p.
>fixation p.
>respiratory p.
>p. in speech

paving stone degeneration
Pavlov
>P. method
>P. theory of schizophrenia

pavlovian conditioning
pavor
>p. diurnus
>p. nocturnus
>p. scleresis

Pavulon
Paxarel
Paxil
Paxipam
payer
>third party p.

Paykel Life Events Scale
paz
P-BAP
>Behavioral Assessment of Pain Questionnaire

PBC
>pregnancy and birth complication

PBG
>porphobilinogen

PBI
>protein-bound iodine

PBMC
>peripheral blood mononuclear cell

PBQ
>Preschool Behavior Questionnaire

PBS
>Pediatric Behavior Scale

PC
>PC subtest
>phrase construction
>picture completion
>>PC subtest (PC)

p.c.
>after meals

PC-2048B positron emission tomograph
PCA
>patient-controlled analgesia
>posterior cerebral artery
>>DAT for PCA

PCAS
>Psychotherapy Competence Assessment Schedule

PCG
>Planning Career Goals

PCI
>Premarital Communication Inventory

PCO₂
>carbon dioxide pressure

PComA
>posterior communicating artery

PCP
>PCP abuse
>PCP intoxication
>PCP intoxication delirium
>PCP use disorder

PCP-induced anxiety disorder
PCP-related disorder, not otherwise specified
PCR
>polymerase chain reaction
>>frataxin gene PCR
>>X25 PCR

PCS
>Priority Counseling Survey

pcs
>preconscious

PCT
>Physiognomic Cue Test

PCV chemotherapy
PD
>panic disorder
>Parkinson disease
>problem drinker
>Process Diagnostic
>psychopathic deviate
>psychotic depression

PDA
>polymorphic delta activity
>>PDA on electroencephalogram

PDD
>pervasive developmental disorder
>primary degenerative dementia
>>PDD NOS

PDDAT
>primary degenerative dementia of Alzheimer type

PDH
>pyruvate dehydrogenase
>>PDH complex

PDI Employment Inventory
PDN
>Prosthetic Disc Nucleus

PDP
>passive-dependent personality

PDQ-R
>Personality Diagnostic Questionnaire-Revised

PDR
>Physicians' Desk Reference

PDS
>pain dysfunction syndrome

PDT
>photodynamic therapy

PE
>physical examination
>probable error

PEA
>phenylethylamine

Peabody
>P. Developmental Motor Scales and Activity Cards
>P. Individual Achievement Test (PIAT)
>P. Mathematics Readiness Test
>P. Picture Vocabulary Test (PPVT)
>P. Vocabulary Test (PVT)

peaceful coexistence

P

peacemaker role
peace tablet
peak
    p. acoustic gain
    p. amplitude variability
    Bragg ionization p.
    p. clipping
    p. experience
    kilovoltage p. (kVp)
    p. level of drug activity
    p. and trough level
peak-dose dyskinesia
peak-to-peak amplitude
Péan
    P. clamp
    P. forceps
peapod intervertebral disk forceps
PEAQ
    Personal Experience and Attitude
        Questionnaire
pear bur
pearl-chain appearance
pearl tumor
pearly neoplasm
pear-shaped nerve hook
PEC
    politico-economic-conservatism
        PEC scale
peccatiphobia, peccatophobia
pecking order
pectoralgia
pectoralgic
    p. migraine
    p. migraine headache
pectoralis major muscle
pectoral reflex
pectoris
    angor p.
    Prinzmetal vasospastic angina p.
peculiar
    p. behavior
    p. personality trait
pedagogy
pedal system
pedantic
pederast
pederasty
pedes (*pl. of* pes)
Pediapred Oral
pediatric
    American Academy of P.'s
    P. Behavior Scale (PBS)
    p. brain stem glioma
    p. C-D hook
    p. Cotrel-Dubousset rod
    P. Early Elementary Examination
    P. Examination of Educational
        Readiness at Middle Childhood
    P. Extended Examination at Three
        (PEET)
    p. growth chart
    p. headrest
    p. moyamoya disease
    p. neuroradiology
    p. psychiatry

    p. psychology
    p. psychopharmacology
    P. Speech Intelligibility Test
    p. supratentorial hemispheric tumor
    p. TSRH hook
pedicle
    adjoining p.
    p. anatomy
    p. axis angle
    p. C-D hook
    p. cortex disruption
    p. diameter
    p. dimensions
    p. entrance point
    p. evaluation
    p. landmark
    p. localization
    p. location
    lower thoracic p.
    lumbar p.
    p. marker
    p. morphometry
    p. screw
    p. screw breakage
    p. screw chord length
    p. screw construct
    p. screw hardware prominence
    p. screw insertion
    p. screw linkage design
    p. screw path length
    p. screw plating
    p. screw pullout strength
    p. screw-rod fixation
    p. sounding probe
    thoracic p.
pedicular fixation
pediculophobia
pedigree
    p. method
    p. study
pedionalgia
pedioneuralgia
pediophobia
pedis (*gen. of* pes)
pedohebephilia
pedologia
pedologist
pedology
pedomorphism
pedophile
    heterosexual p.
    homosexual p.
pedophilia
    adolescent p.
    bisexual p.
    heterosexual p.
    homosexual p.
    middle age p.
    p. paraphilia
    senescent p.
pedophilic
    p. behavior
    p. homosexuality
    p. stimulus
pedophobia

pedotrophy
peduncle
cerebellar p.
cerebral p.
p. of corpus callosum
p. of flocculus
inferior cerebellar p.
inferior thalamic p.
lateral thalamic p.
p. of mamillary body
middle cerebellar p.
olfactory p.
superior cerebellar p.
ventral thalamic p.
peduncular
p. ansa
p. hallucinosis
hallucinosis p.
p. loop
peduncularis ansa p.
peduncularis ansa peduncular
pedunculi (*pl. of* pedunculus)
pedunculopontine
p. cholinergic group
p. neuron
p. nucleus
pedunculotomy
pedunculus, pl. pedunculi
p. cerebellaris inferior
p. cerebellaris medius
p. cerebellaris superior
p. cerebri
p. corporis callosi
p. corporis mamillaris
p. flocculi
p. of pineal body
p. thalami inferior
p. thalami lateralis
p. thalami ventralis
PEEP
positive end-expiratory pressure
peeping Tom
peer
age p.
p. anxiety
conflicts with p.'s
p. criticism
p. group
p. interaction
p. interactional situation
p. likability
P. Nomination Inventory of
Depression
p. ostracism
p. play
p. pressure
P. Profile
p. rating
p. relationship
p. review
p. review organization (PRO)
peer-helping service
PEET
Pediatric Extended Examination at Three
Peet splanchnic resection

peevish
PEF
Psychiatric Evaluation Form
PEG
pericyte edema generation
peg
fibular p.
Peganone
pegboard
grooved p.
Lafayette p.
Peiper-Beyer laminectomy rongeur
pejorative
p. delusion
p. nature
p. voice
pejorism
pelea
mal de p.
peliagroid
peliosis
parenchymal bacillary p.
Pelizaeus-Merzbacher
P.-M. disease
P.-M. leukodystrophy
pellagra
p. dementia
pellagra sine p.
pellagragenic
pellagral
pellagraphobia
pellagrin
pellagroid
pellagrous
pellucidi
cavum septi p. (CSP)
pellucidum
cavity of septum pellucidum
septum p.
pelopsia
Pelorus
P. stereotactic frame
P. surgical system
pelvic
p. fixation
p. ganglia
p. obliquity
p. pain
p. plexus
p. thrusting
pelvis
crossed reflex of p.
pelvofemoral
p. muscular dystrophy
PEMF
pulsating electromagnetic field
pemoline
magnesium p.
pen
p. alignment
p. yan
penal code
penalize
penalty
minor p.

P

penalty, frustration, anxiety, guilt, hostility (PFAGH)
penance
penchant
pencil grip
pencil-grip instrument
pendetide
    satumomab p.
pendular nystagmus
pendulous
penectomy
    self-administered p.
penetrable
penetrance
    lack of p.
penetrating
    p. injury
    p. trauma
penetration
    anterior cortex p.
    antibiotic p.
    finger p.
    p. response
    vertebral body anterior cortex p.
Penfield
    P. dissector
    P. hypothesis
    P. neurodissector
penfluridol
peniaphobia
penicillamine
penicillin
    benzathine p.
    p. G
    p. G benzathine suspension
    p. V
Penicillium
penile
    p. arousal
    p. impotence
    p. plethysmograph
    p. plethysmography
    p. prosthesis
    p. tumescence
penilingus
penis
    artificial p.
    p. captivus
    p. envy
    erector p.
    p. fear
    glans p.
    immissio p.
    p. pride
    squeeze technique of p.
    tenesmus p.
    p. wish
penitent
Penn cube function formula
penology
Penrose drain
pensé
    déjà p.
pensée
    tic de p.

pensee operatoire
penses
    echo des p.
pension neurosis
pentagastrin
pentamidine
pentapeptide
pentastarch
pentazocine
    p. analgesia
    p. compound
pentetrazol
pentobarbital
    p. coma
    p. sodium
pentobarbitone
Pentothal Sodium
pentoxifylline
pentylenetetrazol (PTZ)
penumbra
    ischemic p.
penurious
penury
PEO
    progressive external ophthalmoparesis
peonage
    institutional p.
peotillomania
PEP
    Psychiatric Evaluation Profile
    Psychoeducational Profile
    Psycho-Epistemological Profile
PEPAP
    analog of meperidine
Pepper
    P. neuroblastoma
    P. syndrome
peptic ulcer
peptide
    atrial natriuretic p. (ANP)
    beta amyloid p.
    brain natriuretic p. (BNP)
    calcitonin gene-related p. (CGRP)
    cardioexcitatory p.
    p. cotransmitter
    C-type natriuretic p. (CNP)
    delta sleep-inducing p.
    gastrin-inhibiting p.
    neuroactive p.
    neurohypophyseal p.
    p. neurotransmitter
    opioid p.
    sleep-inducing p.
    tau protein p.
    vasoactive intestinal p. (VIP)
peptidergic
PER
    Periodic Evaluation Record
per
    p. anum
    p. day (/d)
    p. mesem
    p. os
    p. rectum
    p. vaginam

peracute mania
perazine
per capita
perceived
    p. emotional abandonment
    p. interpersonal rejection
    p. loss
    p. neglect
    p. reality
percentile
    Adaptive Behavior Composite p.
    p. norm
    p. rank
    p. score
percept
    body p.
    p. image
perceptible
perception
    aberration of p.
    P. of Ability Scale for Students
      (PASS)
    abnormal p.
    abstract p.
    alteration in time p.
    altered mind-body p.
    altered sensory p.
    auditory space p.
    automorphic p.
    binocular p.
    body-image p.
    clerical p. (Q)
    color p.
    complex visual p.
    conscious p.
    cross-modality p.
    p. deficit
    depth p.
    Developmental Test of Visual P.
      (DTVP)
    Developmental Test of Visual P.,
      Second Edition (DTVP-2)
    p. disorder
    distance p.
    distorted p.
    disturbance of p.
    p. disturbance
    ecological p.
    p. ego
    endopsychic p.
    exaggerated p.
    extrasensory p. (ESP)
    facial p.
    family p.
    figure-ground p.
    fingertip number writing p.
    form p.
    Frostig Developmental Test of
      Visual P. (FDTVP)
    gravity p.
    hallucination of p.
    haptic p.
    hypnagogic p.
    hypnopompic p.
    P. of Illness Scale

    inferential p.
    internal world of p.
    p. inventory
    kinesthetic p.
    p. localized within the body
    LSD-type p.
    motion p.
    obligatory p.
    pain p.
    person p.
    physiognomic p.
    posthallucinogen p.
    proprioceptive p.
    sensory p.
    situational p.
    size p.
    social p.
    p. of sound
    p. of sound inside the head
    p. of sound outside the head
    space p.
    p. of spatial relations
    stereognostic p.
    subconscious p.
    subliminal p.
    substance-induced p.
    tactile p.
    tactile kinesthetic p.
    Test of Visual P.
    time p.
    touch p.
    transactional theory of p.
    true p.
    visual p.
    Weber Advanced Spatial P.
      (WASP)
    weight p.
perception-hallucination
Perception-of-Relationships-Test (PORT)
perceptive
    p. deafness
    p. epilepsy
perceptivity
Percepto-Diagnostic
    Minnesota P.-D. (MPD)
perceptorium
perceptual
    p. abnormality
    p. analysis
    p. anchoring
    p. closure
    p. consciousness
    p. consistency
    p. constancy
    p. cue
    p. cycle
    p. defect
    p. defense
    p. deficit
    p. deprivation
    p. disability
    p. disorder
    p. distortion
    p. disturbance
    p. expansion

P

perceptual *(continued)*
  p. extinction
  p. field
  p. filter
  p. filtering
  p. immaturity
  p. induction
  p. maintenance
  p. masking
  P. Maze Test
  p. motor abilities disturbance
  p. motor ability
  p. motor dysfunction
  p. organization
  p. organizational index
  P. Organization Deviation Quotient (PODQ)
  p. psychology
  p. restructuring
  p. retardation
  p. rivalry
  p. schema
  p. segregation
  p. sensitization
  p. set
  p. skill
  p. sociogram
  p. speed
  p. structure
  p. style
  p. symptoms
  p. synthesis
  p. training
  p. transformation
  p. vigilance
perceptually handicapped
perceptual-motor
  p.-m. abilities impairment
  p.-m. disability
  p.-m. impairment
  p.-m. learning
  p.-m. match
  p.-m. region
  p.-m. skill
percipient
Percocet
Percodan-Demi
Percogesic
Percolone
percussion
  distal tingling on p. (DTP)
  p. hammer
percutaneous
  p. balloon commissurotomy
  p. cabling
  p. cordotomy
  p. discoscope
  p. electrode array
  p. epidural electrode
  p. glycerol rhizolysis (PGR)
  p. intraarterial embolization
  p. laser nucleolysis
  p. radiofrequency gangliolysis
  p. radiofrequency rhizolysis (PRF)

  p. radiofrequency rhizotomy
  p. retrogasserian glycerol chemoneurolysis
  p. retrogasserian glycerol rhizolysis
  p. retrogasserian glycerol rhizotomy
  p. spinal endoscope
  p. stimulation
  p. thecoperitoneal shunt
  p. transluminal coronary angioplasty (PTCA)
  p. transvenous coil embolization
  p. trigeminal nerve compression
perdida del alma
peregrinating problem patient
perencephaly
perennial dream
Perez reflex
perfect
  p. negative relationship
  p. performance
  p. positive relationship
perfectible
perfectionism preoccupation
perfectionistic
perfection state
perfluorocarbon
perfluorooctyl bromide
perforant pathway
perforated space
perforating bur
perforation
  esophageal p.
  vascular p.
perforator
  Acra-Cut cranial p.
  Aesculap skull p.
  cranial p.
  Cushing cranial p.
  Heifetz cranial p.
  Heifetz skull p.
  Hudson p.
  powered automatic skull p.
  Raney p.
performance
  p. abnormality
  p. anxiety
  as-if p.
  p. assessment
  P. Assessment of Syntax Elicited and Spontaneous (PASES)
  automaticity of p.
  p. characteristic
  P. Efficiency Test
  p. fear
  impaired p.
  P. Intelligence Quotient (PIQ)
  P. IQ Score
  P. Levels of a School Program Survey
  motor p.
  p. neurosis
  p. objective
  perfect p.
  psychometric p.
  psychomotor p.

quality of p.
p. requirement
P. Scale Score
school p.
p. score
sexual p.
p. situation
standard of p.
p. task
p. test
performance-intensity function
performative speech
Perf-Plate cranial plate
perfunctory
perfusate drip
perfusion
critical p.
p. deficit
luxury p.
microcirculatory p.
misery p.
p. pressure breakthrough
pergolide mesylate
perhaps neurosis
PERI
Psychiatric Epidemiology Research
Interview
Periactin
perianal
perianeurysmal hemorrhage
periapical abscess
periaqueductal
p. central gray (PAG)
p. gray matter
p. hemorrhage
periarterial sympathectomy
periarteritis nodosa
periatrial disease
periaxonal
periblepsis
pericallosal azygos artery
pericardial reflex
pericarditis
perichareia
perichrome
periciazine
periclaustral lamina
Perico
pericorpuscular synapse
pericranial temporalis flap
pericranii
sinus p.
pericranitis
pericranium
pericyazine
pericyte edema generation (PEG)
pericytosis
peridural
periencephalitis
perifascicular
p. atrophy
p. migration
perifocal edema
periforaminal
perigemmal

peri-ictal headache
perikaryal
perikaryon, pl. **perikarya**
perilesional inhibitory cortex
perilous
periluteal phase dysphoric disorder
perilymphatic
p. duct
fistula p.
p. fistula
perimedullary venous system
perimeningitis
perimesencephalic
p. cistern
p. nonaneurysmal subarachnoid
hemorrhage (PNSH)
perimetry
Goldman p.
perinatal
p. anoxia
p. development
p. history
p. infection
p. morbidity
perineal
p. body
p. fascia
p. post
perineometer
electromyographic p.
perineural
p. anesthesia
p. infiltration
perineuria (*pl. of* perineurium)
perineurial cyst
perineuritis
perineurium, pl. **perineuria**
period
absolute refractory p.
adaptation p.
apneic p.
apneustic p.
child raising p.
chum p.
concrete operations p.
critical p.
depression p.
developmental p.
discrete p.
enactive p.
endogenous circadian p.
fantasy p.
fetal p.
formal operations p.
growth p.
ictal p.
interictal p.
involutional p.
latency p. (LP)
latent p.
menstrual p.
oedipal p.
Oedipus p.
oral biting p.
practicing p.

P

period *(continued)*
    prenatal p.
    preoperational thought p.
    p. prevalence
    prodromal p.
    psychological refractory p.
    readout p.
    refractory p.
    REM p.
    sadness p.
    sensorimotor intelligence p.
    silent p.
    sleep onset REM p.
    storm-and-stress p.
    thought p.
periodic
    p. acid-Schiff (PAS)
    p. acid-Schiff-hematoxylin stain
    p. alternating nystagmus
    p. catatonia
    p. drinker
    p. drinking
    p. edema
    P. Evaluation Record (PER)
    p. insanity
    p. jactitation
    p. lateralizing epileptiform discharge
      (PLED)
    p. limb movement disorder
    p. mania
    p. migrainous neuralgia
    p. paralysis
    p. psychosis of puberty
    p. reinforcement
    p. reinforcement relationship
    p. screening
periodicity theory
periontogenic
perioperative
    p. anoxia
    p. cisternography
    p. reduction
perioptic
    p. meningioma
    p. subarachnoid space
perioral tremor
periorbita
periorbital ecchymosis
periosteal
    p. elevator
    p. reflex
peripachymeningitis
peripapullar astrocyte
peripersonal space
peripheral
    p. anesthesia
    p. apnea
    p. autonomic neuropathy
    p. blood mononuclear cell (PBMC)
    p. chemoreceptor
    p. cue test
    p. deafferentation pain
    p. dysarthria
    p. electromyographic activity

    p. epilepsy
    p. examination
    p. field image
    p. masking
    p. myelin protein 22
    p. nerve
    p. nerve axotomy
    p. nerve disease
    p. nerve entrapment syndrome
    p. nerve fascicle
    p. nerve injury
    p. nerve lesion
    p. nerve level motor impairment
    p. nerve myelin (PNM)
    p. nerve neuroma
    p. nerve pressure palsy
    p. nerve regeneration conduit
    p. nerve sheath tumor
    p. nervous system (PNS)
    p. neuritis
    p. neurofibromatosis
    p. neuropathic pain syndrome
    p. nociceptor activation
    p. sensation
    p. sensory loss
    p. sympathomimetic effect
    p. tabes
    p. vascular disease
peripheralism
peripheralist psychology
periphery dose
periphlebitis retinae
periphrastic
peripneial
peripolar zone
periproctic
perirectal
perirectitis
perirolandic parietal cortex
perispondylitis
peristasis
peristriate
    p. area
    p. cortex
perisylvian cortex
perithelial small cell sarcoma
peritoneal
    p. catheter
    subdural p. (SP)
peritoneum
peritonism
peritorcular meningioma
peritraumatic
    p. dissociation
    P. Dissociation Index
Peritrode
peritumoral
    p. band
    p. brain edema
periurethral
perivaginal
perivascular
    p. cuff
    p. cuffing
    p. mononuclear cell

p. nerve-ending stimulation
p. space
periventricular
p. disease
p. fiber
p. gray
p. gray matter (PVG)
p. hyperintense lesion
p. radiolucency (PVL)
p. white matter
p. white matter lesion
periventricular-intraventricular hemorrhage
Perky effect
Perley-Guze Hysteria Checklist
Perlia nucleus
Perls stain
permanence
p. concept
object p.
permanent
p. disability
p. dominant idea
p. epilation
p. magnet
p. memory
p. planning
p. residual impairment
p. section
p. sympathectomy
p. vegetative state
Permax
permeability
permeable
permeation
permissible dose
permission, limited information, specific suggestion, and intensive therapy (PLISSIT)
permissive
p. environment
p. hypothesis of affective
p. hypothesis of affective disorders
p. parent
p. substrate
Permitil Oral
permutation
perneoscrotal
perneovaginal
pernicious
p. anemia
p. trend
perocephalic edema
peroneal
p. entrapment neuropathy
p. muscular atrophy
p. nerve palsy
p. phenomenon
p. somatosensory evoked potential
peroral
peroration
peroxidation
lipid p.

peroxisomal
p. disease
p. proliferator receptor (PPAR)
peroxisome
peroxynitrite
perpend
perpendicular fasciculus
perpetuate
perpetuating factor
perpetuator of abuse
perpetuity
perphenazine
amitriptyline and p.
p. and amitriptyline hydrochloride
perplexed manic-depressive psychosis
perplexed-type manic-depressive
perplexity
morbid p.
parent p.
parental p.
p. psychosis
p. state
vague p.
Persantine
persecution
p. complex
delirium of p.
delusion of p.
p. delusion
p. ideation
social p.
p. syndrome
p. theme
themes of p.
persecutor
persecutory
p. anxiety
p. delusion
p. delusional disorder
p. delusional system
p. idea
p. paranoia
P. Type
persecutory-type schizophrenia
persenilin gene
perseveration
p. deficit
infantile p.
motor p.
p. set
verbal p.
perseverative
p. error
p. functional autonomy
p. movement
p. response
p. speech
p. trace
Persian
P. Gulf War
P. Gulf War syndrome
persistence
motor p.
persistent
p. clonus

P

persistent *(continued)*
    p. delusion
    p. discomfort
    p. facial palsy
    p. hypersomnia
    p. inappropriate idea
    p. inappropriate image
    p. inappropriate impulse
    p. insomnia
    p. intrusive idea
    p. intrusive image
    p. intrusive impulse
    p. motor activity
    p. partialism
    p. pattern
    p. pattern of conduct
    p. puberism
    p. thought
    p. tremor
    p. vegetative state (PVS)
    p. vegetative state disorder
persisting
    p. dementia
    p. disorder
person
    Attitudes Toward Disabled P.'s (ATDP)
    composite p.
    p. deixis
    displaced p.
    disturbed p.
    dominant p.
    exposure of p.
    inner-directed p.
    other-directed p.
    p. in the patient
    p. perception
    RLS p.
    significant supporting p.
    spectral relationship to famous p.
    street p.
    time, place, and p. (TP&P)
    very important p. (VIP)
    p. with AIDS
persona
    p. grata
    p. non grata
    organic p.
    in propria p.
    symbolic p.
personal
    p. adjustment
    P. Adjustment and Role Skills (PARS)
    P. Adjustment and Role Skills Scale
    p. assault
    P. Assessment for Continuing Education (PACE)
    P. Assessment of Intimacy in Relationships (PAIR)
    P. Attributes Questionnaire (PAQ)
    p. attribution
    p. audit

    p. care
    p. care home
    P. Communication Plan
    p. construct
    p. construct theory
    p. counselor
    p. data inventory
    p. data sheet
    p. demoralization
    p. development
    p. disposition
    p. distance zone
    p. document analysis
    p. dysjunction
    p. effects
    p. equation
    P. Experience and Attitude Questionnaire (PEAQ)
    P. Experience Inventory Defensiveness
    P. Experience Screening Questionnaire (PESQ)
    p. function
    p. growth
    p. growth group
    p. growth laboratory
    p. history (PH)
    p. history questionnaire
    p. hygiene
    p. identity
    p. identity confusion
    p. idiom
    p. image
    p. inadequacy
    p. inadequacy theme
    P. Inventory
    P. Inventory of Needs
    p. judgment
    p. locus of control (PLC)
    p. loss
    p. man
    p. motivation
    p. myth
    p. need
    P. Orientation Inventory (POI)
    P. Preference Scale (PPS)
    P. Problems Checklist (PPC)
    P. Problems Checklist for Adolescents (PPC)
    p. relationship
    P. Relationship Inventory (PRI)
    P. Resource Questionnaire (PRQ)
    p. response
    p. responsibility
    P. and Role Skills (PARS)
    p. satisfaction
    P. Skills Map
    p. and social history (P&SH)
    p. social motive
    p. space
    p. space invasion
    P. Strain Questionnaire (PSQ)
    P. Style Inventory (PSI)
    p. supply of drug
    p. unconscious

p. value
P. Values Abstract (PVA)
P. Values Inventory (PVI)
personalism
personality
    acromegaloid p.
    addiction-prone p. (APP)
    addictive p.
    P. Adjective Check List (PACL)
    affective p.
    aggressive p.
    alexithymic p.
    allotropic p.
    alternating p.
    altruistic p.
    amoral psychopathic p.
    amoral trends psychopathic p.
    anal p.
    anal-retentive p.
    anancastic p.
    antisocial p. (ASP)
    antisocial neurotic p.
    antisocial psychopathic p.
    antisocial trends psychopathic p.
    as-if p.
    asocial p.
    p. assessment
    P. Assessment Inventory (PAI)
    p. assessment system (PAS)
    asthenic p.
    atypical mixed or other p.
    authoritarian p.
    avoidant p.
    basic p.
    borderline p.
    California Test of P. (CTP)
    Cattell factorial theory of p.
    p. change
    p. change due to a general
      medical condition
    P. Change Due to a General
      Medical Condition, Aggressive
      Type
    P. Change Due to a General
      Medical Condition, Apathetic
      Type
    P. Change Due to a General
      Medical Condition, Disinhibited
      Type
    P. Change Due to a General
      Medical Condition, Labile Type
    P. Change Due to a General
      Medical Condition, Paranoid Type
    p. characteristic
    chronic hypomanic p.
    coarctated p.
    co-conscious p.
    codependent p.
    compulsive p.
    cult of p.
    p. cult
    cycloid p.
    cyclothymic p.
    dependent p.
    depressive p.

p. deterioration
p. development
p. deviation
P. Diagnostic Questionnaire-Revised
  (PDQ-R)
diehard p.
p. disintegration
disordered p.
P. Disorder Examination
p. disorder NOS
p. disorders scale
p. disturbance
disturbed p.
dominant p.
double p.
dual p.
dynamic p.
p. dynamics
dyssocial p.
eccentric p.
emotional p.
emotionally unstable p.
epileptic p.
epileptoid p.
exploitative p.
explosive p.
extroverted p.
P. Factor Questionnaire (PFQ)
16 P. Factor Questionnaire (16 PF)
factor theory of p.
fanatic p.
p. feature
p. formation
freudian theory of p.
p. functioning
p. and gender
haltlose-type p.
histrionic p.
hoarding p.
hyperaesthetic p.
hypomanic p.
hysterical p.
hysteroid p.
ideal p.
immature p.
p. impoverishment
inadequate p.
P. Index (PI)
inmate p.
p. integration
interactional theory of p.
interictal epileptic p.
intraconscious p.
introverted schizoid p.
P. Inventory (PI)
P. Inventory for Children (PIC)
Jekyll and Hyde p.
Karolinska Scales of P.
lifetime p.
magnetic p.
maladaptive p.
marketing p.
masochistic p.
melancholic p.
migraine p.

P

personality *(continued)*
 mixed psychopathic p.
 multiple p.
 multiplication of p.
 narcissistic p.
 neurotic p.
 p. neurotic disorder
 obsessional p.
 obsessive p.
 obsessive-compulsive p.
 oral p.
 p. organization
 p. panel
 paranoid p.
 passive p.
 passive-aggressive p. (PAP)
 passive-aggressive neurotic p.
 passive-dependent p. (PDP)
 pathologic p.
 p. pattern
 p. pattern disturbance
 physiological basis of p.
 Polyfactorial Study of P.
 posttraumatic p.
 premorbid p.
 prepsychotic p.
 presenting p.
 pretraumatic p.
 p. problem
 productive p.
 p. profile
 psychoinfantile p.
 p. psychology
 p. psychoneurosis
 psychoneurotic p.
 psychopathic p.
 p. questionnaire
 P. Rating Scale (PRS)
 p. reaction
 receptive p.
 repressive p.
 P. Research Form (PRF)
 role theory of p.
 sadistic p.
 schizoid p.
 schizophrenic p.
 schizothymic p.
 schizotypal schizoid p.
 Schneider definition of p.
 schneiderian criteria for
  depressive p.
 seclusive p.
 secondary p.
 seductive p.
 self-defeating p.
 shut-in p.
 Singer-Loomis Inventory of P.
  (SLIP)
 sociopathic p.
 p. sphere
 split p.
 stable p.
 stormy p.
 p. structure

 p. syndrome
 syntonic p.
 p. test
 P. Test Guilford
 p. trait
 p. trait disturbance
 p. trait stability
 p. trait theory
 p. type
 type A p.
 type B p.
 ulcer p.
 unstable p.
 unusual p.
 viscosity p.
 volatile p.
personalization
personalized interpretation
personate
person-centered theory
person-environment interaction
personification
 eidetic p.
personified self
personify
personnel
 p. date
 p. placement
 p. psychology
 P. Reaction Blank
 P. Security Preview (PSP)
 p. selection
 P. Selection Inventory
 p. test
 P. Tests for Industry (PTI)
 p. training
personologic psychotherapy
personology
person's culture
perspective
 alternating p.
 alternative p.
 atmospheric p.
 categorical p.
 extraspective p.
 humanistic p.
 temporal p.
perspiration artifact
persuasion
 coercive p.
 p. therapy
persuasive communication
Perthes-Bankart lesion
Pertscan 99m
perturbation
pertussis-toxin-catalyzed
 ADP-ribosylation
pervasive
 p. anhedonia
 p. anxiety
 childhood-onset p.
 p. developmental disorder (PDD)
 p. disinhibited type of
  developmental disorder
 p. distrust

p. emotion
p. impairment of development
p. pattern
p. and persistent maladaptive
  personality traits
p. pessimism
p. proneness to guilt
p. self-criticism
p. unhappiness
perversion
excretory p.
polymorphous p.
sex p.
sexual p.
perverted
p. appetite
p. logic
p. sexuality
p. thinking
pervigilium
PES
Pleasant Events Schedule
psychiatric emergency service
pes, gen. **pedis**, pl. **pedes**
p. hippocampi
p. pedunculi
PESQ
Personal Experience Screening
  Questionnaire
pessimism
oral p.
pervasive p.
therapeutic p.
PET
Parent Effectiveness Training
positron emission tomography
Professional Employment Test
psychiatric emergency team
  PET image
  nonstereotactic PET
  PET scan
petechia, pl. **petechiae**
petechial hemorrhage
Peter Principle
PET-FDG
positron emission tomography with [^{18}F]-
  labeled fluorodeoxyglucose
PET-guided stereotactic biopsy
petit
p. mal
p. mal epilepsy
p. mal seizure
p. mal status
p. mal variant seizure
p. pas
P. syndrome
petition of mental illness (PMI)
petrification
petrochemical
petroclinoclival meningioma
petroclival
p. cholesterol granuloma
p. lesion
p. meningioma
p. tumor

petroclivotentorial meningioma
petrooccipitalis
fissura p.
petrosal
p. approach
p. ganglion
p. impression of the pallium
p. nerve
p. neuralgia
p. sinus
p. sinus sampling
petrosectomy
petrositis, petrousitis
petrosphenoidal ligament
petrosquamosal sinus
petrous
p. apex
p. carotid artery
p. carotid-to-intradural carotid
  saphenous vein graft
p. ganglion
p. ridge chemodectoma
petrousitis (*var. of* petrositis)
Pette-Döring disease
petting behavior
peyote
p. cactus
p. dependence
peyotism
Peyronie disease
Peyton brain spatula
PF
Fiorgen PF
16 PF
16 Personality Factor Questionnaire
PFAGH
penalty, frustration, anxiety, guilt,
  hostility
  PFAGH stuttering
Pfeiffer syndrome
PFQ
Personality Factor Questionnaire
PFS
Patient and Family Services
picture frustration study
primary fibromyalgia syndrome
progression-free survival
  Folex PFS
Pfuhl sign
PGR
percutaneous glycerol rhizolysis
psychogalvanic reflex
psychogalvanic response
PGSR
psychogalvanic skin resistance
PGT
play group therapy
PH
past history
personal history
phacoma, phakoma
phacomatosis
Phaedra complex
phagocytosis
phagomania

P

phagophobia (*var. of* pagophobia)
phagotherapy
phakoma (*var. of* phacoma)
phalangeal cell
Phalen
    P. maneuver
    P. sign
    P. test
phallic
    p. character
    p. level
    p. love
    p. mother
    p. overbearance
    p. partner
    p. phase
    p. pride
    p. primacy
    p. sadism
    p. stage
    p. stage psychosexual development
    p. symbol
    p. woman
phallicism, phallism
phallic-narcissistic character
phallic-oedipal phase
phalliform
phallism (*var. of* phallicism)
phallocentric culture
phalloid
phalloides
    Amanita p.
phallometry
phallophobia
phallus envy
phaneromania
phanerothyme
phantasia
phantasm
phantasmagoria
phantasmatomoria
phantasmology
phantasmoscopia
phantasmoscopy
phantastica (*var. of* fantastica)
phantasy (*var. of* fantasy)
phantogeusia
phantom
    p. absence seizure
    p. arm
    p. base
    p. boarders
    Compass stereotactic p.
    p. extremity
    gelatin p.
    hot-spot p.
    p. image
    p. limb
    p. limb pain
    p. lover syndrome
    plexiglas p.
    p. reaction
    p. sensation
    p. speech
    three-dimensional SPECT p.

    p. tooth pain
    p. vision
phantomize
pharmaceutical
    p. alternative
    p. equivalent
pharmacodynamic
    p. change
    p. tolerance
pharmacodynamics
    age-related p.
pharmacoeconomics
pharmacogenetics
pharmacogenic orgasm
pharmacogeriatrics
pharmacokinetic change
pharmacological
    p. antagonism
    p. blockade
    p. experimentation
    p. management
    p. provocation
    p. therapy
    p. treatment
pharmacologic prophylaxis
pharmacology
    nicotine p.
    serotonergic p.
pharmacomania
pharmacopedia
Pharmacopeia
    United States P. (USP)
pharmacophilia
pharmacophobia
pharmacopsychoanalysis
pharmacopsychosis
pharmacotherapeutic
    p. intervention
    p. treatment
pharmacotherapy
pharmacothymia
pharyngeal
    p. anesthesia
    p. cleft
    p. hypophysis
    p. pouch
    p. psychophysiologic reaction
    p. reflex
    p. tubercle
    p. weakness
pharyngismus
pharyngoplegia
pharyngospasm
phase
    absolute construction of p.'s
    active p.
    acute p.
    p. advance
    anal p.
    p. angle
    appetitive p.
    autistic p.
    p. cancellation
    circadian rhythm sleep' disorder, delayed sleep p.

p. coherence
p. cue
p. cycling
p. delay
dementia p.
depressive p.
developmental p.
p. difference
p. disparity
p. effect
p. encoding
endogenous circadian rhythm p.
equatorial p.
excitement p.
extradural p.
follicular p.
genital p.
group p.
illness p.
insomnia p.
p. instability
intradural p.
p. lag on EEG
late luteal p.
latency p.
libidinal p.
p. of life
p. of life problem
p. locking
luteal p.
magic p.
manic p.
p. mapping
moon p.
oedipal p.
opposite p.
oral p.
oral-eroticism p.
oral-incorporative p.
orgasmic p.
phallic p.
phallic-oedipal p.
plateau p.
postambivalent p.
preambivalent p.
pregenital p.
pre-oedipal p.
preoperational p.
presuperego p.
prodromal p.
residual p.
resolution p.
p. reversal
p. reversal potential
rhythm p.
schizophrenia p.
second negative p.
p. of seizure
sensorimotor p.
separation-individuation p.
p. sequence
p. shift
p. shift of sleep-wake cycle
sleep p.
p. spike

p. spike on EEG
symbiotic p.
tonic p.
transverse magnetization p.
urethral p.
vector p.
walking swing p.
phase-contrast
p.-c. map
p.-c. method
p.-c. technique
phased-array
p.-a. coil
p.-a. color-flow ultrasound system
phase-encoding
p.-e. direction
p.-e. gradient
phase-sensitive
p.-s. detector
p.-s. gradient-echo MR imaging
phase-shift effect
phasic
p. activation
p. function
p. nystagmus
p. reflex
phasmophobia
phasophrenia
Phelps Kindergarten Readiness Scale (PKRS)
PHEMA
polyhydroxyethylmethacrylate
Phemetrazine
phenacemide
phenadoxone hydrochloride
phenaglycodol
Phenaphen with codeine
Phenazine
phenazocine
phencyclidine
p. abuse
p. and amphetamine/methamphetamine
analog of p.
cannabis and p.
cannabis, cocaine, heroin and p.
cannabis laced with p.
cannabis laced with cocaine and p.
crack dipped in p.
crack liquid and p.
p. delusional disorder
p. dependence
p. and heroin
p. hydrochloride
p. intoxication
p. intoxication delirium
p. intoxication, with perceptual disturbance
methylenedioxymethamphetamine and p.
p. mixed organic brain
p. mixed organic brain syndrome
p. thiophene
p. use disorder
phencyclidine-associated psychosis

P

phencyclidine-induced
    p.-i. disorder
    p.-i. psychotic disorder with
      delusions
    p.-i. psychotic disorder with
      hallucinations
phencyclidine-like substance
phencyclidine-related
    p.-r. disorder
    p.-r. disorder NOS
phendimetrazine tartrate
Phendry Oral
phenelzine sulfate
Phenerbel-S
Phenergan
phengophobia
pheniprazine
pheniramine
phenmetrazine
phenobarbital
    p. sodium
    very high dose p. (VHDPB)
phenobarbitone
phenobutiodil
phenocopy
phenogenetic
phenol
phenology
phenolphthalein
phenomena (*pl. of* phenomenon)
phenomenal
    p. absolutism
    p. field
    p. motion
    p. pattern
    p. regression
    p. report
    p. self
phenomenalism
phenomenalistic introspection
phenomenistic
    p. causality
    p. thought
phenomenological
    p. analysis
    p. feature
    p. field
    p. reality
    p. subgroup
phenomenology
    existential p.
phenomenon, pl. **phenomena**
    abstinence p.
    alien limb p.
    arm p.
    Aubert p.
    Aubert-Forster p.
    autoscopic p.
    Babinski p.
    baked brain p.
    Bell p.
    Bezold-Brucke p.
    breakaway p.
    breakoff p.
    breakthrough p.

breast-phantom p.
Capgras p.
cervicolumbar p.
choo-choo p.
clasp-knife p.
cogwheel p.
constancy p.
crossed phrenic p.
Cushing p.
déjà vu p.
Dejerine hand p.
Dejerine-Lichtheim p.
dissociative p.
disturbance associated with
    conversion p.
doll's eyes p.
doll's head p.
Doppler p.
Duckworth p.
echo p.
escape p.
extinction p.
facialis p.
Féré p.
finger p.
freezing p.
Fregoli p.
Galassi pupillary p.
gestalt p.
Gibbs p.
Grasset p.
Grasset-Gaussel p.
Gunn p.
halo p.
hesitation p.
hip p.
hip-flexion p.
Hoffmann p.
Hunt paradoxical p.
hypofrontality p.
identification p.
p. identification
implausible p.
interactive p.
interictal p.
intracranial steal p.
Isakower p.
jamais p.
jaw-winking p.
jet lag p.
Kernohan notch p.
knee p.
Kohnstamm p.
Kühne p.
lactate dehydrogenase p.
leg p.
Leichtenstern p.
Lhermitte p.
Marcus Gunn p.
misdirection p.
motoric p.
napping p.
Negro p.
no-reflow p.
normal voluntary napping p.

on-off p.
panic-spectrum p.
panum p.
paradoxical pupillary p.
paranormal p.
paroxysmal p.
pathergy p.
peroneal p.
Pool p.
psi p.
psychic p.
psychomotor p.
Pulfrich p.
radial p.
Raynaud p.
rebound p.
release p.
riddance p.
Ritter-Rollet p.
Rust p.
Schiff-Sherrington p.
Schüller p.
sensory p.
Sherrington p.
split screen p.
staircase p.
steal p.
Strümpell p.
Tarchanoff p.
tibial p.
tip-of-the-tongue p.
toe p.
tongue p.
TOT p.
trailing p.
transference p.
transient visual p.
transvestic p.
Uhthoff p.
voluntary napping p.
Wernicke hemianopic pupillary p.
Westphal p.
Westphal-Piltz p.
Wever-Bray p.
Zeigarnik effect p.
phenomotive
phenoplegia
phenothiazine
p. agent
aliphatic p.
p. derivative
phenotype
DMD p.
myelinating p.
phenotypic expression
phenoxybenzamine
phensuximide
phentermine
p. hydrochloride
p. resin
phentolamine
Phenurone
phenylalanine disorder
phenylbutazone

phenylephrine
phenylethanolamine-N-methyltransferase (PNMP, PNMT)
phenylethylamine (PEA)
phenylketonuria (PKU)
phenylpiperazine
phenyl piperazine
phenylpiperidine
phenylpropanolamine hydrochloride
phenylpropranolamine (PPA)
phenylpropylamine
phenylpyruvic
p. acid
amentia p.
p. amentia
p. imbecility
p. oligophrenia
phenylpyruvica
oligophrenia p.
phenyl-*t*-butyl-nitrone
phenyltoloxamine
acetaminophen and p.
p. citrate
phenytoin (PHT)
phenytoin-induced
p.-i. chorea
p.-i. choreoathetosis
pheochromocytoma and neuroblastoma localization study
pheromone
PHI
physiological hyaluronidase inhibitor
Philadelphia
P. collar
P. halo
P. Head Injury Questionnaire (PHIQ)
P. Multilevel Assessment Instrument
Philippe triangle
Philips
P. Gyroscan S5
P. Gyroscan S15
P. linear accelerator
P. 400 transmission electron microscope
Phillips' Milk of Magnesia
Phillipson reflex
Phillips Scale
Philly bolt
philobat
philology
philomimesia
philoneism
philopatridomania
philoprogenitive
philosophical
p. analysis
p. psychology
philosophobia
philosophy
analytical p.
coercive p.
moral p.
philter, philtre
philtrum

P

PHIQ
   Philadelphia Head Injury Questionnaire
phi rhythm
phlebitis
   sinus p.
phlebography
phlegm
phlegmatic constitutional type
phobanthropy
phobia
   animal p.
   animal/insect p.
   animal-type specific p.
   blood/injection p.
   disease p.
   driving p.
   examination p.
   height p.
   illness p.
   isolated p.
   obsessional p.
   panic-related p.
   protein p.
   p. psychoneurosis
   school p.
   simple p.
   situational specific p.
   sleep p.
   social p.
   specific p.
   universal p.
   water p.
   work p.
phobic
   p. anxiety
   p. attitude
   P. Attitude Evaluation
   p. avoidance
   p. behavior
   p. character
   p. companion
   p. desensitization
   p. disorder
   mixed p.
   p. neurosis
   nongeneral p.
   p. obsessional neurosis
   p. psychoneurotic reaction
   p. situation
   p. state
   p. stimulus
   p. syndrome
   p. trend
phobic-anxiety-depersonalization
Phoenix
   P. ancillary valve
   P. Anti-Blok ventricular catheter
   P. cranial drill
   P. cruciform valve
   P. fifth ventricle system
   P. House
phoesthesia
phonasthenia
phonation
phonatory theory

phoneme
   anterior feature English p.
   back p.
   diffuse p.
phoneme-grapheme association
phonemic
   p. analysis
   p. awareness
phonetically balanced words
phonetic analysis
phonetics
   acoustic p.
phoniatrics
phonic spasm
phonism
phonoangiography
   quantitative spectral p.
phonogram
phonological
   p. agraphia
   p. analysis
   p. disorder
   p. processing
phonologically
   p. irregular words
   p. regular words
phonology
   Bankson-Bernthal Test of P.
   (BBTOP)
phonomania
phonomyoclonus
phonomyography
phonopathy
phonophobia
phonopsia
phonoreceptor
phopathy
phosphatase
   acid p.
   alkaline p.
phosphate
   amphetamine p.
   cellulose sodium p.
   dextroamphetamine p.
   dibasic calcium p.
   disopyramide p.
   Hexadrol P.
   Hydrocortone P.
   p. metabolism
   potassium p.
   potassium phosphate and sodium p.
   sodium p.
   tri-ortho-cresyl p.
phosphate-wasting syndrome
phosphatidylinositol
phosphatidyl inositol system
phosphatidylserine
phosphene
phosphocreatine
phosphocreatinine
   frontal p.
phosphoinositol metabolite
phosphokinase
   creatine p. (CPK)
phospholipid hydroperoxide

phosphoribosyltransferase
phosphorus
    p. nuclear magnetic resonance
      spectroscopy (P-MRS)
    red p.
    serum p.
phosphorus-31
phosphorylase deficiency
phosphorylation
    oxidative p.
    posttranslation p.
    protein tyrosine p.
photalgia
photalgiophobia
photangiophobia
photaugiaphobia, photaugiophobia
photesthesia
photic
    p. driving
    p. epilepsy
    p. stimulation
    p. stimulation activating technique
photism
Photo Articulation Test (PAT)
photoaxis
photochemically-induced graded spinal
  cord infarction
photocoagulation
    in situ p.
photodynamic therapy (PDT)
photodynia
photodysphoria
photoesthetic
photofrin porfimer sodium
photogenic
    p. epilepsy
    p. seizure
photographic memory
photokinetic
photolabile
photoma
photomania
photometrazol test
photomicrograph
photomyoclonic jerk
photomyoclonus
    hereditary p.
photon
    p. beam radiosurgery
    p. ray
photonic radiosurgical system
photopathy
photophobia
photopic vision
photopilic
photopsia
photoptarmosis
photoradiation therapy
photoreceptor
    p. cell
    ocular p.
photosensitive epilepsy
photosensitivity
photosensitizer
phototherapy

photothrombosis
    arterial p.
photothrombotic infarction
phototransduction
    humoral p.
phrase construction (PC)
phren
phrenalgia
phrenectomy
phrenemphraxis
phrenetic
phrenic
    p. ganglia
    p. mononeuropathy
    p. motor nucleus
    p. nerve conduction time
    p. neuropathy
phrenicectomy
phreniclasia
phrenicoexeresis
phreniconeurectomy
phrenicotomy
phrenicotripsy
Phrenilin Forte
phrenitica
    aphrodisia p.
phrenitis
phrenocardia
phrenoglottic
phrenology
phrenoplegia
phrenoplegy
phrenopraxic
phrenospasm
phrenotropic
phrictopathia
phronemomania
phronemophobia
phronesis
PHSQ
    Psychosocial History Screening
      Questionnaire
PHST
    Psychosocial History Screening Test
PHT
    phenytoin
phthinoid
phthiriomania
phthiriophobia
phthisica
phthisicus
    habitus p.
phthisiomania
phthisiophobia
phthisis bulbi
Phycomycetes
phyloanalysis
phylobiology
phylogenesis
phylogenetic
    p. mneme
    p. principle
    p. symptoms
phylogenetically
phylogeny

P

Phynox cobalt alloy clip material
physaliformis
    ecchordosis p.
physaliphorous cell
physiatrics
physiatry
physical
    p. abuse
    p. abuse of adult
    p. abuse of child
    p. aggression
    p. agitation
    p. anergia
    p. anthropology
    p. appearance
    P. and Architectural Features
      Checklist
    p. bondage
    p. capacity
    p. change
    p. concomitant of anxiety
    p. condition
    p. condition organic psychosis
    p. defect
    p. dependence
    p. disorder
    p. environment
    p. examination (PE)
    p. experience
    p. fight
    p. fitness
    p. harm
    history and p. (H&P)
    p. impairment
    p. independence
    p. intersex condition
    p. manifestation of pain
    p. medicine
    P. Self-Maintenance Scale
    p. sensation
    p. sign
    p. signs and symptoms
    p. strain
    p. stress
    p. support
    p. symptom
    p. symptoms adjustment reaction
    p. tension
    p. therapist
    P. Tolerance Profile (PTP)
    p. trauma
physically endangered
physician
    attending p.
    family p.
    house p.
    primary p.
    primary care p.
    resident p.
    P.'s for Social Responsibility
      (PSR)
physician-assisted suicide
physician-patient relationship

Physicians'
    P. Desk Reference (PDR)
    P. Questionnaire
physician's
    p. assistant (PA)
    p. assistant, certified (PA-C)
physicochemical
    p. interaction
    p. principle
physiodrama
physiogenesis
physiogenetic depression
physiogenic
physiognomic
    P. Cue Test (PCT)
    p. perception
    p. thinking
physiognomy
physiognosis
physiologica
    alalia p.
physiological, physiologic
    p. age
    p. amenorrhea
    p. antagonism
    p. artifact
    p. basis
    p. basis of personality
    p. dependence
    p. drive
    p. effect
    p. factor
    p. feedback
    p. functional variation
    p. hyaluronidase inhibitor (PHI)
    p. intoxication
    p. limit
    p. maintenance
    p. manifestation
    p. mechanism
    p. memory
    p. motive
    p. need
    p. norm
    p. paradigm
    p. process
    psychogenic p.
    p. psychology
    p. psychology
    p. reactivity
    p. response
    p. response specificity
    p. self-regulation
    p. sleepiness
    p. sleepiness index
    p. tremor
physiology
    ejaculation p.
    respiratory p.
    sexual p.
physiomedical
physioneurosis
physiopathologic
physiopathology
physioplastic stage

physiopsychic
physiotherapy
physique type
physocephaly
physostigmine
  parenteral p.
phytogenous
phytonadione
PI
  paradoxical intention
  Personality Index
  Personality Inventory
  present illness
  proactive inhibition
  pulsatility index
pi
  p. procedure
  p. rhythm
pia
  p. mater
  p. mater encephali
pia-arachnitis
pia-arachnoid
Piaget cognitive development stage
piagetian
pial
  p. artery
  p. cortical vessel
  p. funnel
pial-glial membrane
pia mater spinalis
pianist's cramp
piano player's cramp
PIAPACS
  psychological information, acquisition,
    processing, and control system
PIAT
  Peabody Individual Achievement Test
piblokto, pibloktog, pibloktoq
  p. syndrome
PIC
  Personality Inventory for Children
PICA
  Porch Index of Communicative Ability
  posterior inferior cerebellar artery
  posterior inferior communicating artery
  posteroinferior cerebellar artery
    PICA aneurysm
    PICA index
pica
  p. disorder
  paper p.
PICAC
  Porch Index of Communicative Ability in
    Children
Picchu
Pices electrode
Picha-Seron Career Analysis
Pick
  P. atrophy
  P. body
  P. bundle
  P. disease

  P. disease dementia
  P. syndrome
Pickford Projectives Picture (PPP)
picking
  orifice p.
  skin p.
pickwickian syndrome
picornavirus
picrotoxin
PICS
  Parent Interview for Child Syndrome
  Patterns of Individual Change Scale
PICSI
  Picture Identification for Children-
    Standardized Index
PICSYMS
  picture symbols
pictogram
pictograph
pictophilia
pictorial
  p. aphasia
  p. imagery
  P. Test of Intelligence (PTI)
picture
  Allen p.
  P. Anomalies Test
  p. arrangement
  p. arrangement subtest
  P. Articulation and Language
    Screening Test (PALST)
  p. assembly
  Blacky p.
  clinical p.
  p. completion (PC)
  p. completion subtest
  concrete p.
  p. frustration study (PFS)
  P. Identification for Children-
    Standardized Index (PICSI)
  P. Identification Test (PIT)
  P. Interest Exploration Survey
    (PIES)
  P. Interpretation Test
  p. inventory
  inward p.
  Pickford Projectives P. (PPP)
  p. in picture technique
  P. Reasoning Test (PRE, PRT)
  P. Story Language Test (PSLT)
  p. symbols (PICSYMS)
  P. World Test
PICU
  psychiatric intensive care unit
piedras
pieds terminaux
Pierre Robin syndrome
**Piers-Harris Children's Self-Concept
  Scale**
PIES
  Picture Interest Exploration Survey
piesesthesia
piezoelectric potential
piezo-resistive transducer

P

PIF
> premorbid inferiority feeling
> prolactin-inhibiting factor

Pigem question

pigment
> acute posterior multifocal
>   placoid p.
> p. epithelial lesion
> melanin p.

pigmentary retinopathy

pigmented
> p. layer of retina
> p. villonodular synovitis (PVNS)

pigmenti
> incontinentia p.

pigmentosa
> retinitis p.

pigmentosum
> xeroderma p.

PIL
> purpose in life
>   PIL Test

pili torti

pill
> birth control p. (BCP)
> morning-after p.
> p. rolling
> sleeping p.

pillar
> anterior p. of fornix
> p. cell of Corti
> Corti p.
> p.'s of fornix
> posterior p. of fornix

pillar-and-post microsurgical retractor

pillow
> Mediflow p.
> Nec-Hugger cervical support p.
> psychological p.

pill-rolling tremor

pilocarpine

pilocytic juvenile astrocytoma

piloerection

piloid
> p. astrocytoma
> p. gliosis

pilojection

pilomatrixoma

pilomotor
> p. fiber
> p. reflex
> p. response

pilonidal sinus

pilot study

Piltz
> P. reflex
> P. sign

pimethixene

pimozide

Pimsleur Language Aptitude Battery

PIN
> posterior interosseous nerve
>   PIN entrapment

pin
> p. fixation headrest

> p. headholder
> Kirschner p.
> Mayfield disposable skull p.
> Mayfield skull cap p.
> Steinmann p.
> Synthes guide p.
> p. test
> torlone fixation p.
> p. yen

pinazepam

pincer grip

pindolol

pineal
> p. body
> p. cell
> p. cell tumor
> p. cyst
> p. gland
> p. habenula
> p. meningioma
> p. parenchymal neoplasm
> p. recess
> p. region
> p. regional choriocarcinoma
> p. region teratoma
> p. substance
> p. therapy

pinealectomy

pinealoblastoma (*var. of* pineoblastoma)

pinealocyte

pinealocytoma

pinealoma
> ectopic p.
> extrapineal p.

pinealopathy

Pinel-Hasiam syndrome

Pinel-Haslam syndrome

Pinel system

pineoblastoma, pinealoblastoma

pineocytoma

ping-pong
> p.-p. appearance
> p.-p. fracture
> p.-p. gaze

piniform

pinion
> p. headholder
> Mayfield p.

pink
> p. disease
> p. noise
> p. spot

pinna

pinocytosis

pinocytotic vesicle

pinpoint pupils

pins-and-needles sensation

pins-sticking sensation

Pinter-Paterson Scale of Performance Test

pinus

pinwheel
> Safe-T-Wheel p.

PIP
> Psychotic Inpatient Profile**

pipamperone
piperacetazine
piperacillin
piperazine
    phenyl p.
piperidine derivative
piperidinediones
piperidyl derivative
pipe stemming of ankle-brachial index
PIPIDA
    technetium 99m P.
PIPIS
    Rhode Island Pupil Identification Scale
pipoglutamic aciduria
Piportil Depot
pipotiazine
pipradrol
PIQ
    Performance Intelligence Quotient
piracetam
piribedil
piriform
    p. area
    p. cortex
piriformis syndrome
pirisudanol
pirlindole
piroxicam
Pisa syndrome
Pisces electrode
pistol grip
pistol-grip instrument
piston
    MTS electrohydraulic p.
PIT
    Picture Identification Test
pit
    central p.
    primitive p.
    snake p.
Pitanguy
    P. oval skin resection
    P. plastic surgery
pitch
    absolute p.
    basal p.
    p. discrimination
pithecoid idiot
pithiatism
pithiatric
Pitocin
Pitowsky Illness Behavior Questionnaire
Pitres
    P. area
    P. law
    P. rule
    P. sign
Pitressin Tannate in Oil
pitting edema
Pittsburgh
    P. gamma knife group
    P. Sleep Quality Index
pituicytoma
pituitary
    p. abscess

p. adamantinoma
p. adenoma
p. apoplexy
p. autoimmunity
p. basophilia
p. cachexia
p. curette
p. dwarfism
p. dysfunction
p. eunuchism
p. forceps
p. gland
p. microadenoma
p. replacement therapy
p. spoon
p. stalk
p. stalk lesion
p. stalk section
p. tumor
pityrodes
    alopecia p.
piuturi
pivazepam
pixelated parietotemporal perfusion deficit
PK
    psychokinesis
    psychokinetic
PKC
    protein kinase C
PKRS
    Phelps Kindergarten Readiness Scale
PKSAP, PKSSAP
    Psychiatric Knowledge and Skills Self-Assessment Program
PKU
    phenylketonuria
PL
    psychosocial-labile
place
    closed p.
    crowded p.
    p. deixis
    p. identity
    4-p. laminectomy
    open p.
    oriented to time and p.
    safe p.
    p. theory
    unfamiliar p.
placebo
    active p.
    balanced p.
    p. effect
    p. medication trial
    p. reactor
placement
    bone graft p.
    clip p.
    p. counseling
    electrode p.
    endosaccular coil p.
    foster p.
    International 10–20 system of electrode p.

P

placement *(continued)*
    job p.
    Kirschner wire p.
    K-wire placement
    personnel p.
    plate p.
    posterolateral bone graft p.
    rod p.
    sacral screw p.
    sheltered workshop p.
    p. test
    variable screw p. (VSP)
placid disposition
Placidyl
placode
    neural p.
placoid pigment epitheliopathy
placophobia
plagiocephalic idiocy
plagiocephaly
    lambdoid p.
plain
    Citanest P.
    p. forceps
    p. radiography
    p. tomography
plain-folks technique
plan
    cottage p.
    game p.
    homicidal p.
    life p.
    multidisciplinary treatment p.
    (MTP)
    organizational p.
    Personal Communication P.
    realistic p.
    subjective, objective, assessment, p.
    (SOAP)
    suicidal p.
    treatment p. (TRPL)
plana
    pars p.
planar
    p. spin imaging
    P. Stereotaxic Atlas of the Human
    Brain
plane
    arachnoid p.
    coronal p.
    frontal p.
    median sagittal p.
    parietal p.
    sagittal p.
    sensitive p.
    subjective p.
    subplatysmal p.
    vertical p.
planigraphy
planned
    p. learning environment
    P. Parenthood
    p. pregnancy

planner
    High School Career-Course P.
    (HSCCP)
planning
    Autism Screening Instrument for
    Educational P.
    career p.
    P. Career Goals (PCG)
    p. disturbance
    image integrated surgery
    treatment p.
    inverse treatment p. (ITP)
    motor p.
    operational p.
    permanent p.
    poor motor p.
    preoperative p.
    social policy p.
    strategic p.
    treatment p.
    uninhibited motor p.
planomania
planophrasia
planotopokinesia
plantalgia
plantar
    p. muscle reflex
    p. nerve
    p. response
planum
    fetal p.
    p. polare
    p. sphenoidale
    p. temporale
    p. temporale asymmetry
    p. temporale morphology
plaque
    AMY p.
    argentophilic p.
    argyrophil p.
    argyrophilic p.
    atherosclerotic p.
    fibrous p.
    Hollenhorst p.
    neuritic p.
    p. reduction assay
    sclerotic p.
    senile p.
    p. shadow
plasma
    p. cell dyscrasia
    p. cortisol
    p. dopamine beta-hydroxylase
    (DBH)
    p. elastase
    p. factor
    p. fibrinolytic enzyme system
    p. homocysteine level
    p. thromboplastin
plasmacytoma
    primary intracranial p.
plasmapheresis
    p. and intravenous immunoglobulin
Plasmatein
plasmatofibrous astrocyte

plasmid
    circular p.
    drug resistance p.
    R p.
plasmin
plasmin-antiplasmin complex
plasminogen activator (PA)
Plasmodium falciparum
plastic
    p. arts therapy
    p. collar
    p. scalp clip
    p. surgery
    p. tonus
plasticity
    decerebrate p.
    functional p.
    hippocampal synaptic p.
    p. of libido
    neural p.
    neuronal p.
    synaptic p.
Plastizote cervical collar
plasty
    aqueductal p.
plate
    alar p.
    alar p. of neural tube
    American Optical Hardy-Rand-
      Rittler color p.
    AO dynamic compression p.
    AO reconstruction p.
    ASIF broad dynamic compression
      bone p.
    ASIF T p.
    basal p. of neural tube
    bone p.
    broad AO dynamic compression p.
    butterfly-shaped monobloc
      vertebral p.
    cartilage p.
    cartilaginous end p.
    Caspar anterior cervical p.
    Caspar trapezoidal p.
    cervical p.
    commissural p.
    contoured anterior spinal p.
    cortical p.
    cranial bone fixation p.
    craniocervical p.
    cranioplasty p.
    cribriform p.
    dorsal p. of neural tube
    3D titanium mini bone p.
    end p.
    E-Z Flap cranial bone p.
    p. fixation
    Hardy-Rand-Rittler p.
    Harm posterior cervical p.
    Howmedica Microfixation cranial p.
    Ishihara p.
    Leibinger 3-D p.
    Leibinger Micro Plus p.
    Leibinger Micro System cranial
      fixation p.
    Lorenz cranial p.
    Lorenz titanium screws and p.
    Luhr micro p.
    Luhr Microfixation cranial p.
    Luhr mini p.
    Luhr pan p.
    medullary p.
    metal p.
    Mini Orbita p.
    Morscher anterior cervical p.
    Morscher titanium cervical p.
    motor end p.
    narrow AO dynamic
      compression p.
    neural p.
    orbital p.
    ORION anterior cervical p.
    Orozco cervical p.
    Perf-Plate cranial p.
    p. placement
    prochordal p.
    Profil-O-Plastic p.
    quadrigeminal p.
    roof p.
    round hole p.
    Roy-Camille p.
    skull p.
    sole p.
    spinous process p.
    stainless steel preformed skull p.
    Steffee p.
    Storz Microsystems cranial
      fixation p.
    symmetrical sacral p.
    symmetrical thoracic vertebral p.
    Synthes cervical p.
    Synthes Microsystem cranial
      fixation p.
    T-p.
    tantalum preformed skull p.
    terminal p.
    thoracolumbosacral p.
    titanium p.
    TSRH p.
    ventral p. of neural tube
    vertebral p.
    Vitallium p.
    wing p.
plateau
    p. in improvement
    p. masking technique
    p. method
    p. phase
    p. speech
platelet
    p. activating factor
    p. count
    p. disorder
    p. glycoprotein Ia/IIa deficiency
    p. monoamine oxidase
    p. thromboxane release
platelet-derived growth factor
platelet-fibrin embolus
platelet-shaped knife

P

plate-screw
p.-s. fixation
p.-s. osteosynthesis
plate-spacer washer
platform
orgasmic p.
positioning p.
plating
anterior spinal p.
Caspar p.
pedicle screw p.
posterior spinal p.
Steffee p.
Platinol
platinum
p. coil
p. microcoil
platinum-Dacron microcoil
platonic
p. friendship
p. love
p. nymphomania
p. relationship
platonism
platonization
platybasia
platysma muscle
Plavix
play
associative p.
dramatic p.
extended p.
fantasy p.
p. the field
free p.
p. the game
games people p.
group p.
p. group psychotherapy
p. group therapy (PGT)
imaginative p.
independent p.
joint p.
make-believe p.
p. on words
organized p.
parallel p.
peer p.
repetitive p.
rough-and-tumble p.
p. session
shadow p.
symbolic p.
p. technique
verbal p.
p. with oneself
playing
activity p.
p. dead
game p.
multiple role p.
role p.
PLC
personal locus of control

plea of insanity
Pleasant Events Schedule (PES)
pleasurable stimuli
pleasure
activity p.
aesthetic p.
p. center
p. ego
p. experience
p. fear
function p.
loss of p.
muscle p.
organ p.
organic p.
p. principle
sensual p.
sexual p.
pleasure-pain principle
PLED
periodic lateralizing epileptiform discharge
synchronous bilateral PLED
pledget
cotton p.
cottonoid p.
Gelfoam p.
latex covered p.
Plegine
pleiotrophin
plenary indulgence
pleniloquence
pleocytosis
cerebrospinal fluid p.
p. of cerebrospinal fluid
mononuclear p.
pleomorphic xanthoastrocytoma (PXA)
pleonasm
pleonexia
Pletal
plethysmograph
penile p.
vaginal p.
plethysmography
air p.
penile p.
pleura
pleurothotonos, pleurothotonus
pleusirs
folie à p.
plexectomy
plexiform
p. layer of cerebral cortex
p. layers of retina
p. neurofibroma
p. neuroma
plexiglas phantom
plexitis
plexopathy
plexus, pl. plexus, plexuses
anterior p.
Auerbach p.
p. autonomici
Batson p.
brachial p.

carotid p.
cavernous p.
celiac p.
p. celiacus
choroid p.
p. of choroid artery
p. choroideus
p. choroideus ventriculi lateralis
p. choroideus ventriculi quarti
p. choroideus ventriculi tertii
choroid p. of fourth ventricle
choroid p. of lateral ventricle
choroid p. of third ventricle
epidural venous p.
Erb-Duchenne-Klumpke injury to brachial p.
Exner p.
lumbar p.
lumbosacral p.
Meissner p.
meningeal p.
p. meningeus
myenteric p.
p. myentericus
nerve p.
p. nervorum spinalium
p. nervosus
paravertebral venous p.
pelvic p.
posterior p.
pterygoid p.
sagittal p.
sciatic p.
spinal nerve p.
p. of spinal nerves
subdermal p.
p. submucosus
sympathetic plexuses
tentorial p.
p. uterovaginalis
venous p.
plica, gen. and pl. **plicae**
p. choroidea
plicamycin
plicata
pars p.
pliers
Howmedica Microfixation System p.
Leibinger Micro System p.
Luhr Microfixation System p.
PLIF
posterior lumbar interbody fusion
PLISSIT
permission, limited information, specific suggestion, and intensive therapy
PLISSIT Model
PLP
proteolipid protein
PLS
Preschool Language Scale
PLSA
posterolateral spinal artery
plucking at clothes

plug
methylmethacrylate cranioplastic p.
soaked fat p.
soaked muscle p.
plugging
Obex p.
plumbism
pluralism marriage
pluralistic utilitarianism
plus
DHC P.
Esgic P.
Extra Strength Bayer P.
Lorcet P.
Siemens Somatom P.
plutocracy
plutomania
PM
polymyositis
Excedrin PM
Midol PM
PMAT
Primary Mental Abilities Test
PM/DM
polymyositis/dermatomyositis
PMH
pure motor hemiparesis
PMI
petition of mental illness
PMJ
progressive multifocal leuko-J encephalopathy
PML
progressive multifocal leukoencephalopathy
P-MRS
phosphorus nuclear magnetic resonance spectroscopy
PMS
premenstrual syndrome
Midol PMS
PMT
Porteus Maze Test
PMTS
premenstrual tension syndrome
PN
pontine nuclei
psychiatry-neurology
psychoneurologist
psychoneurology
psychoneurotic
P&N
psychiatry and neurology
PNAVQ
positive-negative ambivalent quotient
PNET
primary neuroectodermal tumor
primitive neuroectodermal tumor
pneumatic
p. chair lift
p. microscope
pneumatocele
extracranial p.
intracranial p.
pneumatophobia

P

pneumatorhachis
pneumatosis
    epidural p.
pneumobulbar
pneumocele
    extracranial p.
    intracranial p.
pneumocephalus
    epidural p.
    tension p.
pneumococcal meningitis
pneumocranium
Pneumocystis carinii
pneumoencephalogram
pneumoencephalography
pneumogastric nerve
pneumogram
pneumograph
pneumoniae
    Streptococcus p.
pneumoorbitography
pneumophonia
pneumoplethysmography
    ocular p.
pneumorhachis
pneumotachogram
pneumotachograph
pneumotaxic
    p. center of Lumsden
    p. localization
pneumotonometry
pneumoventricle
PNF
    proprioceptive neuromuscular facilitation
    PNF exercise
PNI
    psychoneuroimmunology
pnigerophobia
pnigophobia
PNM
    peripheral nerve myelin
PNMP
    phenylethanolamine-N-methyltransferase
PNMT
    phenylethanolamine-N-methyltransferase
PNP
    psychogenic nocturnal polydipsia
PNS
    parasympathetic nervous system
    peripheral nervous system
PNSH
    perimesencephalic nonaneurysmal
    subarachnoid hemorrhage
Po
    position response
POBE
    Profile of Out-of-Body Experiences
podismus
podospasm, podospasmus
PODQ
    Perceptual Organization Deviation
    Quotient

POEMS
    polyneuropathy, organomegaly,
    endocrinopathy, myeloma, and skin
    change
    POEMS syndrome
Poggendorf illusion
pogonophobia
POI
    Personal Orientation Inventory
poiesis
poikilothermia
poikilothymia
poinephobia
point
    anchoring p.
    anterior commissure-posterior
      commissure reference p.
    apophysary p.
    apophysial p.
    change p.
    choice p.
    critical p.
    Crutchfield drill p.
    end p.
    entry p.
    Erb p.
    p. fear
    fixation p.
    flicker-fusion p.
    3-p. headrest
    p. imaging
    indifference p.
    Keen p.
    Kocher p.
    p. localization
    p. localization test
    motor p.
    multiple sensitive p.
    p. mutation
    p. of no return
    painful p.
    pedicle entrance p.
    powered automatic stopping drill p.
    pressure p.
    p. prevalence
    racial saturation p.
    p. of regard
    p. resolved spectroscopy (PRESS)
    sacral brim target p.
    p. scale
    p. scanning
    self-stopping drill p.
    sensitive p.
    p. of subjective equality (PSE)
    sylvian p.
    tender p.
    trigger p.
    Trousseau p.
    Valleix p.
    p. of view
pointed awl
pointes
    torsades de p.
point-for-point correspondence

pointing
    bone p.
    p. of the bone
    finger p.
Poiseuille
    P. equation
    P. law
poison hemlock
poisoning
    acetaminophen p.
    acute amphetamine p.
    acute lead p.
    alcohol p.
    amphetamine p.
    antifreeze p.
    arsenic p.
    aspirin p.
    barbiturate p.
    blood p.
    bromide p.
    carbon dioxide p.
    carbon monoxide p.
    carbon tetrachloride p.
    cholinesterase inhibitory p.
    chronic lead p.
    curare p.
    cyanide p.
    deadly nightshade p.
    ethylene glycol p.
    food p.
    gas p.
    iron p.
    Jamaica ginger p.
    lead p.
    mercury p.
    methanol p.
    methotrexate p.
    methyl alcohol p.
    muscarine p.
    narcotic p.
    nicotine p.
    nightshade p.
    opiate p.
    opioid p.
    opium p.
    organophosphate pesticide p.
    organophosphorus insecticide p.
    paregoric p.
    pyrimethamine p.
    thallium p.
    valproic acid p.
Poisson distribution
poker spine
pokeweed mitogen
polacrilex
    nicotine p.
polar
    p. artery
    p. coordinate system
    p. opposite
    p. zone
polare
    planum p.
Polaris adjustable spinal cage implant

polarity
    p. response
    reverse p.
    sorting p.'s
polarization
    mass p.
    principle of dynamic p.
    sexual p.
Polar-Mate coagulator
polarographic
pole
    frontal p.
    occipital p.
    temporal p.
poli (*pl. of* polus)
police power
policy
    p. analysis
    P. and Program Information Form
polio
    French p.
polioclastic
poliodystrophia cerebri progressiva
  infantilis
poliodystrophy
    cerebral p.
    progressive cerebral p.
polioencephalitis
    p. infectiva
    inferior p.
    superior hemorrhagic p.
polioencephalomeningomyelitis
polioencephalomyelitis
polioencephalopathy
poliomyelencephalitis (*var. of*
  poliomyeloencephalitis)
poliomyelitis
    acute anterior p.
    acute bulbar p.
    chronic anterior p.
    neonatal p.
    p. treatment
poliomyelitis-induced respiratory failure
poliomyeloencephalitis,
  poliomyelencephalitis
poliomyelopathy
POLIP
    polyneuropathy, ophthalmoplegia,
    leukoencephalopathy, and intestinal
    pseudoobstruction
political
    p. genetics
    p. psychiatry
    p. value
politico-economic-conservatism (PEC)
    p.-e.-c. scale
politicomania
politicophobia
politikon
    zoon p.
Politte Sentence Completion Test
pollicomental reflex
pollodic
polluted environment
Pollyanna-like view

P

Pollyanna mechanism
Polocaine
poltergeist
polus, pl. poli
    p. frontalis cerebri
    p. occipitalis cerebri
    p. temporalis cerebri
polyamine biosynthesis inhibitor
polyandry
polyangiitis
polyanhydride biodegradable polymer
    wafer
polyanhydroglucuronic acid
polyarteritis
    p. nodosa (PAN)
    p. nodosa dementia
    p. nodosa peripheral neuropathy
polyaxial screw
Polybus love
polychondritis
    relapsing p.
Polycillin-N
polycinematosomnography
Polycitra-K
polyclonia
polyclot patty
Polycrates complex
polycratism
polycythemia vera
polydipsia
    hysterical p.
    psychogenic p.
    psychogenic nocturnal p. (PNP)
    psychosis-induced p.
polydrug
    p. abuse
    p. addiction
polydystrophic oligophrenia
polyene thread
polyesthesia
polyethic criteria set
polyethylene
    p. intravenous catheter
    p. sleeve
Polyfactorial Study of Personality
polyganglionic
polygenic
    p. inheritance
    p. trait
polyglot
    p. amnesia
    p. neophasia
polygraph
    Keeler p.
polygynous
polygyny
polygyria
polyhydroxyethylmethacrylate (PHEMA)
polyideic somnambulism
polyleptic
polylogia
polymatric
polymer
    cellulose acetate p.

HTR p.
Hydrolene p.
polymerase chain reaction (PCR)
polymethylmethacrylate
polymicrogyria
polyminimyoclonus
polymorphic delta activity (PDA)
polymorphism
    restriction fragment length p.
    (RFLP)
    sequence p.
polymorphous
    p. layer
    p. perverse disposition
    p. perverse sexuality
    p. perversion
polymyalgia
    p. arteritica
    p. rheumatica
polymyoclonus
polymyositis (PM)
polymyositis/dermatomyositis (PM/DM)
polymyxin
polyneural
polyneuralgia
polyneuritica
    psychosis p.
polyneuritic alcoholic psychosis
polyneuritiformis
    heredopathia atactica p.
polyneuritis
    acute idiopathic p.
    chronic familial p.
    erythredema p.
    infectious p.
polyneuronitis
polyneuropathy
    acute inflammatory p. (AIP)
    acute painful p.
    alcoholic p.
    buckthorn p.
    chronic inflammatory
    demyelinating p. (CIDPN)
    chronic relapsing p.
    critical illness p. (CIP)
    diabetic sensorimotor p.
    distal p.
    dying-back p.
    dysimmune p.
    familial amyloidotic p.
    gait disorder, autoantibody, late-age
    onset, p. (GALOP)
    generalized p.
    gestational p.
    idiopathic p.
    nutritional p.
    recurrent p.
    sarcoid p.
    sensorimotor axonal p.
    subacute p.
    symmetric p.
    symmetrical p.
    thallium p.
    uremic p.

polyneuropathy,
  p. ophthalmoplegia,
    leukoencephalopathy, and intestinal
    pseudoobstruction (POLIP)
  p. organomegaly, endocrinopathy,
    myeloma, and skin change
    (POEMS)
polyomavirus
polyopia
polyparesis
polypeptide
  p. hormone
  p. hormone gene
  neuronal p.
  vasoactive intestinal p. (VIP)
polyphagia
polyphallic
polypharmacy
polyphasic
  p. activity
  p. motor unit
  p. potential
  p. sleep rhythm
polyphobia
polyphrasia
polyphyria
polyplegia
polypnea
polypoid degeneration of true fold
polyposia
polyposis
  intestinal p.
polypropylene suture
polypsychism
polyradiculitis
polyradiculomyopathy
polyradiculoneuropathy
  acute inflammatory demyelinating p.
    (AIDP)
  chronic inflammatory p. (CIP)
  demyelinating p.
  inflammatory demyelinating p.
polyradiculopathy
  acute inflammatory demyelinating p.
    (AIDP)
  chronic inflammatory
    demyelinating p. (CIDP)
  diabetic p.
polyrhythmic activity
polysemous
polysemy
polysensory unit
polyserositis
polysomnogram (PSG, PSM)
polysomnograph (PSG)
polysomnographic
  p. abnormality
  p. study
polysomnography (PSG)
polyspike-and-wave discharge
Polysporin ointment
polysteraxic
polysubstance
  p. abuse

p. addiction
p. dependence
polysubstance-related disorder
polysurgical addiction
polysymptomatic syndrome
polysynaptic
polytetrafluoroethylene
  expanded p. (ePTFE)
polytheism
polythetic
polythiazide
  prazosin and p.
polytomography
polytoxicomanic
polytrophic defect
polytropic defect
polyuria
polyvalent
  antivenin (Crotalidae) p.
polyvinyl
  p. acetate emulsion
  p. alcohol (PVA)
  p. alcohol foam
  p. alcohol particle
polyvitamin therapy
POM
  prescription-only medicine
POMC
  proopiomelanocortin
Pompadour fantasy
Pompe disease
Pompili
POMS
  Profile of Mood States
pond fracture
Pondimin
ponopathy
ponophobia
PONS
  Profile of Nonverbal Sensitivity
pons, pl. pontes
  p. cerebelli
  lower p.
  upper p.
  p. varolii
Ponstel
pontile apoplexy
pontine
  p. angle
  p. angle tumor
  p. artery
  p. cistern
  p. flexure
  p. glioma
  p. gray matter
  p. hemorrhage
  p. hydatid cyst
  p. infarction
  p. lateral gaze center
  p. lesion
  p. nuclei (PN)
  p. paramedian reticular formation
    (PPRF)
  p. parareticular formation (PPRF)
  p. sign

P

pontine *(continued)*
    p. sleep
    p. syndrome
    p. tegmentum
    p. tractotomy
pontis
    basis p.
    brachium p.
Pontocaine With Dextrose Injection
pontocerebellar
    p. angle syndrome
    p. recess
pontomedullary
    p. epidermoid cyst
    p. groove
    p. junction
    p. separation
    p. sulcus
pontomesencephalic
    p. cavernous hemangioma
    p. junction
pooh-pooh theory
pool
    autonomic motor p.
    dirty p.
    gene p.
    P. phenomenon
pooling
Pool-Schlesinger sign
poor
    p. academic preparation
    p. form response
    p. impulse control
    p. insight
    p. judgment
    p. law
    p. motor planning
    p. mouth
    p. peer relationship
    p. quality drug
    p. sleep quality
poorlaw
poorly
    p. defined boundary
    p. groomed
    p. systematized delusion
poorness of fit
popliteal
    p. artery
    p. nerve
Poppen
    P. intervertebral disk laminectomy
      rongeur
    P. ventricular needle
Poppen-Blalock carotid clamp
Poppen-Gelpi laminectomy retractor
pop psychology
popular response
population
    adolescent p.
    p. cage
    clinic patient p.
    community p.
    culturally diverse p.

    p. density
    general p.
    general medical/surgical p.
    p. genetics
    outpatient patient p.
    partial hospital patient p.
    primary care patient p.
    p. research
    p. setting
    p. standard deviation
POR
    problem-oriented record
Porch
    P. Index of Communicative Ability
      (PICA)
    P. Index of Communicative Ability
      in Children (PICAC)
porcine
    p. cell transplantation
    p. dopaminergic cell
porencephalia *(var. of* porencephaly)
porencephalic, porencephalous
    p. cyst
porencephalitis
porencephalopathy
porencephalous *(var. of* porencephalic)
porencephaly, porencephalia
poriomania
poriomanic fugue
pornographic writing
pornographomania
pornography
    child p.
    p. dependence
    dependence on p.
    paraphiliac p.
pornolagnia
porosis, pl. **poroses**
    cerebral p.
porphobilinogen (PBG)
porphyria
    acute intermittent p.
    hepatic p.
    intermittent acute p. (IAP)
    p. peripheral neuropathy
    p. synthesizing enzyme
    variegate p.
porphyric neuropathy
porphyrin metabolism
porphyrinuria
porphyrismus
porphyrophobia
porropsia
PORT
    Perception-of-Relationships-Test
port
    lumbar p.
    p. wine nevus
porta, pl. **portae**
portal
    integrated sideport access p.
    p. systemic encephalopathy (PSE)
porte manteau procedure
Porteus Maze Test (PMT)
portmanteau word

Portnoy
P. DPV device
P. ventricular cannula
P. ventricular catheter
Portuguese-Azorean disease
port-wine stain
porus acusticus
pos
positive
Posey restraint
posiomania
POSIT
Problem-Oriented Screening Instrument
for Teenagers
position
p. agnosia
P. Analysis Questionnaire (PAQ)
angular p.
body p.
brow-down p.
coital p.
cortical thumb p.
depressive p.
fetal p.
information optimization p.
knee-chest p.
lounging p.
observer p.
ordinal p.
paranoid-schizoid p.
park bench p.
prone p.
p. response (Po)
p. of responsibility
reverse Trendelenburg p.
rigid body p.
schizoid p.
semi-Fowler p.
p. sense
sitting p.
subordinate p.
sustained p.
translational p.
Trendelenburg p.
tuck p.
positional
p. nystagmus
p. tremor
p. vertigo
positioning
patient p.
p. platform
proper neck p.
positive (pos)
p. ability
p. acceleration
p. adaptation
p. afterimage
p. attitude change
p. attribute
p. cathexis
p. communication skills
p. comparison
p. conditioned reflex
p. correlation

p. emotion
p. emotionality
p. end-expiratory pressure (PEEP)
p. eugenics
p. event
false p.
p. feedback
p. feeling
p. frontal release sign
guaiac p.
P. Humanitarian Subscale
p. incentive
p. induction
p. ion
p. mental attitude
P. Military Subscale
p. motivation
P. and Negative Stroke Scale
(PANSS)
P. and Negative Symptom Scale
P. and Negative Symptoms of
Schizophrenia Scale
P. and Negative Syndrome Scale
(PANSS)
p. occipital sharp transient
p. occipital sharp transients of
sleep (POSTS)
p. parenting
p. predictive power
p. recency
p. regard
p. reinforcement
p. reinforcement therapy
p. reinforcer
p. relationship
p. response
p. schizophrenic symptoms
p. sharp wave
p. speech content
p. spike pattern
p. symptoms psychosis
p. thought disorder
p. transfer
p. transference
true p.
p. valence
positively bathmotropic
**positive-negative ambivalent quotient
(PNAVQ)**
positivism
logical p.
positivity
p. of Input 1
p. of Input 2
positron
p. emission tomography (PET)
p. emission tomography with [18F]-
labeled fluorodeoxyglucose (PET-
FDG)
possessed by spirit
possessing agent
possession
demonic p.
drug p.
spirit p.

P

possession *(continued)*
    spiritual p.
    p. trance
    p. trance state
    p. trance symptom
possession/trance disorder
possessor-possession
possumus
    non p.
POST
    National Police Officer Selection Test
post
    Caspar retraction p.
    p. hoc testing
    iliac p.
    p. infectious disseminated
      encephalomyelitis
    Isola spinal implant system iliac p.
    Luque-Galveston p.
    perineal p.
postabortion syndrome
postactivation
    exhaustion p.
    p. exhaustion
    p. facilitation
postadrenalectomy syndrome
postambivalence
postambivalent
    p. phase
    p. stage
postanalytic supervision
postanoxic
    p. coma
    p. encephalopathy
    p. epilepsy
postapoplectic
postbasic stare
post-binge anguish
postcentral
    p. area
    p. fissure
    p. gyrus
    p. sulcus
postcoital
    p. euphoria
    p. headache
postconcentration camp syndrome
postconcussion
    p. disorder
    p. headache
    p. neurosis
    p. syndrome
postconcussive amnesia
postcontusional brain syndrome
postcontusion syndrome encephalopathy
postconvulsive stupor
postdiphtheritic paralysis
postdisaster
    p. psychosocial intervention
    p. stress
postdivorce depression
postdormital
    p. chalastic fit

    p. depression
    p. sleep paralysis
postdormitum
post-ECT seizure
postelectroconvulsive
    p. amnesia
    p. therapy
postembolization angiogram
postemotive schizophrenia
postencephalitic
    p. parkinsonism
    p. syndrome
postepileptic
    p. paralysis
    p. twilight state
posterior
    p. alexia
    p. arthrodesis
    p. atlantoaxial arthrodesis
    p. beaten copper appearance
    p. bone graft
    p. callosal vein
    p. canal line
    p. central convolution
    p. central gyrus
    p. cerebellar artery
    p. cerebral artery (PCA)
    p. cerebral commissure
    p. cerebral territory infarction
    p. cervical fixation
    p. cervical spinal instrumentation
    p. cervical spine surgery
    p. choroidal artery
    p. cingulate gyrus
    p. column cordotomy
    p. column lesion
    p. column osteosynthesis
    p. column of spinal cord
    p. communicating artery (PComA)
    p. communicating artery aneurysm
    p. communicating nerve
    p. compartment lesion
    p. construct
    p. cord syndrome
    p. craniocervical junction
    p. decompression
    p. distraction instrumentation
    p. dominant activity
    p. ecchymosis
    p. fixation system biomechanics
    forceps p.
    p. fossa
    p. fossa aneurysm
    p. fossa-atrial shunt
    p. fossa craniotomy
    p. fossa dural arteriovenous fistula
    p. fossa hematoma
    p. fossa lesion
    p. fossa meningioma
    p. fossa syndrome
    p. funiculus
    p. hook-rod spinal instrumentation
    p. horn
    p. hypothalamic nucleus
    p. inferior cerebellar artery (PICA)

p. inferior cerebellar artery syndrome
p. inferior communicating artery (PICA)
p. inferior communicating artery aneurysm
p. intermediate groove
p. interosseous nerve (PIN)
p. interspinous wiring
p. joint syndrome
p. language area lesion
p. language zone
p. limb of internal capsule
p. lobe of hypophysis
p. longitudinal bundle
p. longitudinal ligament
p. lower cervical spine stabilization
p. lower cervical spine surgery
p. lumbar interbody fusion (PLIF)
p. lumbar interbody fusion surgery
p. lumbar spine and sacrum surgery
p. lunate lobule
p. medial nucleus of thalamus
p. median fissure of the medulla oblongata
p. median fissure of spinal cord
p. median sulcus of medulla oblongata
p. median sulcus of spinal cord
p. medullary velum
p. notch of cerebellum
p. occipitocervical approach
p. parietal cortex
p. parolfactory sulcus
p. perforated substance
p. periventricular nucleus
p. pillar of fornix
p. pituitary fossa
p. pituitary gland ectopia
p. plexus
posterioris apex cornus p.
p. primary ramus
p. pyramid of the medulla
rachischisis p.
p. rachischisis
p. rhizotomy
p. rod system
p. root
p. root ganglion
p. segmental fixation
p. semicircular canal
p. spinal artery
p. spinal fusion
p. spinal plating
p. spinal sclerosis
p. spinocerebellar tract
p. surgical exposure of sacrum and coccyx
p. tibial nerve
p. tibial nerve-evoked potential
p. upper cervical spine surgery
p. vein of septum pellucidum
ventralis oralis p. (VOP)
p. vomer

posterior-interbody lumbar spinal fusion
posterioris apex cornus posterior
posterior-lateral lumbar spinal fusion
posterodorsal temporal lobe
posteroinferior cerebellar artery (PICA)
posterolateral
p. approach
p. bone graft
p. bone grafting
p. bone graft placement
p. costotransversectomy incision
p. costotransversectomy technique
p. fissure
p. groove
p. lumbosacral fusion
p. spinal artery (PLSA)
p. sulcus
posterolateralis
nucleus ventralis p.
posteromedialis
nucleus ventralis p.
ventralis p. (VPM)
posteroparietal
posteroperative confusion
posterotemporal artery occlusion
posteroventral
p. pallidotomy (PVP)
p. sensorimotor pallidum
postexertional malaise
postfebrile dementia
postganglionic
p. motor neuron
p. oculosympathetic palsy
posthallucinogen
p. perception
p. perception disorder
posthemiplegic
p. athetosis
p. chorea
posthemorrhagic hydrocephalus
postherpetic neuralgia
posthion
posthippocampal fissure
posthypnotic
p. amnesia
p. psychosis
p. suggestion
posthypophysectomy traction syndrome
posthysterectomy depression
postictal
p. confusion
p. depression
p. depression phase of seizure
p. migrainous headache
p. paresis
p. psychosis
p. state
posticus
p. palsy
p. paralysis
tetanus p.
postinfectious
p. depression
p. hydrocephalus

P

postinfectious *(continued)*
    p. leukoencephalitis
    p. psychosis
postirradiation OVM
postketamine
postlaminectomy
    p. kyphosis
    p. syndrome
    p. two-level spondylolisthesis
postleukotomy syndrome
postlingual fissure
postlobotomy syndrome
post-LP headache
post-lumbar puncture headache
postlunate fissure
postmature
postmeningitic hydrocephalus
postmenopausal seizure
postmortem
postnatal
    p. depression
    p. development
postneuritic atrophy
postoperative
    p. anemia
    p. angiogram
    p. bracing
    p. care
    p. casting
    p. confusion
    p. confusional state
    p. corticosteroid
    p. extubation
    p. immobilization
    p. infection
    p. lumbosacral orthosis
    p. paraplegia
    p. pressure alopecia
    p. psychosis
    p. regimen
    p. skull defect
    p. status
    p. tetany
postparainfectious encephalomyelitis
postparalytic
postpartum
    p. alopecia
    p. blues
    p. major depression
    p. mania
    p. necrosis
    p. pituitary necrosis syndrome
    p. psychosis
postpolio
    p. sequela
    p. syndrome (PPS)
postpoliomyelitis syndrome (PPS)
postprandial (PP)
postpsychotic
    p. depression
    p. depressive disorder
    p. depressive disorder of
      schizophrenia
postpubertal

postpubescent
postpyramidal fissure
postradiation fibrosis
postreceptor
    heterotrimeric p.
    p. information transduction
postrema
    area p.
    p. area posttraumatic
postrhinal fissure
postrolandic
postrotational nystagmus
POSTS
    positive occipital sharp transients of sleep
      POSTS on electroencephalogram
postsaccadic neuronal response
postspike facilitation
poststreptococcal glomerulonephritis
poststress ankle/arm Doppler index
poststroke depression
postsynaptic
    p. cortical neuronal potential
    p. fold
    p. membrane
    p. potential (PSP)
    p. receptor
posttermination
    boundaries p.
    p. boundary
posttetanic potentiation
posttorture syndrome
posttranscriptional
posttranslational modification
posttranslation phosphorylation
posttraumatic
    p. amnesia (PTA)
    p. apoplexy
    p. apoplexy of Bollinger
    p. chronic disability
    p. cortical dysfunction
    p. delirium
    p. dementia
    p. deterioration
    p. disorientation
    p. disturbance
    p. encephalopathy
    p. epilepsy
    p. epileptiform activity
    p. hallucination
    p. headache
    p. hydrocephalus
    p. intradiploic pseudomeningocele
    p. kyphosis
    p. leptomeningeal cyst
    p. neuralgia
    p. neuroma
    p. neurosis
    p. organic psychosis
    p. osteoporosis
    p. pain
    p. patient
    p. personality
    postrema area p.
    p. psychopathic
    p. psychopathic constitution

p. seizure
p. spinal deformity
p. stress disorder (PTSD)
p. stress disorder complex
p. stress disorder by proxy
P. Stress Disorder Scale
P. Stress Disorder Symptom Scale
p. stress syndrome

postural
p. awareness
p. hypotension
p. instability
p. myoneuralgia
p. orthostatic tachycardia syndrome
p. reflex
p. seizure
p. set
p. syncope
p. tremor
p. vertigo

posture
bent p.
bizarre p.
body p.
curled-into-fetal-position p.
decerebrate p.
fetal position p.
inappropriate p.
open p.
rigid p.
sagging p.
p. sense
sleep p.
unusual sleep p.

posturing
catatonic p.
cerebrate p.
decerebrate p.
decorticate p.
dystonic p.

postvaccinal encephalitis
postvaccinial leukoencephalitis
post-Vietnam psychiatric syndrome (PVNPS)
potamophobia
Potasalan
potassium
p. acetate
p. acetate, potassium bicarbonate, and potassium citrate
p. bicarbonate
p. bicarbonate and potassium chloride, effervescent
p. bicarbonate, potassium chloride, and potassium citrate
p. bicarbonate and potassium citrate, effervescent
p. bromide
p. channel gene
p. chloride
p. chloride elixir
p. chloride and potassium gluconate
p. citrate and citric acid
p. citrate and potassium gluconate

p. gluconate
p. phosphate
p. phosphate and sodium phosphate
p. salicylate
serum p.
p. sparing diuretic

potatorum
tremor p.

potato tumor of neck
potence
potency
orgastic p.
sexual p.

Potensan
potent
potential
acoustic evoked p.
acting out p.
action p.
P. for Addiction Index
p. adverse effect
Assessment of Suicide P.
auditory compound actional p.
auditory evoked p. (AEP)
bioelectric p.
biotic p.
biphasic action p.
brain p.
brain evoked p. (BEP)
brainstem auditory evoked p. (BAEP)
brainstem evoked p.
cerebral p.
cochlear microphonic p.
compound motor action p.
compound muscle action p. (CMAP)
compound nerve action p. (CNAP)
cortical evoked p.
cortical somatosensory evoked p. (CSSEP)
p. cumulative trauma disorder
demarcation p.
dermatosensory evoked p.
direct auditory compound actional p.
early latency p.
EEG p.
effective-reaction p.
electrical p.
electromyographic p.
endplate p. (EPP)
p. energy
equal p.
estimated learning p. (ELP)
event-related p. (ERP)
evoked p. (EP)
excitatory postsynaptic p. (EPSP)
p. external award
p. external reward
extreme somatosensory evoked p. (ESEP)
far-field evoked p.
fasciculation p.
fibrillation p.

P

potential *(continued)*
    giant motor unit action p.
    glossokinetic p.
    graded p.
    high tolerance p.
    human p.
    p. impact
    inhibitory postsynaptic p. (IPSP)
    injury p.
    p. intellectual capacity
    latency-evoked p.
    leadership p.
    local p.
    localized evoked p.
    low tolerance p.
    median mixed nerve action p.
    membrane p.
    monophasic action p.
    motor evoked p. (MEP)
    motor unit p. (MUP)
    motor unit action p. (MUAP)
    multimodality evoked p. (MEP)
    myogenic motor evoked p.
    nascent motor unit p.
    nerve action p. (NAP)
    peroneal somatosensory evoked p.
    phase reversal p.
    piezoelectric p.
    polyphasic p.
    p. positive event
    posterior tibial nerve-evoked p.
    postsynaptic p. (PSP)
    postsynaptic cortical neuronal p.
    pudendal somatosensory evoked p.
    Relative Aspects of P. (RAP)
    resource holding p.
    resting p.
    scalp electrical p.
    sensory evoked p. (SEP)
    sensory nerve action p. (SNAP)
    small motor unit p.
    somatosensory evoked p. (SEP, SSEP)
    specific action p.
    spinal sensory evoked p.
    suicidal p.
    sural sensory p.
    System for Testing and Evaluation of P.
    p. target
    Test of Creative P.
    tolerance p.
    trigeminal evoked p. (TEP)
    visual evoked p. (VEP)
potentiation
    long-term p. (LTP)
    posttetanic p.
potentiometer
    angle position p.
potlatch
potomania
potophobia
Pott
    P. abscess

P. disease
P. paralysis
P. paraplegia
P. puffy tumor
potu
    delirium e p.
    mania á p.
potus
    fastidium p.
pouch
    Blake p.
    pharyngeal p.
    Rathke p.
    spinal extradural arachnoid p.
pounding
    p. heart
    p. pain
Pourfour du Petit syndrome
poverty
    clinical p.
    p. of content
    p. of content of speech
    p. of content of thought
    p. delusion
    delusion of p.
    p. of idea
    p. of movement
    psychomotor p.
povidone-iodine
    aqueous p.-i.
POW
    prisoner of war
    POW syndrome
Powassan
    P. encephalitis
    P. virus
powder
    antibiotic p.
    B-C p.
    Dover p.
    Goody's Headache P.'s
powdered opium
power
    p. amplifier
    distribution of p.
    p. drill
    endocratic p.
    inflated p.
    instantaneous p.
    negative predictive p.
    police p.
    positive predictive p.
    processing p.
    resolving p.
    p. router
    special p.
    p. spectral analysis (PSA)
    p. struggle
    p. struggle leadership pattern
    p. test
    p. theme
    war p.
    will to p.

powered
p. automatic skull perforator
p. automatic stopping drill point

pox

PP
postprandial

PPA
phenylpropranolamine
propanolamine

PPAR
peroxisomal proliferator receptor

PPC
Personal Problems Checklist
Personal Problems Checklist for
Adolescents

PPCP
Parent Perception of Child Profile

PPD, Ppd
packs per day

PPMS
Purdue Perceptual-Motor Survey

PPP
Pain Perception Profile
Pickford Projectives Picture

PPPMA
progressive postpolio muscle atrophy

PPRF
pontine paramedian reticular formation
pontine parareticular formation

PPRST
Printing Performance School Readiness
Test

PPS
Personal Preference Scale
postpoliomyelitis syndrome
postpolio syndrome

PPVT
Peabody Picture Vocabulary Test

PR
psychotherapy responder
OncoScint PR

practical
P. Math Assessment
p. reasoning
p. social judgment score

practice
p. effect
massed negative p.
negative p.
programmed p.
reinforced p.
P. Research Network

practicing period

practitioner
nurse p.

Prader-Willi syndrome

praecocissima
dementia p.

praecox
dementia p.
ejaculatio p.
heboid p.
neurasthenia p.
predementia p.

pubertas p.
senium p.

pragmatagnosia

pragmatamnesia

pragmatic
p. aphasia
p. level
P.'s Profile of Early
Communication Skills
P.'s Screening Test
p. structure
p. text

pragmatism

pralidoxime

prameha
sukra p.

pramipexole
p. dihydrochloride tablet

Pranayama

PRAS
Patient Rated Anxiety Scale

Pravachol

pravastatin sodium

praxiology

praxis
ideokinetic p.

prazepam

praziquantel

prazosin and polythiazide

PRE
Parkland Rapid Exam
partial-reinforcement effect
Picture Reasoning Test

preadaptive attitude

preadolescence

pre-AIDs

preambivalence

preambivalent phase

prearchaic thinking

preataxic

preattachment stage

preauricular tag

PREB
Pupil Record of Education Behavior

precausal thinking

precaution
radiation p.
suicide p.

preceding association

precentral
p. area
p. cerebellar vein
p. gyrus
p. seizure
p. sulcus

precession
fast imaging with steady p. (FISP)
Larmor p.
steady-state free p. (SSFP)

precessional frequency

precipitating
p. crisis
p. of epilepsy
p. event
p. factor

P

precipitating *(continued)*
  p. stress
  p. tremor
precipitous mood shift
precision
  coil p.
  law of p.
  p. therapy
preclinical medicine
Preclude
  P. dura substitute prosthesis
  P. spinal membrane
precocious
  p. aging
  p. puberty
precocity
  islet of p.
precollagenous filamentous material
precommissural
  p. bundle
  p. septal area
  p. septum
preconceptual stage
preconscious (pcs)
  p. thinking
precontoured unit rod
preconvulsive
precordial pain
precoronal bur hole
Precose
precuneal
precuneate
precuneus
precursor
  p. load strategy
  neural crest p.
  p. sign to rupture of aneurysm
Pred
  Liquid P.
predation
predator
  sexual p.
Predcor-TBA Injection
predelay reinforcement
predementia praecox
predicate thinking
prediction
  p. of dangerousness
  p. of mortality
  p. study
predictive
  P. Ability Test (PAT)
  P. Screening Test of Articulation
  p. validity
  p. value
predictor
  psychometric p.
  p. variable
predisposed
  p. panic attack
  situationally p.
predisposing factor

predisposition
  biologic p.
  genetic p.
prednisolone
Prednisol TBA Injection
prednisone
predominant
  p. affect
  p. current defense level
  p. mood disturbance
  p. symptom presentation
predominantly
  p. hyperactive-impulse attention
    deficit hyperactivity disorder
  p. inattentive-type attention deficit
    hyperactivity disorder
  p. predormital sleep paralysis
predormital sleep paralysis
predormitum
predorsal bundle
preemployment screening test
preepisode status
preexisiting underlying emotional issue
preexisting
  p. condition
  p. dementia
  p. illness
  p. mental disorder
  p. mental disorder symptom
  p. tremor
preference
  color p.
  conditioned place p. (CPP)
  eye p.
  food p.
  gaze p.
  hand p.
  paraphiliac p.
  risk p.
  sexual p.
preferred
  p. method
  p. representational system
prefixation
prefixed chiasm
prefrontal
  p. activation
  p. area
  p. cortex
  p. cortical activity dysregulation
  p. hyperactivity
  p. hypermetabolism
  p. hypofunction
  p. leukotomy
  p. lobotomy
  p. sonic treatment (PST)
pregabalin
preganglionic motor neuron
pregenital
  p. factor
  p. love
  p. organization
  p. phase
  p. stage

pregnancy
    accidental p.
    adolescent p.
    p. and birth complication (PBC)
    false p.
    hysterical p.
    p. loss
    planned p.
    psychosis in p.
    termination of p.
    unplanned p.
    untimely p.
    unwanted p.
    voluntary interruption of p. (VIP)
prehemiplegic chorea
prehensile
prehension
preictal headache
preindustrial
preinsular gyrus
prejudice
    ethnic p.
    radial p.
preketamine
Preliminary Diagnostic Questionnaire
prelingual deafness
preliterate
prelogical
    p. mind
    p. thinking
Prelone Oral
Prelu-2
Preludin
Premack principle
premaniacal
premarital
    P. Communication Inventory (PCI)
    p. counseling
    p. sex
premature
    p. alopecia
    p. birth
    p. closure
    p. death
    p. ejaculation
    p. ejaculation psychosexual
      dysfunction
    p. female orgasm
    p. male orgasm
    p. orgasm
prematurity
premedication
premeditation
premedullary arteriovenous fistular
premenopausal amenorrhea
premenstrual
    P. Assessment Form (PAF)
    p. dysphoric disorder
    p. syndrome (PMS)
    p. tension
    p. tension state
    p. tension syndrome (PMTS)
premium
    incitement p.
premonition of seizure

premonitory
    p. sigh
    p. sign
    p. symptom
premorality
premorbid
    p. ability
    p. adjustment
    p. asociality
    p. history
    p. inferiority feeling (PIF)
    p. intellectual function
    p. level of functioning
    p. personality
    P. Social Adjustment Scale
    p. state
premotor
    p. area
    p. cortex
    p. syndrome
prenatal
    p. development
    p. diagnosis
    p. history
    p. influence
    p. period
prenodular fissure
prenubile
preoccipital notch
preoccupation
    control p.
    death p.
    defect p.
    details p.
    homicidal p.
    hypochondriacal p.
    lists p.
    obsessive p.
    orderliness p.
    organization p.
    pathologic p.
    perfectionism p.
    rules p.
    schedules p.
    suicidal p.
    p. of thought
    unshakable p.
    p. with death
    p. with defect
    p. with detail
    p. with sameness
pre-oedipal, preoedipal
    p.-o. factor
    p.-o. level
    p.-o. phase
    p.-o. stage
preoperational
    p. phase
    p. thinking
    p. thought
    p. thought period
    p. thought stage
preoperative
    p. angiogram
    p. angiography

P

preoperative *(continued)*
- p. evaluation
- p. planning
- p. preparation
- p. sedation
- p. tomography

preoptic
- p. area
- p. region

preorgasmic
preparalytic
preparation
- academic p.
- facet joint p.
- intermediate-acting insulin p.
- long-acting insulin p.
- marijuana p.
- poor academic p.
- preoperative p.
- rod contour p.
- short-acting insulin p.
- split-brain p.
- wire contour p.

prepared and draped
preparedness
- anxiety p.
- principle of p.

prephallic
prepiriform gyrus
prepontine
- p. cistern
- p. region

prepotent
Pre-Professional Skills Test
preprohormone
prepsychotic
- p. pain
- p. personality
- p. psychosis
- p. schizophrenia

prepubertal
- p. borderline psychosis
- p. child
- p. children
- p. psychopathology

prepuberty
prepubescent
preputial sensation
prepyramidal tract
Pre-Reading Expectancy Screening Scale (PRESS)
pre-Rolandic artery occlusion
prerubral
- p. field
- p. nucleus

prerupture of aneurysm
presacral
- p. neurectomy
- p. sympathectomy

presaturation pulse
presbyacusis, presbycusis
presbyophrenia
presbyophrenic psychosis
preschizophrenic ego

preschool
- P. Behavior Questionnaire (PBQ)
- p. child
- P. Development Inventory
- P. and Kindergarten Interest Descriptor
- P. Language Scale (PLS)
- P. Language Screening Test
- P. Screening Test
- P. Speech and Language Screening Test

preschoolers
- Behavioral Scale for Developmentally Deviant P.
- Miller Assessment for P.

prescience
prescribed treatment
prescription (Rx)
- p. drug
- p. drug abuse
- p. drug-related disorder
- p. medication

prescription-only medicine (POM)
Prescriptive Reading Inventory (PRI)
preselection
- sex p.

presenile
- confusional state p.
- p. dementia
- p. dementia confusional state
- p. mental disorder
- p. organic psychotic state
- p. paraphrenia
- p. psychosis

presenilis
- alopecia p.
- anxietas p.
- dementia p.

presenium
present
- p. distress
- p. illness (PI)
- p. oriented
- P. State Examination (PSE)

presentation
- atypical p.
- catatonic p.
- clinical p.
- conversion disorder with mixed p.
- equivalent symptomatic p.
- heterogeneous clinical p.
- historical p.
- histrionic p.
- mixed p.
- pain p.
- predominant symptom p.
- psychotic p.
- substance-induced p.
- subthreshold p.
- symptom p.
- symptomatic p.

presentational ritual
presenting
- p. characteristic
- p. personality

p. psychopathology
p. symptom
preservation
p. of affect
carotid p.
lordosis p.
lumbar lordosis p.
p. technique
preservative-free normal saline
preserved conduction velocity
presidents test
presigmoid approach
PRESS
point resolved spectroscopy
Pre-Reading Expectancy Screening Scale
pressing thought
pressor
p. fiber
p. nerve
pressoreceptor
p. nerve
p. reflex
p. system
pressure
acoustic p.
ambient air p.
p. anesthesia
p. autoregulation
p. autoregulatory status
blood p.
carbon dioxide p. (PCO_2)
central venous p.
cerebral perfusion p. (CPP)
cerebrospinal p.
closure p.
colloid oncotic p. (COP)
continuous positive airway p.
 (CPAP)
cranial perfusion p. (CPP)
environmental p.
feeding mean arterial p. (FMAP)
p. gauge
group p.
p. of ideas
intracranial p. (ICP)
intracranial epidural p. (ICEDP)
intraocular p.
intraspinal epidural p. (ISEDP)
mean arterial blood p. (MABP)
minimal audible p.
p. necrosis
p. palsy
p. paralysis
partial p.
peer p.
p. point
positive end-expiratory p. (PEEP)
pulmonary capillary wedge p.
regional cerebral perfusion p.
 (rCPP)
p. sense
social p.
p. sore
systolic p. (SP)
tentorial p.

thought p.
time p.
pressured
p. behavior
p. speech
pressure-volume index
prestige suggestion
Preston ligamentum flavum forceps
prestriate area
presumed
p. causality
p. etiology
presumption
tender years p.
presuperego phase
presupposition
presynaptic
p. functional deficit
p. membrane
p. neuron
subsensitization of p.
pretectal
p. area
p. lesion
p. region
p. syndrome
pretectum
pretendica
pretendo
prethymectomy
pretraumatic
p. amnesia
p. personality
pretreatment
prevalence
cross-sectional p.
differential p.
lifetime p.
period p.
point p.
p. rate
suicide p.
treated p.
prevention
accident p.
anxiety p.
Dropout Prediction and P. (DPP)
exposure and response p.
infection p.
primary p.
relapse p.
response p.
rod rotation p.
secondary p.
stress p.
suicide p.
tertiary p.
P. and Treatment of Depression
 (PTD)
preventive
p. intervention
p. medicine
p. psychiatry
prevertebral ganglia

P

655

preview
> Personnel Security P. (PSP)

previous history
previously stabilizing social situations
Prevocational
> P. Assessment and Curriculum Guide (PACG)
> P. Assessment Screen (PAS)

PRF
> percutaneous radiofrequency rhizolysis
> Personality Research Form
> prolactin-releasing factor

PRI
> Partner Relationship Inventory
> Personal Relationship Inventory
> Prescriptive Reading Inventory

priapism
pride
> brute p.
> domesticated p.
> excessive p.
> moral p.
> penis p.
> phallic p.
> p. system

prilocaine
> lidocaine and p.

primacy
> complete genital p.
> early genital p.
> genital p.
> oral p.
> phallic p.

prima donna
primal
> p. anxiety
> p. fantasy
> p. father
> p. libido
> p. repression
> p. sadism
> p. scene
> p. scream
> p. therapy
> p. trauma

primary
> p. ability
> p. affective disorder (PAD)
> p. affective witzelsucht
> p. amebic meningoencephalitis (PAM)
> p. amenorrhea
> p. amentia
> p. aminoaciduria
> p. anesthesia
> p. angiitis of the central nervous system
> p. angiitis of the CNS
> p. antiphospholipid antibody syndrome
> p. antiphospholipid syndrome (PAPS)
> p. anxiety
> p. anxiety disorder
> p. auditory cortex

p. autism
p. autonomous function
p. axotomy
p. behavior
p. behavior disorder
p. brain lymphoma
p. brain vesicle
p. care
P. Care Evaluation of Mental Disorders (PRIME-MD)
p. caregiver
p. care patient population
p. care physician
p. care setting
p. caretaker
p. circular reaction
p. clip
p. CNS lymphoma
p. color
p. complaint
p. defense symptom
p. degenerative dementia (PDD)
p. degenerative dementia of Alzheimer type (PDDAT)
p. diagnosis
p. disorder of sleep
p. disorder of wakefulness
p. drive
p. dysthymia
p. encopresis
p. end-to-end anastomosis
p. epidural cyst
p. factor
p. feeblemindedness
p. fibromyalgia syndrome (PFS)
p. fissure of the cerebellum
p. gain
p. generalized epilepsy
p. hue
p. hydrocephalus
p. hypersomnia
P. Hypersomnia, Recurrent Type
p. ictal automatism
p. identification
p. identity
p. impotence
p. insomnia
p. integration
p. intracranial plasmacytoma
p. intramedullary lymphoma
p. lateral sclerosis
p. leptomeningeal lymphoma
p. mania
p. memory
P. Mental Abilities Test (PMAT)
P. Mental Ability
p. mental image
p. microorchidism
p. motivation
p. motor deficit
p. narcissism
p. need
p. neurasthenia
p. neuroectodermal tumor (PNET)
p. neuronal degeneration

p. nocturnal enuresis
p. object love
p. object-love
p. oppositional attitude
p. optic atrophy
p. orgasmic dysfunction
p. Parkinson disease
p. parkinsonism
p. personality trait
p. physician
p. prevention
p. process thinking
p. progressive amyotrophy
p. progressive cerebellar
  degeneration
p. psychic process
p. quality
p. reinforcement
p. reinforcer
p. relationship
p. repression
p. responsibility
p. retarded ejaculation
p. reward conditioning
p. rhinencephalic psychomotor
  epilepsy
p. schizophrenia
Screening Assessment for Gifted
  Elementary Students, P. (SAGES-
  P)
p. seizure
P. Self-Concept Inventory (PSCI)
p. senile dementia
p. sensation
p. sex character
p. sex characteristic
p. sexual deviation
p. shock
p. Sjögren syndrome (PSS)
p. stress
p. subarachnoid supratentorial
  hemorrhage
p. support group
p. task
P. Test of Cognitive Skills (PTCS)
The P. Language Screen (TPLS)
p. thrombocytopenia idiopathic
p. tic
p. transitional object
p. trunk syndrome
p. visual area
p. visual cortex
P. Visual Motor Test (PVMT)
p. vitreous
p. zone
Primatene
prime of life
PRIME-MD
  Primary Care Evaluation of Mental
  Disorders
primidone
priming memory
primiparas
primitiva
  meninx p.

primitivation
primitive
p. idealization
p. knot
p. lamina terminalis
p. maxillary vein
p. narcissism
p. neuroectodermal tumor (PNET)
p. node
p. otic artery
p. pit
p. psychosomatic language
p. reflex
p. streak
p. superego
p. trigeminal artery
p. trigeminal artery variant
primitivization
primordial
p. delusion
p. inferior hypophyseal artery
p. panic
primum non nocere
principal
p. diagnosis
p. focus
p. investigation
p. objective
p. symptom
principle
p. of anticipatory maturation
anticipatory-maturation p.
authority p.
binary p.
closure p.
communion p.
consistency p.
disuse p.
dynamic p.
p. of dynamic polarization
echo p.
economic p.
epigenetic p.
homeopathic p.
homeostatic p.
image formation p.
p. of inertia
intimacy p.
isopathic p.
least-effort p.
moral p.
morality of self-accepted moral p.
Nirvana p.
optimal-stimulation p.
organizing p.
pain p.
pain-pleasure p.
Pauli exclusion p.
Peter P.
phylogenetic p.
physicochemical p.
pleasure p.
pleasure-pain p.
Premack p.
p. of preparedness

principle *(continued)*
    psychophysiologic p.
    reality p.
    rebus p.
    repetition-compulsion p.
    talion p.
    transfer of p.
    treble safeguard p.
    utilitarian p.
    von Domarus p.
    weighted-harm p.
Pringle disease
**Printing Performance School Readiness
  Test (PPRST)**
Prinzide
Prinzmetal
    P. angina
    P. vasospastic angina pectoris
Priodax
prion disease
prior to admission (PTA)
a priori
priori
    a p.
prioritize
Priority Counseling Survey (PCS)
pris
    parti p.
prism
    Fresnel p.
    Fresnel paste-on p.
prison
    p. neurosis
    p. psychiatry
    p. psychosis
    p. sentence
prisoner
    p. of war (POW)
    p. of war syndrome
Pritikin diet
private
    p. psychiatric hospital
    p. psychosis
privilege
    bathroom p.'s
    lost p.'s (LP)
    testimonial p.
privileged communication
PRL
    prolactin
PRN
    as necessary
PRO
    peer review organization
proaccelerin
proactive inhibition (PI)
Proavil
probabilistic fashion
probability
    conditional p.
    p. curve
    p. learning
    transitional p.
probable error (PE)

proband
    autistic p.
    p. diagnosis
    Down syndrome p.
    p. method
Pro-Banthine
probarbital
probation
probe
    bipolar cautery p. (BICAP)
    Bunnell dissecting p.
    Bunnell forwarding p.
    Dandy p.
    Doppler p.
    EEF p.
    electromagnetic flow p.
    electromagnetic focusing field p.
    extended sector ultrasonic p.
    fluoroptic thermometry p.
    gearshift p.
    hemispherical contact p.
    intraoperative ultrasonic p.
    Jacobson p.
    Jannetta p.
    Laserflo Doppler p.
    LED p.
    monitoring p.
    neuro trend p.
    Nucleotome aspiration p.
    Nucleotome Flex II flexible
      cutting p.
    P3 p.
    pedicle sounding p.
    radiolabeled p.
    right-angle blunt p.
    SpineStat p.
    TCD p.
    Transonics flow p.
    ultrasonic p.
    Vasamedics laser Doppler flow p.
    virtual p.
probenecid
problem
    acculturation p.
    affect intensity p.
    aggregation p.
    alcohol p.
    arithmetic p.
    p. child
    p.'s of childhood
    clinical appraisal of
      psychosocial p.'s (CAPP)
    concurrent psychiatric p.
    developmental learning p. (DLP)
    Differential Test of Conduct and
      Emotional P.'s (DT/CEP)
    disciplinary p.
    p. drinker (PD)
    emotional p.
    environmental p.
    P. Experiences Checklist
    faith conversion p.
    familial aggregation p.
    feeding p.
    gait p.

identity p.
impulse-control p.
integrative p.
International Statistical Classification
 of Diseases and Related
 Health P.'s
language p.
learning p.
life circumstance p.
marital p.
mind-body p.
nuclear p.
occupational p.
orgasmic p.
other interpersonal p.
p. parent
parental control p.
parent-child relational p.
partner relational p.
p. patient
personality p.
phase of life p.
psychological p.
psychophysiological p.
psychosocial p.
questioning faith p.
real-life p.
p.'s related to abuse
p.'s related to abuse or neglect
relational p.
religious or spiritual p.
retrieval p.
school discipline p.
school entering p.
sibling relational p.
social p.
p. solving
P. Solving Inventory
stress-related psychophysiological p.
substance-related legal p.
p.'s with boundary
problem-based learning
problem-oriented
 p.-o. record (POR)
**Problem-Oriented Screening Instrument
 for Teenagers (POSIT)**
problem-solving
 p.-s. communication
 group p.-s.
 p.-s. negotiation
 p.-s. skill
 p.-s. strategy
 p.-s. style
procainamide
procaine
procarbazine hydrochloride
procedure
 ablative central neurosurgical p.
 age correction p.
 Albee shelf p.
 anterior stabilization p.
 attention-focusing p.
 augmented reality p.
 blocking p.

Buschke Free and Cued Selective
 Reminding P.
carotid ablative p.
carotid Amytal p. (CAP)
cervical spine stabilization p.
Cloward p.
Colonna shelf p.
Committee on Standards and
 Survey P.'s
debulking p.
decremental p.
Dewar posterior cervical fixation p.
diagnostic p.
DREZ p.
EDAS p.
EEG activating p.
extracranial-to-intracranial bypass p.
Functional Pragmatic P.
Gill p.
Hacker p.
Halstead-Reitan Neurological Battery
 and Allied P.'s
Heifetz p.
Hoffman and Mohr p.
instillation p.
Jaeger-Hamby p.
Jannetta microvascular
 decompression p.
Koerte p.
LDD p.
Learning Disability Rating P.
Linguistic Analysis and
 Remediation P.
lower cervical spine p.
micro-operative p.
microsurgical p.
Müller-König p.
Multiphasic Environmental
 Assessment P. (MEAP)
non-microsurgical p.
nucleotome p.
pi p.
porte manteau p.
psychological p.
recording p.
retrogasserian p.
Scaramella p.
single bur hole p.
Smith-Robinson p.
standard p.
test orientation p. (TOP)
time-out p.
two-stage p.
upper cervical spine p.
proceeding
 care and protection p.
 incompetency p.
 protection p.
process
 absent spinous p.
 action-group p.
 adaptive p.
 adjustment p.
 analytical p.
 anterior clinoid p.

P

process *(continued)*
apical p.
P. for the Assessment of Effective
Student Functioning
automatic psychological p.
axonal p.
biologic p.
bizarre thought p.
central p.
circumstantial thought p.
clinoid p.
closure p.
cognitive p.
collaborative treatment p.
complexity of mental p. (CMP)
complex learning p.
comprehensive identification p.
(CIP)
computational p.
concrete thought p.
conscious p.
counseling p.
cultural p.
decision-making p.
deficient spinous p.
Deiters p.
dementia p.
dementing p.
dendritic p.
P. Diagnostic (PD)
disease p.
due p.
egocentric thought p.
elementary p.
p. of elimination
emotive p.
empirical p.
ergotropic p.
escalative p.
evidence-based p.
excitatory-inhibitory p.
explicit p.
family p.
fantasy p.
feature contrasts p.
free access to p.
fundamental response p.
goal-oriented p.
group p.
harmony p.
higher mental p.
idiosyncratic p.
imaginal p.
information input p.
intact spinous p.
interpersonal p.
p. issue
judicial p.
Lenhossék p.
lexical p.
linear thought p.
mastoid p.
mental p.
motoric reproduction p.

neurodegenerative p.
neurodevelopmental telencephalic
ontogenic p.
neurotic p.
normative aging p.
odontoid p.
pathologic p.
pathophysiological p.
physiological p.
primary psychic p.
psychobiological p.
psychological p.
p. psychosis
psychosocial p.
psychotic p.
Children's Language P.'s
reactivation p.
revision p.
Ross Test of Higher
Cognitive P.'s
p. schizophrenia
schizophrenic p.
secondary psychic p.
separation-individuation p.
P. Skills Rating Scale (PSRS)
social p.
spinous p.
sublexical p.
switch p.
systematic p.
therapeutic p.
p. thinking
thought p.
transition p.
uncinate p.
unconscious p.
processed cocaine
processing
attentional p.
auditory p.
p. disorder
distributed p.
higher integrative language p.
information p.
language p.
lexical p.
parallel p.
phonological p.
p. power
semantic p.
signal p.
unconscious p.
visual motor p.
visuospatial p.
P. Word Class
processomania
processor
array p.
prochlorperazine maleate
prochordal plate
proctalgia fugax
proctoparalysis
proctophobia, rectophobia
proctoplegia
proctospasm

procursiva
 aura p.
procursive
 p. chorea
 p. epilepsy
procyclidine
prodigy
 child p.
 idiot-p.
prodromal
 p. episode
 p. period
 p. phase
 p. phase of schizophrenia
 p. schizophrenia
 p. symptom
prodromata
prodrome
 epileptic p.
 visual p.
product
 end p.
 gene p.
 NeuroCell-HD neural cell
  transplant p.
 NeuroCell-PD porcine neural cell
  transplant p.
 Valleylab neurosurgical p.
production
 divergent p.
 language comprehension and p.
 Work Skills Series P. (WSS)
productive
 p. love
 p. personality
 p. symptoms
 p. thinking
productivity of thought
product-moment correlation
prodynorphin
proencephalon
proenkephalin
professional
 P. and Administrative Career
  Examination (PACE)
 p. burnout
 p. code
 p. counselor
 p. criticism
 p. distance
 P. Employment Test (PET)
 p. ethics
 p. exploiter
 p. gambling
 p. negligence
 p. neurasthenia
 p. neurosis
 p. patient syndrome
 P. Sexual Role Inventory (PSRI)
 p. spasm
 Staff Burnout Scale for
  Health P.'s
 P. Standards Review Organization
  (PSRO)
professional-family relation

proficiency
 Bruininks-Oseretsky Test of
  Motor P.
 Trainer's Assessment of P. (TAP)
Proficiency Assessment Report (PAR)
profile
 adaptability p.
 P. of Adaptation to Life (PAL)
 AGS Early Screening P.
 Alcohol Assessment and
  Treatment P.
 anxiety p.
 Autistic Behavior Composite
  Checklist and P.
 Behavior Activity P. (BAP)
 Behavioral Deviancy P.
 Behavior Rating P., Second Edition
  (BRP-2)
 Brief Drinker P.
 Child and Adolescent
  Adjustment P.
 clinical p.
 Collis-Romberg Mathematical
  Problem Solving P.
 Comprehensive Drinker P.
 conversion V p.
 criminal p.
 demyelinative spinal fluid p.
 development p.
 Diagnostic Employability P.
 Diagnostic Mathematics P.
 Diversity Awareness P. (DAP)
 Employee Effectiveness P.
 employment p.
 eye-motor-verbal p.
 Five P's: Parent Professional
  Preschool Performance P.
 Follow-up Drinker P.
 Functional Communication P. (FCP)
 Functional Limitation P. (FLP)
 Hawaii Early Learning P.
 Hilson Adolescent P.
 Hypnotic Induction P. (HIP)
 inhibition p.
 Learning Accomplishment P.
 Learning Style P. (LSP)
 left-out sibling p.
 low p.
 Management Development P.
 Management Readiness P.
 metapsychological p.
 microsomal isoenzyme
  metabolism p.
 mood p.
 P. of Mood States (POMS)
 Musical Aptitude P. (MAP)
 neurotic direction p.
 P. of Nonverbal Sensitivity (PONS)
 Nottingham Health P.
 P. of Out-of-Body Experiences
  (POBE)
 Pain Patient P. (P-3)
 Pain Perception P. (PPP)
 Paranoid Sensitivity P.

P

profile *(continued)*
    Parent Perception of Child P. (PPCP)
    Peer P.
    personality p.
    Physical Tolerance P. (PTP)
    Psychiatric Evaluation P. (PEP)
    Psychoeducational P. (PEP)
    Psycho-Epistemological P. (PEP)
    psychotic direction p.
    Psychotic Inpatient P. (PIP)
    Psychotic Reaction P. (PRP)
    Revised Edinburgh Functional Communication P.
    risk p.
    SEED Developmental P.
    Sexuality Preference P. (SPP)
    sibling p.
    Sickness Impact P. (SIP)
    side effect p.
    spiked p.
    STAR P.
    structural p.
    Student Talent and Risk P.
    Test Anxiety P.
    Thackray Reading Readiness P. (TRRP)
    Thinking Good P.
    trait p.
    Validity Indicator P. (VIP)
    velocity p.
    P. VS
Profil-O-Plastic plate
profound
    p. amnesia
    p. dementia
    p. idiocy
    p. idiot
    p. mental retardation
    p. mental subnormality
profoundly retarded
profunda
    cisterna intercruralis p.
progenitor
    temperature-sensitive neural p.
progesterone
progestin
prognathic
prognosis (Px, px)
    direction p.
    extent p.
prognostic value
Prograf
program
    Advanced Placement P. (APP)
    Ann Arbor Learning Inventory and Remediation P.
    P. for Assessing Youth Employment Skills
    Basic Skills Assessment P.
    behavior modification p.
    career planning p. (CPP)
    Child and Adolescent Fear and Anxiety Treatment P.

    community p.
    Comparative Guidance and Placement P. (CGP)
    cooperative institutional research p. (CIRP)
    development p.
    Dole-Nyswauder p.
    drug abuse rehabilitation p.
    dual diagnosis p.
    educational p.
    Employee Assistance P. (EAP)
    enrichment p.
    entitlement p.
    Fast Track P.
    Frostig-Horne training p.
    Head Start p.
    individualized education p.
    infant stimulation p.
    Instructional Leadership Evaluation and Development P. (ILEAD)
    Leksell GammaPlan computerized p.
    Leksell SurgiPlan computerized p.
    Life Skills P.
    Minnesota Comprehensive Epilepsy P. (Mincep)
    National Institute of Mental Health-Epidemiologic Catchment Area P.
    PAR Admissions Testing p.
    parent therapist p.
    Psychiatric Knowledge and Skills Self-Assessment P. (PKSAP, PKSSAP)
    standard bone algorithm p.
    12-step p.
    Steps Up Developmental Screening P.
    supported employment p.
    Thematic Content Modification P. (TCMP)
    therapeutic p.
    Transformational Leadership Development P.
    transitional p.
    Treatment of Depression Collaborative Research P.
    weight-control p.
    work-study p.
programmable
    p. pulse generator
    p. valve
programmed
    p. cell death
    p. practice
    p. therapy
programming
    genotypic p.
progredient neurosis
progress
    P. Assessment Chart of Social and Personal Development (PAC)
    p. chart
    Monitoring Basic Skills P. (MBSP)

progression
    obstinate p.
progression-free survival (PFS)
progressiva
    dysbasia lordotica p.
    dyssynergia cerebellaris p.
    leukodystrophia cerebri p.
    ophthalmoplegia p.
progressive
    P. Achievement Tests of Listening
      Comprehension (PATLC)
    P. Achievement Tests of Reading
    p. assimilation
    p. bulbar palsy
    p. bulbar paralysis
    p. cerebellar tremor
    p. cerebral poliodystrophy
    p. degenerative
    p. degenerative disease
    p. degenerative subcortical
    p. dementia
    p. dementing illness
    p. deterioration
    p. disability
    p. disease
    p. dysarthria
    p. education
    p. external ophthalmoparesis (PEO)
    p. external ophthalmoplegia
    p. extraocular paresis
    p. flaccid quadriparesis
    p. hypertrophic interstitial
      neuropathy
    p. hypertrophic neuropathy
    p. leptomeningeal fibrosis
    p. lingual hemiatrophy
    p. multifocal leukoencephalopathy
      (PML)
    p. multifocal leuko-J
      encephalopathy (PMJ)
    p. muscular dystrophy
    p. muscular relaxation
    p. neuropathic muscle atrophy
    p. nuclear amyotrophy
    p. paratonia
    p. paratonia dementia
    p. posthemorrhagic ventriculomegaly
    p. postpolio muscle atrophy
      (PPPMA)
    p. psychosis
    p. relaxation
    p. rubella panencephalitis
    p. spinal amyotrophy
    p. subcortical encephalopathy
    p. subcortical gliosis
    p. supranuclear palsy (PSP)
    p. teleologic regression
    p. torsion spasm
    p. traumatic encephalopathy
    p. ventricular dilation
ProHance
prohormone
project
    Aptitude Research P. (ARP)
    Human Genome P.

    Menninger Clinic Treatment
      Intervention P.
    Oregon Adolescent Depression P.
    Stony Brook High Risk P.
projected jealousy
projectile vomiting
projection
    anteroposterior p.
    applied extrasensory p. (AESP)
    astral p.
    axial p.
    Caldwell p.
    p. defense mechanism
    delusional p.
    eccentric p.
    p. fiber
    filtered-back p.
    impersonal p.
    lateral p.
    p. neuron
    optical p.
    sagittal p.
    p. system
    thalamocortical p.
    ventral amygdaloid fugal p.
projectional paranoia
projective
    P. Assessment of Aging Method
    P. Human Figure Drawing Test
    p. identification
    p. personality assessment
    p. technique
prolactin (PRL)
    p. response
    serum p.
prolactin-inhibiting factor (PIF)
prolactinoma
prolactin-producing adenoma
prolactin-releasing factor (PRF)
prolapse
    mitral valve p. (MVP)
Prolene suture
proliferation
    cell p.
    control cell p.
    fibroblastic p.
    smooth muscle p.
    T-cell p.
proliferative malignant glial cell
Prolixin
    P. Decanoate
    P. Decanoate Injection
    P. enanthate
    P. Enanthate Injection
    P. Oral
Proloid
prolongata
    alalia p.
prolongation
    pulse repetition time p.
prolongatus
    coitus p.
prolonged
    p. depressive reaction
    p. grief

P

prolonged *(continued)*
    p. grief reaction
    p. nocturnal sleep episode
    p. posttraumatic stress disorder
    p. prodrome of schizophrenia
    p. situational depression
    p. sleep latency
    p. sleep therapy
    p. sleep treatment
    p. transition to fully awake state
promazine
promethazine
    p. hydrochloride
    meperidine and p.
prominence
    pedicle screw hardware p.
prominent
    p. anxiety
    p. aspect
    p. deterioration
    p. grimacing
    p. hallucination
    p. irritable mood
    p. mood symptom
Prominol
promiscuity
    ego-dystonic p.
    protracted p.
    sexual p.
    sexual pleasure sexual p.
promiscuous
    p. sex
    p. sexual behavior
Promit
promoter
    endogenous chromosomal p.
promotion neurosis
pronator
    p. reflex
    p. teres syndrome
proneness to addiction
prone position
Pronestyl
pronoun
    anaphoric p.
    bound p.
proof
    forensic p.
    incontrovertible p.
    obvious p.
    p. of paternity
proopiomelanocortin (POMC)
prop
    Oberto mouth p.
Propacet
propagation of activity
propallylonal
propanolamine (PPA)
propantheline
proparacaine hydrochloride
Propavan
propensity
propentofylline

proper
    ego p.
    p. fasciculi
    p. neck positioning
    p. repression
property
    anticholinergic p.
    destruction of p.
    field p.
    hebbian p.
prophase
prophecy
    self-fulfilling p.
prophetic dream
prophylactic
    p. hypertensive hypervolemic
      hemodilution
    p. treatment
prophylaxis
    anaphylactic shock p.
    anticonvulsant p.
    antimicrobial p.
    pharmacologic p.
propiomazine
Propionibacterium acnes
propizepine
Proplast
proplexus
propofol infusion
proportion
    delusional p.
    p. of survivors affected (PSA)
proposagnosia
propositus
propoxyphene
    p. and acetaminophen
    p. and aspirin
    p. dependence
    p. hydrochloride
    p. napsylate and acetaminophen
propranolamine
propranolol
    p. hydrochloride
    p. and hydrochlorothiazide
propria
    dura p.
propriem
proprioception deficit
proprioceptive
    p. feedback
    p. neuromuscular facilitation (PNF)
    p. perception
    p. reflex
    p. sensation
    p. sensibility
    p. sensory deficit
    p. vertigo
proprioceptor
proprionic acidemia
propriospinal myoclonus
proptosis
propulsion
propylene glycol toxicity
propyliodone
Prorex

prosencephalon
prosodic feature
prosody
prosopagnosia
prosopalgia
prosopodiplegia
prosoponeuralgia
prosoplegia
prosopospasm
prospective study
prospermia
prostacyclin
prostaglandin
Prostaphlin
ProStep Patch
prosternation
prosthesis
    acrylic p.
    behavioral p.
    neural p.
    NeuroCybernetic p. (NCP)
    penile p.
    Preclude dura substitute p.
    sacral segmental nerve stimulation
      implantable neural p.
prosthetic
    P. Disc Nucleus (PDN)
    P. Disc Nucleus device
    p. heart valve
Prostigmin
prostigmin test
protagonist
Protamine
    P. Zinc and Iletin I
    P. Zinc Insulin
protaxic mode
protease
protection
    airway p.
    cerebral p.
    p. factor
    p. proceeding
protective
    p. barrier
    p. glasses
    p. laryngeal reflex
    p. survival strategy
protector
    Adson dural p.
    p. identity
    MouthGuard oral p.
    p. role
protein
    p. 2
    amyloid precursor p.
    antiglial fibrillary acidic p.
    argyrophil organizer region p.
      (AgNOR)
    Bence Jones p.
    beta-amyloid p.
    p. C deficiency
    cerebrospinal fluid p.
    connexin 32 p.
    C-reactive p. (CRP)

    cyclin-dependent kinase
      inhibitory p.
    cytoskeletal p.
    p. electrophoresis
    G p.
    gamma carboxylated p.
    glial fibrillary acidic p. (GFAP)
    growth-associated p. (GAP)
    heat shock p.
    hemostasis-related p.
    heterotrimeric G p.
    homeodomain p.
    huntingtin p.
    inhibitory p.
    56 kD p.
    p. kinase
    p. kinase C (PKC)
    microtubule-associated p.
    myelin basic p. (MBP)
    myelin/oligodendrocyte-specific p.
      (MOSP)
    N p.
    Nurrl p.
    opioid precursor p.
    peripheral myelin p. 22
    p. phobia
    proteolipid p. (PLP)
    S-100 p.
    p. S deficiency
    serum p.
    signal-transducing guanine-nucleotide
      binding p.
    tau p.
    p. tyrosine phosphorylation
    voltage-sensitive p.
    p. zero
proteinaceous infectious particle
proteinase
    aspartic p.
    cysteine p.
    serine p.
protein-bound iodine (PBI)
proteinphobia
proteinuria
protensity
proteoglycan
    chondroitin sulfate p.
    disk matrix p.
proteolipid protein (PLP)
proteolysis
proteolytic fragment
protest
    body p.
    masculine p.
    p. psychosis
Protestant
    white Anglo-Saxon P. (WASP)
Proteus syndrome
Prothiaden
prothipendyl
prothrombin time (pro-time, PT)
prothymia
pro-time
    prothrombin time
protirelin

P

protocol
> fractionation p.
> Gliadel wafer treatment p.
> Managed Care Appropriateness P.
> test p.

protomasochism

proton
> p. beam
> p. density
> p. density weighting
> p. imaging
> p. nuclear magnetic resonance
> spectroscopy
> p. relaxation time
> p. spectrum

proton-electron dipole-dipole interaction

protoneuron

proton-weighted image

proto-oncogene

Protopam

protopathic sensibility

protophallic

protoplasmic
> p. astrocyte
> p. astrocytoma

protoporphyrin IX

protospasm

prototaxic mode

prototypical course pattern

protozoan infection

protracted
> p. difficulty
> p. promiscuity
> p. reactive paranoid psychosis
> p. withdrawal syndrome

protracts
> catatonia p.

protriptyline

protruded disk

protrusio defect

protrusion
> medullary p.
> pseudopodial p.

protuberans
> dermatofibrosarcoma p.

protuberantia occipitalis interna

Proventil

proverb interpretation test

Providence scoliosis system

provisional diagnosis

proviso
> parapathetic p.

provocateur
> agent p.

provocation
> aggression without p.
> minimal p.
> pharmacological p.
> sexual p.

provocative
> p. behavior
> p. diagnosis
> p. testing

provoked anxiety

provoking
> p. stimulus
> thought p.

prowazekii
> *Rochalimaea p.*

prowess
> sexual p.

proxemics

proxibarbal

proximal
> p. balloon occlusion
> p. carotid ring
> p. clipping
> latency p.
> p. myopathy
> p. receptor
> p. segment retraction

proximity
> mother-infant p.

proximoataxia

proxy
> factitious disorder by p.
> Munchausen disease by p.
> posttraumatic stress disorder by p.

proxy-for-deficit syndrome

Prozac

Prozine-50

PRP
> Psychotic Reaction Profile

PRQ
> Personal Resource Questionnaire

PRS
> Personality Rating Scale
> Pupil Rating Scale

PRT
> OISE Picture Reasoning Test
> Pantomime Recognition Test
> Picture Reasoning Test
> psychotic trigger reaction

Pruitt-Inahara shunt

pruning
> neuronal p.

pruritic
> p. disorder
> p. exanthema

pruritus
> p. ani
> generalized p.
> localized p.
> psychogenic p.
> p. vulvae

PS
> psychiatric
> PS Medical Flow Control valve

PSA
> pathologic spontaneous activity
> power spectral analysis
> proportion of survivors affected

psalterial

psalterium, pl. psalteria

psammocarcinoma

psammoma
> p. body
> Virchow p.

psammomatoid ossifying fibroma

psammomatous
p. meningioma
psammous
PSAN, PsAn
psychoanalysis
psychoanalyst
PSCI
Primary Self-Concept Inventory
PSE
point of subjective equality
portal systemic encephalopathy
Present State Examination
Lactulose PSE
pselaphesis, pselaphesia
psellism
pseudagraphia
pseudaphia
pseudarthrosis
documented p.
failed back syndrome with
documented p.
p. rate
p. repair
pseudesthesia
pseudoabducens
p. nerve paresis
p. palsy
pseudoaggression
pseudoagrammatism
pseudoagraphia
pseudoamnesia
pseudoaneurysm
pseudoapoplexy
pseudoapraxia
pseudo-Argyll Robertson pupil
pseudoarthritis
pseudo as-if
pseudoataxia
pseudoathetosis
pseudoautosomal locus for schizophrenia
pseudo-battered child syndrome
pseudobulbar
p. palsy
p. paralysis
p. speech
pseudocatatonia
traumatic p.
pseudocele
pseudocephalocele
pseudocholinsterase
pseudochorea
pseudochromesthesia
pseudoclonus
pseudocoma
pseudocombat
p. fatigability
p. fatigue
pseudoconvulsion
pseudocyesis syndrome
pseudocyst
secreting glial p.
pseudocystic hypodense lesion
pseudodelirium

pseudodementia
p. of depression
hysterical p.
pseudodepression
pseudoephedrine and ibuprofen
pseudoepileptic seizures
pseudoepileptiform activity
pseudoesthesia
pseudoflexibilitas
pseudofracture
pseudoganglion
pseudogeusesthesia
pseudogeusia
pseudogiftedness
pseudo-Graefe sign
pseudographia
pseudohallucination
ego dystonic p.
imaged p.
manipulative p.
pseudohermaphrodite
pseudohomosexual
pseudohydrocephaly
pseudohydrophobia
pseudohypersexuality
pseudohypertrophic
p. muscular atrophy
p. muscular dystrophy
p. muscular paralysis
pseudohypnosis
pseudohypoparathyroidism
pseudoidentification
pseudoillusion
pseudoimbecility
pseudoinclusion
nuclear p.
pseudoinsomnia
pseudo-internuclear ophthalmoplegia
pseudointoxication
pseudolalia
pseudolobulated
pseudologia fantastica
pseudologue
pseudomalignancy
pseudomania
pseudomasturbation
pseudomedial longitudinal fasciculus
lesion
pseudomelancholia
pseudomelia paraesthetica
pseudomembranous colitis
pseudomemory
pseudomeningitis
pseudomeningocele
posttraumatic intradiploic p.
traumatic p.
pseudomnesia
Pseudomonas
P. aeruginosa
P. exotoxin
pseudomuscular hypertrophy
pseudomyasthenia
ocular p.

P

pseudomyotonia
    Debré-Sémélaigne p.
    p. disease
pseudonarcotic
pseudonarcotism
pseudonecrophilia
pseudoneoplasm
pseudoneurogenic bladder
pseudoneurological
    p. symptom grouping
    p. symptoms
pseudoneuroma
pseudoneurotic schizophrenia
pseudonym
pseudoobstruction
    polyneuropathy, ophthalmoplegia,
    leukoencephalopathy, and
    intestinal p. (POLIP)
pseudopalisading astrocytoma
pseudoparalysis
    arthritic general p.
    congenital atonic p.
pseudoparameter
pseudoparanoia
pseudoparaplegia
    Basedow p.
pseudoparesis
    alcoholic p.
pseudoparkinsonism
pseudopellagra
pseudoperitonitis
pseudopersonality
pseudophotesthesia
pseudoplegia
pseudopodial protrusion
pseudopsammoma body
pseudopsia
pseudopsychopathic schizophrenia
pseudopsychosis
pseudoptosis
pseudopuberty
pseudoquerulant
pseudorosette
pseudoschizophrenia
pseudoscience
pseudosclerosis
    Westphal p.
    Westphal-Strümpell p.
pseudoseizure
pseudosenility
pseudosexuality
pseudosmia
pseudosocial personality disorder
pseudosplenium
pseudotabes
    diabetic p.
    pupillotonic p.
pseudotransference
pseudotumor
    p. cerebri
    idiopathic orbital p.
    orbital p.
pseudotumoral lymphocytic hypophysitis

pseudounipolar
    p. cell
    p. neuron
pseudoventricle
pseudoxanthoma elasticum
PSG
    polysomnogram
    polysomnograph
    polysomnography
    Albert Grass Heritage PSG
P&SH
    personal and social history
PSI
    Personal Style Inventory
    Psychological Screening Inventory
    psychosomatic inventory
    PSI Basic Skills Test for Business,
    Industry and Government
psi
    p. phenomenon
    p. system
Psicronizer
psilocin
psilocybin dependence
psittacism
psittacosis encephalitis
PSLT
    Picture Story Language Test
PSM
    polysomnogram
PSMed
    psychosomatic medicine
psoas
    p. abscess
    p. muscle
psopholalia
psoriasis
    p. spondylitica
psoriatic arthritis
PSP
    Personnel Security Preview
    postsynaptic potential
    progressive supranuclear palsy
PSQ
    Personal Strain Questionnaire
PSR
    Physicians for Social Responsibility
PSRI
    Professional Sexual Role Inventory
PSRO
    Professional Standards Review
    Organization
PSRS
    Process Skills Rating Scale
PSS
    primary Sjögren syndrome
    psychiatric services section
    Psychiatric Status Schedule
PSS:NICU
    Parental Stressor Scale: Neonatal
    Intensive Care Unit
PST
    prefrontal sonic treatment
PSTO
    Purdue Student-Teacher Opinionnaire

psuedoperiodic discharge
PSV
   psychological, social, and vocational
Psy, psy
   psychiatry
   psychology
PSYCH, psych
   psychiatry
psychagogy
psychal
psychalgia, psychalgalia
psychalgic
psychalia
psychanalysis
psychanopsia
psychasthene
psychasthenia
   compulsive p.
   mixed compulsive p.
   mixed compulsive states p.
   obsession p.
   P. "7" Scale
   p. scale
psychasthenic
   p. delirium
   p. neurosis
psychataxia
psychauditory
psyche
   contrasexual component of p.
psycheclampsia
psychedelic
   p. agent
   p. agent dependence
   p. therapy
psycheism
psychelytic
psychentonia
psychephoric
psycheplastic
psycherhexic
psychezymic
psychiat
   psychiatric
psychiatric (PS, psychiat)
   p. anaphylaxis
   p. assistant
   p. case register
   p. chemistry
   p. comorbidity
   p. deviance
   p. diagnosis
   P. Diagnostic Interview
   p. disability
   p. disease
   p. disturbance
   p. education
   p. emergency
   p. emergency service (PES)
   p. emergency team (PET)
   P. Epidemiology Research Interview
   (PERI)
   p. evaluation
   P. Evaluation Form (PEF)
   P. Evaluation Profile (PEP)

p. examination
p. genetics
p. ghetto
p. history
p. hospital
p. illness
p. intensive care unit (PICU)
p. interview
P. Knowledge and Skills Self-
   Assessment Program (PKSAP,
   PKSSAP)
p. manifestation
p. nomenclature
p. nosology
p. nurse
p. patient
p. rating scale
p. reacting scale
p. services section (PSS)
p. social work
p. social worker
p. somatic therapy
p. statistics
P. Status Rating Scale
P. Status Schedule (PSS)
p. system interface disorder
p. technician
p. treatment
p. trend
p. unit
p. ward
psychiatrically disabled
psychiatrism
psychiatrist
   board certified p.
   board eligible p.
   child p.
   forensic p.
psychiatrize
psychiatry (Psy, psy, PSYCH, psych)
   academic p.
   addiction p.
   administrative p.
   adolescent p.
   adulthood p.
   analytic p.
   asylum p.
   behavioral p.
   biologic p.
   biologic p.
   child p. (CHP, CP)
   clinical p.
   Clunis inquiry forensic p.
   common sense p.
   community p.
   comparative p.
   consultation p.
   consultation liaison p.
   contractual p.
   correctional p.
   criminal p.
   cross-cultural p.
   cultural p.
   descriptive p.
   dynamic p.

psychiatry *(continued)*
    ecological p.
    existential p.
    experimental p.
    folk p.
    forensic p.
    geriatric p.
    gerontologic p.
    gerontological p.
    hospital-based p.
    hospital and community p.
    industrial p.
    infant p.
    interpersonal p.
    legal p.
    liaison p.
    military forensic p.
    minority group p.
    molecular p.
    multidisciplinary group p.
    p. and neurology (P&N)
    occupational p.
    old-age p.
    organic p.
    organized-care p.
    orthomolecular p.
    outpatient-based p.
    pastoral p.
    pediatric p.
    political p.
    preventive p.
    prison p.
    psychoanalytic p.
    psychopharmacologic p.
    public p.
    rehabilitation p.
    rural p.
    schools of p.
    social p.
    Standard System of P. (SSOP)
    transcultural p.
    urban p.
    Washington School of P.
psychiatry-neurology (PN)
psychic
    p. ability
    p. aftershock
    p. anaphylaxis
    p. apparatus
    p. blindness
    p. censor
    p. contagion
    p. deafness
    p. dependence
    p. determinism
    p. disorder
    p. disturbance
    p. divorce
    p. dualism
    p. energizer
    p. energy
    p. epilepsy
    p. equivalent
    p. experience

    p. factor
    p. force
    p. helplessness
    p. impotence
    p. inertia
    p. masturbation
    p. numbing
    p. numbness
    p. ontogeny
    p. organization
    p. overtone
    p. pain
    p. phenomenon
    p. reflex
    p. scar
    p. seizure
    p. shock
    p. shock syndrome
    p. suicide
    p. tic
    p. trauma
    p. vaginismus
psychical
    p. manner
    p. reality
psychicism
psychinosis
psychism
psychnosia
psychoacoustic
    p. test (PAT)
    P. Testing (PAT)
psychoactive
    p. disorder
    p. drug
    p. drug abuse
    p. effect
    p. medication
    p. substance
    p. substance abuse
    p. substance delirium
    p. substance dementia
    p. substance dependence
    p. substance hallucinosis
    p. substance-induced organic
    p. substance intoxication
    p. substance withdrawal
psychoaffective disorder (PAD)
psychoallergy
psychoanaleptica
psychoanalysis (PA, PSAN, PsAn)
    active p.
    adlerian p.
    applied p.
    boundaries in p.
    existential p.
    freudian p.
    fundamental rule of p.
    jungian p.
    wild p.
psychoanalyst (PA, PSAN, PsAn)
psychoanalytic
    p. group
    p. group psychotherapy
    p. interpretation

p. neurosis
p. pathography
p. psychiatry
p. situation
p. technique
p. therapy
psychoanalytical
p. pathography
p. theory
psychoanalyze
psychoanopsia
psychoasthenics
psychoataxia
psychoauditory
psychobacillosis
psychobioanalysis
psychobiogram
psychobiological
p. process
p. process of dementia
psychobiology
clinical p.
development p.
objective p.
psychocardiac
psychocardic reflex
psychocatharsis
psychocentric
psychochemistry
psychochrome
psychochromesthesia
psychocinesia
psychocoma
psychocortical center
psychocutaneous
psychodiagnosis
psychodiagnostics
psychodietetics
psychodometer
psychodometry
psychodrama
forms of p.
p. group therapy
psychodramatic
p. catharsis
p. shock
psychodynamic
adaptational p.
p. approach
p. cerebral system
p. concept
p. conflict
p. formulation
p. interpretation
p. interpretation and treatment
p. orientation
p. psychotherapy
p. research orientation
p. theory
psychodynamic-experiential model
psychodysleptic drug
psychoeducational
p. evaluation
P. Profile (PEP)
p. test

psychoeducation group therapy
psychoendocrinology
psychoepilepsy
psychoepileptic episode
Psycho-Epistemological Profile (PEP)
psychoexploration
psychogalvanic
p. reflex (PGR)
p. response (PGR)
p. skin reaction
p. skin resistance (PGSR)
psychogalvanometer
psychogender
psychogenesis
psychogenia
psychogenic
p. air hunger
p. alopecia
p. amnesia
p. anxiety
p. aphagia
p. aphasia
p. aspermia (PA)
p. asthenia
p. ataxia
p. backache
p. cardiac nondisease
p. cardiospasm
p. confusion
p. constipation
p. cough
p. cyclical vomiting
p. deafness
p. depression
p. depressive psychosis
p. dermatitis
p. diarrhea
p. disorder
p. drug
p. dysmenorrhea
p. dyspareunia
p. dyspepsia
p. dystonia
p. dysuria
p. eczema
p. enuresis
p. excitation
p. excoriation
p. fatigability
p. fatigue
p. fugue
gastrointestinal functional p.
p. headache
p. hearing loss
p. hiccup
p. hyperventilation
p. illness
p. impotence
p. megacolon
p. nocturnal polydipsia (PNP)
p. nocturnal polydipsia syndrome
p. obesity
p. oculogyric crisis
p. origin
p. overlay

P

psychogenic *(continued)*
    p. painful coitus
    p. painful erection
    p. painful menstruation
    p. paralysis
    p. paranoid nonorganic
    p. paranoid nonorganic psychosis
    p. paroxysmal
    p. paroxysmal tachycardia
    p. penis pain
    p. physical symptom
    p. physiological
    p. physiological manifestation
    p. polydipsia
    p. pruritus
    p. purpura syndrome
    p. reaction
    p. retention
    p. rumination
    p. seizure
    p. stupor
    p. testicular pain
    p. testis pain
    p. tic
    p. torticollis
    p. twilight state
    p. ulcer
    p. urticaria
    p. uterus pain
    p. vertigo
    p. vomiting
    p. yawning
psychogeny
psychogeriatrics
psychogerontology
psychogeusic
psychognosia
psychognosis
psychogogic
psychogonical
psychogony
psychogram
psychograph
psychographic disturbance
psychography
psychohistory
psychoimmunology
psychoinfantile personality
psychoinfantilism
psychokinesia
psychokinesis (PK)
psychokinetic (PK)
psychokym
psycholagny
psycholepsis
psycholepsy
psycholeptica
psycholeptic episode
psycholinguistic
    p. ability
    P. Rating Scale
    p. test
    p. theory
psycholinguistics

psychologic
    p. defense system
    p. desensitization
    p. factor affecting physical condition
    p. medicine
    p. programming therapy
    p. rating scale
    p. testing
    p. tremor
psychological
    p. abuse
    p. acculturation
    p. addiction
    p. adjustment
    p. basis
    p. capacity
    p. change
    p. debriefing
    p. defense system
    p. deprivation
    p. distortion
    p. distress
    P. Distress Inventory
    p. dysfunction
    p. dysfunction symptom
    p. evaluation
    p. examination
    p. factor
    p. factors affecting a mental condition
    p. field
    p. game
    p. information, acquisition, processing, and control system (PIAPACS)
    p. intervention
    p. interview
    p. inventory
    p. loaner
    p. loner
    p. management
    p. marker
    p. mindedness
    p. model
    p. motivation
    p. need
    p. pain
    p. pillow
    p. problem
    p. procedure
    p. process
    p. rapport
    p. reaction
    p. refractory period
    p. related symptoms
    P. Screening Inventory (PSI)
    p. signs and symptoms
    p. strain
    p. stress
    p. syndrome
    p. technique
    p. test
    p. testing
    p. theory

p. therapy
p. toner
p. trauma depressive
p. trauma depressive psychosis
p. warfare (PW)
psychologically mediated response
psychological, social, and vocational (PSV)
psychologist
clinical p.
consulting p.
counseling p.
engineering p.
environmental p.
licensed p.
social p.
psychology (Psy, psy)
abnormal p.
p. act
adlerian p.
adolescent p.
advertising p.
analytical p.
animal p.
applied p.
atomistic p.
behavioral p.
behavioristic p.
blame p.
centralist p.
child p. (CP)
clinical p.
cognitive p.
community p.
comparative p.
constitutional p.
consumer p.
content p.
correctional p.
counseling p.
courtroom p.
criminal p.
depth p.
developmental p.
dynamic p.
educational p.
ego p.
engineering p.
environmental p.
existential p.
experimental p.
faculty p.
folk p.
forensic p.
functional p.
genetic p.
geriatric p.
gestalt p.
health-related p.
holistic p.
human factor p.
humanistic p.
id p.
individual p.
industrial p.

interbehavioral p.
jungian p.
legal p.
mass p.
medical p.
military p.
mob p.
objective p.
organismic p.
organizational p.
pediatric p.
perceptual p.
peripheralist p.
personality p.
personnel p.
philosophical p.
physiological p.
physiological p.
pop p.
rational p.
schizophrenic p.
self p.
social p.
subjective p.
topographical p.
topological p.
transpersonal p.
uprooted p.
victim p.
psychomathematics
psychometer
psychometric
p. evaluation
p. performance
p. performance characteristic
p. predictor
p. test
p. testing
psychometrician
psychometry
psychomimetic
psychomimic syndrome
psychomotility
psychomotor
p. activity
p. agitation
p. attack
p. behavior
p. change
p. convulsion
p. development
p. disorder
p. disturbance
p. disturbance stress reaction
p. epilepsy
p. excitement
p. fit
p. intelligence
p. measurement
p. overactivity
p. performance
p. phenomenon
p. poverty
p. restlessness
p. retardation

P

psychomotor *(continued)*
   p. seizure
   p. slowing
   p. speed
   p. stimulant
   p. symptom
   p. test
psychoneural parallelism
psychoneuroendocrinology
psychoneuroid
psychoneuroimmunological research
psychoneuroimmunology (PNI)
psychoneurologist (PN)
psychoneurology (PN)
psychoneurosis, pl. **psychoneuroses**
   anxiety p.
   battle p.
   climacteric p.
   compensation p.
   compulsion p.
   conversion hysteria p.
   defense p.
   depersonalization p.
   depressive-type p.
   dissociative hysteria p.
   hypochondriacal p.
   hysteria p.
   p. maidica
   mixed p.
   neurasthenic p.
   obsessional p.
   obsessive-compulsive p.
   occupational p.
   paranoid p.
   personality p.
   phobia p.
   senile p.
psychoneurotic (PN)
   depersonalization p.
   p. depression
   p. mental disorder
   p. personality
   p. reaction
psychonoetism
psychonomic
psychonomy
psychonosis
psychonosology
psychonoxious
psychooncology
psychooptical reflex control
psychoorganic
   p. brain syndrome
   nonpsychotic severity p.
psychoparesis
psychopath
   criminal sexual p. (CSP)
   sexual p.
psychopathia
   p. martialis
   p. partialis
   p. sexualis
psychopathic
   antisocial trends p.

   p. constitution
   p. deviance
   P. Deviance "4" Scale
   p. deviance scale
   p. deviate (PD)
   p. diathesis
   p. inferiority
   mixed-type p.
   p. personality
   posttraumatic p.
   p. state
Psychopathological Rating Scale
psychopathologist
psychopathology
   p. of epilepsy
   impulsive/compulsive p.
   p. level
   prepubertal p.
   presenting p.
   related p.
   retardation p.
   p. of retardation
psychopathosis
psychopathy
   autistic p.
   benign p.
   passive parasitic p.
psychopedagogy
psychopenetration test
psychopetal
psychopharmaceutical intervention
psychopharmacological
   p. therapy
   p. treatment
psychopharmacologic psychiatry
psychopharmacology
   P. Bulletin
   clinical p.
   gender-sensitive p.
   geriatric p.
   pediatric p.
psychopharmacotherapy
psychophobia
psychophonasthenia
psychophylaxis
psychophysical
   p. function
   p. parallelism
psychophysics
psychophysiologic
   p. correlate
   p. manifestation
   p. principle
   p. reaction
psychophysiological
   p. change
   p. disorder
   p. insomnia
   p. problem
   p. test
psychophysiology
psychoplegia
psychopneumatology
psychopolitics
psychoprophylactic treatment

psychoprophylaxis
psychoreaction
psychorelaxation
psychorhythm
psychorhythmia (*var. of*
  psychorrhythmia)
psychormic
psychorrhagia
psychorrhea
psychorrhexis
psychorrhythmia, psychorhythmia
psychosedation
psychosedative
psychosensorial
psychosensory
    p. aphasia
    p. epilepsy
    p. stimulus
    p. symptom
psychose passionelle
psychoses (*pl. of* psychosis)
psychosexual
    p. development
    p. disorder
    p. dysfunction
    p. factor
    p. history
    p. identity
    p. identity crisis
    inhibited female orgasm p.
    inhibited male orgasm p.
    inhibited sexual desire p.
    p. moratorium
    p. sphere
    p. stage
    p. symptom
psychosexuality
psychosis, pl. **psychoses**
    abstinence syndrome alcoholic p.
    accidental p.
    acute p.
    addiction organic p.
    addiction-type organic p.
    affective p.
    affective paranoid organic p.
    akinetic p.
    alcoholic Korsakoff p.
    alcoholic liver disease-type
     organic p.
    alcoholism organic p.
    alternating p.
    alternative p.
    amnestic confabulatory alcoholic p.
    amnestic syndrome alcoholic p.
    amnestic syndrome drug p.
    amphetamine p.
    anergastic organic p.
    anxiety-blissfulness p.
    arteriosclerotic brain disease-type
     organic p.
    arteriosclerotic organic p.
    p. of association
    atypical p.
    autistic p.
    autoscopic p.

barbed-wire p.
biogenic p.
bipolar affective p.
birth brain trauma organic p.
black patch p.
borderline p.
brain disease organic p.
brain infection organic p.
brain trauma organic p.
brief reactive p.
bromide p.
buffoonery p.
cannabis p.
cardiac p.
cerebral glucose metabolic-type
  organic p.
cerebrovascular disease organic p.
cerebrovascular ischemia-type
  organic p.
Cheyne-Stokes p.
child p.
p. in childbirth
childbirth organic p.
childhood p.
p. of childhood
childhood-onset p.
chronic p.
circular p.
circulatory p.
climacteric paranoid p.
cocaine p.
collective p.
confusional p.
confusion reactive p.
conjugal p.
constitutional p.
cycloid p.
degeneration p.
degenerative p.
delirious transient organic p.
delirium state drug p.
delirium transient organic p.
delirium tremens alcoholic p.
delusional syndrome drug p.
delusional transient organic p.
dementia state drug p.
dependence organic p.
dependence-type organic p.
depressed bipolar affective p.
depressive p.
disintegrative childhood p.
drug p.
drug-induced p.
p. due to physical condition
dysmnesic p.
electrical current brain trauma
  organic p.
embarrassment p.
emotional stress depressive p.
endocrine disease organic p.
epilepsy organic p.
epileptic transient organic p.
excitative p.
excitative-type nonorganic p.
exhaustion p.

P

psychosis *(continued)*
exhaustive p.
exogenous p.
exotic p.
familial p.
febrile p.
functional p.
furlough p.
gender ambiguity p.
gestational p.
governess p.
group p.
hallucinatory state drug p.
hallucinatory transient organic p.
hallucinosis alcoholic p.
heredofamilial p.
housewife p.
Huntington chorea organic p.
hypochondriacal p.
hypomanic p.
hyposomnia associated with p.
hysteria p.
hysterical p.
iatrogenic p.
ICU p.
idiopathic p.
idiophrenic p.
incipient schizophrenic p.
induced p.
infantile p.
infection-exhaustion p.
infection organic p.
infectious-exhaustive p.
infective p.
influenced p.
insomnia associated with p.
interactional childhood p.
interictal p.
intermittent p.
interval p.
intoxication organic p.
intoxication-type organic p.
intracranial infection organic p.
invocational p.
involutional p.
ischemia organic p.
Jakob-Creutzfeldt disease organic p.
juvenile p.
koro p.
Korsakoff p.
Korsakoff alcoholic p.
Korsakoff nonalcoholic p.
kraepelinian view of p.
K's p.
latent p.
liver disease organic p.
major depressive affective p.
malignant p.
manic p.
manic-depressive affective p.
marijuana p.
melancholia affective p.
meningismus p.
menopausal paranoid p.

metabolic disease organic p.
migration p.
mixed bipolar affective p.
mixed manic-depressive p.
model p.
monosymptomatic
  hypochondriacal p.
mood swings affective p.
motility p.
motor p.
multi-infarct p.
multiple sclerosis organic p.
nonorganic p.
organic p.
paranoiac p.
paranoic p.
paranoid p.
paranoid/affective organic p.
paretic p.
paroxysmal p.
pathologic drug intoxication
  drug p.
pathologic intoxication alcoholic p.
perplexed manic-depressive p.
perplexity p.
phencyclidine-associated p.
physical condition organic p.
p. polyneuritica
polyneuritic alcoholic p.
positive symptoms p.
posthypnotic p.
postictal p.
postinfectious p.
postoperative p.
postpartum p.
posttraumatic organic p.
p. in pregnancy
prepsychotic p.
prepubertal borderline p.
presbyophrenic p.
presenile p.
prison p.
private p.
process p.
progressive p.
protest p.
protracted reactive paranoid p.
psychogenic depressive p.
psychogenic paranoid nonorganic p.
psychological trauma depressive p.
puerperal p.
p. in puerperium
purpose p.
reactive confusion nonorganic p.
reactive depressive p.
reactive paranoid p.
recurrent episode depressive p.
scale of p. (SP)
schizoaffective p.
schizophrenia p.
schizophrenic/affective p.
schizophrenic paranoid p.
schizophreniform p.
semantic p.
senile p.

senility organic p.
sensory p.
septicemia p.
shock p.
simple deterioration senile p.
simple-type arteriosclerotic p.
single episode depressive p.
situational p.
sleeplessness associated with p.
somatic p.
status epilepticus organic p.
stigmata p.
stigmata of p.
stress p.
stuporous manic-depressive p.
subacute p.
substance-induced chronic p.
surgical brain trauma organic p.
symbiotic infantile p.
symptomatic p.
p. of syphilis
tabetic p.
toxic p.
toxic-infectious p.
transient organic p.
transitory p.
trauma organic p.
traumatic p.
uncomplicated arteriosclerotic p.
unipolar manic-depressive p.
Windigo p.
withdrawal syndrome alcoholic p.
withdrawal syndrome drug p.
p. with mental retardation
Wittigo p.
zoophil p.
zoophile p.
psychosis-induced polydipsia
psychosocial
P. Adjustment to Illness Scale (PAIS)
p. assessment (PA)
P. Assessment of Childhood Experiences (PACE)
p. complication
p. deprivation
p. development
p. dwarfism
p. event
p. factor
P. Factor Evaluation
p. function
p. functioning
p. history
P. History Screening Questionnaire (PHSQ)
P. History Screening Test (PHST)
p. intervention
p. moratorium
p. pain
p. pathology
p. problem
p. process
p. rehabilitation
p. retardation

p. setting
p. skill acquisition
p. stigmata
p. stress
p. stressor
p. treatment
psychosocial-environmental
psychosocial-labile (PL)
psychosocially determined short stature
psychosolytic
psychosoma
psychosomatic
p. disorder
p. illness
p. inventory (PSI)
p. medicine (PSMed)
p. reaction
p. symptom
psychosomimetic
psychostimulant
p. dependence
p. drug
psychosuggestive
psychosurgeon
psychosurgery
seed p.
psychosyndrome
algogenic p.
focal organic p.
organic p.
partial organic p.
psychosynthesis
psychotaxis
psychotechnics
psychotherapeusis
psychotherapeutic
p. drug
p. measure
p. spectrum
p. treatment
psychotherapy
active analytical p.
activity group p.
activity-interview group p. (A-IGP)
adlerian p.
adolescent p.
anaclitic p.
analytic group p.
autonomous p.
behavioral p.
brief p.
client-centered p.
cognitive p.
cognitive-behavioral p.
P. Competence Assessment Schedule (PCAS)
contractual p.
cooperative p.
crisis-intervention group p.
didactic group p.
directive p.
dyadic p.
dynamic p.
educational p.
ego p.

P

psychotherapy *(continued)*
    emergency p.
    existential p.
    experiential p.
    exploratory insight-oriented p. (EIO)
    family p.
    family and systemic p.
    focal p.
    freudian p.
    gestalt p.
    group analytic p.
    heteronomous p.
    hypnotic p.
    individual p.
    insight-oriented p.
    intensive p.
    interactional group p.
    Internet p.
    interpersonal p. (IPT)
    interview group p.
    long-term p.
    marathon group p.
    medical p.
    Morita p.
    multiple p.
    nondirective p.
    objective p.
    patterning p.
    personologic p.
    play group p.
    psychoanalytic group p.
    psychodynamic p.
    rational p.
    rational-emotive p.
    reciprocal inhibition p.
    reconstructive p.
    regressive-inspirational group p.
    relationship p.
    remedial p.
    p. responder (PR)
    short-contact p.
    short-term anxiety-provoking p.
    (STAPP)
    structured interactional group p.
    suggestive p.
    superficial p.
    P. Supervisory Inventory
    supportive-expressive p.
    terminal reinforcement p.
    time-limited p. (TLP)
    traditional p.
    transactional p.
psychothymia
psychotic
    p. attack
    p. behavior
    p. break
    p. choreoathetosis
    p. delusion
    p. delusions scale
    p. denial
    p. depression (PD)
    p. depression scale
    p. direction

    p. direction profile
    p. disease
    p. disorder
    p. disorder due to a general
      medical condition
    p. disorder with delusions
    p. disorder with hallucinations
    p. disorganization
    p. disorganization in schizophrenia
    p. distortion
    p. disturbance
    electroshock-induced p.
    p. exacerbation
    p. factor
    p. feature
    p. fugue
    p. illness
    P. Inpatient Profile (PIP)
    p. manifestation
    p. posttraumatic brain syndrome
    p. presentation
    p. process
    P. Reaction Profile (PRP)
    recurrent episode p.
    p. schizophrenic episode
    p. speech
    p. state
    p. symptom
    p. symptomatology
    p. thinking
    p. thinking scale
    p. trigger reaction (PRT, PTR)
psychoticism
psychotogen
psychotoid
psychotomimetic
    p. agent
    p. agent dependence
    p. drug
psychotonic
psychotoxicomania
psychotropic drug (PTD)
psychovisual therapy
psychroalgia
psychroesthesia
psychrophobia
psyllium
psyoma
PT
    prothrombin time
pt
    patient
PTA
    posttraumatic amnesia
    prior to admission
    pure tone average
PTCA
    percutaneous transluminal coronary
      angioplasty
PTCS
    Primary Test of Cognitive Skills
PTD
    Prevention and Treatment of Depression
    psychotropic drug
pterion

pterional
- p. approach
- p. craniotomy

pteronophobia
pterygoid plexus
pterygopalatine
- p. fossa
- p. ganglion
- p. neuralgia

PTH
parathyroid hormone
PTI
Personnel Tests for Industry
Pictorial Test of Intelligence
PTO
Purdue Teacher Opinionnaire
ptosis, pl. **ptoses**
- cerebral p.
- p. sympathetica

PTP
Physical Tolerance Profile
PTQ
Parent-Teacher Questionnaire
Purdue Teacher Questionnaire
PTR
psychotic trigger reaction
PTSD
posttraumatic stress disorder
PTS-Ultrason
PTT
partial thromboplastin time
PTZ
pentylenetetrazol
puberal
puberism
persistent p.
pubertal
- p. sexual recapitulation
- p. stage

pubertas praecox
puberty
- atypical p.
- p. melancholia
- periodic psychosis of p.
- precocious p.
- p. rite

pubescent
public
- p. display of emotion
- p. drunkenness
- p. health model
- p. psychiatry

Pucci pediatrics hand orthoses
pudding opium
pudendal
- p. nerve
- p. SEP
- p. somatosensory evoked potential

pudendum, pl. **pudenda**
Pudenz
- P. shunt
- P. valve
- P. ventricular catheter

Pudenz-Heyer shunt system
puer eternus

puericulture
puerile
puerilism
hysterical p.
puerperal
- p. convulsion
- p. delirium
- p. dementia
- p. eclampsia
- p. mania
- p. melancholia
- p. psychosis
- p. seizure

puerperium
psychosis in p.
puesto
mal p.
pugilistica
dementia p.
Puka
Pulfrich phenomenon
pulling
- p. of clothes
- ear p.
- hair p.

pullout
- screw p.
- p. strength

pull test
Pulmonair 40 bed
pulmonary
- p. arteriovenous shunt
- p. capillary wedge pressure
- p. edema
- p. embolism
- p. encephalopathy

pulmonocoronary reflex
pulp
vertebral p.
pulposus
- herniated nucleus p.
- nucleus p.

pulsatility
- Gosling p.
- p. index (PI)

pulsating
- p. electromagnetic field (PEMF)
- p. headache
- p. neurasthenia
- p. pain
- p. visual halo

pulsation
- p. artifact
- carotid p.

pulse
- alternating p.
- chest p.
- p. flip angle
- p. generator
- p. length
- ocular p.
- p. oximeter
- p. oximetry
- presaturation p.
- radiofrequency p.

P

pulse *(continued)*
    p. repetition time
    p. repetition time prolongation
    RF p.
    p. sequence
    p. synchronous sound
    p. timing diagram
    p. wave artifact
    p. wave Doppler
    p. waveform
    p. width
pulsed
    p. Doppler
    p. Doppler imaging
    p. fluorography
    p. gradient
pulsed-field gel electrophoresis
pulsed-range gated Doppler instrument
pulseless disease
pulveratum
    opium p.
pulvinar
pulvinotomy
Pulvules
    Darvon Compound-65 P.
pump
    Cordis Secor implantable p.
    drug infusion p.
    implanted infusion p.
    Infusaid M400 constant flow p.
    infusion p.
    intra-ortic balloon p. (IABP)
    Medtronic SynchroMed
      implantable p.
    Shiley-Infusaid p.
    SynchroMed model 8611H
      prototype implantable p.
    volumetric infusion p.
punch
    bone p.
    Cone skull p.
    disk p.
    dural p.
    Fehling TOP ejector p.
    Ferris Smith-Kerrison p.
    Hajek-Koffler p.
    Hajek laminectomy p.
    Hardy sellar p.
    intervertebral p.
    Kerrison bone p.
    Raney laminectomy p.
    p. rongeur
    Roton sellar p.
    sellar p.
    skull p.
punch-drunk
    punch-drunk encephalopathy
    punch-drunk syndrome
puncta (*pl. of* punctum)
punctata
    rhizomelic chondrodysplasia p.
punctate white matter hyperintensity
punctum, gen. **puncti**, pl. **puncta**
    p. dolorosum

    p. luteum
    p. vasculosum
puncture
    Bernard p.
    brain p.
    cistern p.
    cisternal p.
    diabetic p.
    lumbar p. (LP)
    Quincke p.
    spinal p.
    stereotactic p.
    sternal p.
    suboccipital p.
    ventricular p.
punishment
    contingent p.
    corporal p.
    deserved p.
    p. dream
    expiatory p.
    Midas p.
    need for p.
    reciprocal p.
    unconscious need for p.
punning
Puno-Winter-Byrd (PWB)
    P.-W.-B. system
pupil
    absent p.
    Adie-Holmes p.
    Adie tonic p.
    Argyll Robertson p.
    blown p.
    consensual response p.
    constricted p.
    corn-picker's p.
    dilated p.'s
    fixed p.
    Holmes-Adie p.
    Hutchinson p.
    inverse Argyll Robertson p.
    isocoric p.
    Marcus Gunn p.
    myotonic p.
    paradoxical p.
    pinpoint p.'s
    pseudo-Argyll Robertson p.
    P. Rating Scale (PRS)
    P. Rating Scale: Screening for
      Learning Disabilities
    P. Record of Education Behavior
      (PREB)
    rigid p.
    Robertson p.
    tonic p.
    tonically dilated p.
    tonohaptic reaction of p.
pupillary
    p. abnormality
    p. constriction
    p. light reflex
    p. reaction
    p. skin reflex
pupillomotor

pupilloplegia
pupillotonia
pupillotonic pseudotabes
pupil-teacher fit
puppy love
purchase
    bony p.
    p. drug
    p. fake drug
Purdue
    P. Pegboard Dexterity Test
    P. Perceptual-Motor Survey (PPMS)
    P. Student-Teacher Opinionnaire (PSTO)
    P. Teacher Opinionnaire (PTO)
    P. Teacher Questionnaire (PTQ)
pure
    p. absence
    p. agraphia
    p. alexia
    p. aphasia
    p. aphemia
    p. athetoid palsy
    p. hemisensory stroke
    p. limb apraxia
    p. line
    p. mania
    p. mood
    p. motor hemiparesis (PMH)
    p. motor hemiplegia
    p. obsession
    p. sensory neuropathy
    p. sensory stroke
    p. spastic palsy
    p. tone audiogram
    p. tone average (PTA)
    p. tone discrimination
    p. tone hearing
    p. word deafness
    p. word mutism
pure-tone audiometry
purgation
purge
    binge and p.
    bulimic p.
purging
    eating and p.
    p. method
purified pleasure ego
purine metabolism
purist
    language p.
Purkinje
    P. afterimage
    P. cell
    P. corpuscle
    P. layer
Purmann method
purple
    p. heart
    p. ozoline
    p. people syndrome
purpose
    p. in life (PIL)

    P. in Life Test
    p. psychosis
purposeful
    p. behavior
    p. movement
purposeless
    p. agitation
    p. motor activity
    p. movement
purposive movement
purpura
    Henoch-Schönlein p.
    p. simplex
    thrombotic thrombocytopenic p.
pursing
    lip p.
pursuit
    p. abnormality
    p. defect
    p. eye movement
    family p.
    saccadic p.
    smooth p.
    p. system
purulent encephalitis
pusher
    Jacobson suture p.
putamen
    ventral p.
putaminal hemorrhage
putative
    p. adoptee
    p. adoptee vulnerability
    p. endogenous ligand
    p. index
    p. neurotransmitter
Putnam-Dana syndrome
putty
    Bishop p.
    Silly P.
PVA
    Personal Values Abstract
    polyvinyl alcohol
p value
PVG
    periventricular gray matter
PVI
    Personal Values Inventory
PVL
    periventricular radiolucency
PVMT
    Primary Visual Motor Test
PVNPS
    post-Vietnam psychiatric syndrome
PVNS
    pigmented villonodular synovitis
PvO2
    partial venous gas tension of oxygen
PVP
    posteroventral pallidotomy
PVS
    Beery Picture Vocabulary Screening
    persistent vegetative state
PVT
    Peabody Vocabulary Test

PW
psychological warfare
PWB
Puno-Winter-Byrd
PWP
Parents Without Partners
Px, px
prognosis
PXA
pleomorphic xanthoastrocytoma
pycnic (*var. of* pyknic)
pyelography
pyencephalus
Pygmalion effect
pygmalionism
pyknic, pycnic
p. constitutional type
pyknoepilepsy, pyknolepsy
pyknophrasia
pyla
pylar
pyloric stenosis
pylorospasm
pyocephalus
circumscribed p.
external p.
internal p.
pyogenes
Streptococcus p.
pyogenic
p. discitis
p. osteomyelitis
p. pachymeningitis
pyogenica
encephalitis p.
pyramid
anterior p.
cerebellar p.
Malacarne p.
p. of medulla oblongata
olfactory p.
posterior p. of the medulla
P. Scale
syndrome of the p.
pyramidal
p. cell
p. cell dendritic spines
p. cell layer

p. cerebral palsy
p. decussation
p. fiber
p. neuron
p. pathway
p. radiation
p. sign
p. system
p. tract
p. tractotomy
p. trocar
pyramidotomy
medullary p.
spinal p.
pyramis, pl. pyramides
p. medullae oblongatae
p. vermis
pyranocarboxylic acid class
pyrazinamide
pyrexiophobia
pyridostigmine bromide
pyridoxine
pyriform cortex
pyrilamine maleate
pyrimethamine
p. poisoning
p. sulfadoxine
pyrimidine metabolism
pyritinol
pyrolagnia
pyromania
p. disorder
erotic p.
pyrophobia
pyrophosphate
technetium 99m p.
technetium stannous p.
pyroptothymia
pyrosis
pyruvate
p. carboxylase
p. carboxylase deficiency
p. dehydrogenase (PDH)
p. dehydrogenase complex
pyschasthenia
pyschoplegia
Pythium

Q
clerical perception
quantitative test
Q data
Q method
Q methodology
Q sort
Q technique
Q test

q
every
quartile deviation

QA
quality assurance

QALE
quality-adjusted life expectancy

QALY
quality-adjusted life year

QCL
quadrigeminal cistern lipoma

QEEG
quantitative electroencephalogram
quantitative electroencephalography

qi-gong psychotic reaction

QLQ
Quality of Life Questionnaire

QNS
quantity not sufficient

QOL
quality of life

QOLI
Quality of Life Interview
Quality of Life Inventory

QPVT
Quick Picture Vocabulary Test

Q&Q   drug

Q-SART
Quantitative Sudomotor Axon Reflex
Test

Q-Set
California Child Q-S

Q-Sort
California Q.-S.

QT
Quick Test

qt
quiet

Quaalude

quad

quader

Quadramet

quadrangular
q. lobule
q. therapy

quadrantanopia

quadrantanopsia

quadrate
q. gyrus
q. lobe
q. lobule

quadrature detector

quadriceps
q. myopathy
q. reflex

quadrigemina
corpora q.

quadrigeminal
q. arachnoid cyst
q. body
q. cistern
q. cistern lipoma (QCL)
q. plate

quadrigeminum

Quadrilite 6000 fiberoptic headlight

quadriparesis
progressive flaccid q.

quadripedal extensor reflex

quadriplegia
spastic q.

qualitative
q. approach
q. difference
q. impairment in communication
q. judgment

quality
q. adjusted life-year (QUALY)
q. assurance (QA)
q. of caring
determining q.
q. drug
exaggerated negative q.
exaggerated positive q.
q. factor
image q.
q. of life (QOL)
Q. of Life Enjoyment and
 Satisfaction Questionnaire
Q. of Life Interview (QOLI)
Q. of Life Inventory (QOLI)
Q. of Life Questionnaire (QLQ)
q. of life rehabilitation assessment
q. of mood
negative q.
q. of obsession
q. of performance
poor sleep q.
primary q.
semiautomatic q.
q. of sexual functioning
q. of sleep
q. of speech
q. time
uncontrollable q.
Q. of Well-Being Scale

quality-adjusted
q.-a. life expectancy (QALE)
q.-a. life year (QALY)

QUALY
quality adjusted life-year

quandrantic hemianopia

quanta (*pl. of* quantum)

quantal hypothesis

quantified cognitive assessment

quantitative
  q. approach
  q. EEG analysis
  q. electroencephalogram (QEEG)
  q. electroencephalography (QEEG)
  q. electrophysiological battery
  q. imaging
  q. judgment
  q. motor unit potential analysis
  q. receptor autoradiography
  q. score
  q. semantics
  q. spectral phonoangiography
  Q. Sudomotor Axon Reflex Test
    (Q-SART)
  q. test (Q)
  q. variable
quantity
  absolute q.
  drug q.
  q. not sufficient (QNS)
  q. of speech
  sufficient q.
quantum, pl. **quanta**
  libido q.
  q. mechanics
  q. number
  q. theory
quarta
  macula cribrosa q.
quarter-way house
quarti
  apertura lateralis ventriculi q.
  apertura mediana ventriculi q.
quartile deviation (q)
quartz
Quartzo device
quasi-action
quasi-contract
quasi-experimental
  q.-e. design
  q.-e. research
quasi-expert
Quasimodo complex
quasi-need
quasi-purposive movement
quasi-representative
quasi-rhythmic
quaternity
quazepam
Queckenstedt-Stookey test
Queckenstedt test
quench
  magnet q.
querulans
  paranoia q.
querulent
querulous paranoia
quest
  Chronicle Career Q. (CCQ)
question
  closed-ended q.
  key q.
  open-ended q.
  Pigem q.

  q. stage
  yes-no q.
questioning
  q. faith problem
  socratic q.
questionnaire
  Abbreviated Conners Teacher Q.
  Adolescent Life Change Event Q.
    (ALCEQ)
  Adolescent Self-Report Trauma Q.
  Adult Neuropsychological Q.
    (ANQ)
  Adult Suicidal Ideation Q. (ASIQ)
  Agoraphobic Cognitions Q.
  Albany Panic and Phobia Q.
  Alcohol Usage Q. (AUQ)
  Andresen Six-Basic-Factors-
    Model Q. (A-SBFM)
  Anorectic Attitude Q.
  Anxiety Scale Q. (ASQ)
  assessment q.
  Attitude to School Q. (ASQ)
  Attributional Style Q.
  Q. of Basic Personality Support
  Beck Q.
  Behavioral Assessment of Pain Q.
    (P-BAP)
  Behavior Style Q. (BSQ)
  Big Five Q. (BFQ)
  Body Image and Eating Q.
  Body Sensations Q.
  Body Shape Q.
  Brief Disability Q.
  CAGE alcohol use q.
  Cattell Personality Factor Q.
  Change Agent Q. (CAQ)
  Childhood Antecedents Q.
  Child Neuropsychological Q. (CNQ)
  Children's Personality Q. (CPQ)
  Classroom Atmosphere Q. (CAQ)
  Clinical Analysis Q. (CAQ)
  Close Persons Q.
  Cognitive Failures Q. (CFQ)
  College Student Q. (CSQ)
  College Student Satisfaction Q.
    (CSSQ)
  Community College Student
    Experiences Q. (CCSEQ)
  Conners Abbreviated Symptom Q.
  Conners Parent Q. (CPQ)
  Conners Parent and Teacher
    Symptom Q.
  Conners Teacher Q. (CTQ)
  depression q.
  Depressive Experiences Q. (DEQ)
  description q.
  Desert Storm Trauma Q.
  development q.
  Diagnostic Symptom Q.
  Dimensional Assessment of
    Personality Pathology-Basic Q.
    (DAPP-BQ)
  Early School Personality Q.
    (ESPQ)
  Eight State Q.

Q

everyday memory q.
Extended Personal Attributes Q. (EPAQ)
Eysenck Personality Q. (EPQ)
Fagerstrom Tolerance Q.
Family Aptitudes Q. (FAQ)
Family Attitudes Q. (FAQ)
Fatigue Q.
Fear Q.
Frost Self-Description Q. (FSDQ)
Functional Status Q. (FSQ)
Functional Time Estimation Q. (FTEQ)
General Health Q. (GHQ)
General High Altitude Q. (GHAG, GHAQ)
Health Assessment Q. (HAQ)
Health Care Q.
High School Personality Q. (HSPQ)
Holmes-Rahe q.
Home Environment Q.
Home School Situations Q.-Revised
Home Screening Q.
Hostility and Direction of Hostility Q. (HDHQ)
Illness Behavior Q. (IBQ)
Insight to Treatment Q.
Insight and Treatment Attitudes Q. (ITAQ)
Intermediate Personality Q. (IPQ)
International Version of the Mental Status Q.
Intrex Q.
Kenney Self-Care Q.
Lambeth Disability Screening Q.
Leader Behavior Description Q. (LBDQ)
Leadership Opinion Q. (LOQ)
Leatherman Leadership Q. (LLQ)
Levine-Pilowsky Depression Q.
Managerial Style Q. (MSQ)
McGill Pain Q. (MPQ)
McMaster Health Index Q.
memory q.
Menstrual Distress Q. (MDQ)
Mental Status Q. (MSQ)
Minnesota Importance Q. (MIQ)
Minnesota Job Description Q. (MJDQ)
Minnesota Satisfaction Q. (MSQ)
Modified Health Assessment Q. (MHAQ)
modified McGill Pain Q.
Movement Disorder Q.
Multifactor Leadership Q. (MLQ)
NEO personality q.
Neuroticism/Extroversion/Openness to Experience personality q.
Neuroticism Scale Q. (NSQ)
OARS Multidimensional Functional Assessment Q. (OMFAQ)
Occupational Roles Q. (ORQ)
Offer Parent-Adolescent Q.
Offer Self-Image Q. (OSIQ)

Q. on Resources and Stress for Families with Chronically Ill or Handicapped
opinion q.
Organizational Value Dimensions Q. (OVDQ)
pain q.
Panic-Agoraphobic Spectrum Q.
Parental Acceptance-Rejection Q.
Parent-Teacher Q. (PTQ)
Patient Satisfaction Q.-III
Personal Attributes Q. (PAQ)
Personal Experience and Attitude Q. (PEAQ)
Personal Experience Screening Q. (PESQ)
personal history q.
personality q.
Personality Diagnostic Q.-Revised (PDQ-R)
Personality Factor Q. (PFQ)
16 Personality Factor Q. (16 PF)
Personal Resource Q. (PRQ)
Personal Strain Q. (PSQ)
Philadelphia Head Injury Q. (PHIQ)
Physicians' Q.
Pitowsky Illness Behavior Q.
Position Analysis Q. (PAQ)
Preliminary Diagnostic Q.
Preschool Behavior Q. (PBQ)
Psychosocial History Screening Q. (PHSQ)
Purdue Teacher Q. (PTQ)
Transitional Object Q.
Quality of Life Q. (QLQ)
Quality of Life Enjoyment and Satisfaction Q.
RAND Patient Satisfaction Q.
Revised Childhood Experiences Q.
Revised Denver Prescreening Development Q. (R-PDQ)
Rutter-B Q.
Rutter Child Behaviour Q.
Sales Personality Q. (SPQ)
Scale Q.
School Atmosphere Q. (SAQ)
Screening Q.
Seasonal Pattern Assessment Q. (SPAQ)
Self-Administered Dependency Q. (SADQ)
Self-Description Q. II (SDQII)
Self-Esteem Q.
Sense of Coherence Q.
Sexual Experiences Q.
Sexual and Physical Abuse Q.
Short Portable Mental Status Q. (SPMSQ)
Sixteen Personality Factor Q.
Smoking Behavior Q. (SBQ)
Social Adjustment Self-Report Q.
Speech Q.
Speech and Language Screening Q. (SLSQ)

questionnaire *(continued)*
 status q.
 Street Survival Skills Q.
 Student Adaptation to College Q.
 (SACQ)
 Subjective Response Q.
 Substance Abuse Q. (SAQ)
 Suicide Opinion Q. (SOQ)
 Teacher Feedback Q.
 Three-Factor Eating Q.
 Toronto Functional Capacity Q.
 (TFCQ)
 Tourette Syndrome Q.
 Traumatic Antecedents Q.
 Tridimensional Personality Q.
 Verbalizer-Visualization Q. (VVQ)
 Vocational Interest Q. (VIQ)
 Waring Intimacy Q. (WIQ)
 Work Attitudes Q. (WAQ)
quetiapine fumarate
Quick
 Q. Neurological Screening Test
 Q. Picture Vocabulary Test
 (QPVT)
 Q. Screening of Mental
 Development
 Q. Test (QT)
 Q. Word Test
quickening
Quick-Pep
Quick-Score Achievement Test
Quickscreen
quicksilver
quiescent
Quiess
quiet (qt)
 q. biting attack
 q. sleep
 wakefulness q.
 q. wakefulness mode
quieting
quietism
**QuietLite Quadrilite 6000 fiberoptic
 headlight**
quietude
quinalbarbitone
Quinamm
Quincke
 Q. disease
 Q. edema
 Q. puncture
 Q. spinal needle
quinethazone
quinidine
quinine
 q. ascorbate
 q. sulfate
quinolone
quintana
 Rochalimaea q.

quintessential
quinuclidinyl benzilate
quinupramine
quiritarian epilepsy
Quitaxon
Quiver
Quixote
 Don Q.
quixotic
quixotism
quo
 status q. (SQ)
quotient
 accomplishment q. (AQ)
 achievement q. (AQ)
 activity q.
 adolescent language q.
 ambivalent q.
 aphasia q. (AQ)
 brain age q.
 cognitive laterality q. (CLQ)
 Custody Q.
 custody q.
 deterioration q.
 deviation q.
 education q. (EQ)
 educational q. (EQ)
 expressive language q.
 Freedom from Distractibility
 Deviation Q. (FDDQ)
 Full-Scale Intelligence Q. (FSIQ)
 grammar language q.
 Hilson Personnel Profile/Success Q.
 (HPP/SQ)
 intelligence q. (IQ)
 Intimacy Potential Q. (IPQ)
 language q.
 listening language q.
 memory q. (MQ)
 open q.
 Perceptual Organization
 Deviation Q. (PODQ)
 Performance Intelligence Q. (PIQ)
 positive-negative ambivalent q.
 (PNAVQ)
 reading language q.
 receptive language-processing q.
 social q. (SQ)
 speed q.
 spoken language q.
 Verbal Comprehension Deviation Q.
 (VCDQ)
 Verbal Intelligence Q. (VIQ)
 verbal language q.
 vocabulary language q.
 Wechsler Memory
 Scale/Memory Q. (WMS-MQ)
 written language q.

R
relapse
relation
remission
R plasmid
90-R
RAATE score
RAB
remote afterloading brachytherapy
rabbit syndrome
rabid
rabies
r. encephalitis
r. virus
Rabiner neurological hammer
Rabot disease
raccoon eye
racemic amphetamine
rachial
rachicentesis
rachidial
rachidian
rachigraph
rachilysis
rachiocentesis
rachiochysis
rachiometer
rachiopathy
rachioplegia
rachioscoliosis
rachiotome
rachiotomy
rachischisis
r. partialis
posterior r.
r. posterior
r. totalis
rachitome
rachitomy
racial
r. discrimination
r. memory
R. Perceptions Inventory (RPI)
r. saturation point
racism
aversive r.
raclopride
radial
r. artery
r. artery graft
r. glia
r. nerve
r. phenomenon
r. prejudice
r. reflex
radian
radiant
radiate crown
radiatio, pl. **radiationes**
r. acustica
r. corporis callosi

r. optica
r. pyramidalis
radiation
acoustic r.
r. angiopathy
auditory r.
r. beam
beta-emitting r.
Bragg-peak r.
r. of corpus callosum
r. effect
electromagnetic r.
fibrosis r.
geniculocalcarine r.
Gratiolet r.
r. injury
leukoencephalopathy r.
low-energy gamma r.
r. myelopathy
r. necrosis
r. neuropathy
occipitothalamic r.
optic r.
r. precaution
pyramidal r.
r. retinopathy
single-fraction r.
stereotactic gamma r.
temporal lobe r.
r. therapy
r. vasculitis
visual r.
Wernicke r.
radiation-induced
r.-i. glioma
r.-i. mental deterioration
r.-i. vasculopathy
radiation-injury headache
radical
r. behaviorism
r. decompressive craniotomy
diflavin free r.
free r.
hydroxyl r.
r. prefrontal lobotomy
r. therapy
radices (*pl. of* radix)
radicis (*gen. of* radix)
radicotomy
radiculalgia
radicular
r. deficit
r. distribution of pain
r. hyporeflexia
r. motor deficit
r. neuropathy
r. syndrome
r. vein
radiculectomy
radiculitis
acute brachial r.
brachial r.

R

radiculoganglionitis
radiculomedullary
    r. fistula
    r. syndrome
radiculomeningeal spinal vascular
  malformation
radiculomeningomyelitis
radiculomyelopathy
radiculoneuropathy
radiculopathy
    cervical r.
    lumbosacral r.
radiculospinal artery
radii of angulation
radioactive iodide
radiobicipital reflex
radiocapitellar joint ganglion
radiofluoroscopy
    televised r.
Radiofocus introducer B kit
radiofrequency (RF, rf)
    r. coil
    r. eddy current
    r. electromagnetic field
    r. generator
    r. heating
    r. homogeneity pattern
    r. lesion
    r. lesioning
    r. needle electrode system
    r. pulse
    r. rhizotomy
    r. spoiling
    r. thermocoagulation
    r. thoracic sympathectomy
    r. transmitter
radiofrequency-induced echo
radiograph
radiography
    plain r.
radiohumeral joint
radioimmunoassay
radioimmunometric assay
radioimmunoprecipitation (RIP)
radioimmunotherapy
radioisotope
    r. brain scanning
    r. cisternogram
    r. cisternography
    r. scan
radiolabeled probe
radioligand
radiological
    chemical, bacteriological, r. (CBR)
    r. pressure-volume index
radiology
    interventional r.
radiolucency
    hydrocephalic periventricular r.
    periventricular r. (PVL)
radiolucent
    r. cranial pin headholder
    r. operating room table extension
radionecrosis
radioneuritis

Radionics
    R. bipolar coagulation unit
    R. bipolar instrument
    R. CRW stereotactic head frame
    R. RF lesion generator
radionucleotide scanning
radionuclide
    r. cisternography
    r. imaging
    r. study
radiopaque fiducial
radioperiosteal reflex
radiophobia
radioreceptor
radiosensitizer
radiosignal line
radiosurgery
    advanced design LINAC r.
    (ADLR)
    Bragg peak r.
    charged particle r.
    cranial r.
    extracranial r.
    gamma knife r.
    LINAC r.
    linear accelerator r.
    multiarc LINAC r.
    particle beam r.
    photon beam r.
    repeat r.
    stereotactic r.
    stereotactic r.
radiotherapy (RT, XRT)
    r. brain mapping
    fractionated r.
    heavy particle r.
    hyperfractionated r.
    interstitial r.
    mathematical optimization and
    logical dimensioning for r.
    (MOLDR)
    stereotactic linear accelerator r.
radius of angulation
radix, gen. radicis, pl. radices
    r. anterior
    r. brevis ganglii ciliaris
    r. cochlearis
    radices craniales
    r. dorsalis
    r. facialis
    r. inferior ansae cervicalis
    r. inferior nervi vestibulocochlearis
    r. lateralis nervi mediani
    r. lateralis tractus optici
    r. longa ganglii ciliaris
    r. medialis nervi mediani
    r. medialis tractus optici
    r. motoria
    r. nasociliaris
    r. nervi facialis
    radices nervi trigemini
    r. oculomotoria ganglii ciliaris
    r. parasympathica ganglii ciliaris
    r. posterior
    r. sensoria nervi trigemini

radices spinales
r. superior ansae cervicalis
r. superior nervi vestibulocochlearis
r. sympathica ganglii ciliaris
r. ventralis
r. vestibularis
Rado view of depressive disorder
RADS
Reynolds Adolescent Depression Scale
Raeder
R. paratrigeminal neuralgia
R. paratrigeminal syndrome
rage
r. attack
defiant r.
driver's r.
explosive r.
jealous r.
narcissistic r.
retroflexed r.
road r.
sham r.
unconscious r.
rageful feeling
ragged red fiber (RRF)
Ragin' Cajun disease
railroad neurosis
railway nystagmus
Raimondi
R. infant scalp hemostatic forceps
R. low pressure shunt
R. spring catheter
R. ventricular catheter
Rainin clip-bending spatula
rainy day woman
raison d'être
RALT
Riley Articulation and Language Test
RAM
rapid alternating movement
Rambaud syndrome
rambling
r. flow of thought
r. speech
rami (*pl. of* ramus)
ramicotomy
ramisection
ramitis
ramp stimulation
Ramsay Hunt
R. H. syndrome
R. H. type of inherited
dentatorubral degeneration
ramus, pl. rami
rami ad pontem
rami centrales anteromediales
rami choroidei
r. choroidei posteriores laterales
r. choroidei posteriores mediales
r. choroidei ventriculi lateralis
r. choroidei ventriculi quarti
r. choroidei ventriculi tertii
r. communicans
r. communicans cum nervo
glossopharyngeo

rami communicantes
dorsal rami
posterior primary r.
r. sinus carotici
rancorous
Rand
R. Functional Limitations Battery
R. Physical Capacities Battery
R. Social Health Battery
random
r. activity
r. assignment
R. Letter Test
R. Letter Test Raskin Severity of
Depression Scale
r. mating
r. model
r. movement
r. noise
r. observation
r. sample
r. variable
r. wave
randomization
randomized
r. clinical trial (RCT)
r. group design
**RAND Patient Satisfaction
Questionnaire**
Raney
R. coagulating forceps
R. laminectomy punch
R. laminectomy rongeur
R. perforator
R. rongeur forceps
R. scalp clip
R. scalp clip applier
R. scalp clip-applying forceps
R. stirrup-loop curette
range
r. of affect
affect within normal r.
alpha frequency r.
borderline r.
bright normal r.
dull normal r.
dynamic r.
emotional r.
r. of feeling
frequency r.
r. of interests
some degree of r.
tolerance r.
wide r.
ranging
wide r.
ranitidine
rank
r. correlation
r. order
percentile r.
rank-difference correlation
rankian
r. theory
r. therapy

R

ranking
    merit r.
Ransford loop
Ranvier
    R. cross
    R. disk
    node of R.
    R. node
    R. segment
RAP
    Relative Aspects of Potential
rap
    r. group
    r. session
rape
    r. act
    R. Aftermath Symptom Test
    anal r.
    r. crisis center
    date r.
    r. fantasy
    gang r.
    homosexual r.
    male r.
    sadistic act of r.
    spouse r.
    statutory r.
    r. trauma syndrome
raphe
    r. corporis callosi
    dorsal r.
    medullary r.
    r. nuclei
    r. pontis
    serotonergic dorsal r.
    Stilling r.
rapid
    r. acquisition radiofrequency-echo
      steady state imaging
    r. alternating movement (RAM)
    r. change in activity
    r. cycler
    r. cycling
    r. eye movement (REM)
    r. eye movement latency
    r. eye movement sleep
    r. eye movement state
    r. eye therapy
    r. fine movement
    r. motor movement
    r. neuroleptization
    r. nystagmus
    r. plasma reagin (RPR)
    r. repetitive movement
    r. speech
    r. tremor
    r. vocalization
rapid-change theory
rapid-cycling
    r.-c. bipolar disorder
    r.-c. course
    r.-c. pattern
rapidity
    r. of analyzing information

    r. of assimilating information
    r. of reinforcement
rapid-smoking theory
rapid-time-zone-change syndrome
rapport
    en r.
    inadequate r.
    interpersonal r.
    psychological r.
rapprochement
    r. crisis
    r. subphase
rapture-of-the-deep syndrome
raptus
    r. action
    r. of attention
    impulsive r.
    r. melancholicus
    status r.
rare detail response (Dr)
rarefaction
    r. stimulation
    r. stimulus
RAS
    reality-adaptive supportive
    reticular activating system
rasa
    tabula r.
rasagiline
rash
    butterfly r.
    glue sniffer's r.
    heliotrope r.
Raskin
    R. Depression Scale
    R. Severity of Depression Scale
Rasmussen
    R. encephalitis
    R. syndrome
ras **oncogene**
rasp
    Filtzer interbody r.
    Jansen r.
    Nicola r.
    Olivecrona r.
    Yasargil r.
ras signaling pathway
RAT
    Remote Associates Test
RATC
    Robert Apperception Test for Children
ratchet rigidity
rate
    accelerated heart r.
    alternate motion r. (AMR)
    basal metabolic r. (BMR)
    base r.
    birth r.
    case fatality r.
    concordance r.
    r. control
    cure r.
    death r.
    diadochokinesia r.
    divorce r.

R

erythrocyte sedimentation r. (ESR)
r. of fluency disturbance
fusion nonunion r.
implant survival r.
incidence r.
intrathecal IgG synthetic r.
limbic neuronal firing r.
long-term mortality r.
maturation r.
mentation r.
mortality r.
mutation r.
nonunion r.
prevalence r.
r. of production of speech
pseudarthrosis r.
response r.
specific absorption r.
suicide r.
transverse relaxation r.
T2 relaxation r.
vertebral osteosynthesis fusion r.

Rated
R. Anxiety Scale
R. Overall Life Impairment
Rathke
R. cleft cyst
R. pouch
R. pouch cyst
R. pouch tumor
Rathus Assertiveness Test
ratification theory
rating
Arithmetic Grade R.
behavior r.
Bunney-Hamburg nurse r.
Clinical Dementia R. (CDR)
daily symptom r.
evaluative r.
Flight Aptitude R. (FAR)
global r.
grade r.
internalized-state r.
R. Inventory for Screening
    Kindergartners
maturity r.
merit r.
peer r.
Reading Grade R.
risk rescue r. (RRR)
r. scale
R. Scale of Communication in
    Cognitive Decline (RSCCD)
sexual maturity r.
Spelling Grade R.
subjective unit of distress r.
symptom r.
Tanner sexual maturity r.
three-factor model of global r.
trait r.
ratio
absolute terminal innervation r.
achievement r. (AR)
affective r.
affectivity r.

age r.
association sensation r.
bicaudate r.
brain-to-plasma r.
CD4/CD8 r.
Cho:NAA r.
contrast-to-noise r. (CNR)
correlation r.
critical r.
dopamine r.
Evans r.
extinction r.
fixed r. (FR)
functional terminal innervation r.
guanine/cytosine r.
gyromagnetic r.
high affectivity r.
H/M r.
International Normalized R. (INR)
oral-nasal acoustic r. (TONAR)
r. scale
sex r.
signal-to-noise r. (SNR)
stimulation r.
^{99m}Tc HMPAO T/C r.
tumor:cerebellum r.
tumor:healthy tissue r.
variable r. (VR)
ventricle-to-brain r. (VBR)
rational
r. emotive therapy (RET)
r. medicine
r. psychology
r. psychotherapy
r. suicide
r. therapy (RT)
rational/cognitive coping
rationale
reduction r.
rational-emotive psychotherapy
rationalization defense mechanism
Ratliff avascular necrosis classification
rattle
death r.
rattlesnake bite
Raudixin
Rauverid
Rauwolfia
R. serpentina
rauwolfia
r. alkaloid
r. serpentina
Raven
R. Colored Progressive Matrices
    Test (RCPMT)
R. Standard Progressive Matrices
    (RSPM)
raving madness
RAVLT
Rey Auditory Verbal Learning Test
ray
R. brain spatula
R. brain spatula spoon
gamma r.
R. mania

ray *(continued)*
    photon r.
    R. pituitary curette
    R. syndrome
    R. Threaded Fusion Cage
Raybar 75
Raymond
    R. apoplexy
    R. syndrome
Raymond-Cestan syndrome
Raynaud
    R. phenomenon
    R. syndrome
rayon
Rayport
    R. dural dissector and knife
    R. dural and knife dissector
Ray-Tec sponge
Rayvist
RBD
    REM behavior disorder
RBE
    relative biological effectiveness
RBH Test of Learning Ability
RBMT
    Rivermead Behavioral Memory Test
RBRVS
    Resource-Based Relative Value Scale
rCBF
    regional cerebral blood flow
RCDS
    Revised Children's Depression Scale
    Reynolds Child Depression Scale
RCPMT
    Raven Colored Progressive Matrices Test
rCPP
    regional cerebral perfusion pressure
RCRS
    Rehabilitation Client Rating Scale
RCS
    Reality Check Survey
RCT
    randomized clinical trial
    Rorschach Content Test
RD
    reaction of degeneration
        DR or RD
RDA
    recommended daily allowance
RDC
    Research Diagnostic Criteria
RDI
    Retirement Descriptive Index
RDM, Rdm
    readmission
rea
    mens r.
reach
    grasp and r.
reactance
    inductive r.
reacting scale
reaction
    Abderhalden-Fauser r.

accelerated r.
acute paranoid schizophrenic r.
  (APSR)
acute stress situational r.
acute undifferentiated
  schizophrenic r. (AU/SR)
adaptation r.
adjustment r.
r. of adolescence
adolescent turmoil r.
adult situational stress r. (ASSR)
adverse drug r. (ADR)
affective depressive r.
aggressive r.
alarm r. (AR)
alcohol-Antabuse r.
allergic r.
all-or-none r.
amplification r.
anaphylactoid r.
anergastic r.
anesthetic conversion r.
anger r.
angry r.
anniversary r.
antigen-antibody r.
antisocial r.
anxiety r.
anxious mood adjustment r.
arousal r.
arrest r.
aseptic meningeal r.
associative r.
asthenic r.
astrocytic r.
autonomic conversion r.
aversion r.
behavior r.
r.'s biography
brief depressive r.
brief psychotic r.
cancer r.
cardiac r.
catastrophic r.
r. of childhood
choice r.
chronic paranoid schizophrenic r.
  (CPSR)
chronic stress r.
chronic undifferentiated
  schizophrenic r.
circular r.
civilian-catastrophe r.
climacteric paranoid r.
combat r.
compulsive psychoneurotic r.
conduct disturbance adjustment r.
confusional psychotic r.
consciousness disturbance stress r.
consensual r.
conversion psychoneurotic r.
cutaneous r.
dangerous behavior r.
r. to death
defense r.

defensive r.
deferred r.
r. of degeneration (RD)
dehydration r.
delayed hypersensitivity r.
delirious r.
dental-patient r.
depersonalization psychoneurotic r.
depressed mood adjustment r.
depressive r.
dissociate-dysmnesic substitution r.
dissociative r.
doll's eye r.
drug r.
duplicative r.
dysergastic r.
dyssocial r.
dysthymic adjustment r.
dystonic r.
echo r.
elective mutism adjustment r.
emotional r.
emotional conflicts or r.
emotional disturbance adjustment r.
emotional disturbance stress r.
emotionally unstable immaturity r.
emotions-conduct adjustment r.
escape r.
excitation psychotic r.
exogenous r.
fear r.
Fenton r.
fight-or-flight r.
fixation r.
r. formation
r. formation defense mechanism
galvanic skin r.
gemistocytic r.
general adaptation r.
glial r.
grief r.
gross stress r.
group delinquent r.
group stress r.
hand-to-mouth r.
heel-tap r.
hyperkinetic conversion r.
hypochondriacal psychoneurotic r.
hypomanic r.
hypomanic-depressive r.
hypomanic manic-depressive r.
hysterical conversion r. (HCR)
hysterical psychoneurotic r.
idiosyncratic r.
immaturity r.
intensity of r.
intermittent emotional conflicts
  or r.
involutional r.
Jarisch-Herxheimer fever r.
Jolly r.
justifiable r.
laryngeal psychophysiologic r.
late r.
latent schizophrenic r.

lengthening r.
R. Level Scale (RLS)
R. to Loss Inventory
LSD r.
magnet r.
maladaptive r.
maniacal grief r.
manic r.
manic-depressive r.
melancholic involutional r.
menopausal paranoid r.
r. to minor stimuli
mixed conduct/emotional disturbance
  adjustment r.
mixed disturbance stress r.
mixed emotions/conduct
  adjustment r.
mixed paralytic conversion r.
mixed stress r.
mobilization r.
MRZ r.
Much-Holzmann r.
myasthenic r.
neurasthenic psychoneurotic r.
neurogenic r.
neurotic r.
neurotic-depressive r.
nonpathological r.
obsessional psychoneurotic r.
obsessive r.
obsessive-compulsive r.
obsessive psychoneurotic r.
ocular tilt r.
organic r.
overanxious r.
pain r.
paradoxical r.
paranoid r.
paresthetic conversion r.
passive r.
passive-aggressive r.
passive-dependent r.
pathologic grief r.
personality r.
phantom r.
pharyngeal psychophysiologic r.
phobic psychoneurotic r.
physical symptoms adjustment r.
polymerase chain r. (PCR)
primary circular r.
prolonged depressive r.
prolonged grief r.
psychogalvanic skin r.
psychogenic r.
psychological r.
psychomotor disturbance stress r.
psychoneurotic r.
psychophysiologic r.
psychosomatic r.
psychotic trigger r. (PRT, PTR)
pupillary r.
qi-gong psychotic r.
recurrent episode psychotic r.
repetition r.
retrograde axon r.

reaction *(continued)*
    runaway r.
    r. scale
    schizophrenic r. (SR, S/R)
    schizophrenic reaction circular r.
    senile paranoid r.
    shock r.
    shortening r.
    simple paranoid r.
    single-episode psychotic r.
    situational r.
    socialized runaway r.
    somatization r.
    spite r.
    spoiled-child r.
    startle r.
    stress situational r.
    subacute organic r.
    suspected adverse drug r. (SADR)
    sympathetic stress r.
    symptomatically r.
    task-oriented r.
    tension state psychoneurotic r.
    tertiary circular r.
    r. test
    therapeutic r. (TR)
    thymonoic r.
    r. time (RT)
    toxic r.
    transference r.
    transient depressive r.
    transplantation r.
    trigger r.
    r. type
    unaggressive undersocialized r.
    undersocialized nonaggressive r.
    visual disorientation r.
    Wernicke r.
    withdrawal adjustment r.
reaction-type deterioration
reactivation process
reactive
    r. alcoholism
    r. astrocyte
    r. attachment disorder
    r. attachment disorder of infancy
    R. Attachment Disorder of Infancy or Early Childhood
    R. Attachment Disorder of Infancy or Early Childhood, Disinhibited Type
    R. Attachment Disorder of Infancy or Early Childhood, Inhibited Type
    r. bowel
    r. cell
    r. confusion
    r. confusional state
    r. confusion nonorganic psychosis
    r. depression and anxiety
    r. depressive psychosis
    r. disorder
    r. ego alteration
    r. epilepsy

    r. exaltation
    r. excitation
    r. excitement
    r. gliosis
    r. inhibition
    r. mania
    r. measure
    r. melancholia
    r. mental excitement
    r. paranoid psychosis
    r. psychotic depression
    r. reinforcement
    r. response
    r. schizophrenia
    symptomatically r.
    r. thought
reactivity
    affective r.
    automatic r.
    autonomic r.
    lack of r.
    mood r.
    physiological r.
reactor
    placebo r.
readaptation
    neurobehavioral r.
readiness
    Anton Brenner Developmental Gestalt Test of School R.
    complex r.
    explosion r.
    r. inventory
    Lollipop Test: A Diagnostic Screening Test of School R.
    reading r.
    R. Scale - Self Rating and Manager Rating Forms
    Screening Test of Academic R.
    Slosson Test of Reading R. (STRR)
    r. test
reading
    r. achievement
    r. backwardness
    R. Comprehension Battery for Aphasia
    r. comprehension impairment
    R. Comprehension Inventory
    delusions of mind r.
    r. developmental delay disorder
    Diagnostic Assessments of R. (DAR)
    r. disability
    r. epilepsy
    r. grade equivalent
    R. Grade Rating
    Individualized Criterion Reference Testing R. (ICRTR)
    r. language quotient
    lip r.
    mind r.
    R. Miscue Inventory (RMI)
    Progressive Achievement Tests of R.

r. readiness
R. Sight Vocabulary Standard
  Score
r. skills acquisition
r. skills learning retardation
thought r.
reading/everyday activities in life
Reading-Free Vocational Interest
  Inventory (RFVII)
reading, writing and repetition
readjust
readmission (RDM, Rdm)
readout
r. delay
r. gradient
r. period
reaffirm
reagin
rapid plasma r. (RPR)
real
r. abandonment
r. anxiety
r. external stimulus
r. image
r. life
r. loss
r. origin
r. self
realignment
circadian r.
realism
experimental r.
moral r.
mundane r.
realistic
r. plan
r. thinking
reality
r. ability testing
r. adaptation
r. anxiety
r. assumption
r. awareness
break with r.
R. Check Survey (RCS)
r. confrontation
contact with r.
r. denial
denial of external r.
disconnection with r.
r. ego
escape from r.
external r.
flight from r.
independent physical r.
r. issue
r. life of ego
objective r.
r. orientation (RO)
r. oriented (RO)
r. oriented therapy
out of touch with r.
perceived r.
phenomenological r.
r. principle

psychical r.
relativity of r.
retreat from r.
sense of r.
r. system
r. test
r. testing
r. testing ability
r. ties
ties with r.
reality-adaptive supportive (RAS)
reality-oriented supportive strategy
realization
symbolic r.
real-life
r.-l. circumstance
r.-l. problem
real-time
r.-t. color Doppler imaging
r.-t. guidance
r.-t. monitoring
real-world setting
reaming awl
reanalysis strategy
reanalyzed data
reanimation
facial r.
reason
R.'s for Living Inventory (RLI)
r. for visit
reasonable
r. ego
r. fear
reasoning
r. ability
abstract r.
age of r.
arithmetical r.
Arlin Test of Formal R.
deductive r.
r. disturbance
dynamic r.
evaluative r.
exonerative moral r.
hypothetical-deductive r.
idiosyncratic r.
illogical r.
inductive r.
r. mania
r. and memory skills
Nonverbal R.
practical r.
Similarities Test of Verbal
  Abstract R.
syllogistic r.
verbal, numerical, and r. (VNR)
reassessment
attitude r.
sexual attitude r. (SAR)
reassignment
gender r.
hormonal sexual r.
sexual r.
surgical sex r.
reassociation

reassurance sensitivity
reassuring explanation
reattribution technique
rebelliousness
Rebif MS
rebirth fantasy
rebleed
    aneurysmal r.
rebleeding of aneurysm
rebound
    r. insomnia
    r. mood swing
    r. nystagmus
    r. phenomenon
    REM sleep r.
reboxetine mesylate
rebus principle
recalcitrant pain
recalibrate
recall
    body-image r.
    delayed r.
    digit r.
    diminished r.
    dream r.
    free r.
    inconsistent r.
    r. of information test
    r. 5 items after 5 minutes test
    r. memory
    memory r.
    r. method
    recognition vs. r.
    recollection and r.
    retention and r.
    rote r.
    total r.
    verbatim r.
    vivid dream r.
recall-generated emotion
recalling new information disturbance
recanalization
    angiographic r.
    TCD r.
recant
recapitulation
    pubertal sexual r.
recapture
recathexis
recede
receiver
    r. bandwidth
    r. coil
    r. limitation
    r. operating characteristic (ROC)
    r. overflow
    r. overload
    r. saturation
receiving type
recency
    positive r.
recent
    r. life event (RLE)
    r. past memory

receptive
    r. aphasia
    r. character
    r. dysphagia
    r. dysphasia
    r. function
    r. language development
    r. language disorder
    r. language-processing
    r. language-processing quotient
    R. One Word Picture Vocabulary
      Test (ROWPVT)
    r. orientation
    r. personality
receptive-expressive
    R.-e. Emergent Language (REEL)
    R.-e. Emergent Language scale
    r.-e. observation (REO)
    R.-e. Observation Scale
receptoma
receptor
    acetylcholine r. (AChR)
    acetylcholine cholinergic r.
    ACh r.
    adrenergic r.
    all-trans retinoic acid r.
    alpha adrenergic r.
    r. alteration
    beta adrenergic r.
    cholinergic r.
    9-cis retinoic acid r. (RXR)
    delta opiate r.
    r. density
    r. dimerization
    distance r.
    dopamine r.
    epidermal growth factor r. (EGFR)
    epsilon opiate r.
    excitatory amino acid r.
    extrasynaptic r.
    r. functioning
    heterodimeric r.
    5-HT2 r.
    5-HT3 r.
    5HTIA r.
    kappa opiate r.
    r. ligand
    mu opiate r.
    muscarinic cholinergic r.
    neurotransmitter r.
    nicotinic acetylcholine r.
    nicotinic cholinergic r.
    NMDA r.
    N-methyl-D-aspartate r.
    noradrenergic r.
    opiate r.
    opioid r.
    pain r.
    peroxisomal proliferator r. (PPAR)
    postsynaptic r.
    proximal r.
    sensory r.
    serotonergic r.
    sigma r.
    signal transducing r.

stretch r.
tumor necrosis factor r. (TNFR)
tyrosine-kinase r.
unencapsulated joint r.
vitamin D r. (VDR)

recess
cerebellopontine r.
cochlear r.
infundibular r.
lateral r. of fourth ventricle
optic r.
pineal r.
pontocerebellar r.
Reichert cochlear r.
suprapineal r.
triangular r.

recessive
autosomal r.
r. dystonia musculorum deformans
r. gene
r. trait

recessus, pl. recessus
r. anterior
r. cochlearis
r. infundibuli
r. lateralis ventriculi quarti
r. opticus
r. pinealis
r. posterior
r. suprapinealis
r. triangularis

Rechtschaffen
criteria of R.

recidivation
recidivism
r. in schizophrenia
victim r.

recipient
action r.

recipiomotor
reciprocal
r. agreement
r. assimilation
r. communication
r. determinism
r. inhibition
r. inhibition and desensitization
r. inhibition psychotherapy
r. parenting
r. punishment
r. regulation
r. social interaction

reciprocity
emotional r.
overadequate-inadequate r.

recitative
recite
survey, question, read, review, r.
(SQ3R)

reckless behavior
Recklinghausen disease
recognition
facial r.
r. memory
R. Memory Test

pattern r.
Reitan-Klove Tactile Form R.
r. site
r. time
visual pattern r.
r. vs. recall
r. in wit

recognize, empathize, think, hear, integrate, notice, keep (RETHINK)
recollection
intrusive r.
r. and recall
r. of trauma

recombinant
r. DNA technique
r. human tumor necrosis factor-α
r. tau isoform
r. tissue plasminogen activator

recommencement
mania of r.
r. mania

recommended daily allowance (RDA)
reconciliation attempt
reconditioning
orgasmic r.
r. therapy

reconstituted family
reconstruction
craniofacial r.
r. dream
maximum intensity pixel r.
r. method
pathology-induced memory r.
split bone graft r.
three-dimensional r.

reconstructive
r. psychotherapy
r. therapy

record
activity r.
automated clinical r.
Bayley Behavior R.
behavior r.
chronological drinking r.
cumulative r.
far-field r.
Functional Performance R. (FPR)
infant behavior r.
Kuder Preference R.
Kuder Preference R.-Vocational
(KPR-V)
Manager Profile R.
medical r.
near-field r.
Periodic Evaluation R. (PER)
problem-oriented r. (POR)
Supervisory Profile R.

recording
ambulatory EEG r.
behavior-specimen r.
continuous electromyographic r.
continuous on-line r.
depth r.
microelectrode r.
nonreference r.

recording *(continued)*
    paired electrode r.
    r. procedure
    videocassette r.
recovery
    r. from delinquency
    full interepisode r.
    r. of function
    interepisode r.
    inversion r.
    language r.
    partial r.
    r. and reorganization
    saturation r.
    short-tau inversion r. (STIR)
    short time inversion r.
    social r.
    spontaneous r.
    r. stage
    uncomplicated r.
    r. wish
recreation
    active r.
    passive r.
    therapeutic r.
recreational
    r. drinking
    r. drug
    r. drug use
    r. therapy (RT)
recruiting response
recruitment
    r. line
    r. pattern
rectal
    r. disease
    r. psychogenic disorder
    RMS R.
rectangle
    Hartshill r.
    Luque r.
rectangular
    r. awl
    r. brain spatula
rectocardiac reflex
rectolaryngeal reflex
rectophobia *(var. of* proctophobia)
rectosigmoidal endoscopic
rectum
    per r.
rectus
    gyrus r.
    r. paralysis
recurrent
    r. artery of Heubner
    r. brief depressive disorder
    r. depersonalization
    r. dream
    r. encephalopathy
    r. enteric cyst
    r. episode
    r. episode chronic mania
    r. episode depressive psychosis
    r. episode psychotic

    r. episode psychotic depression
    r. episode psychotic reaction
    r. illusion
    r. laryngeal nerve
    major depressive disorder, r.
    r. mania
    r. melancholia
    r. migraine headache
    r. motor movement
    r. pain
    r. panic attack
    r. perforating artery
    r. polyneuropathy
    r. seizure
    r. suicidal ideation
    r. thought
    r. tumor
    r. vocalization
recurring
    r. dream
    r. headache
    r. idea
    r. theme
recursion
recursive autoassociative memory
recycled air
recycling
    lipid r.
red
    r. man syndrome
    r. neck syndrome
    r. neuralgia
    r. nucleus
    r. phosphorus
    r. rubber catheter
redifferentiation
redirection
redness of eye
reduced
    r. attention ability
    r. level of consciousness
    r. rapid eye movement latency
    r. responsiveness
    r. sodium diet restricted diet
    r. verbal output
reducer
    Cloward cervical dislocation r.
reductase
    aldose r.
reduction
    accident r.
    r. of amplitude
    anxiety r.
    r. of anxiety
    cluster r.
    contrast sensitivity r.
    cue r.
    drive r.
    R.'s in Eating Attitudes Test
    r. fixation
    fracture r.
    fracture-dislocation r.
    r. method
    pain threshold r.
    perioperative r.

r. rationale
risk r.
spondylolisthesis r.
r. stabilization
stress r.
swan neck deformity r.
r. technique
tension r.
T12-L1 fracture-dislocation r.
reductive
redundancy
correlation r.
genetic r.
r. rule
redundant neuron
Redupax
reduplicated babbling
reduplicative paramnesia
Redutemp
Redux
reeducation
emotional r.
reeducative therapy
REEL
Receptive-Expressive Emergent
Language
REEL scale
reemergence
reenactment
emotional r.
trauma-specific r.
reevaluation counseling
reexperienced traumatic event
reexperiencing
r. perceptual symptom
r. trauma
reference
cultural frame of r.
delusion of r.
r. electrode
frame of r.
r. group
idea of r.
r. measurement
memory r.
r. montage
Physicians' Desk R. (PDR)
rotating frame of r.
standard r.
transient ideas of r.
r. zero level
referencing
dynamic r.
optical image guided surgery
system with dynamic r.
referential
r. attitude
r. delusion
r. function
r. idea
r. index
r. semantics
referred
r. pain
r. sensation

ReFix
R. noninvasive fixation
R. stereotactic head fixator
R. stereotactic head holder
reflectance spectrophotometry
reflection
factor r.
r. of feeling
reflex, pl. **reflexes**
A r.
abdominal r.
absent r.
accommodation r.
r. accommodation
Achilles tendon r.
acoustic r.
acousticopalpebral r.
acquired r.
acromial r.
r. act
acute affective r.
adductor r.
r. akinesia
allied r.
r. amaurosis
anal r.
ankle r.
r. anosmia
antagonistic r.
aponeurotic r.
r. arc
r. asymmetry
attention r.
attitudinal r.
auditory oculogyric r.
auriculopalpebral r.
auropalpebral r. (APR)
autoaggressive behavior r.
axon r.
Babinski r.
back of foot r.
bar r.
Barkman r.
basal joint r.
Bechterew-Mendel r.
behavior r.
Benedek r.
Bezold-Jarisch r.
biceps femoris r.
Bing r.
bladder r.
blink r.
body righting r.
bone r.
brachioradial r.
Brain r.
brainstem r.
bregmocardiac r.
brisk r.
Brissaud r.
bulbocavernosus r.
bulbomimic r.
carotid sinus r.
r. center
cephalic r.

R

reflex *(continued)*
  cephalopalpebral r.
  cervicocollic r.
  Chaddock r.
  chain r.
  r. change
  chin r.
  Chodzko r.
  ciliospinal r.
  cochleo-orbicular r.
  cochleopalpebral r.
  cochleopupillary r.
  cochleostapedial r.
  conditioned r.
  consensual r.
  contralateral r.
  r. control
  r. convulsion
  convulsive r.
  coordinated r.
  corneal r.
  costal arch r.
  costopectoral r.
  cough r.
  craniocardiac r.
  cremasteric r.
  crossed adductor r.
  crossed extension r.
  crossed knee r.
  crossed r. of pelvis
  crossed spinoadductor r.
  cry r.
  cuboidodigital r.
  cutaneous pupillary r.
  darwinian r.
  r. decay
  deep abdominal r.
  deep tendon r. (DTR)
  defecation r.
  defense r.
  deglutition r.
  Dejerine r.
  delayed r.
  depressed r.
  detrusor r.
  diffused r.
  digital r.
  diminished r.
  r. disorder
  diving r.
  doll's eye r.
  dorsal r.
  dorsocuboidal r.
  dorsum of foot r.
  dorsum pedis r.
  ejaculatory r.
  elbow r.
  emptying r.
  enterogastric r.
  epigastric r.
  erector-spinal r.
  esophagosalivary r.
  external oblique r.
  eye-closure r.

  r. eye movement
  facial r.
  faucial r.
  femoral r.
  femoroabdominal r.
  finger-thumb r.
  flexion r.
  flexor r.
  forced grasping r.
  front-tap r.
  gag r.
  Galant r.
  galvanic skin r.
  gastrocolic r.
  gastroileac r.
  Geigel r.
  Gifford r.
  glabella tap r.
  gluteal r.
  Golda r.
  Golgi r.
  Gordon r.
  grasping r.
  grasping and groping r.
  great toe r.
  Guillain-Barré r.
  gustatory-sudorific r.
  H r.
  r. hallucination
  hand-to-mouth r.
  r. headache
  heart r.
  Hering-Breuer r.
  Hoffmann r.
  hypochondrial r.
  hypogastric r.
  r. incontinence
  r. inhibition of epilepsy
  innate r.
  interscapular r.
  intersegmental r.
  intrasegmental r.
  intrinsic r.
  inverted radial r.
  investigatory r.
  ipsilateral r.
  r. iridoplegia
  Jacobson r.
  jaw r.
  jaw-closing muscle r.
  jaw winking r.
  jaw-working r.
  Joffroy r.
  Kisch r.
  knee-jerk r.
  labyrinthine righting r.
  lacrimal r.
  lacrimogustatory r.
  Landau r.
  laryngospastic r.
  r. latency
  latent r.
  laughter r.
  Liddell-Sherrington r.
  lip r.

Lovén r.
lower abdominal periosteal r.
magnet r.
mandibular r.
mass r.
masseter r.
Mayer r.
McCarthy r.
mediopubic r.
Mendel-Bechterew r.
Mendel instep r.
metacarpohypothenar r.
metacarpothenar r.
metatarsal r.
micturition r.
milk-ejection r.
Mondonesi r.
Moro r.
muscle stretch r.
muscular r.
Myerson r.
myotatic r.
myxedema r.
nasomental r.
neck r.
r. neurogenic bladder
r. neurologic activity
nociceptive r.
nocifensor r.
nose-bridge-lid r.
nose-eye r.
nuchocephalic r.
oculocardiac r.
oculocephalic r.
oculocephalogyric r.
oculovestibular r.
olecranon r.
Oppenheim r.
optical righting r.
opticofacial r.
orbicularis oculi r.
orbicularis pupillary r.
orienting r.
oropharyngeal r.
palatal r.
palatine r.
palmar r.
palm-chin r.
palmomental r.
parachute r.
paradoxical extensor r.
patellar tendon r.
patelloadductor r.
pathologic r.
r. pattern
pectoral r.
Perez r.
pericardial r.
periosteal r.
pharyngeal r.
phasic r.
Phillipson r.
pilomotor r.
Piltz r.
plantar muscle r.

pollicomental r.
positive conditioned r.
postural r.
pressoreceptor r.
primitive r.
pronator r.
proprioceptive r.
protective laryngeal r.
psychic r.
psychocardic r.
psychogalvanic r. (PGR)
pulmonocoronary r.
pupillary light r.
pupillary skin r.
quadriceps r.
quadripedal extensor r.
radial r.
radiobicipital r.
radioperiosteal r.
rectocardiac r.
rectolaryngeal r.
Remak r.
respiratory r.
riddance r.
righting r.
Roger r.
rooting r.
Rossolimo r.
scapular r.
scapulohumeral r.
scapuloperiosteal r.
Schäffer r.
scrotal r.
r. seizure
semimembranosus r.
semitendinosus r.
r. sensation
sensitivity prediction from the
  acoustic r. (SPAR)
sinus r.
skin r.
skin-muscle r.
skin-pupillary r.
snapping r.
snout r.
sole tap r.
r. spasm
spinal r.
spinoadductor r.
stapes r.
Starling r.
startle r.
static r.
statokinetic r.
statotonic r.
sternobrachial r.
sternutatory r.
stress-altered startle r.
stretch r.
Strümpell r.
styloradial r.
sucking r.
superficial r.
supination r.
supinator longus r.

reflex *(continued)*
    supraorbital r.
    suprapatellar r.
    supraumbilical r.
    swallowing r.
    r. sympathetic dystrophy (RSD)
    r. sympathetic dystrophy syndrome
      (RSDS)
    synchronous r.
    tarsophalangeal r.
    tendo Achillis r.
    tendon r.
    r. therapy
    threat r.
    r. threshold
    thumb r.
    thumb-chin r.
    r. time
    toe r.
    tonic foot r.
    tonic neck r.
    trace conditioned r.
    trained r.
    triceps surae r.
    trigeminofacial r.
    trochanter r.
    Trömner r.
    ulnar r.
    unconditioned r. (UCR)
    upper abdominal periosteal r.
    urinary r.
    utricular r.
    vasopressor r.
    venorespiratory r.
    vesical r.
    vestibuloocular r. (VOR)
    vestibulospinal r.
    viscerogenic r.
    visceromotor r.
    viscerosensory r.
    visual orbicularis r.
    vomiting r.
    Wartenberg r.
    Weingrow r.
    Westphal pupillary r.
    wink r.
    withdrawal r.
    wrist clonus r.
reflexive movement
reflexogenic zone
reflexogenous
reflexograph
reflexology
reflexometer
reflexophil, reflexophile
reflexotherapy
reflux
    ejaculation r.
    r. management
    sleep-related gastroesophageal r.
reform
    thought r.
reformation
reformatory paranoia

reformatted image
reformist delusion
reformulation
refractoriness to treatment
refractory
    r. period
    r. state
    r. status epilepticus (RSE)
    treatment r.
refraining
reframing
    context r.
    meaning r.
refreshing sleep attack
refrigerator parenting
Refsum
    R. disease
    R. peripheral neuropathy
    R. syndrome
refusal
    school r.
    r. of treatment
regard
    field of r.
    mutual r.
    point of r.
    positive r.
    unconditional positive r.
regeneration
    aberrant r.
    axon r.
    axonal r.
    neural r.
    neuronal r.
regimen
    birth control r.
    postoperative r.
region
    brain r.
    bridge r.
    craniocervical r.
    critical r.
    dorsolateral r.
    germ-cell tumor with synchronous
      lesions in pineal and
      suprasellar r. (GCTSPS)
    hyaluron-binding r.
    r. of interest (ROI)
    motoric r.
    occipitonuchal r.
    orbitofrontal r.
    paramedian r.
    paranodal r.
    perceptual-motor r.
    pineal r.
    preoptic r.
    prepontine r.
    pretectal r.
    subicular r.
    temporal speech r.
    temporomesial r. (TMR)
    transentorhinal r.
    watershed r.
    Wernicke r.

R

regional
- r. background
- r. cerebral blood flow (rCBF)
- r. cerebral blood flow scintigraphy
- r. cerebral metabolic rate of oxygen
- r. cerebral perfusion pressure (rCPP)
- r. differentiation
- r. enteritis
- r. epilepsy
- r. hypothermia
- r. ileitis
- r. oxygen extraction fraction

register
- case r.
- psychiatric case r.

registered
- Activities Therapist, R. (ATR)
- Music Therapist, R. (MTR)
- r. nurse
- r. recreation therapist

registration
- r. error
- r. menu
- segmental r.
- surface vessel r.

registry
- Acoustic Neuroma R.
- Brain Tumor R.
- Clozaril National R.
- Mayo Alzheimer Disease Center/Alzheimer Disease Patient R.

Regitine
regnancy
Regonol Injection
regression
- age r.
- r. analysis
- atavistic r.
- r. defense mechanism
- Galton law of r.
- logistic r.
- multiple r.
- r. neurosis
- partial r.
- past-life hypnotic r.
- phenomenal r.
- progressive teleologic r.
- spontaneous r.
- teleologic r.

regressive
- r. alcoholism
- r. assimilation
- r. behavior
- r. electroshock treatment (REST)
- r. infantilism
- r. schizophrenia
- r. substitute
- r. symptoms of schizophrenia
- r. transference neurosis

regressive-inspirational
- r.-i. group
- r.-i. group psychotherapy

regressive-reconstructive approach
regrowth
- axon r.

regular
- r. diet
- R. Iletin I
- R. Strength Bayer Enteric 500 Aspirin

regulation
- cerebrovascular r.
- immune system r.
- impulse r.
- reciprocal r.
- sexual r.
- volume r.

regulator
- suction Regugauge r.

regulatory
Regulus frameless stereotactic system
regurgitant lesion
regurgitation
rehabilitation
- acoupedic r.
- alcoholic r.
- aquatic r.
- r. assessment
- r. behavior
- Boston University Model of Psychiatric R.
- R. Client Rating Scale (RCRS)
- cognitive r.
- r. counselor
- r. evaluation
- r. facility
- geriatric r.
- R. Indicator (RIs)
- neurologic r.
- neuromuscular r.
- occupational r.
- r. psychiatry
- psychosocial r.
- sexual r.
- social r.
- r. stage
- testing, orientation, and work evaluation for r. (TOWER)
- r. treatment
- vocational r. (VR)

Rehbein rib spreader
rehearsal
- behavior r.
- behavioral r.
- cognitive r.
- obsessional r.
- thought r.

Reichert
- R. cochlear recess
- R. stereotaxy system

Reichert-Mundinger
- R.-M. stereotactic head frame
- R.-M. syndrome

Reichert-Mundinger-Fischer stereotactic head frame
Reid
- R. base line

Reid *(continued)*
> R. baseline
> R. Report

reign of terror
Reiki
Reil
> R. ansa
> R. band
> R. ribbon
> R. triangle

rein
> free r.

reincarnation
reindoctrination
reinforced
> r. practice
> r. thought

reinforcement
> adventitious r.
> aperiodic r.
> chained r.
> concurrent r.
> conjunctive r.
> contingency r.
> continuous r.
> r. counseling
> covert r.
> delayed r.
> differential r.
> fixed r.
> homogeneous r.
> intermittent r.
> interval r.
> mixed r.
> multiple r.
> negative r.
> partial r.
> periodic r.
> positive r.
> predelay r.
> primary r.
> rapidity of r.
> reactive r.
> schedule of r.
> r. schedule
> secondary r.
> self-managed r.
> social r.
> systematic r.
> tandem r.
> Teflon mesh r.
> terminal r.
> time out from r.
> variable r.
> verbal r.

reinforcer
> conditioned r.
> negative r.
> positive r.
> primary r.
> secondary r.

reinnervation of target organ
reinsert
reinstinctualization

reintegration
Reintegration to Normal Living Index
reinterpret
reintrojection
Reissner
> R. fiber
> R. membrane

Reitan
> R. (and Selz) rules to assess
> R. Evaluation of Hemispheric
> Abilities and Brain Improvement
> Training

Reitan-Indiana
> R.-I. Aphasia Screening Test
> (RIAST)
> R.-I. Neuropsychological Test
> Battery for Adults
> R.-I. Neuropsychological Test
> Battery for Children

Reitan-Klove
> R.-K. Lateral Dominance
> Examination
> R.-K. Sensory Perceptual
> Examination
> R.-K. Tactile Form Recognition
> R.-K. Tactile Form Recognition
> Test

reiterate
Reiter syndrome
rejecting-neglecting parent
rejecting parent
rejection
> r. fear
> fear of r.
> feelings of r.
> interpersonal r.
> maternal r.
> parental r.
> perceived interpersonal r.
> r. sensitivity

rejuvenation fantasy
relabeling
Relafen
relapse (R)
> full r.
> impending r.
> r. prevention

relapse-prevention technique
relapsing
> r. hypertrophic neuritis
> r. neuropathy
> r. polychondritis

related
> alcohol r. (AR)
> drug r.
> r. psychopathology
> r. sleep disorder
> transformational r.
> transformationally r.

relatedness
> developmentally inappropriate
> social r.
> disturbed social r.
> failure to develop r.
> functional r.

inappropriate social r.
semantic r.
social r.
symbiotic r.
relating
disordered r.
forms of satisfactory r.
r. to others
time periods of satisfactory r.
relation (R)
r. to age
community-institutional r.'s
court of domestic r.'s
extramarital r.'s
family r.
human r.
intergenerational r.
interinstitutional r.
interpersonal r.
interprofessional r.
object r.
perception of spatial r.'s
professional-family r.
sexual r.
sibling r.
step r.
r.'s test
relational
r. behavior
r. opposite
r. problem
r. threshold
r. unit
relationship
addiction r.
r. addiction
anaclitic r.
appropriate r.
causal r.
cause-effect r.
chewing-speech r.
chronological r.
clearly demarcated r.
competent r.
conflictual r.
consistent r.
counseling r.
counterintuitive r.
demarcated r.
destructive r.
detachment from social r.
disrupted r.
disturbed interpersonal r.'s (DIR)
doctor-patient r.
dysfunctional r.
early r.
etiological r.
failure to sustain a monogamous r.
family r.
helping r.
r. history
hypnotic r.
I-it r.
impaired r.

impersonal r.
incestual r.
instability in interpersonal r.
intense r.
interpersonal r.
interpsychic r.
intrafamilial r.
r. inventory
inverse r.
inversion r.
I-thou r.
meaningful interpersonal r.
monogamous r.
mother-child r. (MCR)
mother-infant r.
negative r.
no-win r.
object r.
optimal r.
parent-child r.
peer r.
perfect negative r.
perfect positive r.
periodic reinforcement r.
personal r.
Personal Assessment of Intimacy
in R.'s (PAIR)
physician-patient r.
platonic r.
poor peer r.
positive r.
primary r.
r. problems of childhood
r. psychotherapy
replacement r.
required r.
sadomasochistic r.
semantic r.
spectral r.
stress-strain r.
temporal r.
therapeutic r.
r. therapy
transference r.
troubled r.
trusting r.
unsatisfying r.
unstable r.
working r.
relative
r. afferent pupillary defect
R. Aspects of Potential (RAP)
r. band amplitude
r. biological effectiveness (RBE)
r. dementia
r. elective mutism
first-degree biological r.'s
r. frequency
r. hyperemia
r. impotence
r. risk
r. scotoma
r. slow-wave sleep stability
R. Value Scale

relativism
    cultural r.
    moral r.
relativity
    law of r.
    r. of reality
    special theory of r.
relaxant
    depolarizing muscle r.
    muscle r.
    skeletal muscle r.
relaxation
    r. constant
    differential r.
    dipole-dipole r.
    intramolecular r.
    longitudinal r.
    nuclear r.
    paramagnetic r.
    progressive r.
    progressive muscular r.
    r. rate enhancement
    r. response
    spin-lattice r.
    spin-spin r.
    stress r.
    T1 r.
    T2 r.
    r. technique
    r. technique training
    r. theory
    therapeutic r.
    r. therapy
    r. time
    transverse r.
relaxation-induced anxiety (RIA)
relaxed
    squarely (face person), open
        posture, lean (toward person), eye
        (contact), r. (SOLER)
relay
    thalamocortical r. (TCR)
relearning method
release
    emotional r.
    neurotransmitter r.
    orgastic r.
    r. phenomenon
    platelet thromboxane r.
    r. therapy
Relefact TRH injection
relevant
    r. diagnostic criteria
    r. diagnostic criterion
reliability
    r. coefficient
    equivalent form r.
    index of r.
    interjudge r.
    interobserver r.
    interrater r.
    test-retest r.
reliable history
reliance
    hemispheric r.

relief
    pain r.
    Solarcaine Aloe Extra Burn R.
    Tylenol Extended R.
reliever
    Arthritis Foundation Pain R.
    Cama Arthritis Pain R.
religiosa
    melancholia r.
religious
    r. activity
    r. affiliation
    r. cult
    r. delusion
    r. ecstasy
    r. faith
    r. insanity
    r. institution
    r. mania
    r. obsession
    r. orthodoxy factor
    r. or spiritual problem
    r. values
Relton-Hall frame
REM
    rapid eye movement
        REM activity
        REM behavior disorder (RBD)
        REM density
        REM latency
        REM period
        REM sleep
        REM sleep behavior
        REM sleep behavior disorder
        REM sleep efficiency
        REM sleep rebound
        REM state
remacemide
Remak
    R. fiber
    R. ganglia
    R. reflex
    R. sign
remark
    derogatory r.
    self-deprecatory r.
remedial
    r. intervention
    r. psychotherapy
    r. teaching
remediation
    cognitive r.
Remeron
remifentanil
remilitarize
reminder
    traumatic r.
reminisce
reminiscence therapy
reminiscent
    r. aura
    r. neuralgia
Reminyl
remission (R)
    early full r.

partial r.
spontaneous r.
sustained full r.
sustained partial r.
transference r.
remitting
r. dementia
r. schizophrenia
remodeled forehead
remodeling
craniofacial r.
neural foramen r.
REM-onset sleep
remorse
lack of r.
remote
r. afterloading brachytherapy (RAB)
R. Associates Test (RAT)
r. memory
r. symptomatic seizure
remotivation
removal
Arana-Iniquez intracranial cyst r.
Dowling intracranial cyst r.
implant r.
metastatic tumor r.
rib r.
transsphenoidal r.
removed affect
remuneration
remyelinate
renal
r. failure
r. ganglia
Rendu-Osler angiomatosis
Rendu-Osler-Weber disease
renege
renegotiable
Renese
Renografin
R.-60
R.-76
Reno-M
R.-M-30
R.-M-60
R.-M-Dip
Renovist II
Renovue
Renpenning syndrome
Renshaw cell
renunciation
instinctual r.
REO
receptive-expressive observation
REO Scale
reorganization
cortical r.
recovery and r.
reorient
repair
Gardner meningocele r.
pseudarthrosis r.
rod fracture r.
Repan
reparation

reparenting
repartee
repeat
microtubule-binding r.
r. offender
r. radiosurgery
r. tendency
trinucleotide r.
repeated
r. FID
r. heavy drinker
r. infarct dementia
r. painful experience
r. REM sleep interruptions
r. substance self-administration
R. Test of Sustained Wakefulness
(RTSW)
repeater
accident r.
repeating ritual
repentant
repercussion
repersonalization
repertoire
behavioral r.
Repertory Test
repetition
r. compulsion
compulsive r.
r. by imitation
needless r.
r. reaction
reading, writing and r.
senseless imitative word r.
sentence r. (SR)
r. of sound
stereotyped r.
r. test
r. time (TR)
trauma-related r.
repetition-compulsion principle
repetitious
r. activity
r. behavior
r. request
repetitive
r. checking behavior
r. convulsion
r. idea
r. imitative movement
r. impulse disorder
r. lying
r. motor activity
r. nerve stimulation (RNS)
r. partial seizure
r. pattern
r. pattern of behavior
r. play
r. task
rephasing
even-echo r.
r. gradient
replaceable
replacement
electrolyte r.

R

replacement *(continued)*
    facet r.
    r. formation
    hard tissue r. (HTR)
    r. memory
    r. relationship
    r. therapy
    tile plate facet r.
repletion
replication
reply
    latency of r.
report
    case r.
    Conners Preliminary Parent R.
    Conners Teacher Preliminary
      School R.
    mental status examination r.
      (MSER)
    Parent Daily R.
    paucity of r.'s
    phenomenal r.
    Proficiency Assessment R. (PAR)
    Reid R.
Reposans-10 Oral
reprehend
representation
    Cartesian coordinate r.
    coitus r.
    collective r.
    concrete r.
    spherical coordinate r.
representational
    abstract versus r.
    r. system
representative
    r. intelligence
    r. sample
repressed
    r. feeling
    r. impulse
    r. instinctual drive
    r. need
    return of the r.
repression
    cognitive approaches to dreaming
      and r.
    emotional r.
    organic r.
    primal r.
    primary r.
    proper r.
    r. resistance
    r. scale
    secondary r.
repression-sensitization scale
repressive
    r. behavior
    r. personality
reprocessing
    eye movement desensitization
      and r. (EMDR)
reproducible target imaging

reproduction
    chain r.
    visual r.
reproductive
    r. assimilation
    r. facilitation
    r. failure
    r. mortality
reptilian stare
repulsive axon guidance signal
request
    repetitious r.
Requip
required
    r. relationship
    r. task
requirement
    energy r.
    job r.
    performance r.
rerupture of aneurysm
RES
    reticuloendothelial system
rescind
rescission
Rescriptor
Rescudose
    Roxanol R.
rescue fantasy
research
    action r.
    advocacy r.
    applied r.
    behavioral r.
    brain r.
    comparative r.
    construct r.
    R. Diagnostic Criteria (RDC)
    evaluation r.
    ex post facto r.
    field r.
    genetic r.
    infancy r.
    intervention r.
    motivation r.
    neurochemical r.
    nonspecific r.
    normatological r.
    operational r.
    operations r. (OR)
    population r.
    psychoneuroimmunological r.
    quasi-experimental r.
    specificity of r.
resection
    anteromedial temporal lobe r.
      (AMTR)
    Badgley iliac wing r.
    caudal lamina r.
    cesarean r.
    condyle r.
    cortical r.
    iliac crest r.
    intracranial meningioma r.
    lateral temporal r.

R

neural arch r.
nonlesional cortical r.
odontoid process r.
Peet splanchnic r.
Pitanguy oval skin r.
r. of pituitary tumor, transfacial
  approach
seizure foci r.
surgical r.
transcranial r.
transoral odontoid r.
transthoracic vertebral body r.
tumor r.
vertebral r.
volumetric r.
Resectisol Irrigation Solution
resective surgery
resentment
covert r.
reserpine
chlorothiazide and r.
hydralazine, hydrochlorothiazide,
  and r.
hydrochlorothiazide and r.
hydroflumethiazide and r.
reservatus
coitus r.
reserve
cognitive r.
cross-flow r.
operant r.
reservoir
Accu-Flo CSF r.
Braden flushing r.
McKenzie r.
Ommaya r.
on-off flushing r.
retromastoid Ommaya r.
Rickham r.
Salmon Rickham ventriculostomy r.
side-port flat-bottomed Ommaya r.
r. sign
suboccipital Ommaya r.
ventricular catheter r.
ventricular Ommaya r.
residence
intensive-care community r.
residential
r. setting
r. treatment
r. treatment center (RTC)
r. treatment facility
resident physician
Resident and Staff Information Form
residual
r. amnesia
r. autoparalytic syndrome
r. dense nasal defect
r. disability
r. hemiparesis
r. impairment
least-square r.
r. pain
r. paralysis
r. phase

r. phase of schizophrenia
r. psychotic symptom
r. schizophrenia
r. schizophrenic
r. state
r. type schizophrenic disorder
residue
archaic r.
daunosamine r.
day r.
night r.
resignation
neurotic r.
resilience
resin
cannabis r.
phentermine r.
Spurr epoxy r.
resistance
analysis of the r.
character r.
compliance masking covert r.
conscious r.
covert r.
ego r.
estimated cerebrovascular r. (eCVR)
galvanic skin r.
id r.
least r.
level of r.
r. level
motiveless r.
overt compliance masking covert r.
passive r.
patient r.
psychogalvanic skin r. (PGSR)
repression r.
social r.
state of r.
superego r.
r. to thyroid hormone (RTH)
transference r.
unconscious r.
resistant
r. attachment
r. depression
seizure r. (SR)
resistentiae
locus minoris r.
resistive magnet
resistiveness
resistor
variable r.
resolution
anxiety r.
conflict r.
crisis r.
r. of crisis
r. phase
r. phase of sexual response cycle
spatial r.
resolve conflict
resolving
r. conflict skills
r. power

resonance
acoustic r.
r. disorder
fast-scan magnetic r.
localized magnetic r. (LMR)
magnetic r. (MR)
nuclear magnetic r. (NMR)
resonant frequency
resonator
birdcage r.
resource
community r.'s
r. holding potential
human r.'s
intellectual r.
mental health r.
r. state
Resource-Based Relative Value Scale (RBRVS)
respiration
abdominal-diaphragmatic r.
ataxic r.
Biot r.
bronchial r.
Cheyne-Stokes r.
corneal r.
diffusion r.
electrophrenic r.
internal r.
opposition r.
temperature, pulse, r. (TPR)
tissue r.
respirator
r. brain
Drinker tank r.
respiratory
r. acidosis
r. alkalosis
r. anosmia
r. care
r. center
r. chain
r. embarrassment
r. impairment sleep disorder
r. pause
r. physiology
r. reflex
r. system
respondeat superior
respondent
r. behavior
r. conditioning
respond to environment
responder
psychotherapy r. (PR)
response
abnormal muscle r. (AMR)
achromatic color r.
r. acquiescence
acute genomic r.
adaptive r.
affect r.
anamnestic r.
angiogenic r.
anticipatory r.

antidromic r.
antiparkinsonian r.
anxiety relief r.
anxiolytic r.
appropriate r.
appropriateness of emotional r.
auditory brainstem r. (ABR)
auditory evoked r.
autonomic r.
average evoked r. (AER)
aversion r.
avoidance r.
axon r.
barrier r.
blink r.
blunted r.
brainstem auditory evoked r. (BAER)
bulldog r.
catastrophic r.
cellular immunologic r.
center-surround r.
chaining r.
chromatic r.
circular-pattern r.
clasp-knife r.
clerical r.
color r.
conditioned r.
conditioned emotional r. (CER)
conditioned escape r.
confabulated detail r. (dD)
confabulated whole r. (DW)
cortical-evoked r.
covert r.
criminal r.
culturally sanctioned r.
culturally unsanctioned r.
cumulative r.
r. curve
Cushing r.
delayed r.
r. deviation
differential r.
r. dispersion
dorsal horn neuronal r.
dysphoric r.
dyspnea r.
electrodermal r. (EDR)
electromyographic r.
emotional r.
r. to environment
evoked r. (ER)
evoked cortical r. (ECR)
evoked potential r. (EPR)
evoked somatosensory r.
exaggerated startle r.
extensor plantar r.
F r.
fabulized r.
false-negative r.
false-positive r.
fastigial pressor r. (FPR)
fear r.
fetal r.

R

flight or fight r.
form r. (F)
free r.
frequency r.
frustration r.
galvanic skin r. (GSR)
generalization r.
r. generalization general learning
  ability
good form r. (F+)
hedonic r.
r. hierarchy
hostile r.
human r. (h)
human figure parts r. (Hd)
human movement r.
humoral immune r.
hyperadrenergic r.
hyperemic r.
hypnotic r.
hypoxic ventilatory r.
immune r.
implicit r.
impunitive r.
inadequate r.
inappropriate r.
incompatible r.
r. index
individual r.
inhibited sexual r.
instrumental r.
intropunitive r.
involuntary r.
Janz r.
latency of r.
latent r.
level of r.
local r.
long latency r.
maladaptive r.
marriage r.
mediated r.
monosynaptic segmental reflex r.
morbid r.
negative r.
negativistic r.
neuroplastic r.
oculomotor r.
orienting r.
original r.
overt r.
r. to pain
paradigmatic r.
paradoxical r.
r. pattern
penetration r.
perseverative r.
personal r.
physiological r.
pilomotor r.
plantar r.
polarity r.
poor form r.
popular r.
position r. (Po)

positive r.
postsaccadic neuronal r.
r. prevention
prolactin r.
psychogalvanic r. (PGR)
psychologically mediated r.
rare detail r. (Dr)
r. rate
reactive r.
recruiting r.
relaxation r.
satiety r.
segmentary r.
r. set
sexual r.
shading r. (ShR)
skin conductance orienting r.
  (SCOR)
small detail r.
somatosensory evoked r. (SER)
sonomotor r.
space r.
r. specificity
startle r.
stimulus r.
stress r.
stress effect and immune r.
stress-related physiological r.
supramaximal r.
sympathetic skin r. (SSR)
syntagmatic r.
r. system
target r.
texture r.
r. theory
r. time
total r. (lz R)
treatment r.
unconditioned r. (UCR)
unexpected r.
unsanctioned r.
unusual detail r. (Dd)
unusual rare detail r. (dr)
vibrotactile r.
vista r.
visual evoked r. (VER)
whole r. (W, WR)
response-produced cue
response-specificity
  individual r.-s.
responsibility
  ascriptive r.
  assigned r.
  criminal r.
  diminished r.
  distribution of r.
  generational r.
  homemaking r.
  household r.
  increased r.
  R. and Independence Scale for
    Adolescents (RISA)
  individual r.
  interpersonal r.
  legal r.

responsibility (*continued*)
    limited r.
    new r.
    noxious r.
    patient r.
    personal r.
    Physicians for Social R. (PSR)
    position of r.
    primary r.
    serotonergic r.
    sexual r.
    social r.
    test of criminal r.
responsiveness
    abnormal r.
    affective r.
    diminished r.
    emotional r.
    facial r.
    mutual affective r.
    reduced r.
    threshold of r.
responsivity
    neuroleptic r.
REST
    regressive electroshock treatment
    Restricted Environment Stimulation
        Therapy
rest
    aneurysmal r.
    r. pain
    r. tremor
Restcue bed
rest-cure technique
restiform
    r. body
    r. eminence
resting
    r. ankle/arm Doppler index
    r. energy expenditure
    r. potential
    r. tremor
    wakefulness r.
restitution
    cognitive r.
    neurologic r.
restitutional
    r. schizophrenia
    r. symptoms of schizophrenia
restitutive therapy
restless
    r. behavior
    r. leg
    r. legs syndrome
    r. pacing
restlessness
    motor r.
    psychomotor r.
Reston
    R. dressing
    R. foam-padded headrest
restorative neurology
Restoril
restraining therapy

restraint
    chemical r.
    chest r.
    compulsive r.
    four-point r.
    lack of r.
    leather r.
    Posey r.
    seclusion and r. (S&R)
    situational r.
    soft r.
    wrist r.
restricted
    r. activity
    r. behavior
    r. diet
    R. Environment Stimulation
        Therapy (REST)
    r. range of affect
    r. range of emotional expression
restricting behavior
restriction
    activity r.
    building r.
    close watch r.
    ego r.
    r. endonuclease
    r. fragment length polymorphism
        (RFLP)
    gown r.
    r. of inward gaze
    open seclusion r.
    shoe r.
    unit r.
restrictive behavior
restructuring
    attitude r.
    cognitive r.
    perceptual r.
    sexual attitude r. (SAR)
    systematic rational r. (SRR)
restzustand schizophrenia
Resume electrode
resuscitate
    do not r. (DNR)
resuscitation
    cardiopulmonary r.
resuscitative snores
resymbolization
RET
    rational emotive therapy
Ret, ret
    retarded
retardate
    ejaculatio r.
    Screening Tests for Young
        Children and R.'s (STYCAR)
retardation
    Amsterdam-type r.
    arithmetical learning r.
    arithmetical skills learning r.
    borderline r.
    borderline mental r.
    cultural-familial mental r.
    developmental r.

r. developmental delay disorder
familial r.
idiopathic language r.
incidental learning language r.
language r.
language skills learning r.
learning r.
mental r. (MR)
mild mental r.
moderate mental r.
perceptual r.
profound mental r.
psychomotor r.
r. psychopathology
psychopathology of r.
psychosis with mental r.
psychosocial r.
reading skills learning r.
severe mental r.
simple r.
trichorrhexis nodosa with mental r.
unspecified mental r.
retarded (Ret, ret)
r. depression
r. development
educable mentally r. (EMR)
educationally mentally r. (EMR)
r. ejaculation
r. maturation
mentally r.
profoundly r.
r. schizophrenia
TMR Performance Profile for the Severely and Moderately R.
trainable mentally r. (TMR)
rete
carotid r.
r. mirabile
r. mirabile caroticum
retention
anal r.
brain r.
r. control training
r. defect
fluid r.
informal r.
involuntary r.
memory r.
psychogenic r.
r. and recall
selective r.
voluntary r.
RETHINK
recognize, empathize, think, hear, integrate, notice, keep
reticula (*pl. of* reticulum)
reticular
r. activating system (RAS)
r. formation
r. nuclei of the brainstem
r. nucleus of thalamus
r. substance
r. thalamic nucleus
reticularis
livedo r. (LR)

reticulata
pars r.
substantia nigra pars r. (Snr)
reticulocortical pathway
reticulocyte count
reticulocytosis
cerebroside r.
reticuloendothelial system (RES)
reticulospinal tract
reticulotomy
reticulum, pl. reticula
r. cell sarcoma
endoplasmic r.
Kölliker r.
smooth endoplasmic r.
r. stain
retina, gen. retinae, pl. retinae
blood and thunder r.
macula retinae
periphlebitis retinae
retinaculatome
Paine r.
retinal
r. angioma
r. cone
r. cyst
r. degeneration
r. detachment
r. embolism
r. infarction
r. migraine
r. migraine headache
r. pathway
r. pigment epitheliopathy
r. pigment epithelium
r. stroke
r. vasculitis
retinitis pigmentosa
retinoblastoma
ectopic intracranial r.
r. gene
retinocerebral angiomatosis
retinocochleocerebral arteriolopathy
retinofugal target
retinoneuropathy
toxic r.
retinopathy
arterial-occlusive r.
hypotensive r.
infectious r.
pigmentary r.
radiation r.
stasis r.
venous stasis r.
retirement
R. Descriptive Index (RDI)
r. neurosis
r. syndrome
retracted
anteriorly r.
retracting suture
retraction
brain r.
cerebellar r.
r. injury

R

Tew cranial spinal r.
titanium wound r.
Tuffier laminectomy r.
Tuffier-Raney r.
Valin hemilaminectomy r.
Weary nerve root r.
Weitlaner r.
Weitlaner-Beckman r.
Wiltse-Gelpi r.
Yasargil r.
Yasargil-Leyla brain r.

retreat
r. from reality
vegetative r.
York r.

retrenchment
ego r.

retrieval
information r.
limited-capacity r.
r. problem
r. task

retroactive
r. amnesia
r. displacement
r. inhibition (RI)

retroanterograde amnesia
retroauricular edema
retrobulbar
r. hemorrhage
r. injection
r. neuritis
r. orbital metastasis

retrochiasmal
r. lesion
r. visual pathway

retrochiasmatic lesion
retrocochlear
r. deafness
r. lesion

retrocollic spasm
retrocollis
retrocursive absence
retroflexed rage
retroflex fasciculus
retroflexion
retrogasserian
r. anhydrous glycerol injection
  therapy
r. injection
r. neurectomy
r. neurotomy
r. procedure

retrogenesis
law of r.

retrognathic
retrograde
r. amnesia
r. axon reaction
r. blood flow
r. chromatolysis
r. degeneration
r. ejaculation
r. fast component neuropathy
r. loss of memory

r. memory
r. memory interference

retrography
retrogression
retrogressive differentiation
retrolabyrinthine-presigmoid approach
retrolabyrinthine-transsigmoid approach
retrolental
retrolenticular limb of internal capsule
retrolisthesis
retromastoid
r. approach
r. craniotomy
r. Ommaya reservoir
r. suboccipital craniectomy

retromembranous hematoma
retroocular
retroorbital pain
retroperitoneal
r. approach
r. fibrosis

retropharyngeal
r. abscess
r. approach
r. hematoma
r. space

retropulsed bone excision
retropulsion of gait
retropulsive epilepsy
retrosigmoid
r. approach
r. craniectomy

retrospect
retrospective
r. falsification
r. gaps in memory
r. study

retrosplenial cingulate
Retrovir
retrovirus
retrusion
midface r.

Rett
R. disorder
R. syndrome

Retter aneurysm needle
return
law of diminishing r.
point of no r.
r. of the repressed

Retzius
R. fiber
R. foramen
R. gyrus

reuniens
nucleus r.

reuptake
dopamine r.
r. inhibitor
neuronal r.

reus
actus r.

revascularization
brain r.
cerebral r.

R

revenant
revenge
    desire for r.
    r. obsession
reverberating circuit
reverence
reverie
    hypnagogic r.
reversal
    r. of affect
    behavior r.
    deficit r.
    r. formation
    habit r.
    homuncular organization phase r.
    r. learning
    phase r.
    role r.
    sex r.
    r. test
reverse
    r. digit span recall test
    r. discrimination
    r. diurnal variation
    r. ocular bobbing
    r. polarity
    r. Trendelenburg position
    r. vegetative symptoms
reverse-angled curette
reversed
    r. optokinetic nystagmus
    r. orientation
reversible
    r. affective disorder syndrome
    r. amnesia
    r. C-arm
    r. cholinesterase inhibitor
    r. decortication
    dementia r.
    r. ischemic neurological deficit
    (RIND)
    r. ischemic neurologic disability
    (RIND)
    r. memory impairment
    r. motor neuron disease
    r. schizophrenia
    r. shock
reversion
Reversol Injection
revert
Revex
ReVia
review
    claims r.
    comprehensive r.
    concurrent r.
    continued-stay r. (CSR)
    contract r.
    critical r.
    drug use r. (DUR)
    empirical r.
    extended-care r.
    extended-stay r.
    medical r.
    r. method

    peer r.
    systematic r.
    r. of systems (ROS)
    utilization r. (UR)
Revilliod sign
Revised
    R. Behavior Problem Checklist
    R. Childhood Experiences
    Questionnaire
    R. Children's Depression Scale
    (RCDS)
    R. Children's Manifest Anxiety
    Scale
    R. Denver Prescreening
    Development Questionnaire (R-
    PDQ)
    R. Diagnostic Interview for
    Borderlines
    R. Edinburgh Functional
    Communication Profile
    R. Evaluating Acquired Skills in
    Communication
    R. NEO Personality Inventory
    R. Ontario Child Health Study
    Scale
    R. Token Test
    R. Trauma Score (RTS)
    R. Ways of Coping Checklist
revision
    r. process
    secondary r.
revivication
revocable
revoke
revolution
    sexual r.
revulsion
    sexual stimuli r.
reward
    delayed r.
    r. dependence
    external r.
    extrinsic r.
    intrinsic r.
    potential external r.
    r. by the superego
    token r.
    token economy r.
rewinder gradient
Rexed lamina
Rey
    R. Auditory Verbal Learning Test
    (RAVLT)
    R. Complex Figure Test
    R. and Taylor Complex Figure
    Test
Reye syndrome
Reynell-Zinkin Scales: Developmental
Scales for Young Handicapped
Children
Reynolds
    R. Adolescent Depression Scale
    (RADS)
    R. Adolescent Scale
    R. Child Depression Scale (RCDS)

R. number
R. skull traction tongs
Rey-Osterrieth
R.-O. complex
R.-O. Complex Figure Copy
R.-O. Complex Figure Copy and
Delayed Recall Test
R.-O. Complex Figure Design
Rezine
RF, rf
radiofrequency
RF coil
RF electrocoagulation
RF pulse
RFG-3C radiofrequency lesion generator system
RFLP
restriction fragment length polymorphism
RFVII
Reading-Free Vocational Interest
Inventory
R-Gel
RGEPS
Rucker-Gable Educational Programming
Scale
rhabdoid tumor
rhabdomancy
rhabdomyolysis
rhabdomyoma
rhabdomyosarcoma
rhabdophobia
rhabdovirus infection
rhathymia
rhembasmus
rhenium-186
rheobase
rheoencephalogram
rheoencephalography
rheologic therapy
rheumatic
r. carditis
r. chorea
r. disorder
r. heart disease
r. tetany
r. torticollis
rheumatica
polymyalgia r.
tetania r.
rheumatism
lumbar r.
rheumatoid
r. arteritis
r. arthritis
r. disease
r. disorder
r. factor
r. neuropathy
r. spondylitis
Rheumatrex
rhigosis
rhigotic
rhinal
r. fissure
r. sulcus

Rh incompatibility
rhinencephalic mamillary body
rhinencephalon
rhinitis
vasomotor r.
viral r.
rhinolalia
r. aperta
r. clausa
rhinoplasty
external r.
rhinorrhea
cerebrospinal fluid r.
rhinoseptal approach
rhinosinusitis
rhinotomy
lateral r.
rhizolysis
percutaneous glycerol r. (PGR)
percutaneous radiofrequency r.
(PRF)
percutaneous retrogasserian
glycerol r.
rhizomelic chondrodysplasia punctata
rhizomeningomyelitis
rhizopathy
Rhizopus **infection**
rhizotomy
anterior r.
bilateral ventral r.
Dana posterior r.
dorsal r.
facet r.
Frazier-Spiller r.
glycerol r.
intracranial r.
percutaneous radiofrequency r.
percutaneous retrogasserian
glycerol r.
posterior r.
radiofrequency r.
selective dorsal r. (SDR)
thermal r.
trigeminal r.
Rhode Island Pupil Identification Scale (PIPIS, RIPIS)
Rhodesian trypanosomiasis
Rhodococcus rodochrous
rhombencephalic
r. gustatory nucleus
r. isthmus
r. sleep
rhombencephalitis
rhombencephalon
ventricle of r.
rhombencephalosynapsis
rhombic
rhombocele
rhomboidalis
sinus r.
rhomboidal sinus
rhomboid fossa
rhombomere
rhotacism

Rhoton
R. ball dissector
R. dissecting forceps
R. forceps
R. loop curette
R. micro curette
R. microdissector
R. spatula
R. spoon curette
R. suction tip
Rhoton-Cushing forceps
Rhoton-Merz suction tube
Rhoton-Tew bipolar forceps
rho wave
RHV
rotating hemostatic valve
rhyming
r. delirium
r. slang
word r.
rhypophagy
rhypophobia, rupophobia
rhythm
alpha r.
background r.
Berger r.
beta r.
bicircadian r.
biologic r.
breach r.
cardiac r.
circadian r.
circannual r.
circaseptan r.
delta r.
EEG alpha r.
endogenous r.
erratic speech r.
fast field-potential r.
focal slowing of background r.
infradian r.
r. method
r. method of contraception
mu r.
r. phase
phi r.
pi r.
polyphasic sleep r.
rolandic mu r.
sleep-wake r.
r. test
theta r.
ultradian r.
wicket r.
rhythmic
r. artifact
r. chorea
r. contraction
r. sensory bombardment therapy (RSBT)
r. slow eye movement
r. spindle-shaped activity
r. tremor

rhythmical
r. midtemporal discharge (RMTD)
r. twitch
rhythmicity of tremor
RI
retroactive inhibition
RIA
relaxation-induced anxiety
RIAST
Reitan-Indiana Aphasia Screening Test
rib
r. cranioplasty
r. fracture
r. graft
r. removal
ribavirin
ribbed hook
ribbon
r. blade
r. encephaloduromyosynangiosis
Reil r.
Ribes ganglion
RIBLS
Riley Inventory of Basic Learning Skills
ribonucleic acid (RNA)
rich
Rolaids Calcium R.
Richards
R. curette
R. tamp
Richardson-Steele-Olszewski syndrome
Richards-Rundel syndrome
Richards-Rundle syndrome
riche
nouveau r.
Richmond
R. bolt
R. subarachnoid screw instrument
Richter laminectomy punch forceps
ricin
rickets
tumor-associated r.
rickettsial infection
rickettsii
Rochalimaea r.
Rickham reservoir
riddance
r. phenomenon
r. reflex
ridden
instinct r.
Ridenol
ridge
apical ectodermal r. (AER)
supraorbital r.
ridging
spondylitic r.
Ridley
R. circle
R. sinus
Riedel thyroiditis
Rienhoff-Finochietto rib spreader
Rienhoff rib spreader
Riese hearing
rifampin

Rift Valley fever
right (rt)
    bill of r.'s
    civil r.'s
    r. frontal craniotomy for gross
      total resection of tumor
    r. frontal lobe
    r. frontoparietal infarct
    gay r.'s
    r. hemiplegia
    r. hemisphere
    r. hemisphere cognitive skills
    r. hemisphere dominance
    mentally retarded persons' r.'s
    moral r.
    r.'s of others
    parental r.'s
    r. parietal lobe syndrome
    r. parietal occipital vertex
      craniotomy
    patient r.'s
    r. to refuse treatment
    r. temporoparietal craniotomy
    r. thoracic curve
    r. thoracic curve scoliosis
    r. thoracic curve with hypokyphosis
    r. thoracic curve with junctional
      kyphosis
    r. thoracic left lumbar curve
      pattern
    r. thoracic left lumbar scoliosis
    r. thoracic left thoracolumbar
      scoliosis
    r. thoracic minor curve pattern
    r. to treatment
    r. ventricle
    visitation r.'s
right-angle
    r.-a. bipolar cautery
    r.-a. blunt probe
    r.-a. booster clip
    r.-a. drill
    r.-a. screwdriver
right-ankle bur
right-bearing nystagmus
right-footed
right-hand dominant
right-handed
right-handedness
righting reflex
right-left
    r.-l. confusion
    r.-l. discrimination
    r.-l. disorientation
    R.-l. Orientation Test (RLO)
right-sided
    r.-s. submandibular transverse
      incision
    r.-s. thoracotomy
right-to-left shunt
Right-Wing Authoritarianism scale
right-wrong test
rigid
    r. attitude
    r. body position

    r. body transformation matrix
    r. cerebral palsy
    r. control
    r. curve
    r. curve scoliosis
    r. family
    r. internal fixation
    r. pedicle screw
    r. posture
    r. pupil
    r. spine syndrome
    r. ventriculoscope
rigid-akinetic syndrome
rigidity
    affective r.
    catatonic r.
    C-D instrumentation r.
    cerebellar r.
    clasp-knife r.
    cogwheel r.
    Cotrel pedicle screw r.
    decerebrate r.
    decorticate r.
    r. decorticate
    excessive r.
    extensor r.
    intellectual r.
    lead-pipe r.
    muscle r.
    mydriatic r.
    nuchal r.
    parkinsonian muscular r.
    ratchet r.
    spinal fixation r.
Riley
    R. Articulation and Language Test
      (RALT)
    R. Inventory of Basic Learning
      Skills (RIBLS)
    R. Motor Problems Inventory
    R. Preschool Developmental
      Screening Inventory (RPDSI)
Riley-Day syndrome
Rilutek
riluzole
rim
    supraorbital r.
RIND
    reversible ischemic neurological deficit
    reversible ischemic neurologic disability
ring
    r. block anesthesia
    Brown-Roberts-Wells base r.
    Budde halo r.
    carotid r.
    r. chromosome
    Cosman-Roberts-Wells stereotactic r.
    cricoid r.
    r. curette
    dural r.
    enhancing r.
    Gibbs r.
    halo r.
    head r.
    Kayser-Fleischer r.

ring *(continued)*
    Luque r.
    R. and Peg Tests of Behavior
      Development
    proximal carotid r.
    tentorial r.
    V1 halo r.
ringed formed forceps
Ringer lactate
ring-wall lesion
Rinne test
Rio Bravo virus
Riopan
riot gun
RIP
    radioimmunoprecipitation
RIPIS
    Rhode Island Pupil Identification Scale
Rip van Winkle
RIs
    Rehabilitation Indicator
RISA
    Responsibility and Independence Scale
      for Adolescents
RISB
    Rotter Incomplete Sentences Blank
risedronate
rise time
risk
    accident r.
    r. activity
    addictive r.
    at r.
    attributable r.
    depression r.
    elevated r.
    empiric r.
    r. factor
    health r.
    high r.
    r. indicator
    infant at r.
    r. inventory
    r. level
    level of r.
    lifetime r.
    minimal r.
    morbid r.
    operative r.
    r. preference
    r. profile
    r. reduction
    relative r.
    r. rescue rating (RRR)
    schizophrenia r.
    Screening Instrument for Targeting
      Educational R. (SIFTER)
    significant r.
    suicide r.
    r. of suicide attempt
    violence r.
risk-taking
    r.-t. behavior

    sex-related r.-t.
    sexual r.-t.
Risk-Taking, Attitude, Values Inventory
    (RTAVI)
risky behavior
Risperdal
risperidone
Risser-Cotrel body cast
Risser localizer
risus
    r. caninus
    r. sardonicus
Ritalin-SR
ritanserin
Ritchie index
rite
    r. of passage
    puberty r.
ritonavir
Ritter
    R. law
    R. opening tetanus
Ritter-Rollet phenomenon
ritual
    r. abuse
    ADHD r.'s
    r. behavior
    centro r.
    checking and touching r.'s
    compulsive r.
    degrading r.
    handwashing r.
    healing r.
    marriage r.
    masochistic r.
    painful r.'s
    presentational r.
    repeating r.
    touching r.'s
ritualistic
    r. behavior
    r. thinking
ritualized makeup application
Ritvo-Freeman Real Life Rating Scale
    for Autism
rivalry
    perceptual r.
    sibling r.
Rivermead
    R. ADL index
    R. ADL Test
    R. Behavioral Memory Test
      (RBMT)
    R. Behavioural Memory Test
    R. Mobility Index (RMI)
    R. Motor Assessment
    R. Perceptual Assessment Battery
      (RPAB)
rizatriptan
RLE
    recent life event
RLI
    Reasons for Living Inventory
RLO
    Right-Left Orientation Test

RLS
  Reaction Level Scale
  RLS person
RMI
  Reading Miscue Inventory
  Rivermead Mobility Index
RMS Rectal
RMTD
  rhythmical midtemporal discharge
  RMTD on electroencephalogram
RNA
  ribonucleic acid
  RNA expression
  heterogeneous nuclear RNA
   (hnRNA)
  messenger RNA
  RNA virus
RNS
  repetitive nerve stimulation
RN scanning
RO
  reality orientation
  reality oriented
R/O
  rule out
roached out
road
   r. rage
   yellow brick r. (YBR)
Robaxin
Robaxisal
Robert Apperception Test for Children
  (RATC)
Robertson pupil
robin complex
Robinow syndrome
Robinson
  R. anterior cervical discectomy
  R. anterior cervical fusion
robot
   Grenoble stereotactic r.
   Kwoh-Young stereotactic r.
   Lausanne stereotactic r.
   Long Beach stereotactic r.
   Mayo Clinic stereotactic r.
   neurosurgical stereotactic r.
   stereotactic r.
ROC
  receiver operating characteristic
Rocaltrol
Rochalimaea
   R. akari
   R. henselae
   R. mooseri
   R. prowazekii
   R. quintana
   R. rickettsii
   R. tsutsugamushi
Rochester
   R. lamina dissector
   R. method
rock
   r. attack
   r. cocaine

rocking
   body r.
   sheet r.
Rocky
   R. Mountain spotted fever
   R. Mountain spotted fever
    meningoencephalitis
rod
   aluminum master r.
   r. bending
   r. cell of retina
   cerebellomesoencephalic fissure
    Perspex r.
   compression r.
   compressive r.
   r. contour preparation
   Corti r.
   Cotrel-Dubousset r.
   Delrin r.
   distraction r.
   double-L spinal r.
   Edwards-Levine r.
   Edwards modular system
    universal r.
   r. fiber
   r. fracture repair
   Harrington r.
   Hartshill rectangle r.
   Isola spinal implant system eye r.
   Jacobs locking hook spinal r.
   Knodt r.
   Kostuik r.
   r. linkage
   Luque r.
   r. migration
   modified Harrington r.
   Moe r.
   pediatric Cotrel-Dubousset r.
   r. placement
   precontoured unit r.
   r. rotation prevention
   screw alignment r.
   spinal r.
   unit spinal r.
   Wiltse system aluminum master r.
   Wiltse system spinal r.
rod-hook construct
rodochrous
   Rhodococcus r.
rodomontade
rodonalgia
rod-sleeve
   Edwards modular system spinal r.-
    s.
Roeder
   R. Manipulative Aptitude Test
   R. manipulative aptitude test device
roentgen knife
roentgenogram
   biplane r.
   lateral r.
roentgenographic opaque marker
rogerian
   r. group therapy
   r. theory

Roger reflex
Rogers Criminal Responsibility Scale
Rogozinski spinal rod system
Rohypnol
ROI
    region of interest
Rokeach Value Survey (RVS)
Rolaids Calcium Rich
rolandic
    r. cortex
    r. epilepsy
    r. epileptiform discharge
    r. fissure
    r. line
    r. mu rhythm
    r. paroxysmal focus
    r. seizure
Rolando
    R. angle
    R. area
    R. cell
    R. column
    fissure of R.
    R. gelatinous substance
    R. tubercle
    R. zone
rolandoparietal glioma
role
    adultomorphic behavior r.
    alternating r.
    altruistic r.
    r. ambiguity
    anticipation of r.
    attacker r.
    behavior r.
    r. boundary
    caretaking r.
    community r.
    complementary r.
    r. conflict
    r. confusion
    R. Construct Repertory Test
    contributing r.
    cross-sex r.
    cultural r.
    r. demand
    dependent patient r.
    r. deprivation
    r. deviance
    r. diffusion
    discomfort with gender r.
    r. experimentation
    explicit r.
    feminine social r.
    r. fixation
    follower r.
    r. function
    gender r.
    helper r.
    implicit r.
    r. insufficiency
    interpersonal r.
    interpreter r.
    intrinsic transverse connector r.
    leader r.

    leadership r.
    masculine social r.
    maternal r.
    r. model
    noncomplementary r.
    r. obligation
    r. obsolescence
    parentified r.
    r. pattern
    peacemaker r.
    r. playing
    protector r.
    r. reversal
    sex r.
    r. shift
    sick r.
    social r.
    r. specialization
    spectator r.
    stereotypical r.
    stereotypical gender r.'s
    thematic r.
    r. theory of personality
    therapeutic r.
    r. therapy
    victim r.
    women's r.
role-enactment theory
role-playing
roll
    chest r.
    FLUFTEX gauze r.
    laminectomy r.
    Spiegel eye r.
roller-coaster emotion
Roller nucleus
rolling
    head r.
    pill r.
roll-off filter
romance
    family r.
    r. fantasy
    memory r.
Roman holiday
Romano-Ward syndrome
romantic fantasy
Romazicon
Romberg
    R. disease
    R. sign
    R. symptom
    R. syndrome
    R. test
    R. trophoneurosis
Romberg-Howship symptom
rombergism
rongeur
    Adson cranial r.
    Bacon cranial r.
    Beyer laminectomy r.
    bone-biting r.
    Bucy laminectomy r.
    Cherry-Kerrison laminectomy r.
    Cloward disk r.

Cloward-English laminectomy r.
Codman-Harper laminectomy r.
Codman-Kerrison laminectomy r.
Codman-Leksell laminectomy r.
Codman-Schlesinger cervical
  laminectomy r.
Codman-Schlesinger laminectomy r.
Colclough-Scheicher laminectomy r.
cranial r.
Cushing cranial r.
Cushing disk r.
Cushing intervertebral disk r.
Dahlgren cranial r.
DeVilbiss cranial r.
disk r.
double-action r.
Echlin laminectomy r.
Echlin-Luer r.
Elekta Leksell r.
Ferris Smith-Kerrison
  laminectomy r.
Fulton laminectomy r.
gooseneck r.
Gruenwald neurosurgical r.
Hajek-Koffler laminectomy r.
Hoen intervertebral disk r.
Hoen pituitary r.
Horsley r.
Hudson cranial r.
Husk bone r.
Jansen r.
Jansen-Middleton r.
Jarit-Kerrison laminectomy r.
Jarit-Liston bone r.
Jarit-Ruskin bone r.
Kerrison r.
Leksell r.
Love-Gruenwald cranial r.
Love-Gruenwald disk r.
Love-Gruenwald pituitary r.
Love-Kerrison laminectomy r.
Love pituitary r.
Mayfield r.
micropituitary r.
Mount laminectomy r.
narrow-bite bone r.
needle-nose r.
Nicola pituitary r.
Oldberg intervertebral disk r.
Oldberg pituitary r.
Olivecrona r.
Peiper-Beyer laminectomy r.
Poppen intervertebral disk
  laminectomy r.
punch r.
Raney laminectomy r.
Schlesinger intervertebral disk r.
Schlesinger laminectomy r.
Selverstone intervertebral disk r.
Smith-Petersen laminectomy r.
Spence intervertebral disk r.
Spurling-Kerrison laminectomy r.
Stille-Luer r.
Stookey cranial r.
Tiedmann r.

upbiting/downbiting pituitary r.
Watson-Williams intervertebral
  disk r.
Weil-Blakesley intervertebral disk r.
Whitcomb-Kerrison laminectomy r.
Yasargil pituitary r.
roof
  r. of fourth ventricle
  r. nucleus
  orbital r.
  r. plate
roof-patch graft
roofplate
room
  behavior control r. (BCR)
  r. and board
  dead r.
  emergency r. (ER)
  free field r.
  locked r.
  padded r.
  semiprivate r.
Roos brachial plexus root retractor
Roosen clamp
root
  addiction r.
  anterior r.
  cochlear r. of vestibulocochlear
    nerve
  conjoined nerve r.
  cranial r.
  cultural r.
  developmental r.
  r. doctor
  dorsal r.
  entering r.
  r. entry-zone lesion
  facial r.
  r. of facial nerve
  inferior r. of cervical loop
  inferior r. of vestibulocochlear
    nerve
  lateral r. of median nerve
  lateral r. of optic tract
  r. level motor impairment
  long r. of ciliary ganglion
  r. mean square error
  medial r. of median nerve
  medial r. of optic tract
  motor r. of ciliary ganglion
  motor r. of trigeminal nerve
  nasociliary r.
  nerve r.
  olfactory r.
  r.'s of olfactory tract, lateral and
    medial
  posterior r.
  sensory r. of ciliary ganglion
  sensory r. of trigeminal nerve
  short r. of ciliary ganglion
  r. sign
  r. sleeve fibrosis
  spinal nerve r.
  superior r. of cervical loop

R

root *(continued)*
> superior r. of vestibulocochlear nerve
> symptomatic r.
> r. syndrome
> trigeminal r.
> r.'s of trigeminal nerve
> ventral r.
> vestibular r. of vestibulocochlear nerve

rootedness need
rooted obsession
rooting reflex
rootwork
ropinirole hydrochloride
ropivacaine
roples
Rorschach
> R. card
> R. Content Test (RCT)
> R. Index of Primitive Thought
> R. Inkblot Test
> R. Projective Technique

ROS
> review of systems

rosa
> mal de la r.

rose
> r. bengal test
> R. cephalic tetanus

rose-colored glasses
Rosen
> R. bur
> R. Drawing Test

Rosenbach law
Rosenberg
> R. Draw-A-Person Technique
> R. Draw-A-Person Test
> R. Self-Esteem Scale (RSES)

Rosenmüller
> fossa of R.

Rosenthal
> basal vein of R. (BVR)
> R. fiber
> R. fiber formation
> R. syndrome
> R. vein

Rosenzweig Picture-Frustration Study (RPFS)
Ross
> R. Information Processing Assessment
> R. Test of Higher Cognitive Processes

Rosser crypt hook
rosso
> mal r.

Rossolimo
> R. contraction
> R. reflex
> R. sign

rostra *(pl. of* rostrum)
rostrad

rostral
> r. basilar artery syndrome
> r. brainstem
> r. brain stem ischemia
> caudal to r.
> r. cingulotomy
> r. interstitial nucleus
> r. lamina
> r. layer
> r. midbrain
> r. neuropore
> r. subcortical target
> r. transtentorial herniation

rostralis
rostrocaudal
> r. contact array
> r. epidural array

rostrum, pl. **rostra, rostrums**
> r. corporis callosi
> sphenoid r.

Rotablator rotating bur
rotary
> r. nystagmus
> r. vertigo

rotating
> r. frame of reference
> r. hemostatic valve (RHV)
> r. mechanism

rotation
> factor r.
> gantry r.
> r. test

rotational
> r. correction
> r. injury

rotationally
> r. induced shear-strain injury
> r. induced shear-strain lesion

rotator
> Jarit r.

rotatoria
> chorea r.

rotatory
> r. luxation
> r. nystagmus
> r. spasm
> r. tic

rote
> r. learning
> r. memory
> r. recall

Roth
> R. disease
> R. spot

Roth-Bernhardt disease
Rothwell-Miller Interest Blank
Roton sellar punch
rotoscoliosis
rotted obsession
Rotter
> I-E Scale of R.
> R. Incomplete Sentences Blank (RISB)
> R. Sentence Completion Test (RSCT)

rotunda
fenestra r.
rotundum
foramen r.
Rouget muscle
rough-and-tumble play
rough hoarseness
rouleaux formation
round
r. bur
r. eminence
r. hole plate
round-handled forceps
round-tipped periosteal elevator
Roussy-Dejerine syndrome
Roussy-Lévy
R.-L. disease
R.-L. hereditary areflexic dystasia
R.-L. syndrome
router
power r.
routine
agreed-on r.
family r.
grimly adhered-to r.
negligible r.
r. skill
rover
roving
r. eye movement
r. ocular movement
row
death r.
skid r.
Rowland
criteria of R.
ROWPVT
Receptive One Word Picture Vocabulary
Test
Roxanol
R. Oral
R. Rescudose
R. SR Oral
Roxiam
Roxicet 5/500
Roxicodone
Roxilox
Roxiprin
royal blues
Roy-Camille
R.-C. plate
R.-C. posterior screw plate fixation
R.-C. posterior screw plate fixation
biomechanics
R.-C. technique
RPAB
Rivermead Perceptual Assessment
Battery
R-PDQ
Revised Denver Prescreening
Development Questionnaire
RPDSI
Riley Preschool Developmental
Screening Inventory

RPFS
Rosenzweig Picture-Frustration Study
RPI
Racial Perceptions Inventory
RPR
rapid plasma reagin
RPR test
RRF
ragged red fiber
RRR
risk rescue rating
RSBT
rhythmic sensory bombardment therapy
RSCCD
Rating Scale of Communication in
Cognitive Decline
RSCT
Rotter Sentence Completion Test
RSD
reflex sympathetic dystrophy
RSDS
reflex sympathetic dystrophy syndrome
RSE
refractory status epilepticus
RSES
Rosenberg Self-Esteem Scale
RSPM
Raven Standard Progressive Matrices
RT
radiotherapy
rational therapy
reaction time
recreational therapy
rt
right
RTAVI
Risk-Taking, Attitude, Values Inventory
RTC
residential treatment center
RTH
resistance to thyroid hormone
RTS
Revised Trauma Score
RTSW
Repeated Test of Sustained Wakefulness
rubber
burning r.
r. button
r. cement
r. sheeting
silicone r.
rubbing
coin r.
rubella
r. panencephalitis
r. virus
rubeosis iridis
ruber
nucleus r.
Rubinstein-Taybi syndrome
rubral tremor
rubric
rubrobulbar tract
rubroreticular tract

rubrospinal
    r. decussation
    r. tract
Rucker-Gable Educational Programming Scale (RGEPS)
ruderalis
rudimentary paranoia
rudimentum, pl. **rudimenta**
    r. hippocampi
Ruffini
    R. corpuscle
    R. mechanoreceptor
Ruggles Surgical Instruments
rule
    r. of abstinence
    American Law Institute r.
    analytic r.
    Anstie r.
    assimilation r.
    base r.
    basic r.
    r. bending
    disregard for r.'s
    dissimilation r.
    Durham r.
    R. Eleven Psych Evaluation
    r.'s of evidence
    Grandma r.
    ground r.
    group r.
    Hebb r.
    house r.
    inverse square r.
    Jackson r.
    mature minor r.
    M'Naghten r.
    morphological r.
    neutralization r.
    New Hampshire r.
    r. out (R/O)
    Pitres r.
    r.'s preoccupation
    redundancy r.
    sequencing r.
    serious violations of r.'s
    R. skills
    r. of Spence
    syntactic r.
    Tarasoff r.
    r. of thumb
    transformational r.
    r. of two
    r. utilitarianism
    violations of r.'s
ruling
rumination
    anxious r.
    behavioral theory of r.
    r. disorder
    r. disorder of infancy
    homicidal r.
    morbid r.
    neurotic r.
    obsessional r.
    obsessive r.

    psychogenic r.
    suicidal r.
    r. syndrome
ruminative
    r. idea
    r. tension state
    r. thought
Rum-K
runaway
    habitual r.
    r. hotline
    r. reaction
runners
    intrinsic-negative r.
    intrinsic-positive r.
running
    r. commentary
    r. fit
    r. stitch
runs
    r. of activity
    r. in family
rupophobia (*var. of* rhypophobia)
rupture
    aneurysmal r.
    annular radial r.
    intervertebral disk r.
    intraoperative r.
    longitudinal ligament r.
    vein patch r.
ruptured
    r. aneurysm
    r. disk
ruralist
rural psychiatry
Russell
    R. sign
    R. syndrome
    R. variant of the Wechsler Memory Scale
    R. Version Wechsler Memory Scale
    R. viper venom time
Russell-Rubinstein cerebrovascular malformation classification
Russian
    R. autumn encephalitis
    R. spring-summer encephalitis (Eastern or Western subtype)
    R. tick-borne encephalitis
russomania
russophobia
Rust
    R. disease
    R. Inventory of Schizotypal Cognitions
    R. phenomenon
Rutler-Graham Psychiatric Interview
Rutter-B Questionnaire
Rutter Child Behaviour Questionnaire
Ruvalcaba-Myhre syndrome
Ru-Vert-M
RVS
    Rokeach Value Survey
RWA scale

Rx
  prescription
  therapy
  treatment

RXR
  9-cis retinoic acid receptor
rypophobla

R

S

    S factor
    S incision
    S phase cell

S-100

    S-100 protein
    S-100 tumor marker

S-44

    Grass stimulator S.

7's

    serial sevens test

SA

    self-analysis
    sensory awareness
    social acquiescence
    social age
    suicide attempt

sa

    social acquiescence
    social age

SAAST

    self-administered alcohol screening test

SAB

    short-acting block
    SAB anesthesia

sabeluzole
Saber CBF-ICP trauma sensor
Sabin-Feldman dye test
sabotage

    masochistic s.

saboteur
sabulous
sac

    endolymphatic s. (ELS)
    nasal mucosal s.
    thecal s.

saccade

    contrapulsion of s.'s
    s. impairment
    s. paralysis
    s. velocity
    visually-guided s.

saccadic

    s. abnormality
    s. contraversive head turning
    s. eye movement
    s. overshooting
    s. palsy
    s. pursuit
    s. slowing
    s. tracking

saccharate

    dextroamphetamine s.

saccharopinuria
saccular

    s. aneurysm
    s. spot

sacculus, pl. sacculi

    s. communis
    macula sacculi

sacerdotal

Sachs

    S. brain suction tip
    S. brain suction tube
    S. dural hook
    S. dural separator
    S. nerve separator-spatula
    S. nerve spatula

SACL

    Sales Attitude Check List

SACQ

    Student Adaptation to College
     Questionnaire

sacral

    s. agenesis
    s. alar screw
    s. brim target point
    s. dimple
    s. foraminal approach
    s. ganglia
    s. hemangioma
    s. meningocele
    s. nerve
    s. nerve root cyst
    s. nerve stimulation (SNS)
    s. nerve stimulation therapy
    s. pedicle screw
    s. pedicle screw fixation
    s. plexus avulsion
    s. screw placement
    s. segmental nerve stimulation
     implantable neural prosthesis
    s. spine
    s. spine decompression
    s. spine fixation
    s. spine fusion
    s. spine modular instrumentation
    s. spine stabilization
    s. spine universal instrumentation

sacramental
sacrificial
sacrilege
sacrococcygeal

    s. agenesis
    s. myxopapillary ependymoma
    s. spine
    s. teratoma

sacroiliac joint
sacroiliitis
sacrolisthesis
sacrum fusion screw fixation
SAD

    seasonal affective disorder
    Self-Assessment Depression
    separation anxiety disorder
    social avoidance and distress
     SAD scale

SADD

    Standardized Assessment of Depressive
     Disorders
    Students Against Drunk Driving

saddle

    Cloward surgical s.

saddle *(continued)*
 s. coil
 s. nose deformity
 tubercle of s.
saddle-area sensory loss
saddle-shaped anesthesia
SADIA
 small angle double incidence angiogram
sadism
 anal s.
 id s.
 infantile s.
 larval s.
 manual s.
 s. and masochism
 omnipotent infantile s.
 oral s.
 phallic s.
 primal s.
 sexual s.
 superego s.
sadism/masochism (S/M)
sadist
sadistic
 s. abuse
 s. act of rape
 s. behavior
 s. mutilation
 s. personality
 s. personality disorder
 s. rape act
SADL, SADLs
 simulated activities of daily living
sadness period
sadomasochism (SM, S&M, S/M)
 sexual s.
sadomasochistic
 s. personality disorder
 s. relationship
SADQ
 Self-Administered Dependency
 Questionnaire
SADR
 suspected adverse drug reaction
SADS
 Schedule for Affective Disorders and
 Schizophrenia
 seasonal affective disorder syndrome
 Shipman Anxiety Depression Scale
SADS-C
 Schedule for Affective Disorders and
 Schizophrenia-Change
SADS-L
 Schedule for Affective Disorders and
 Schizophrenia-Lifetime
Saenger sign
Saethre-Chotzen syndrome
safe place
Safe-T-Wheel pinwheel
safety
 s. device
 s. of ego
 s. motive
 s. valve

Safil synthetic absorbable surgical
 suture
Safran Student's Interest Inventory
 (SSII)
safrazine
SAFTEE
 Systematic Assessment for Treatment of
 Emergent Events
SAGES-P
 Screening Assessment for Gifted
 Elementary Students, Primary
sagging posture
sagittal
 s. anatomic alignment
 s. deformity
 s. groove
 s. orientation
 s. pedicle angle
 s. pedicle diameter
 s. plane
 s. plane instability
 s. plexus
 s. projection
 s. sinus
 s. sinus thrombosis
 s. slice fracture
 s. spin-echo image
 s. synostosis
 s. T1-weighted SE image
SAH
 subarachnoid hemorrhage
 angiogram-negative SAH
SAHS
 sleep apnea hypersomnolence syndrome
SAHS-UAO
 sleep apnea hypersomnolence syndrome
 associated with upper airway
 obstruction
SAI
 Schedule for Assessment of Insight
 Social Adequacy Index
 Student Adjustment Inventory
SAID
 sexually acquired immunodeficiency
Saint
 S. Anthony fire
 S. Anthony's dance
 S. Dymphna disease
 S. John's dance
 S. Joseph Adult Chewable Aspirin
 S. Louis Criteria for Schizophrenia
 S. Louis encephalitis
 S. Louis encephalitis virus (SLEV)
 S. Martin disease
 S. Mathurin disease
 S. Vitus dance
Sakoda complex
salaam
 s. attack
 s. convulsion
 s. seizure
 s. spasm
salad
 word s.

Salamon-Conte Life Satisfaction in the Elderly Scale (LSES)
salax
    paroneiria s.
salbutamol
sales
    S. Attitude Check List (SACL)
    S. Personality Questionnaire (SPQ)
    S. Style Diagnostic Test
Saleto
    S.-200
    S.-400
    S.-600
    S.-800
Salflex
Salgesic
Salibi carotid artery clamp
salicylamide
salicylate
    ammonium s.
    amyl s.
    choline s.
    ethyl s.
    magnesium s.
    potassium s.
    serum s.
    sodium s.
    triethanolamine s.
Salience Inventory (SI)
saline
    s. injection
    preservative-free normal s.
    s. torch
saline-soaked sponge
salivary
    s. gland
    s. gland dysfunction
saliva smearing
Salla disease
Salmonella
Salmonine Injection
Salmon Rickham ventriculostomy reservoir
Salpix
salsalate
Salsitab
saltation
saltatoria
    chorea s.
saltatory
    s. chorea
    s. conduction
    s. evolution
    s. spasm
salt-free diet
salts
    Earle s.
salt wasting
salubrious
Saluron
salute
    allergic s.
Salutensin
SAM
    sex arousal mechanism

samarium cobalt
samarium-EDTMP
sameness
    preoccupation with s.
same-sex
    s.-s. marriage
    s.-s. orientation
sample
    Life Study S. (LSS)
    Linguistic Analysis of Speech S.'s (LASS)
    random s.
    representative s.
    s. standard deviation
sampling
    area s.
    behavior s.
    block s.
    controlled s.
    petrosal sinus s.
SAMS
    Study Attitudes and Methods Survey
samsara
Samuels-Weck Hemoclip
SAN
    slept all night
sanatorium, sanitarium
    s. disease
sanction
    legal s.
    social s.
sanctioned
    culturally s.
sand
    s. body
    brain s.
    s. tumor
sandbox marriage
Sander disease
Sandhoff disease
Sandifer syndrome
Sandler
    S. triad
    S. view of depressive disorder
sandwich
    fascia-muscle-fascia s.
    s. generation
Sanfilippo
    S. disease
    S. syndrome
sangue dormido
sanguine constitutional type
sanitarium (*var. of* sanatorium)
Sano clip applier
Sanorex
SANS
    Scale for the Assessment of Negative Symptoms
Sansert
Santavuori disease
Santavuori-Haltia disease
Santavuori-Haltia-Hagberg disease
SAPD
    self-administration of psychoactive drug

S

saphenous
  s. vein
  s. vein bypass graft
  s. vein patch graft
sapience
sapphism
Sapporo shunt tube
SAPS
  Scale for the Assessment of Positive
  Symptoms
SAQ
  School Atmosphere Questionnaire
  Substance Abuse Questionnaire
saquinavir
SAR
  sexual attitude reassessment
  sexual attitude restructuring
Sarason General Anxiety and Test
  Anxiety Scale
sarcoglia
sarcoid
  s. neuropathy
  s. polyneuropathy
sarcoidosis
  intracranial s.
  s. peripheral neuropathy
sarcolemma membrane
sarcoma
  angiolithic s.
  Ewing s.
  fibrous s.
  granulocytic s.
  juxtacortical s.
  Kaposi s.
  orbital granulocytic s.
  osteogenic s.
  perithelial small cell s.
  reticulum cell s.
sarcomatous tumor
sarcosinemia
Sardinian multiple sclerosis
sardonic
  s. grin
  s. laugh
sardonicus
  risus s.
  trismus s.
sarmassation
saroten
SAS
  School Assessment Survey
  School Attitude Survey
  self-rating anxiety scale
  Situational Attitude Scale
  sleep apnea syndrome
  Social Adaptation Status
SASI
  Separation Anxiety Symptom Inventory
SASRS, SAS-RS
  Social Adjustment Self-Report Scale
SASSI
  Substance Abuse Subtle Screening
  Inventory
Sassouni analysis

SAT
  Scholastic Aptitude Test
  School Ability Test
  School Attitude Test
  Senior Apperception Technique
  Senior Apperception Test
  Shapes Analysis Test
  Stanford Achievement Test
  systematized assertive therapy
SATA
  Scholastic Abilities Test for Adults
satanic
  s. cult
  s. worship
satanism
satanophobia
satan's secret
Satan worship
SATB
  Special Aptitude Test Battery
satellite
  s. cell
  s. housing
satellitosis
satiation
  eating without s.
  food s.
satiety
  s. center
  s. response
satisfaction
  Index of Work S. (IWS)
  s. inventory
  job s.
  patient s.
  personal s.
sativa
  Cannabis s.
satumomab pendetide
saturation
  arterial oxygen s.
  jugular bulb venous oxygen s.
  jugular venous oxygen s. (SjO$_2$)
  partial s.
  receiver s.
  s. recovery
  s. transfer
Saturday night palsy
saturnine
  s. encephalopathy
  s. tremor
satyriasis
satyrism
satyromania
Saunders cervical HomeTrac
Saunders-Sutton syndrome
savant
  idiot s.
  linguistic s.
saver
  Cell S.
  intraoperative cell s.
savoir faire
saw
  Adson wire s.

Bier s.
Cushing s.
DeMartel wire s.
Gigli s.
Midas Rex craniotomy s.
Olivecrona-Gigli s.
Olivecrona wire s.
spinal s.
undercutting s.

Saxonius
coitus S.

Sayk preparation of cerebrospinal fluid

SB, S-B
Stanford-Binet
SB intelligence test
SB test

SBAI
Social Behavior Assessment Inventory

SBB
stimulation-bound behavior

SBD
Supervisory Behavior Description

SBIS
Stanford-Binet Intelligence Scale

SBQ
Smoking Behavior Questionnaire

SBS
social breakdown syndrome

scabiophobia

scaffolding

SCAL
Self-Concept as a Learner
SCAL scale

scala, pl. **scalae**
Löwenberg s.
s. media

SCALE
Scaled Curriculum Achievement Levels
Test
Scales of Creativity and Learning
Environment

scale
A s.
Abbreviated Conners Teacher
Rating S. (ACTRS)
Abnormal Involuntary
Movements S. (AIMS)
absolute rating s.
Academic Orientation s.
Academic Readiness S. (ARS)
Acceptance of Disability S.
achromatic-chromatic s.
Acuity of Psychiatric Illness s.
AD S.
Adaptive Behavior S. (ABS)
Adaptive Behavior Evaluation S.
(ABES)
ADD-H: Comprehensive Teacher's
Rating S., Second Edition
(ACTeRS)
ADL s.
Adult Self-Expression S. (ASES)
Affect Balance S.
age s.
age equivalent s.

aggressive s.
alcohol abuse s.
Alzheimer Disease Assessment S.
(ADAS)
Alzheimer Disease Rating S.
(ADRS)
American Musculoskeletal Tumor
Society rating s.
Amphetamine Interview Rating S.
(AIRS)
Annett hand preference s.
Anorexic Behavior S.
antisocial s.
anxiety s.
anxiety rating s.
Aphasia Language Performance S.
(ALPS)
Arizona Sexual Experience S.
A-S s.
Ashworth s.
assessment s.
S. for the Assessment of Negative
Symptoms (SANS)
S. for the Assessment of Positive
Symptoms (SAPS)
S. for Assessment of Thought,
Language, and Communication
S. for the Assessment of
Unawareness of Mental Disorder
(SUMD)
Attention Deficit Disorder Behavior
Rating S. (ADDBRS)
Attention Deficit Disorder
Comprehensive Teacher Rating S.
Attention Deficit Disorders
Evaluation S. (ADDES)
Attitudes Toward Mainstreaming S.
(ATMS)
autonomy s.
avoidant s.
balance s.
Balthazar S.'s of Adaptive
Behavior (BSAB)
Balthazar S.'s for Adaptive
Behavior I: Scales of Functional
Independence
Barnes Akathisia S.
Barron-Welsh Art S. (BWAS)
Beck Depression S.
Beck Hopelessness S. (BHS)
Beck Suicide Intent S.
Beck Suicide Lethality S.
Bedford Life Events and
Difficulties S.
BEHAVE-AD Rating S.
Behavioral Pathology in Alzheimer
Disease Rating S.
Behavioral Problems S.
behavioral rating s.
Behavior Disorders Identification S.
(BDIS)
Behavior Evaluation S. (BES-2)
behavior rating s.
behind the s.
Binet s.

S

scale (continued)
Binet-Simon s.
Birth to Three Developmental S.
Blessed Behavior S.
Blessed Dementia Rating S. (BDRS)
Blessed-Roth Dementia S. (BRDS)
borderline s.
Bracken Basic Concept S.
Brazelton Neonatal Behavioral Assessment S.
Brief Cognitive Rating S. (BCRS)
Brief Outpatient Psychopathology S.
Brief Psychiatric Rating S. (BPRS)
Bristol Language Development S. (BLADES)
British Ability S. (BAS)
British Ability Scales: Spelling S.
Brown Assessment of Beliefs S.
Bunney-Hamburg Rating S.
Burks Behavior Rating S. (BBRS)
Bzoch-League Receptive-Expressive Emergent Language S.
Caine-Levine Social Competency S.
California F S.
California Preschool Social Competency S. (CPSCS)
Callier-Azusa S.
Canadian Neurological S.
Catell Infant S.
Cattell Infant Intelligence S.
CDR S.
Center for Epidemiologic Studies-Depression S.
CES-D S.
CGI S.
Chapman S.
Child Anxiety S.
Child "At Risk" for Drug Abuse Rating S.
Child Health Self-Concept S.
Childhood Autism Rating S. (CARS)
Child Personality S. (CPS)
Children's Affective Rating S. (CARS)
Children's Depression S. (CDS)
Children's Depression Rating S.-Revised
Children's Global Assessment S. (CGAS)
Children's Hypnotic Susceptibility S.
Children's Manifest Anxiety S. (CMAS)
Children's Psychiatric Rating S. (CPRS)
Children's Self-Concept S. (CSCS)
Children's Version/Family Environmental S.
Children's Yale-Brown Obsessive Compulsive S. (CY-BOCS)
chromatic s.
Classroom Environmental S. (CES)

clinical s.
Clinical Adaptive Test/Clinical Linguistic Auditory Milestone S. (CAT/CLAMS)
Clinical Dementia Rating S.
Clinical Global Impressions S.
Clinical Global Improvement S.
Clinical Rating S. (CRS)
Clinician-Administered PTSD S.
Clinician Rated Anxiety S. (CRAS)
Clinician Rated Overall Life Impairment S.
Clinician's Global Rating S. (CGRS)
Clyde Mood S. (CMS)
Cognitive Behavior Rating S.'s
Collaborative Study Psychotherapy Rating S.
College and University Environment S.'s (CUES)
Columbia Mental Maturity S. (CMMS)
coma s.
Combat Exposure S.
communication s.
Community-Oriented Programs Environment S. (COPES)
Comprehensive Career Assessment S. (CCAS)
Comprehensive Level of Consciousness S. (CLCS)
Comprehensive Psychiatric Rating S. (CPRS)
Comprehensive Psychopathological Rating S.
compulsive s.
Comrey Personality S. (CPS)
Concept-Specific Anxiety S. (CAS)
Conflict in Marriage S. (CIMS)
Conflict Tactics S.
Conners Parent Rating S.
Conners Parent-Teacher Rating S.
Conners Teacher Rating S. (CRS-39, CTRS-28)
content s.
Cook-Medley Hostility S.
Cooper-Farran Behavioral Rating S. (CFBRS)
Cornell Depression S.
Correctional Institutions Environment S. (CIES)
Covi Anxiety S.
Craving Analog S.
S.'s of Creativity and Learning Environment (SCALE)
Cultural Attitude S. (CAS)
cumulative s.
Cumulative Illness Rating S.
Cumulative Illness Rating S.-Geriatric
Current and Past Psychopathology S. (CAPPS)
Curtis Interest S.
DBD S.
Death Anxiety S. (DAS)

Defensive Functioning S. (DFS)
Dementia Behavior Disturbance S.
Dementia Mood Assessment S.
(DMAS)
Dementia Rating S.
dependent s.
depression s.
Depression Rating S.
Derogatis Affects Balance S.
(DABS)
Description of Body S.
deterioration s.
development s.
developmental s.
development language s.
Devereux Adolescent Behavior
Rating S.
Devereux Elementary School
Behavior Rating S. II (DESBRS-
II)
dichotomous s.
Differential Ability S.
digital vernier s.
Dimensions of Delusional
Experience S.
Direct Assessment of Functional
Status S.
disability status s. (DSS)
discrepancy s.
Dissociative Disorders Interview S.
Dissociative Experience S. (DES)
drug abuse s.
Duke Severity of Illness S.
Dyadic Adjustment S.
dysthymia s.
E s.
Early Language Milestone S.
Early Social Communication S.
(ESCS)
Edinburgh 2 Coma S. (E2CS)
Edinburgh Postnatal Depression S.
Edinburgh Rehabilitation Status S.
E-F s.
Ego Development S. (EDS)
ego strength s.
Emotional and Behavior
Problem S. (EBPS)
S. for Emotional Blunting (SEB)
Endler Multidimensional Anxiety S.
(EMAS)
Environment S.
equal-interval s.
ethnocentrism s.
Everyday Worries S.
EVM grading of Glasgow
Coma S.
experiences s.
Extended Merrill-Palmer S.
Extrapyramidal Symptom Rating S.
Fagerstrom Nicotine Addiction S.
Family Adaptability and Cohesion
Evaluation S. III (FACES III)
Family Drawing Depression S.
(FDDS)
Family Environment S. (FES)

family evaluation s.
Family Satisfaction S.
Fazekas S.
Fels Parent Behavior Rating S.
fish s.'s
Fixity of Beliefs S.
Flint Infant Security S. (FISS)
Folstein Mini-Mental S.
Frankel s.
Functional Ergonomic Prolo S.
Functional Life S. (FLS)
Functional Systems S. (FSS)
GAF s.
GAF s.
Gait Abnormality Rating S.
(GARS)
GARF s.
Gastrointestinal Symptom Rating S.
Generalized Contentment S. (GCS)
Geriatric Depression S.
Gesell Child Development Age S.
(GCDAS)
Gesell Developmental S.
Gesell Infant S.
Gifted Evaluation S. (GES)
Glasgow Coma S. (GCS)
Glasgow Outcome S. (GOS)
Global Assessment S. (GAS)
Global Assessment of
Functioning S.
Global Assessment of Relational
Functioning S.
Global Clinical Judgments S.
Global Deterioration S. (GDS)
Global Obsessive Compulsive S.
global ward behavior s. (GWBS)
Goal Attainment S. (GAS)
grade s.
graphic rating s.
Grief Measurement S.
Group Encounter S. (GES)
Group Environment S. (GES)
Hachinski Ischemia S.
Hahnemann Elementary School
Behavior Rating S.
Hahnemann High School Behavior
Rating S.
Hamilton Anxiety S. (HAMA)
Hamilton Anxiety Rating S.
(HARS)
Hamilton Depression S. (HAMD)
Hamilton Depression Rating S.
(HDRS)
Haptic Intelligence S.
Hasegawa Dementia S.
Hess School Readiness S. (HSRS)
Hillside Akathisia S.
histrionic s.
Hoehn and Yahr s.
Hoge 10-Item Intrinsic
Religiosity S.
Hospital Anxiety and Depression S.
(HADS)
House-Brackmann S.

S

scale *(continued)*

House-Brackmann facial nerve
  function grading s.
House-Brackmann Grading S.
How-I-See-Myself S. (HISMS)
Hunt-Hess subarachnoid
  hemorrhage s.
hypochondriasis s. (Hs)
hypomania s.
hypomanic s.
hysteria s.
I-E S.
Impact of Events S.
Impulsive Nonconformity S.
S. of Independent Behavior
Infant/Toddler Environment
  Rating S. (ITERS)
inferred Self-Concept S.
infrequency s.
Injury Severity S. (ISS)
Inpatient Multidimensional
  Psychiatric S. (IMPS)
intelligence s.
interest s.
internal versus external s.
Interpersonal Perception S. (IPS)
interval s.
Intra- and Interpersonal
  Relations S.
introversion-extroversion s. (IES)
Introvertive Anhedonia S.
Iowa Conners Rating S.
Iowa Stuttering S.
IPAT Anxiety S.
IPAT Depression S.
Irritability/Depression and
  Anxiety S.
Job Attitude S. (JAS)
Karnofsky Performance S.
Karnofsky Rating S.
Katz Adjustment S. (KAS)
Kaufman Development S.
Kaufman Infant and Preschool S.
Kent Infant Development S.
Kurtzke Expanded Disability
  Status S.
language s.
Leadership Evaluation and
  Department S.
Learning Disability Evaluation S.
  (LDES)
Leiter Adult Intelligence S.
Leiter International Performance S.
  (LIPS)
Leiter Recidivism S.
lethality s.
lie s.
life change rating s.
Likert s.
Lincoln-Oseretsky Motor
  Development S.
Lock Wallace Short Marital
  Adjustment S.
Locus of Control of Behavior S.

London Psychogeriatric S. (LPS)
Lorr S.
Luborsky Health-Sickness Rating S.
MacAndrew Addiction S. (MAS)
Mach S.
Major Role Adjustment S. II
Major Symptoms of
  Schizophrenia S.
Management Philosophies S. (I-V)
  (MPS)
Mandel Social Adjustment S.
  (MSAS)
Mania "9" S.
Mania Rating S. (MRS)
Manic-State Rating S.
Manifest Anxiety S. (MAS)
manual vernier s.
Marital Communication S.
Marks-Sheehan Phobia S.
Marlow-Crowne S. (MCS)
masculinity-femininity s.
Maternal Attitude S. (MAS)
Mathematics Anxiety Rating S.
  (MARS)
Mathematics Anxiety Rating S.-
  Adolescents (MARS-A)
Mattis Dementia Rating S.
Mattis-Kovner S.
maturity s.
McAndrews Alcoholism S. (MAC)
Medical Outcomes Study Short-
  Form General Health Survey
  Physical Functioning S.
Meffill-Palmer S.
memory s.
Memory Assessment S.'s (MAS)
mental s.
Merrill-Palmer S.
Mill Hill Vocabulary S.
Minnesota Cocaine Craving S.
  (MCCS)
Minnesota Preschool S.
Minnesota Satisfaction S. (MSS)
Miskimins Self-Goal-Other
  Discrepancy S.
Modified Rankin S.
Modified Simpson Dyskinesia S.
Montgomery-Asberg Depression
  Rating S. (MADRS)
Mood and Physical Symptoms S.
  (MPSS)
Moos Family Environment S.
movement s.
Multidimensional Self Concept S.
  (MSCS)
narcissistic s.
National Institute of Mental
  Health-Global Obsessive
  Compulsive S. (NIMH-OC)
National Institutes of Health
  Stroke S.
Naylor-Harwood Adult
  Intelligence S. (NHAIS)
Naylor-Harwood Intelligence S.
  (NHIS)

Need for Cognition S.
Neonatal Behavioral Assessment S. (NBAS)
Neurosurgical Cervical Spine S.
New York University Parkinson Disease S.
NGI S.
NIH Stroke S.
NIMH Global Obsessive-Compulsive S.
Nottingham Ten-Point ADL S.
Nurse's Global Impressions S.
Objective Opiate Withdrawal S.
Object Sorting S. (OSS)
Obsessive-Compulsive Drinking S. (OCDS)
Obsessive-Compulsive Subscale of the Comprehensive Psychopathological Rating S.
Oral-Motor/Feeding Rating S.
Overcontrolled Hostility S. (OHS)
Overt Aggression S.
Oxford STA s.
Panic Disorder Severity S.
Paranoia "6" S.
paranoid s.
Parent-Adolescent Communication S.
Parental Stressor S.
Parent Attitude S. (PAS)
PARS S.
passive-aggressive s.
Patient Rated Anxiety S. (PRAS)
Patient Rated Disability S.
Patient Rated Impairment S.
Pattern Misfit S.
Patterns of Individual Change S. (PICS)
Paykel Life Events S.
PEC s.
Pediatric Behavior S. (PBS)
Perception of Illness S.
Personal Adjustment and Role Skills S.
personality disorders s.
Personality Rating S. (PRS)
Personal Preference S. (PPS)
Phelps Kindergarten Readiness S. (PKRS)
Phillips S.
Physical Self-Maintenance S.
Piers-Harris Children's Self-Concept S.
point s.
politico-economic-conservatism s.
Positive and Negative Stroke S. (PANSS)
Positive and Negative Symptom S.
Positive and Negative Symptoms of Schizophrenia S.
Positive and Negative Syndrome S. (PANSS)
Posttraumatic Stress Disorder S.
Posttraumatic Stress Disorder Symptom S.
Premorbid Social Adjustment S.

Pre-Reading Expectancy Screening S. (PRESS)
Preschool Language S. (PLS)
Process Skills Rating S. (PSRS)
Psychasthenia "7" S.
psychasthenia s.
psychiatric rating s.
psychiatric reacting s.
Psychiatric Status Rating S.
Psycholinguistic Rating S.
psychologic rating s.
Psychopathic Deviance "4" S.
psychopathic deviance s.
Psychopathological Rating S.
s. of psychosis (SP)
Psychosocial Adjustment to Illness S. (PAIS)
psychotic delusions s.
psychotic depression s.
psychotic thinking s.
Pupil Rating S. (PRS)
Pyramid S.
Quality of Well-Being S.
S. Questionnaire
Random Letter Test Raskin Severity of Depression S.
Raskin Depression S.
Raskin Severity of Depression S.
Rated Anxiety S.
rating s.
ratio s.
reacting s.
reaction s.
Reaction Level S. (RLS)
Receptive-Expressive Emergent Language s.
Receptive-Expressive Observation S.
REEL s.
Rehabilitation Client Rating S. (RCRS)
Relative Value S.
REO S.
repression s.
repression-sensitization s.
Resource-Based Relative Value S. (RBRVS)
Revised Children's Depression S. (RCDS)
Revised Children's Manifest Anxiety S.
Revised Ontario Child Health Study S.
Reynolds Adolescent S.
Reynolds Adolescent Depression S. (RADS)
Reynolds Child Depression S. (RCDS)
Rhode Island Pupil Identification S. (PIPIS, RIPIS)
Right-Wing Authoritarianism s.
Rogers Criminal Responsibility S.
Rosenberg Self-Esteem S. (RSES)
Rucker-Gable Educational Programming S. (RGEPS)

S

scale *(continued)*
Russell variant of the Wechsler Memory S.
Russell Version Wechsler Memory S.
RWA s.
SAD s.
Salamon-Conte Life Satisfaction in the Elderly S. (LSES)
Sarason General Anxiety and Test Anxiety S.
SCAL s.
schizoid s.
Schizophrenia "8" S.
schizophrenia s.
schizotypal s.
School Handicap Condition S. (SEH)
school readiness s.
School Social skills Rating S.
Schwab and England Activities of Daily Living S.
s. scores subtest
Screening for Learning Disabilities, Pupil Rating S.
SEC S.
Self-Assessment Depression S.
Self-Concept S.
Self-Concept as a Learner s.
Self-Consciousness S.
Self-Control S. (SCS)
self-esteem s.
self-rating anxiety s. (SAS)
Self-Rating Depression S. (SDS, SRDS)
Sensation-Seeking S. (SSS)
sensory s.
Severity of Psychiatric Illness S.
Severity of Psychosocial Stressors S.
sexual differentiation s. (SDS)
Sheehan Disability S.
Sheltered Care Environment S.
Shipley-Hartford S.
Shipley Institute of Living S. (SILS)
Shipman Anxiety Depression S. (SADS)
Simpson S.
Simpson-Angus S.
Simpson-Angus Rating S.
Situational Attitude S. (SAS)
Sleep and Breathing Problems S.
Sleepiness S.
Slosson Children's Version Family Environment S.
Smith-Johnson nonverbal Performance S.
Social Adjustment S.
Social Adjustment S. II
Social Adjustment Self-Report S. (SASRS, SAS-RS)
Social Avoidance and Distress S.
Social Climate S. (SCS)

S. of Social Development
Social Disability S.
Social-Emotional Dimension S.
Social Interaction S.
social introversion s.
Social and Occupational Functioning Assessment S.
Social Readjustment Rating S. (SRRS)
social readjustment rating s.
Social Reintegration S.
Social Reticence S.
Social Support S.
sociotropy s.
Somatic "3" S.
somatoform s.
special s.
Spelling S.
Spetzler-Martin grading s.
Spielberger Anger Expression S.
Spiritual Well-Being S. (SWBS)
Stanford-Binet Intelligence S. (SBIS)
Stanford Hypnotic Susceptibility S. (SHSS)
Stanford Sleepiness S.
State-Trait Anger S. (STAS)
status s.
Stress Impact S. (SIS)
Stress Response S.
Subjective High Assessment S.
Subjective Opiate Withdrawal S.
Subjective Symptoms S.
Subjective Treatment Emergent Side Effects S.
Subjective Units of Distress S. (SUDS)
Subject Treatment Emergent Symptom S.
Suicide Intent S.
Suicide Probability S.
Suinn Test Anxiety Behavior S. (STABS)
suppressor s.
Swanson, Nolan, and Pelham Rating S.
Symptom Rating S. (SRS)
Task Assessment S.
Taylor Manifest Anxiety S. (TMAS)
Teacher Evaluation S. (TES)
Teasdale and Jennett s.
Tennessee Self-Concept S. (TSCS)
Test Anxiety S.
test point s.
The Instructional Environment S. (TIES)
Thorndike Handwriting S.
Thurstone Attitude S.
Timed Stereotypes Rating S.
TMJ S.
Toronto Alexithymia S.
Tourette Syndrome Association Unified Tic Rating S.
Tourette Syndrome Global S.

Tourette Syndrome Severity S.
Transition Behavior S. (TBS)
tridimensional evaluational s. (TES)
Unified Parkinson Disease
  Rating S. (UPDRS)
University Residence
  Environment S. (URES)
Uzgiris-Hunt S.
validity s.
Vane Evaluation of Language S.
  (VELS)
verbal s. (VS)
Verbal Language Development S.
Verdun Depression Rating S.
  (VDRS)
Verdun Target Symptom Rating S.
  (VTSRS)
Vineland Adaptive Behavior S.
Vineland percentile s.
Vineland Social Maturity S.
  (VSMS)
visual analog s. (VAS)
vocabulary s.
Vocabulary Comprehension S.
Waldrop S.
Ward Atmosphere S. (WAS)
Ward Behavior Rating S. (WBRS)
Ways of Coping S.
Weak Opiate Withdrawal S.
  (WOWS)
Wechsler Adult Intelligence S.
  (WAIS)
Wechsler Adult Intelligence S.-
  Revised
Wechsler Adult Intelligence S.-
  Third Edition (WAIS-III)
Wechsler-Bellevue S. (WBS)
Wechsler Intelligence S.
Wechsler Intelligence S. for
  Children-Revised (WISC-R)
Wechsler Intelligence S. for
  Children, Revised Version and
  Version III
Wechsler Intelligence S. for
  Children-Third Edition (WISC-III)
Wechsler IQ S.
Wechsler Memory S. (WMS)
Wechsler Memory S. - Revised
  (WMS-R)
well-being s.
Wender Utah Rating S.
WHO Handicap S.
Wiggins Content S. (WCS)
Wing Negative Symptom S.
Wittenborn Psychiatric Rating S.
  (WITT, WPRS)
Wood Assessment S.
Work Environment S. (WES)
Work and Social Adjustment S.
Worse Premorbid Adjustment S.
Wortman Social Support S.
Yale-Brown Obsessive
  Compulsive S. (YBOCS)
Yale Global Tic Severity S.
Young Mania Rating S.

Zung Anxiety S.
Zung Depression S. (ZDS)
Zung Self-Rating Depression S.

scaled
  S. Curriculum Achievement Levels
    Test (SCALE)
  s. stereotactic atlas section

scalene
scalenectomy
scalenotomy
scalenus
  s. anterior syndrome
  s. anticus
  s. anticus muscle

scaling
  age-grade s.
  item s.

scalp
  s. clip
  s. clip applicator
  s. clip forceps
  s. closure
  s. contusion
  s. EEG monitoring
  s. electrical potential
  s. electroencephalography
  s. flap
  s. flap forceps
  s. hematoma
  s. incision
  s. infection
  s. laceration
  s. lock
  s. tenderness

scalp-sphenoidal electroencephalography
(SSEEG)
SCAMI, SCAMIN
  Self-Concept and Motivation Inventory
SCAN
  suspected child abuse/neglect
scan
  attenuation coefficient on MRI s.
  attenuation value on MRI s.
  bone-window CT s.
  brain s.
  contrast-enhanced CT s.
  CT s.
  emission tomography s.
  eye s.
  fluorodopa positron emission
    tomographic s.
  gallium s.
  instant s.
  MRI s.
  nuclear MR s.
  PET s.
  radioisotope s.
  sequential computed tomographic s.
  SPECT s.
  technetium s.
  1.5-Tesla General Electric signa s.
  s. time
  tomography s.
  triple phase bone s.
  T1-weighted inversion recovery s.

S

scanner
s. assisted target localization
ATL real-time Neurosector s.
General Electric CT 9800 s.
General Electric Hispeed Advantage helical s.
General Electric signa 1.5-Tesla magnetic resonance s.
OctreoScan s.
Siemens Magnetom s.
SilkTouch CO_2 laser s.
SwiftLase s.
Vista American Health 0.5 Tesla MRI s.

scanning
CAT s.
s. communication board
comparative s.
computerized axial tomography s.
confocal laser s. (CLSM)
diffusion-weighted s.
duplex s.
s. electron microscopy (SEM)
eye s.
functional activation PET s.
line s.
point s.
radioisotope brain s.
radionucleotide s.
RN s.
s. speech
s. visage
XeCT s.
xenon CT s.

SCAN-TRON Reading Test
scapegoated subsystem
scapegoating communication pattern
scaphocephalic idiocy
scaphocephaly
scaphohydrocephalus, scaphohydrocephaly
scapulae
levator s.

scapular
s. nerve
s. reflex

scapulohumeral
s. atrophy
s. reflex

scapuloperiosteal reflex
scapuloperoneal
s. muscular atrophy
s. muscular dystrophy
s. syndrome

scar
emotional s.
hemosiderin s.
psychic s.

Scaramella procedure
scarify
scarlet letter
SCARMD
severe childhood autosomal recessive muscular dystrophy

Scarpa
S. ganglion
S. method

scarring
glial s.

SCAT
School and College Ability Test

scatologia
telephone s.

scatological language
scatology
scatophagy
scatophobia
scatter
s. child
s. diagram
intratest s.

scattered
s. dysrhythmic slow activity
s. dysrhythmic slow activity on EEG

scattergram
scattering
Compton s.

scavenger
free radical s.

SCBF
spinal cord blood flow

SCD
sequential compression device
service-connected disability

Scedosporium apiospermum
scelalgia
scelerophobia
scelotyrbe
scene
primal s.
traumatic s.

Sceratti arc
Schacher ganglion
schadenfreude
Schaffer
S. collateral
S. collateral cell

Schäffer reflex
Schaie-Thurstone Adult Mental Abilities Test
Schaltenbrand-Wahren stereotactic atlas
Scharff microbipolar and suction forceps
Schaumberg disease
schedule
abnormal sleep-wake s.
S. for Affective Disorders and Schizophrenia (SADS)
S. for Affective Disorders and Schizophrenia-Change (SADS-C)
S. for Affective Disorders and Schizophrenia - Change
S. for Affective Disorders and Schizophrenia-Lifetime (SADS-L)
S. for Affective Disorders and Schizophrenia Lifetime Version
S. for Affective Disorders and Schizophrenia for School-Age

Children (KIDDIE-SADS, K-SADS)
S. for Affective Disorders and Schizophrenia for School Age Children
S. for Affective Disorders and Schizophrenia for School-Age Children-Epidemiologic Version (K-SADS-E)
S. for Affective Disorders and Schizophrenia for School-Age Children-Present Episode (K-SADS-P)
Anxiety Disorders Interview S.
S. for Assessment of Insight (SAI)
Brown and Harris Life Event and Difficulty S.
California Life Goals Evaluation S.
Child Assessment S. (CAS)
continuous reinforcement s.
developmental s.
Diagnostic Interview S. (DIS)
Dissociative Disorders Interview S.
s. drug
Edwards Personal Preference S. (EPPS)
Family History Research Diagnostic Criteria S.
Fear Survey S. (FSS)
fixed-interval reinforcement s.
fixed-ratio reinforcement s.
Gesell Developmental S.'s
Glasgow Assessment S.
S. of Growing Skills
S. I
S. II
S. III
Illness and Symptom History S.
interest s.
intermittent reinforcement s.
S. IV
Laterality Preference S.
medical taper s.
mental status s. (MSS)
Neuropsychiatric Rating S.
Past History S.
Pleasant Events S. (PES)
s.'s preoccupation
Psychiatric Status S. (PSS)
Psychotherapy Competence Assessment S. (PCAS)
S. of Recent Experience (SRE)
s. of reinforcement
reinforcement s.
shifting sleep-work s.
sleep-wake s.
Social Behavior Assessment S.
Social Maladjustment S.
status s.
Thurstone Interest S.
Thurstone Temperament S.
Unpleasant Events S. (UES)
variable-interval reinforcement s.
vocational interest s. (VIS)

Work Environment Preference S. (WEPS)
Yale Revised Developmental S.
Scheicker laminectomy punch forceps
Scheid
cyanotic syndrome of S.
S. cyanotic syndrome
Scheie
S. disease
S. syndrome
schema, pl. **schemata**
body s.
cognitive s.
perceptual s.
schematic
scheme
Integrated Child Development S. (ICDS)
schenckii
Sporothrix s.
Scheuermann
S. disease
S. kyphosis
Schicksal analysis
Schiefferdecker disk
Schiff-Sherrington phenomenon
Schilder
S. aminoaciduria
S. disease
S. encephalitis
Schilling test
Schirmer
S. syndrome
S. test
schism
marital s.
schismatic
schistorrhachis
Schistosoma mansoni
schistosomiasis
schizaxon
schizencephalic microcephaly
schizencephaly
schizoaffective
s. disorder
s. episode
s. psychosis
s. schizophrenia
schizobipolar
schizocaria
schizogen
schizogyria
schizoid
s. disorder
s. disorder of childhood
s. fantasy
s. feature
s. personality
s. personality disorder
s. position
s. scale
schizoidia
schizoidism
schizoid-schizotypal personality disorder (SSPD)

S

schizomania
schizomimetic
schizophasia
schizophrene
schizophrenese
schizophrenia (SZ)
    active phase of s.
    active-phase symptoms of s.
    acute s.
    agitation catatonic s.
    alternative dimensional descriptors
      for s.
    ambulatory s.
    arrest of s.
    atypical s.
    behavioral disorganization in s.
    borderline s. (BS)
    burned-out anergic s.
    catalepsy s.
    catastrophic s.
    catatonic s.
    s., catatonic type
    cenesthesiopathic s.
    cenesthopathic s.
    Chestnut Lodge Prognostic Scale
      for Chronic S.
    childhood s.
    chronic s.
    chronic undifferentiated s.
    compensation s.
    cyclic s.
    s. deliriosa
    depressed schizoaffective s.
    diathesis-stress theory of s.
    disorganized factor in s.
    disorganized speech in s.
    s., disorganized type
    disorganized-type s.
    distorted communication in s.
    distorted language in s.
    double bind theory of s.
    early-onset s.
    engrafted s.
    exaggerated communication in s.
    exaggerated inferential thinking
      in s.
    excited catatonic s.
    excited schizoaffective s.
    3-factor dimensional model of s.
    familial s.
    familial transmission of s.
    Finnish Adoptive Family Study
      of S.
    first-episode s.
    flexibilitas cerea s.
    fragmentary hallucinations in s.
    grandiose-type s.
    hebephrenic s.
    iatrogenic s.
    incipient s.
    s. index
    individual with S.
    induced s.
    International Pilot Study of S.
      (IPSS)

jealous-type s.
larval s.
latent s.
late-onset s.
mixed s.
mixed-type s.
negative-symptom s.
nondeficit s.
non-kraepelinian chronic s.
nonregressive s.
nonsystematic s.
nuclear s.
oneiroid s.
paranoid s.
s., paranoid type
paraphrenic s.
Pavlov theory of s.
persecutory-type s.
s. phase
postemotive s.
postpsychotic depressive disorder
    of s.
prepsychotic s.
primary s.
process s.
prodromal s.
prodromal phase of s.
prolonged prodrome of s.
pseudoautosomal locus for s.
pseudoneurotic s.
pseudopsychopathic s.
s. psychosis
psychotic disorganization in s.
reactive s.
recidivism in s.
regressive s.
regressive symptoms of s.
remitting s.
residual s.
residual phase of s.
s., residual type
restitutional s.
restitutional symptoms of s.
restzustand s.
retarded s.
reversible s.
s. risk
Saint Louis Criteria for S.
S. "8" Scale
s. scale
Schedule for Affective Disorders
    and S. (SADS)
Schedule for Affective Disorders
    and S.-Change (SADS-C)
Schedule for Affective Disorders
    and S.-Lifetime (SADS-L)
schizoaffective s.
schizophreniform s.
Schneider diagnostic system for s.
Selvini-Palazzoli model of s.
simple s.
s. simplex
somatic s.
stupor catatonic s.
subchronic s.

s. symptom
systematic s.
three-day s.
total push treatment of s.
toxic s.
treatment-refractory s.
treatment-resistant s.
undifferentiated s.
s., undifferentiated type
unspecified s.
water balance in s.
withdrawn catatonic s.
s. with premorbid asociality (SPA)
s. with premorbid association
(SPA)

schizophrenic
s. affect
anergic s.
S.'s Anonymous
s. attack
burned-out s.
s. catalepsy
s. catatonia
s. defect state
s. dementia
s. disorder
disorganized-type s.
s. episode
s. exacerbation
s. excitement
s. factor
s. genotype
neuroleptic-resistant s.
s. paranoid psychosis
s. personality
s. process
s. psychology
s. reaction (SR, S/R)
s. reaction, acute, paranoid
(SR/AP)
s. reaction, acute undifferentiated
(SR/AU)
s. reaction, acute, undifferentiated
s. reaction, chronic, paranoid
(SR/CP)
s. reaction, chronic, undifferentiated
(SR/CU)
s. reaction circular reaction
residual s.
s. residual state (SRS)
s. spectrum (SS)
s. surrender
s. syndrome
s. syndrome of childhood
treatment-resistant s.

schizophrenic/affective psychosis
schizophreniform
s. attack
confusional s.
s. disorder
s. psychosis
s. schizophrenia

schizophrenogenic mother
schizophrenoides
delirium s.

schizophrenosis
schizotaxia
schizothyme
schizothymia
introverted s.
schizotypal s.

schizothymic personality
schizotonia
schizotypal
s. personality disorder
s. scale
s. schizoid personality
s. schizothymia

Schlesinger
S. intervertebral disk rongeur
S. laminectomy rongeur
S. sign

Schlichter test
Schloffer operation
Schmeden dural scissors
Schmidt-Fischer angle
Schmidt-Lanterman
S.-L. clefts
S.-L. incisure

Schmidt vagoaccessory syndrome
Schmieden-Taylor dissector
Schmitt disease
Schmorl
S. node
S. nodule

Schneider
S. definition of personality
S. diagnostic system for
schizophrenia

schneiderian
s. criteria for depressive personality
s. delusion
s. first-rank symptom

Schnidt clamp
Scholastic
S. Abilities Test for Adults
(SATA)
S. Aptitude Test (SAT)
S. Level Exam (SLE)

scholionophobia
Scholz disease
school
S. Ability Test (SAT)
s. achievement
s. adjustment
S. Administrator Assessment Survey
alternative s.
S. Apperception Method
S. Assessment Survey (SAS)
S. Atmosphere Questionnaire (SAQ)
S. Attitude Survey (SAS)
S. Attitude Test (SAT)
s. aversion
S. Climate Inventory
S. and College Ability Test
(SCAT)
s. counselor
day s.
s. difficulty
s. discipline problem

school *(continued)*
    s. drop-out
    s. dysfunction
    s. entering problem
    S. Environment Preference Survey
    existential s.
    s. functioning
    s. functioning impairment
    s. handicap condition (SEC)
    S. Handicap Condition Scale (SEH)
    s. history
    humanistic s.
    S. Interest Inventory
    s. language
    S. Library/Media Skills Test
    S. Motivation Analysis Test (SMAT)
    Multidimensional Assessment of Gains in S. (MAGS)
    s. performance
    s. phobia
    S. Problem Screening Inventory (SPSI)
    s.'s of psychiatry
    s. readiness scale
    S. Readiness Screening Test
    S. Readiness Survey
    s. refusal
    s. refusal syndrome
    S. Situation Survey (SSS)
    S. Social skills Rating Scale
    Test of Attitude Toward S. (TAS)
    s. truancy
    Zurich s.
school-age testing
schoolcraft
Schooler-Kane criteria
schoolsickness
Schreber case
Schrötter chorea
Schubert General Ability Battery
Schuele sign
Schüller-Christian syndrome
Schüller phenomenon
Schultze
    S. bundle
    S. cell
    S. sign
Schütz
    S. bundle
    S. Measures
Schwabach Test
Schwab and England Activities of Daily Living Scale
Schwalbe nucleus
Schwann
    S. cell
    S. cell body
    S. cell differentiation
    S. cell marker
    S. cell origin
    S. white substance
Schwann-cell implant

schwannoma
    acoustic s.
    cerebellopontine angle s.
    intraosseous s.
    spinal intradural s.
    synchronous facial s.
    vestibular s. (VS)
schwannosis
Schwartz
    S. aneurysm clip
    S. laminectomy retractor
    S. temporary intracranial artery clamp
    S. tractotomy
Schwartz-Jampel syndrome
sciaphobia
sciatic
    s. nerve
    s. nerve lesion
    s. neuralgia
    s. neuritis
    s. notch syndrome
    s. pain
    s. plexus
    s. scoliosis
sciatica
SCID
    Structured Clinical Interview for DSM-III-R
    Structured Clinical Interview for DSM-IV
SCID-CV
    Structured Clinical Interview for DSM-IV Axis I Disorders: Clinician Version
SCID-D
    Structured Clinical Interview for DSM-III-R Dissociative Disorders
    Structured Clinical Interview for DSM-IV Dissociative Disorders
SCID-II
    Structured Clinical Interview for DSM-IV Axis II Personality Disorders
SCID-IV
    Structured Clinical Interview for DSM-IV Dissociative Disorders
SCID-P
    Structured Clinical Interview for DSM-III-R-Patient Version
SCID-PD
    Structured Clinical Interview for DSM-III-R Psychotic Disorders
science
    behavioral s.
    cognitive s.
    S. Research Associates (SRA)
    S. Research Associates Mechanical Aptitude
scientific method
scientism
SCII
    Strong-Campbell Interest Inventory
scintiangiography
scintigram
    ^{99m}Tc-HMPAO leukocyte s.

scintigraphy
 Ga s.
 indium-111 octreotide s.
 leukocyte s.
 regional cerebral blood flow s.
 ^{99m}Tc-HMPAO leukocyte s.
 ^{201}Tl s.
scintillating scotoma
scintillation camera
scintiphoto
sciolism
sciophobia
sciosophy
scissor gait
scissoring
scissors
 Adson ganglion s.
 alligator MacCarty s.
 Aslan endoscopic s.
 bipolar cautery s.
 Codman s.
 Dandy neurological s.
 Dandy neurosurgical s.
 Dandy trigeminal nerve s.
 DeBakey endarterectomy s.
 Decker alligator s.
 Decker microsurgical s.
 dural s.
 Frazier dural s.
 Harrington s.
 Jacobson microneurosurgical s.
 Jannetta-Kurze dissecting s.
 Jansen-Middleton s.
 Kurze dissection s.
 Malis bipolar cautery s.
 Malis neurological s.
 Mayo s.
 Metzenbaum s.
 Micro-Two s.
 Nicola s.
 Olivecrona dura s.
 Olivecrona trigeminal s.
 Schmeden dural s.
 Smellie s.
 Strully dural s.
 Strully neurological s.
 Sweet pituitary s.
 Taylor brain s.
 Taylor dural s.
 Toennis dissecting s.
 Yasargil bayonet s.
SCIWORA
 spinal cord injury without radiological
  abnormality
scleractinian coral
sclerencephaly, sclerencephalia
scleresis
 pavor s.
scleritis
sclerneuropsia
sclerodactyly, sclerodactylia
scleroderma
sclerodermatomyositis
scleropia

sclerosing
 s. encephalitis
 s. panencephalitis
sclerosis, pl. scleroses
 Alzheimer s.
 Ammon horn s.
 amyotrophic lateral s. (ALS)
 Baló s.
 Baló concentric s.
 Canavan s.
 cerebral s.
 combined s.
 congenital hippocampal s.
 diffuse cerebral s.
 diffuse infantile familial s.
 discogenic s.
 disseminated s.
 Evers diet for multiple s.
 familial amyotrophic lateral s.
 familial forms of amyotrophic
  lateral s. (FALS)
 focal s.
 hippocampal s.
 insular s.
 ipsilateral mesial temporal s.
 Krabbe diffuse s.
 laminar cortical s.
 lateral spinal s.
 lobar s.
 MacDougall diet for multiple s.
 mantle s.
 mesial temporal s. (MTS)
 multiple s. (MS)
 posterior spinal s.
 primary lateral s.
 Sardinian multiple s.
 secondary-progressive multiple s.
 subchondral s.
 systemic s.
 tuberous s.
 s. of white matter
sclerotic
 s. area
 s. plaque
sclerotica
 eutonia s.
scleroticans
 encephaloleukopathia s.
sclerotome area
SCL-90-R
 Symptom Checklist-90-Revised
SCM
 split-cord malformation
scoleciphobia
scoliosis
 adult s.
 compensatory s.
 congenital s.
 degenerative lumbar s.
 double major curve s.
 double thoracic curve s.
 fracture with s.
 idiopathic s.
 King type II s.
 King type V s.

S

scoliosis *(continued)*
    lumbar s.
    neuromuscular s.
    osteopathic s.
    paralytic s.
    right thoracic curve s.
    right thoracic left lumbar s.
    right thoracic left thoracolumbar s.
    rigid curve s.
    sciatic s.
    thoracic curve s.
    thoracolumbar idiopathic s.
    thoracolumbar spine s.
scoliotic curve fixation
scoop
    Cushing pituitary s.
    Scoville intervertebral disk s.
    Yasargil s.
SCOPE
    systematic, complete, objective, practical,
    empirical
scope
    VM900 Smart S.
scopolagnia
scopolamine
    transdermal s.
scopomorphinism
scopophilia
scopophobia, scoptophobia
SCOR
    skin conductance orienting response
scoracratia
score
    Abbreviated Injury S. (AIS)
    Acute Physiology S.
    age s.
    Apgar s.
    ASA s.
    Beck depression inventory s.
    Champion Trauma S. (CTS)
    Children's Coma S. (CCS)
    Chronic Disease S.
    clinical performance s. (CPS)
    com s.
    critical s.
    dichotomization of s.
    s. discrimination
    finger-tapping s.
    Full Scale IQ s.
    Hachinski ischemic s.
    Hamilton Depression S.
    Hopkins Symptom Checklist-90
      Total S. (HSCL-90 T)
    House-Brackmann S.
    Injury Severity S. (ISS)
    intelligence s.
    ipsative s.
    Karnofsky performance s. (KPS)
    K-corrected raw s.
    Lahey s.
    Least Preferred Coworker S.
    LOCI s.
    LOD s.
    Maternal Trait Anxiety S. (MTAS)

    memory s.
    PAD s.
    pain and distress s.
    percentile s.
    performance s.
    Performance IQ S.
    Performance Scale S.
    practical social judgment s.
    quantitative s.
    RAATE s.
    Reading Sight Vocabulary
      Standard S.
    Revised Trauma S. (RTS)
    social judgment s.
    speech discrimination s. (SDS)
    subclinical s.
    subtest scale s.
    summary s.
    Verbal IQ s.
    Verbal Scale S.
    Visual Memory S. (VMS)
    word discrimination s.
    z s.
scoring
    objective s.
scotoma, pl. **scotomata**
    absolute s.
    scotomata of action
    bilateral centrocecal s.
    cecocentral s.
    central s.
    dense s.
    flittering s.
    fortification s.
    hemianopic s.
    homogenous scintillating s.
    homonymous scintillating s.
    mental s.
    negative s.
    paracentral s.
    relative s.
    scintillating s.
scotomization
scotophilia
scotophobia
Scott
    S. cannula
    S. Mental Alertness Test
    S. silicone ventricular catheter
Scoville
    S. blade
    S. brain clip-applying forceps
    S. brain spatula
    S. brain spatula forceps
    S. cervical disk retractor
    S. clip
    S. clip-applying forceps
    S. disk curette
    S. dissector
    S. hemilaminectomy retractor
    S. intervertebral disk scoop
    S. nerve root hook
    S. nerve root retractor
    S. ruptured disk curette
    S. skull trephine

S. spatula forceps
S. ventricular needle
Scoville-Haverfield hemilaminectomy
retractor
Scoville-Richter laminectomy retractor
scratch fear
scratching automatism
scream
primal s.
SCREEN
Screening Children for Related Early
Educational Needs
screen
Basic School Skills Inventory-S.
blood drug s.
S. for Child Anxiety Related
Emotional Disorders
Communication Abilities Diagnostic
Test and S.
s. defense
dream s.
drug s.
Early Years Easy S. (EYES)
ether s.
s. fantasy
heavy metal s.
Lancaster red-green s.
memory s.
s. memory
s. out irrelevant stimulus
Prevocational Assessment S. (PAS)
Test of Articulation
Performance, S. (TAP-S)
The Primary Language S. (TPLS)
urine drug s.
screener
Basic Achievement Skills
Individual S.
Bayley Infant
Neurodevelopmental S. (BINS)
Voc-Tech Quick S. (VTQS)
screening
S. Assessment for Gifted
Elementary Students, Primary
(SAGES-P)
Beery Picture Vocabulary S. (PVS)
Bexley-Maudsley Automated
Psychological S.
S. Children for Related Early
Educational Needs (SCREEN)
developmental s.
Ewing & Rooss four-question
alcohol s. (CAGE)
s. examination
fetal s.
genetic s.
S. Instrument for Targeting
Educational Risk (SIFTER)
s. inventory
S. Kit of Language Development
(SKOLD)
language s.
S. for Learning Disabilities
S. for Learning Disabilities, Pupil
Rating Scale

Mother/Infant Communication S.
(MICS)
organicity s.
periodic s.
S. Questionnaire
s. test
S. Test of Academic Readiness
S. Test of Adolescent Language
S. Test for the Assignment of
Remedial Treatment (STaRT)
S. Test for Auditory
Comprehension of Language
(STACL)
S. Test for Educational Prerequisite
Skills (STEPS)
S. Tests for Young Children and
Retardates (STYCAR)
screw
alar s.
s. alignment bar
s. alignment rod
s. angulation
s. backout
bone s.
s. breakage
Camino subdural s.
cancellous s.
Caspar cervical s.
cortical s.
Cotrel pedicle s.
Edwards sacral s.
s. fixation
iliac s.
iliosacral s.
s. implantation
s. insertion
s. insertion technique
Isola spinal implant system iliac s.
KLS-Martin center-drive s.
Kostuik s.
Leibinger Micro Plus s.
s. loosening
Lorenz cranial s.
lumbar pedicle s.
Micro Plus s.
mille pattes s.
Mini Würzburg s.
pedicle s.
s. plate approach
polyaxial s.
s. position perioperative monitoring
s. pullout
rigid pedicle s.
sacral alar s.
sacral pedicle s.
set s.
s. stabilization
stainless steel s.
Steinhauser cranial s.
s. stripout
subarachnoid s.
subdural pressure s.
superior thoracic pedicle s.
Synthes s.

S

screw *(continued)*
　　Texas Scottish Rite Hospital
　　　pedicle s.
　　thoracolumbar pedicle s.
　　TiMesh s.
　　transarticular s.
　　transpedicular s.
　　triangulated pedicle s.
　　tulip pedicle s.
　　Vari-angle s.
screwdriver
　　right-angle s.
　　Stab-and-Grab s.
screw-to-screw compression construct
scribblemania
scribomania
script
　　s. analysis
　　life s.
　　sexual s.
　　S. Stat, Inc. dispensing system
scriptorius
　　calamus s.
　　tic s.
scrivener's palsy
scrotal
　　s. pain
　　s. reflex
scruple
　　decoration s.
　　virginity s.
scrupulosity
SCS
　　Self-Control Scale
　　Social Climate Scale
　　spinal cord stimulation
　　subacute confusional state
SCT
　　Sentence Completion Test
　　Sexual Compatibility Test
sculpting
　　family s.
scurrilous
SD
　　senile dementia
　　severe disability
　　social desirability
　　socialized delinquency
　　socialized dementia
　　spreading depression
　　standard deviation
　　sudden death
　　suicide-depression
S-D
　　suicide-depression
　　　S-D Proneness Checklist
Sd
　　stimulus drive
SDAT
　　senile dementia of Alzheimer type
SDAVF
　　spinal dural arteriovenous fistula
SDB
　　sleep disordered breathing

SDD
　　specific developmental disorder
　　sporadic depressive disease
SDEEG
　　stereotactic depth electroencephalogram
SDI
　　Self-Description Inventory
SDL
　　self-directed learning
SDMT
　　Symbol Digit Modalities Test
SDPC
　　Suicide-Depression Proneness Checklist
SDQII
　　Self-Description Questionnaire II
SDR
　　selective dorsal rhizotomy
SDRI
　　small, deep, recent infarction
SDRT
　　Stanford Diagnostic Reading Test
SDS
　　Self-Directed Search
　　Self-Rating Depression Scale
　　sensory deprivation syndrome
　　sexual differentiation scale
　　speech discrimination score
　　Student Disability Survey
　　sudden death syndrome
SDS-PAGE
　　sodium dodecyl sulfate-polyacrylamide
　　　gel electrophoresis
SE
　　spin-echo
　　standard error
　　supportive-expressive
SEA
　　spinal epidural abscess
　　Survey of Employee Access
sealant
　　tissue fibrin s.
seaman mania
seamstress's cramp
search
　　Self-Directed S. (SDS)
　　transderivational s.
　　s. warrant
　　Word S.
**SEARCH: A Scanning Instrument for
the Identification of Potential
Learning Disability**
searing pain
Seashore Rhythm Test (SRT)
seasonal
　　s. affective disorder (SAD)
　　s. affective disorder syndrome
　　　(SADS)
　　s. energy syndrome
　　s. migraine
　　s. migraine headache
　　s. mood disorder
　　s. pattern
　　S. Pattern Assessment Questionnaire
　　　(SPAQ)
seasonal-related psychosocial stressor

season of birth
seat
    Wayne laminectomy s.
seatbelt fracture
SEB
    Scale for Emotional Blunting
sebaceous adenoma
sebaceus nevus
seborrheic keratosis
SEC
    school handicap condition
    spontaneous echo contrast
    SEC Scale
secandi
    mania s.
Sechrist monoplace hyperbaric chamber
Seckel syndrome
seclusion
    locked s.
    s. need
    office s.
    s. and restraint (S&R)
seclusive personality
secobarbital
    amobarbital and s.
    s. sodium
Seconal Injection
second
    s. cervical nerve
    s. childhood
    s. cranial nerve
    s. messenger
    s. messenger system
    s. negative phase
    seizure s.'s
    s. signaling system
    s. temporal convolution
secondary
    s. amenorrhea
    s. amine
    s. autism
    s. autoerotism
    s. axotomy
    s. defense symptom
    s. degeneration
    s. dementia
    s. depression
    s. deviance
    s. drive
    s. elaboration
    s. elaboration of dream
    s. encephalitis
    s. environment
    s. fantasy
    s. fissure of the cerebellum
    s. gain
    s. generalized epilepsy
    s. hydrocephalus
    s. identification
    s. impotence
    s. integration
    s. mania
    s. mental deficiency
    s. motivation
    s. narcissism

    s. pain
    s. personality
    s. personality trait
    s. post-traumatic syringomyelia
    s. prevention
    s. process thinking
    s. psychic process
    s. reinforcement
    s. reinforcer
    s. repression
    s. retarded ejaculation
    s. revision
    s. reward conditioning
    s. self
    s. sensation
    s. sensory cortex
    s. sensory nuclei
    s. sex character
    s. sex characteristic
    s. sleep disorder
    s. stress
    s. syphilis
    s. transitional object
    s. visual area
    s. visual cortex
secondary-progressive multiple sclerosis
second-messenger molecule
second-order conditioning
Secor system
secret
    s. control
    s. curette
    satan's s.
    s. society
secretin
secreting glial pseudocyst
secretion
    cortisol s.
    syndrome of inappropriate s. of
      antidiuretic hormone (SIADH)
secretive manner
secretory
    s. function
    s. nerve
sectio, pl. **sectiones**
section
    attached cranial s.
    coronal s.
    detached cranial s.
    frozen s.
    permanent s.
    pituitary stalk s.
    psychiatric services s. (PSS)
    scaled stereotactic atlas s.
    vestibular nerve s.
sectioning
    cryomicrotome s.
SECTL
    single enhancing CT lesion
sector
sectoranopia
secular trend
secure
    s. attachment

secure *(continued)*
s. base effect
s. environment
SecureStrand
S. cable
S. cervical fusion system
security
s. blanket
emotional s.
s. operation
Social S. (SS)
Sedabamate
Sedan cannula
Sedan-Nashold needle
Sedan-Vallicioni cannula
Sedapap-10
sedate
sedation
daytime s.
preoperative s.
s. threshold
sedative
s. abuse
s. addiction
Battley s.
s. delirium
s. dependence
s. drug
s. effect
hypnotic s.
s., hypnotic, or anxiolytic-induced anxiety disorder
s., hypnotic, or anxiolytic-induced persisting dementia
s., hypnotic, or anxiolytic-induced sexual dysfunction
s. intoxication
s. occupation
s. use disorder
s. withdrawal
sedative-hypnotic
s.-h. agent
s.-h. drug
s.-h. withdrawal symptom
sedative-induced
s.-i. anxiety
s.-i. disorder
s.-i. persisting dementia
s.-i. psychotic disorder with delusions
s.-i. psychotic disorder with hallucinations
sedativism
Seddon classification of nerve injuries
sedentary lifestyle
sedimentation
seduction
infantile s.
seductive
s. behavior
s. personality
s. personality disorder
s. tendency

seed
^{125}I s.
s. psychosurgery
SEED Developmental Profile
seeding
subarachnoid s.
surgical s.
SEEG
stereotactic electroencephalogram
seeker
care s.
fact s.
seeking
S. of Noetic Goals Test
novelty s.
Seeligmüller sign
seesaw nystagmus
segment
clinoidal s. (ClinSeg)
exiting s.
interannular s.
internodal s.
intradural s.
Lanterman s.
M s.
motion s.
neural s.
ophthalmic s. (OphSeg)
P s.
Ranvier s.
s.'s of spinal cord
sympathetic s.
traversing s.
segmenta (*pl. of* segmentum)
segmental
s. analysis
s. anesthesia
s. arterial disorganization
s. compression construct
s. fixation
s. neuritis
s. neurofibromatosis
s. neuropathy
s. registration
s. spinal instrumentation (SSI)
segmentary response
segmentation
volume s.
segmentum, pl. segmenta
s. internodale
segmenta medullae spinalis
s. medullae spinalis cervicalia
s. medullae spinalis coccygea
s. medullae spinalis lumbalis
s. medullae spinalis sacralis
s. medullae spinalis thoracica
segregation
administrative s.
s. analysis study
disciplinary s.
s. hypothesis
mitotic s.
perceptual s.
SEH
School Handicap Condition Scale

severe emotional handicap
subdural effusion with hydrocephalus
SEI
Self-Esteem Index
Self-Esteem Inventory
Seitelberger disease
seizure
absence s.
s. activity
acute s.
affective symptom of s.
akinetic s.
alcohol as cause of s.
alcohol-related s.
alcohol withdrawal s.
alimentary s.
anosognosic s.
aphasic s.
apneic s.
apoplectiform s.
asteric s.
asymptomatic s.
atonic absence s.
atypical absence s.
audiogenic s.
auditory s.
automatic s.
autonomic s.
benign neonatal familial s.
bilateral myoclonic s.
brain s.
cardiovascular s.
catamenial s.
central s.
centrencephalic s.
cephalic s.
cerebellar fits s.
cerebral s.
cerebrospinal s.
clonic s.
clonicotonic s.
clonic-tonic-clonic s.
complex partial s. (CPS)
continuing petit mal s.
conversion s.
convulsive s.
coordinate s.
cryptogenic s.
diencephalic s.
drug-induced s.
drug withdrawal s.
s. dyscontrol
eclamptic s.
electrodecremental s.
elementary partial s.
emotional cause of s.
encephalotrigeminal angiomatosis s.
epilepsia partialis continua s.
s. epilepsy
epileptic s.
epileptiform s.
erotic s.
essential s.
febrile s.
fluent aphasic s.

focal s.
s. foci resection
fragmentary s.
s. frequency (SF)
generalized tonic-clonic s.
grand mal s.
gustatory s.
hippocampal s.
s. history
HIV-related s.
hysterical s.
iatrogenic s.
ictal confusional s.
ictal depression phase of s.
idiopathic s.
infantile s.
jackknife s.
jacksonian s.
Janz juvenile myoclonic s.
Lennon-Gastaut s.
major motor s.
massive s.
maximal electroshock s. (MES)
mimetic s.
mimic s.
myoclonic s.
neonatal familial s.
new-onset s.
nonfluent aphasic s.
olfactory psychomotor s.
paroxysmal s.
partial complex s.
partial sensory s.
partial tonic s.
petit mal s.
petit mal variant s.
phantom absence s.
phase of s.
photogenic s.
post-ECT s.
postictal depression phase of s.
postmenopausal s.
posttraumatic s.
postural s.
precentral s.
premonition of s.
primary s.
pseudoepileptic s.'s
psychic s.
psychogenic s.
psychomotor s.
puerperal s.
recurrent s.
reflex s.
remote symptomatic s.
repetitive partial s.
s. resistant (SR)
rolandic s.
salaam s.
s. seconds
s. sensitive (SS)
sensory-evoked s.
simple partial s. (SPS)
single s.
situation-related s.

S

seizure *(continued)*
    sleep-related epileptic s.
    somatosensory s.
    spasmodic s.
    spontaneous s.
    subclinical s.
    subjective s.
    sylvian s.
    symptomatic s.
    temporal lobe s.
    tetanic s.
    s. threshold
    tonic s.
    tonic-clonic s.
    traumatic s.
    typical absence s.
    uncinate s.
    unilateral s.
    uremic s.
    vertiginous s.
    visual s.
    withdrawal s.
sejunctiva
    dementia s.
selaphobia
Seldane
Seldinger
    S. angiogram
    S. method
    S. retrograde wire/intubation
        technique
selection
    adverse s.
    s. bias
    bone plate s.
    Edwards modular system
        construct s.
    item s.
    natural s.
    personnel s.
    slice s.
selective
    s. amnesia
    s. attachment
    s. attention
    s. auditory agnosia
    s. deafness
    s. dorsal rhizotomy (SDR)
    s. embolization
    s. excitation
    s. focusing on environmental
        stimuli
    s. imaging and graphics for
        stereotactic surgery (SIGSS)
    s. inattention
    s. irradiation
    s. memory
    s. microadenomectomy
    s. mutism
    s. phosphodiesterase inhibitor
    s. preventive intervention
    s. relaxation enhancement
    S. Reminding Test
    s. retention

    s. serotonin reuptake inhibitor
        (SSRI)
    s. silence
    s. thoracic spine fusion
    s. T2 shortening
selectivity
    motivational s.
selector
    Leksell s.
    S. ultrasonic aspirator
selegiline
selenophobia
Seletz-Gelpi laminectomy retractor
Seletz nonrigid ventricular catheter
self
    actual s.
    aniled sense of s.
    bad s.
    s. concept
    creative s.
    dangerous to one's s.
    deformation of s.
    disturbed sense of s.
    empirical s.
    ethical s.
    s. experience
    glorified s.
    harming s.
    hidden s.
    idealized s.
    looking-glass s.
    nonturning against s. (NTS)
    personified s.
    phenomenal s.
    s. psychology
    real s.
    secondary s.
    sense of s.
    subconscious s.
    subliminal s.
    Tests of Perception of Scientists
        and S. (TOPOSS)
    true s.
    turning against s. (TAS)
self-absorbed tendency
self-absorption
    intimacy versus s.-a.
self-accusation
    delusion of s.-a.
self-adhering electrode
Self-Administered
    S.-A. Dependency Questionnaire
        (SADQ)
self-administered
    s.-a. alcohol screening test
        (SAAST)
    s.-a. penectomy
self-administration
    s.-a. of psychoactive drug (SAPD)
    repeated substance s.-a.
self-analysis (SA)
Self-Assessment
    S.-A. Depression (SAD)
    S.-A. Depression Scale
    S.-A. in Writing Skills

self-attaching electrode
self-attribution of guilt
self-awareness
    objective s.-a.
self-blaming depression
self-care
    s.-c. activity
    s.-c. dysfunction
    s.-c. skill
self-centered attitude
self-comparison
    negative s.-c.
Self-Concept
    S.-C. as a Learner (SCAL)
    S.-C. as a Learner scale
    S.-C. and Motivation Inventory
    (SCAMI, SCAMIN)
    S.-C. Scale
self-confidence
    lack of s.-c.
    low s.-c.
self-conflict
    undisciplined s.-c.
Self-Consciousness Scale
Self-Control
    S.-C. Inventory
    S.-C. Scale (SCS)
self-control
    s.-c. technique
    s.-c. therapy
self-criticism
    pervasive s.-c.
self-damaging
    s.-d. behavior
    s.-d. impulsivity
self-defeating
    s.-d. behavior
    s.-d. personality
    s.-d. personality disorder
    s.-d. thinking
    s.-d. trait
self-deprecating thought
self-deprecatory remark
self-derogatory
    s.-d. concept
    s.-d. content
    s.-d. theme
Self-Description
    S.-D. Inventory (SDI)
    S.-D. Questionnaire II (SDQII)
self-destructive
    s.-d. behavior
    s.-d. hallucination
    s.-d. patient
self-directed
    s.-d. exposure
    s.-d. learning (SDL)
Self-Directed Search (SDS)
self-dramatizing behavior
Self-Esteem
    S.-E. Index (SEI)
    S.-E. Inventory (SEI)
    S.-E. Questionnaire
self-esteem
    Behavioral Academic S.-e.

    Children's Inventory of S.-e.
    (CISE)
    denigrated s.-e.
    s.-e. scale
self-fellator
self-fulfilling prophecy
self-handicapping strategy
self-harm
    deliberate s.-h. (DSH)
self-help
    belief system of s.-h.
    s.-h. group
    s.-h. skill
self-helper
    inner s.-h.
self-image
    negative s.-i.
    unstable s.-i.
self-induced
    s.-i. alopecia
    s.-i. hair loss
    s.-i. injury
    s.-i. vomiting
self-inflicted (SI)
    s.-i. bodily injury
    s.-i. wound (SIW)
self-injurious behavior (SIB)
self-injury
    motivation for s.-i.
self-managed reinforcement
self-mutilating behavior
self-mutilation (SM)
self-peeping
    narcissistic s.-p.
Self-Perception
    S.-P. Inventory (SPI)
    S.-P. Profile for Children
self-pitying constellation
self-punishing behavior
self-punishment
    expiatory s.-p.
    illness as s.-p.
Self-Rating
    S.-R. Depression Scale (SDS,
    SRDS)
self-rating
    s.-r. anxiety scale (SAS)
    s.-r. test
self-regulation
    physiological s.-r.
self-regulatory capacity
self-reinforcement
    cognitive s.-r.
self-reliance training
self-report
    s.-r. personalities inventory
    s.-r. psychological inventory
    Young Adult s.-r.
    Youth s.-r.
self-retaining
    s.-r. brain retractor
    s.-r. brain retractor frame
self-role concept
self-stimulatory behavior
self-stopping drill point

S

self-treatment
    hormonal s.-t.
Seligman view of depressive disorder
sella, sellae, pl. **sellae**
    ballooning of the s.
    diaphragm of s.
    diaphragma sellae
    empty s.
    s. punch forceps
    tuberculum sellae
    s. turcica
sellar
    s. aneurysm
    s. cyst
    s. entrance
    s. gangliocytoma
    s. punch
    s. tumor
Selter disease
Selverstone
    S. clamp
    S. cordotomy hook
    S. intervertebral disk rongeur
Selvini-Palazzoli model of schizophrenia
Selye
    adaptation syndrome of S.
Selz and Reitan rules to assess learning disorders
SEM
    scanning electron microscopy
    standard error of the mean
semantic
    s. aberration
    s. activation
    s. aphasia
    s. argument
    s. argument communication pattern
    s.'s of autism
    behavioral s.'s
    s. category
    s. clustering
    s. cue
    s. cueing
    s. dementia
    s. differential
    s. dissociation
    extension s.'s
    general s.'s
    generative s.'s
    s. jargon
    s. memory
    s. pragmatic disorder
    s. processing
    s. psychosis
    quantitative s.'s
    referential s.'s
    s. relatedness
    s. relationship
    s. therapy
semantogenic disorder
semeiology (*var. of* semiology)
semeiopathic, semiopathic
semeiosis, semiosis
semeiotic (*var. of* semiotic)

semen
    s. fear
    loss of s.
    s. loss
semialdehyde
    succinic s.
semiautomated spatial normalization technique
semiautomatic quality
semi-autonomous systems concept of brain function
semicircular
    s. canal
    s. duct
semicomatose
semiconscious
semicretinism
semidominant
semierect
semi-Fowler position
Semilente Iletin I
semilunar
    s. fasciculus
    s. ganglion
    s. notch
    s. nucleus of Flechsig
semimembranosus reflex
seminarcosis
seminoma
    intracranial s.
seminomad
semiobsession à deux
semiology, semeiology
semiopathic (*var. of* semeiopathic)
semiosis (*var. of* semeiosis)
semiotic, semeiotic
    s. function
semioval center
semipermeable
semipornographic
semiprivate room
semipurposeful behavior
semiquantitative
semispinalis capitis
Semi-Structured Assessment for the Genetics of Alcoholism
semistructured diagnostic interview
semisynthetic sphingolipid
semitendinosus reflex
semitendinous
Semmes curette
Semmes-Weinstein esthesiometer
Semon-Hering theory
Semon law
Semon-Rosenbach law
semustine
senescence
senescent
    s. fibroblast
    s. forgetfulness
    s. pedophilia
senile
    s. brain syndrome
    s. chorea
    s. degeneration**

s. delirium
s. dementia (SD)
s. dementia of Alzheimer type (SDAT)
s. dementia confusional state
s. depression
s. deterioration
s. epilepsy
s. gait disorder
s. imbecility
s. insanity
s. involution
s. mania
s. melancholia
s. memory
s. neurosis
s. organic psychotic state
s. osteoporosis
s. paranoia
s. paranoid reaction
s. paraplegia
s. plaque
s. psychoneurosis
s. psychosis
s. psychotic mental disorder
s. tremor

senilis
alopecia s.
paranoia s.
sexualitas s.

senility organic psychosis
Senior
S. Apperception Technique (SAT)
S. Apperception Test (SAT)

senium praecox
Senn retractor
Senoussi Multiphasic Marital Inventory (SMMI)
sensate
s. focus
s. focus learning

sensate-focus-oriented therapy
sensation
altered s.
buzzing s.
cincture s.
creeping-crawling s.
delayed s.
diminished s.
drug-induced floating s.
dysesthesic s.
s. of ejaculatory inevitability
epicritic s.
facial s.
feeling s.
fine tactile s.
girdle s.
s. increment
kinesthetic s.
light touch s.
loss of s.
numbing s.
objective s.
out-of-body s.
out-of-mind s.

peripheral s.
phantom s.
physical s.
pins-and-needles s.
pins-sticking s.
preputial s.
primary s.
proprioceptive s.
referred s.
reflex s.
secondary s.
sexual s.
smothering s.
special s.
sticking s.
subjective s.
superficial s.
tactile s.
taste s.
temperature s.
tingling s.
touch s.
transferred s.
visual s.

sensation-focused apprehension
Sensation-Seeking
S.-S. Scale (SSS)
sensation-seeking trait
sense
s. of apprehension
s. of arousal
s. of attachment
s. of bodily change
chemical s.
S. of Coherence Questionnaire
s. of commitment
s. of concern
s. of detachment
s. of entitlement
equilibratory s.
s. of equilibrium
external s.
s. of humor
s. of identity
s. of impending doom
internalized s.
joint s.
kinesthetic s.
labyrinthine s.
muscular s.
obstacle s.
s. organ
position s.
posture s.
pressure s.
s. of reality
s. of self
seventh s.
sixth s.
space s.
special s.
special s.
static s.
stimulation of s. (SOS)
street s.

S

sense *(continued)*
    tactile s.
    temperature s.
    thermal s.
    thermic s.
    time s.
    touch s.
    visceral s.
    s. of well-being
senseless imitative word repetition
sensibilia
sensibility
    articular s.
    bone s.
    cortical s.
    deep s.
    dissociation s.
    electromuscular s.
    epicritic s.
    mesoblastic s.
    pallesthetic s.
    proprioceptive s.
    protopathic s.
    splanchnesthetic s.
    vibratory s.
sensible hemideficit
sensiferous
sensigenous
sensimeter
sensitiva
sensitive
    s. Beziehungswahn paranoid
    phase-s.
    s. plane
    s. point
    seizure s. (SS)
    s. volume
sensitiver Beziehungswahn paranoid
state
sensitivity
    absolute s.
    anxiety s. (AS)
    contrast s.
    cosmic s.
    deep-pressure s.
    dopamine receptor s.
    general stress s.
    s. group
    s. prediction from the acoustic
      reflex (SPAR)
    Profile of Nonverbal S. (PONS)
    s. reaction of adolescence
    s. reaction of childhood
    reassurance s.
    rejection s.
    separation s.
    substance s.
    s. training
sensitivity-training group
sensitization
    behavioral s.
    covert s.
    overt s.
    perceptual s.

sensomobility
sensomotor
sensor
    CardioSearch s.
    DC SQUID s.
    DermaTemp infrared
      thermographic s.
    disposable Doppler-constant
      thermocouple s.
    MEG s.
    s. operation
    Paratrend 7 s.
    s. position indicator (SPI)
    Saber CBF-ICP trauma s.
    telemetric intracranial pressure s.
    zero drift of the s.
Sensorcaine
Sensorcaine-MPF
sensoria (*pl. of* sensorium)
sensorial
    s. area
    s. epilepsy
    s. idiocy
sensoriglandular
sensorimotor
    s. act
    s. arc
    s. area
    s. axonal polyneuropathy
    s. development
    s. intelligence period
    s. peripheral neuropathy
    s. phase
    s. skill
    s. stage
    s. system
    s. theory
sensorimuscular
sensorineural
    s. acuity level masking technique
    s. deafness
sensorium, pl. **sensoria, sensoriums**
    clear s.
    clouded s.
    cloudy s.
sensorivascular
sensorivasomotor
sensory
    s. acuity
    s. alexia
    s. amusia
    s. anesthesia
    s. aphasia
    s. apraxia
    s. area
    s. ataxia
    s. aura
    s. awareness (SA)
    s. bondage
    s. charge
    s. conversion symptoms
    s. cortex
    s. crossway
    s. decussation of medulla oblongata
    s. defect

s. deficit
s. deprivation
s. deprivation syndrome (SDS)
s. difficulty
s. discrimination
s. dissociation
s. dissociation syndrome
s. distribution
s. disturbance
s. environment
s. evoked potential (SEP)
s. experience
s. extinction
s. function
s. functioning
s. ganglion
s. image
s. impairment
s. impression
s. inattention
s. integration
S. Integration and Praxis Tests (SIPT)
s. jacksonian attack
s. level
s. loss
s. modality
s. neglect
s. nerve
s. nerve action potential (SNAP)
s. nerve action potential amplitude
s. neurogenic arthropathy
s. neuron
s. neuronopathy
s. neuropathy
s. nucleus
s. paralysis
s. perception
S. Perceptual Examination (SPE)
s. phenomenon
s. precipitated epilepsy
s. psychosis
s. receptor
s. root of ciliary ganglion
s. root of trigeminal nerve
s. scale
s. shock
s. speech center
s. stimulation
s. stimulus
s. threshold
s. tract
transcortical s.
sensory-deprivation nystagmus
sensory-evoked seizure
sensory-induced epilepsy
sensory-motor
s.-m. strip
s.-m. stroke
sensory-motor-autonomic neuropathy
sensory/motor behavior
sensory-perceptual test
sensual
s. dysarthria
s. pleasure

sensuous
sentence
S. Closure Test
s. completion
S. Completion Test (SCT)
complex s.
death s.
jail s.
life s.
prison s.
s. repetition (SR)
sentence-closure task
sentience
sentient
SentiLite
S. EEG monitor
S. neurological monitor
sentimental value
sentinel
s. activity
s. leak
s. spinous process fracture
S. system
Sentinel-4 neurological monitor
Seoul virus
SEP
sensory evoked potential
somatosensory evoked potential
pudendal SEP
separated
s. from spouse
legally s. (LS)
separation
affective s.
s. agreement
s. anxiety
anxiety s.
s. anxiety disorder (SAD)
s. anxiety disorder of childhood
S. Anxiety Symptom Inventory (SASI)
articular mass s.
atlantoaxial s.
atlantooccipital s.
s. distress
family s.
pontomedullary s.
s. sensitivity
sibling s.
traumatic s.
trial s.
twin s.
separation-individuation
s.-i. phase
s.-i. process
separative
separator
Davis dural s.
Davis nerve s.
Dorsey dural s.
dural s.
Frazier dural s.
Hoen dural s.
Horsley dural s.
Hunter dural s.

S

separator *(continued)*
    Sachs dural s.
    s. state
    synovial s.
    Woodson dural s.
separator-spatula
    Davis nerve s.-s.
    Sachs nerve s.-s.
    Woodson dural s.-s.
septa *(pl. of* septum)
septal area
septation
    intraventricular s.
septi *(gen. of* septum)
septic
    s. embolus
    s. shock
    s. thrombosis
    s. venous vasculitis
septicemia psychosis
septomarginal
    s. fasciculus
    s. tract
septooptic dysplasia
septostomy
septuagenarian
septum, gen. **septi,** pl. **septa**
    s. cervicale intermedium
    s. linguae
    s. lucidum
    nucleus accumbens septi
    s. pellucidum
    precommissural s.
    s. of tongue
    transparent s.
    transverse s.
sequela, pl. **sequelae**
    postpolio s.
sequence
    Carr-Purcell s.
    Carr-Purcell-Meiboom-Gill s.
    elaborate dream s.
    s. of events
    genetic s.
    gradient-refocused s.
    hemisphere s.
    s. memory
    phase s.
    s. polymorphism
    pulse s.
    short-tau inversion recovery MRI s.
    spin-warp pulse s.
    stimulated spin-echo s. (STEAM)
    STIR s.
    storylike dream s.
    three-dimensional spoiled GRASS s.
    s. time
sequenced
    S. Inventory of Communication Development (SICD)
    S. Inventory of Language Development (SILD)
sequencing
    s. ability

    auditory s.
    s. deletion breakpoint
    s. disability
    s. rule
sequential
    S. Assessment of Mathematics Inventories: Standardized Inventory
    s. compression device (SCD)
    s. computed tomographic scan
    s. gradient-recalled acquisition in the steady state
    s. GRASS
    s. memory
    s. multiple analysis (SMA)
    s. plane imaging
    s. point imaging
    S. Tests of Educational Progress, Series III (STEP-III)
    S. Tests of Educational Study (STEP)
    s. ultrasonography
sequester
sequestrated disk
sequestration
sequitur
    non s.
SER
    somatosensory evoked response
Ser-Ap-Es
Serax
Serenid Forte
Serentil
serial
    s. assaulter
    s. CT
    s. epilepsy
    s. list learning
    s. murderer
    s. observation
    s. percutaneous needle drainage
    s. sevens test (7's)
    s. sexual killer
    s. 7's (sevens)
seriatim function
series
    ACER Test of Basic Skills - Blue S.
    ACER Test of Basic Skills - Green S.
    Aptitude-Intelligence Test S.
    Beery Picture Vocabulary Screening S.
    Beery Picture Vocabulary Test and Beery Picture Vocabulary Screening S.
    Comprehensive Assessment Program: Achievement S.
    Educational Development S.
    experimental s.
    Hogan Personnel Selection S.
    I.P.I Aptitude-Intelligence Test S.
    Leksell gamma knife target s.

Missouri Children's Picture S.
(MCPS)
Somatic Inkblot S.
serine proteinase
serious
s. assaultive act
s. consequence
s. impairment
s. traumatic stress
s. violations of rules
seriously wounded in action (SWA)
Serlect
sermon fear
Sernyl
seroepidemiological study (SES)
serologic test
serology
Seromycin
seronegative spondyloarthropathy
Seroquel
serosa
s. meningitis
meninx s.
serositis
serostatus
serotonergic
s. activity
s. anxiolytic
s. deficiency hypothesis
s. deficit
s. dorsal raphe
s. neuron
s. neurotransmission
s. pharmacology
s. raphe nuclei
s. receptor
s. responsibility
s. synapse
s. tract
serotonin
s. level
s. receptor assay
s. reuptake inhibitor (SRI)
s. syndrome
serotonin-dopamine
serous
s. apoplexy
s. meningitis
Serpasil
serpentina
Rauwolfia s.
rauwolfia s.
serpentine aneurysm
serpiginous mass
serrati
Serratia
serration
dentated s.
sertindole
Sertraline
sertraline
s. HCl
s. hydrochloride
serum
s. amylase

antilymphocyte s. (ALS)
s. bicarbonate
s. bromide
s. caffeine level
s. calcium
s. ceruloplasmin
s. chloride
s. copper
s. cotinine
s. diagnosis
s. enzyme determination
s. ferritin
s. folate
s. folic acid
s. glutamic oxaloacetic transaminase (SGOT)
s. glutamic-pyruvic transaminase (SGPT)
s. glutamyl transaminase
s. heavy metal intoxication
s. iron
s. magnesium
s. neopterin
s. phosphorus
s. potassium
s. prolactin
s. protein
s. salicylate
s. sickness
s. sickness peripheral neuropathy
s. sodium
s. testosterone
s. vitamin A
s. vitamin B12
service
access to health care s.'s
ACT Evaluation/Survey S.
Adult Protective S.'s (APS)
American Psychiatry Association/Center for Mental Health S.'s
Anticoagulation S.
Center for Mental Health S.'s (CMHS)
Children's Protective S. (CPS)
Civilian Health and Medical Program of the Uniformed S. (CHAMPUS)
consultation-liaison s.
Council on Psychiatric S.'s
counseling s.
Crisis Evaluation Referral S. (CERS)
Department of Health and Human S.'s (DHHS)
disability determination s. (DDS)
Educational Testing S. (ETS)
environment-centered s.
Guidelines for Adolescent Preventive S.'s (GAPS)
Health and Human S.'s
Memphis Educational Model Providing Handicapped Infant S.'s (MEMPHIS)
mutual-help s.'s

S

service *(continued)*
    outreach s.'s
    patient-centered s.'s
    Patient and Family S.'s (PFS)
    peer-helping s.
    psychiatric emergency s. (PES)
    social s. (SS)
    Social and Rehabilitation S. (SRS)
    System to Plan Early
      Childhood S.'s (SPECS)
    United States Public Health S.
      (USPHS)
    Vocational Rehabilitation S.'s
      (VRS)
service-connected disability (SCD)
Serzone
SES
    seroepidemiological study
    socioeconomic status
session
    adjunctive individual s.
    dyadic s.
    fixed-ended s.
    four-way s.
    group s.
    learning s.
    marathon s.
    open-ended s.
    orientation s.
    play s.
    rap s.
    skull s.
    therapy s.
sestamibi
    technetium 99m s.
SET
    support, empathy and truth
    SET therapy
set
    s. s.
    abract s.
    acquiescent-response s.
    aluminum contouring template s.
    Bremer halo crown traction s.
    data s.
    difficulty in changing response s.
    Greenberg retractor s.
    Health Plan Employer Data and
      Information S. (HEDIS)
    Hudson cranial drill s.
    jet s.
    learning s.
    mental s.
    Mira Mark III cranial drill s.
    Mira Mark V craniotome s.
    s. in motion
    Mullan percutaneous trigeminal
      ganglion microcompression s.
    s. in one's ways
    perceptual s.
    perseveration s.
    polyethic criteria s.
    postural s.
    response s.

    s. screw
    single criteria s.
    substance-specific intoxication
      criteria s.'s
    substance-specific withdrawal
      criteria s.'s
    V. Mueller McCulloch universal
      instrument s.
setter
    fire s. (FS)
setting
    behavior s.
    clinical s.
    community s.
    Consortium on Special Psychiatric
      Delivery S.
    dimensional s.
    educational s.
    fire s.
    forensic s.
    goal s.
    group s.
    home s.
    inpatient psychiatric s.
    intentional fire s.
    juvenile fire s.
    limit s.
    outpatient mental health clinic s.
    partial hospital s.
    population s.
    primary care s.
    psychosocial s.
    real-world s.
    residential s.
    social s.
settling
    cranial s.
sevens
    serial 7's (s.)
seventh
    s. cranial nerve
    s. cranial nerve transposition
    s. nerve palsy
    s. sense
sever
severe
    s. anxiety
    s. ataxia
    s. childhood autosomal recessive
      muscular dystrophy (SCARMD)
    s. degenerative disk disease
    s. dementia
    s. depression
    s. diffuse brain dysfunction
    s. disability (SD)
    s. dissociative symptom
    s. emotional handicap (SEH)
    s. environmental deprivation
    s. head injury (SHI)
    s. intoxication
    s. kyphoscoliosis
    s. life stress
    s. mental retardation

s. mental subnormality
s. rigid right thoracic curve
severely mentally impaired (SMI)
severity
APACHE II measure of disease s.
S. of Psychiatric Illness Scale
S. of Psychosocial Stressors Scale
s. specifier
sewing spasm
sex
s. addict
anal s.
s. appeal
s. arousal mechanism (SAM)
assigned s.
biologic s.
s. change
s. characteristic
s. chromatin
s. chromosome
compulsive s.
s. counseling
s. determination
s. deviant
s. differentiation
s. drive
s. education
extramarital s.
fair s.
s. fear
forced s.
s. headache
indeterminate s.
s. infantilism
s. interest
intermediate s.
Internet s.
s. inventory (SI)
S. Knowledge and Attitude Test
(SKAT)
s. limitation
s. linkage
900 number s.
s. object
s. offender (SO)
s. offense
online s.
opposite biological s.
oral s.
orogenital s.
s. perversion
premarital s.
s. preselection
promiscuous s.
s. ratio
s. reassignment surgery (SRS)
s. reversal
s. role
s. role inversion
s. steroid
s. and stroke psychiatric syndrome
s. symbol
telephone s.
s. therapy
third s.

trading s.
s. typing
unprotected s.
sexagenarian
sex-conditioned character
sexism
sexist
sexless
sex-limited character
sex-linkage
sex-linked character
sexological examination
sexology
sexopathy
sexploitation
sex-reassignment
hormonal s.-r.
sex-related risk-taking
sex-role behavior
sexual
s. aberration
s. abstinence
s. abuse
s. abuse of adult
s. abuse of child
S. Abuse Interview
s. acting out
s. activity
s. addiction
s. adjustment
s. aid
s. anesthesia
s. anomaly
s. anxiety
s. arousal
s. assault
s. attitude
s. attitude reassessment (SAR)
s. attitude restructuring (SAR)
s. aversion
s. aversion disorder
s. behavior
s. boundary violation
s. climax
s. coercion
S. Compatibility Test (SCT)
s. concern
s. contact
s. curiosity
s. delusion
s. desire disorder
s. desire disturbance
s. development
s. deviance
s. deviance disorder
s. deviation
s. deviation neurotic disorder
s. differentiation scale (SDS)
s. dimorphism
s. discrimination
s. disorder
s. domination
s. drive
s. dysfunction

S

sexual *(continued)*
s. dysfunction due to a general medical condition
s. energy
s. erethism
s. escapade
s. excitement
s. exhibition
s. experience
S. Experiences Questionnaire
s. expression
s. fantasy
s. fear
s. frigidity
s. functioning
S. Functioning Index (SFI)
s. and gender identity disorder
s. gratification
s. harassment (SH)
s. history
s. identity
s. impotence
s. inappropriateness
s. indifference
s. indiscretion
s. infantilism
s. inhibition
s. instinct
s. interaction
s. intercourse
s. interest
s. intimacy
s. inversion
s. learning
s. libido
s. life
s. love
s. maladjustment
s. masochism
s. maturity rating
s. melancholia
s. mores
s. motivation
s. myth (SM)
s. negativism
s. neurasthenia
s. neurosis
s. obsession
s. opportunity
s. orientation
s. orientation distress
s. orientation disturbance
s. pain
s. performance
s. perversion
S. and Physical Abuse Questionnaire
s. physiology
s. pleasure
s. pleasure sexual promiscuity
s. polarization
s. potency
s. predation behavior
s. predator

s. preference
s. promiscuity
s. provocation
s. prowess
s. psychopath
s. reassignment
s. regulation
s. rehabilitation
s. relation
s. response
s. response cycle
s. responsibility
s. revolution
s. risk-taking
s. sadism
s. sadomasochism
s. script
s. sensation
s. soliloquy
s. stimulation
s. stimuli revulsion
s. stimulus
s. surrogate
s. symptom
s. symptom grouping
s. synergism
s. tension
s. trauma
s. urge
s. vandalism

sexualis
psychopathia s.
sexualism
sexualitas senilis
sexuality
index of s. (IS)
s. index
infantile s.
pathologic s.
perverted s.
polymorphous perverse s.
S. Preference Profile (SPP)
three essays on the theory of s.
sexualization
sexually
s. acquired immunodeficiency (SAID)
s. arousing behavior
s. arousing fantasy
s. dimorphic
s. transmitted condition (STC)
s. transmitted disease (STD)
SF
seizure frequency
Kaochlor SF
SF-36
Short Form-36 General Health Survey
SFEMG
single-fiber electromyography
SFI
Sexual Functioning Index
Social Function Index
SFLE
stress from life experience

SFTAA
Short Form Test of Academic Aptitude
SGLPG
sulfate-3-glucuronyllactosaminyl
paragloboside
SGOT
serum glutamic oxaloacetic transaminase
SGPG
sulfate-3-glucuronyl paragloboside
SGPT
serum glutamic-pyruvic transaminase
SH
sexual harassment
social history
state hospital
P & SH
S&H
speech and hearing
sha
gwa s.
shading
emotional s.
s. response (ShR)
s. response to black areas (Fc)
s. response to gray areas (Fc)
shadow
s. dance
object s.
plaque s.
s. play
shadowing
acoustical s.
s. masking technique
shagreen patch
shaking
hand s.
s. palsy
s. tremor
s. voice
shallow
s. affect
s. expression
shallowness of affect
sham
s. disorder
s. feeding
s. rage
shaman
shamanism
shamanistic thought disorder
shame-aversion therapy
shamefaced
shamelessness
sham-movement vertigo
shampoo
chlorhexidine s.
shanghai
shank clipping
Shannon bur
shape
S.'s Analysis Test (SAT)
body s.
good s.
shaping
behavior s.

Shapiro-Wilk test
shared
s. delusional belief
s. mechanism
s. paranoid disorder
s. phenomenological feature
s. psychotic disorder
s. thought pattern
s. understanding
sharing
Edwards modular system load s.
s. of values
Sharplan
S. laser
S. Ultra ultrasonic aspirator
shaving cramp
Shaw
S. aneurysm needle
S. catheter
SHCU
state hospital children's unit
SHE
spinal epidural hemorrhage
Shealy theory
shearing injury
shear-strain deformation
shear stress
sheath
arachnoid s.
carotid s.
dural s.
femoral introducer s.
ganglionic cyst in synovial
tendon s.
Henle s.
s. of Key and Retzius
Mauthner s.
medullary s.
myelin s.
outer mesaxon of the myelin s.
s. of Schwann
Sheehan
S. Disability Scale
S. syndrome
sheet
personal data s.
s. rocking
s. sign
timed behavioral rating s. (TBRS)
sheeting
rubber s.
Sheffield
S. collimator helmet
S. gamma unit
Sheldon hemilaminectomy retractor
Sheldon-Spatz vertebral arteriogram
needle
shellacking
shell shock
shell-shocked
sheltered
S. Care Environment Scale
s. home
s. life

sheltered *(continued)*
    s. workshop
    s. workshop placement
shelve
shenjing shuairuo
shen-k'uei, shenkui
Sherrington
    S. law
    S. phenomenon
SHI
    severe head injury
shield
    AME PinSite s.
    designs for vision side s.
    Faraday s.
    gray s.
    ideational s.
shielding
    magnet s.
shift
    s. ability
    abrupt topic s.
    binaural s.
    biobehavioral s.
    brain s.
    chemical s.
    Doppler s.
    fat/water chemical s.
    field s.
    frequency s.
    functional s.
    gaze refixational s.
    gradual topic s.
    s. masking technique
    midline s.
    mood s.
    paradigm s.
    paradigmatic s.
    phase s.
    precipitous mood s.
    s. referential index
    role s.
    temporary threshold s. (TTS)
    transmembrane ionic s.
    s. work-type dyssomnia
shifting
    associative s.
    idiosyncratic topic s.
    s. sleep-work schedule
    topic s.
Shiley
    S. catheter
    S. catheter distention system
    S. distention kit
Shiley-Infusaid pump
shim coil
shimmering light with aura
shin-byung
shinkeishitsu
Shipley
    S. Abstraction Test
    S. Institute of Living Scale (SILS)
    S. Personal Inventory (SPI)

Shipley-Hartford Scale
Shipman Anxiety Depression Scale
    (SADS)
Shirley drain
shock
    anaphylactic s.
    break s.
    cardiogenic s.
    cultural s.
    culture s.
    deferred s.
    delayed s.
    delirious s.
    electrical s.
    electric skin s.
    electroconvulsive s. (ECS)
    erethismic s.
    s. exhibitionism
    s. fear
    future s.
    hypovolemic s.
    insulin s.
    irreversible s.
    mental s.
    neurogenic s.
    primary s.
    psychic s.
    psychodramatic s.
    s. psychosis
    s. reaction
    reversible s.
    sensory s.
    septic s.
    shell s.
    spinal s.
    s. stage
    s. syndrome
    s. therapy (ST)
    transplantation s.
    s. treatment
    s. troops
    vasogenic s.
shoe
    s. fetish
    s. restriction
shook yong
shoot for
shooting pain
short
    S. Category Test
    s. cycle
    s. EEG epoch FFT analysis
    S. Employment Tests
    S. Form-36 General Health Survey
    (SF-36)
    S. Form Test of Academic
    Aptitude (SFTAA)
    s. gyri of the insula
    S. Imaginal Processes Inventory
    (SIPI)
    S. Increment Sensitivity Index
    (SISI)
    s. insular gyrus
    s. inversion recovery imaging
    (STIR)

S. Michigan Alcoholism Screening Test (SMAST)
s. orientation-memory-concentration test (OMC)
S. Portable Mental Status Questionnaire (SPMSQ)
s. pulse repetition time/echo time
s. pulse repetition time/echo time image
s. pulse repetition time/short echo time
s. REM latency
s. root of ciliary ganglion
s. segment spinal fusion
s. sleep duration
s. sleep latency
s. stare epilepsy
s. stature
S. Term Auditory Retrieval and Storage (STARS)
S. Test for Use with Cerebral Palsy Children
s. time inversion recovery
short-acting
s.-a. block (SAB)
s.-a. insulin preparation
shortcoming
short-contact psychotherapy
Shortened Edinburgh Reading Tests
shortening
s. reaction
selective T2 s.
T2 s.
Short-Form Health Survey
short-latency SSEP
short-lived schizophrenic affect
shortness of breath
short-tau
s.-t. inversion recovery (STIR)
s.-t. inversion recovery MRI sequence
short-term
s.-t. anxiety-provoking psychotherapy (STAPP)
s.-t. care facility
s.-t. commitment
s.-t. goal (STG)
s.-t. hospitalization
s.-t. memory (STM)
s.-t. psychotherapy technique
s.-t. visual memory
shot
s. in the arm
fast low angle s. (FLASH)
shotgun
s. marriage
s. wedding
shoulder
cold s.
stooped s.'s
shoulder-girdle syndrome
shoulder-hand syndrome (SHS)
ShR
shading response
shrapnel

shredded Teflon felt
shrinkage
neuronal s.
shrinking retrograde amnesia
SHS
shoulder-hand syndrome
SHSS
Stanford Hypnotic Susceptibility Scale
SHT
STYCAR Hearing Test
shuairuo
shenjing s.
shuffling
s. gait
s. steps
shuk yang
shunt
Accura s.
artery-to-vein s.
s. blockage
cerebrospinal fluid s.
CSF s.
cystoatrial s.
Denver hydrocephalus s.
Edwards/Barbaro syringo-peritoneal s.
s. filter
Hakin-Cortis ventriculoperitoneal s.
Heyer-Schulte neurosurgical s.
Javid s.
lumbar arachnoid peritoneal s.
lumbar-peritoneal s.
lumboperitoneal s.
s. nephritis
Ommaya ventriculoperitoneal s.
percutaneous thecoperitoneal s.
posterior fossa-atrial s.
Pruitt-Inahara s.
Pudenz s.
pulmonary arteriovenous s.
Raimondi low pressure s.
right-to-left s.
Spetzler lumbar-peritoneal s.
Spetzler lumboperitoneal s.
subdural-pleural s.
subduroperitoneal s.
Sundt carotid s.
Sundt loop s.
syringoperitoneal s.
syringosubarachnoid s.
syrinx s.
s. tap
thecoperitoneal Pudenz-Schulte s.
Torkildsen s.
T-shaped Edwards-Barbaro syringeal s.
T-tube s.
UNI-SHUNT hydrocephalus s.
ventriculoatrial s.
ventriculoperitoneal s.
VJ s.
VP s.
zero ICP ventricle s. (ZIPS)
shunted hydrocephalus

S

shunting
  lumbar-peritoneal s.
  syringosubarachnoid s. (SS)
  ventricular peritoneal s.
  ventriculoamniotic s.
  ventriculoperitoneal s.
shut
  s. in
  s. out
shut-in personality
Shy-Drager
  S.-D. neuropathy
  S.-D. syndrome
shyness disorder of childhood
SI
  Salience Inventory
  self-inflicted
  sex inventory
  social introversion
  stimulation index
  structure of intellect
  Systematic Inquiry
SIADH
  syndrome of inappropriate secretion of
  antidiuretic hormone
sialic acid
sialidosis
sialoaerophagy
sialorrhea
Siamese twin
SIB
  self-injurious behavior
sibling
  s. bond
  s. jealousy
  s. profile
  s. relation
  s. relational problem
  s. rivalry
  s. separation
  s.'s subsystem
siboroxime
  technetium 99m s.
sibship method
sibutramine
sicca
  keratoconjunctivitis s.
sicchasia
SICD
  Sequenced Inventory of Communication
  Development
sick
  s. headache
  s. leave
  s. role
  s. sinus syndrome
sickle
  s. cell anemia
  s. cell disease
  s. flap
sickness
  acute African sleeping s.
  African sleeping s.
  altitude s.
  chronic African sleeping s.

decompression s.
East African sleeping s.
falling s.
ghost s.
S. Impact Profile (SIP)
Jamaican vomiting s.
laughing s.
motion s.
serum s.
sleeping s.
West African sleeping s.
side
  s. effect
  s. effect profile
side-cutting cannula
side-opening laminar hook
**side-port flat-bottomed Ommaya
  reservoir**
sideration
siderodromomania
siderodromophobia
siderophobia
siderosis
SIDS
  sudden infant death syndrome
Siegert sign
Siemens
  S. couch
  S. Magnetom scanner
  S. somatoma plus DCT system
  S. Somatom Plus
  S. Sonoline SL-2 echocardiograph
Siemerling-Creutzfeldt disease
SIFTER
  Screening Instrument for Targeting
  Educational Risk
sigh
  premonitory s.
sighing dyspnea
sightedness
  close s.
SIGI
  System for Interactive Guidance
  Information
sigil
sigma
  s. activity
  s. receptor
sigmatism
sigmoid
  s. sinus
  s. sinus ligation
  s. sinus retraction
sign
  Abadie s. of tabes dorsalis
  accessory s.
  alien hand s.
  arithmetic s.
  autonomic hyperactivity s.
  Babinski s.
  Bamberger s.
  Barré s.
  Battle s.
  Bechterew s.
  Beevor s.

Biernacki s.
s. blindness
Bonhoeffer s.
brainstem s.
brim s.
Brudzinski s.
buckling s.
Cantelli s.
cardinal s.
Castellani-Low s.
cerebellar s.
cerebral s.
Chaddock s.
characteristic s.
Chvostek s.
Claude hyperkinesis s.
Collier s.
contralateral s.
conventional s.
Crichton-Browne s.
crossed adductor s.
Dejerine s.
s. depression
doll's eye s.
double fragment s.
Duchenne s.
echo s.
empty delta s.
empty sella s.
empty triangle s.
Erb s.
Erb-Westphal s.
Escherich s.
external malleolar s.
eyelash s.
eye-roll s.
false localizing s.
fan s.
focal neurologic s.
focal nonextrapyramidal
  neurologic s.
Froment s.
frontal release s.
Goldstein toe s.
Gordon s.
Gorlin s.
Gowers s.
Graefe s.
Grasset s.
Griesinger s.
Hoffmann s.
Homans s.
Hoover s.
iconic s.
indexical s.
ipsilateral cerebellar s.
ipsilateral corticospinal tract s.
Jackson s.
Joffroy s.
Kernig s.
s. language
Lasègue s.
Legendre s.
Leichtenstern s.
Leri s.

Leser-Trélat s.
Lhermitte s.
Lichtheim s.
local s.
Macewen s.
Magendie-Hertwig s.
Magnan s.
Mannkopf s.
Marcus Gunn s.
Masini s.
Mayerson s.
medullary s.
meningeal s.
mesencephalic s.
mirror s.
Myerson s.
neck s.
Néri s.
neurological soft s.
neurovegetative s.
nonextrapyramidal neurologic s.
objective s.
Omega s.
operational s.
s. of the orbicularis
s. out
Parinaud s.
pathognomonic s.
Pfuhl s.
Phalen s.
physical s.
Piltz s.
Pitres s.
pontine s.
Pool-Schlesinger s.
positive frontal release s.
premonitory s.
pseudo-Graefe s.
pyramidal s.
Remak s.
reservoir s.
Revilliod s.
Romberg s.
root s.
Rossolimo s.
Russell s.
Saenger s.
Schlesinger s.
Schuele s.
Schultze s.
Seeligmüller s.
sheet s.
Siegert s.
Signorelli s.
Simon s.
soft neurologic s.
spine s.
Spurling s.
Stellwag s.
Stewart-Holmes s.
Straus s.
string s.
Tinel s.
toe s.
tram track s.

S

sign *(continued)*
    Trousseau s.
    Uhthoff s.
    vital s. (VS)
    von Graefe s.
    Weber s.
    Weiss s.
    Wernicke s.
    Westphal s.
    Westphal-Erb s.
    withdrawal s.
    Woltman s.
signal
    acoustic s.
    s. analysis
    anchorage-dependent s.
    s. anxiety
    astrocytic s.
    bilateral contralateral routing of s.'s
      (BICROS)
    contralateral routing of s.'s (CROS)
    s. filtering
    focal contralateral routing of s.'s
      (FOCALCROS)
    free induction s.
    high-density transient s.'s (HITS)
    high-intensity s.
    ideomotor s.
    s. intensity
    s. intensity curve
    intracellular s.
    ipsilateral frontal routing of s.'s
      (IFROS)
    ipsilateral frontal routing of s.'s
      (IFROS)
    s. loss
    magnetic resonance s.
    neuronal s.
    nuclear s.
    s. processing
    s. recognition particle (SRP)
    repulsive axon guidance s.
    s. strength
    s. transducing receptor
    s. transducing receptor component
    s. transduction pathway
    s. void
    s. voltage waveform
signaling
    inside-out s.
    intraceptive s.
    outside-in s.
signalize
signalment
signal-to-noise
    s.-t.-n. ratio (SNR)
    s.-t.-n. threshold
signal-transducing
    s.-t. guanine-nucleotide binding
      protein
Signa 1.5 Tesla unit
signed out against medical advice
  (SOAMA)

significance
    s. level
    monoclonal gammopathies of
      undetermined s. (MGUS)
    monoclonal gammopathy of
      unknown s. (MUGUS)
    nonparametric tests of s.
    parametric test of s.
    statistical s.
    test of s.
significant
    clinically s.
    s. conflict
    s. deterioration
    s. difference
    s. displacement
    s. impairment
    s. loss
    not s. (NS)
    s. other
    s. risk
    s. risk factor
    s. subjective distortion
    s. supporting person
signify
Signorelli sign
signs of alcohol intoxication
SIGSS
    selective imaging and graphics for
      stereotactic surgery
siknis
    grisi s.
Siladryl Oral
Silapap
    Children's S.
    Infants' S.
Silastic
    S. catheter
    S. device
    S. sponge
    S. stent
    S. tube
    S. wick
SILD
    Sequenced Inventory of Language
      Development
sildenafil citrate
silence
    s. communication pattern
    electrocerebral s. (ECS)
    selective s.
    teen s.
    tyranny of s.
silent
    s. area
    s. blocking in speech
    s. cerebral infarction
    s. microembolism
    s. period
    s. speech blockade
    s. stroke
    s. treatment
silicone
    s. balloon
    s. implant

s. rubber
s. sponge
SilkTouch CO₂ laser scanner
silliness
childlike s.
silly
s. affect
S. Putty
silok
SILS
Shipley Institute of Living Scale
silver
s. bullet
s. cord syndrome
Silverman placement of electrode
simethicone
aluminum hydroxide with
magnesium hydroxide and s.
simiae
Herpesvirus s.
simian
s. crease
s. fissure
s. line
similarities
s. mental status test
s. subtest
S. Test of Verbal Abstract
Reasoning
similarity
assumed s.
s. disorder of aphasia
vocabulary, information, block
design, s. (VIBS)
Similes Test
Simmons
S. cervical spine fusion
S. plating system
Simon sign
simple
s. absence
s. affective depression
s. alcoholic drunkenness
s. aphasia
s. confrontation
s. decompression
s. depressive dementia
s. deterioration
s. deterioration senile psychosis
s. deteriorative disorder
s. drunkenness
s. figure
s. hallucination
s. lobule
s. membranous limb of
semicircular duct
s. motor tic
s. obesity
s. paranoid reaction
s. paranoid state
s. partial seizure (SPS)
s. phobia
s. retardation
s. schizophrenia
s. senile dementia

s. skull fracture
s. task
s. vocal tic
simpleminded
simple-type arteriosclerotic psychosis
simplex
herpes s.
melancholia s.
paranoia s.
purpura s.
schizophrenia s.
toxoplasmosis, other infections,
rubella, cytomegalovirus, and
herpes s. (TORCH)
Simpson
S. catheter
S. Grade
S. grading
S. Scale
Simpson-Angus
S.-A. Rating Scale
S.-A. Scale
simulant
simulate
simulated
s. activities of daily living (SADL,
SADLs)
s. presence therapy
simulator
BTE Work S.
simultanagnosia, simultagnosia
simultaneous
s. insanity
s. volume imaging
simvastatin
sin
capital s.
cardinal s.
deadly s.
mortal s.
venial s.
sincalide
sine
s. delirio
s. wave
s. wave unilateral ECT
Sine-Aid IB
Sinemet CR
Sinequan Oral
**Singer-Loomis Inventory of Personality
(SLIP)**
single
s. bur hole procedure
s. combat
s. criteria set
s. custody
S. and Double Simultaneous
Stimulation Test
s. enhancing CT lesion (SECTL)
s. episode
s. episode chronic mania
s. episode depressive psychosis
s. hook retractor
s. photon emission computed
tomography (SPECT)

single *(continued)*
    s. point mutation
    s. seizure
    s. word stage
single-episode
    s.-e. psychotic depression
    s.-e. psychotic reaction
single-fiber electromyography (SFEMG)
single-fraction radiation
single-level
    s.-l. decompressive laminectomy
    s.-l. spinal fusion
single-major-locus (SML)
    s.-m.-l. model
single-parent
    s.-p. family
    s.-p. home
single-rod construct
singsong fashion
singularity
singultus
sinister
sinistrad
sinistral
sinistrocerebral
sinistromanual
sinistropedal
sinkage
sinking feeling
sinodural angle
sinogenic meningitis
Sinografin
sinography
sinonasal
    s. cavity
    s. psammomatoid ossifying fibroma
sinophobia
sinovenous
    s. occlusion
    s. stroke
    s. thrombosis
sinsemillan marijuana
Sintoclar
sinus, pl. **sinus, sinuses**
    Breschet s.
    s. cavernosus
    cavernous s.
    cerebral s.
    circular s.
    s. circularis
    confluence of sinuses
    cranial dermal s.
    dilated intercavernous s.
    s. durae matris
    dural venous s.
    sinuses of dura mater
    endodermal s.
    ethmoid s.
    s. headache
    intercavernous s.
    intracranial venous s.
    lateral s.
    marginal s.
    maxillary s.

    Motrin IB S.
    nasal s.
    s. nerve of Hering
    occluded s.
    s. occlusion
    paranasal s.
    parasinoidal sinuses
    s. pericranii
    petrosal s.
    petrosquamosal s.
    s. phlebitis
    pilonidal s.
    s. rectus
    s. reflex
    rhomboidal s.
    s. rhomboidalis
    Ridley s.
    sagittal s.
    sigmoid s.
    space of the cavernous s. (SpoCS)
    sphenoid s.
    sphenoparietal s.
    sphenotemporal s.
    spinal dermal s.
    straight s.
    superior petrosal s.
    tentorial s.
    Tylenol Allergy S.
    venous s.
sinusitis
sinus-vein thrombosis (SVT)
sinuum
    confluens s.
sinuvertebral nerve
Sinvastatin Survival Study
SIP
    Sickness Impact Profile
SIPI
    Short Imaginal Processes Inventory
SIPS
    sympathetically independent pain
      syndrome
SIPT
    Sensory Integration and Praxis Tests
SIRS
    Structured Interview of Reported
      Symptoms
SIS
    Stress Impact Scale
SISI
    Short Increment Sensitivity Index
sissified
sissyish behavior
Sisyphus dream
SIT
    Slosson Intelligence Test
    stress inoculation training
sit
    s. in
    s. out
site
    graft s.
    high-affinity binding s.
    hook s.
    recognition s.

sitiophobia, sitophobia
sitomania, sitiomania
sitophobia, sitiophobia
sitting
    s. balance
    s. fear
    s. position
situation
    s. anxiety
    Asch s.
    Behavioral Performance S.
    cluster of s.'s
    s. cluster
    conflictual s.
    direful s.
    dreaded s.
    educational s.
    either-or s.
    emotion-laden s.
    family s.
    feared s.
    feared single performance s.
    histrionic s.
    low-activity s.
    low-stimulation s.
    oedipal s.
    one-to-one s.
    open-cue s.
    peer interactional s.
    performance s.
    phobic s.
    previously stabilizing social s.'s
    psychoanalytic s.
    social s.
    stabilizing social s.'s
    triage s.
situational
    acute maladjustment s.
    S. Attitude Scale (SAS)
    s. attribution
    s. crisis
    s. depression
    s. disturbance
    s. ethics
    s. homosexuality
    s. hypoactive sexual desire
    s. insomnia
    s. perception
    s. posttraumatic neurosis
    s. psychosis
    s. reaction
    s. restraint
    s. sexual dysfunction
    s. specific phobia
    s. stressor
    s. test
    s. therapy
    s. trigger
situationally
    s. appropriate atmosphere
    s. bound
    s. bound panic attack
    s. optimistic atmosphere
    s. predisposed
    s. predisposed panic attack

situational-type
    s.-t. disorder
    s.-t. dyspareunia
    s.-t. female orgasmic disorder
    s.-t. female sexual arousal disorder
situation-related
    s.-r. epilepsy
    s.-r. seizure
situs analysis
SIV
    Survey of Interpersonal Values
SIW
    self-inflicted wound
Six-Hour Retarded Child
Sixteen Personality Factor Questionnaire
sixth
    s. cranial nerve
    s. nerve palsy
    s. sense
    s. ventricle
size
    s. perception
    ventricle s.
SjO$_2$
    jugular venous oxygen saturation
Sjögren-Larssen syndrome
Sjögren syndrome (SS)
Sjöqvist tractotomy
SKAT
    Sex Knowledge and Attitude Test
skateboarding accident
skein
    choroid s.
Skelaxin
skeletal
    s. amyloidosis
    s. deformity
    s. muscle relaxant
skeletonize
skeptic
skew
    s. deviation
    s. distribution
    marital s.
SKI
    Skill Indicators
skid-row
    s.-r. bum
    s.-r. derelict
skid row
skill
    ACO: Improving Writing, Thinking
      and Reading S.'s
    activities of daily living s.'s
    adaptation s.
    adaptive s.
    Adult Personal Adjustment and
      Role S.'s
    ambulation s.'s
    Analysis of Readiness S.'s
    s. area
    assertiveness s.
    attentional s.'s
    auditory s.'s
    calculation s.

S

skill *(continued)*
California Test of Basic S.'s (CTBS)
Canadian Tests of Basic S.'s (CTBS)
Checklist of Adaptive Living S.'s (CALS)
conceptual s.
coping s.
core mindfulness s.'s
Criterion Test of Basic S.'s
decision-making s.
decoding s.
developmental s.'s
ego-coping s.
encoding s.
Evaluating the Participant's Employability S.'s
expressive language s.
fine motor s.
functional s.
generic s.
gross motor s.
higher level s.
S. Indicators (SKI)
intellectual s.
interpersonal effectiveness s.
s. inventory
Inventory of Perceptual S.'s (IPS)
Iowa Tests of Basic S.'s
Kaufman Survey of Early Academic and Language S.'s (K-SEALS)
Kent Series of Emergency S.'s
leisure s.
Life S.'s, Forms 1 & 2
Martinez Assessment of the Basic S.'s
mathematical s.
memory s.
Missouri Kindergarten Inventory of Developmental S.'s
motor s.
negotiating goals s.'s
negotiating routines s.'s
negotiating rules s.'s
neuropsychologic s.
New Jersey Test of Reasoning S.'s
numerical reasoning s.'s
organizational s.'s
parenting s.
perceptual s.
perceptual-motor s.
Personal Adjustment and Role S.'s (PARS)
Personal and Role S.'s (PARS)
positive communication s.'s
Pragmatics Profile of Early Communication S.'s
Primary Test of Cognitive S.'s (PTCS)
problem-solving s.
Program for Assessing Youth Employment S.'s

reasoning and memory s.'s
resolving conflict s.'s
right hemisphere cognitive s.'s
Riley Inventory of Basic Learning S.'s (RIBLS)
routine s.
rules s.'s
S. Scan for Management Development
Schedule of Growing S.'s
Screening Test for Educational Prerequisite S.'s (STEPS)
Self-Assessment in Writing S.'s
self-care s.
self-help s.
sensorimotor s.
social s.
socialization s.'s
stress adaptability s.'s
s. training
uncoordinated motor s.'s
unrefined motor s.
visual perceptual s.
visuoconstruction s.
visuospatial s.
word-attack s.
word-finding s.
word-recognition s.

skilled
s. nursing care (SNC)
s. worker
skill-less
skin
clammy s.
s. conductance orienting response (SCOR)
s. depth
s. disease
s. disease fear
s. erotism
s. flap
glossy s.
s. graft harvesting pain
s. incision
s. injury fear
s. lesion
on the s.
s. picking
s. reflex
under the s.
skin-muscle reflex
Skinner box
skinnerian conditioning
skin-pupillary reflex
Skiodan
skip
s. bail
s. class
s. meals
s. out
skipping
grade s.
skirt the issue
SKOLD
Screening Kit of Language Development

Skoog release of Dupuytren contracture
skull
s. asymmetry
s. base
s. bone graft
cloverleaf s.
s. fracture
maplike s.
s. plate
s. punch
s. session
steeple s.
tower s.
SKY
spectral karyotyping
skyscraper fear
Skytron bed
slanderous
slang
rhyming s.
slant
antimongoloid s.
slave
s. driver
s. system component
Slavson Activity Interview Therapy
SLC
sociopolitical locus of control
SLE
Scholastic Level Exam
systemic lupus erythematosus
sleep
abnormal behavior during s.
s. abnormality
abnormal physiological event
during s.
activated s.
active s.
s. activity
alcohol-induced nighttime s.
s. apnea
s. apnea hypersomnolence syndrome
(SAHS)
s. apnea hypersomnolence syndrome
associated with upper airway
obstruction (SAHS-UAO)
s. apnea syndrome (SAS)
s. architecture
s. arousal
arousal from s.
s. attack
s. behavior disorder
benign epileptiform transient of s.
(BETS)
S. and Breathing Problems Scale
circadian phase of s.
s. complaint
confusional arousals from s.
consolidated s.
s. continuity
s. continuity disturbance
continuous s.
crescendo s.
s. cycle
deep s.

delta-wave s.
s. deprivation
s. deprived EEG
depth of s.
s. disorder
s. disorder due to a general
medical condition
s. disordered breathing (SDB)
disorder of initiating and
maintaining s. (DIMS)
s. disorder insomnia
s. disruption
s. dissociation
dreamless s.
s. drunkenness
s. dysfunction
easily disturbed s.
s. efficiency
electric s.
electrotherapeutic s.
environmental disturbance of s.
s. epilepsy
s. fear
fitful s.
forced s.
fragmentation of nocturnal s.
fragmented nighttime s.
s. hygiene
hypnotic s.
indeterminate s.
insufficient nocturnal s.
s. interference
s. inversion
irresistible s.
s. latency
light s. (LS)
s. loss
s. mechanism
s. movement
negative conditioning for s.
nonrapid eye movement s.
non-REM s.
nonrestorative s.
NREM s.
s. numbness
onset of s.
s. onset REM period
s. organization
overconcern with s.
paradoxical s.
s. paralysis
paroxysmal s.
s. pattern
s. phase
s. phase dyssomnia
s. phase syndrome
s. phobia
pontine s.
positive occipital sharp transients
of s. (POSTS)
s. posture
primary disorder of s.
quality of s.
quiet s.
rapid eye movement s.

S

sleep *(continued)*
    REM s.
    REM-onset s.
    rhombencephalic s.
    S. Screening Questionnaire for
      Parents
    slow-wave s. (SWS)
    s. spindle
    s. spindle on EEG
    s. stage
    s. state
    s. state misperception
    s. technique
    telencephalic s.
    s. tendency
    s. terror
    s. terror episode
    s. therapy
    thrombencephalic s.
    transitional s. (TS)
    s. treatment
    twilight s.
    undisturbed nocturnal s.
    unintended s.
    yen s.
sleep-electroshock therapy
Sleep-eze 3 Oral
Sleepinal
sleep-induced
    s.-i. apnea
    s.-i. respiratory impairment
sleep-inducing peptide
sleepiness
    daytime s.
    disorder of excessive s.
    excessive daytime s. (EDS)
    pathologic s.
    physiological s.
    S. Scale
sleeping
    s. drunkenness
    s. erection
    s. partner
    s. pill
    s. sickness
sleeplessness
    s. associated with acute
    s. associated with anxiety
    s. associated with psychosis
sleep-onset
    s.-o. episode
    s.-o. insomnia
sleep-related
    s.-r. abnormal swallowing syndrome
    s.-r. asthma
    s.-r. bruxism
    s.-r. cluster headache
    s.-r. epilepsy
    s.-r. epileptic seizure
    s.-r. gastroesophageal reflux
    s.-r. hallucination
    s.-r. head banging
    s.-r. hemolysis
    s.-r. myoclonus syndrome

sleep-terror event
sleep-wake
    s.-w. abnormality
    s.-w. cycle
    s.-w. rhythm
    s.-w. schedule
    s.-w. schedule disorder
    s.-w. syndrome
    s.-w. system
    s.-w. transition
sleepwalking
    s. behavior
    s. disorder
Sleepwell 2-nite
sleeve
    arachnoid s.
    arachnoidal root s.
    s. graft
    polyethylene s.
SLEM
    slow lateral eye movement
    SLEM on electroencephalogram
slender
    s. fasciculus
    s. lobule
slept all night (SAN)
SLEV
    Saint Louis encephalitis virus
SLI
    speech and language impaired
slice
    digital subtraction venous
      angiography s.
    s. fracture
    s. selection
slice-select encoding gradient
sliding of meanings
slight
    s. defect
    inner s.
Slimline clip
sling
    clip-reinforced cotton s.
    fascia lata s.
Slingerland Screening Tests (SST)
sling/wrapping technique
SLIP
    Singer-Loomis Inventory of Personality
slip
    freudian s.
    s. of (the) tongue
slippage
    cognitive s.
slit
    s. hemorrhage
    s. valve
    s. ventricle
    s. ventricle syndrome
sloppy appearance
Slosson
    S. Children's Version Family
      Environment Scale
    S. Drawing Coordination Test
    S. Intelligence Test (SIT)

S. Test of Reading Readiness
(STRR)

slot
s. fracture
s. machine

slotted
s. hammer
s. suction tip

slough over

slow
s. component neuropathy
s. lateral eye movement (SLEM)
s. learner
s. rate of language development
s. speech
s. virus
s. wave activity

slow-acting viral encephalitis

slowed gait

slow-frequency EEG activity

slowing
cognitive s.
motoric s.
psychomotor s.
saccadic s.

Slow-K

Slow-Mag

slowness
obsessional s.
s. of thought

slow-virus infection

slow-wave
s.-w. sleep (SWS)
s.-w. sleep stability

SLSQ
Speech and Language Screening
Questionnaire

SLT
STYCAR Language Test

Sluder neuralgia

slumber
affective s.

slurred speech

Sluyter-Mehta thermocouple electrode

Sly disease

SM
sadomasochism
self-mutilation
sexual myth

S/M
sadism/masochism
sadomasochism

S&M
sadomasochism

SMA
sequential multiple analysis
spinal muscular atrophy
supplementary motor area

smacking
lip s.

small
s. angle double incidence
angiogram (SADIA)
s. detail response
s. mindedness

s. motor unit potential
s. penis complex
s. sharp spike (SSS)

small-amplitude rapid tremor

small-bowel carcinoid tumor

small, deep, recent infarction (SDRI)

SMAST
Short Michigan Alcoholism Screening
Test

SMAT
School Motivation Analysis Test

SMD
stereotypic movement disorder

smear
blood s.
Tzanck s.

smearing
saliva s.

smell
s. blindness
s. disorder
S. Identification Test
s. imagery
organ of s.

smell-brain

Smellie scissors

SMH
state mental hospital

SMI
severely mentally impaired
Style of Mind Inventory
SMI 3000 bed
SMI 5000 bed

smile
endogenous s.
exogenous s.
forced s.
social s.

Smiley-Williams arteriogram needle

Smith
S. air craniotome
S. nerve root suction retractor

**Smith-Johnson nonverbal Performance
Scale**

Smith-Lemli-Opitz syndrome

Smith-Petersen laminectomy rongeur

Smith-Robinson
S.-R. operation
S.-R. procedure
S.-R. technique

Smithwick
S. button hook
S. dissector
S. ganglion hook
S. sympathectomy
S. sympathectomy hook

**SMK C5 with a 2-mm exposed tip
cannula**

SML
single-major-locus
SML model

SMMI
Senoussi Multiphasic Marital Inventory

smokable amphetamine

S

smoker
    chain s.
smoker's
    s. stroke
    s. syndrome
smoking
    S. Behavior Questionnaire (SBQ)
    s. cessation
    s. gun
SMON
    subacute myelo-optic neuropathy
smooth
    s. endoplasmic reticulum
    s. muscle proliferation
    s. muscle tumor
    s. pursuit
    s. pursuit defect
    s. pursuit eye movement (SPEM)
smothering sensation
smother love
SMPS
    sympathetically mediated pain syndrome
SMS
    stiff-man syndrome
snake
    s. bite
    s. pit
    s. symbol
SNAP
    sensory nerve action potential
    SNAP amplitude
    SNAP on electromyogram
snap finger
snapping reflex
SNC
    skilled nursing care
Snc
    substantia nigra pars compacta
Sneddon syndrome
Snellen letter
sniffing
    s. death
    glue sniffing
    inhalant sniffing
snob appeal
snooping
    data s.
Snooze Fast
snore
    resuscitative s.
snorting
Sno-Traks wheelchair chains
snout reflex
snow
    s. fear
    s. job
snowshoe hare virus
SNR
    signal-to-noise ratio
Snr
    substantia nigra pars reticulata
SNS
    sacral nerve stimulation
    sympathetic nervous system

snuffbox
    anatomical s.
SO
    sex offender
soaked
    s. fat plug
    s. muscle plug
SOAMA
    signed out against medical advice
SOAP
    subjective, objective, assessment, plan
sobriety
    s. test
    white knuckling s.
    Youth Enjoying S. (YES)
sob story
SOC
    state of consciousness
social
    s. abulia
    s. acquiescence (SA, sa)
    s. activity
    s. adaptation
    S. Adaptation Status (SAS)
    S. Adequacy Index (SAI)
    s. adjustment measure
    S. Adjustment Scale
    S. Adjustment Scale II
    S. Adjustment Self-Report
      Questionnaire
    S. Adjustment Self-Report Scale
      (SASRS, SAS-RS)
    s. age (SA, sa)
    s. alienation
    s. anorexia
    s. anxiety
    s. anxiety disorder
    s. apprehensiveness
    s. attachment
    s. avoidance and distortion
    s. avoidance and distress (SAD)
    S. Avoidance and Distress Scale
    s. babbling
    s. barrier
    s. behavior
    S. Behavior Assessment Inventory
      (SBAI)
    S. Behavior Assessment Schedule
    s. breakdown syndrome (SBS)
    s. casework
    s. causation theory
    s. class and mental illness
    S. Climate Scale (SCS)
    s. communication
    s. competence
    s. compliance
    s. conformity
    s. consciousness
    s. control
    s. cripple
    s. cue
    s. darwinism
    s. dependence
    s. deprivation
    s. desirability (SD)

s. detachment
s. development
s. deviance
s. diagnosis
s. disability
S. Disability Scale
s. disability syndrome
s. disconnection
s. disease
s. distance
s. dominance
s. dominance theory
s. drinker
s. drinking
s. dyad
s. dysfunction
s. engineering
s. environment
s. evaluation
s. facilitation
s. function
S. Function Index (SFI)
s. functioning
s. functioning impairment
s. functioning level
s. gambling
s. gesture speech
s. hierarchy
s. history (SH)
s. hunger
s. identification
s. immaturity
s. inappropriateness
s. ineptness
s. inhibition
s. insecurity
s. instinct
s. integration
s. integration-disintegration
s. integration-disintegration model
s. intelligence
S. Intelligence Test
s. interaction
S. Interaction Scale
s. interaction therapy
s. interest
s. introversion (SI)
s. introversion scale
s. island
s. isolate
s. isolation
s. judgment
s. judgment score
s. learning group therapy
s. maladjustment
S. Maladjustment Schedule
s. masochism
s. medicine
s. minded
s. mores
s. network therapy
s. norm
S. and Occupational Functioning Assessment (SOFAS)

S. and Occupational Functioning Assessment Scale
s. organization
s. outcast
s. overdependence
s. perception
s. persecution
s. phobia
s. phobia experience
s. phobic-like behavior
s. policy planning
s. pressure
S. and Prevocational Information Battery (SPIB)
s. problem
s. process
s. psychiatry
s. psychologist
s. psychology
s. quotient (SQ)
S. Readjustment Rating Scale (SRRS)
s. readjustment rating scale
s. recovery
s. reference group
s. rehabilitation
S. and Rehabilitation Service (SRS)
s. reinforcement
S. Reintegration Scale
s. relatedness
s. relatedness disturbance
S. Relations Test (SRT)
s. resistance
s. responsibility
S. Reticence Scale
s. role
s. sanction
S. Security (SS)
S. Security Administration (SSA)
S. Security Disability (SSD)
s. selection theory
s. service (SS)
s. service agency
s. service consultation
s. setting
s. situation
s. skill
s. skills deficit
s. skills deterioration
S. Skills Rating System (SSRS)
s. skills training (SST)
s. smile
s. standard
s. stereotypical behavior
s. stimulation
s. stress
s. stress and functionability inventory (SSFI)
s. stressor
s. structure
s. support
S. Support Scale
s. tension
s. tolerance
s. trap

social *(continued)*
    s. type
    s. value
    s. welfare organization
    s. withdrawal
    s. withdrawal of childhood
    s. work
    s. worker
    s. zone
Social-Emotional
    S.-E. Dimension Scale
social-emotional functioning
socialization skills
socialized
    s. childhood truancy
    s. conduct disorder
    s. delinquency (SD)
    s. dementia (SD)
    s. disturbance
    s. medicine
    s. runaway reaction
socially
    s. acceptable behavior
    s. disruptive environment
    s. effective
    s. intimate model
    s. unacceptable behavior
social phobia
societal
    s. bias
    s. norm
    s. reaction theory
    s. structure
society
    demands of s.
    Hemlock S.
    International Headache S.
    s. level
    majority s.
    Orphan Train Heritage S.
    secret s.
    traditional s.
    Vienna Psychoanalytic S.
    Wednesday Evening S.
sociobiology
sociocenter
sociocentric
sociocentrism
sociocosm
sociocultural
    s. background
    s. milieu
sociodemographic feature
socioeconomic
    s. group
    s. life change
    s. status (SES)
socioenvironmental therapy
sociofugal space
sociogenesis
sociogram
    objective s.
    perceptual s.
sociolinguistics

sociologese
sociological
sociology
    clinical s.
    industrial s.
    medical s.
sociomedical
sociometric distance
sociometrist
sociometry
sociopath
sociopathic
    s. behavior
    s. personality
    s. personality disorder (SPD)
    s. personality disturbance (SPD)
sociopathology
sociopathy
sociopolitical locus of control (SLC)
sociopsychological
socioreligious
sociosexual
sociotaxis
sociotherapy
sociotropy scale
socratic questioning
SOD
    superoxide dismutase
sodium
    s. acetate
    s. aminobenzoate
    amobarbital s.
    ampicillin s.
    Amytal S.
    s. amytal
    s. ascorbate
    s. barbital
    s. bicarbonate
    s. bromide
    s. butabarbital
    butabarbital s.
    Butisol S.
    cefalothin s.
    cefoxitin s.
    s. chloride
    citicoline s.
    danaparoid s.
    dantrolene s.
    Diphenylan S.
    divalproex s.
    s. dodecyl sulfate-polyacrylamide gel electrophoresis (SDS-PAGE)
    indigotin disulfonate s.
    ioxaglate s.
    s. lactate
    s. lactate induced flashback
    levothyroxine s.
    liothyronine s.
    meclofenamate s.
    methicillin s.
    methohexital s.
    methotrexate s.
    nafcillin s.
    s. nitroprusside
    s. oxylate

pentobarbital s.
Pentothal S.
phenobarbital s.
s. phosphate
photofrin porfimer s.
s. polystyrene sulfonate
pravastatin s.
s. salicylate
secobarbital s.
serum s.
technetium 99m pertechnetate s.
thiopental s.
s. thiosalicylate
s. thiosulfate
s. valproate
vinbarbital s.
warfarin s.
zomepirac s.
sodium-responsive periodic paralysis
sodomist, sodomite
sodomize
sodomy
Soemmering
S. ganglion
S. spot
SOF
superior orbital fissure
Sofamor spinal instrument device
SOFAS
Social and Occupational Functioning
Assessment
Sof-Rol dressing
Sofsilk nonabsorbable silk suture
SOFT
Sorting of Figures Test
soft
s. diet
s. disk herniation
s. neurologic sign
s. palate retraction
s. restraint
s. speech
s. spot
s. tissue abnormality
s. tissue dissection
s. tissue injury
s. tissue stretching
s. touch
Softab
Bucladin-S S.
softliner
Softplate
Sof-Wick dressing
SOF'WIRE spinal fixation
SOI
Student Opinion Inventory
SOI-Learning Abilities Test: Screening Form for Gifted
Sokoda complex
solace
Solarcaine Aloe Extra Burn Relief
solar ganglia
soldier of fortune
soldier's heart

sole
s. nuclei
s. plate
s. tap reflex
solemn
s. affect
s. vow
solenoid coil
sole-plate ending
SOLER
squarely (face person), open posture, lean
(toward person), eye (contact), relaxed
Solfoton
solicitation
solicitous
solicitude
solidarity
solidify
solid state coagulator
solid-state instrument
soliloquy
sexual s.
solipsism
solitariness
solitarius
nucleus s.
solitary
s. activity
s. aggressive type conduct
s. aggressive-type conduct disorder
s. bundle
s. confinement
s. extranodal lymphoma
s. fibrous tumor
s. hunter syndrome
s. hydatid cyst
s. neurofibroma
s. stealing
s. tract
solitude
solitudinarian
solium
Taenia s.
Solomon-Bloembergen equation
SOLST
Stephens Oral Language Screening Test
Solu-Biloptin
Solu-Cortef
Solu-Medrol Injection
Solurex L.A.
solute transport
solution
10% acetylcysteine 0.05%
isoproterenol hydrochloride s.
s. analysis
auxiliary s.
Avitene s.
bacitracin s.
Betadine Helafoam s.
comprehensive s.
expansive s.
ferumoxide injectable s.
$[^{18}F]$ fluoride s.
hydroxyethyl methacrylate
polymerizing s.

S

solution *(continued)*
    image guided s.
    Resectisol Irrigation S.
    Zenker s.
Solutrast
solvable
solvent
    s. (inhalation) dependence
    organic s.
    volatile s.
solving
    failure of problem s.
    frontal-lobe abstraction/problem s.
    inductive problem s.
    interpersonal cognitive problem s.
    (ICPS)
    problem s.
    Test of Problem S.
    visuospatial problem s.
Soma Compound
Somanetics
    S. INVOS 3100 cerebral oximeter
    S. INVOS cerebral oximeter device
SomaSensor device
somatagnosia agnosia
somatalgia
somatesthesia
somatesthetic
somatic
    s. block
    s. cell
    s. complaint
    s. delusion
    s. focus
    s. hallucination
    S. Inkblot Series
    s. memory
    S.'s monitoring electrode
    s. motor neuron
    s. motor nuclei
    s. obsession
    s. pain
    s. paranoid disorder
    s. psychosis
    S. "3" Scale
    s. schizophrenia
    s. sensory cortex
    s. symptom
    s. therapy
    s. treatment
    s. treatment for depression
    s. type
somatist
somatization
    s. neurotic disorder
    s. pain symptoms
    s. pseudoneurological symptoms
    s. reaction
    s. sexual symptoms
    s. tendency
somatizing
    s. clinical depression
    s. disorders
somatochrome

somatoform
    s. interface disorder
    s. pain disorder
    s. scale
somatognosia
somatology
Somatom DR1
somatomedin C
somatometry
somatomotor epilepsy
somatopathic drinking
somatophrenia
somatopsychiatric comorbidity
somatopsychic disorder
somatopsychosis
somatosensory
    s. cortex
    s. cued task
    s. epilepsy
    s. evoked potential (SEP, SSEP)
    s. evoked potential monitoring
    s. evoked response (SER)
    s. mapping
    s. seizure
    s. system
somatosexual
somatostatin
somatotherapy
somatotonia
somatotopagnosia
somatotopic
somatotopy
somatotroph
    s. cell
    s. hyperplasia
somatotropin
somatotype
somatron table
somber mood
some degree of range
somesthesia
somesthetic
    s. area
    s. dysarthria
    s. neuron
    s. relay nucleus
    s. system
SOMI
    sternal occipital mandibular
    immobilization
    SOMI brace
    SOMI Jr. brace
Sominex Oral
somite
    embryonic cervical s.
somnambulic epilepsy
somnambulism
    cataleptic s.
    monoideic s.
    polyideic s.
somnambulistic trance
somnial
somnifacient
somniferous

somniferum
    Papaver s.
somnific
somnifugous
somniloquence, somniloquism
somniloquist
somniloquy
somnipathist
somnipathy
somnocinematograph
somnolence, somnolency
    daytime s.
    disorders of excessive s. (DOES)
    excessive s.
    s. syndrome
somnolent detachment
somnolentia
somnolescent
somnolism
somopsychosis
SOMPA
    System of Multicultural Pluralistic
        Assessment
SOMT
    Spatial Orientation Memory Test
song and dance
Songer
    S. cable
    S. cable system
sonic stereometry
Sonneberg neurectomy
Sonocut ultrasonic aspirator
sonogram
sonography
    color-flow Doppler s.
    Doppler s.
    TCD s.
    transcranial color-coded s.
    transcranial color-coded real-time s.
        (TCCS)
sonomotor response
sonophobia
Sono-Stat Plus sound device
sophism
sophistic
sophistry
sophomania
**Sophy mini programmable pressure
    valve**
sopiet
soporiferous
soporifical
soporific drug dependence
soporose, soporous
SOQ
    Suicide Opinion Questionnaire
sorbitol
    Actidose With S.
sorcerous
sore
    pressure s.
    venereal s.
sort
    Missouri Occupational Card S.
    Q s.

sorter
    Keirsey Temperament s.
sorting
    S. of Figures Test (SOFT)
    s. polarities
SOS
    stimulation of sense
    Student Orientations Survey
SOT
    stream of thought
Soteira House
Sotos syndrome
soul
    s. blindness
    folk s.
    s. folk
    s. loss
    negative ruler of the s.
    s. pain
    world s.
sound
    abnormal stoppage of s.
    air-blade s.
    s. analysis
    attention to s.
    s. blending
    coconut s.
    contralateral routing of s. (CROS)
    s. fear
    s. inside the head
    opening s.
    s. outside the head
    perception of s.
    pulse synchronous s.
    repetition of s.
    s. symbolism
    s. therapy
sounding board
soundless voice
sound-symbol association
source
    Arclite 20,000 light s.
    collateral s.'s
    s. derivation
    s. image
    interstitial radiation s.
    Maxenon 300 watt xenon light s.
    Maxillume 250 watt quartz halogen
        light s.
    Minimax 200 watt light s.
    Zeiss Super Lux 40 light s.
201-source
    201-s. cobalt-60 gamma knife
    201-s. cobalt-60 gamma unit
sour-grapes mechanism
sourness fear
South
    S. African tick-bite fever
    S. Oaks Gambling Screen for
        Adolescents
Southern
    S. blot
    S. blot analysis
    S. California Postrotary Nystagmus
        Test

S

Southern *(continued)*
    S. California Sensory Integration
      Tests
SP
    scale of psychosis
    subdural peritoneal
    systolic pressure
SPA
    schizophrenia with premorbid asociality
    schizophrenia with premorbid association
space
    anterior cavernous sinus s.
    arachnoid s.
    s. base
    s. of the cavernous sinus (SpoCS)
    craniospinal s.
    dead s.
    defensible s.
    disk s.
    dorsal subcutaneous s.
    epidural s.
    ethological models of personal s.
    extracellular s. (ECS)
    extradural s.
    extrapersonal s.
    frontal interhemispheric s.
    His perivascular s.
    incisural s.
    inner s.
    intrapersonal s.
    k-s.
    life s.
    L5-S1 disk s.
    Malacarne s.
    s. perception
    perforated s.
    perioptic subarachnoid s.
    peripersonal s.
    perivascular s.
    personal s.
    s. response
    retropharyngeal s.
    s. sense
    sociofugal s.
    subarachnoid s.
    subdural s.
    subgaleal s.
    synaptic s.
    Tarin s.
    Virchow-Robin s.
space-occupying brain lesion
3-SPACE Polhemus digitizing system
spacer
    ceramic vertebral s.
    methylmethacrylate s.
Spadafore Diagnostic Reading Test
SPAMM
    spatial modulation of magnetization
span
    apprehension s.
    s. of attention
    attention s.
    auditory memory s. (AMS)
    comprehension s.
    digit s. (DS)
    eye-voice s.
    Language-Structured Auditory
      Retention S. (LARS)
    memory s.
    s. recall test
    visual memory s. (VMS)
    Wechsler digit s.
SPAQ
    Seasonal Pattern Assessment
      Questionnaire
SPAR
    sensitivity prediction from the acoustic
      reflex
    SPAR Spelling and Reading Test
Sparine
sparing
    macular s.
    music ability s.
spark-gap instrument
spasm
    affect s.
    anorectal s.
    Bell s.
    canine s.
    carpopedal s.
    clonic s.
    convergence s.
    cryptogenic hemifacial s.
    cynic s.
    dancing s.
    facial habit s.
    functional s.
    habit s.
    hemifacial s. (HFS)
    histrionic s.
    infantile s.
    intention s.
    masticatory s.
    mimic s.
    mobile s.
    muscle s.
    near reflex s.
    nictitating s.
    nodding s.
    occupational s.
    paraplegic s.
    phonic s.
    professional s.
    progressive torsion s.
    reflex s.
    retrocollic s.
    rotatory s.
    salaam s.
    saltatory s.
    sewing s.
    synclonic s.
    tailor's s.
    s. tic
    s. and tic
    tonic s.
    tonoclonic s.
    tooth s.
    torsion s.

vasomotor s.
winking s.

spasmodic
    s. apoplexy
    s. convulsion
    s. diathesis
    s. laughter
    s. laughter syndrome
    s. mydriasis
    s. seizure
    s. tic
    s. torticollis
    s. winking syndrome

spasmodica
    dysarthria syllabaris s.
    tabes s.

spasmodicus
spasmogen
spasmology
spasmolygmus
spasmolysis
spasmolytic
spasmophemia
spasmophenia
spasmophilia
spasmophilic diathesis
spasmus
    s. agitans
    s. caninus
    s. coordinatus
    s. nictitans
    s. nutans

spastic
    s. abasia
    s. amaurotic axonal idiocy
    s. aphonia
    s. cerebral palsy
    s. diplegia
    s. dysarthria
    s. dysphonia
    s. dystonia
    s. gait
    s. hemiparesis
    s. hemiplegia
    s. hyperreflexia
    s. micosis
    s. miosis
    s. mydriasis
    s. paraparesis
    s. paraparesis of middle life
    s. paraplegia
    s. quadriplegia
    s. spinal paralysis
    s. state

spastica
    dysphonia s.
    torticollis s.

spasticity
    Ashworth score of muscle s.
    clasp-knife s.
    s. of conjugate gaze
    flexor s.
    sphincter s.

spatia (*pl. of* spatium)

spatial
    s. ability
    s. agnosia
    s. agraphia
    s. aptitude
    s. balance
    s. behavior
    s. contiguity
    s. disorganization
    s. disorientation
    s. distortion
    s. frequency
    s. homogeneity
    s. localization
    s. modulation of magnetization (SPAMM)
    s. neglect
    s. nonrecognition
    s. organization
    s. orientation
    S. Orientation Memory Test (SOMT)
    s. resolution
    S. Span Test
    s. summation
    s. task

spatially
spatium, pl. **spatia**
    s. subdurale

spatula
    brain s.
    Children's Hospital brain s.
    curved-tipped s.
    Cushing brain s.
    Davis brain s.
    Davis nerve s.
    D'Errico brain s.
    s. dissector
    double-vector brain s.
    duck-billed anodized s.
    House-Fisch dural s.
    Jacobson endarterectomy s.
    Mayfield brain s.
    Olivecrona brain s.
    Peyton brain s.
    Rainin clip-bending s.
    Ray brain s.
    rectangular brain s.
    Rhoton s.
    Sachs nerve s.
    Scoville brain s.
    S-shaped brain s.
    tapered brain s.
    Weary brain s.

SPD
    sociopathic personality disorder
    sociopathic personality disturbance

SPE
    Sensory Perceptual Examination

speaking
    avoidance s.
    s. capacity

speak out
Speare dural hook
Spearman correlation coefficient

S

special
 s. ability
 S. Aptitude Test Battery (SATB)
 s. education
 s. jury
 s. power
 s. relationship to deity theme
 s. relationship to famous person
  theme
 s. scale
 s. sensation
 s. sense
 s. somatic afferent column
 s. theory of relativity
 s. visceral column
 s. visceral efferent nuclei
 s. visceral motor nuclei
specialist
 learning-disabilities s.
specialization
 role s.
specialized language assessment
species
 allopathic s.
specific
 s. absorption rate
 s. academic or work inhibition
 s. action potential
 S. Aptitude Test Battery
 s. culture, age, and gender feature
 s. culture feature
 s. curve
 s. delay
 s. developmental disorder (SDD)
 s. dynamic pattern
 s. gender feature
 s. neurotransmitter
 s. pathophysiological mechanism
 s. phobia
 s. situational stressor
specificity
 s. hypothesis
 I-R s.
 physiological response s.
 s. of research
 response s.
 stimulus s.
 symptom s.
 treatment s.
specified
 not otherwise s. (NOS)
specifier
 course s.
 longitudinal course s.
 severity s.
 subtype and/or s.
 type s.
specimen
 flash-frozen tumor s.
 s. staining
SPECS
 System to Plan Early Childhood Services
SPECT
 single photon emission computed
  tomography

SPECT analysis
dual-isotope SPECT
SPECT image
SPECT scan
^{99m}Tc HMPAO SPECT
^{201}Tl SPECT
spectator
 s. role
 s. therapy
spectin
 brain s.
spectra (*pl. of* spectrum)
spectral
 s. analysis
 s. density
 s. density function
 s. karyotyping (SKY)
 s. peak frequency of activity
 s. relationship
 s. relationship to deity
 s. relationship to famous person
 s. velocity
spectrometer
 mass s.
spectrometry
 gas chromatography mass s.
spectrophobia
spectrophotometry
 reflectance s.
spectroscopy
 Fourier s.
 laser-Doppler s.
 magnetic resonance s. (MRS)
 MR s.
 phosphorus nuclear magnetic
  resonance s. (P-MRS)
 point resolved s. (PRESS)
 proton nuclear magnetic
  resonance s.
 in vivo $'$H magnetic resonance s.
 in vivo optical s. (INVOS)
spectrum, pl. **spectra, spectrums**
 acoustic s.
 band s.
 bulimic-anorexic s.
 Doppler frequency s.
 fortification s.
 panic-agoraphobic s.
 proton s.
 psychotherapeutic s.
 schizophrenic s. (SS)
 Structured Clinical Interview for
  the Panic-Agoraphobic S.
 in vitro spectra
**SPECTRUM-I: A Test of Adult Work
 Motivation**
speculum
 bivalved s.
 Cushing-Landolt s.
 Halle s.
 Halle nasal s.
 Hardy bivalve s.
 Killian septum s.
 Landolt pituitary s.
 transsphenoidal s.

speech

accelerated s.
s. act
agrammatic s.
alaryngeal s.
alteration in rate of s.
antiexpectancy s.
s. apraxia
aprosody of s.
s. aprosody
arrest of s.
s. arrest
articulation of s.
s. aspect
Assessment of Intelligibility of Dysarthric S.
ataxic s.
audible blocking in s.
automatic s.
s. behavior
Bell Visible S.
bilateral s.
blocked s.
buccal s.
cerebellar s.
circumstantial s.
cleft-palate s.
clipped s.
confused s.
s. content
cued s.
delayed s.
s. derailment
s. developmental delay disorder
s. difficulty
s. disability
disconnect s.
s. discrimination score (SDS)
s. discrimination test
s. disfluency
s. disorder
disorganized s.
s. disorientation
distractible s.
s. disturbance
disturbance in s.
dramatic s.
s. in dream
droning s.
dysarthric s.
s. dysfunction
s. dyspraxia
dysrhythmic s.
echo s.
egocentric s.
emotional s.
emotive s.
emphatic s.
euphoric s.
excessively impressionistic s.
excessively loud s.
excessively soft s.
executive s.
explosive s.
fast s.

figure of s.
flaccid s.
s. fluency
fluent aphasic s.
fluent paraphasic s.
halting s.
s. and hearing (S&H)
hesitant s.
hyperkinetic s.
hypokinetic s.
imitative s.
impoverished s.
incessant s.
incoherent s.
incomprehensible s.
infantile s.
s. intention center
internalized s.
involuntary pauses in s.
labyrinthine s.
lack of s.
laconic s.
s. and language behavior
s. and language disorder
s. and language impaired (SLI)
S. and Language Screening Questionnaire (SLSQ)
loud s.
manic s.
s. mannerism
mimic s.
mirror s.
s. monitoring center
monosyllabic s.
monotone s.
monotonous s.
s. and motor mapping
nonfluent aphasic s.
nonsensical s.
odd s.
organ s.
organic s.
overabstract s.
overconcrete s.
over-elaborate s.
parasocial s.
parkinsonian s.
paucity of s.
pause in s.
performative s.
perseverative s.
phantom s.
plateau s.
poverty of content of s.
pressured s.
pseudobulbar s.
psychotic s.
quality of s.
quantity of s.
S. Questionnaire
rambling s.
rapid s.
rate of production of s.
s. reading aphasia
s. reception threshold (SRT)

S

speech *(continued)*
 s. recognition threshold
 scanning s.
 silent blocking in s.
 slow s.
 slurred s.
 social gesture s.
 soft s.
 spontaneous s.
 staccato s.
 stilted s.
 subvocal s.
 syllabic s.
 tangential s.
 s. therapy
 tremulous s.
 underproductive s.
 unintelligible s.
 vague s.
 well-articulated s.
 whispered s.
 S. with Alternating Masking Index
 (SWAMI)
**Speech-Language Pathology Evaluation
Assessment**
speech-motor deficit
Speech-Sound Perception Test (SSPT)
speed
 s. of information processing
 disturbance
 motor s.
 perceptual s.
 psychomotor s.
 s. quotient
 s. of thought
 verbal perceptual s.
 visual perceptual s.
SpeedReducer instrument
spelencephaly
spell
 akinetic s.
 akinetic drop s.
 crying s.
 dizzy s.
 doubting s.
 s.'s of doubting and brooding
 s. out
 vacant s.
spell-a-word-backwards test
spelling
 s. dyspraxia
 finger s.
 s. grade equivalent
 S. Grade Rating
 S. Scale
 Test of Written S.
SPELT-P
 Structured Photographic Expressive
 Language Test-II
SPEM
 smooth pursuit eye movement
Spence
 S. intervertebral disk rongeur
 rule of S.

Spencer
 S. biopsy forceps
 S. probe depth electrode
Spens syndrome
spermatophobia, spermophobia
Spetzler
 S. lumbar-peritoneal shunt
 S. lumboperitoneal shunt
 S. Microvac suction tube
 S. system
Spetzler-Martin
 S.-M. classification
 S.-M. classification of arteriovenous
 malformation
 S.-M. grade
 S.-M. Grade III medium-size lesion
 with deep venous drainage
 S.-M. Grade II small lesion with
 deep venous drainage
 S.-M. grading scale
SpF spinal fusion stimulator
SpF-XL stimulator
S-phase fraction
sphecidophobia
spheksophobia
sphenocavernous syndrome
sphenoethmoidal
 s. encephalocele
 s. meningoencephalocele
sphenoethmoidectomy
sphenoid
 s. encephalocele
 s. mucocele
 s. ridge meningioma
 s. rostrum
 s. sinus
 s. wing
 s. wing dysplasia
 s. wing meningioma
sphenoidal
 s. electrode insertion
 s. fossa
 s. herniation
sphenoidale
 planum s.
sphenoidectomy
sphenoiditis
sphenoidostomy
sphenoidotomy
sphenomaxillary encephalocele
sphenooccipitalis
 fissura s.-o.
sphenoorbital
 s. encephalocele
 s. meningioma
 s. meningoencephalocele
sphenopalatine
 s. ganglion
 s. ganglionectomy
 s. neuralgia
sphenoparietal sinus
sphenopharyngeal meningoencephalocele
sphenotemporal sinus
sphere
 conflict-free s.

oriented in all s.'s
personality s.
psychosexual s.
spheresthesia
spherical
s. bur
s. coordinate representation
s. nucleus
sphincter
anal s.
s. control
s. morality
s. spasticity
urinary s.
sphingolipid
semisynthetic s.
sphingolipidosis
cerebral s.
sphingomyelin lipidosis
sphingosine
Sphrintzen syndrome
SPI
Self-Perception Inventory
sensor position indicator
Shipley Personal Inventory
SPIB
Social and Prevocational Information
Battery
spicule
spider
s. bite
s. cell
s. fantasy
spider's web test
Spiegelberg epidural balloon
Spiegel eye roll
Spiegel-Wycis human apparatus
Spielberger
S. Anger Expression Scale
S. Anxiety Inventory
S. State-Trait Anger Expression
Inventory
S. State-Trait Anxiety Inventory
Spielmeyer acute swelling
Spielmeyer-Sjögren disease
Spielmeyer-Vogt disease
Spielmeyer-Vogt-Sjögren disease
spike
centrotemporal s.
s. discharge
interictal epileptiform s.
phase s.
small sharp s. (SSS)
train of s.
spike-and-wave complex
spiked
s. hair
s. profile
spike-like artifact
spiking activity
Spiller-Frazier
S.-F. neurotomy
S.-F. technique
spin
s. density

s. echo
s. magnetization
nuclear s.
s. velocity
spina, gen. and pl. **spinae**
s. bifida
s. bifida aperta
s. bifida cystica
s. bifida manifesta
s. bifida myelomeningocele
s. bifida occulta
s. dorsalis
spinal
s. accessory nerve
s. accessory nerve-facial nerve
anastomosis
s. accessory palsy
s. anesthesia
s. angiography
s. apoplexy
s. arteriography
s. arteritis
s. ataxia
s. blastomycosis
s. block
s. canal
s. canal hydatid cyst
s. catheter
s. column
s. cord
s. cord arachnoiditis
s. cord arteritis
s. cord artery
s. cord blood flow (SCBF)
s. cord blood supply
s. cord compression
s. cord concussion
s. cord disease
s. cord function intraoperative
monitoring
s. cord hemorrhage
s. cord infarction
s. cord infection
s. cord injury
s. cord injury without radiological
abnormality (SCIWORA)
S. Cord Motor Index and Sensory
Indices
s. cord neoplasm
s. cord pain
s. cord stimulation (SCS)
s. cord tumor
s. cord white matter blood flow
s. coronal plane deformity
s. decompression
s. deformity
s. deformity/instability
s. deformity treatment
s. dermal sinus
s. dermal sinus tract
s. drainage
s. dural arteriovenous fistula
(SDAVF)
s. dysraphism
s. endodermal cyst

spinal *(continued)*
s. ependymoma
s. epidural abscess (SEA)
s. epidural angiolipoma
s. epidural hematoma
s. epidural hemorrhage (SHE)
s. extradural arachnoid pouch
s. fixation
s. fixation rigidity
S. Fixation Study Group
s. fusion
s. fusion gouge
s. fusion pathomechanics
s. fusion technique
s. ganglion
s. hemiplegia
s. implant design
s. implant load to failure
s. infection
s. injury operative stabilization
s. instrumentation
s. intradural schwannoma
s. lesion
s. level
s. lipoma
s. mechanics
s. metastasis
s. metastatic disease
s. muscular atrophy (SMA)
s. needle
s. nerve level motor impairment
s. nerve plexus
s. nerve root
s. neurenteric cyst
s. neurofibroma
s. nucleus of accessory nerve
s. nucleus of the trigeminus
s. osteomyelitis
s. osteotomy stabilization
s. paralysis
s. perforating forceps
s. puncture
s. puncture headache
s. pyramidotomy
s. range of motion (SROM)
s. reflex
s. reflex arc
s. rod
s. rod cross-bracing
s. saw
s. segmental myoclonus
s. sensory evoked potential
s. shock
s. stenosis
s. streak
s. stroke
s. subarachnoid hemorrhage
s. subdural hemorrhage (SSH)
s. tap
s. tractotomy
s. tract of trigeminal nerve
s. trigeminal nucleus
s. tuberculosis
ventral derotating s. (VDS)

SpinaLase neodymium:yytrium-aluminum-garnet (Nd:YAG) surgical laser system
spinale
tache s.
spinalis
arachnoidea s.
commotio s.
dura mater spinalis
hydrocele s.
medulla s.
meningitis serous s.
tabes s.
spinant
spindle
alpha s.
s. cell
s. coma
EEG alpha s.
Kühne s.
muscle s.
neuromuscular s.
neurotendinous s.
sleep s.
sleep s.
spindle-celled layer
spindle-cell tumor
spindle-shaped cyst
spine
bamboo s.
caroticojugular s.
cervical s.
cleft s.
dendritic s.
dorsal s.
Henle s.
internal fixation of s.
kinetic cervical s.
laminectomized s.
lower cervical s.
lower lumbar s.
lower thoracic s.
lumbar s.
lumbosacral s.
osteoporotic s.
poker s.
pyramidal cell dendritic s.'s
sacral s.
sacrococcygeal s.
s. sign
thoracic s.
thoracolumbar s.
tumor metastatic to s.
upper thoracic s.
variable screw placement system-instrumented lumbar s.
spin-echo (SE)
s.-e. imaging
long pulse repetition time/long echo time s.-e.
SpineLink system
spinescope
Clarus s.
SpineStat probe
spinifugal

spinipetal
spin-lattice
    s.-l. relaxation
    s.-l. relaxation time
spinoadductor reflex
spinobulbar
spinocerebellar
    s. ataxia
    s. degeneration
    s. tract
spinocerebellum
spinocollicular
spinocranial meningioma
spinogalvanization
spinography
    digitized s.
spinolamellar line
spino-olivary tract
spinopontine degeneration
spinoreticular tract
spinoreticulothalamic pathway
spinospinalis tract
spinosum
    foramen s.
spinotectal tract
spinothalamic
    s. cordotomy
    s. tract
    s. tractotomy
spinous
    s. interlaminar line
    s. process
    s. process fracture
    s. process plate
    s. process-splitting laminoplasty
    s. process wire
    s. process wiring
spin-spin
    s.-s. coupling
    s.-s. relaxation
    s.-s. relaxation time
spin-warp
    s.-w. imaging
    s.-w. pulse sequence
spiny neuron
spiperone
spiral
    cochlear s.
    s. foraminous tract
    s. ganglion of cochlea
    s. membrane
    s. organ
spirit
    acquisitive s.
    ancestral s.
    controlling external s.
    ether s.
    external s.
    neutral s.
    possessed by s.
    s. possession
    s. writing
spiritual
    s. counselor
    s. factor

    s. function
    s. medium
    s. possession
    s. possession experience
    S. Well-Being Scale (SWBS)
spirochetal aneurysm
spirochete
spirohydantoin
spirometry
spiromustine
spironolactone
    hydrochlorothiazide and s.
spiroperidol
spite reaction
Spitz-Holter shunt system
Spitzka
    S. marginal tract
    S. marginal zone
    S. nucleus
Spitz nevus
splanchnesthesia
splanchnesthetic sensibility
splanchnic
    s. anesthesia
    s. ganglion
splanchnicectomy
splanchnicotomy
spleen injury
splenetic
splenial
    s. artery
    s. gyrus
splenium, pl. splenia
    callosal s.
    s. corporis callosi
splenius
    s. capitus
    s. cervicis
splenomegaly
splicing
    exon s.
    gene s.
splinter
    s. function
    s. group
    s. hemorrhage
split
    s. bone graft reconstruction
    s. brain
    s. brain syndrome
    s. calvarial graft
    s. custody
    s. in the ego
    s. half reliability coefficient
    s. notochord syndrome
    palatal s.
    s. personality
    s. screen phenomenon
    vermian s.
split-brain preparation
split-cord malformation (SCM)
split-thickness calvarial graft
splitting
    s. behavior

S

splitting *(continued)*
    ego s.
    time s.
SPMSQ
    Short Portable Mental Status
    Questionnaire
SpoCS
    space of the cavernous sinus
spoiled-child reaction
spoiling
    radiofrequency s.
spoken
    s. language
    s. language quotient
Spondee Picture Test (SPT)
spondylalgia
spondylarthritis
spondylectomy
spondylitica
    psoriasis s.
spondylitic ridging
spondylitis
    ankylosing s.
    cryptococcal s.
    s. deformans
    Kümmell s.
    rheumatoid s.
    tuberculous s.
spondyloarthropathy
    seronegative s.
spondylocace
spondylo construct
spondylodesis
    ventral derotation s. (VDS)
spondylodiskitis
spondylolisthesis
    degenerative s.
    grade IV s.
    high-grade s.
    postlaminectomy two-level s.
    s. reduction
    s. reduction fixation
    symptomatic s.
    s. with significant displacement
spondylolisthetic crisis
spondylolysis
spondylomalacia
spondylopathy
spondyloptosis
spondylopyosis
spondyloschisis
spondylosis
    cervical s.
    degenerative s.
    hyperostotic s.
    lumbar s.
    thoracolumbar s.
spondylosyndesis
spondylotic myelopathy
spondylotomy
sponge
    absorbable gelatin s.
    s. count
    gelatin s.

    Ivalon embolic s.
    NeuroCol neurosurgical s.
    Ray-Tec s.
    saline-soaked s.
    Silastic s.
    silicone s.
    s. stick
sponge-holding forceps
spongiform virus encephalopathy
spongioblast
spongioblastoma
spongiocyte
spongiosum
    corpus s.
spongiosus
    status s.
spongy
    s. degeneration
    s. degeneration leukodystrophy
spontaneity
    parental s.
    s. state
    s. test
    s. training
spontaneous
    s. abortion
    s. activity
    s. convulsion
    s. dyskinesia
    s. echo contrast (SEC)
    s. imitation
    s. intracranial hypotension
    s. laughter
    s. movement
    s. narrative discourse
    s. neuronal hyperactivity
    s. occlusion of the circle of Willis
    Performance Assessment of Syntax
    Elicited and S. (PASES)
    s. recovery
    s. regression
    s. remission
    s. seizure
    s. speech
    s. spinal epidural hematoma
    (SSEH)
spoon
    brain s.
    Cushing brain spatula s.
    Cushing pituitary s.
    Cushing spatula s.
    Hardy pituitary s.
    pituitary s.
    Ray brain spatula s.
spoonerism
sporadic
    s. ataxia
    s. depressive disease (SDD)
Sporothrix schenckii
Sportscreme
spot
    blind s.
    Brushfield s.
    café au lait s.
    central direct current bright s.

cherry-red s.
cold s.
cotton wool s.
figurative blind s.
Graefe s.
hypnogenic s.
mental blind s.
pink s.
Roth s.
saccular s.
Soemmering s.
soft s.
temperature s.
touch s.
Trousseau s.
utricular s.
yellow s.

spotted fever
spouse
s. abuse
s. abuse index
s. abuser
battered s.
dominant s.
s. rape
separated from s.
s.'s subsystem

SPP
Sexuality Preference Profile

SPQ
Sales Personality Questionnaire

spray
air plasma s. (APS)
butorphanol tartrate nasal s.
dihydroergotamine mesylate nasal s.
Fluori-Methane Topical S.
Miacalcin Nasal S.
Migranal Nasal S.
Nicotrol NS Nasal S.
oxymetazoline nasal s.

spread
centripetal s.

spreader
Bailey rib s.
Blount laminar s.
Bobechko s.
Burford-Finochietto rib s.
Caspar disk space s.
Cloward cervical vertebra s.
Cloward lamina s.
Davis rib s.
DeBakey rib s.
Doyen rib s.
Favaloro-Morse sternal s.
Finochietto rib s.
Gerbode-Burford rib s.
Haight-Finochietto rib s.
Haight rib s.
Harken rib s.
Harrington s.
Inge cervical lamina s.
Inge laminectomy s.
lamina s.
Landolt s.
Lemmon sternal s.

Lilienthal rib s.
Miltex rib s.
Morse sternal s.
Nelson rib s.
Rehbein rib s.
Rienhoff-Finochietto rib s.
Rienhoff rib s.
Texas Scottish Rite Hospital
eyebolt s.
Tuffier rib s.
vertebrae s.
Weinberg rib s.
Wilson rib s.
Wiltberger spinous process s.

spreading
s. cortical depression theory
s. depression (SD)

spring
coiled s.
compression s.
s. finger
Gruca-Weiss s.
internal fixation s.
s. mechanism

springing mydriasis
spring-loaded electrode
spring-summer
Kozhevnikov s.-s. encephalitis
Russian s.-s. encephalitis (Eastern
or Western subtype)

Sprotte
S. epidural needle
S. spinal needle

sprouting
neuronal s.

spruce
Belyando s.

sprue peripheral neuropathy
SPS
simple partial seizure

SPSI
School Problem Screening Inventory

SPT
Spondee Picture Test
Supervisory Practices Test
Symbolic Play Test

spur
Morand s.
traction s.

spurious
s. meningocele
s. torticollis

Spurling
S. maneuver
S. nerve root retractor
S. sign

Spurling-Kerrison laminectomy rongeur
Spurr epoxy resin
spurt
end s.
initial s.

SQ
social quotient
status quo

S

SQ3R
  survey, question, read, review, recite
square-ended hook
squarely (face person), open posture, lean (toward person), eye (contact), relaxed (SOLER)
square wave
square-wave jerk
squeeze technique of penis
SR
  schizophrenic reaction
  seizure resistant
  sentence repetition
    Indocin SR
    Oramorph SR
    Ritalin SR
    Wellbutrin SR
S/R
  schizophrenic reaction
S&R
  seclusion and restraint
SRA
  Science Research Associates
    SRA Arithmetic Test
    SRA Pictorial Reasoning Test
    SRA Reading Test
SR/AP
  schizophrenic reaction, acute, paranoid
SR/AU
  schizophrenic reaction, acute undifferentiated
SRC
  Student Reactions to College
SR/CP
  schizophrenic reaction, chronic, paranoid
SR/CU
  schizophrenic reaction, chronic, undifferentiated
SRDS
  Self-Rating Depression Scale
SRE
  Schedule of Recent Experience
SREDA
  subclinical rhythmic epileptiform discharge of adult
    SREDA on electroencephalogram
SRI
  serotonin reuptake inhibitor
S-R Inventory of Anxiousness
SROM
  spinal range of motion
SRP
  signal recognition particle
SRR
  systematic rational restructuring
SRRS
  Social Readjustment Rating Scale
SRS
  schizophrenic residual state
  sex reassignment surgery
  Social and Rehabilitation Service
  Symptom Rating Scale
SRT
  Seashore Rhythm Test

  Social Relations Test
  speech reception threshold
SS
  schizophrenic spectrum
  seizure sensitive
  Sjögren syndrome
  Social Security
  social service
  syringosubarachnoid shunting
SSA
  Social Security Administration
SS-B/La
SSC
  Stein Sentence Completion
    SSC test
SSD
  Social Security Disability
SSEEG
  scalp-sphenoidal electroencephalography
SSEH
  spontaneous spinal epidural hematoma
SSEP
  somatosensory evoked potential
    short-latency SSEP
SSFI
  social stress and functionability inventory
SSFP
  steady-state free precession
SSH
  spinal subdural hemorrhage
SSHA
  Survey of Study Habits and Attitudes
S-shaped brain spatula
SSI
  segmental spinal instrumentation
  Supplemental Security Income
    anterior-posterior fusion with SSI
SSIAM
  Structured and Scaled Interview to Assess Maladjustment
SSII
  Safran Student's Interest Inventory
SSOP
  Standard System of Psychiatry
SSPD
  schizoid-schizotypal personality disorder
SSPE
  subacute sclerosing panencephalitis
SSPT
  Speech-Sound Perception Test
SSR
  sympathetic skin response
    SSR on electromyogram
SSRI
  selective serotonin reuptake inhibitor
SSRS
  Social Skills Rating System
SSS
  School Situation Survey
  Sensation-Seeking Scale
  small sharp spike
    SSS on electroencephalogram
SST
  Slingerland Screening Tests
  social skills training

ST
    shock therapy
    standardized test
STA
    superficial temporal artery
Stab-and-Grab screwdriver
stabbing pain
stabilimeter
stability
    s. of ego
    emotional s.
    family s.
    lumbar spine rotational s.
    marital s.
    mental s.
    occupational s.
    personality trait s.
    relative slow-wave sleep s.
    slow-wave sleep s.
    temporal s.
    Test of Work Competency and S.
      (TWCS)
stabilization
    anterior internal s.
    anterior short-segment s.
    s. approach
    atlantoaxial s.
    atlantooccipital s.
    cervical spine s.
    cervicothoracic junction s.
    flexion-compression spine injury s.
    fracture s.
    iliac crest bone graft s.
    lower cervical spine posterior s.
    lumbar spine s.
    occipitocervical s.
    odontoid fracture s.
    posterior lower cervical spine s.
    sacral spine s.
    screw s.
    spinal injury operative s.
    spinal osteotomy s.
    subluxation s.
    thoracolumbar spine s.
    TSRH crosslink s.
    wire s.
stabilizer
    mood s.
stabilizing social situations
stable
    s. cervical spine injury
    s. ego structure
    s. personality
    s. sleep difficulty
    s. sleep-wake pattern
    s. xenon CT
STABS
    Suinn Test Anxiety Behavior Scale
staccato speech
stacking anchor
STACL
    Screening Test for Auditory
      Comprehension of Language
Staderini nucleus
Stadol NS

Staff Burnout Scale for Health Professionals
stage
    adolescence developmental s.
    adulthood developmental s.
    alarm reaction s.
    anal s.
    anal-expulsive s.
    attending to language s.
    autonomous s.
    bereavement s.
    biting s.
    childhood developmental s.
    cognitive development s.
    cognitive development s.'s (Period
      I–IV)
    concrete operations s.
    dementia s.
    developmental s.
    equality s.
    equity s.
    s. of exhaustion
    exhaustion s.
    formal operations s.
    functional assessment s.
    genital s.
    grammar development s.
    grammar formation s.
    group s.
    heteronomous s.
    HIV illness s.
    ideoplastic s.
    individuation s.
    infancy developmental s.
    intuitive s.
    late life developmental s.
    latency s.
    life s.
    locomotor-genital s.
    s. 3 mania
    muscular-anal s.
    oedipal s.
    oral s.
    oral-sensory s.
    phallic s.
    physioplastic s.
    Piaget cognitive development s.
    postambivalent s.
    preattachment s.
    preconceptual s.
    pregenital s.
    pre-oedipal s.
    preoperational thought s.
    psychosexual s.
    pubertal s.
    question s.
    recovery s.
    rehabilitation s.
    sensorimotor s.
    shock s.
    single word s.
    sleep s.
    symbiotic s.
    symptom experience s.
    Tanner s.

S

stage *(continued)*
    toddler s.
    true communication s.
    two-word messages s.
    urethral s.
staged
    s. bilateral stereotactic thalamotomy
    s. embolization
Stagesic
staggering gait
staging
    neuraxis s.
stagnant hypoxia
stagnation
    generativity versus s.
STAI
    State-Trait Anxiety Inventory
STAIC
    State-Trait Anxiety Inventory for
    Children
stain
    Elastica-Masson s.
    Elastica van Gieson s.
    Fite s.
    Gomori trichome s.
    Grocott s.
    hematoxylin-eosin s.
    Masson-Fontana s.
    Masson trichrome s.
    periodic acid-Schiff-hematoxylin s.
    Perls s.
    port-wine s.
    reticulum s.
    trichrome s.
staining
    CD34 s.
    Golgi s.
    immunoperoxidase s.
    Nissl s.
    specimen s.
    Sudan black s.
    Weigert s.
stainless
    s. steel equipment
    s. steel preformed skull plate
    s. steel screw
staircase phenomenon
STAI-Y
stake
stalemate
    analytic s.
stalk
    infundibular s.
    pituitary s.
stalking behavior
STA-MCA
    superficial temporal artery-middle
    cerebral artery
        STA-MCA anastomosis
        STA-MCA bypass
stammering of the bladder
stamp
    digit s.

stance
    adultomorphic s.
    approach-avoidance s.
    defensive adultomorphic s.
    norm-assertive s.
    walking s.
stand
    Brown-Roberts-Wells floor s.
    Contraves s.
    s. out
    Yasargil OptiMat floor s.
standard
    s. behavior
    s. bone algorithm program
    competency s.
    s. deviation (SD)
    double s.
    s. error (SE)
    s. error of difference
    s. error of the mean (SEM)
    foreign s.
    legal s.
    s. of living
    living s.
    s. of performance
    s. procedure
    S. Progressive Matrices
    s. psychiatric nomenclature
    s. reference
    s. retroperitoneal flank approach
    s. retroperitoneal flank incision
    social s.
    S. System of Psychiatry (SSOP)
    s. thoracotomy
    s. Würzburg titanium mini-plating
    system
standardization of a test
standardized
    S. Assessment of Depressive
    Disorders (SADD)
    s. cognitive assessment technique
    s. test (ST)
    S. Test of Computer Literacy
    (STCL)
standing balance
Stanford
    S. Achievement Test (SAT)
    S. Diagnostic Arithmetic Test
    S. Diagnostic Reading Test
    (SDRT)
    S. Early School Achievement Test
    S. Hypnotic Clinical Scale and
    Children
    S. Hypnotic Susceptibility Scale
    (SHSS)
    S. Sleepiness Scale
Stanford-Binet (SB, S-B)
    S.-B. Intelligence Scale (SBIS)
    S.-B. intelligence test
Stanford-Terman Study
Stangyl
Stanton Survey

STA-PCA
  superficial temporal artery-posterior
  cerebral artery
   STA-PCA bypass
stapedial artery
stapedius muscle fatigue
stapes
  footplate of the s.
  s. reflex
Staphcillin
staphylococcal meningitis
Staphylococcus
  S. *aureus*
  S. *epidermidis*
staphyloma
staphyloplegia
STAPP
  short-term anxiety-provoking
  psychotherapy
starch eating
stare
  blank s.
  empty s.
  postbasic s.
  reptilian s.
  vacant s.
star fear
staring
  s. face
  s. facial expression
Starling reflex
STAR Profile
STARS
  Short Term Auditory Retrieval and
  Storage
STaRT
  Screening Test for the Assignment of
  Remedial Treatment
  stereotactic-assisted radiation therapy
  fractionated StaRT
START kit
startle
  s. abnormality
  acoustic s.
  s. disease
  s. epilepsy
  s. reaction
  s. reflex
  s. response
  s. syndrome
  s. technique
startling stimulus
starvation fasting
STAS
  State-Trait Anger Scale
STA-SCA
  superficial temporal artery-superior
  cerebellar artery
   STA-SCA bypass
stasibasiphobia
stasiphobia
stasis
  libido s.
  s. retinopathy
  venous s.

STAT
  Suprathreshold Adaptation Test
state
  absent s.
  across identity s.
  activated s.
  acute confusional s. (ACS)
  adrenergic-response s.
  adult ego s.
  affect s.
  affective and paranoid s.
  agitated s.
  alcoholic confusional s.
  alcoholic paranoid s.
  alcoholic twilight s.
  alcohol-induced paranoid s.
  alert awake s.
  s. of alertness
  alpha s.
  altered s.
  amnesic s.
  amnestic s.
  anxiety s. (AS)
  anxiety tension s. (ATS)
  apallic s.
  apprehension s.
  arousal s.
  arteriosclerotic dementia
  confusional s.
  arteriosclerotic paranoid s.
  arteriosclerotic psychosis
  confusional s.
  atypical neurotic anxiety s.
  awake s.
  borderline s.
  break s.
  catatonic s.
  central excitatory s.
  central motive s.
  chronic deficit s.
  chronic delusional s.
  clear twilight s.
  climacteric paranoid s.
  clouded s.
  confusional twilight s.
  conscious s.
  consciousness s.
  s. of consciousness (SOC)
  constitutional psychopathic s. (CPS)
  convulsive s.
  crepuscular s.
  delirium-like s.
  s. dependence
  depressed s.
  depressive s.
  dietary s.'s
  diffusional s.
  disorganized s.
  dissociated s.
  dissociative s.
  dream s.
  dreamlike s.
  dreamy s.
  drug-induced confusional s.
  drug psychosis hallucinatory s.

S

state *(continued)*
    dysequilibrium s.
    ego s.
    emotional s.
    end s.
    epileptic confusional s. (ECS)
    erotomanic delusional s.
    euthymic s.
    excited s.
    exhaustion s.
    fatigue s.
    fluctuating ego s.
    fugue s.
    fusion s.
    generalized neurotic anxiety s.
    global attractor s.
    Golombok-Rust Inventory of
        Marital S. (GRIMS)
    gradient-recalled acquisition in the
        steady s. (GRASS)
    hallucinatory s.
    heightened attention s.
    s. of heightened attention
    heightened awareness s.
    s. of heightened awareness
    hospital (SH)
    s. hospital children's unit (SHCU)
    hypercoagulable s.
    hyperdopaminergic s.
    hypereridic s.
    hypnagogic s.
    hypnoid s.
    hypnopompic s.
    hypnotic s.
    hypodopaminergic s.
    hysterical fugue s.
    hysteric coma-like s.
    identity s.
    immobile s.
    internal s.
    involutional paranoid s.
    lacunar s.
    litigious delusional s.
    local excitatory s.
    locked in s.
    manic s.
    marasmic s.
    s. markers of heavy drinking
    menopausal paranoid s.
    mental s.
    s. mental hospital (SMH)
    merger s.
    s. of mind
    mixed-mood s.
    mixed paranoid/affective organic
        psychotic s.
    moribund s.
    multiple ego s.
    mute s.
    negative mood s.
    neurotic s.
    nonresponsive s.
    obsessional s.
    obsessive-ruminative tension s.

oneiroid s.
opposite affect s.
oral s.
organic psychotic s.
oxidation s.
pain s.
panic s.
panic attack neurotic anxiety s.
paranoia paranoid s.
paranoia querulans paranoid s.
paranoid litigious s.
paraphonic s.
paraphrenia paranoid s.
parasomniac conscious s.
perfection s.
permanent vegetative s.
perplexity s.
persistent vegetative s. (PVS)
phobic s.
possession trance s.
postepileptic twilight s.
postictal s.
postoperative confusional s.
premenstrual tension s.
premorbid s.
presenile dementia confusional s.
presenile organic psychotic s.
Profile of Mood S.'s (POMS)
prolonged transition to fully
    awake s.
psychogenic twilight s.
psychopathic s.
psychotic s.
rapid eye movement s.
reactive confusional s.
refractory s.
REM s.
residual s.
s. of resistance
resource s.
ruminative tension s.
schizophrenic defect s.
schizophrenic residual s. (SRS)
senile dementia confusional s.
senile organic psychotic s.
sensitiver Beziehungswahn
    paranoid s.
separator s.
sequential gradient-recalled
    acquisition in the steady s.
simple paranoid s.
sleep s.
spastic s.
spontaneity s.
steady s.
subacute confusional s. (SCS)
subdelirious s.
substance-induced s.
subsyndromal s.
tension s.
toxic confusional s.
trance s.
transcendental s.
transient postictal confusional s.
traumatic defect s.

twilight confusional s.
unresponsive s.
vegetative s.
wakeful s.
withdrawal s.

stated
s. age
s. desire

state-dependent
s.-d. learning
s.-d. memory

statement
"I" s.
nonsensical s.

State-Trait
S.-T. Anger Expression Inventory (STAXI)
S.-T. Anger Scale (STAS)
S.-T. Anxiety Index
S.-T. Anxiety Inventory (STAI)
S.-T. Anxiety Inventory for Children (STAIC)
S.-T. Anxiety Inventory for Stein Sentence Completion test
S.-T. Personality Inventory (STPI)

static
s. acoustic impedance
s. ataxia
s. convulsion
s. dementia
s. demography
s. and dynamic sitting balance
s. and dynamic standing balance
s. encephalopathy
s. infantilism
s. intervention
s. magnetic field
s. reflex
s. sense
s. standing balance
s. tremor

station
Sun Sparc S. 10
s. test

stationary visual stimuli
statistical
s. deviation
s. inference
s. mean
s. median
s. significance
s. trend

statistics
descriptive s.
inferential s.
National Center for Health S.
psychiatric s.
vital s.

statoacusticus
nervus s.

statokinetic reflex
statotonic reflex
stature
psychosocially determined short s.
short s.

status
absence s.
altered mental s.
ambulatory s.
s. aura
biologic s.
s. choreicus
clinical s.
confident s.
s. convulsivus
s. cribrosus
s. criticus
current cognitive s.
Current, Global, Psychiatric-Social S. (CGPS)
degenerative s.
s. degenerativus
s. deterioration
disordered mental s.
s. dysgraphicus
s. dysmyelinisatus
s. dysraphicus
elopement s. (ES)
s. epilepsy
s. epilepticus
s. epilepticus organic psychosis
s. examination
female biological s.
grand mal s.
s. hemicranicus
higher s.
s. hypnoticus
s. hypoplasticus
immigrant s.
s. index
S. Indicators
Karnofsky Performance S.
s. lacunaris
male biological s.
s. marmoratus
mental s.
s. nervosus
s. offender
open-ward s.
petit mal s.
s. post commotio cerebri
postoperative s.
preepisode s.
pressure autoregulatory s.
s. questionnaire
s. quo (SQ)
s. raptus
s. scale
s. schedule
Social Adaptation S. (SAS)
socioeconomic s. (SES)
s. spongiosus
symptomatic s.
temporal lobe s.
s. typhosus
uncertain biological s.
s. value
s. vertiginosus

S

statutory
>   s. offense
>   s. rape

statuvolence
statuvolent
Stauder lethal catatonia
stauroplegia
staurosporine
stavudine
STAXI
>   State-Trait Anger Expression Inventory

stay
>   estimated length of s.
>   length of s. (LOS)
>   length of patient s. (LOPS)

STC
>   sexually transmitted condition

STCL
>   Standardized Test of Computer Literacy

STD
>   sexually transmitted disease

steady
>   s. gait
>   s. state

steady-state free precession (SSFP)
steal
>   cerebral ischemia s.
>   s. index
>   intracerebral s.
>   s. phenomenon
>   subclavian s.
>   s. to support a habit

stealing
>   s. an anchor
>   compulsive s.
>   s. impulse
>   solitary s.

StealStation image guided surgery system
Stealth angioplasty balloon catheter
StealthStation
>   S. image-interactive system
>   S. system real-time guidance

STEAM
>   stimulated spin-echo sequence

steam autoclavable
steam-shaping mandrel
Stearns alcoholic amentia
steatosis
>   hepatic s.
>   microvesicular s.

Stecher arachnoid knife
Steele-Richardson-Olszewski
>   S.-R.-O. disease
>   S.-R.-O. syndrome

steep-dose gradient
steeple skull
Steering Committee on Practice Guidelines
Steffee
>   S. instrumentation
>   S. pedicle screw-plate system
>   S. plate
>   S. plating

stege

Stegreif theater
Stein
>   S. Sentence Completion (SSC)
>   S. Sentence Completion Test

Steinert
>   S. disease
>   S. myotonic dystrophy

Steinhauser cranial screw
Steinmann pin
Stelazine
stellate
>   s. astrocyte
>   s. cell of cerebral cortex
>   s. ganglion
>   s. neuron
>   s. skull fracture

stellectomy
Stellwag sign
stem
>   gaze mechanism in brain s.
>   infundibular s.
>   s. serotonergic cell

sten
Stenger Test
stenogyria
stenophobia
Stenosimeter
stenosis, pl. stenoses
>   acquired spinal s.
>   aqueductal s.
>   artery s.
>   asymptomatic carotid artery s. (ACAS)
>   carotid s.
>   cervical spinal s.
>   foraminal s.
>   high-grade s.
>   lateral recess s.
>   lumbar spinal s.
>   pyloric s.
>   spinal s.
>   thoracolumbar spinal canal s.

stenostenosis
Stensen duct
stent
>   Silastic s.

STEP
>   Sequential Tests of Educational Study

step
>   12-s. program
>   s. relation

stepdown connector
Stephenson-Gibbs reference electrode
Stephens Oral Language Screening Test (SOLST)
STEP-III
>   Sequential Tests of Educational Progress, Series III

steppage gait
steppingstone theory
STEPS
>   Screening Test for Educational Prerequisite Skills

steps
>   shuffling s.

S. Up Developmental Screening
  Program
stepwise deterioration
stercoralis
  Strongyloides s.
stereoadapter
  Laitinen s.
stereoagnosis
stereoanesthesia
stereoelectroencephalography
stereoencephalometry
stereoencephalotomy
stereognosis
  oral s.
stereognostic perception
stereoguide collimator
stereomagnification angiography
stereometry
  sonic s.
stereopathy
stereopsyche
stereoscopic vision
stereotactic, stereotaxic
  s. anatomic target localization
  s. angiography
  s. anteroposterior and lateral
    metrizamide ventriculography
  s. arc
  s. aspiration
  s. atlas
  s. biopsy
  s. biopsy exploration
  s. brachytherapy
  s. catheter drainage
  s. cingulotomy
  s. cordotomy
  s. depth electroencephalogram
    (SDEEG)
  s. electroencephalogram (SEEG)
  s. focused-radiation therapy
  s. frame
  s. gamma radiation
  s. gamma unit
  s. guidance
  s. guide
  s. instrument
  s. instrumentation
  s. intracystic injection
  s. intratumoral photodynamic
    therapy
  s. irradiation
  s. linear accelerator
  s. linear accelerator radiotherapy
  s. localization
  s. microsurgical approach
  s. microsurgical craniotomy
  s. neurosurgery
  s. operation
  s. pallidotomy
  s. PET image
  s. puncture
  s. radiation therapy treatment
  s. radiosurgery
  s. radiosurgery
  s. retractor

  s. robot
  s. surgery
  s. surgery
  s. surgical ablation
  s. thalamotomy
  s. thermocoagulation
  s. tractotomy
  s. VL thalamotomy
stereotactic-assisted
  s.-a. radiation therapy (STaRT)
  s.-a. radiation therapy kit
stereotactic-guided craniotomy
stereotaxic (*var. of* stereotactic)
stereotaxis
stereotaxy
  frame s.
  functional s.
stereotyped
  s. activity
  s. attitude
  s. body movement
  s. interest
  s. motor movement
  s. pattern of behavior
  s. repetition
  s. stress
  s. vocalization
stereotypic
  s. motor movement
  s. movement disorder (SMD)
stereotypical
  s. behavior
  s. gender roles
  s. role
stereotypy
  s. and habit disorder
  oral s.
Steri-Dent dry heat sterilizer
sterile
  s. abscess
  s. meningoencephalitis
sterility
  elective s.
sterilizer
  Steri-Dent dry heat s.
Steripaque
  S.-BR
  S.-V
Steri-Strips
Steritek ICP mini monitor
sternal
  s. occipital mandibular
    immobilization (SOMI)
  s. puncture
sternobrachial reflex
sternocleidomastoid
  s. muscle
  s. muscle weakness
sternohyoid muscle
sternomastoid muscle
sternooccipitomanubrial immobilizer
sternothyroid muscle
sternotomy
sternum-splitting approach

S

sternutatory
> s. absence
> s. reflex

steroid
> anabolic s.
> lumbar epidural s.
> sex s.
> s. withdrawal syndrome

steroid-sensitive neuropathy
stethoparalysis
stethospasm
Stevens-Johnson syndrome
Stewart-Holmes sign
Stewart-Morel syndrome
STG
> short-term goal

STGC
> syncytiotrophoblastic giant cell

stick
> needle s.
> sponge s.

sticking sensation
sticky platelet syndrome
stiff-man syndrome (SMS)
stiff neck
stiffness
> axial s.
> fusion s.
> hemiparkinsonian s.
> torsional s.

stigmata, stigma, stigmas
> external s.
> s. psychosis
> s. of psychosis
> psychosocial s.

stigmatic
stiletto
stillborn
Stille bur
Stille-Luer rongeur
Stilling
> S. column
> S. gelatinous substance
> S. nucleus
> S. raphe

stilted
> s. attitude
> s. speech
> s. view

Stimson dressing
stimulant
> s. abuse
> beta s.
> central nervous system s.
> s. challenge test
> CNS s.
> s. effect
> psychomotor s.

stimulant-induced
> s.-i. insomnia
> s.-i. postural tremor

stimulated spin-echo sequence (STEAM)
stimulating
> s. environment

> s. experience
> s. occupation

stimulation
> amygdaloid s.
> audiobrain s.
> autogenital s.
> brain s.
> chemical s.
> chimeric s.
> click s.
> cognitive s.
> condensation s.
> deep brain s. (DBS)
> direct brain s. (DBS)
> dorsal column s.
> dorsal cord s. (DCS)
> double simultaneous s. (DSS)
> electrical intracranial s.
> electrical transcranial s. (ETS)
> electrophysiological s.
> endogenous s.
> environmental s.
> epileptogenic s.
> exogenous s.
> external s.
> fast-frequency repetitive transcranial magnetic s. (FFr-TMS)
> s. fatigability
> s. fatigue
> functional electrical s. (FES)
> genital s.
> high-intensity click s.
> s. index (SI)
> insufficient s.
> intracranial s. (ICS)
> intraoperative electrical s.
> intraoperative electrical cortical s. (IOECS)
> macro s.
> magnetoelectric s.
> manual s.
> s. mapping
> neuromuscular electrical s. (NMES)
> noncoital s.
> olfactory s.
> oral s.
> pathway s.
> percutaneous s.
> perivascular nerve-ending s.
> photic s.
> ramp s.
> rarefaction s.
> s. ratio
> repetitive nerve s. (RNS)
> sacral nerve s. (SNS)
> s. of sense (SOS)
> sensory s.
> sexual s.
> social s.
> spinal cord s. (SCS)
> subliminal s.
> synesthetic s.
> tactile genital s.
> tetanic s.
> thalamic s.

therapeutic electrical s. (TES)
transcranial high-frequency repetitive
  electrical s.
transcranial magnetic s. (TMS)
transcutaneous electrical nerve s.
  (TENS)
vagus nerve s. (VAS, VNS)
visual s.
stimulation-bound behavior (SBB)
stimulator
  Axostim nerve s.
  constant current s.
  dorsal column s. (DCS)
  EMG s.
  Hilger facial nerve s.
  Itrel II spinal cord s.
  magnetic s.
  Micro-Z neuromuscular s.
  nerve s.
  OCS-1 cortical s.
  SpF spinal fusion s.
  SpF-XL s.
  Toennis ES standalone constant-
    current electrical s.
stimulus, pl. stimuli
  accidental stimuli
  adequate s.
  alerting s.
  angry reaction to minor stimuli
  anxiogenic stimuli
  s. artifact
  auditory s.
  aversive s.
  chemical s.
  conditioned s. (CS)
  s. control
  discriminative s.
  distracting stimuli
  dream s.
  s. drive (Sd)
  s. duration
  effective s.
  emotional s.
  emotionally provoking s.
  emotion-related feedback s.
  environmental s.
  epileptogenic s.
  erotic s.
  external s.
  s. fading
  fatness s.
  frightening s.
  s. generalization
  heterologous s.
  homologous s.
  inadequate s.
  incidental s.
  ineffective s.
  internal s.
  irrelevant external stimuli
  liminal s.
  masking s.
  maximal s.
  method of constant stimuli
  minor s.

musical s.
neutral s.
novel s.
noxious s.
outside s.
s. overload
painful s.
paraphiliac s.
pedophilic s.
phobic s.
pleasurable stimuli
provoking s.
psychosensory s.
rarefaction s.
reaction to minor stimuli
real external s.
s. response
screen out irrelevant s.
selective focusing on environmental
  stimuli
s. sensitive myoclonus
sensory s.
sexual s.
s. specificity
startling s.
stationary visual stimuli
subliminal s.
s. substitution
subthreshold s.
summation of stimuli
supramaximal s.
tactile s.
target s.
s. tension
terrifying s.
test s.
s. therapy
thermal s.
threshold s.
s. threshold
train-of-four s.
triggering s.
unconditioned s. (UCS)
visual s.
visuospatial s.
stimulus-bound
Stimulus-Recognition Test
stimulus-response
  s.-r. theory
stinging pain
STIR
  short inversion recovery imaging
  short-tau inversion recovery
    STIR sequence
stir fever
Stirling County study
stitch
  running s.
STM
  short-term memory
STN
  subthalamic nucleus
stock
  bone s.
Stockholm syndrome

S

stocking anesthesia
stocking-glove
    s.-g. anesthesia
    s.-g. distribution
    s.-g. sensory loss
stockings
    Orthawear antiembolism s.
    Vairox high compression
    vascular s.
Stoffel operation
stoker's cramp
Stokes-Adams
    S.-A. attack
    S.-A. disease
    S.-A. syndrome
Stokes law
stoma blast
stomach psychogenic disorder
stomatitis
    aphthous s.
stomodeum
stone
    S. and Neale Daily Coping
      Assessment
    s. wall
Stony Brook High Risk Project
Stookey cranial rongeur
Stookey-Scarff operation
stooped shoulders
stop-and-think technique
stopcock
    Luer-Lok s.
stop, look and listen intervention
storage
    iconic s.
    memory s.
    Short Term Auditory Retrieval
      and S. (STARS)
stories (pl. of story)
storiform
    s. pattern
    s. whorl
stork leg
storm
    emotional s.
    Operation Desert S. (ODS)
storm-and-stress period
stormed defense
stormy personality
story, pl. stories
    s. fear
    Make-A-Picture-S. (MAPS)
    Michigan Picture Stories
    sob s.
storylike dream sequence
Storz
    S. Microsystem microplate
    S. Microsystems cranial fixation
    plate
    S. Microsystems drill bit
STPI
    State-Trait Personality Inventory
strabismus
    Braid s.
    kinetic s.

StrAbs
    striated muscle
Strachan syndrome
straight
    s. aneurysm clip
    s. cannula with locking dilator
    s. connector
    s. filament
    s. gyrus
    s. incision
    s. knot-tying forceps
    s. leg raising test
    s. line bayonet forceps
    s. microscissors
    s. needle
    s. needle electrode
    s. nerve hook
    s. ring curette
    s. sinus
straightening cannula
straight-in ventriculostomy
strain
    alpha wave s.
    s. gauge
    interpersonal s.
    physical s.
    psychological s.
    vocational s.
straitjacket
    chemical s.
strait jacket
strammonium
strangalesthesia
strangeness fear
stranger
    s. anxiety
    s. fear
strangulated affect
strap
    Flushmesh s.
    s. muscle
strata (pl. of stratum)
strategic
    s. compliance
    s. family therapy
    s. intervention
    s. planning
strategy
    antisense s.
    bibliotherapeutic s.
    challenge s.
    cognitive s.
    conflict-resolution s.
    coping s.
    data reanalysis s.
    defense s.
    empirical-rational s.
    gambling s.
    hockey-stick s.
    inference s.
    learning s.
    mnemonic s.
    precursor load s.
    problem-solving s.
    protective survival s.

reality-oriented supportive s.
reanalysis s.
self-handicapping s.
survival s.
treatment evaluation s.
treatment package s.

stratification
Davidoff age s.

stratum, gen. **strati,** pl. **strata**
s. album profundum
s. cérébrale retinae
s. cinereum colliculi superioris
s. ganglionare nervi optici
s. ganglionare retinae
s. gangliosum cerebelli
s. granulosum cerebelli
s. griseum colliculi superioris
s. griseum medium
s. griseum profundum
s. griseum superficiale
s. interolivare lemnisci
s. lemnisci
s. moleculare
s. moleculare cerebelli
s. moleculare retinae
s. neuroepitheliale retinae
s. neuronorum piriformium
s. nucleare externum et internum retinae
s. nucleare externum retinae
s. nucleare internum retinae
s. opticum
s. pigmenti bulbi
s. pigmenti retinae
s. plexiforme externum et internum retinae
s. zonale

Straus sign
Strauss syndrome
streak
angioid s.
fatty s.
meningitic s.
primitive s.
spinal s.

stream
breath s.
s. of consciousness
s. of mental activity
s. of thought (SOT)

streaming
intravascular s.

street
s. drug
s. fear
s. gang
s. person
s. sense
S. Survival Skills Questionnaire

street-drug culture
strength
antagonistic muscle s.
Aspirin Free Anacin Maximum S.
associative s.
axial gripping s.

Bayer Low Adult S.
bending s.
bone-screw interface s.
C-D instrumentation fixation s.
Cotrel pedicle screw fixation s.
Ecotrin Low Adult S.
effective-habit s.
ego s. (ES)
Excedrin, Extra S.
fatigue s.
field s.
S. of Grip Test
habit s.
masseter s.
motor s.
pedicle screw pullout s.
pullout s.
signal s.
torsional gripping s.

strephosymbolia
streptococcal meningitis
Streptococcus
S. pneumoniae
S. pyogenes
S. viridans

streptococcus
beta-hemolytic s.
group A β-hemolytic s. (GABHS)
group B s. (GBS)

streptokinase
streptomycin
stress
adaptability to s.
s. adaptability skills
S. Audit
biologic s.
catastrophic s.
causative s.
chronic s.
combat s.
contrastive s.
disabling s.
s. disorder
s. effect and immune response
s. effect in old age
s. effect on adult
s. effect on adult thinking
s. effect on learning
s. effect on memory
ego s.
emotional s.
environmental s.
S. Evaluation Inventory
exceptional s.
excessive s.
executive s.
exogenous s.
family s.
fatigue s.
s. from life experience (SFLE)
s. and functionability inventory
heat s.
iambic s.
identifiable s.
s. immunity

stress *(continued)*
  S. Impact Scale (SIS)
  s. inoculation
  s. inoculation training (SIT)
  s. interview
  s. inventory
  job s.
  Level of Psychosocial S.
  life s.
  maternal s.
  measured s.
  medical s.
  mental s.
  nonspecific s.
  occupational s.
  oxidative s.
  physical s.
  postdisaster s.
  precipitating s.
  s. precipitating tremor
  s. prevention
  primary s.
  psychological s.
  s. psychosis
  psychosocial s.
  s. reduction
  s. relaxation
  s. response
  S. Response Scale
  s. response syndrome
  secondary s.
  serious traumatic s.
  severe life s.
  shear s.
  s. situational reaction
  social s.
  stereotyped s.
  temporary s.
  tensile s.
  tertiary s.
  traumatic s.
  trochaic s.
  s. ulcer
  war-related s.
  weak s.
stress-altered startle reflex
stress-diathesis model
stress-driven diathesis
stressful life experience
stress-induced
  s.-i. alopecia
  s.-i. reactive bowel
stressor
  accidents as major childhood s.
  brief reactive psychosis with
    marked s.
  external s.
  extreme s.
  identifiable s.
  internal s.
  life's s.
  maladaptive reaction to a s.
  psychosocial s.
  seasonal-related psychosocial s.

situational s.
social s.
specific situational s.
traumatic s.
s. uncontrollability
stress-related
  s.-r. amenorrhea
  s.-r. disorder
  s.-r. disturbance
  s.-r. paranoid ideation
  s.-r. physiological response
  s.-r. psychophysiological problem
stress-relaxation
  intraoperative s.-r.
stress-strain relationship
stretch
  s. receptor
  s. reflex
  s. reflex pathway
stretching
  soft tissue s.
stria, gen. and pl. **striae**
  acoustic s.
  auditory striae
  striae distensae
  s. fornicis
  Gennari s.
  striae lancisi
  lateral longitudinal s.
  s. longitudinalis lateralis
  s. longitudinalis medialis
  medial longitudinal s.
  striae medullares ventriculi quarti
  s. medullaris thalami
  medullary striae of the fourth
    ventricle
  medullary s. of the thalamus
  striae olfactoriae
  olfactory striae
  s. tecta
  terminal s.
  s. terminalis
  s. ventriculi tertii
striatal
  s. dopamine
  s. dopamine transporter density
  s. hand
  s. hypometabolism
  s. lesion
  s. neuron
  s. target
  s. toe
striate
  s. area
  s. body
  s. cortex
  s. hemorrhage
  s. vein
striated muscle (StrAbs)
striatocapsular infarction
striatocerebellar tremor
striatocerebral tremor
striatonigral degeneration
striatopallidothalamocortical pathway
striatopetal fiber

striatum
corpus s.
ventral s.
strict parent
stricture
clip-induced s.
strident
stridor
string sign
striosome patch
strip
AdTech electrode s.
motor s.
sensory-motor s.
Telfa s.
stripe of Gennari
stripout
screw s.
stripper
striving
conative appetitive s.
emancipatory s.
maintenance s.
superiority s.
stroboscope
stroboscopic light activating technique
stroke
acute s.
anterior circulation s.
brainstem s.
cardioembolic s.
embolic s.
hemisphere s.
s.-in-evolution
ipsilateral s.
ischemic s.
lacunar s.
migraine-induced s.
pure hemisensory s.
pure sensory s.
retinal s.
sensory-motor s.
silent s.
sinovenous s.
smoker's s.
spinal s.
s. syndrome
stroking
stroma
tumor s.
Strong
S. Vocational Interest Blank
(SVIB)
S. vocational interest test
Strong-Campbell Interest Inventory
(SCII)
strongly held idea
Strongyloides stercoralis
strongyloidiasis
strontium-89
Stroop
S. Color-Word Interference Test
S. effect
S. Interference Test

STRR
Slosson Test of Reading Readiness
structural
s. ambiguity
s. analysis of social behavior
s. atrophy
s. balance
s. brain abnormality
s. brain imaging
s. diagnosis
s. integration
s. malformation
s. pathology
s. profile
structuralism
structural-strategic therapy
structure
abnormal brain s.
base s.
character s.
cognitive s.
cooperative reward s.
deep s.
ego s.
endopsychic s.
external s.
extrapyramidal s.
field s.
functional superego s.
group s.
hierarchial s.
hierarchical s.
individualistic reward s.
initiating s.
s. of intellect (SI)
S. of Intellect Learning Abilities
Test, From P
intermediate s.
intraarachnoid neurovascular s.
lack of s.
mental s.
mesencephalic premotor s.
mesial cerebral s.
organizational s.
perceptual s.
personality s.
pragmatic s.
social s.
societal s.
stable ego s.
subcortical s.
superego s.
surface s.
underlying s.
Wachs Analysis of Cognitive S.'s
structured
S. Clinical Interview for DSM-III-
R (SCID)
S. Clinical Interview for DSM-III-
R Dissociative Disorders (SCID-
D)
S. Clinical Interview for DSM-III-
R-Patient Version (SCID-P)
S. Clinical Interview for DSM-III-
R Psychotic Disorders (SCID-PD)

S

structured *(continued)*
    S. Clinical Interview for DSM-IV (SCID)
    S. Clinical Interview for DSM-IV Axis I Disorders: Clinician Version (SCID-CV)
    S. Clinical Interview for DSM-IV Axis II Personality Disorders (SCID-II)
    S. Clinical Interview for DSM-IV Dissociative Disorders (SCID-D, SCID-IV)
    S. Clinical Interview for DSM-IV Patient Edition
    S. Clinical Interview for the Panic-Agoraphobic Spectrum
    S. Composite International Diagnostic Interview for Psychological Disorders
    s. hallucination
    s. interactional group
    s. interactional group psychotherapy
    s. interview
    S. Interview of Reported Symptoms (SIRS)
    s. milieu
    S. Photographic Expressive Language Test-II (SPELT-P)
    S. and Scaled Interview to Assess Maladjustment (SSIAM)
    s. task

struggle
    s. behavior
    leadership power s.
    power s.

Strully
    S. dural hook
    S. dural scissors
    S. neurological scissors

Strümpell
    S. disease
    S. phenomenon
    S. reflex

Strümpell-Leichtenstern encephalitis
Strümpell-Lorrain disease
Strümpell-Marie disease
Strümpell-Westphal disease
strut
    allograft s.
    corticocancellous s.
    s. fusion technique
    s. graft
    s. grafting
    miniplate s.

Struthers ligament
strychnine
    aloin, belladonna, s. (ABS)
    lysergic acid diethylamide and s.

strychninism
strychnomania
Stryker
    S. bed
    S. drill
    S. frame

Stuart-Power factor
stuck
    s. finger
    S. laminectomy retractor

student
    above-average s.
    S. Adaptation to College Questionnaire (SACQ)
    S. Adjustment Inventory (SAI)
    S.'s Against Drunk Driving (SADD)
    below-average s.
    S. Disability Survey (SDS)
    s. disease
    Evaluating Educational Programs for Intellectually Gifted S.'s
    S. Opinion Inventory (SOI)
    S. Orientations Survey (SOS)
    Perception of Ability Scale for S.'s (PASS)
    S. Reactions to College (SRC)
    S. Talent and Risk Profile
    S. *t* test

study, pl. **studies**
    adoption s.
    air contrast s.
    Allport A-S Reaction S.
    analog s.
    antidromic conduction studies
    antiphospholipid antibodies in stroke s. (APASS)
    asymptomatic carotid atherosclerosis s. (ACAS)
    S. Attitudes and Methods Survey (SAMS)
    bidirectional selection s.
    blind s.
    brain imaging s.
    Brain Matters Stroke Initiative Edinburgh Artery S.
    brain perfusion s.
    Bronx Aging S.
    California Relative Value Studies (CRVS, CVRS)
    carotid artery stenosis with asymptomatic narrowing: operation versus aspirin s.
    CASANOVA s.
    case control s.
    case history s.
    Center for Epidemiologic Studies-Depression (CES-D)
    Children's Health S. (CHS)
    chromosome s.
    clinical s.
    cohort s.
    community s.
    correlation s.
    crossover s.
    cross sectional s.
    s. design
    diachronic s.
    double-blind s.
    Dunedin Multidisciplinary Health and Development S.

ecological s.
efficacy s.
electrodiagnostic s.
emotional fatigue s.
Epidemiological Catchment Area S.
ethological s.
family studies
family risk s.
followup s.
Framingham Heart S.
genetic linkage s.
Global Burden of Disease S.
s. group
high-risk s.
hysteria s.
ICA-occluded stable Xe/CT CBF s.
International Society for Traumatic
  Stress Studies
Interpersonal Behavior S. (IBS)
longitudinal s.
Mayo Asymptomatic Carotid
  Endarterectomy S.
Medical Outcomes S.
metrizamide contrast s.
Midtown Manhattan S.
Minnesota Twin Family S.
MIRAGE s.
moon-phase s.
multivariate s.
nerve conduction s. (NCS)
neural crest tumor localization s.
neural imaging s.
neuroendocrine tumor localization s.
neuroimaging studies
New Haven s.
nocturnal penile tumescence s.
nonphantom s.
Northern Manhattan Stroke S.
studies on hysteria
Operation Versus Aspirin s.
parametric s.
pedigree s.
pheochromocytoma and
  neuroblastoma localization s.
picture frustration s. (PFS)
pilot s.
polysomnographic s.
prediction s.
prospective s.
radionuclide s.
retrospective s.
Rosenzweig Picture-Frustration S.
  (RPFS)
segregation analysis s.
Sequential Tests of Educational S.
  (STEP)
seroepidemiological s. (SES)
Sinvastatin Survival S.
Stanford-Terman S.
Stirling County s.
synchronic s.
systematic s.
time and motion s.
Trail of Nonpharmacologic
  Interventions in the Elderly S.

twin studies
United States-United Kingdom S.
S. of Values (SV)
Xe/CT CBF s.
stumbling
  syllable s.
stump
  distal sympathetic s.
  s. embolization syndrome
  s. hallucination
  jumpy s.
  nerve s.
  s. neuralgia
stun gun
stupefacient, stupefactive
stupemania
stupor
  affective s.
  akinetic s.
  alcoholic s.
  anergic s.
  benign s.
  Cairns s.
  catatonic s.
  s. catatonic schizophrenia
  delusion s.
  depressive s.
  diencephalic s.
  emotional s.
  epileptic s.
  examination s.
  exhaustive s.
  idiopathic recurring s. (IRS)
  lethargic s.
  malignant s.
  s. mania
  manic s.
  postconvulsive s.
  psychogenic s.
stuporosa
  melancholia s.
stuporous
  s. catatonia
  s. depression
  s. manic-depressive psychosis
  s. melancholia
  s. patient
Sturge disease
Sturge-Kalischer-Weber syndrome
Sturge-Weber
  S.-W. disease
  S.-W. syndrome
Sturge-Weber-Dimitri syndrome
stuttering
  s. block theory
  s. gait
  gait s.
  hysterical s.
  labiochoreic s.
  PFAGH s.
  urinary s.
STYCAR
  Screening Tests for Young Children and
  Retardates
    STYCAR Hearing Test (SHT)

STYCAR *(continued)*
    STYCAR Language Test (SLT)
    STYCAR Vision Test (SVT)
stygiophobia
style
    adaptive s.
    analysis of coping s.
    cognitive s.
    coping s.
    deception s.
    dramatic interpersonal s.
    dysfunctional personality s.
    extratensive personality s.
    interpersonal s.
    introintensive personality s.
    introtensive problem-solving s.
    S. of Leadership and Management
    S. of Leadership Survey
    S. of Management Inventory
    S. of Mind Inventory (SMI)
    parenting s.
    perceptual s.
    problem-solving s.
    Test of Attentional S.
    Vocational Learning S.'s (LSV2)
stylet, stylette
    Frazier s.
stylomastoid foramen
styloradial reflex
stylus-type sensor wand
subacute
    s. cerebellar degeneration
    s. combined degeneration of the
      spinal cord
    s. confusional insanity
    s. confusional state (SCS)
    s. delirium
    s. demyelinating neuropathy
    s. hemorrhage
    s. inclusion body encephalitis
    s. measles encephalitis
    s. meningitis
    s. myelo-optic neuropathy (SMON)
    s. necrotic myelopathy
    s. necrotizing encephalopathy
    s. necrotizing myelitis
    s. necrotizing myelopathy
    s. organic reaction
    s. polyneuropathy
    s. psychoorganic syndrome
    s. psychosis
    s. sclerosing leukoencephalitis
    s. sclerosing leukoencephalopathy
    s. sclerosing panencephalitis (SSPE)
    s. spongiform encephalopathy
subaffective dysthymia
subanesthetic
subantigen
subarachnoid
    s. bolt
    s. cavity
    s. cysticerci
    s. hemorrhage (SAH)
    s. lipoma

    s. screw
    s. seeding
    s. space
subarachnoidal cistern
subaverage
    s. academic function
    s. academic functioning
    s. intellectual functioning
    s. motor coordination
subcalcarine
    subcallosa area s.
subcallosa area subcalcarine
subcallosal
    s. area
    s. fasciculus
    s. gyrus
subcapsular
subcaudate tractotomy
subcellular localization
subception
subchondral sclerosis
subchoroidal approach
subchronic schizophrenia
subclassification
    subclavia ansa s.
subclavia ansa subclassification
subclavian
    s. artery
    s. loop
    s. steal
    s. steal syndrome
subclinical
    s. absence
    s. neuropathy
    s. rhythmic epileptiform discharge
      of adult (SREDA)
    s. score
    s. seizure
subcollateral gyrus
subcoma
    s. insulin treatment
    s. therapy
subcommissural organ
subconjunctival hemorrhage
subconscious
    s. awareness
    s. memory
    s. mind
    s. perception
    s. self
subconsciousness
subcortex
subcortical
    s. alexia
    s. arteriosclerotic
    s. arteriosclerotic encephalopathy
    s. atrophy
    s. brain involvement
    s. dementia
    s. dysequilibrium
    s. encephalomalacia
    s. hemorrhage
    s. lesion
    s. motor aphasia
    progressive degenerative s.

s. protoplasmic astrocytoma
s. sensory aphasia
s. structure
s. syndrome
s. vascular encephalopathy
s. white matter
subcorticalis chronica encephalitis
subcranial
subcultural language
subculture norm
subcutaneous
s. injection
s. sacrococcygeal myxopapillary
ependymoma
subdelirious state
subdelirium
subdermal plexus
subdue
subdural
s. abscess
s. button
s. cavity
s. effusion with hydrocephalus
(SEH)
s. empyema
s. grid
s. grid electrode
s. grid implantation
s. hematoma
s. hematorrhachis
s. hemorrhage
s. hygroma
s. ICP monitoring
s. meningioma
s. peritoneal (SP)
s. pressure screw
s. space
s. strip electrode
s. tap
s. tumor
subdural-pleural shunt
subduroperitoneal shunt
subendocardial myocardial infarction
subendymal
subependymal
s. extension
s. giant cell astrocytoma
s. glomerate astrocytoma
s. hamartoma
s. hemorrhage
s. mixed glioma
s. tuber
s. tumor
subependymoma
subepicranium
subfalcial herniation
subfalcine herniation
subfissure
subfolium
subfrontal
s. craniotomy
s. meningioma
s. transbasal approach
subgaleal
s. abscess

s. drain
s. emphysema
s. hematoma
s. hemorrhage
s. space
subglial cerebrospinal fluid
subgroup
cultural s.
phenomenological s.
subgrundation
subhyaloid hemorrhage
subicular region
subiculum, pl. **subicula**
subintimal hemorrhage
subject
ego s.
s. homoerotic
S. Treatment Emergent Symptom
Scale
subjective
s. distress
s. doubles
s. drive
s. equality
s. error
s. experience
s. fear
s. feeling
S. High Assessment Scale
s. insomnia complaint
s. manifestation
s. mentation
S. Opiate Withdrawal Scale
s. orientation
s. pain
s. plane
s. psychology
S. Response Questionnaire
s. seizure
s. sensation
s. symptoms
S. Symptoms Scale
S. Treatment Emergent Side
Effects Scale
s. unit of distress rating
S. Units of Distress Scale (SUDS)
s. vertigo
s. vision
subjective, objective, assessment, plan
(SOAP)
subjectivism factor
subjectivity
overwhelmed s.
subject-verb agreement
subjugate
subjunctive mood
sublabial
s. midline rhinoseptal approach
s. transseptal transsphenoidal
approach
sublaminar
s. fixation
s. wire
s. wiring
sublenticular limb of internal capsule

sublexical process
subligamentous disk herniation
sublimate
sublimation
    s. defense mechanism
    s. difficulty
Sublimaze Injection
sublime
subliminal
    s. behavior
    s. consciousness
    s. excitation
    s. fringe
    s. learning
    s. message
    s. perception
    s. self
    s. stimulation
    s. stimulus
    s. suggestion
    s. thirst
sublingual
    s. ganglion
    s. medication
subluxation
    atlantoaxial s.
    degenerative s.
    s. stabilization
    unilateral interfacetal dislocation
       or s. (UID/S)
    vertebral s.
submachine gun
submandibular ganglion
submania
submaxillary ganglion
submerge
submerged individual need
submission
    authoritarian s.
submissive behavior
submodalities
    critical s.
subnormal
    educationally s. (ESN)
subnormality
    mental s.
    mild mental s.
    moderate mental s.
    profound mental s.
    severe mental s.
subnucleus caudalis
suboccipital
    s. craniectomy
    s. craniotomy
    s. decompression
    s. encephalocele
    s. headache
    s. neuralgia
    s. neuritis
    s. Ommaya reservoir
    s. posterior fossa approach
    s. puncture
    s. transmeatal approach
suboccipitale
    malum vertebrale s.

subordinate
    s. association
    s. position
subparietal sulcus
subperiosteal
    s. corticotomy
    s. cyst
    s. dissection
    s. hematoma
subphase
    rapprochement s.
subpial
subplate zone
subplatysmal plane
subpoena duces tecum
subpotent
subpsyche
subscale
    ADAS noncognitive s.
    Alzheimer disease noncognitive s.
    dichotomized MMPI s.
    low-magnitude stressor s.
    noncognitive s.
    Positive Humanitarian S.
    Positive Military S.
    vegetative s.
    War Zone Exposure S.
subsensitization of presynaptic
subsequent
    s. amnesia
    s. development
subshock therapy
subsidiation
subsistence diet
subsocial
subsonic
substance
    s. abuse
    s. abuse counselor
    s. abuse and dependence
    s. abuse and dependence disorder
    S. Abuse Problem Checklist
    S. Abuse Questionnaire (SAQ)
    s. abuser
    S. Abuse Subtle Screening
       Inventory (SASSI)
    s. addiction
    amphetamine-like s.
    anterior perforated s.
    anxiolytic s.
    basophil s.
    behavior-altering s.
    central gray s.
    chromophil s.
    controlled s.
    ego s.
    endogenously produced s.
    gelatinous s.
    gray s.
    s. group
    illicit psychoactive s.
    innominate s.
    s. intoxication
    s. intoxication or withdrawal
    s. K

long-half-life anxiolytic s.
medullary s.
methamphetamine-like s.
mood-altering s.
neurosecretory s.
Nissl s.
nontoxic s.
s. P
phencyclidine-like s.
pineal s.
posterior perforated s.
psychoactive s.
reticular s.
Rolando gelatinous s.
Schwann white s.
s. sensitivity
Stilling gelatinous s.
tigroid s.
s. tolerance
toxic s.
transmitter s.
s. use disorder
white s.
s. withdrawal tremor
substance-abuse persisting dementia
substance-induced
s.-i. anxiety
s.-i. chronic psychosis
s.-i. delirium
s.-i. disorder
s.-i. dystonia
s.-i. etiology
s.-i. intoxication
s.-i. manic episode
s.-i. perception
s.-i. persisting dementia
s.-i. presentation
s.-i. sexual dysfunction
s.-i. state
s.-i. symptomatology
s.-i. syndrome
substance-related
s.-r. cause
s.-r. disorder
s.-r. legal problem
substance-seeking behavior
substance-specific
s.-s. intoxication criteria sets
s.-s. withdrawal
s.-s. withdrawal criteria sets
substantia, pl. **substantiae**
s. alba
s. basophilia
s. cinerea
s. ferruginea
s. gelatinosa
s. gelatinosa centralis
s. grisea
s. grisea centralis
s. innominata
s. intermedia centralis et lateralis
s. medullaris
s. nigra
s. nigra disorder
s. nigra pars compacta (Snc)

s. nigra pars reticulata (Snr)
s. perforata anterior
s. perforata posterior
s. reticularis
substantial comorbidity
substantive universals
substitute
displacement s.
father s.
s. formation
human dural s.
mother s.
s. object
opioid s.
regressive s.
substituted
s. amphetamine
s. benzamide
substituting
s. behavior
s. feeling
s. thought
substitution
s. analysis
creeping s.
s. defense mechanism
s. disorder
dissociate-dysmnesic s.
stimulus s.
symptom s.
substitutive
s. medication
s. reaction type
substrate
permissive s.
s. transport
subsultus
s. clonus
s. tendinum
subsyndromal
s. depressive symptom
s. state
s. thought disorder
subsystem
s. boundary
depreciated s.
individuals s.
parents s.
scapegoated s.
siblings s.
spouses s.
visual s.
subtalar arthralgia
subteen
subtemporal
s. decompression
s. dissection
s. infratemporal approach
s. keyhole approach
subtentorial lesion
subtest
arithmetic s.
block design s.
comprehension s.
digit span s.

S

subtest *(continued)*
    Halstead-Reitan category s.
    information s.
    Logical Memory and Visual
      Reproduction s. Russell's revised
    OA s. (OA)
    object assembly s.
    PA s.
    s. PA
    PC s. (PC)
    picture arrangement s.
    picture completion s.
    s. scale score
    scale scores s.
    similarities s.
    Word Discrimination s.
subtetanic
subthalamic nucleus (STN)
subthalamus
subthreshold
    s. presentation
    s. stimulus
subtle
    s. gesture
    s. meaning
subtraction
    s. imaging
    s. technique
subtype
    s. and/or specifier
    Central European s.
    diagnostic s.
    disorganized s.
    Eastern s.
    kraepelinian s.
    male alcoholism s.
    Western s.
subunit
    beta s.
    glutamide receptor s. (GluR1)
subventricular zone
subversion
subversive
subvocal speech
subwaking
succedaneum
    caput s.
success
    cumulative probability of s. (CPS)
    s. experience
    failure through s.
    s. neurosis
successful suicide
successive approximation
succimer
    technetium 99m s.
succinate
    chloramphenicol sodium s.
    cortisol and sodium s.
    loxapine s.
    methylprednisolone and sodium s.
    sumatriptan s.
succinct
succinic semialdehyde

succinylcholine
succorance need
succubus
sucker
    malleable s.
sucking
    s. behavior
    finger s.
    s. reflex
    s. technique
suckling
    eternal s.
sucralfate
suction
    s. cautery
    s. dissection
    Ferguson s.
    s. injury
    s. ophthalmodynamometry
    s. Regugauge regulator
    s. tube
suction-irrigator
    Brackmann s.-i.
    Kurze s.-i.
Sudan black staining
sudanophilic leukodystrophy
sudden
    s. death (SD)
    s. death syndrome (SDS)
    s. fear
    s. infant death syndrome (SIDS)
    s. insight
    s. motor movement
    s. onset
    s. unexplained nocturnal death
      syndrome
    s. vocalization
sudden-onset headache
Sudeck
    S. atrophy
    S. syndrome
sudomotor fiber
SUDS
    Subjective Units of Distress Scale
Suetens-Gybels-Vandermeulen
    angiographic localizer
Sufenta Injection
sufentanil
suffering
    s. death
    ego s.
suffering-hero daydream
sufficient
    s. quantity
    quantity not s. (QNS)
suffocating attachment
suffocation
    corneal s.
    s. fear
    s. hysterics
    s. panicker
    traumatic s.
suffrage
    female s.

sugar
s. block
blood s.
white s.
suggestibility
disturbance in s.
s. effect
suggestion
affective s.
s. hypnosis
hypnotic s.
posthypnotic s.
prestige s.
subliminal s.
s. therapy
s. under hypnosis
verbal s.
suggestive
s. medicine
s. psychotherapy
s. therapeutics
Sugita
S. fork
S. head clamp
S. headframe
S. head holder
S. headholder
S. multipurpose head frame
S. retractor
S. side-curved bayonet clip
S. temporary straight clip
Sugita-Ikakogyo clip
suicidal
s. behavior
s. crisis
s. gesture
s. ideation
s. intent
s. melancholia
s. plan
s. potential
s. preoccupation
s. rumination
s. thinking
s. thought
suicide
accidental s.
accomplished s.
s. act
adolescent s.
alcohol-related risk for s.
altruistic s.
anomic s.
assisted s.
s. attempt (SA)
s. attempt history
s. cluster
cluster s.'s
collective s.
completed s.
copy-cat s.
Durkheim theory of s.
egotistic s.
focal s.
half-hearted attempt at s.

s. hotline
s. incidence
Index of Potential S.
S. Intent Scale
S. Intervention Response Inventory
s. inventory
s. method
s. motivation
S. Opinion Questionnaire (SOQ)
s. pact
physician-assisted s.
s. precaution
s. prevalence
s. prevention
s. prevention center
S. Probability Scale
psychic s.
s. rate
rational s.
s. risk
successful s.
teenage s.
s. tendency
suicide-depression (SD, S-D)
Suicide-Depression Proneness Checklist (SDPC)
suicide-risk factor
suicidogenic
suicidology
suigenderism
Suinn Test Anxiety Behavior Scale (STABS)
sukra prameha
sulazepam
sulbactam
sulcal
s. atrophy
s. enlargement
sulci (*gen. and pl. of* sulcus)
sulcocommissural artery
sulcomarginal tract
sulcus, gen. and pl. sulci
anterior parolfactory s.
anterolateral s.
basilar s.
s. basilaris pontis
calcarine s.
s. calcarinus
callosal s.
s. callosomarginalis
central s.
s. centralis
cerebellar sulci
cerebral s.
sulci cerebri
cingulate s.
s. cinguli
s. of cingulum
s. circularis insulae
circular s. of Reil
collateral s.
s. collateralis
s. corporis callosi
s. of corpus callosum
cortical s.

S

sulcus *(continued)*
s. effacement
fimbriodentate s.
s. fimbriodentatus
frontal s.
s. frontalis inferior
s. frontalis medius
s. frontalis superior
s. frontomarginalis
s. hippocampi
hypothalamic s.
s. hypothalamicus
inferior frontal s.
inferior temporal s.
s. intermedius anterior
s. intermedius posterior
interparietal s.
s. intragracilis
intraparietal s.
s. intraparietalis
intraparietal s. of Turner
lateral s.
lateral cerebral s.
s. lateralis anterior
s. lateralis cerebri
s. lateralis posterior
lateral occipital s.
s. limitans
s. limitans fossae rhomboideae
limiting s. of Reil
limiting s. of rhomboid fossa
lunate s.
s. lunatus cerebri
s. medialis cruris cerebri
median s. of fourth ventricle
median frontal s.
s. medianus posterior medullae
   oblongatae
s. medianus posterior medullae
   spinalis
s. medianus ventriculi quarti
middle frontal s.
middle temporal s.
Monro s.
s. nervi oculomotorii
occipital s.
s. occipitalis lateralis
s. occipitalis superior
s. occipitalis transversus
occipitotemporal s.
s. occipitotemporalis
s. olfactorius
olfactory s.
orbital sulci
sulci orbitales
parietooccipital s.
s. parieto-occipitalis
s. parolfactorius anterior
s. parolfactorius posterior
pontomedullary s.
postcentral s.
s. postcentralis
posterior median s. of medulla
   oblongata

posterior median s. of spinal cord
posterior parolfactory s.
posterolateral s.
precentral s.
s. precentralis
rhinal s.
s. rhinalis
subparietal s.
s. subparietalis
superior frontal s.
superior occipital s.
superior temporal s.
temporal s.
sulci temporales transversi
s. temporalis inferior
s. temporalis medius
s. temporalis superior
terminal s.
transverse occipital s.
transverse temporal sulci
Turner s.
s. ventralis
s. verticalis
sulfadiazine
sulfadoxine
pyrimethamine s.
sulfamethoxazole
sulfatase
s. A
s. A deficiency
cerebroside s.
sulfate
amikacin s.
amphetamine s.
barium s.
bleomycin s.
butabarbital s.
butacaine s.
dehydroepiandrosterone s. (DHEA-S)
dextroamphetamine s.
ephedrine s.
gentamicin s.
guanethidine s.
heparin s.
hyoscyamine s.
keratan s.
magnesium s.
metaproterenol s.
morphine s.
morphinium s.
phenelzine s.
quinine s.
tobramycin s.
vinblastine s.
vincristine s.
sulfate-3-glucuronyllactosaminyl
   paragloboside (SGLPG)
sulfate-3-glucuronyl paragloboside
   (SGPG)
sulfatide lipidosis
sulfatidosis
sulfinpyrazone
sulfite oxidase deficiency aminoaciduria
sulfonamide peripheral neuropathy

sulfonate
    sodium polystyrene s.
sulforidazine
sulfosuccinate
    dioctyl sodium s.
sulfoxide
    dimethyl s. (DMSO)
sulindac
sulpiride
sultorpride
sumatriptan
    s. succinate
    s. succinate injection
SUMD
    Scale for the Assessment of Unawareness
    of Mental Disorder
summary score
summation
    spatial s.
    s. of stimuli
Sun
    S. microsystem
    S. Sparc Station 10
sunburst mechanism
Sunday neurosis
sundowner syndrome
sundown syndrome
Sundt
    S. AVM microclip system
    S. booster clip
    S. carotid shunt
    S. carotid ulceration classification
    S. loop shunt
    S. straddling clip
Sundt-Kees
    S.-K. encircling patch clip
    S.-K. graft clip
    S.-K. Slimline clip
sunlight fear
sunrise fear
SUN workstation
suo yang
super
    s. acid
    s. joint
superantigen
superconducting
    s. magnet
    0.5-T s. magnet
superconductor
    Type 2 s.
superego
    s. anxiety
    autonomous s.
    s. control
    s. disturbance
    double s.
    group s.
    heteronomous s.
    s. lacuna
    parasites of the s.
    parasitic s.
    primitive s.
    s. resistance
    reward by the s.

    s. sadism
    s. structure
superexcitation
superficial
    s. affect
    s. idiot
    s. middle cerebral vein
    s. origin
    s. pain
    s. petrosal nerve
    s. psychotherapy
    s. reflex
    s. sensation
    s. siderosis of the central nervous
    system
    s. temporal artery (STA)
    s. temporal artery-middle cerebral
    artery (STA-MCA)
    s. temporal artery-posterior cerebral
    artery (STA-PCA)
    s. temporal artery to posterior
    cerebral artery bypass
    s. temporal artery-superior
    cerebellar artery (STA-SCA)
    s. temporal vein
superfine fiberscope
superimposed
    s. delirium
    s. dementia
superior
    s. alternating hemiplegia
    s. anastomotic vein
    area vestibularis s.
    s. cerebellar artery
    s. cerebellar artery syndrome
    s. cerebellar peduncle
    s. cervical ganglion
    s. cervical ganglionectomy
    s. colliculus
    s. frontal convolution
    s. frontal gyrus
    s. frontal sulcus
    s. functioning
    s. ganglion of glossopharyngeal
    nerve
    s. ganglion of the vagus nerve
    s. hemorrhagic polioencephalitis
    s. hypophyseal artery (SupHypArt)
    s. intelligence
    s. intradural approach
    s. laryngeal artery
    s. laryngeal nerve
    s. laryngeal nerve external branch
    s. longitudinal fasciculus
    macula cribrosa s.
    s. manner
    s. medullary velum
    s. mesenteric artery syndrome
    s. mesenteric ganglion
    s. oblique tendon sheath syndrome
    s. occipital gyrus
    s. occipital sulcus
    oliva s.
    s. olivary nucleus
    s. olive

S

superior *(continued)*
  s. ophthalmic vein approach
  s. orbital fissure (SOF)
  s. paraplegia
  s. parietal gyrus
  s. parietal lobule
  s. part of vestibulocochlear nerve
  s. petrosal sinus
  s. pontine syndrome
  s. pulmonary sulcus tumor
  s. quadrigeminal brachium
  s. rectus muscle
  respondeat s.
  s. root of cervical loop
  s. root of vestibulocochlear nerve
  s. sagittal sinus occlusion
  s. salivary nucleus
  s. semilunar lobule
  s. surface of cerebellar hemisphere
  s. temporal convolution
  s. temporal fissure
  s. temporal gyrus
  s. temporal sulcus
  s. thoracic pedicle screw
  s. thyroid artery
  s. thyroid vein
  s. vein of cerebellar hemisphere
  s. vena cava syndrome
  s. vestibular area
  s. vestibular nucleus
superior-inferior submucous tunnel
superiority
  s. complex
  s. feeling
  s. striving
superlative
supermotility
supernaturalism
supernumerary
superolateral surface of cerebrum
superordinate
superoxide dismutase (SOD)
superparamagnetic iron oxide
superparamagnetism
superpersonal unconscious
superposition
superselective
  s. angiography
  s. embolization
supersensory
superstitious
  s. behavior
  s. control
supervalent thought
supervision
  boundaries in postanalytic s.
  one-on-one s.
  postanalytic s.
Supervisory
  S. Behavior Description (SBD)
  S. Practices Inventory
  S. Practices Test (SPT)
  S. Profile Record

SupHypArt
  superior hypophyseal artery
supination reflex
supinator
  s. jerk
  s. longus reflex
supplement
  Electrolyte S.
  Neonatal Behavioral Assessment Scale with Kansas S.'s (NBAS-K)
Supplemental Security Income (SSI)
supplementary
  s. motor area (SMA)
  s. motor cortex
  s. motor epilepsy
supplicate
supply
  cochlear vascular s.
  drug s.
  emotional s.
  spinal cord blood s.
support
  child s.
  community s.
  considerable external s.
  decision s.
  emotional s.
  s., empathy and truth (SET)
  s., empathy and truth therapy
  empirical s.
  environmental s.
  external s.
  family s.
  s. group
  informational s.
  instrumental s.
  limited s.
  Olympia VACPAC s.
  physical s.
  Questionnaire of Basic Personality S.
  social s.
  VACPAC s.
supported employment program
supporter
  Malis vessel s.
supportive
  s. ego
  s. group therapy
  reality-adaptive s. (RAS)
supportive-expressive (SE)
  s.-e. psychotherapy
suppressant
  appetite s.
  vestibular s.
suppression
  bone marrow s.
  conditioned s.
  s. neurosis
  s. test
  vestibuloocular reflex s.
suppressive therapy
suppressor scale

Supprettes
    Aquachloral S.
    B&O S.
suppurative
    s. cerebritis
    s. encephalitis
supracallosal gyrus
supracerebellar
    s. approach
    infratentorial s.
supracerebral
suprachiasmatic nuclei
supraclavicular approach
supraclinoid
    s. aneurysm
    s. carotid artery
    s. internal carotid artery
supraindividual
supraliminal
supramarginal
    s. convolution
    s. gyrus
supramarginal/angular cortex
supramaximal
    s. response
    s. stimulus
supranuclear
    s. gaze palsy
    s. lesion
    s. ophthalmoplegia
    s. paralysis
    s. vertical gaze impairment
supraoptic
    s. commissure
    s. nucleus
supraopticohypophysial tract
supraorbital
    s. nerve
    s. neuralgia
    s. pericranial flap
    s. pterional approach
    s. reflex
    s. ridge
    s. rim
suprapatellar reflex
suprapineal recess
suprarational
suprascapular
    s. nerve
    s. nerve entrapment
suprasegmental analysis
suprasellar
    s. adenoma
    s. capsule
    s. cistern
    s. cyst
    s. extension
    s. lesion
    s. mass
    s. meningioma
suprastriate layer
suprasylvian
supratentorial
    s. approach
    s. arteriovenous malformation

    s. astrocytoma
    s. brain
    s. cavernous angioma
    s. craniotomy
    s. glioma
    s. lobar ependymoma
    s. mass
    s. overlay
    s. primary malignant brain tumor
    s. primitive neuroectodermal tumor
    s. structural lesion
    s. subdural hemorrhage
suprathreshold
    S. Adaptation Test (STAT)
    s. ECT
supraumbilical reflex
supremacist
    white s.
supreme
    s. being
    s. court
    s. intercostal artery
suprofen
Suprol
sural
    s. nerve
    s. nerve biopsy
    s. nerve bridge graft
    s. nerve cable graft
    s. sensory potential
surd
surdimutism
surface
    s. coil
    s. coil array
    s. coil MR
    s. coil spectroscopic imaging
    s. ego
    s. epitope
    s. fiducial marker
    inferior s. of cerebellar hemisphere
    s. landmark
    medial s. of cerebral hemisphere
    s. structure
    superior s. of cerebellar hemisphere
    superolateral s. of cerebrum
    s. vessel registration
surfeit
surgency
surgent growth
surgery
    adult scoliosis s.
    anterior cervical spine s.
    anterior cervicothoracic junction s.
    anterior cranial fossa s.
    anterior lower cervical spine s.
    cervical decompression s.
    cervicothoracic junction s.
    computer-assisted stereotactic s.
    (CASS)
    craniofacial s.
    cytoreductive s.
    decompressive s.
    DREZ s.
    ECA-PCA bypass s.

S

surgery *(continued)*
  endoscopic sinus s.
  epilepsy s.
  extracranial-intracranial bypass s.
  hypotensive s.
  International Cooperative Study on
    the Timing of Aneurysm S.
  intradural tumor s.
  intraorbital s.
  keyhole s.
  laser s.
  lower posterior lumbar spine and
    sacrum s.
  minimum incision s. (MIS)
  nasal s.
  neuronavigator-guided brain s.
  Pitanguy plastic s.
  plastic s.
  posterior cervical spine s.
  posterior lower cervical spine s.
  posterior lumbar interbody fusion s.
  posterior lumbar spine and
    sacrum s.
  posterior upper cervical spine s.
  resective s.
  selective imaging and graphics for
    stereotactic s. (SIGSS)
  sex reassignment s. (SRS)
  stereotactic s.
  stereotactic s.
  thoracic and thoracolumbar spine s.
  transsphenoidal s.
  vascular s.
Surgica K6 laser
surgical
  s. addiction
  s. anatomy
  s. brain trauma organic psychosis
  s. correction
  s. decompression
  s. dressing
  s. epilepsy
  s. exposure
  s. hearing loss
  s. microscope
  s. resection
  s. seeding
  s. sex reassignment
  s. technique
Surgicel
  S. fibrillator absorbable hemostat
  S. Nu-Knit dressing
Surgi-Spec telescope
Surgivac drain
Surmontil
surrealism
surrender
  schizophrenic s.
  will to s.
surreptitious
surrogate
  father s.
  s. father
  human s.

  mother s.
  s. mother
  s. parent
  s. partner
  sexual s.
  s. sexual partner
surroundings
  familiar s.
  indifferent to s.
  oblivious to s.
surveillance
survey
  Access Management S. (AMS)
  Adult Performance Level S.
    (APLS)
  American Drug and Alcohol S.
  Aptitude Survey and Interest
    Schedule-Interest S.
  attitude s.
  California Occupational
    Preference S. (COPS)
  Campbell Interest and Skill S.
    (CISS)
  Campbell Organizational S.
  Carlson Psychological S.
  Chicago area s.
  Children's Attention and
    Adjustment S. (CAAS)
  Clarke Reading Self-Assessment S.
  Conflict Management S. (CMS)
  Creativity Attitude S. (CAS)
  s. data
  Dyslexia Screening S.
  S. of Employee Access (SEA)
  Executive Profile S.
  Fleishman Job Analysis S. (F-JAS)
  Gardner Analysis of Personality S.
    (GAP)
  Gifted Program Evaluation S.
  Group Encounter S. (GES)
  Guilford-Zimmerman Aptitude S.
    (GZAS)
  Guilford-Zimmerman
    Temperament S. (GZTS)
  Hereford Parental Attitude s.
    (HPA)
  Human Information Processing S.
  Incomplete Sentences S.
  indirect s.
  interest s.
  Interpersonal Behavior S. (IBS)
  S. of Interpersonal Values (SIV)
  Jackson Vocational Interest S.
    (JVIS)
  Jenkins Activity S. (JAS)
  Kuder General Interest S., Form E
  Kuder Occupational Interest S.
    (KOIS)
  Life Experience S. (LES)
  Management Appraisal S. (MAS)
  Marriage and Family Attitude S.
  Maryland Parent Attitude S.
  Meyer-Kendall Assessment S.
    (MKAS)
  National Comorbidity S.

needs-assessment s.
Ohio Vocational Interest S. (OVIS)
Organization Health S.
Parent Awareness Skills S. (PASS)
Performance Levels of a School
  Program S.
S. of Personal Values
Picture Interest Exploration S.
  (PIES)
Priority Counseling S. (PCS)
Purdue Perceptual-Motor S. (PPMS)
Reality Check S. (RCS)
Rokeach Value S. (RVS)
School Administrator Assessment S.
School Assessment S. (SAS)
School Attitude S. (SAS)
S. of School Attitudes
School Environment Preference S.
School Readiness S.
School Situation S. (SSS)
Short Form-36 General Health S.
  (SF-36)
Short-Form Health S.
Stanton S.
Student Disability S. (SDS)
Student Orientations S. (SOS)
Study Attitudes and Methods S.
  (SAMS)
S. of Study Habits and Attitudes
  (SSHA)
Style of Leadership S.
Team Effectiveness S. (TES)
temperament s.
Transactional Analysis Life
  Position S. (TALPS)
Vocational Interest S.
Vocational Interest Inventory and
  Exploration S.
S. of Work Values, Revised, Form
  U

surveyor
Occupational Interests S. (OIS)
survey, question, read, review, recite
  (SQ3R)
survival
s. of the fittest
s. guilt
nerve cell s.
overall s. (OS)
progression-free s. (PFS)
s. skills workshop
s. strategy
survivor
s. of child abuse
s. of death
s. guilt
s. of neglect
s. syndrome
Susac syndrome
susceptibility
s. agent
s. artifact
s. effect

Harvard Group Scale of
  Hypnotic S. (HGSHS)
magnetic s.
suspected
s. adverse drug reaction (SADR)
s. awareness
s. child abuse/neglect (SCAN)
s. disease
suspended
s. animation
s. embryonic astrocyte
suspension
Alksne iron s.
Children's Advil Oral S.
Children's Motrin Oral S.
magnesium hydroxide s.
penicillin G benzathine s.
suspicious
s. behavior
s. ideation
Sustacal
sustained
s. ankle clonus
s. belief
s. emotion
s. fatigability
s. fatigue
s. full remission
s. manner
s. partial remission
s. position
sustenance
sustentacular fiber of retina
sustentation
sustention/intention tremor
Sustiva
susto
suture
American silk s.
Bondek s.
s. clamp
coronal s.
cranial s.
Czerny s.
s. diastasis
dural tack-up s.
lambdoidal s.
metopic s.
Millipore s.
nerve s.
Nurolon s.
nylon s.
occipitomastoid s.
parietosquamous s.
polypropylene s.
Prolene s.
retracting s.
Safil synthetic absorbable
  surgical s.
Sofsilk nonabsorbable silk s.
tacking s.
tension s.
tentalum wire tension s.
tympanosquamous s.
Vicryl Rapide s.

S

suturectomy
SV
Study of Values
SVIB
Strong Vocational Interest Blank
SVT
sinus-vein thrombosis
STYCAR Vision Test
SWA
seriously wounded in action
swallow-belch method
swallowing
air s.
s. automatism
s. disorder
s. reflex
SWAMI
Speech with Alternating Masking Index
swan
s. neck deformity
s. neck deformity reduction
Swan-Ganz catheter
Swanson, Nolan, and Pelham Rating Scale
Swanson scaphoid awl
swastika
swaying
body s.
s. gait
SWBS
Spiritual Well-Being Scale
sweating test
Swedish gamma knife group
sweep-cheek test
Sweet
S. pituitary scissors
S. two-point discrimination
sweetheart contract
sweet-lemon mechanism
swelled head
swelling
blennorrhagic s.
brain s.
Spielmeyer acute s.
SwiftLase scanner
swimmer's view
swimming
s. head
s. in the head
swindler
epileptic s.
pathologic s.
swing
compensatory mood s.
cyclic mood s.
decreased arm s.
energy s.
mood s.
s. phase control
rebound mood s.
swinging-flashlight test
Swinging Story Test
switch
s. process
s. referential index

SWS
slow-wave sleep
Sx
symptom
sycophant
Sydenham
S. chorea
S. disease
Sydney line
syllabic
s. blindness
s. speech
syllable stumbling
sylleptic argument
syllogism
syllogistic reasoning
sylvian
s. angle
s. approach
s. aqueduct
s. aqueduct syndrome
s. dissection
s. fissure
s. hematoma
s. line
s. operculum
s. point
s. seizure
s. ventricle
sylvian/rolandic junction
sylvii
aqueductus s.
cistern s.
cisterna fossae s.
Sylvius
aqueduct of S.
fissure of Sylvius
fossa of S.
Symadine
symbion, symbiont
symbiosis
dyadic s.
triadic s.
symbiotic
s. attachment
s. infantile psychosis
s. marriage
s. phase
s. psychosis of childhood
s. relatedness
s. stage
symbol
association of sounds and s.'s
digit s. (DS)
S. Digit Modalities Test (SDMT)
mathematical s.
memory s.
phallic s.
picture s.'s (PICSYMS)
sex s.
snake s.
universal s.
Wing s.
symbolia

symbolic
    s. categorization
    s. computation
    s. displacement
    s. elaboration
    s. function
    s. loss
    s. masturbation
    s. meaning
    s. persona
    s. play
    S. Play Test (SPT)
    s. realization
    s. thinking
    s. thought
    s. value
    s. wounding
symbolism
    anagogic s.
    cryptogenic s.
    cryptophoric s.
    dream s.
    functional s.
    material s.
    metaphoric s.
    sound s.
    threshold s.
    true s.
symbolization
    s. defense mechanism
    Visual-Tactile System of
      Phonetic S.
symbolophobia
Symmetrel
symmetric
    s. distal neuropathy
    s. polyneuropathy
symmetrical
    s. diffuse neuropathy
    s. polyneuropathy
    s. sacral plate
    s. thoracic vertebral plate
symmetromania
symmetrophobia
symmetry
    Hermetian s.
    s. obsession
Symonds headache
sympathectomy, sympathetectomy
    cervical perivascular s.
    chemical s.
    s. effect
    Leriche s.
    lumbar s.
    periarterial s.
    permanent s.
    presacral s.
    radiofrequency thoracic s.
    Smithwick s.
    visceral s.
sympathetic
    s. dysfunction
    s. dystrophy syndrome
    s. epilepsy
    s. ganglia

    s. hypertonia
    s. imbalance
    s. iridoplegia
    s. meningitis
    s. nerve
    s. nervous system (SNS)
    s. part
    s. plexuses
    s. reflex dystrophy
    s. segment
    s. skin response (SSR)
    s. stress reaction
    s. trunk
sympathetica
    ptosis s.
sympathetically
    s. independent pain syndrome
    (SIPS)
    s. mediated pain syndrome (SMPS)
sympathetoblastoma
sympathicectomy
sympathicoblastoma
sympathicogonioma
sympathiconeuritis
sympathicopathy
sympathicotonia
sympathicotonic
sympathicotripsy
sympathism
sympathoadrenal
sympathoblastoma
sympathogonioma
sympatholytic drug
sympathomimetic
    s. abuse
    s. addiction
    s. delirium
    s. delusional disorder
    s. drug
    s. effect
    s. intoxication
    s. withdrawal
sympathotonic orthostatic hypotension
sympathy seeking symptom
symptom (Sx)
    abstinence s.
    accessory s.
    active-phase s.
    active psychotic s.
    adjustment reaction physical s.
    alcoholic s.
    anchor s.
    anxiety s.
    Assessment of Positive S.
    attention-deficit s.
    atypical factitious disorder with
      physical s.'s
    auditory s.
    autoplastic s.
    avoidance s.
    baseline s.
    behavioral dysfunction s.
    biologic dysfunction s.
    biphasic s.
    cardiac s.'s

S

symptom *(continued)*
    catatonic s.
    S. Checklist-90-Revised (SCL-90-R)
    s. cluster
    s. complex
    compulsive s.
    constellation of signs and s.'s
    conversion s.
    s. criteria
    culturally sanctioned s.
    cyclical pattern of s.'s
    deficit s.
    delusion s.
    depression s.
    s. diary
    disorganization dimension of
      positive schizophrenic s.'s
    dissociative s.
    eclamptic s.'s
    emotional s.
    Epstein s.
    equivalent s.
    s.'s evaluation
    exacerbated s.'s
    s. experience stage
    extrapyramidal s. (EPS)
    fatigue s.
    feigned s.
    first rank s. (FRS)
    florid s.'s
    s. formation
    frank psychotic s.'s
    s. free
    Frenkel s.
    fundamental s.
    Gordon s.
    gramophone s.
    s. group
    s. grouping
    Haenel s.
    hypnotic withdrawal s.
    hypochondriacal s.
    impairment s.
    insomnia s.
    intentionally produced s.
    intentional production of s.'s
    Kerandel s.
    localization of s.'s
    Macewen s.
    manic s.
    minimal residual s.
    mood s.
    motor conversion s.
    movement s.
    negative s.
    s. neurosis
    neurovegetative s.
    nonbizarre s.'s
    nonpsychotic onset of s.'s
    objective s.
    onset of s.'s
    pain s.
    painful s.
    perceptual s.'s

    phylogenetic s.'s
    physical s.
    physical signs and s.'s
    positive schizophrenic s.'s
    possession trance s.
    preexisting mental disorder s.
    premonitory s.
    s. presentation
    presenting s.
    primary defense s.
    principal s.
    prodromal s.
    productive s.'s
    prominent mood s.
    pseudoneurological s.'s
    psychogenic physical s.
    psychological dysfunction s.
    psychological related s.'s
    psychological signs and s.'s
    psychomotor s.
    psychosensory s.
    psychosexual s.
    psychosomatic s.
    psychotic s.
    s. rating
    S. Rating Scale (SRS)
    reexperiencing perceptual s.
    s. relief through hypnosis
    residual psychotic s.
    s. response pattern
    reverse vegetative s.'s
    Romberg s.
    Romberg-Howship s.
    Scale for the Assessment of
      Negative S.'s (SANS)
    Scale for the Assessment of
      Positive S.'s (SAPS)
    schizophrenia s.
    schneiderian first-rank s.
    secondary defense s.
    sedative-hypnotic withdrawal s.
    sensory conversion s.'s
    severe dissociative s.
    sexual s.
    somatic s.
    somatization pain s.'s
    somatization pseudoneurological s.'s
    somatization sexual s.'s
    s. specificity
    Structured Interview of
      Reported S.'s (SIRS)
    subjective s.'s
    s. substitution
    subsyndromal depressive s.
    sympathy seeking s.
    target s.
    Trendelenburg s.
    Ulthoff s.
    unintentionally produced s.
    vegetative s.
    visual s.
    Wartenberg s.
    withdrawal s.
symptomatic
    s. act

s. dystonia
s. epilepsy
s. headache
s. hydrocephalus
s. impotence
s. indication
s. neuralgia
s. paramyotonia
s. presentation
s. psychosis
s. root
s. seizure
s. spondylolisthesis
s. status
s. therapy
s. torticollis
s. treatment
symptomatica
alopecia s.
indicatio s.
symptomatically
s. reaction
s. reactive
symptomatize
symptomatology
depressive s.
mood s.
panic s.
psychotic s.
substance-induced s.
symptom-sparing
extrapyramidal s.-s.
synalgia
synalgic
Synalgos
Synalgos-DC
synangiosis
synaphoceptor
synapse, pl. **synapses**
adrenergic s.
axoaxonic s.
axodendritic s.
axosomatic s.
chemical s.
cholinergic s.
conjoint s.
dendrodendritic s.
dopaminergic s.
electrical s.
electrotonic s.
excitatory s.
hebbian potentiation of s.
humoral s.
noradrenergic s.
pericorpuscular s.
serotonergic s.
synaptic
s. bouton
s. cleft
s. compartment
s. compensation
s. degeneration
s. ending
s. knob
s. pathway

s. plasticity
s. space
s. terminal
s. transmission
s. trough
s. vesicle
synaptobrevin
synaptogenesis
synaptology
synaptophysin
synaptosome
synaptotagmin
syncheiria, synchiria
synchondrosis
synchrocyclotron operation
SynchroMed
S. drug administration device
S. model 8611H prototype
implantable pump
synchronic study
synchronous
s. bilateral PLED
s. facial schwannoma
s. lesion
s. reflex
synchrony
bilateral s.
interhemispheric s.
synclonic spasm
synclonus
syncopal
s. migraine
s. migraine headache
syncope
cardiac s.
cardiac catheterization cardiac s.
carotid sinus s.
convulsive s.
hysterical s.
laryngeal s.
local s.
micturition s.
near s.
neurocardiogenic s.
postural s.
tussive s.
vasomotor s.
vasopressor s.
vasovagal s.
syncopic
syncretic
s. thinking
s. thought
syncretism
syncytial island
syncytiotrophoblastic giant cell (STGC)
syncytium
syndactyly
syndesmosis
syndromal
s. depression
s. pattern
syndrome
Aarskog s.
aberrant motivational s.

S

syndrome *(continued)*

abolic s.
absence s.
abstinence s.
abused-child s.
acarinatum s.
Acosta s.
acquired hepatocerebral s.
acquired immunodeficiency s. (AIDS)
acroparesthesia s.
acute brain s. (ABS)
Adams-Stokes s.
adaptation s.
addiction s.
Adie tonic pupil s.
adiposogenital s.
adrenogenital s.
adult respiratory distress s. (ARDS)
adult Reye s.
advanced sleep-phase s.
affective disorder s.
aggressive behavior s.
Aicardi s.
air pollution s. (APS)
akinetic-abulic s.
alcoholic brain s.
alcoholic malabsorption s.
alcohol-induced organic mental s.
alcohol withdrawal s.
Alice in Wonderland s.
ALS-like s.
Alstrom s.
Alström-Haligren s.
alveolar hypoventilation s.
Alzheimer s.
amnesic-confabulatory s.
amnestic-confabulatory s.
amok s.
amotivational s.
androgen insensitivity s.
Angelman s.
Angelucci s.
anger and violence psychiatric s.
angry woman s.
anterior bulb s.
anterior cervical cord s.
anterior cingulate prefrontal s.
anterior spinal artery s.
anticholinergic s.
antimotivational s.
antiphospholipid s. (APS)
Anton s.
anxiety-related psychiatric s.
aortic arch s.
apallic s.
apathy s.
Apert s.
s. aphasia
approximate answers s.
s. of approximate relevant answers
Arigelucci s.
Arnold-Chiari s.
Asperger s.

asphyctic s.
attention problems s.
atypical or mixed organic brain s.
auriculotemporal nerve s.
Autley-Bixler s.
autoerythrocyte sensitization s.
autoscopic s.
Avellis s.
aviator's effort s.
avoidance s.
axonopathic neurogenic thoracic outlet s.
Babinski s.
Babinski-Nageotte s.
Balint s.
Baller-Gerold s.
Baltic s.
Bannayan s.
Bannwarth s.
Bardet-Biedl s.
Barlow s.
Barré-Lieou s.
Bartschi-Rochaix s.
Bartter s.
basal cell nevus s.
basal ganglia s.
basilar artery thrombosis s.
Bassen-Kornzweig s.
Basser s.
battered child s. (BCS)
battered infant s.
battered spouse s.
battered woman s. (BWS)
Beckwith-Wiedemann s.
behavioral reaction brain s.
Behçet s.
Behr s.
Benedikt s.
Bernard-Horner s.
Bernhardt-Roth s.
Bessman-Baldwin s.
Beuren s.
Bianchi s.
Biedl-Moon-Laurence s.
Biemond s.
bilateral acoustic neuroma s.
Bing-Horton s.
Bing-Neel s.
biopercular s.
black patch s.
blue velvet s.
Bonnet-Dechaume-Blanc s.
Bonnevie-Ulrich s.
Bonnier s.
Börjeson-Forssman-Lehmann s.
brachial-basilar insufficiency s.
bradykinetic s.
brain death s.
brain psychoorganic s.
brainstem s.
Briquet s.
Brissaud s.
Brissaud-Marie s.
Bristowe s.
Broca s.

Brown s.
Brown-Séquard s.
Bruns s.
buffoonery s.
burning feet s.
burnout s.
C2 s.
callosal disconnection s.
Capgras s.
capsulothalamic s.
cardiopulmonary-obesity s.
carinatum s.
carotid sinus s.
carpal tunnel s.
Carpenter s.
cataract-oligophrenia s.
catastrophic ancataplexy s.
catatonic s.
cat-cry s.
cat's-eye s.
cauda equina s. (CES)
caudal regression s.
cavernous sinus s.
central hypoventilation s.
cerebellar hemisphere s.
cerebellar hemorrhage s.
cerebellomedullary malformation s.
cerebellopontine angle s.
cerebral-blast s.
cerebral salt wasting s.
cerebral steal s.
cerebrohepatorenal s.
cerebrovascular s.
cervical compression s.
cervical fusion s.
cervical rib s.
cervical tension s.
Cestan-Chenais s.
characteristic withdrawal s.
Charcot-Weiss-Baker s.
Chavany-Brunhes s.
Chediak-Higashi s.
cherry-red spot myoclonus s.
Chiari II s.
chiasma s.
child abuse s.
childhood Tourette s.
China s.
choreic s.
choreiform s.
Chotzen s.
chromosome 21-trisomy s.
chronic alcoholic brain s. (CABS)
chronic brain s. (CBS)
chronic fatigue s. (CFS)
chronic fatigue and immune
  dysfunction s. (CFIDS)
Churg-Strauss s.
Cinderella s.
Citelli s.
Claude s.
Clerambault erotomania s.
clinically isolated s. (CIS)
clinical poverty s.
cloverleaf skull s.

clumsiness s.
Cobb s.
Cockayne s.
Cogan s.
Cohen s.
Collet-Sicard s.
compartment s.
complex regional pain s. (CRPS)
compression s.
compulsive swearing s.
concentration camp s. (CCS)
concussion s.
confused language s. (CLS)
congenital Horner s.
Conradi s.
contralateral neglect s.
cord s.
Cornelia de Lange s.
corpus callosum s.
cortical s.
Costen s.
costoclavicular s.
Cotard s.
CREST s.
Creutzfeldt-Jakob s.
cri-du-chat s.
Crigler-Najjar s.
crocodile tears s.
Crouzon s.
Crow-Fukase s.
crush s.
cubital tunnel s.
culture-bound s.
culture-specific s.
Cushing s.
DaCosta s.
Dandy-Walker s.
Davidoff-Dyke-Masson s.
deafferentation pain s.
de Clerambault s.
deficit s.
Dejerine anterior bulb s.
Dejerine-Roussy s.
de Lange s.
delayed sleep phase s.
Delilah s.
delusional s.
dementia-aphonia s.
dementia-related psychiatric s.
de Morsier s.
denervation pain s.
denial visual hallucination s.
Denis Browne s.
Denis Browne, Foley s.
Dennie-Marfan s.
dependence s.
depersonalization s.
depression-related psychiatric s.
depressive-type psychoorganic s.
deprivation s.
De Sanctis-Cacchione s.
s. of deviously relevant answers
dialysis dysequilibrium s.
dialysis encephalopathy s.
diencephalic s. of infancy

S

syndrome *(continued)*
dietary chaos s.
DiMauro s.
disconnection s.
disinhibition psychiatric s.
disk s.
disorganization s.
displaced child s.
dissociation s.
Ditthomska s.
DNA repletion s.
Don Juan s.
Doose s.
dorsal mesencephalic s.
dorsal midbrain s.
dorsolateral convexity s.
dorsolateral prefrontal s.
dorsomedial mesencephalic s.
Down s.
drug abstinence s.
drug withdrawal s.
dry eye s.
Duane retraction s.
Dubowitz s.
Duchenne s.
Duncan s.
dysarthria-clumsy hand s.
dysmnesic s.
dyspraxia s.
Eagle s.
Eaton-Lambert s.
ectopic ACTH s.
Edwards s.
effort s.
Ehlers-Danlos s.
Ehret s.
Eisenlohr s.
Ekbom s.
electroshock-induced psychotic s.
Elpenor s.
elusive s.
empty nest s.
empty sella s.
encephalotrigeminal vascular s.
endogenomorphic s.
enzyme deficiency s.
eosinophilia-myalgia s. (EMS)
epileptic automatism s.
episodic dyscontrol s.
Epstein-Barr s.
Erb-Duchenne s.
Escobar s.
exhaustion s. (EPS)
extrapyramidal s. (EPS)
facet s.
Fahr s.
failed back surgery s. (FBSS)
failure-to-grow s.
failure-to-thrive s.
false memory s.
Fanconi s.
fatigue s.
FAV s.
Fazio-Londe s.

Felty s.
feminizing-testes s.
fetal alcohol s. (FAS)
fetal hydantoin s.
FG s.
fibromyalgia s.
fibrositis/fibromyalgia s.
Figueira s.
Fisher s.
flashing pain s.
flat back s.
floppy head s.
floppy infant s.
fluid retention s. (FRS)
flu-like s.
Flynn-Aird s.
focal brain s.
Foix s.
Foix-Alajouanine s.
Foster Kennedy s.
Foville s.
fragile X s.
Franceschetti s.
Fregoli s.
Freud s.
Frey s.
Fröhlich s.
Froin s.
frontal lobe s.
Ganser s.
Garcin s.
Gardner s.
G-D s.
Gélineau s.
gender difference psychiatric s.
gender dysphoria s.
general adaptation s. (GAS)
Gerstmann s.
Gerstmann-Sträussler s. (GSS)
Giessing s.
Gilles de la Tourette s.
Gjessing s.
Goldenhar s.
Gorlin s.
Gowers s.
Gradenigo s.
gray-out s.
Greig cephalopolysyndactyly s.
Gubler s.
Guillain-Barré s. (GBS)
Guillain-Barré-Strohl s.
Guillain-Garcin s.
Gunn s.
gustatory sweating s.
Haddad s.
Hajdu-Cheney s.
Hakim s.
Hallervorden s.
Hallervorden-Spatz s.
hallucinatory-type psychoorganic s.
happy puppet s.
Harris s.
headache s.
head-bobbing doll s.
Heller s.

hemibasal s.
hemichorea-hemiballism s.
hemineglect s.
hemisensory s.
hemispheric disconnection s.
hepatorenal s.
hereditary spinocerebellar ataxia s.
Herrmann s.
HHE s.
Hinman s.
holiday s.
Holmes-Adie s.
Hopkins s.
Horner s.
hospital addiction s.
housewife s.
Hunt s.
Hunter s.
Hurler s.
hyperabduction s.
hyperactive child s. (HACS)
hypereosinophilic s.
hyperkinetic s.
hyperperfusion s.
hypersensitivity s.
hypertrophied frenula s.
hyperventilation s. (HVS)
hyperviscosity s.
hypokinetic s.
hypophysial s.
hypophysiosphenoidal s.
idiopathic Parsonage-Turner s.
iliac crest s.
immune deficiency s.
impostor s.
s. of inappropriate secretion of
  antidiuretic hormone (SIADH)
indifference to pain s.
infectious-exhaustive s.
infectious polyneuritis s.
inferior pontine s.
infratentorial neoplastic s.
infratentorial structural s.
insular-opercular s.
intensive care s.
intermediate brain s.
intermediolateral mesencephalic s.
internal capsule s.
intoxication s.
intracranial steal s.
inverse Anton s.
irritable bowel s.
Isaacs s.
isolation s.
Jackson s.
Jackson-Weiss s.
Jacod s.
Jahnke s.
Jarcho-Levin s.
jaw-winking s.
jet lag s.
Joubert s.
jugular foramen s.
jumping Frenchmen of Maine s.
Kahn s.

Kallmann s.
Kanner s.
Kasabach-Merritt s.
Kearns-Sayre s. (KSS)
Kennedy s.
Kernohan notch s.
Kiloh-Nevin s.
Kiver-Bucy s.
Kleine-Levin s.
Klinefelter s.
Klippel-Feil s.
Klippel-Trenaunay s.
Klippel-Trenaunay-Weber s.
Klover-Bucy s.
Klumpke-Dejerine s.
Klüver-Bucy s.
Kocher-Debré-Semelaigne s.
Koerber-Salus-Elschnig s.
koro s.
Korsakoff s.
Krabbe s.
K's s.
Kugelberg-Welander s.
Labbé neurocirculatory s.
labyrinthine concussion s.
lacunar s.
Lambert-Eaton myasthenic s.
  (LEMS)
Lance-Adams s.
Landau s.
Landau-Kleffner s.
Landry s.
Landry-Guillain-Barré s.
Landry-Guillain-Barré-Strohl s.
Lasègue s. II
latah s.
late whiplash s.
Laurence-Biedl s.
Laurence-Moon s.
Laurence-Moon-Bardet-Biedl s.
Laurence-Moon-Biedl s.
Lawford s.
laxative abuse s. (LAS)
Leigh s.
Lennox s.
Lennox-Gastaut s.
Leriche s.
Lesch-Nyhan s.
Levine-Critchley s.
Li-Fraumeni s.
linear nevus sebaceous s.
lissencephalic s.
lobotomy s.
locked-in s.
loculation s.
Louis-Bar s.
low back s. (LBS)
Lowe s.
lower motor neuron s.
lumbar flat back s.
lumbar theco-peritoneal shunt s.
luxury perfusion s.
MacKenzie s.
Madame Butterfly s.
Mad Hatter s.

S

syndrome *(continued)*
Maffucci s.
Magenblase s.
Magendie-Hertwig s.
MAGIC s.
Main s.
male climacteric s.
malignant neuroleptic s.
Malin s.
manic-depressive s.
Marcus Gunn s.
Marfan s.
Marie-Robinson s.
Marin Amat s.
Marinesco-Garland s.
Marinesco-Sjögren s.
Maroteaux-Lamy s.
Martin-Bell s.
Mast s.
May-White s.
McLeod s.
Meckel-Gruber s.
medical s.
medullary s.
Meige s.
MELAS s.
Melkersson-Rosenthal s.
Ménière s.
Menkes kinky hair s.
menstrual-associated s.
MERRF s.
MERRLA s.
microphthalmos-corneal opacity-
    spasticity s.
middle radicular s.
midline s.
midpontine s.
migraine equivalent
    Miller-Fisher s.
migrainous s.
Millard-Gubler s.
Miller-Dieker s.
Miller-Fisher variant of Guillain-
    Barré s.
Milles s.
Möbius s.
Monakow s.
mood swing s.
Moore s.
Morgagni s.
Morgagni-Adams-Stokes s.
morning glory s.
Morquio s.
moyamoya s.
Moynahan s.
mtDNA depletion s.
Muenzer-Rosenthal s.
multi-impulsivity s.
multiple mucosal neuroma s.
multiple operations s.
Munchausen s.
Munchausen by proxy s.
myasthenic s.
myelopathy s.

myofascial pain s.
Naffziger s.
Nager Miller s.
narcolepsy cataplexy s.
neglect s.
Nelson s.
nest s.
Neumann s.
neural crest s.
neurobehavioral s.
neurocutaneous s.
neurogenic shock s.
neuroleptic malignant s. (NMS)
neuromusculoskeletal s.
neurotic reaction brain s.
Nielsen s.
night-eating s.
nocturnal drinking s.
nocturnal eating s.
non-24-hour sleep-wake s.
nonlacunar s.
nonpsychotic severity
    psychoorganic s.
nonsense s.
nonspecific s.
Noonan s.
Nothnagel s.
numb-chin s.
obsessional s.
obstructive sleep apnea s.
ocular ischemic s.
ocular motor s.
oculocerebrorenal s.
Oden s.
olfactory reference s.
Omersch-Woltman s.
one-and-a-half s.
opiate abstinence s.
Oppenheim s.
opsoclonus-myoclonus s. (OMS)
optic chiasmal s.
opticocerebral s.
opticopyramidal s.
optic tract s.
oral-facial-digital s. (OFD)
orbital apex s.
orbitofrontal s.
orbitomedial s.
organic s.
organic brain s. (OBS)
organic mental s. (OMS)
oriental nightmare-death s.
orofaciodigital s.
osmotic demyelination s.
Othello s.
overdrainage s.
pain dysfunction s. (PDS)
pain, touch and stroke
    psychiatric s.
paleostriatal s.
pallidal s.
Pancoast s.
panic-agoraphobic s.
paramedian mesencephalic s.
paraneoplastic pain s.

paranoia and delusions
  psychiatric s.
Parent Interview for Child S.
  (PICS)
parietal lobe s.
Parinaud s.
Parsonage-Aldren-Turner s.
Parsonage-Turner s.
s. pattern
Pepper s.
peripheral nerve entrapment s.
peripheral neuropathic pain s.
persecution s.
Persian Gulf War s.
personality s.
Petit s.
Pfeiffer s.
phantom lover s.
phencyclidine mixed organic
  brain s.
phobic s.
phosphate-wasting s.
piblokto s.
Pick s.
pickwickian s.
Pierre Robin s.
Pinel-Hasiam s.
Pinel-Haslam s.
piriformis s.
Pisa s.
POEMS s.
polysymptomatic s.
pontine s.
pontocerebellar angle s.
postabortion s.
postadrenalectomy s.
postconcentration camp s.
postconcussion s.
postcontusional brain s.
postencephalitic s.
posterior cord s.
posterior fossa s.
posterior inferior cerebellar
  artery s.
posterior joint s.
posthypophysectomy traction s.
postlaminectomy s.
postleukotomy s.
postlobotomy s.
postpartum pituitary necrosis s.
postpolio s. (PPS)
postpoliomyelitis s. (PPS)
posttorture s.
posttraumatic stress s.
postural orthostatic tachycardia s.
post-Vietnam psychiatric s.
  (PVNPS)
Pourfour du Petit s.
POW s.
Prader-Willi s.
premenstrual s. (PMS)
premenstrual tension s. (PMTS)
premotor s.
pretectal s.
primary antiphospholipid s. (PAPS)

primary antiphospholipid antibody s.
primary fibromyalgia s. (PFS)
primary Sjögren s. (PSS)
primary trunk s.
prisoner of war s.
professional patient s.
pronator teres s.
Proteus s.
protracted withdrawal s.
proxy-for-deficit s.
pseudo-battered child s.
pseudocyesis s.
psychic shock s.
psychogenic nocturnal polydipsia s.
psychogenic purpura s.
psychological s.
psychomimic s.
psychoorganic brain s.
psychotic posttraumatic brain s.
punch-drunk s.
purple people s.
Putnam-Dana s.
s. of the pyramid
rabbit s.
radicular s.
radiculomedullary s.
Raeder paratrigeminal s.
Rambaud s.
Ramsay Hunt s.
rape trauma s.
rapid-time-zone-change s.
rapture-of-the-deep s.
Rasmussen s.
Ray s.
Raymond s.
Raymond-Cestan s.
Raynaud s.
red man s.
red neck s.
reflex sympathetic dystrophy s.
  (RSDS)
Refsum s.
Reichert-Mundinger s.
Reiter s.
Renpenning s.
residual autoparalytic s.
restless legs s.
retirement s.
Rett s.
reversible affective disorder s.
Reye s.
Richardson-Steele-Olszewski s.
Richards-Rundel s.
right parietal lobe s.
rigid-akinetic s.
rigid spine s.
Riley-Day s.
Robinow s.
Romano-Ward s.
Romberg s.
root s.
Rosenthal s.
rostral basilar artery s.
Roussy-Dejerine s.
Roussy-Lévy s.

S

syndrome *(continued)*
    Rubinstein-Taybi s.
    rumination s.
    Russell s.
    Ruvalcaba-Myhre s.
    Saethre-Chotzen s.
    Sandifer s.
    Sanfilippo s.
    Saunders-Sutton s.
    scalenus anterior s.
    scapuloperoneal s.
    Scheid cyanotic s.
    Scheie s.
    Schirmer s.
    schizophrenic s.
    Schmidt vagoaccessory s.
    school refusal s.
    Schüller-Christian s.
    Schwartz-Jampel s.
    sciatic notch s.
    seasonal affective disorder s.
     (SADS)
    seasonal energy s.
    Seckel s.
    senile brain s.
    sensory deprivation s. (SDS)
    sensory dissociation s.
    serotonin s.
    sex and stroke psychiatric s.
    Sheehan s.
    shock s.
    shoulder-girdle s.
    shoulder-hand s. (SHS)
    Shy-Drager s.
    sick sinus s.
    silver cord s.
    Sjögren s. (SS)
    Sjögren-Larssen s.
    sleep apnea s. (SAS)
    sleep apnea hypersomnolence s.
     (SAHS)
    sleep phase s.
    sleep-related abnormal
     swallowing s.
    sleep-related myoclonus s.
    sleep-wake s.
    slit ventricle s.
    Smith-Lemli-Opitz s.
    smoker's s.
    Sneddon s.
    social breakdown s. (SBS)
    social disability s.
    solitary hunter s.
    somnolence s.
    Sotos s.
    spasmodic laughter s.
    spasmodic winking s.
    Spens s.
    sphenocavernous s.
    Sphrintzen s.
    split brain s.
    split notochord s.
    startle s.
    Steele-Richardson-Olszewski s.

    steroid withdrawal s.
    Stevens-Johnson s.
    Stewart-Morel s.
    sticky platelet s.
    stiff-man s. (SMS)
    Stockholm s.
    Stokes-Adams s.
    Strachan s.
    Strauss s.
    stress response s.
    stroke s.
    stump embolization s.
    Sturge-Kalischer-Weber s.
    Sturge-Weber s.
    Sturge-Weber-Dimitri s.
    subacute psychoorganic s.
    subclavian steal s.
    subcortical s.
    substance-induced s.
    sudden death s. (SDS)
    sudden infant death s. (SIDS)
    sudden unexplained nocturnal
     death s.
    Sudeck s.
    sundown s.
    sundowner s.
    superior cerebellar artery s.
    superior mesenteric artery s.
    superior oblique tendon sheath s.
    superior pontine s.
    superior pontine s.
    superior vena cava s.
    survivor s.
    Susac s.
    sylvian aqueduct s.
    sympathetically independent pain s.
     (SIPS)
    sympathetically mediated pain s.
     (SMPS)
    sympathetic dystrophy s.
    syringomyelic cord s.
    tabagism s.
    Taijin-kyofusho s.
    Tapia s.
    tardive Tourette s.
    tarsal tunnel s.
    tea and toast s.
    tegmental s.
    temporal lobe s.
    teratogenic s.
    Terson s.
    testicular feminization s. (TFS)
    tethered spinal cord s.
    thalamic pain s.
    thyrohypophysial s.
    tight filum terminale s.
    time-zone-change s.
    Todeserwartung s.
    Tolosa-Hunt s.
    top of the basilar s.
    TORCH s.
    Torré s.
    Torsten Sjögren s.
    Tourette s. (TS)
    toxic shock s.

trait-like s.
trapped ventricle s.
Treacher Collins s.
s. of the trephined
triangular s.
trisomy s.
trisomy 8 s.
trisomy 13 s.
trisomy 20 s.
trisomy C s.
trisomy D s.
Trousseau s.
Turcot s.
Turner s.
Unverricht-Lundborg s.
upper radicular s.
Usher s.
uveomeningoencephalic s.
vagoaccessory s.
van der Knaap s.
vasovagal s.
velocardiofacial s.
ventral medial mesencephalic s.
Vernet s.
vertebrogenic pain s.
very low-density s.
vesica pudica s.
vibration s.
victim s.
Villaret s.
Villaret-Mackenzie s.
VIP s.
visual hallucination denial s.
visual paraneoplastic s.
Vogt s.
Vogt-Koyanagi-Harada s.
von Hippel-Lindau s.
vulnerable child s.
Waardenburg s.
Walker-Warburg s.
Wallenberg s.
Warburg s.
warfarin s.
Waring blender s.
Weber s.
Weber-Leyden s.
Wermer s.
Wernicke s.
Wernicke-Korsakoff s.
Werther s.
West s.
Westphal-Leyden s.
wet brain s.
whiteout s.
Williams s.
Wilson s.
Windigo culture-specific s.
winking spasmodic s.
withdrawal emergent s.
Wittmaak-Ekbom s.
women who fail s.
wounded victim s.
Wyburn-Mason s.
X-linked lymphoproliferative s.
XXXX s.

XXXXX s.
XXXXY s.
XXXY s.
XXY s.
XXYY s.
XYY s.
yo-yo s.
Zange-Kindler s.
Zanoli-Vecchi s.
Zappert s.
Zellweger cerebrohepatorenal s.
Zieve s.
Zollinger-Ellison s.

synecdoche
synencephalocele
synergetic
synergic
    s. control
    s. marriage
synergism
    sexual s.
synergistic divergence
synergy
synesthesia
    s. algica
    auditory s.
synesthesialgia
synesthetic stimulation
synkinesia
synkinesis
synkinetic motor movement
synostosis
    coronal s.
    lambdoid s.
    metopic s.
    sagittal s.
    tribasilar s.
    unicoronal s. (UCS)
synovial
    s. cyst
    s. separator
synovitis
    pigmented villonodular s. (PVNS)
syntactic
    s. aphasia
    s. category
    s. complexity
    s. rule
syntactical aphasia
syntagmatic response
syntality
syntax
syntaxic
    s. language
    s. mode of experience
    s. thought
syntaxin
synthase
    endothelial nitric oxide s. (eNOS)
    immunologic nitric oxide s. (iNOS)
    neuronal nitric oxide s. (nNOS)
    nitric oxide s. (NOS)
Synthes
    S. cervical plate
    S. guide pin

S

Synthes *(continued)*
    S. Microsystem cranial fixation
      plate
    S. Microsystem drill bit
    S. Microsystem microplate
    S. screw
synthesis
    analysis by s.
    analysis and s.
    distributive analysis and s.
    fibronectin s.
    Fourier s.
    perceptual s.
synthesizing ability
synthetase
    alanyl-tRNA s.
synthetic
    s. corticotropin-releasing factor
    s. drug dependence
    s. function
    s. heroin dependence
    s. method
    S. Sentence Identification Test
Synthroid
syntonic
    ego s.
    s. personality
syntropic
syntropy
syphiliphobia, syphilophobia
syphilis
    cerebral s.
    CNS s.
    meningovascular s.
    psychosis of s.
    secondary s.
    tertiary s.
syphilitic
    s. alopecia
    s. amyotrophy
    s. cerebral hypertrophic
      pachymeningitis
    s. cirrhosis
    s. dementia
    s. meningitis
    s. meningoencephalitis
    s. osteonecrosis
    s. paralytic dementia
    s. progressive dementia
syphilitica
    alopecia s.
syphilology
syphilomania
syphilophobia *(var. of* syphiliphobia)
syphilopsychosis
Syracuse
    S. anterior I-plate
    S. anterior I-plate insertion
syringe
    bulb s.
    glass s.
    s. grip
syringeal
syringes (*pl. of* syrinx)

syringobulbia
syringocele
syringocephalus
syringocisternostomy
syringocystadenoma
syringoencephalomyelia
syringohydromyelia
syringoid
syringomeningocele
syringomyelia
    ape hand of s.
    secondary post-traumatic s.
    traumatic s.
syringomyelia-Chiari complex
syringomyelic
    s. cavity
    s. cord syndrome
    s. dissociation
    s. hemorrhage
syringomyelocele
syringomyelomeningocele
syringomyelus
syringoperitoneal shunt
syringopontia
syringosubarachnoid
    s. shunt
    s. shunting (SS)
syrinx, pl. **syringes**
    s. cavity
    s. drainage
    s. formation
    s. shunt
syrup
    glutethimide and codeine cough s.
    pancakes and s.
system
    Academic Instruction
      Measurement S.
    Accusway balance measurement s.
    Acra-clip s.
    Acra-gun s.
    action s.
    Activa tremor control s.
    activity s.
    adrenergic s.
    Aesculap ABC cervical plating s.
    angiographic reference s. (ARS)
    AngioJet rapid thrombectomy s.
    ANSER S.
    Anspach 65K instrument s.
    Anspach 65K neuro s.
    anterior Kostuik-Harrington
      distraction s.
    antireward s.
    arc-centered guidance s.
    arc-quadrant stereotactic s.
    arc radius s.
    Ariel computerized exercise s.
    ascending reticular activating s.
      (ARAS)
    ascending reticular arousal s.
    Aspen ultrasound s.
    association s.
    auditory s.
    autonomic nervous s. (ANS)

axial spinal s.
Barry Five Slate S.
behavioral activation s. (BAS)
Behavioral Health S.'s (BHS)
behavioral inhibition s. (BIS)
Betaseron needle-free delivery s.
bilateral variable screw
 placement s.
Biojector 2000 needle-free injection
 management s.
biophysical s.
BIOWARE software for Biodex
 isokinetic exercise s.
Birth to Three Assessment and
 Intervention S.
Bleuler diagnostic s.
boarding-out s.
Boston Classification S.
Bowen Family S.'s
Braille Telecaption s.
BrainSCAN computer planning s.
BrainSCAN Linac radiosurgery s.
Bremer halo crown s.
Brown-Roberts-Wells arc s.
Brown Schools Behavioral
 Health S.
Bruker Biospec s.
Bruker S 200 MR s.
Budde halo retractor s.
Budde surgical s.
bulbosacral s.
BWM spine s.
Camino intracranial pressure
 monitoring s.
CASS whole-brain mapping s.
categorical s.
central nervous s. (CNS)
Central Texas Veterans Health
 Care S. (CTVHCS)
centrencephalic integrating s.
cerebrospinal s.
circadian s.
closed-loop feedback s.
CMS AccuProbe 450 s.
Codman anterior cervical plate s.
Codman neurological headrest s.
Committee on Information S.'s
COMPASS arc-quadrant
 stereotactic s.
COMPASS frame-based
 stereotactic s.
computer-controlled neurological
 stimulation s.
conceptual nervous s.
Cordis-Hakim shunt s.
Cosman-Roberts-Wells stereotactic s.
Cotrel-Dubousset distraction s.
Cotrel-Dubousset screw-rod s.
cranial osteosynthesis s.
cranial plating s.
craniomaxillofacial plating s.
craniosacral s.
CRW arc s.
CRW stereotactic s.
CUSA CEM s.

DALE S.
data acquisition s.
Daumas-Duport s.
decision support s.
delusional s.
Diastat Rectal Delivery S.
dimensional s.
Dingman oral retraction s.
direct motor s.
disposition s.
double-pore vent s.
Dual Quattrode spinal cord
 stimulation s.
Dyadic Parent-Child Interaction
 Coding S.
DYNA-LOC anterior fixation s.
EasyGuide Neuro image-guided
 surgery s.
Education and Career
 Exploration S. (ECES)
Edwards modular s.
Elan-E electronic motor s.
Electri-Cool cold therapy s.
Embolyx liquid embolic s.
endocrine s.
entorhinal-hippocampal s.
epicritic s.
Epstein staging s.
Equinox EEG neuromonitoring s.
ergotropic s.
esthesiodic s.
Exner Scoring S.
expert s.
exterofective s.
extrapyramidal s. (EPS)
E-Z flap cranial flap fixation s.
Facial Action Coding S. (FACS)
family support s.
Family Tracking S. (FTS)
feedback s.
feeding s.
first-signal s.
Fischer stereotaxy s.
five-axis s.
fixed delusional s.
flavin-containing mono-oxygenase
 metabolic s. (FMO)
F.L. Fischer modular stereotaxy s.
fluoroptic thermometry s.
focus of delusional s.
Freehand neuroprosthetic s.
Galassi classification s.
gamma efferent s.
gamma motor s.
Gardner and Robertson
 classification s.
GE 9800 CT s.
gNomos stereotactic s.
Golgi s.
granulomatous angiitis of the
 central nervous s. (GANS)
Greenberg retracting s.
Haid universal bone plate s.
Halifax interlaminar clamp s.
halo retractor s.

S

system *(continued)*
  Halstead Russell Neuropsychological
    Evaluation S. (HRNES)
  Hannover s.
  haptic s.
  Harrington rod and hook s.
  heads-up imaging s.
  Hematome s.
  hepatobiliary s.
  Hermetic external ventricular
    drainage s.
  Hermetic II drainage
    management s.
  Hermetic lumbar drainage s.
  high-force Sundt clip s.
  high-resolution brain SPECT s.
  Howmedica VSF fixation s.
  humoral immune s.
  Hunt-Hess aneurysm grading s.
  hypothalamohypophysial portal s.
  immune s.
  incentive s.
  Indiana tome carpal tunnel
    release s.
  indirect motor s.
  innate response s.
  Instatrak guidance s.
  Integrated Assessment S. (IAS)
  S. for Interactive Guidance
    Information (SIGI)
  Interest Determination, Exploration
    and Assessment S. (IDEAS)
  internal fixation plate-screw s.
  internal second messenger s.
  interofective s.
  intracellular second messenger s.
  intraspinal drug infusion s.
  involuntary nervous s.
  INVOS 3100 cerebral oximeter
    monitoring s.
  irrigation bipolar s.
  Isola spinal implant s.
  isolated angiitis of the central
    nervous s.
  Itrel II spinal cord stimulation s.
  Itrel 3 spinal cord stimulation s.
  Jackson Evaluation S.
  Kaneda anterior spinal/scoliosis s.
    (KASS)
  Kelly-Goerss COMPASS
    stereotactic s.
  Kelly stereotactic s.
  Kernohan s.
  kinship s.
  knowledge information processing s.
    (KIPS)
  Kostuik-Harrington distraction s.
  Kraepelin diagnostic s.
  Ladd fiberoptic s.
  Laitinen stereotactic s.
  lateralized brain language s.
  LDD delivery s.
  Leibinger titanium mini-Würzburg
    implant s.

Leksell Micro-Stereotactic s.
life support s.
limbic s.
LINAC s.
LINAC-based radiosurgical s.
Linac radiosurgery s.
linear accelerator s.
Liquid Embolic S. (LES)
Lorenz Neuro/skull base titanium
  osteosynthesis s.
3M Agee carpal tunnel release s.
Magerl hook-plate s.
Magerl plate-screw s.
MAGNES MEG s.
Magnetom SP 4000 1.5-Tesla s.
magnocellular visual s.
Malis CMC-III electrosurgical s.
man-machine s.
massive parallel processing s.
  (MPPS)
maxillofacial plating s.
Mayfield headrest s.
Mayfield surgical s.
MED s.
MED^{next} bone dissecting s.
Medisorb drug delivery s.
MEG head-based coordinate s.
mesolimbic dopamine s.
metameric nervous s.
microcatheter s.
MicroChoice electric powered
  surgical s.
microendoscopic discectomy s.
microMax drill s.
Micro-Plus titanium plating s.
Midas Rex power s.
miniature s.
Mini Würzburg implant s.
Minnesota Occupational
  Classification S. (MOCS-III)
MKM stereotactic image-guided s.
mnemonic s.
Moe s.
monocular heads-up display
  imaging s.
motor s.
MPM I multi-parameter
  monitoring s.
multiaxial classification s.
S. of Multicultural Pluralistic
  Assessment (SOMPA)
MultiDop XS s.
multistate information s. (MSIS)
NCP S.
NECYSYS home neck care s.
needle trephination s.
nervous s.
NeuroCybernetic Prosthesis S.
neuroendocrine s.
NeuroLink II EEG data
  acquisition s.
Neuropak 8 s.
Neuropak Four EMG/Evoked
  Response Measuring S. Model
  MEM-4104K

neurotransmitter s.
Neurotrend continuous multiparameter s.
Neuroview integrated visualization s.
Nicolet Viking II electrophysiologic s.
nigrostriatal dopaminergic s.
Nishioka s.
nonspecific s.
noradrenergic s.
norepinephrine neurotransmitter s.'s
NS2000 bipolar generator s.
oculomotor s.
ophthalmic s.
OSI modular table s.
paranoid belief s.
Parastep I S.
parasympathetic nervous s. (PNS)
Patil stereotactic s. II
pedal s.
Pelorus surgical s.
perimedullary venous s.
peripheral nervous s. (PNS)
persecutory delusional s.
personality assessment s. (PAS)
phased-array color-flow ultrasound s.
Phoenix fifth ventricle s.
phosphatidyl inositol s.
photonic radiosurgical s.
Pinel s.
S. to Plan Early Childhood Services (SPECS)
plasma fibrinolytic enzyme s.
polar coordinate s.
posterior rod s.
preferred representational s.
pressoreceptor s.
pride s.
primary angiitis of the central nervous s.
projection s.
Providence scoliosis s.
psi s.
psychodynamic cerebral s.
psychological defense s.
psychological information, acquisition, processing, and control s. (PIAPACS)
psychologic defense s.
Pudenz-Heyer shunt s.
Puno-Winter-Byrd s.
pursuit s.
pyramidal s.
radiofrequency needle electrode s.
reality s.
Regulus frameless stereotactic s.
Reichert stereotaxy s.
representational s.
respiratory s.
response s.
reticular activating s. (RAS)
reticuloendothelial s. (RES)
review of s.'s (ROS)

RFG-3C radiofrequency lesion generator s.
Rogozinski spinal rod s.
Script Stat, Inc. dispensing s.
second messenger s.
second signaling s.
Secor s.
SecureStrand cervical fusion s.
sensorimotor s.
Sentinel s.
Shiley catheter distention s.
Siemens somatoma plus DCT s.
Simmons plating s.
sleep-wake s.
Social Skills Rating S. (SSRS)
somatosensory s.
somesthetic s.
Songer cable s.
3-SPACE Polhemus digitizing s.
Spetzler s.
SpinaLase neodymium:yyttrium-aluminum-garnet (Nd:YAG) surgical laser s.
SpineLink s.
Spitz-Holter shunt s.
standard Würzburg titanium mini-plating s.
StealStation image guided surgery s.
StealthStation image-interactive s.
Steffee pedicle screw-plate s.
Sundt AVM microclip s.
superficial siderosis of the central nervous s.
sympathetic nervous s. (SNS)
table-fixed retractor s.
Talairach bicommissural reference s.
Talairach stereotactic s.
Talairach/Tournoux s.
TARC Assessment S.
Taylor and Abrams diagnostic s.
Tech-Attach connection s.
Telefactor beehive s.
temporolimbic s.
Tesla MRI s.
S. for Testing and Evaluation of Potential
Texas Scottish Rite Hospital cross-link s.
Texas Scottish Rite Hospital screw-rod s.
thalamic reticular activating s.
theoretical s.
third nervous s.
Thompson-Farley spinal retractor s.
thoracolumbar s.
thoracolumbosacroiliac implant s.
TiMesh titanium bone plating s.
titanium hollow screw plate s.
titanium micro s.
TSRH universal spinal instrumentation s.
UltraPower basic drill s.
UltraPower revision drill s.
UltraPower surgical drill s.

S

system *(continued)*
unilateral variable screw
placement s.
Valleylab CUSA CEM s.
valve s. (VS)
variable screw placement s.
Varigrip spine fixation s.
vegetative nervous s.
venous s.
ventricular s.
Ventrix fiberoptic ventricular
drainage s.
Ventrix fiberoptic ventricular
monitoring s.
Ventrix tunnelable ventricular ICP
monitoring and drainage s.
Ventrix tunnelable ventricular
intracranial pressure monitoring s.
vergence s.
VertAlign spinal support s.
vertebrobasilar s.
vestibular s.
Viewing Wand image guided s.
villa s.
viral vector s.
visceral nervous s.
visual s.
well-systematized delusional s.
wet bipolar s.
whole-cortex MEG/EEG s.
Wiltse s.
Würzburg implant s.
Würzburg titanium plating s.
X-Trel spinal cord stimulation s.
ZD stereotactic s.
Zeiss Image Guided S.
Zeiss OpMi CS-NC2 surgical
microscope s.
Zeppelin micro-motor s.
Z-plate fixation s.

systema
s. nervosum

s. nervosum autonomicum
s. nervosum centrale
s. nervosum periphericum

systematic
S. Assessment for Treatment of
Emergent Events (SAFTEE)
s. desensitization
S. Inquiry (SI)
s. method
s. process
s. rational restructuring (SRR)
s. reinforcement
s. review
s. schizophrenia
s. study
s. vertigo

systematica
paraphrenia s.

**systematic, complete, objective, practical,
empirical (SCOPE)**

systematization

systematized
s. amnesia
s. assertive therapy (SAT)
s. delusion

systemic
s. assertive therapy
s. desensitization
s. family
s. giant cell disorder
s. lupus erythematosus (SLE)
s. mastocytosis
s. multifocal fibrosclerosis
s. myelitis
s. sclerosis
s. vasculature
s. vasculitis

systolic pressure (SP)

SZ
schizophrenia

Szondi Test

T
tesla
    T group
    T myelotomy

T1
    T1 relaxation
    T1 weighting

T2
    T2 relaxation
    T2 relaxation rate
    T2 shortening
    T2 weighting

T$_4$
levothyroxine
thyroxine

T$_3$
triiodothyronine

T11-L5 thoracolumbar burst fracture
T12-L1 fracture-dislocation reduction
T8-L3 thoracolumbar burst fracture
TA
test age
Transactional Analysis
TAB
therapeutic abortion
tabagism syndrome
tabes
    t. diabetica
    t. dorsalis
    t. ergotica
    juvenile t.
    peripheral t.
    t. spasmodica
    t. spinalis
tabetic
    t. arthropathy
    t. crisis
    t. cuirass
    t. dissociation
    t. form paralytic dementia
    t. neurosyphilis
    t. psychosis
tabetiform
tabic
tabid
table
    activator t.
    American Sterilizer operating t.
    life t.
    somatron t.
table-fixed retractor system
tablet
    aspirin, phenacetin, and
      caffeine t.'s
    cannabis t.
    Depakote T.'s
    Koala Pad graphics t.
    mirtazapine t.
    peace t.
    pramipexole dihydrochloride t.
    Tums E-X Extra Strength T.

taboo, tabu
    incest t.
    totem and t.
    virginity t.
taboparesis
tabophobia
tabu (*var. of* taboo)
tabula
    t. interna
    t. rasa
tabular index
tabulation
    allophone t.
Tac
    T. gel for EMS unit
    T. gel for TENS unit
Tac-40
tache
    t. cérébrale
    t. méningéale
    t. spinale
tachistoscope
tachistoscopy viewing
tachophobia
tachyathetosis
tachycardia
    paroxysmal t.
    psychogenic paroxysmal t.
    ventricular t. (VT)
tachykinin
tachylalia
tachylogia
tachyphagia
tachyphasia
tachyphemia
tachyphrasia
tachyphrenia
tachyphylaxis
tachypnea
tachypneic
tachypragia
tachypsychia
tachytrophism
tacking suture
TACL
Test for Auditory Comprehension of
    Language
TACL-R
Tests for Auditory Comprehension of
    Language-Revised
tacrine HCl
tacrolimus
tactical maneuver
TACTICON peripheral neuropathy
  screening device
tactile
    t. agnosia
    t. alexia
    t. amnesia
    t. anesthesia
    t. anomia
    t. aphasia

T

tactile *(continued)*
    t. aphonia
    t. bisection task
    t. corpuscle
    t. disk
    t. extinction
    t. feedback
    T. Finger Recognition Test (TFRT)
    T. Form Recognition Test (TFRT)
    t. genital stimulation
    t. hallucination
    t. hyperesthesia
    t. illusion
    t. image
    t. imagery
    t. kinesthetic perception
    t. meniscus
    T. Naming Test
    t. perception
    T. Performance Test (TPT)
    t. pricklings with aura
    t. sensation
    t. sense
    t. sensory difficulty
    t. sensory modality
    t. stimulus
    t. transfer deficit
tactile-perceptual disorder
tactility
tactometer
tact operant
tactor
tactual hallucination
tactus
    meniscus t.
TAD
    Test of Auditory Discrimination
Tadoma method
Taenia solium
taeniophobia
taftian
    t. theory
    t. therapy
tag
    preauricular t.
Tagamet
TAI
tai chi
taijin kyofusho
Taijin-kyofusho syndrome
tail
    t. of caudate nucleus
    t. of dentate gyrus
    dural t.
tailor's
    t. cramp
    t. spasm
taima
Takayasu
    T. arteritis
    T. disease
take
    t. advantage

    t. issue
    t. out
taking control
Takkouri
Talacen
Talairach
    T. bicommissural reference system
    T. stereotactic frame
    T. stereotactic system
    T. whole-brain mapping
Talairach/Tournoux system
talbutal
talc
tale
    tall t.'s
    tell a t. (TAT)
talent
    creative t.
    Group Inventory for Finding
      Creative T.
talion
    t. dread
    t. law
    t. principle
talionis
    lex t.
talipes spasmodicus
talisman
talk
    t. out
    t. over
    t. therapy
talk-down from overdose
talking
    t. cure
    t. fear
    t. it out
tall tales
Talma disease
talocalcaneal
    anteroposterior t. (APTC)
TALPS
    Transactional Analysis Life Position
    Survey
Talwin
    T. Compound
    T. NX
TAM
    tamoxifen
tamoxifen (TAM)
    t. therapy
tamp
    Richards t.
tampon
    Merocel t.
Tanacetum parthenium
tandem
    t. clipping technique
    t. connector
    t. double mutation
    t. reinforcement
tanescin
tangent
    t. screen examination

tangential
- t. association
- t. incision
- t. layer
- t. speech
- t. thinking

tangentiality

Tangier
- T. disease
- T. peripheral neuropathy

tangle
- Alzheimer t.'s
- t. fragment
- intraneural neurofibrillary t.
- intraneuronal fibrillary t.'s
- neurofibrillary t.
- neurofibrillatory t. (NFT)

tannate
- vasopressin t.

Tanner
- T. sexual maturity rating
- T. stage

tantalum
- t. cranioplasty
- t. mesh
- t. powder contrast agent
- t. preformed skull plate

tantalum-178

tantra

tantric yoga

tanycyte

TAP
- Trainer's Assessment of Proficiency

tap
- heel t.
- shunt t.
- spinal t.
- subdural t.

TAP-D
- Test of Articulation Performance - Diagnostic

tape
- Mersiline t.

tapered
- t. blade
- t. brain spatula

tapetum, pl. tapeta
- t. nigrum
- t. oculi

tapeworm fear

taphephobia, taphophobia

taphophilia

Tapia
- T. syndrome
- T. vagohypoglossal palsy

tapinophobia

tapir
- bouche de t.
- t. mouth

TAP-S
- Test of Articulation Performance, Screen

tarantism

Tarasoff
- T. case
- T. decision
- T. rule
- T. warning

TARC Assessment System

Tarchanoff phenomenon

tarda
- epilepsia t.
- neurosis t.
- neurosis t.

tardive
- t. dementia
- t. dyskinesia
- t. dystonia
- forme t.
- myoclonus t.
- t. myoclonus
- t. oral dyskinesia
- t. orobuccal dyskinesia
- t. tic
- t. Tourette syndrome
- t. tremor

tardy epilepsy

target
- t. acquisition
- t. behavior
- brain t.
- t. language
- t. localization
- t. localization error
- t. multiplicity
- t. organ
- t. patient
- potential t.
- t. response
- retinofugal t.
- rostral subcortical t.
- t. stimulus
- striatal t.
- t. symptom

targeted
- t. brain biopsy
- t. medication

targeting
- angiographic t.
- multiple t.

targetry
- angiographic t.

Tarin
- T. space
- T. tenia
- T. valve

Tarlov cyst

tarot card

tarsal
- t. tunnel
- t. tunnel syndrome

tarsophalangeal
- t. reflex

tarsorrhaphy
- bilateral temporary t.
- lateral t.

tartrate
- belladonna, phenobarbital, and ergotamine t.
- butorphanol t.
- ergotamine t.

T

tartrate *(continued)*
    levallorphan t.
    levorphanol t.
    metoprolol t.
    phendimetrazine t.
    thorium t.
    zolpidem t.
TAS
    Test of Attitude Toward School
    turning against self
TASB
    Teacher Assessment of Social Behavior
T-ASI
    Teen Addiction Severity Index
task
    t. analysis
    T. Assessment Scale
    cognitive t.
    t. completion
    complex multistep t.
    Continuous Performance T.
    dichotic listening t.
    T.'s of Emotional Development
      (TED)
    forced-choice span of
      apprehension t.
    T. Force on Electroconvulsive
      Therapy
    T. Force on Local Arrangements
    T. Force on Nicotine Dependence
    T. Force on Sexually Dangerous
      Offenders
    Free and Cued Selective
      Reminding T.
    Incomplete Sentences T.
    instrumental t.
    t. inventory
    lateralized rapid activating t.
    light-prompted button t.
    linguistic content of t.
    manipulatory t.
    mental status cognitive t.
    modal adaptive t.
    multistep t.
    necessary t.
    nine-digit t.
    nonverbal t.
    particular t.
    performance t.
    t. performance and analysis
    primary t.
    repetitive t.
    required t.
    retrieval t.
    sentence-closure t.
    simple t.
    somatosensory cued t.
    spatial t.
    structured t.
    tactile bisection t.
    three-step t.
    visual memory span t.
    visual-motor t.

task-oriented
    t.-o. approach
    t.-o. assessment
    t.-o. group
    t.-o. reaction
Tasmar
taste
    t. blindness
    t. cell
    color t.
    t. disorder
    t. fear
    t. imagery
    organ of t.
    t. sensation
    t. threshold
TAT
    tell a tale
    Thematic Apperception Test
    Thematic Aptitude Test
tau
    fetal t.
    t. protein
    t. protein peptide
Taube neurological percussion hammer
tau-negative nerve cell
taurine
taurophobia
taut
tautologous
tautomeric
    t. fiber
tautophone
Tavistock Clinic
TAWF
    Test of Adolescent/Adult Word Finding
Taxilan
Taxol
taxonomy
    biologic t.
Taylor
    T. and Abrams diagnostic system
    T. brain scissors
    T. dural scissors
    T. halter device
    T. Manifest Anxiety Scale (TMAS)
    T. percussion hammer
    T. retractor
taylorism
Taylor-Johnson Temperament Analysis (T-JTA, TJTA)
Tay-Sachs disease
TBI
    traumatic brain injury
TBNAA
    total body neutron activation analysis
TBRS
    timed behavioral rating sheet
TBS
    Transition Behavior Scale
TC
    therapeutic community
    thermocouple
Tc
    technetium

^{99m}Tc
  ^{99m}technetium
  technetium-99m
    ^{99m}Tc HMPAO SPECT
    ^{99m}Tc HMPAO T/C ratio
Tc-99m HMPAO cerebral perfusion SPECT imaging
TCA
  tricyclic antidepressant
  tricyclic antipsychotic
TCAD
  tricyclic antidepressant drug
^{99m}TcCEA
TCCS
  transcranial color-coded real-time sonography
TCD
  transcerebellar diameter
    TCD probe
    TCD pulsatility index
    TCD recanalization
    TCD sonography
    TCD ultrasound
TCDB
  Traumatic Coma Data Bank
TCE
  trichloroethanol
T-cell
  T.-c. proliferation
TCET
  transcerebral electrotherapy
^{99m}Tc-hexamethylpropyleneamine oxime (^{99m}Tc-HMPAO)
TcHIDA
^{99m}Tc-HMPAO
  ^{99m}Tc-hexamethylpropyleneamine oxime
    ^{99m}Tc-HMPAO leukocyte scintigram
    ^{99m}Tc-HMPAO leukocyte scintigraphy
    ^{99m}Tc-HMPAO SPECT imaging
TCMP
  Thematic Content Modification Program
TCNB
  Tru-Cut needle biopsy
TCR
  thalamocortical relay
    TCR neuron
TCSM
  Test of Cognitive Style in Mathematics
TCSW
  thinking creatively with sounds and words
TCU
  Test of Concept Utilization
TD
  threshold of discomfort
TDE
  thiamine deficiency encephalopathy
TDF
  thinking disturbance factor
TE
  echo time
T&E
  testing and evaluation

Te
  tellurium
  tetanic contraction
teacher
  T. Assessment of Social Behavior (TASB)
  t. attitude inventory
  T. Evaluation Scale (TES)
  T. Feedback Questionnaire
  t. inventory
  T. Opinion Inventory
  T. and Parent Separation Anxiety Rating Scales for Preschool Children
  T. School Readiness Inventory (TSRI)
  T. Stress Inventory
teacher-child-parent
teacher's reading global improvement (TRGI)
teacher-student model
teaching
  clinical t.
  diagnostic t.
  remedial t.
  T. Style Inventory
team
  crisis t.
  T. Effectiveness Survey (TES)
  interdisciplinary t. (IDT)
  t. leader (TL)
  t. member (TM)
  psychiatric emergency t. (PET)
  two-person interview t.
tear
  crocodile t.'s
  t. gas
  intraoperative dural t.
teardrop
  t. dissector
  t. fracture
tearfulness
  breakthrough t.
tearful outburst
Teasdale and Jennett scale
tea and toast syndrome
teboroxime
  technetium 99m t.
TECA-TD20 EMG machine
tecate
Tech-Attach connection system
Techneplex
Technescan MAG3
technetium (Tc)
  t. albumin colloid
  t. etidronate
  t. 99m albumin aggregated
  t. 99m bicisate
  t. 99m disofenin
  t. 99m ferpentetate
  t. 99m furifosmin
  t. 99m glucepate
  t. 99m HIDA
  t. 99m iron-ascorbate-DTPA
  t. 99m lidofenin

T

technetium *(continued)*
t. 99m macroaggregated albumin
t. 99m medronate
t. 99m mertiatide
t. 99m, or 99mTc
t. 99m oxidronate
t. 99m pertechnetate sodium
t. 99m PIPIDA
t. 99m pyrophosphate
t. 99m sestamibi
t. 99m siboroxime
t. 99m succimer
t. 99m sulfur colloid
t. 99m teboroxime
t. 99m tetrofosmin
t. scan
t. stannous pyrophosphate
^{99m}**technetium** (^{99m}**Tc**)
technetium-gagged Cardiolite
technetium-99m (^{99m}**Tc**)
technician
emergency medical t. (EMT)
psychiatric t.
technique
Abbott fluorescence polarization
immunoassay t.
activation t.
active daydream t.
adaptive t.
Agee t.
Alexander t.
angiographic road-mapping t.
Animal and Opposite Drawing T.
(AODT)
Arana-Iniquez intracranial cyst
removal t.
arousal reduction t.
ascending t.
Asher physical build assessment t.
assets-liabilities t.
average evoked response t.
avidin-biotin stain t.
backward making t.
ballet t.
Barbour t.
behavioral t.
bell and pad t.
biportal t.
blind matching t.
Bohlman cervical fusion t.
boost irradiation t.
brief stimuli t.
Brooks t.
capping t.
carotid preservation t.
cervical screw insertion t.
cervical spondylotic myelopathy
fusion t.
Cloward t.
Cobb t.
cognitive-behavioral t.
compensatory t.
composite addition t.
Cone-Grant t.

continuous-wave t.
contoured anterior spinal plate t.
corrective t.
critical-incident t.
Cushing t.
decortication t.
descending t.
destructive interference t.
direct screw fixation t.
Dolenc t.
double-rod t.
Dowling intracranial cyst
removal t.
Drake tandem clipping t.
drilling t.
Drummond spinous wiring t.
effort-shape t.
empty-chair t.
endovascular t.
facet excision t.
fat-suppression t.
feeding t.
finger fracture t.
fixation t.
Flamm t.
flow detection t.
Fourier transform t.
frameless stereotactic t.
fusion t.
Gallie-Rodgers t.
Gallie wiring t.
glissando t.
gradient recalled echo t. (GRE)
graphomotor t.
Håkanson t.
Halstead modified t.
Harriluque t.
Hartel t.
head turn t.
Hirsch endonasal t.
Holtzman Inkblot T. (HIT)
Hood masking t.
hot-seat t.
House-Tree-Person T.
Hunt-Early t.
hyperventilation activating t.
immunoelectrotransfer blot t.
interspinous segmental spinal
instrumentation t.
interview t.
intravenous oxygen-15 water
bolus t.
ipsilateral transcallosal t.
Jacobs locking hook spinal rod t.
Kennerdell-Maroon t.
kinesthetic t.
Lamaze t.
Leksell t.
Levy Draw-and-Tell-a-Story T.
loss-of-resistance t.
Luque instrumentation concave t.
Luque instrumentation convex t.
Luque sublaminar wiring t.
Luria t.
macroelectrode t.

mandibular swing t.
manipulative t.
Meyer sublaminar wiring t.
microelectrode t.
midface degloving t.
mille pattes t.
mirror t.
t. of Miyazaki and Kato
modified Gilsbach t.
multiple regression t.
Object Relations T.
observation t.
operative t.
Ouchterlony double diffusion t.
paradoxical t.
phase-contrast t.
photic stimulation activating t.
picture in picture t.
plain-folks t.
plateau masking t.
play t.
posterolateral costotransversectomy t.
preservation t.
projective t.
psychoanalytic t.
psychological t.
Q t.
reattribution t.
recombinant DNA t.
reduction t.
relapse-prevention t.
relaxation t.
rest-cure t.
Rorschach Projective T.
Rosenberg Draw-A-Person T.
Roy-Camille t.
screw insertion t.
Seldinger retrograde
  wire/intubation t.
self-control t.
semiautomated spatial
  normalization t.
Senior Apperception T. (SAT)
sensorineural acuity level
  masking t.
shadowing masking t.
shift masking t.
short-term psychotherapy t.
sleep t.
sling/wrapping t.
Smith-Robinson t.
Spiller-Frazier t.
spinal fusion t.
standardized cognitive assessment t.
startle t.
stop-and-think t.
stroboscopic light activating t.
strut fusion t.
subtraction t.
sucking t.
surgical t.
tandem clipping t.
thin-slab acquisition t.
thoracolumbar spondylosis
  surgical t.

threshold shift-masking t.
tilted optimized nonsaturating
  excitation t.
time-of-flight t.
time-out t.
transcortical t.
triple-wire t.
uncovering t.
utilization t.
verbal t.
WAY t.
Whitesides-Kell cervical t.
Who Are You? t.
wire removal t.
word association t.
^{133}Xe intravenous injection t.
technological
  t. detection of deceit
  t. illiteracy
technology
  Cogent microillumination t.
  genetic t.
tecta (*pl. of* tectum)
tectal
  t. glioma
  t. lesion
  t. lipoma
  t. plate tumor
tectobulbar tract
tectopontine tract
tectospinal
  t. decussation
  t. tract
tectum, pl. **tecta**
  t. mesencephali
  optic t.
tecum
  subpoena duces t.
TED
  Tasks of Emotional Development
TEEM
  Test for Examining Expressive
  Morphology
Teen
  T. Addiction Severity Index (T-
  ASI)
teenager
  Problem-Oriented Screening
  Instrument for T.'s (POSIT)
teenage suicide
teen silence
teeth grinding
teetotaler, teetotaller
Teflon
  T. felt
  T. liner
  T. mesh
  T. mesh reinforcement
  T. tube graft
Teflon-coated brain retractor
tefludazine
tegmen, gen. **tegminis**, pl. **tegmina**
  t. cruris
  t. ventriculi quarti
tegmenta (*pl. of* tegmentum)

T

tegmental
t. decussation
t. field of Forel
t. syndrome
tegmentotomy
tegmentum, pl. **tegmenta**
lateral dorsal t.
t. mesencephali
mesencephalic t.
midbrain t.
t. of pons
pontine t.
t. rhombencephali
t. of rhombencephalon
tegmina (*pl. of* tegmen)
tegminis (*gen. of* tegmen)
Tegopen
Tegretol
Tegretol-XR
teichopsia
TEL
Test of Economic Literacy
tela, gen. and pl. **telae**
t. choroidea
t. choroidea inferior
t. choroidea superior
t. choroidea ventriculi quarti
t. choroidea ventriculi tertii
choroid t. of fourth ventricle
choroid t. of third ventricle
t. vasculosa
telalgia
telangiectasia
ataxia t.
calcinosis, Raynaud phenomenon,
esophageal dysmotility,
sclerodactyly, and t. (CREST)
capillary t.
cephalooculocutaneous t.
hereditary hemorrhagic t.
telangiectasis, pl. **telangiectases**
telangiectatic
t. angiomatosis
t. change
t. glioma
telangiectodes
glioma t.
neuroma t.
telangiectatic glioma
TELD
Test of Early Language Development
TELD-2
Test of Early Language Development,
Second Edition
Telebrix
teleceptor
teledendrite
Telefactor beehive system
telegnosis
telegrammatism
telekinesis
telemetric intracranial pressure sensor
telencephalic
t. flexure
t. fusion

t. sleep
t. vein
t. ventriculofugal artery
t. vesicle
telencephalization
telencephalon
teleoanalysis
teleologic
t. hallucination
t. regression
teleological
teleology
teleonomic
teleonomy
teleophobia
teleopsia
Telepaque
telepathic dream
telephone
t. scatologia
t. sex
telephonophobia
teleplasm
teleradiotherapy unit
telergy
telescope
High-Vision surgical t.
Luxtec illuminated surgical t.
Surgi-Spec t.
telescopia
telesensor
Cosman T.
in-line t.
Osaka t.
telesis
telesthesia
Telestill photo adapter
teletactor
teletherapy
televised
t. radiofluoroscopic control
t. radiofluoroscopy
television
closed-circuit t. (CCTV)
television-induced epilepsy
Telfa
T. dressing
T. strip
Tell-Me-A-Story (TEMAS)
tell a tale (TAT)
tellurium (Te)
telodendria
telodendron
telophobia
telovelotonsillar
TEMAS
Tell-Me-A-Story
temazepam
Temodal
temozolomide
temper
t. dyscontrol
t. outburst
temperament
T. Assessment Battery for children

hyperthymic t.
manic t.
t. survey
t. trait
T. and Values Inventory (TVI)
temperance
temperature
ambient t.
basal t.
t. biofeedback
core body t.
t. effect
t. erotism
t. sensation
t. sense
t. spot
temporalis muscle t. (TMT)
temperature, pulse, respiration (TPR)
temperature-sensitive neural progenitor
template
Damasio and Damasio t.
Marchac forehead t.
Temple-Fay laminectomy retractor
tempo
conceptual t.
temporal
t. arachnoid cyst
t. arteritis
t. artery
t. association
t. bone
t. contiguity
t. cortex
t. cortices
t. fossa
t. fossa floor
t. gyrus
t. hallucination
t. headache
t. horn
t. horn atrophy
t. horn neoplasm
t. integration deficit
t. lobe
t. lobectomy
t. lobe epilepsy (TLE)
t. lobe herniation
t. lobe illusion
t. lobe infarction
t. lobe radiation
t. lobe retraction
t. lobe seizure
t. lobe status
t. lobe syndrome
medial superior t. (MST)
t. operculum
t. organization
t. orientation
t. perspective
t. pole
t. relationship
t. speech region
t. stability
t. sulcus
temporal-cerebral arterial anastomosis

temporale
planum t.
temporalis
t. muscle
t. muscle temperature (TMT)
Tutoplast fascia t.
temporal-occipital junction
temporal, occipital, parietal (TOP)
temporal-perceptual disorder
temporarily disabled
temporary
t. admission
t. clip
t. commitment
t. deafness
t. disability
t. epilation
t. habit
t. percutaneous SCS electrode
t. stress
t. threshold shift (TTS)
temporizer
temporofrontal tract
temporolimbic
t. epilepsy
t. system
temporomandibular
t. joint (TMJ)
t. joint arthralgia
t. joint dislocation
t. joint pain
temporomesial region (TMR)
temporooccipital craniotomy
temporoparietal
t. aphasia
t. intrasylvian cortex
temporopolar artery (TPA)
temporopontine tract
temporosuboccipital bone graft
Tempra
temptation
fits of horrific t.
horrific t.
tenascin
Tencet
Tencon
tendency, pl. **tendencies**
acting out t.
t. of action
anagogic t.
antisocial t.
central t.
dependence t.
destructive t.
evasive t.
excitement-seeking t.
familial t.
final t.
hypomanic t.
impulsive t.
insightless t.
introversive t.
katagogic t.
measure of central t.
narcissistic t.

T

tendency *(continued)*
    paranoid t.
    repeat t.
    seductive t.
    self-absorbed t.
    sleep t.
    somatization t.
    suicide t.
    tender-minded t.
    tough-minded t.
    t. toward amelioration
    t. wit
tendentious apperception
tender
    t. line
    t. loving care (TLC)
    t. point
    t. years presumption
    t. zone
tender-minded tendency
tenderness
    scalp t.
tendineus
    annulus t.
tendinum
    subsultus t.
    tremor t.
tendo Achillis reflex
tendon
    t. reflex
    Tutoplast anterior tibialis t.
tenens
    locum t.
tenesmus penis
tenia, pl. **teniae**
    teniae acusticae
    t. choroidea
    t. fimbriae
    t. fornicis
    t. of the fornix
    t. of fourth ventricle
    t. hippocampi
    medullary teniae
    t. semicircularis
    Tarin t.
    t. tecta
    t. telae
    t. terminalis
    t. thalami
    thalamic t.
    t. ventriculi quarti
    t. ventriculi tertii
teniola corporis callosi
Ten-K
Tennessee Self-Concept Scale (TSCS)
Tenoretic
Tenormin
tenosynovectomy
tenoxicam
TENS
    transcutaneous electrical nerve
      stimulation
tense gaze
tensile stress

Tensilon
    T. Injection
    T. test
tension
    combat t.
    emotional t.
    inner t.
    instinctual t.
    marked t.
    mental t.
    t. migraine
    t. migraine headache
    muscular t.
    need t.
    nervous t.
    oxygen t.
    physical t.
    t. pneumocephalus
    premenstrual t.
    t. reduction
    t. reduction therapy
    sexual t.
    social t.
    t. state
    t. state psychoneurotic reaction
    stimulus t.
    t. suture
tension-reduction theory
tension-vascular headache
tensity
tentalum wire tension suture
tenth cranial nerve
tentorial
    t. angle
    t. apex meningioma
    t. herniation
    t. hiatus
    t. incisura
    t. leaf meningioma
    t. plexus
    t. pressure
    t. ring
    t. sinus
    t. traversal
tentorium, pl. **tentoria**
    t. cerebelli
    t. of hypophysis
    notch of t.
Tenuate Dospan
tenuis
    meninx t.
tenuous
TENVAD
    Test of Nonverbal Auditory
      Discrimination
teonanactl
TEP
    trigeminal evoked potential
Tepanil
tephromalacia
tephrylometer
TEPP
    tetraethylpyrophosphate
teratogen
teratogenic syndrome

teratoid tumor
teratological defect
teratology
    mammalian t.
teratoma
    atypical t.
    HcG-secreting suprasellar
      immature t.
    malignant t.
    pineal region t.
    sacrococcygeal t.
teratophobia
Terazoff Act
terbutaline
terebrant, terebrating
terephthalate
    oxycodone t.
teres major muscle
terfenadine
tergiversation
tergo
    coitus á t.
Teridax
terminal
    t. achievement behavior
    t. anoxia
    axon t.
    t. bouton
    t. dementia
    t. filum
    t. ganglion
    t. insomnia
    t. lag
    t. myelocystocele
    t. nerve corpuscle
    t. neuronal field
    t. nuclei
    t. plate
    t. reinforcement
    t. reinforcement psychotherapy
    t. stria
    t. sulcus
    synaptic t.
    t. thread
    t. tremor
    t. vein
    t. ventricle
    t. ventriculostomy
terminale
    filum t.
terminalis
    lamina t.
    primitive lamina t.
    stria t.
    ventriculus t.
terminally ill
terminatio, pl. **terminationes**
    terminationes nervorum liberae
termination
    t. issue
    t. of pregnancy
    t. of therapy
terminological obfuscation

terpin
    t. hydrate elixir
    t. hydrate with codeine
terra firma
terrible
    enfant t.
terrifying
    t. experience
    t. stimulus
territorial
    t. aggression
    t. dominance
territory
    interaction t.
    vascular t.
terror
    current night t.
    day t.
    t. dream
    night t.
    reign of t.
    sleep t.
terrorism behavior
Terson syndrome
tertiary
    t. amine tricyclic antidepressant
      drug
    t. circular reaction
    t. gain
    t. prevention
    t. stress
    t. syphilis
tertiary-process thinking
TES
    Teacher Evaluation Scale
    Team Effectiveness Survey
    therapeutic electrical stimulation
    tridimensional evaluational scale
tesla (T)
    1.5-T. General Electric signa scan
Tesla MRI system
Tessier osteotomy
test
    Ability-to-Benefit Admissions T.
    ABLA t.
    absurdities t.
    Academic Alertness T.
    Academic Aptitude T. (AAT)
    Accounting Program Admission T.
      (APAT)
    accuracy t.
    ACE T.
    ACER Advanced T. B90
    ACER Applied Reading T.
    Achenbach Child Behavior T.
    achievement t. (AT)
    acid t.
    acoustic immittance measurement t.
    Ad7C cerebrospinal fluid t.
    ADL t.
    T. of Adolescent/Adult Word
      Finding (TAWF)
    T. of Adolescent Language
      (TOAL)
    Adolescent Language Screening T.

T

test (continued)
Adolescent Separation Anxiety T.
adrenalin-mecholyl t.
Adson t.
t. age (TA)
Age Projection T. (APT)
AH4 Group Intelligence T.
aiming t.
Ainsworth Strange Situation T.
air conduction t.
Akerfeldt T.
Alcadd T.
Alcock t.
Allen t.
Allied Health Professions
  Admission T.
alpha verbal t.
alternate binaural loudness
  balance t.
alternate response t.
alternate uses t.
American Law Institute T.
Ammons quick t.
amphetamine challenge t.
analyst anchor t.
anchor t.
t. anxiety
t. anxiety inventory
T. Anxiety Profile
T. Anxiety Scale
Aphasia Screening T. (AST)
apperception t.
apprehension t.
Aptitude Research Project T.
Armed Forces Qualification T.
  (AFQT)
Army General Classification T.
  (AGCT)
ARS art t.
art t.
Arthur Point Scale of
  Performance T.
articulation t.
T. of Articulation Performance -
  Diagnostic (TAP-D)
T. of Articulation Performance,
  Screen (TAP-S)
Assigning Structure Stages T.
association t.
attention alertness t.
T. of Attentional Style
T. of Attitude Toward School
  (TAS)
Auditory Apperception T. (AAT)
T. for Auditory Comprehension of
  Language (TACL)
T.'s for Auditory Comprehension
  of Language-Revised (TACL-R)
Auditory Discrimination T. (ADT)
T. of Auditory Discrimination
  (TAD)
Aussage t.
axial manual traction t.
ball-and-field t.

balloon occlusion t.
Bankson Language T.-2 (BLT-2)
Bankson Language Screening T.
  (BLST)
Bárány t.
Barranquilla Rapid Survey
  Intelligence T. (BARSIT)
Basic Educational Skills T.
t.'s of basic experience (TOBE)
Basic Language Concepts T.
Basic Occupational Literacy T.
  (BOLT)
Basic School Skills Inventory
battery t.
t. battery
battery t.
Beery-Buktinica Developmental T.
Beery Visual Motor T.
Behavioral Assessment T.
Behavioral Inattention T. (BIT)
Behn-Rorschach T.
Bekesy Functionality Detection T.
  (BFDT)
Bender-Gestalt T. (BGT)
Bender-Gestalt Visual Motor T.
Bender Visual-Motor Gestalt T.
  (BVMGT)
Bender Visual Retention T.
Bennett Mechanical
  Comprehension T.
Benton Face Recognition T.
Benton Line Orientation T.
Benton Revised Visual
  Retention T.
Benton Visual Retention T.
  (BVRT)
Bero T.
beta t.
Bielschowsky head tilt t.
Bilingual Syntax Measure II T.
  (BSM)
Binet t.
Binet-Simon t.
Bingham Button T. (BBT)
binomial t.
Blessed IMC T.
Blessed Information and
  Concentration T.
Blessed Information-Memory-
  Concentration T.
Blind Learning Aptitude T.
block design t.
blood t.
blood screen for drugs t.
Bloom Analogies T.
Bolgar-Fischer Word T.
Boston Famous Faces T.
Boston Naming T.
brain t.
Brief Alcoholism Screening T.
bromocriptine t.
Brook Reaction T. (BRT)
Bruininks-Oseretsky T.
Bruininks-Oseretsky Standardized T.
Bryant-Schwan Design T. (BSDT)

Buschke Free and Cued Selective
  Reminding T.
Buschke-Fuld Selective Memory T.
Buschke Selective Reminding T.
Buschke Short-Term Recall T.
calculation t.
California Achievement T. (CAT)
California Achievement T., Fifth
  Edition (CAT/5)
California Critical Thinking
  Skills T. (CCTST)
California T. of Mental Maturity,
  Short-Form
California Motor Accuracy T.,
  Southern Revised
California Psychological
  Inventory T. (CPIT)
California Verbal Learning T.
  (CVLT)
caloric t.
Canadian Cognitive Abilities T.
  (CCAT)
cancellation t.
Canter Background Interference
  Procedure for the Bender
  Gestalt T.
cardiac function t.
card-sorting t.
carotid ultrasound t.
Carrell Discrimination T.
Carrow Receptive Language T.
t. case
Category T. (CT)
cause-and-effect t.
ceruloplasmin t.
challenge t.
Charteris Reading T.
Children of Alcoholism
  Screening T. (CAST)
Children's Apperception T. (CAT)
Children's Apperceptive Story-
  Telling T. (CAST)
Children's Articulation T. (CAT)
Children's Auditory Verbal
  Learning T.-2 (CAVLT-2)
Children's Embedded Figures T.
  (CEFT)
chi square t.
chloride t.
cholecystokinin t.
city and state t.
classification t.
clock face t.
Clymer-Barrett Readiness T.
Cochran-Mantel-Haenszel T.
code t.
Cognitive Abilities T. (CAT)
T. of Cognitive Style in
  Mathematics (TCSM)
CO$_2$ inhalation t.
College Ability T. (CAT)
color sorting t.
combining power t. (CPT)
Communication Abilities
  Diagnostic T. (CADT)

completion, arithmetic, vocabulary,
  and directions t.
Complex Figure T. (CFT)
complex thematic pictures t.
Comprehensive T. of Basic Skills,
  Forms U and V
Computerized Reaction Time T.
Concentration Performance T.
  (CPT)
concentration performance t.
Concept Mastery T. (CMT)
Conceptual Systems T. (CST)
T. of Concept Utilization (TCU)
t. condition
confrontation naming t.
Continuous Performance T. (CPT)
Continuous Visual Memory T.
  (CVMT)
Coombs t.
Cooperative Primary T. (CPT)
Cooper-MacGuire Diagnostic Word
  Analysis T.
Coping with Stress T.
copy geometric designs t.
copy intersecting pentagons t.
could not t. (CNT)
count backwards from 100 t.
countercurrent
  immunoelectrophoresis t.
CO$_2$-withdrawal seizure t.
C-reactive protein t.
T. of Creative Potential
creativity t.
t. of criminal responsibility
criterion-referenced t.
Crithidia IFA t.
Critical Reasoning T. (CRT)
Cultural Literacy T.
Culture Fair Intelligence T. (CFIT)
Culture Free T. (CFT)
Culture Free Intelligence T. (CFIT)
cumulative t.
DAP T.
day of month t.
Decoding Skills T.
delayed-alteration t.
delayed-matching t.
Del Rio Language Screening T.
  (DRLST)
Denver Developmental Screening T.
  (DDST)
Denver II t.
development t.
Developmental Articulation T.
  (DAT)
developmental hand-function t.
  (DHFT)
Developmental Sentence Scoring T.
dexamethasone suppression t. (DST,
  DXM)
Deyerle sciatic tension t.
Differential Aptitude T. (DAT)
Digital Finger Tapping T. (DFTT)
digit repetition t.
digit reversal t.

T

test *(continued)*

digits t.
Digit Span Distractibility T.
Digit Symbol T.
Dix-Hallpike t.
dominance t.
Draw-A-Bicycle T.
Draw-A-Clock-Face T.
Draw-A-Family T.
Draw-A-Flower T.
Draw-A-House T.
Draw-A-Man T.
Draw-A-Person T.
Draw-A-Picture-From-Memory T.
drawing t.
Dunnett t.
Durham t.
Dyslexia Determination T.
T. of Early Language Development (TELD)
T. of Early Language Development, Second Edition (TELD-2)
Early Speech Perception T. (ESP)
Eating Attitudes T.
Ebbinghaus curve of retention t.
T. of Economic Literacy (TEL)
Edinburgh Articulation T. (EAT)
Edinburgh Picture T.
Edinburgh Reading T.
edrophonium chloride t.
educational t.
Education Apperception T. (EAT)
Effective Reading T.
Ego-Ideal and Conscience Development T. (EICDT)
Eidetic Parents T. (EPT)
Elihorn Maze T.
ELISA t.
Embedded Figures T. (EFT)
empirical t.
Employee Aptitude Survey T.
essay t.
Examining for Aphasia T.
T. for Examining Expressive Morphology (TEEM)
excitability t.
Expressive One Word Picture Vocabulary T.
Expressive One-Word Picture Vocabulary T., Upper Extension
fables t.
Face-Hand T.
Facial Recognition T.
Fairview Language Evaluation T. (FLET)
Family Apperception T. (FAT)
Family Attitudes T. (FAT)
Family Relations T. (FRT)
Famous Sayings T.
ferritin t.
FES figure-drawing t.
Figurative Language Interpretation T. (FLIT)

figure-drawing t.
Filtered Audiometer Speech T. (FAST)
Finckh T.
Finger Localization T.
finger-nose t.
Finger Oscillation T. (FOT)
Finger Tapping T.
finger-to-finger t.
Fisher exact t.
Flanagan Aptitude Classification T. (FACT)
Flanagan Industrial T. (FIT)
fluorescent treponemal antibody absorption t. (FTA-ABS)
Fölling t.
forced choice of recognition t.
Forer Structured Sentence Completion T.
Fournier t.
Four Picture T.
Franck Drawing Completion T. (FDCT)
Freeman Anxiety Neurosis and Psychosomatic T. (FANPT)
Frenchay Aphasia Screening T. (FAST)
Fuld Object Memory T.
fund of information t.
Funkenstein t.
Fused Rhymed Dichotic Words T.
F-wave t.
Galveston Orientation and Awareness T. (GOAT)
Gates-MacGinitie Reading T.
Gates-McKillop-Horowitz Reading Diagnostic T.
General Clerical T. (GCT)
Gerontological Apperception T. (GAT)
Gesell Preschool T.
Gesell School Readiness T.
glycerol t.
Goldman-Fristoe-Woodcock T.
Goldscheider t.
Goodenough Animal T.
Goodenough Draw-A-Man T.
Goodenough Draw-A-Person T.
Goodenough-Harris Drawings T.
good and evil t.
Gordon Diagnostic System T.
Graded Naming T.
Graded Word Spelling T.
Graduate Record Examination Aptitude T. (GREAT)
Grassi Block Substitution T.
Gray Oral Reading T.
Gray Oral Reading T., Third Edition (GORT-3)
grip strength t.
Grooved Pegboard T.
Group Embedded Figures T. (GEFT)
Group Reading T. (GRT)

Guilford-Zimmerman Personality T.
(GZPT)
Guthrie t.
Hallpike t.
Halstead Aphasia T. (HAT)
Halstead Category T.
Halstead-Wepman Aphasia
Screening T.
hand t. (HT)
Hand Dynamometer T. (HDT)
Hanfmann-Kasanin Concept
Formation T.
Harding W87 T.
head-dropping t.
Healy Pictorial Completion T.
heel-tap t.
heel-to-knee t.
Henderson-Moriarty ESL/Literacy
Placement T.
Hendler t.
Henmon-Nelson Ability T.,
Canadian Edition
Henmon-Nelson Ability T.,
Canadian Edition
hidden clue t.
hidden figures t.
Hirschberg t.
Hodkinson Mental T. (HMT)
Hollander t.
Holter monitor t.
Hooper Visual Organization T.
Horn-Hellersberg Drawing
Completion T.
House-Tree T. (HT)
House-Tree-Person T.
Howell Prekindergarten
Screening T.
HTP t.
Hundred Pictures Naming T.
(HPNT)
H-wave t.
hyperventilation t.
IDEA Oral Language
Proficiency T. II
identification t.
IER t.
Illinois Children's language
Assessment T.
immediate memory t.
immunofluorescence t.
Improving Writing, Thinking and
Reading Skills t.
incomplete-pictures t.
incomplete-sentence t.
incomplete sentence blank t.
individual t.
infant and preschool t.
Infant Reading T.
Informal Reading Comprehension
Placement T.
information t.
inkblot t. (IBT)
Institute of Educational
Research T.

Institute for Personality and
Ability T.
Instrument Timbre Preference T.
insulin hypoglycemia t.
Integration T.
Intelligence Quotient t.
intelligibility t.
interest t.
Intermediate Booklet Category T.
internal carotid balloon t.
Interpersonal Reaction T. (IPRT)
Inter-Person Perception T. (IPPT)
t. interpretation
interpretation t.
inventory t.
Iowa Algebra Aptitude T. (IAAT)
Iowa T.'s of Educational
Development, Forms X-8 and Y-
8
Iowa Pressure Articulation T.
(IPAT)
IQ T.
Irresistible Impulse T.
ischemic forearm exercise t.
isoproterenol tilt table t.
Item Counseling Evaluation T.
48-Item Counseling Evaluation T.
(ICET)
15-Item Memorization T.
James Language Dominance T.
Janet t.
Jenkins Non-Verbal T.
job-specific t.
Johnson-Kenney Screening T.
(JKST)
Jolly t.
Jordan Left-Right Reversal T.
Joseph Pre-School and Primary
Self-Concept Screening T.
Jung association t.
Kahn Intelligence T. (KIT)
Kasanin-Hanfmann Concept
Formation T.
Katzman t.
Kaufman Adolescent and Adult
Intelligence T. (KAIT)
Kaufman Brief Intelligence T. (K-
BIT)
Kent EGY T.
Kent-Rosanoff T.
Kernig t.
Kindergarten Auditory Screening T.
(KAST)
Kindergarten Language
Screening T. (KLST)
Kindergarten Readiness T. (KRT)
knowledge t.
Knowledge of Occupations T.
(KOT)
Knox Cube T.
Kohnstamm T.
Kohs Block T.
Kohs Block-Design T.
Krimsky t.
Kveim t.

T

test *(continued)*
    laboratory t.
    labyrinthine fistula t.
    lactate dehydrogenase t.
    T. of Language Competence (TLC)
    T. of Language Competence for Children (TLC-C)
    T. of Language Development (TOLD)
    T. of Language Development - Intermediate, Second Edition (TOLD-I:2)
    T. of Language Development - Primary, Second Edition (TOLD-P:2)
    Language Processing T.
    Language Screening T.
    Lasègue t.
    L-dopa stimulation t.
    learning t.
    T. of Learning Accuracy in Children (TLAC)
    Learning Efficiency T.-II (LET-II)
    leg-raising t.
    lidocaine t.
    Lincoln-Oseretsky Motor Performance T. (LOMPT)
    Lindamood Auditory Conceptualization T. (LACT)
    T. of Listening Accuracy in Children (TLAC)
    Listening Comprehension T. (LCT)
    literacy t.
    liver function t.
    Loevinger's Washington University Sentence Completion T.
    logical memory t.
    Lombard T.
    Lorge-Thorndike Cognitive Abilities T.
    Lorge-Thorndike Intelligence T.
    LOTE Reading and Listening T.
    Luria T.
    Machover Draw-A-Person T. (MDAP)
    Macmillan Graded Word Reading T.
    making change t.
    Male Impotence T. (MIT)
    Management Position Analysis T.
    Manipulative Aptitude T. (MAT)
    Mann-Whitney t.
    Mann-Whitney U T.
    Mantel-Haenszel T.
    Matas t.
    matching t.
    Matching Familiar Figures T. (MFFT)
    Matrix Analogies T.
    Maudsley Mentation T. (MaMT)
    maze t.
    McCarthy Screening T.
    Medical College Admission T. (MCAT)

Meeting Street School Screening T. (MSSST)
melatonin t.
memory t.
Memory-for-Designs T.
mental status t.
Merrill-Palmer Scale of Mental T.'s
Mertens Visual Perception T. (MVPT)
methylphenidate challenge t.
Metropolitan Achievement T. (MAT)
Metropolitan Achievement T., Seventh Edition (MAT7)
Metropolitan Language Instructional T.
Metropolitan Readiness T. (MRT)
metyrapone t.
MFD T.
Michigan Alcoholism Screening T. (MAST)
MicroFet 2 muscle t.
Miller Analogies T. (MAT)
Miller-Fisher t.
Miller-Yoder Language Comprehension T.
Minimum Essentials T. (MET)
Minnesota Clerical T. (MCT)
Minnesota Clerical Aptitude T. (MCAT)
Minnesota Engineering Analogies T. (MEAT)
Minnesota Mechanical Assembly T. (MMAT)
Minnesota Paper Form Board T. (MPFBT)
Minnesota Percepto-Diagnostic T. (MPDT)
Minnesota Rate of Manipulation T.
Minnesota Scholastic Aptitude T. (MSAT)
Minnesota Spatial Relations T. (MSRT)
misplaced objects t.
missing-parts t.
Missouri Auditory Learning T.
M'Naghten t.
Modern Occupational Skills T. (MOST)
Modified Vygotsky Concept Formation T.
Modified Word Learning T. (MWLT)
Monotic Word Memory T. (MWMT)
Mooney T.
Mooney Faces Closure T.
morphine-naloxone t.
Mosaic T.
Motivation Analysis T. (MAT)
Motor-Free Visual Perception T. (MVPT)
Motor Impersistence T. (MIT)
motor performance t.

multi-item t.
Multiple Aptitude T.
Multiple Sleep Latency T. (MSLT)
multiplication table t.
Myers-Briggs psychological t.
Myokinetic Psychodiagnosis T.
Naffziger t.
Nalline t.
name the date t.
Names Learning T. (NLT)
naming common objects t.
National Adult Reading T. (NART)
National Attention T. (NAT)
National Educational
  Development T.
National Police Officer
  Selection T. (POST)
need a sentence t.
neostigmine t.
neuroendocrine t.
neuropsychiatric t.
neuropsychologic t.
neuropsychometric t.
Neurotic Personality Factor T.
  (NPFT)
Newman-Keuls T.
New Mexico Attitude Toward
  Work T. (NMATWT)
New Mexico Career Planning T.
  (NMCPT)
New Mexico Job Application
  Procedures T. (NMJAPT)
New Mexico Knowledge of
  Occupations T. (NMKOT)
nicotine t.
nocturnal penile tumescence t.
Non-Language Learning T.
Non-Language Multi-Mental T.
Non-Reading Intelligence T., Levels
  1-3 (NRIT)
Nonverbal Ability T. (NAT)
T. of Nonverbal Auditory
  Discrimination (TENVAD,
  TNVAD)
T. of Nonverbal Intelligence
  (TONI)
Norris Educational Achievement T.
  (NEAT)
Northwestern Syntax Screening T.
  (NSST)
Northwestern University Children's
  Perception of Speech T.
NUM t.
number 3 traced on patient's
  palm t.
Numerical Attention T. (NAT)
Nymox urinary t.
object t. (OT)
t. object
Object Classification T. (OCT)
objective t. (OT)
Object Sorting T. (OST)
O'Brien Vocabulary Placement T.
occupational t.

Occupational Test Series-Basic
  Skills T.
oculocephalic t.
Office Skills T.
OISE Picture Reasoning T. (PRT)
Oliphant Auditory Discrimination
  Memory T. (OADMT)
Oliphant Auditory Synthesizing T.
  (OAST)
One Word Receptive Picture
  Vocabulary T.
opposites t.
oral t.
Oral Language Sentence Imitation
  Screening T. (OLSIST)
Oral Verbal Intelligence T. (OVIT)
Organic Integrity T. (OIT)
orientation-memory-concentration t.
t. orientation procedure (TOP)
Orleans-Hanna Algebra
  Prognosis T.
Otis-Lennon Mental Ability T.
  (OLMAT)
Otis-Lennon School Ability T.
Otis Quick Scoring Mental
  Abilities T.
Paced Auditory Serial Addition T.
  (PASAT)
Pachon t.
Pain Apperception T. (PAT)
palmomental t.
Pantomime Recognition T. (PRT)
paragraph-meaning t.
paragraph recall t.
paternity t.
Patrick t.
Peabody Individual Achievement T.
  (PIAT)
Peabody Mathematics Readiness T.
Peabody Picture Vocabulary T.
  (PPVT)
Peabody Vocabulary T. (PVT)
Pediatric Speech Intelligibility T.
T.'s of Perception of Scientists
  and Self (TOPOSS)
Perceptual Maze T.
performance t.
Performance Efficiency T.
peripheral cue t.
personality t.
personnel t.
Phalen t.
Photo Articulation T. (PAT)
photometrazol t.
Physiognomic Cue T. (PCT)
Picture Anomalies T.
Picture Articulation and Language
  Screening T. (PALST)
Picture Identification T. (PIT)
Picture Interpretation T.
Picture Reasoning T. (PRE, PRT)
Picture Story Language T. (PSLT)
Picture World T.
PIL T.
pin t.

T

test *(continued)*

Pinter-Paterson Scale of Performance T.
placement t.
point localization t.
t. point scale
Politte Sentence Completion T.
Porteus Maze T. (PMT)
power t.
T. of Pragmatic Language (TOPL)
Pragmatics Screening T.
Predictive Ability T. (PAT)
preemployment screening t.
Pre-Professional Skills T.
Preschool Language Screening T.
Preschool Screening T.
Preschool Speech and Language Screening T.
presidents t.
Primary Mental Abilities T. (PMAT)
Primary Visual Motor T. (PVMT)
Printing Performance School Readiness T. (PPRST)
T. of Problem Solving
Professional Employment T. (PET)
Projective Human Figure Drawing T.
prostigmin t.
t. protocol
proverb interpretation t.
psychoacoustic t. (PAT)
psychoeducational t.
psycholinguistic t.
psychological t.
psychometric t.
psychomotor t.
psychopenetration t.
psychophysiological t.
Psychosocial History Screening T. (PHST)
pull t.
Purdue Pegboard Dexterity T.
Purpose in Life T.
Q t.
quantitative t. (Q)
Quantitative Sudomotor Axon Reflex T. (Q-SART)
Queckenstedt t.
Queckenstedt-Stookey t.
Quick T. (QT)
Quick Neurological Screening T.
Quick Picture Vocabulary T. (QPVT)
Quick-Score Achievement T.
Quick Word T.
Random Letter T.
Rape Aftermath Symptom T.
Rathus Assertiveness T.
Raven Colored Progressive Matrices T. (RCPMT)
reaction t.
readiness t.
reality t.

recall of information t.
recall 5 items after 5 minutes t.
Receptive One Word Picture Vocabulary T. (ROWPVT)
Recognition Memory T.
Reductions in Eating Attitudes T.
Reitan-Indiana Aphasia Screening T. (RIAST)
Reitan-Klove Tactile Form Recognition T.
relations t.
Remote Associates T. (RAT)
Repertory T.
repetition t.
reversal t.
reverse digit span recall t.
Revised Token T.
Rey Auditory Verbal Learning T. (RAVLT)
Rey Complex Figure T.
Rey-Osterrieth Complex Figure Copy and Delayed Recall T.
Rey and Taylor Complex Figure T.
rhythm t.
Right-Left Orientation T. (RLO)
right-wrong t.
Riley Articulation and Language T. (RALT)
Rinne t.
Rivermead ADL T.
Rivermead Behavioral Memory T. (RBMT)
Rivermead Behavioural Memory T.
Roeder Manipulative Aptitude T.
Role Construct Repertory T.
Romberg t.
Rorschach Content T. (RCT)
Rorschach Inkblot T.
rose bengal t.
Rosenberg Draw-A-Person T.
Rosen Drawing T.
rotation t.
Rotter Sentence Completion T. (RSCT)
RPR t.
3-R's T.
Sabin-Feldman dye t.
Sales Style Diagnostic T.
SB t.
SB intelligence t.
Scaled Curriculum Achievement Levels T. (SCALE)
SCAN-TRON Reading T.
Schaie-Thurstone Adult Mental Abilities T.
Schilling t.
Schirmer t.
Schlichter t.
Scholastic Aptitude T. (SAT)
School Ability T. (SAT)
School Attitude T. (SAT)
School and College Ability T. (SCAT)
School Library/Media Skills T.

School Motivation Analysis T. (SMAT)
School Readiness Screening T.
Schwabach T.
Scott Mental Alertness T.
screening t.
Seashore Rhythm T. (SRT)
Seeking of Noetic Goals T.
Selective Reminding T.
self-administered alcohol screening t. (SAAST)
self-rating t.
Senior Apperception T. (SAT)
Sensory Integration and Praxis T.'s (SIPT)
sensory-perceptual t.
Sentence Closure T.
Sentence Completion T. (SCT)
Sequential T.'s of Educational Progress, Series III (STEP-III)
serial sevens t. (7's)
serologic t.
Sex Knowledge and Attitude T. (SKAT)
Sexual Compatibility T. (SCT)
Shapes Analysis T. (SAT)
Shapiro-Wilk t.
Shipley Abstraction T.
Short Category T.
Short Employment T.'s
Shortened Edinburgh Reading T.'s
Short Michigan Alcoholism Screening T. (SMAST)
short orientation-memory-concentration t. (OMC)
t. of significance
similarities mental status t.
Similes T.
Single and Double Simultaneous Stimulation T.
situational t.
Slingerland Screening T.'s (SST)
Slosson Drawing Coordination T.
Slosson Intelligence T. (SIT)
Smell Identification T.
sobriety t.
T. of Social Inferences (TSI)
Social Intelligence T.
Social Relations T. (SRT)
Sorting of Figures T. (SOFT)
Southern California Postrotary Nystagmus T.
Southern California Sensory Integration T.'s
Spadafore Diagnostic Reading T.
span recall t.
SPAR Spelling and Reading T.
Spatial Orientation Memory T. (SOMT)
Spatial Span T.
speech discrimination t.
Speech-Sound Perception T. (SSPT)
spell-a-word-backwards t.
spider's web t.
Spondee Picture T. (SPT)

spontaneity t.
SRA Arithmetic T.
SRA Pictorial Reasoning T.
SRA Reading T.
SSC t.
standardization of a t.
standardized t. (ST)
Stanford Achievement T. (SAT)
Stanford-Binet intelligence t.
Stanford Diagnostic Arithmetic T.
Stanford Diagnostic Reading T. (SDRT)
Stanford Early School Achievement T.
State-Trait Anxiety Inventory for Stein Sentence Completion t.
station t.
Stein Sentence Completion T.
Stenger T.
Stephens Oral Language Screening T. (SOLST)
stimulant challenge t.
t. stimulus
Stimulus-Recognition T.
straight leg raising t.
Strength of Grip T.
Strong vocational interest t.
Stroop Color-Word Interference T.
Stroop Interference T.
Structured Photographic Expressive Language T.-II (SPELT-P)
Structure of Intellect Learning Abilities T., From P
Student *t* t.
STYCAR Hearing T. (SHT)
STYCAR Language T. (SLT)
STYCAR Vision T. (SVT)
Supervisory Practices T. (SPT)
suppression t.
Suprathreshold Adaptation T. (STAT)
sweating t.
sweep-cheek t.
swinging-flashlight t.
Swinging Story T.
Symbol Digit Modalities T. (SDMT)
Symbolic Play T. (SPT)
T. of Syntactic Ability (TSA)
Synthetic Sentence Identification T.
Szondi T.
t t.
Tactile Finger Recognition T. (TFRT)
Tactile Form Recognition T. (TFRT)
Tactile Naming T.
Tactile Performance T. (TPT)
Tensilon t.
theatrical t.
Thematic Apperception T. (TAT)
Thematic Aptitude T. (TAT)
thematic picture t.
The Mega T.
thenar weakness t.

T

test *(continued)*
This I Believe T.
Three-Dimensional Block
  Construction T. (3DBCT)
Three Minute Reasoning T.
three-stage command t.
three-tube t.
three-word recall t.
thyroid function t. (TFT)
TIB T. (TIB)
Time Sense T.
Tinker Toy T.
tolerance t.
Tomkins-Horn Picture
  Arrangement T.
TPI t.
Trail Making T. (TMT)
Treponema pallidum
  immobilization t.
Tukey t.
tuning fork t.
Twenty Statements T. (TST)
tyramine challenge t.
T. of Variables of Attention
  (TOVA)
VASC t.
VDRL t.
Venereal Disease Research
  Laboratory t.
Verbal-Auditory Screen for
  Children t.
Verbal-Auditory Screen for
  Children T.
Verbal Fluency T.
Verbal Meaning T.
Vigotsky T.
visual choice reaction time t.
visual distortion t. (VDT)
visual evoked response t.
Visual Form Discrimination T.
  (VFDT)
Visual Motor T.
Visual-Motor Gestalt T. (VMGT)
T. of Visual Motor Integration
Visual-Motor Integration T. (VMIT)
Visual-Motor Sequencing T.
  (VMST)
Visual Neglect T.
Visual Pattern Completion t.
Visual Perception T.
T. of Visual Perception
Visual Retention T.
Visual Search and Attention T.
  (VSAT)
visual threat t.
vocabulary t.
Vocational Apperception T. (VAT)
von Frey t.
Vygotsky Concept Formation T.,
  Modified
Wada t.
WAIS-R Block Design T.
Warrington Recognition Memory T.

Washington Speech Sound
  Discrimination T. (WSSDT)
Washington University Sentence
  Completion T. (WUSCT)
WAY t.
Weber t.
Weinstein Enhanced Sensory T.
  (WEST)
Weiss Comprehensive
  Articulation T.
Weiss Intelligibility T.
Welsh Figure Preference T.
Wepman Auditory
  Discrimination T.
Wesman Personnel Classification T.
Western blot t.
Who Are You? t.
Wide Range Achievement T.
  (WRAT)
Wide Range Achievement T.-
  Revised (WRAT, WRAT-R)
Wide Range Employment
  Sample T. (WREST)
Wide Range Intelligence and
  Personality T. (WRIPT)
Wide Range Interest-Opinion T.
  (WRIOT)
Wiggly Block T.
Wilcoxon rank sum t.
Wisconsin Card-Sorting T. (WCST)
Wisconsin Scoring T.
Wittenborn Psychiatric Rating
  Scale T.
Wonderlic Personnel T.
Woodcock-Johnson Achievement T.
  (WJAT)
Woodcock Reading Mastery T.
Word Association T.
word-building t.
T. of Word Finding (TWF)
Word Finding T.
T. of Word Finding in Discourse
  (TWFD)
Word Fluency T.
Word-in-Context T.
Word Processing T.
Word Recognition T.
T. of Work Competency and
  Stability (TWCS)
work-limit t.
T. of Written Language (TOWL)
T. of Written spelling
X-O t.
Yerkes-Bridges T. (YBT)
Zimmerman Personality T.
Zulliger T.
testamentary capacity
tester
West hand and foot nerve t.
testes (*pl. of* testis)
testicular
t. atrophy
t. feminization mutation (TFM)
t. feminization syndrome (TFS)

t. hypofunction
t. insufficiency
testimonial privilege
testimony
expert t.
testing
adaptive t.
air conduction t.
American College of T. (ACT)
Amsler grid t.
attention t.
autoantibody assay t.
biomechanical t.
caloric t.
cerebellar aggregation culture for
  teratogenicity t.
conduction t.
confrontation t.
cortical t.
cross-cultural t.
cultural t.
demarcation in sensory t.
Diamox challenge t.
diminished reality t.
electrodiagnostic t.
t. and evaluation (T&E)
functional gain t.
gross impairment of reality t.
hypothesis t.
Individualized Criterion
  Referenced T. (ICRT)
Institute of Personality and
  Ability T. (IPAT)
intraarterial Amytal t.
intracarotid sodium Amytal
  memory t.
intracorporeal pharmacological t.
mental t.
motivation analysis t.
National Occupation Competency T.
  (NOCT)
neurophysiological t.
neuropsychologic t.
t., orientation, and work
t., orientation, and work evaluation
  for rehabilitation (TOWER)
post hoc t.
provocative t.
Psychoacoustic T. (PAT)
psychologic t.
psychological t.
psychometric t.
reality t.
reality ability t.
school-age t.
**Testing-Teaching Module of Auditory
Discrimination (TTMAD)**
testis, pl. **testes**
irritable t.
testophobia
testosterone
t. enanthate
serum t.
testosterone-estradiol-binding globulin

test-retest
t.-r. reliability
t.-r. reliability coefficient
Tesuloid
tetani
Clostridium t.
tetania
t. epidemica
t. gastrica
t. gravidarum
t. neonatorum
t. parathyreopriva
t. rheumatica
tetanic
t. contraction (Te)
t. convulsion
t. seizure
t. stimulation
tetaniform
tetanigenous
tetanilla
tetanism
tetanization
tetanode
tetanoid
t. chorea
t. epilepsy
t. paraplegia
tetanometer
tetanomotor
tetanus
t. anticus
apyretic t.
benign t.
cephalic t.
cerebral t.
t. completus
t. dorsalis
drug t.
extensor t.
flexor t.
generalized t.
head t.
hydrophobic t.
imitative t.
intermittent t.
local t.
t. neonatorum
t. posticus
Ritter opening t.
Rose cephalic t.
toxic t.
t. toxoid
traumatic t.
tetany
t. of alkalosis
duration t. (DT)
epidemic t.
gastric t.
hyperventilation t.
hypoparathyroid t.
infantile t.
latent t.
manifest t.
neonatal t.

T

tetany *(continued)*
    parathyroid t.
    parathyroprival t.
    postoperative t.
    rheumatic t.
tetchy
tête-à-tête
tethered
    t. spinal cord
    t. spinal cord syndrome
tethering
tetrabenazine
tetrabromophenolphthalein
tetracaine and dextrose
tetrachloride
    carbon t.
tetracyclic antidepressant
tetracycline
tetrad
    narcoleptic t.
tetraethylpyrophosphate (TEPP)
tetraethylthiuram disulfide
tetrahydroaminoacridine (THA)
tetrahydrobiopterin
tetrahydrocannabinol dependence
tetrahydronaphthalene
tetrahydropyridine
    1-methyl-4-phenyl-1,2,3,6-t.
    N-methyl-4-phenyl-1,2,3,6-t.
tetraiodophenolphthalein
tetraparalysis
tetraparesis
tetrapeptide
    cholecystokinin t. (CCK-4)
tetraplegia
tetrasomy
tetrofosmin
    technetium 99m t.
teutonomania
teutonophobia, teutophobia
Tew cranial spinal retractor
Texas
    T. Revised Inventory of Grief
    T. Scottish Rite Hospital (TSRH)
    T. Scottish Rite Hospital corkscrew device
    T. Scottish Rite Hospital crosslink
    T. Scottish Rite Hospital cross-link system
    T. Scottish Rite Hospital eyebolt spreader
    T. Scottish Rite Hospital hook holder
    T. Scottish Rite Hospital hook inserter
    T. Scottish Rite Hospital I-bolt
    T. Scottish Rite Hospital mini-corkscrew device
    T. Scottish Rite Hospital pedicle screw
    T. Scottish Rite Hospital rod fixation
    T. Scottish Rite Hospital screw-rod system

    T. Scottish Rite Hospital trial hook
    T. Scottish Rite Hospital wrench
text
    t. blindness
    pragmatic t.
textbook case
textual description
texture
    causal t.
    t. response
TF
    transvestic fetishism
TFC
    threaded fusion cage
TFCQ
    Toronto Functional Capacity Questionnaire
TFM
    testicular feminization mutation
TFNE
    transient focal neurologic event
TFRT
    Tactile Finger Recognition Test
    Tactile Form Recognition Test
TFS
    testicular feminization syndrome
TFT
    thyroid function test
6TG
    6-thioguanine
TGA
    transient global amnesia
T-Gesic
T-group
    training group
THA
    tetrahydroaminoacridine
    transient hemisphere attack
thaasophobia
Thackray Reading Readiness Profile (TRRP)
thalamectomy
thalamencephalic
thalamencephalon
thalami (*pl. of* thalamus)
thalamic
    t. aphasia
    t. astrocytoma
    t. circulation
    t. dementia
    t. epilepsy
    t. glioma
    t. gustatory nucleus
    t. hemorrhage
    t. hyperesthetic anesthesia
    t. infarction
    t. lesion
    t. neglect
    t. pain
    t. pain syndrome
    t. reticular activating system
    t. stimulation
    t. tenia
    t. tumor

thalamic-subthalamic hemorrhage
thalamocaudate
    t. arteriovenous malformation
    t. artery
thalamocortical
    t. activity
    t. pathway
    t. projection
    t. relay (TCR)
thalamogeniculate artery
thalamopeduncular infarction
thalamoperforating artery
thalamoperforator
thalamostriate vein
thalamotomy
    gamma t.
    staged bilateral stereotactic t.
    stereotactic t.
    stereotactic VL t.
    ventrolateralis t.
    Vim t.
    VL t.
thalamus, pl. thalami
    anterior nuclei of t.
    motor t.
    nuclei anteriores thalami
    nuclei intralaminares thalami
    nucleus arcuatus thalami
    nucleus centralis lateralis thalami
    nucleus lateralis thalami
    nucleus medialis thalami
    nucleus medialis centralis thalami
    nucleus paracentralis thalami
    nucleus reticularis thalami
    nucleus ventralis anterior thalami
    nucleus ventralis intermedius
     thalami
    nucleus ventralis posterior thalami
    nucleus ventralis posterior
     intermedius thalami
    nucleus ventralis posterolateralis
     thalami
    paramedian t.
thalassemia
thalassomania
thalassophobia
thalassoposia
thalectomy
thalidomide
Thalitone
thallium
    t. peripheral neuropathy
    t. poisoning
    t. polyneuropathy
thallium-201 (^{201}Tl)
THAM-E Injection
THAM Injection
thanatography
thanatology
thanatomania
thanatophobia
thanatopsia
thanatopsy
thanatos
thanatotic

T-handle
    T.-h. bone awl
    T.-h. Jacob chuck
    T.-h. nut wrench
    T.-h. screw wrench
Thane method
thank-you theory
thaumaturgic
thaumaturgy
THC dependence
theater
    Stegreif t.
theatrical test
theatrics
theatromania
theatrophobia
theca, pl. thecae
    t. vertebralis
thecal
    t. abscess
    t. sac
    t. sac compression
thecoperitoneal Pudenz-Schulte shunt
theism
thematic
    T. Apperception Test (TAT)
    T. Aptitude Test (TAT)
    T. Content Modification Program
     (TCMP)
    t. paralogia
    t. paraphasia
    t. paraphrasia
    t. picture test
    t. role
thematically related groups
theme
    central t.
    common t.
    death t.
    depressed mood t.
    deserved punishment t.
    disease t.
    grandiose t.
    guilt t.
    identity t.
    inflated worth t.
    t. interference
    knowledge t.
    manic mood t.
    mythological t.
    nihilism t.
    persecution t.
    t.'s of persecution
    personal inadequacy t.
    power t.
    recurring t.
    self-derogatory t.
    special relationship to deity t.
    special relationship to famous
     person t.
    typical t.
themomatic paralogia
thenar
    t. eminence
    t. weakness test

T

theocracy
theologian
theologize
theology
    natural t.
theomania
theonomous
theophobia
theophylamine
theophylline
theorem
    central-limit t.
theoretical
    t. assumption
    t. system
theorist
    defect t.
theory
    abstract t.
    adaptation level t.
    Adler t.
    adlerian t.
    affective-arousal t.
    aggressive behavior t.
    aging t.
    allenian t.
    Allport group relations t.
    Allport personality trait t.
    t. of anxiety
    anxiety sensitivity t.
    arousal t.
    attachment t.
    attitude t.
    attribution t.
    balance t.
    behavioral t.
    behavior-constraint t.
    biofeedback t.
    biolinguistic t.
    biolinguistic language t.
    biologic t.
    biosocial t.
    Burn and Rand t.
    Cannon t.
    Cannon-Bard t.
    catastrophe t.
    classical psychoanalytical t.
    cloacal t.
    t. of cognition
    cognitive dissonance t.
    cognitive learning t.
    color t.
    communication t.
    t. of constitutional bisexuality
    constitutional bisexuality t.
    continuum t.
    crisis t.
    cross-linkage t.
    cybernetic t.
    decay t.
    decision t.
    degeneracy t.
    developmental t.
    dietary t.
    ding-dong t.

    double blind t.
    drive reduction t.
    dual-instinct t.
    dual-process t.
    ego alter t.
    emergency t.
    empiricist t.
    environmental learning t.
    environmental load t.
    environmental stress t.
    epigenetic t.
    equity t.
    ERG t.
    evolution t.
    exclamation t.
    existence, relatedness, and
      growth t.
    expectancy t.
    factor t.
    family systems t.
    field t.
    Flourens t.
    flow t.
    focal conflict t.
    Freud t.
    freudian t.
    game t.
    gate t.
    gate-control t.
    gating t.
    general systems t.
    genetic t.
    gestalt t.
    group relations t.
    hearing t.
    humanistic t.
    human-motivation t.
    humoral t.
    iceblock t.
    immanence t.
    implicit personality t.
    incentive t.
    information t.
    injury-healing t.
    innateness t.
    interference t.
    interpersonal t.
    item response t. (IRT)
    James-Lange t.
    James-Lange-Sutherland t.
    Jung t.
    jungian t.
    Klein suffocation alarm t.
    labeling t.
    lamarckian t.
    language t.
    leadership t.
    learning t.
    libido t.
    life cycle t.
    life-event stress t.
    mass action t.
    McLone and Knepper etiological t.
    Melzack and Wall gate t.
    memory t.

Meyer t.
miasma t.
mixture t.
mnemenic t.
motor learning t.
nativist t.
object relations t.
observational learning t.
periodicity t.
personal construct t.
personality trait t.
person-centered t.
phonatory t.
place t.
pooh-pooh t.
psychoanalytical t.
psychodynamic t.
psycholinguistic t.
psychological t.
quantum t.
rankian t.
rapid-change t.
rapid-smoking t.
ratification t.
relaxation t.
response t.
rogerian t.
role-enactment t.
Semon-Hering t.
sensorimotor t.
Shealy t.
social causation t.
social dominance t.
t. of social dominance
social selection t.
societal reaction t.
spreading cortical depression t.
steppingstone t.
stimulus-response t.
stuttering block t.
taftian t.
tension-reduction t.
thank-you t.
three-component t.
topographical t.
total composite t.
trace-decay t.
trait t.
understimulation t.
vasogenic t.
violence t.
vulnerability t.
watchspring t.
Wolff vasogenic t.
Wollaston t.
X-bar t.
yo-he-ho t.
theosophy
theotherapy
Thera
T. Cane
T. Pulse bed
therapeusis
therapeutic
t. abortion (TAB)

t. agent
t. alliance
t. atmosphere
t. blood level
t. botulinum neurotoxin
t. communication
t. community (TC)
t. crisis
differential t.'s
t. dose
t. dose dependence
t. drug holiday
t. effect
t. electrical stimulation (TES)
t. embolism
t. embolization
t. environment
t. exercise
t. failure
t. group analysis
t. impasse
t. index
t. intervention
t. malaria
t. matrix
t. milieu
t. modality
t. neutrality
t. nihilism
t. optimism
t. pessimism
t. play group (TPG)
t. process
t. program
t. reaction (TR)
t. recreation
t. relationship
t. relaxation
t. role
suggestive t.'s
t. trial
t. trial visit (TTV)
t. window
therapeutic-agent related neuropathy
therapeutist
therapist
active t.
activities t.
auxiliary t.
corrective t.
educational t.
language t.
Licensed Marriage and Family T. (LMFT)
monkey t.
t. obligation
occupational t. (OT)
passive t.
physical t.
registered recreation t.
therapy, therapia (Rx)
aboriginal t.
Activa tremor control t.
active t.
activity group t. (AGT)

T

therapy *(continued)*

acute t.
adaptation-promoting t.
adjunctive t.
adjustment t.
adjuvant whole-brain radiation t.
administrative t.
adolescent group t.
adult group t.
agonist t.
albendazole t.
allenian t.
anaclitic t.
analytical play t.
antiandrogen t.
anticoagulation t.
anticonvulsant t.
antifibrinolytic t.
antimigraine t.
antiplatelet t.
apotreptic t.
art t.
assertion structured t.
assignment t.
atropine coma t. (ACT)
attitude t.
aversion t.
aversive t.
avoidance t.
ballet t.
behavioral couples group t.
behavioral marital t. (BMT)
bioenergetic t.
biologic t.
biomedical t.
body t.
boron neutron capture t. (BNCT)
Bragg peak proton beam t.
brain gene t.
branching steps in t.
brief group t.
brief stimulus t. (BST)
carbon dioxide t.
cerebral protective t.
chelation t.
chemical aversion t.
child group t.
child-guidance t.
clay-modeling t.
client-centered t.
cognitive t.
cognitive behavior t. (CBT)
cognitive-physiological t.
cognitive remediation t.
collaborative t.
color t.
coma t.
combined t.
common sense t.
communication t.
concurrent t.
conditioned-reflex t.
conditioning t.
conjoint t.

contextual t.
continuation t.
continuous-sleep t.
contract t.
convulsive shock t.
cooperative t.
corrective t. (CT)
corticoid t.
counselor-centered t.
couples group t.
couples sex t.
crisis t.
dance t.
delay t.
delayed t.
deliberate t.
dependence on t.
depot medication injection t.
depth t.
deterrent t.
diagnostic t.
dialectical behavior t.
directed group t.
diversional t.
divorce t.
drug t.
dual t.
dual-sex t.
dual transference t.
ego-state t.
elective t.
electric differential t. (EdiT)
electric shock t. (EST, est)
electroconvulsive t. (ECT)
electroconvulsive shock t. (ECST)
electroshock t. (ECT, EST, est)
electrosleep t. (ETS)
electrotherapeutic sleep t.
emotive t.
endocrine t.
endovascular t.
environmental t.
estrogen replacement t. (ERT)
exercise t.
existential-humanistic t.
experiential t.
experimental t.
exploratory t.
exposure-based cognitive behavior t.
expressive t.
extended family t. (EFT)
family member t.
family unit t.
filial t.
fluency shaping t.
focused expressive t.
focused radiation t.
food t.
gene t.
Gerson t.
gestalt t.
global gene replacement t.
goal-limited adjustment t.
graphic-arts t.
grief t.

group adjustment t. (GAT)
helper t.
heroin antagonist and learning t. (HALT)
highly active antiretroviral t. (HAART)
humanistic t.
hypertensive, hypervolemic, hemodilutional t.
imagery t.
immunosuppressive t.
implosive t.
indirect method of t.
individual t. (IT)
Indoklon t.
industrial t.
insight t.
inspirational group t.
instigation t.
insulin coma t. (ICT)
integrated psychological t.
intensity modulated radiation t.
interaction-oriented group t.
interpersonal t. (IPT)
interpretive t.
interstitial radiation t. (IRT)
interview t.
intravenous immune globulin humoral t.
irritation t.
IT-MS infusion t.
language enrichment t. (LET)
leaderless group t.
light t.
lithium t.
localized restorative central nervous system gene t.
long-term t.
maintenance drug t.
major role t. (MRT)
marital couples group t.
marriage t.
mass t.
megavitamin t.
Metrazol shock t.
milieu t.
minimum-change t.
modified ECT t.
Morita t.
morning bright light t.
movement t.
multimodal behavior t.
multiple t.
multiple family t.
music t. (MT)
musical t.
myofunctional t.
narrative t.
network t.
nonconfrontive t.
nondirective t.
nonphobic anxiety behavior t.
nutritional t.
occupational t. (OT)
old-age t.

operant t.
organic t.
orgone t.
orthomolecular t.
outcome-based t.
oxygen t.
paradoxical t.
paraverbal t.
passive t.
permission, limited information, specific suggestion, and intensive t. (PLISSIT)
persuasion t.
pharmacological t.
photodynamic t. (PDT)
photoradiation t.
pineal t.
pituitary replacement t.
plastic arts t.
play group t. (PGT)
polyvitamin t.
positive reinforcement t.
postelectroconvulsive t.
precision t.
primal t.
programmed t.
prolonged sleep t.
psychedelic t.
psychiatric somatic t.
psychoanalytic t.
psychodrama group t.
psychoeducation group t.
psychological t.
psychologic programming t.
psychopharmacological t.
psychovisual t.
quadrangular t.
radiation t.
radical t.
rankian t.
rapid eye t.
rational t. (RT)
rational emotive t. (RET)
reality oriented t.
reconditioning t.
reconstructive t.
recreational t. (RT)
reeducative t.
reflex t.
relationship t.
relaxation t.
release t.
reminiscence t.
replacement t.
restitutive t.
restraining t.
Restricted Environment Stimulation T. (REST)
retrogasserian anhydrous glycerol injection t.
rheologic t.
rhythmic sensory bombardment t. (RSBT)
rogerian group t.
role t.

T

therapy *(continued)*
  sacral nerve stimulation t.
  self-control t.
  semantic t.
  sensate-focus-oriented t.
  t. session
  SET t.
  sex t.
  shame-aversion t.
  shock t. (ST)
  simulated presence t.
  situational t.
  Slavson Activity Interview T.
  sleep t.
  sleep-electroshock t.
  social interaction t.
  social learning group t.
  social network t.
  socioenvironmental t.
  somatic t.
  sound t.
  spectator t.
  speech t.
  stereotactic-assisted radiation t.
   (STaRT)
  stereotactic focused-radiation t.
  stereotactic intratumoral
   photodynamic t.
  stimulus t.
  strategic family t.
  structural-strategic t.
  subcoma t.
  subshock t.
  suggestion t.
  support, empathy and truth t.
  supportive group t.
  suppressive t.
  symptomatic t.
  systematized assertive t. (SAT)
  systemic assertive t.
  taftian t.
  talk t.
  tamoxifen t.
  Task Force on Electroconvulsive T.
  tension reduction t.
  termination of t.
  theta-criterion t.
  third-force t.
  thought field t.
  three-cornered t.
  thrombolytic t.
  time-extended t.
  total push t.
  transvenous t.
  triadic t.
  triangular t.
  Triple-H t.
  ultrasonic t.
  unmodified ECT t.
  validation t.
  verbal aversion t.
  viral vector-mediated t.
  vitamin t.
  weight loss t.

  Weir Mitchell t.
  whole-brain radiation t. (WBRT)
  will t.
  work t.
  Zen t.
there-and-then approach
theriomorphism
thermal
  t. anesthesia
  t. blanket
  t. rhizotomy
  t. sense
  t. stimulus
thermalgesia, thermoalgesia
thermalgia
thermanalgesia, thermoanalgesia
thermanesthesia *(var. of*
  thermoanesthesia)
thermesthesia, thermoesthesia
thermesthesiometer *(var. of*
  thermoesthesiometer)
thermic
  t. anesthesia
  t. sense
Thermistor needle
thermoalgesia *(var. of* thermalgesia)
thermoanalgesia *(var. of* thermanalgesia)
thermoanesthesia, thermanesthesia
thermocoagulation
  radiofrequency t.
  stereotactic t.
thermocouple (TC)
  copper-constantan t.
thermoesthesia *(var. of* thermesthesia)
thermoesthesiometer, thermesthesiometer
thermogenic action
thermography
thermohyperalgesia
thermohyperesthesia
thermohypesthesia, thermohypoesthesia
thermoluminescent dosimeter
thermometer
  Fear T.
thermoneurosis
thermophobia
thermoplastic
thermoreceptor
thermoregulation
thermorhizotomy
theroid
theta
  t. activity
  t. criterion
  t. index
  t. level
  t. rhythm
  t. wave
  t. wave on EEG
theta-criterion therapy
theurgist
theurgy
thiabendazole
thiamine, thiamin
  t. deficiency
  t. deficiency encephalopathy (TDE)

thiamylal
thiazesim
thiazide diuretic
thiazide-induced hypokalemia
thickening
    hyaline t.
    myxomatous t.
thickness
    lumbosacral junction cortical t.
thigh
    driver's t.
    Heilbronner t.
thigh-high alternating compression air
  boot
thigmesthesia
thinking
    t. ability
    abstract t.
    adolescent t.
    allusive t.
    alogical t.
    animistic t.
    archaic-paralogical t.
    associative t.
    asyndetic t.
    autistic t.
    black-and-white t.
    categorical t.
    circular t.
    combinative t.
    t. compulsion
    conceptual t.
    concrete t.
    concretistic t.
    convergent t.
    creative t.
    T. Creatively in Action and
      Motion
    t. creatively with sounds and
      words (TCSW)
    critical t.
    delusional t.
    dereistic t.
    dichotomous t.
    directed t.
    t. disorder
    disordered t.
    disorganized t.
    distorted inferential t.
    distortion of inferential t.
    t. disturbance factor (TDF)
    disturbance in form of t.
    divergent t.
    eccentric t.
    egocentric t.
    either-or t.
    erratic t.
    t. fear
    fragmentation of t.
    futuristic t.
    Goldstein-Scheerer Tests of
      Abstract and Concrete t.
    T. Good Profile
    hypothetical deductive t.
    idiosyncratic t.

illogical t.
impoverishment in t.
incomprehensible t.
inferential t.
janusian t.
magical t.
marginal t.
numerical t.
oppositional t.
paleologic t.
paralogical t.
perverted t.
physiognomic t.
prearchaic t.
precausal t.
preconscious t.
predicate t.
prelogical t.
preoperational t.
primary process t.
process t.
productive t.
psychotic t.
realistic t.
ritualistic t.
secondary process t.
self-defeating t.
stress effect on adult t.
suicidal t.
symbolic t.
syncretic t.
tangential t.
tertiary-process t.
Torrance Tests of Creative t.
  (TTCT)
t. type
undirected t.
Whitaker Index of Schizophrenic t.
  (WIST)
wishful t.
thin-layer agarose gel electrophoresis
thin-section image
thin-slab acquisition technique
thin-wall introducer catheter
thiocyclidine
6-thioguanine (6TG)
thiopental sodium
thiophene
    analog of phencyclidine t.
    phencyclidine t.
thiopropazate
thioproperazine
thioridazine
thiosalicylate
    sodium t.
thiosulfate
    sodium t.
thiothixene hydrochloride
thioxanthene
    t. antipsychotic
    t. derivative
third
    t. cranial nerve
    t. ear
    t. nerve avulsion

T

third *(continued)*
    t. nerve palsy
    t. nervous system
    t. party payer
    t. sex
    t. temporal convolution
    t. ventricle
    t. ventricular hemangioblastoma
    t. ventriculostomy
third-degree continuous spontaneous nystagmus
third-force therapy
third-generation cephalosporin
thirdhand information
thirst
    t. drive
    insensible t.
    morbid t.
    subliminal t.
    twilight t.
this
    T. I Believe (TIB)
    T. I Believe Test
Thixokon
thixophobia
Thompson carotid clamp
Thompson-Farley spinal retractor system
Thomsen
    T. disease
    T. dystrophy
thoracic
    t. curve scoliosis
    t. discectomy
    t. disk herniation
    t. duct injury
    t. ganglia
    t. hypokyphosis
    t. interspace
    t. kyphosis
    t. meningioma
    t. nerve
    t. nucleus
    t. outlet
    t. pedicle
    t. pedicle marker
    t. spinal fusion
    t. spine
    t. spine biopsy
    t. spine decompression
    t. spine fracture
    t. spine lordosis
    t. spine pedicle diameter
    t. spine scoliotic deformity
    t. spine vertebral osteosynthesis
    t. and thoracolumbar spine surgery
    t. tumor
    t. vertebra
thoracoabdominal approach
thoracolumbar
    t. burst fracture
    t. curve
    t. degenerative disease
    t. idiopathic scoliosis

    t. junction
    t. junction surgical exposure
    t. kyphoscoliosis
    t. kyphosis
    t. pedicle screw
    t. retroperitoneal approach
    t. spinal canal stenosis
    t. spine
    t. spine anterior exposure
    t. spine decompression
    t. spine flexion-distraction injury
    t. spine fracture-dislocation
    t. spine scoliosis
    t. spine stabilization
    t. spine vertebral osteosynthesis
    t. spondylosis
    t. spondylosis surgical technique
    t. standing orthosis
    t. system
    t. trauma
    t. vertebra
thoracolumbosacral
    t. orthosis (TLSO)
    t. plate
thoracolumbosacroiliac implant system
thoracostomy
thoracotomy
    left-sided t.
    right-sided t.
    standard t.
Thorazine
thorium
    t. dioxide
    t. tartrate
thorn
    dendritic t.
Thorndike
    T. Handwriting Scale
    T. law of effect
    T. trial-and-error
    T. trial-and-error learning
Thorndike-Lorge criteria
Thornton-Griggs-Moxley disease
Thorotrast
thoroughness, reliability, efficiency, analytic ability (TREA)
Thor-Prom
thought
    abstract logical t.
    adaptive control of t. (ACT)
    alien t.
    archaic t.
    audible t.
    automatic t.
    blasphemous t.
    t. blockade
    t. blocking
    t. broadcasting
    t. broadcasting delusion
    categorical t.
    coherent stream of t.
    compulsive t.
    considered t.
    constraint of t.
    t. constraint

constriction of t.
t. content
content of t.
t. control
t.'s of death
t. deletion
delusional t.
t. deprivation
t. derailment
diminution of t.
disconnected t.
T. Disorder Index
t. disorganization
t. disorientation
distressing t.
t. disturbance
disturbance in content of t.
disturbing t.
t. echoing
emotional t.
errant t.
t. fear
t. field therapy
fluency of t.
focus of t.
t. form
t. hearing
imageless t.
impoverished t.
inappropriate t.
incomprehensible t.
increased speed of t.
Index of Primitive T.
inelasticity of t.
t. insertion
t. insertion delusion
interruption of t.
intrusive t.
latent t.
maladaptive t.
motor theory of t.
multifocal t.
obsessional t.
t. obstruction
omnipotence of t.
t. omnipotence
operational t.
t. pattern
t. period
persistent t.
phenomenistic t.
poverty of content of t.
preoccupation of t.
preoperational t.
pressing t.
t. pressure
t. process
t. process disorder
productivity of t.
t. provoking
rambling flow of t.
reactive t.
t. reading
recurrent t.

t. reform
t. rehearsal
reinforced t.
Rorschach Index of Primitive T.
ruminative t.
self-deprecating t.
slowness of t.
speed of t.
stream of t. (SOT)
substituting t.
suicidal t.
supervalent t.
symbolic t.
syncretic t.
syntaxic t.
t. transference
trend of t.
unacceptable t.
uncontrollable t.
unemotional t.
unrelated t.
unsocialized disturbance of t.
wandering t.
wide circles of t.
t. wit
t. withdrawal
**thousand-hands Kannon universal
  headframe**
thread
neuropil t.
polyene t.
terminal t.
threaded fusion cage (TFC)
thready
threat
t. of death
t. of job loss
t. reflex
threatening
t. behavior
t. comment
t. hallucination
t. voice
threctia
three
t. axis gradient coil
t. bromides elixir
t. dimensional (3D)
t. dimensionality
t. essays on the theory of
  sexuality
T. Fears
T. Mile Island
T. Minute Reasoning Test
oriented and alert times t.
Pediatric Extended Examination
  at T. (PEET)
t. times a day
three-column
t.-c. cervical spine injury
t.-c. concept
three-component theory
three-cornered therapy
three-day schizophrenia

T

Three-Dimensional
>T.-D. Block Construction Test (3DBCT)

three-dimensional
>t.-d. analysis
>t.-d. digitizer neuronavigator
>t.-d. fast low-angle shot imaging
>t.-d. Fourier transform (3DFT)
>t.-d. Fourier transform gradient-echo imaging
>t.-d. Fourier transform imaging
>t.-d. neuroimaging
>t.-d. reconstruction
>t.-d. sonic digitizer
>t.-d. SPECT phantom
>t.-d. spoiled GRASS sequence
>t.-d. target definition

Three-Factor
>T.-F. Eating Questionnaire

three-factor model of global rating

three-point
>t.-p. bending moment
>t.-p. head holder
>t.-p. skull clamp

three-repeat isoform
three-stage command test
three-step task
three-tube test
three-word recall test
threonine
threonyl
threshold
>absolute t.
>acoustic reflex t.
>afterdischarge t.
>auditory t.
>awareness t.
>blackout t.
>brightness t.
>t. of consciousness
>convulsant t.
>detectability t.
>detection t.
>differential t.
>t. differential
>t. of discomfort (TD)
>discomfort t.
>double-point t.
>false t.
>intelligibility t.
>pain t.
>reflex t.
>relational t.
>t. of responsiveness
>sedation t.
>seizure t.
>sensory t.
>t. shift-masking technique
>signal-to-noise t.
>speech reception t. (SRT)
>speech recognition t.
>stimulus t.
>t. stimulus
>t. symbolism
>taste t.

>tickle t.
>vibrotactile t.
>vulnerability t.

thrive
>failure to t. (FTT)

throat pain
throbbing headache
thrombencephalic sleep
thrombin
>topical t.

Thrombinar
thrombin-soaked Gelfoam
thromboangiitis obliterans
thrombocythemia
thrombocytopenia venous-sinus
thrombocytosis
>essential t.

thromboembolectomy
thromboembolism
thromboendophlebitis
Thrombogen
thrombogenic
>t. coil
>t. ferrous mixture

thrombolysis
>intraluminal t.

thrombolytic therapy
thrombophlebitis
>cavernous sinus t.

thromboplastin
>plasma t.

thrombosed
>t. aneurysm
>t. thick-walled vein

thrombosis, pl. thromboses
>cavernous sinus t.
>cerebral t. (CT)
>deep venous t. (DVT)
>dural sinus t.
>fistula-induced sinus t.
>iliofemoral t.
>sagittal sinus t.
>septic t.
>sinovenous t.
>sinus-vein t. (SVT)
>wire t.

Thrombostat
thrombotic
>t. apoplexy
>t. hydrocephalus
>t. thrombocytopenic purpura

thromboxane
thrombus
>chronic t.
>mural t.

throw
>t. out
>t. over

throwaway
throwback
thrust
>extensor t.

thrusting
>pelvic t.

thumb
    cerebral t.
    t. reflex
    rule of t.
thumb-chin reflex
thumbprinting appearance
Thumb-Saver introducer clamp
thunderclap headache
Thurstone
    T. Attitude Scale
    T. Interest Schedule
    T. Temperament Schedule
Thymapad stimulus electrode
thymectomy
thymergasia
thymic
    t. alymphoplasia
    t. myoid cell
thymine
thymocyte apoptosis
thymogenic drinking
thymoleptic
thymoma
thymonoic reaction
thymopathy
Thypinone
thyrocervical trunk of subclavian artery
thyroglobulin
thyrohypophysial syndrome
thyroid
    t. augmentation
    t. cartilage
    t. delirium
    desiccated t.
    t. disorder
    t. function test (TFT)
    t. gland
    t. orbitopathy
    t. response element (TRE)
    t. stimulating hormone (TSH)
thyroiditis
    autoimmune t.
    Riedel t.
thyrotoxic
    t. coma
    t. encephalopathy
    t. myopathy
    t. periodic paralysis
thyrotoxicosis
    apathetic t.
    endogenous t.
thyrotoxicosis-induced
    t.-i. chorea
    t.-i. choreoathetosis
thyrotroph cell
thyrotropin
thyrotropin-producing adenoma
thyrotropin-releasing hormone (TRH)
thyrotropin-stimulating hormone (TSH)
thyroxine (T$_4$)
Thytropar
TI
    inversion time
TIA
    transient ischemic attack

tiagabine hydrochloride
TIB
    This I Believe
    TIB Test
        TIB Test (TIB)
Tibex
tibial
    t. nerve
    t. phenomenon
tic
    articulatory t.
    attitude t.
    atypical t.
    body t.
    breathing t.
    child problem t.
    chronic motor t.
    chronic spasm t.
    comorbid t.
    complex motor t.
    complex vocal t.
    compulsive psychogenic t.
    t. convulsif with coprolalia
    convulsive t.
    current t.
    t. de Guinon
    t. de pensée
    t. disorder
    t. disorder of organic origin
    t. douloureux
    facial t.
    glossopharyngeal t.
    habit t.
    lid t.
    local t.
    mimic t.
    motor t.
    motor-verbal t.
    t. nondouloureux
    occupational t.
    t. orbicularis
    past t.
    primary t.
    psychic t.
    psychogenic t.
    rotatory t.
    t. scriptorius
    simple motor t.
    simple vocal t.
    spasm and t.
    spasm t.
    spasmodic t.
    tardive t.
    tonic t.
    Tourette t.
    vocal t.
TICA
    traumatic intracranial aneurysm
ticarcillin
tick-borne
    t.-b. encephalitis (Central European
        or Eastern subtype)
    t.-b. meningopolyneuritis
ticklers
    brain t.

T

tickle threshold
tickling
tick paralysis
Ticlid
tic-like
    t.-l. behavior
    t.-l. facial grimace
ticlopidine
    t. HCl
    t. hydrochloride
tidal air
Tiedmann rongeur
tier
    Adson knot t.
TIES
    The Instructional Environment Scale
ties
    incestuous t.
    reality t.
    t. with reality
Tigan
tight
    t. brain
    t. filum terminale syndrome
    t. junctioned endothelium
tightener
    Love-Adson wire t.
tigretier
tigroid
    t. body
    t. substance
tigrolysis
TIL
    tumor-infiltrating lymphocyte
Tilcotil
tile plate facet replacement
tilt
    head t.
    T. and Turn Paragon bed
tilted optimized nonsaturating excitation
  technique
tilting of visual images
tiludronate
timbromania
time
    acquisition t.
    adaptation t.
    t. agnosia
    association reaction t.
    t. axis
    biologic t.
    bleeding t.
    central reflex t.
    central somatosensory conduction t.
      (CSCT)
    cochlear response t.
    t. confusion
    t. consciousness
    t. constant
    correlation t.
    t. deixis
    t. disorientation
    t. distortion
    t. dominance

    dream t.
    echo t. (TE)
    t. error
    t. faction
    t. fear
    image acquisition t.
    inertia t.
    interhemispheric propagation t.
    interpulse t.
    inversion t. (TI)
    kaolin clotting t.
    t. killer
    leisure t.
    long pulse repetition time/long
      echo t.
    losing t.
    mass doubling t.
    t. of maximum concentration
    t. and motion study
    oriented to person, place, and t.
    t. out from reinforcement
    partial thromboplastin t. (PTT)
    t. perception
    T. Perception Inventory
    t. periods of satisfactory relating
    phrenic nerve conduction t.
    t. pressure
    T. Problems Inventory
    prothrombin t. (pro-time, PT)
    proton relaxation t.
    pulse repetition t.
    quality t.
    reaction t. (RT)
    recognition t.
    reflex t.
    relaxation t.
    repetition t. (TR)
    response t.
    t. and rhythm disorder
    rise t.
    Russell viper venom t.
    scan t.
    t. sense
    T. Sense Test
    sequence t.
    short pulse repetition time/echo t.
    short pulse repetition time/short
      echo t.
    spin-lattice relaxation t.
    spin-spin relaxation t.
    t. splitting
    total sleep t. (TST)
    T. Use Analyzer
    wake t.
    t. zone
timed
    t. behavioral rating sheet (TBRS)
    T. Stereotypes Rating Scale
time-density curve
time-extended therapy
time-limited psychotherapy (TLP)
timely death
time-of-flight
    t.-o.-f. effect

t.-o.-f. positron emission
tomographic camera
t.-o.-f. technique
time-out
t.-o. procedure
t.-o. technique
time, place, and person (TP&P)
time-sample behavioral checklist (TSBC)
time-series design
TiMesh
T. hardware
T. screw
T. titanium bone plating system
time-zone change
time-zone-change syndrome
timing of decompression
timolol maleate
Timoptic
timorous
tincture
opium t.
Tinel sign
tinge
tingling
t. sensation
t. with aura
Tinker Toy Test
tinnitus
tiotixene
tip
Adson brain suction t.
bipolar diathermy forceps t.
CUSA t.
Ferguson brain suction t.
forceps t.
Frazier suction t.
Japanese suction t.
multipore suction t.
t. of posterior horn
Rhoton suction t.
Sachs brain suction t.
slotted suction t.
tip-of-the-tongue (TOT)
t.-o.-t.-t. phenomenon
Tipramine
tiqueur
tirilazad
tirilazed mesylate (TM)
Tissucol
tissue
arachnoid t.
autologous adrenal medullary t.
brain t.
cortical t.
t. culture flask
distensible t.
fetal mesencephalic t. (FMT)
t. fibrin sealant
t. forceps
t. hyperperfusion
t. implant
t. magnetic susceptibility artifact
mammalian t.
t. plane dissector
t. plasminogen activator (t-PA)

t. respiration
t. transplantation
t. welding
tissue-based monoamine oxidase assay
Tissue-Guard bovine pericardial patch
tissue-type PA (t-PA)
titanium
t. alloy needle
t. aneurysm clip
t. cable
t. construct
t. hollow screw plate system
t. microconnector
t. micromesh
t. micro system
t. mini bur hole cover
t. miniplate
t. plate
t. wire
t. wound retractor
titration
titubation
tizanidine
t. hydrochloride
T-JTA, TJTA
Taylor-Johnson Temperament Analysis
TL
team leader
tolerance level
^{201}Tl
thallium-201
^{201}Tl chloride
^{201}Tl scintigraphy
^{201}Tl SPECT
TLAC
Test of Learning Accuracy in Children
Test of Listening Accuracy in Children
TLC
tender loving care
Test of Language Competence
TLC-C
Test of Language Competence for
Children
TLC-Learning Preference Inventory
TLE
temporal lobe epilepsy
TLP
time-limited psychotherapy
TLSO
thoracolumbosacral orthosis
TM
team member
tirilazed mesylate
Transcendental Meditation
TMAS
Taylor Manifest Anxiety Scale
TMB
total monocular blindness
TMH
trainable mentally handicapped
TMJ
temporomandibular joint
TMJ pain
TMJ Scale

T

TMR
temporomesial region
trainable mentally retarded
TMR Performance Profile for the Severely and Moderately Retarded
TMS
transcranial magnetic stimulation
TMT
temporalis muscle temperature
Trail Making Test
TN
trigeminal neuralgia
TNF
tumor necrosis factor
TNFR
tumor necrosis factor receptor
TNVAD
Test of Nonverbal Auditory Discrimination
TOAL
Test of Adolescent Language
to-and-fro tremor
tobacco
t. abuse
t. addiction
t. amblyopia
t. dependence
t. use disorder
t. withdrawal
tobacco-alcohol amblyopia
tobagism
TOBE
tests of basic experience
tobramycin sulfate
tocainide
tocomania
tocopherol
alpha t.
tocophobia
toddler
t. negativism
t. stage
Todd postepileptic paralysis
Todd-Wells stereotactic frame
Todeserwartung syndrome
toe
t. clonus
t. drop
t. phenomenon
t. reflex
t. sign
striatal t.
TOEFL Test of Written English
Toennis
T. dissecting scissors
T. dura dissector
T. dura knife
T. dural hook
T. ES standalone constant-current electrical stimulator
T. tumor forceps
Toennis-Adson dissector
toewalking
Tofranil
Tofranil-PM

Toft spinal correction treatment
togetherness need
toilet
t. training
t. water
token
t. economy
t. economy reward
t. reward
T. Test for Aphasia
T. Test for Children
T. Test for Receptive Disturbances in Aphasia
tolazamide
tolbutamide
tolcapone
TOLD
Test of Language Development
TOLD-I:2
Test of Language Development - Intermediate, Second Edition
TOLD-P:2
Test of Language Development - Primary, Second Edition
Tolectin DS
tolerance
acute t.
ambiguity t.
anxiety t.
barbiturate t.
benzodiazepine t.
caffeine t.
cross t.
dispositional t.
t. dose
drug t.
frustration t.
t. level (TL)
level of pain t.
metabolic t.
opioid t.
pain t.
pharmacodynamic t.
t. potential
t. range
social t.
substance t.
t. test
tolfenamic acid
Tolinase
Tolman purposive behaviorism
tolmetin
Tolosa-Hunt syndrome
toluene
toluidine blue-stained
Tom
peeping T.
Uncle T.
tomaculous neuropathy
tomboy behavior
Tomism
Uncle T.
Tomkins-Horn Picture Arrangement Test
tommy gun

tomogram
open-mouthed anteroposterior t.
tomograph
CTI/Siemens 933 t.
PC-2048B positron emission t.
Tomomatic 64 single photon
emission computed t.
tomography
automate computed axial t.
computed t. (CT)
computerized axial t. (CAT)
cranial computed t. (CCT)
dynamic computed t. (DCT)
dynamic single photon emission
computed t.
emission computed t.
fluorodopa positron emission t.
infusion computed t.
plain t.
positron emission t. (PET)
preoperative t.
t. scan
single photon emission computed t.
(SPECT)
volumetric computed t.
xenon computed t. (Xe-CT)
xenon enhanced computed t.
(XeCT, Xe-CT)
tomomania
Tomomatic 64 single photon emission
computed tomograph
tomophobia
tonaphasia
TONAR
oral-nasal acoustic ratio
tone
affective t.
biofeedback t.'s
complex t.
t. deafness
depressed t.
emotional t.
episodic bilateral loss of muscle t.
feeling t.
t. of feeling
fundamental t.
inhibitory t.
muscle t.
viscerosomatic t.
t. of voice
toner
psychological t.
tongs
Cherry traction t.
Cone skull traction t.
Crutchfield-Raney skull traction t.
Crutchfield skeletal traction t.
Crutchfield skull traction t.
Edmonton extension t.
Gardner-Wells t.
Mayfield t.
Reynolds skull traction t.
tongue
apex of t.
bifid t.

blade of t.
t. of cerebellum
t. clucking
forked t.
t. phenomenon
septum of t.
slip of (the) t.
tongue-in-groove operation
TONI
Test of Nonverbal Intelligence
tonic
t. block
t. control
t. convulsion
t. epilepsy
t. foot reflex
t. neck reflex
t. phase
t. pupil
t. seizure
t. spasm
t. tic
tonically dilated pupil
tonic-clonic
t.-c. conversion
generalized t.-c. seizure
t.-c. movement
t.-c. seizure
tonicity
tonitrophobia
tonoclonic spasm
tonogeny
tonohaptic reaction of pupil
tonometry
tonotopic
tonsil
cerebellar t.
tonsilla, pl. tonsillae
t. cerebelli
tonsillar herniation
tonus
plastic t.
tool-using behavior
tooth
t. fear
t. grinding
t. spasm
TOP
temporal, occipital, parietal
test orientation procedure
top
t. of the basilar syndrome
t. gun
topalgia
Topamax
topectomy
top-entry (open body) hook
topesthesia
tophus
topic
change of t.
emotionally laden t.
t. shifting
topical
t. clonidine

T

topical *(continued)*
t. flight
t. thrombin
topiramate
TOPL
Test of Pragmatic Language
topoanesthesia
topognosis, topognosia
topographagnosia
topographic
t. hypothesis
t. mapping
topographical
t. agnosia
t. disorientation
t. organization
t. psychology
t. theory
topography
mental t.
topological psychology
topology
toponarcosis
toponeurosis
topophobia
toposcope
toposcopic catheter
TOPOSS
Tests of Perception of Scientists and Self
topothermesthesiometer
Toradol
T. Injection
T. Oral
TORCH
toxoplasmosis, other infections, rubella, cytomegalovirus, and herpes simplex
TORCH syndrome
torch
saline t.
torcida
boca t.
torcular
t. herophili
t. meningioma
Toriello-Carey agnesis
Torkildsen
T. shunt
T. ventriculocisternostomy
torlone fixation pin
tornado epilepsy
Toronto
T. Alexithymia Scale
T. Functional Capacity Questionnaire (TFCQ)
torpedoing
torpent
torpid
t. idiocy
t. idiot
torpor
torque
unwanted screw t.

torr
Torrance Tests of Creative thinking (TTCT)
Torré syndrome
torsades de pointes
torsemide
torsion
t. dystonia
t. neurosis
t. spasm
torsional
t. abnormality
t. gripping strength
t. nystagmus
t. stiffness
torsionometer
Torsten Sjögren syndrome
torti
pili t.
torticollis
benign paroxysmal t.
dermatogenic t.
dystonic t.
fixed t.
intermittent t.
labyrinthine t.
ocular t.
psychogenic t.
rheumatic t.
spasmodic t.
t. spastica
spurious t.
symptomatic t.
tortuous
torture
toruloma
TOT
tip-of-the-tongue
TOT phenomenon
total
t. agenesis
t. aphasia
t. battery composite
t. body neutron activation analysis (TBNAA)
t. communication
t. composite theory
t. disability
Full-Scale Score T. (FSST)
t. hypophysectomy
t. mergent
t. monocular blindness (TMB)
t. parenteral nutrition (TPN)
t. phobic anxiety (TPA)
t. pituitary ablation
t. push therapy
t. push treatment of schizophrenia
t. recall
t. response (lz R)
t. response index (TRI)
t. sleep time (TST)
totalis
alopecia t.
alopecia capitis t.

ophthalmoplegia t.
rachischisis t.
totalism
totality of possible events
totally disabled
totem and taboo
toto
in t.
pars pro t.
touch
t. corpuscle
organ of t.
out of t.
t. perception
t. sensation
t. sense
soft t.
t. spot
touching
t. communication pattern
t. rituals
tough love
tough-minded tendency
Tourette
T. disease
T. disorder
Gilles de la T.
T. syndrome (TS)
T. Syndrome Association Unified
Tic Rating Scale
T. Syndrome Global Scale
T. Syndrome Questionnaire
T. Syndrome Severity Scale
T. Syndrome Symptom List
T. tic
tourniquet
Drake t.
t. ischemia
TOVA
Test of Variables of Attention
towel clip
TOWER
testing, orientation, and work evaluation
for rehabilitation
tower skull
TOWL
Test of Written Language
toxic
t. action
t. amaurosis
t. amblyopia
t. cirrhosis
t. confusional state
t. convulsion
t. deafness
t. delirium
t. dementia
t. disorder
t. dose
t. edema
t. effect
t. effects of alcohol
t. encephalopathy
t. epidermal necrolysis
t. exposure

t. hepatitis
t. hydrocephalus
t. hypoxia
t. ingredient
t. injury
t. insanity
t. level
t. lithium tremor
t. myocarditis
t. neuritis
t. nystagmus
t. psychosis
t. reaction
t. retinoneuropathy
t. schizophrenia
t. shock syndrome
t. substance
t. tetanus
toxica
alopecia t.
toxic-infectious psychosis
toxicity
acute drug t.
acute neuronal t.
behavioral t.
central anticholinergic t.
drug t.
glutamate t.
lithium t.
manganese t.
mercury t.
methyl alcohol t.
propylene glycol t.
toxicological analysis
toxicomania
toxicus
Gambierdiscus t.
toximetabolic encephalopathy
toxin
bacterial t.
botulinum A t.
botulinum t. type A
dietary t.
t. exposure
exposure to t.'s
manganese t.
mercury t.
methyl alcohol t.
toxin-provoked amnesia
toxiphobia
toxocariasis
toxoid
tetanus t.
Toxoplasma gondii
toxoplasmic
t. encephalitis
t. encephalomyelitis
toxoplasmosis
acquired t.
AIDS-related t.
intramedullary t.
toxoplasmosis, other infections, rubella,
cytomegalovirus, and herpes simplex
(TORCH)

T

875

TPA
temporopolar artery
total phobic anxiety
t-PA
tissue plasminogen activator
tissue-type PA
TPG
therapeutic play group
TPI
Treponema pallidum immobilization
TPI test
TPLS
The Primary Language Screen
TPN
total parenteral nutrition
TP&P
time, place, and person
TPR
temperature, pulse, respiration
TPT
Tactile Performance Test
TR
repetition time
therapeutic reaction
trabajando la causa
trabecula
nondecalcified t.
trace
t. conditioned reflex
t. conditioning
memory t.
mnemonic t.
perseverative t.
trace-decay theory
trachea
tracheal injury
trachelagra
trachelism, trachelismus
trachelocyrtosis
trachelodynia
trachelokyphosis
trachelology
tracheostomy
tracing
abnormal EEG t.
dipole t. (DT)
EEG t.
I t.
interrupted t.
track
CD t.
half t.
needle t.
Tracker
T. infusion catheter
T. microcatheter
Tracker-10 catheter
Tracker-18 catheter
tracking
saccadic t.
visual t.
Tracrium
tract
Arnold t.
association t.

auditory t.
Burdach t.
census t.
central tegmental t. (CTT)
cerebellorubral t.
cerebellothalamic t.
cholinergic t.
Collier t.
comma t. of Schultze
corticobulbar t.
corticopontine t.
corticospinal t. (CST)
crossed pyramidal t.
cuneocerebellar t.
deiterospinal t.
dentatothalamic t.
descending t. of trigeminal nerve
direct pyramidal t.
dopaminergic t.
dorsal spinocerebellar t.
dorsolateral t.
extrapyramidal t.
fastigiobulbar t.
Flechsig t.
frontopontine t.
frontotemporal t.
geniculocalcarine t.
genitourinary t.
t. of Goll
Gowers t.
habenulointerpeduncular t.
Hoche t.
hypothalamohypophysial t.
Lissauer t.
Loewenthal t.
mamillothalamic t.
Marchi t.
medullary solitary t.
mesencephalic t. of trigeminal
nerve
mesolimbic-mesocortical t.
Monakos t.
t. of Münzer and Wiener
myelinated axonal t.
nerve t.
nigrostriatal t.
occipitocollicular t.
occipitopontine t.
occipitotectal t.
olfactory t.
olivocerebellar t.
olivospinal t.
optic t.
parietopontine t.
posterior spinocerebellar t.
prepyramidal t.
pyramidal t.
reticulospinal t.
rubrobulbar t.
rubroreticular t.
rubrospinal t.
t. of Schütz
sensory t.
septomarginal t.
serotonergic t.

solitary t.
spinal dermal sinus t.
spinal t. of trigeminal nerve
spinocerebellar t.
spino-olivary t.
spinoreticular t.
spinospinalis t.
spinotectal t.
spinothalamic t.
spiral foraminous t.
Spitzka marginal t.
sulcomarginal t.
supraopticohypophysial t.
tectobulbar t.
tectopontine t.
tectospinal t.
temporofrontal t.
temporopontine t.
tuberoinfundibular t.
Türck t.
urinary t.
ventral spinocerebellar t.
ventral spinothalamic t.
vestibulospinal t.
Waldeyer t.

traction
Ace Trippi-Wells tong cervical t.
Ace universal tong cervical t.
t. alopecia
t. anchor
axial t.
bipolar vertebral t.
Bremer halo crown t.
Crile head t.
device for transverse t. (DTT)
t. neuritis
t. spur
transverse t.

tractotomy
anterolateral t.
bulbar t.
bulbar cephalic pain t.
intramedullary t.
mesencephalic t.
pontine t.
pyramidal t.
Schwartz t.
Sjöqvist t.
spinal t.
spinothalamic t.
stereotactic t.
subcaudate t.
trigeminal t.
Walker t.

tractus, gen. and pl. **tractus**
t. centralis tegmenti
t. cerebellorubralis
t. cerebellothalamicus
t. corticobulbaris
t. corticopontini
t. corticospinalis
t. corticospinalis anterior
t. corticospinalis lateralis
t. descendens nervi trigemini
t. dorsolateralis

t. fastigiobulbaris
t. frontopontinus
t. habenulopeduncularis
t. mesencephalicus nervi trigemini
t. occipitopontinus
t. olfactorius
t. olivocerebellaris
t. opticus
t. parietopontinus
t. pyramidalis
t. pyramidalis anterior
t. pyramidalis lateralis
t. reticulospinalis
t. rubrospinalis
t. solitarius
t. spinalis nervi trigemini
t. spinocerebellaris anterior
t. spinocerebellaris posterior
t. spinotectalis
t. spinothalamicus
t. spinothalamicus anterior
t. spinothalamicus lateralis
t. spiralis foraminosus
t. spiralis foraminulosus
t. supraopticohypophysialis
t. tectobulbaris
t. tectopontinus
t. tectospinalis
t. tegmentalis centralis
t. temporopontinus
t. tuberoinfundibularis
t. vestibulospinalis

trading sex
traditional
t. belief
t. phonetic analysis
t. psychotherapy
t. society
t. value

tradition directed
traffic court
Trager method
tragus
ipsilateral t.

Trail
T. Making Test (TMT)
T. of Nonpharmacologic
Interventions in the Elderly Study

trailing
t. image
t. phenomenon

train
t. fear
t. of spike

trainability
trainable
t. mentally handicapped (TMH)
t. mentally retarded (TMR)

trained reflex
Trainer's Assessment of Proficiency (TAP)
training
alpha wave t.
t. analysis
anxiety control t. (ACT)

T

training *(continued)*
    Anxiety Management T. (AMT)
    assertive t.
    assertiveness t.
    audiovisual t.
    auditory t.
    autogenic t.
    aversive t.
    biofeedback t.
    bladder t.
    bowel t.
    clinical t.
    cognitive self-hypnosis t.
    cooperative t.
    cultural t.
    delayed toilet t.
    t. discrimination
    Erhard Seminar T. (EST, est)
    escape t.
    evaluation of t.
    general relaxation t.
    t. group (T-group)
    habit t.
    human-relations t.
    hypnotic relaxation technique t.
    improvement t.
    interviewer t.
    laboratory t.
    Language Sampling, Analysis
      and T.
    leadership t.
    memory t.
    neurofeedback t. (NT)
    occupational skill t.
    Parent Effectiveness T. (PET)
    perceptual t.
    personnel t.
    Reitan Evaluation of Hemispheric
      Abilities and Brain
      Improvement T.
    relaxation technique t.
    retention control t.
    self-reliance t.
    sensitivity t.
    skill t.
    social skills t. (SST)
    spontaneity t.
    stress inoculation t. (SIT)
    toilet t.
    trait factor t.
    t. transfer
    transfer of t.
    t. unit
    visual t.
    vocational t.
train-of-four stimulus
trait
    t. anxiety
    anxious-neurotic personality t.
    cardinal t.
    t. carrier
    central t.
    character t.
    cognitive personality t.

    common t.
    compensatory t.
    culture t.
    t. dependent
    dominant t.
    egosyntonic t.
    environmental mold t.
    ergic t.
    T. Evaluation Index
    t. factor
    t. factor training
    inflexible personality t.
    interpersonal personality t.
    intrapsychic personality t.
    introversive t.
    maladaptive personality t.
    novelty-seeking t.
    t. organization
    paranoid t.
    pathologic t.
    peculiar personality t.
    personality t.
    pervasive and persistent maladaptive
      personality t.'s
    polygenic t.
    primary personality t.
    t. profile
    t. rating
    recessive t.
    secondary personality t.
    self-defeating t.
    sensation-seeking t.
    temperament t.
    t. theory
    unique t.
    t. variability
trait-like syndrome
trajectory
    operative t.
tramadol
tram track sign
trance
    amnesia after t.
    t. coma
    death t.
    deep t.
    dissociative t.
    ecstatic t.
    hypnotic t.
    hysterical t.
    induced t.
    involuntary state of t.
    light t.
    t. logic
    medium t.
    possession t.
    somnambulistic t.
    t. state
trancelike behavior
trance-possession disorder
tranexamic acid
tranquilize
tranquilizer
    t. abuse
    animal t.

t. chair
t. drug dependence
major t.
minor t.
tranquilosedative
transaction
ulterior t.
transactional
T. Analysis (TA)
T. Analysis Life Position Survey (TALPS)
t. evaluation
t. psychotherapy
t. theory of perception
transaminase
alanine t. (ALT)
GABA t. (GABA-T)
glutamyl t.
serum glutamic oxaloacetic t. (SGOT)
serum glutamic-pyruvic t. (SGPT)
serum glutamyl t.
transantral
t. ethmoidal approach
t. ethmoidal orbital decompression
transarterial platinum coil embolization
transarticular screw
transaxial
transcallosal
t. interforniceal corridor
t. interhemispheric
t. transforaminal approach
transcarbamoylase
ornithine t.
transcatheter obliteration
transcavernous transpetrous apex approach
transcendence
ego t.
t. need
Transcendental
T. Meditation (TM)
transcendental state
transcerebellar
t. diameter (TCD)
t. hemispheric approach
transcerebral electrotherapy (TCET)
transcervical
transchoroidal approach
transcochlear approach
transcortical
t. aphasia
t. apraxia
t. incision
t. motor
t. sensory
t. technique
t. transventricular approach
transcranial
t. B-mode ultrasound
t. color-coded real-time sonography (TCCS)
t. color-coded sonography
t. Doppler TCD
t. Doppler ultrasonography

t. frontofacial advancement
t. frontotemporoorbital approach
t. high-frequency repetitive electrical stimulation
t. magnetic stimulation (TMS)
t. orbital exploration
t. real-time color Doppler imaging
t. resection
transcription
broad phonemic t.
transcubital approach
transcultural psychiatry
transcutaneous electrical nerve stimulation (TENS)
transcytosis
blood-brain t.
bulk flow t.
transderivational search
transdermal
t. absorption
Duragesic T.
t. scopolamine
Transderm Scop Patch
transdominance
transducer
bur hole t.
t. cell
Combitrans t.
Drager MTC t.
force t.
neuro convex t.
piezo-resistive t.
transducer-tipped catheter
transduction
pain t.
postreceptor information t.
transection
fiber tract t.
multiple subpial t.
transendothelial migration
transentorhinal region
transesophageal echocardiography
transethmoidal encephalocele
transethmosphenoidal hypophysectomy
transfacial transclival approach
transfected fibroblast
transfemoral catheter
transfer
bilateral t.
correctional t. (CT)
t. deficit
general t.
t. by generalization
interhemispheric t.
intersensory t.
t. of learning
linear energy t. (LET)
memory t.
positive t.
t. of principle
saturation t.
training t.
t. of training
virus-mediated gene t.
transferase

T

transference
    affectionate t.
    aim t.
    analysis of t.
    t. behavior
    collective t.
    t. cure
    t. dilution
    erotic t.
    extrasensory thought t.
    t. feeling
    floating t.
    hostile t.
    identification t.
    t. improvement
    institutional t.
    libidinal t.
    t. love
    mirror t.
    mirroring the t.
    narcissistic t.
    negative t.
    t. neurosis
    t. paradigm
    t. phenomenon
    positive t.
    t. reaction
    t. relationship
    t. remission
    t. resistance
    thought t.
    traumatic t.
transference-countertransference
transferential
transferred
    t. meaning
    t. sensation
transferrin
    anti-human t.
    carbohydrate-deficient t. (CDT)
transfontanel Doppler ultrasound
transform
    fast-Fourier t.
    Fourier t.
    isotropic three-dimensional
      Fourier t.
    multidimensional Fourier t.
    three-dimensional Fourier t. (3DFT)
    two-dimensional Fourier t. (2DFT)
transformation
    t. of affect
    perceptual t.
    t. theory of anxiety
transformational
    T. Leadership Development
      Program
    t. related
    t. rule
transformationally related
transforming
    t. agent
    t. growth factor beta
transfrontal approach
transfrontonasoorbital approach

transfusion
    albumin t.
    autologous blood t.
    blood t.
    fetal t.
transgenderism
transgene
    nonselective expression of t.
transgenerational role of giving
transgenic
transgression
    behavioral t.
transient
    t. auditory hallucination
    t. auditory illusion
    t. blindness
    t. brain stem ischemia
    t. channel activation
    t. depressive reaction
    t. distortion
    t. ego ideal
    t. focal neurologic event (TFNE)
    t. global amnesia (TGA)
    t. group
    t. hallucinatory experience
    t. hemisphere attack (THA)
    t. hypersomnia
    t. ideas of reference
    t. ideation
    t. image
    t. insomnia
    t. ischemic attack (TIA)
    t. monocular visual loss
    t. nystagmus
    t. organic psychosis
    t. plexus injury
    positive occipital sharp t.
    t. postictal confusional state
    t. signal abnormality
    t. situational disturbance
    t. situational personality disorder
    t. spasm tic disorder of childhood
    t. stress-related paranoid ideation
    t. tactile hallucination
    t. tactile illusion
    t. tic disorder
    t. tremor
    t. visual hallucination
    t. visual illusion
    t. visual phenomenon
    t. voltage
transilient
transilluminate
transinstitutionalization
transinsular
transisthmian
transition
    age t.
    T. Behavior Scale (TBS)
    high-intensity t.
    life-cycle t.
    normal t.
    t. process
    sleep-wake t.
    t. zone

transitional
    t. change
    t. convolution
    t. employment workshop
    t. gyrus
    t. halfway house
    t. meningioma
    t. object
    T. Object Questionnaire
    t. probability
    t. program
    t. sleep (TS)
    t. vertebra
transitory
    t. mania
    t. psychosis
translabyrinthine
    t. and suboccipital approach
    t. transotic approach
translation
    coronal plane deformity sagittal t.
translational
    t. fracture
    t. position
translocation
    chromosomal t.
    t. mongolism
translucent
transluminal angioplasty
transmandibular glossopharyngeal
  approach
transmaxillosphenoidal approach
transmembrane ionic shift
transmethylation
transmigrate
transmissible
    t. agent
    t. spongiform viral encephalopathy
    t. virus dementia (TVD)
transmission
    cultural t.
    diffusion t.
    duplex t.
    ephaptic t.
    extrastriatal dopamine t.
    fetal AIDS t.
    intergenerational t.
    neurohumoral t.
    neuromuscular t.
    nonsynaptic t.
    synaptic t.
    vertical t.
    volume t.
transmitter
    chemical t.
    radiofrequency t.
    t. substance
transmutation
transnasal
    t. approach
    t. biopsy
transnasoorbital approach
transneuronal atrophy
Transonics flow probe

transoral
    t. approach
    t. odontoid resection
transorbital
    t. leukotomy
    t. lobectomy
    t. lobotomy
transosseous
    t. venography
transpalatal approach
transparent septum
transpedicular
    t. approach
    t. fixation effective pedicle
      diameter
    t. fixation system design
    t. screw
    t. screw-rod fixation
    t. spinal instrumentation
transpeptidase
    gamma glutamyl t. (GGT)
transperitoneal approach
transpersonal psychology
transphenoidal cryohypophysectomy
transpicuous
transplant
    chromaffin cell t.
    fetal neural t.
transplantation
    adrenal medulla t.
    brain t.
    core assessment program for
      intracerebral t. (CAPIT)
    fetal cell t.
    intracranial-extracranial t.
    liver t.
    organ t.
    porcine cell t.
    t. reaction
    t. shock
    tissue t.
transport
    active t.
    axoplasmic t.
    passive t.
    solute t.
    substrate t.
transporter
    amino acid t.
transposition
    t. of affect
    Müller-König t.
    seventh cranial nerve t.
    vertebral artery t.
transsexual (TS)
    nuclear t.
    t. voice
transsexualism
transsinus approach
transsphenoidal
    t. approach
    t. bipolar forceps
    t. chiasmapexy
    t. curette
    t. encephalocele

T

transsphenoidal *(continued)*
t. evacuation
t. hook
t. hypophysectomy
t. meningoencephalocele
t. removal
t. selective adenomectomy
t. speculum
t. surgery
transsternal
transsylvian approach
transsynaptic
t. chromatolysis
t. degeneration
transtemporal approach
transtentorial
t. approach
occipital t.
t. uncal herniation
transthalamic
transthoracic
t. approach
t. discectomy
t. vertebral body resection
transtorcular
t. approach
t. embolization
t. occlusion
transuncodiscal approach
transvenous
t. approach
t. therapy
transventricular approach
transverse
t. atlantal ligament
t. connector
t. cord lesion
t. crest
t. fiber of pons
t. fissure of cerebellum
t. fissure of cerebrum
t. fixation
t. fixator application
t. fornix
t. gradient coil
t. hermaphroditism
t. incision
t. magnetization
t. magnetization phase
t. myelitis
t. occipital sulcus
t. orientation
t. pedicle angle
t. pedicle diameter
t. relaxation
t. relaxation rate
t. rhombencephalic flexure
t. septum
t. temporal convolutions
t. temporal gyrus
t. temporal sulci
t. traction
t. tripolar epidural array
transversectomy

transvestic
t. fetishism (TF)
t. phenomenon
transvestism paraphilia
transvestite
marginal t.
nuclear t.
transvestitism
Transylvania effect
transzygomatic approach
Tranxene
Tranxene-SD
tranylcypromine
trap
death t.
social t.
trap-door type flap
trapezius muscle
trapezoid body
trapped ventricle syndrome
trapping
aneurysm t.
t. of aneurysm
Trasylol
Traube-Hering-Mayer
T.-H.-M. wave
T.-H.-M. waves in cerebrospinal
fluid
trauma, pl. **traumas, traumata**
abdominal t.
acoustic t.
acute head t.
aftermath of t.
birth t.
brain t.
cerebral t.
cervical spine t.
childhood t.
closed head t.
CNS t.
cranial t.
t. craniocerebral
craniocerebral drug t.
dementia due to head t.
emotional t.
extreme t.
head t.
intestinal t.
late-age t.
lumbar spine t.
maxillofacial t.
nonpenetrating t.
occult head t.
t. organic psychosis
penetrating t.
physical t.
primal t.
psychic t.
recollection of t.
reexperiencing t.
sexual t.
thoracolumbar t.
type 1 t.
type 2 t.
TraumaCal

trauma-induced
    t.-i. delirium
    t.-i. fistula
trauma-related repetition
traumas (*pl. of* trauma)
trauma-specific reenactment
traumasthenia
Trauma Symptom Checklist for Children Ages 8–15
traumata (*pl. of* trauma)
traumatic
    t. alopecia
    t. amblyopia
    t. amnesia
    t. anesthesia
    T. Antecedents Questionnaire
    t. anxiety
    t. aphasia
    t. asphyxia
    t. bereavement
    t. brain injury (TBI)
    t. cervical discopathy
    t. cervical disk herniation
    T. Coma Data Bank (TCDB)
    t. defect state
    t. delirium
    t. dementia
    t. disorder
    t. displacement
    t. encephalitis
    t. epilepsy
    t. event
    T. Events Booklet
    t. experience
    t. grief
    t. headache
    t. hematoma
    t. idiocy
    t. intracranial aneurysm (TICA)
    t. memory
    t. meningeal hemorrhage
    t. meningocele
    t. mutism
    t. neurasthenia
    t. neuritis
    t. neuroma
    t. neuropathy
    t. neurosis
    t. progressive encephalopathy
    t. pseudocatatonia
    t. pseudomeningocele
    t. psychosis
    t. reminder
    t. scene
    t. seizure
    t. separation
    t. stress
    t. stressor
    t. subarachnoid hemorrhage (TSAH, tSAH)
    t. suffocation
    t. syringomyelia
    t. tetanus
    t. transference

traumatica
    amnesia t.
traumatism
traumatization of the libido
traumatize
traumatology
traumatophilia
traumatophilic diathesis
traumatophobia
Travasorb
traversal
    tentorial t.
traverse jury
traversing segment
travesty in wit
tray
    ONE TIME sharp debridement t.
trazodone hydrochloride
TRE
    thyroid response element
TREA
    thoroughness, reliability, efficiency, analytic ability
Treacher Collins syndrome
treated prevalence
treatise
treatment (Rx)
    achievement through counseling and t. (ACT)
    acidification t.
    active t.
    acute intensive t. (AIT)
    adequate t.
    adjunctive t.
    alternative t.
    analytic t.
    antidepressant t.
    appropriate t.
    Aschner t.
    behavioral t.
    coercive t.
    cognitive-behavioral t.
    cognitive-linguistic t.
    cold-pack t.
    communication/cognition t.
    community-based t.
    compression rod t.
    conservative t.
    continuous bath t.
    course of t.
    day care residential t.
    Depression: Awareness, Recognition, and T. (D/ART)
    T. of Depression Collaborative Research Program
    diet t.
    distraction/compression scoliosis t.
    D-penicillamine t.
    t. driven
    drug maintenance t.
    dual compression scoliosis t.
    early t.
    early and periodic screening, diagnosis, and t. (EPSDT)
    educational t.

T

treatment *(continued)*
    electric shock t. (EST, est)
    electroconvulsive t. (ECT)
    electroconvulsive shock t. (ECST)
    electroshock t. (EST, est)
    t. emergent
    empiric drug t.
    endovascular t.
    enforced t.
    ethanol t.
    t. evaluation strategy
    exercise t.
    t. facility
    family t.
    forced t.
    format t.
    frequency of t.
    gamma-interferon t.
    habit t.
    hazardous t.
    holistic t.
    hypervolemic t.
    ineffective t.
    inhalation convulsive t.
    initiation of t.
    inpatient t.
    insight-oriented t.
    insulin coma t.
    t. interference
    intravenous t.
    intrusive t.
    invasive t.
    involuntary t.
    light t.
    long-term t.
    maintenance t.
    medical t.
    methadone maintenance t.
    Metrazol shock t.
    micro-operative t.
    Mitchell t.
    t. modality
    moral t.
    multimonitored electroconvulsive t.
      (MMECT)
    neuroleptic t.
    neuromuscular scoliosis orthotic t.
    noncompliance with medical t.
    nutrition t.
    obesity t.
    ongoing t.
    opioid t.
    orthomolecular t.
    overly stimulating t.
    t. package strategy
    pharmacological t.
    pharmacotherapeutic t.
    t. plan (TRPL)
    t. planning
    poliomyelitis t.
    prefrontal sonic t. (PST)
    prescribed t.
    prolonged sleep t.
    prophylactic t.

    psychiatric t.
    psychodynamic interpretation and t.
    psychopharmacological t.
    psychoprophylactic t.
    psychosocial t.
    psychotherapeutic t.
    refractoriness to t.
    t. refractory
    refusal of t.
    regressive electroshock t. (REST)
    rehabilitation t.
    residential t.
    t. response
    right to t.
    right to refuse t.
    Screening Test for the Assignment
      of Remedial T. (STaRT)
    shock t.
    silent t.
    sleep t.
    somatic t.
    t. specificity
    spinal deformity t.
    stereotactic radiation therapy t.
    subcoma insulin t.
    symptomatic t.
    Toft spinal correction t.
    ultrasound t.
    t. unit
    Weir Mitchell t.
treatment-refractory schizophrenia
treatment-resistant
    t.-r. schizophrenia
    t.-r. schizophrenic
treble safeguard principle
tredecaphobia
tree
    axodendritic t.
    BTE Assembly T.
    decision t.
    neurovascular t.
trefoil tendon deformation
Trélate-Charlin neuralgia
T_2 **relaxation constant**
T_1 **relaxation constant**
trembling
    t. abasia
    t. palsy
    t. voice
tremens
    alcoholic delirium t.
    delirium t. (DT)
tremogram
tremograph
tremolo massage
tremophobia
tremor
    action t.
    acute cerebral t.
    alternating t.
    anticonvulsant medication-induced
      postural t.
    antidepressant medication-induced
      postural t.
    arsenical t.

t. artuum
benign essential t.
beta-adrenergic medication-induced
  postural t.
cerebellar t.
cerebral outflow t.
coarse t.
continuous t.
counting money t.
cycles per second t.
dopaminergic medication-induced
  postural t.
dystonic t.
emotional stress precipitating t.
end point t.
essential t. (ET)
facial t.
familial t.
fibrillary t.
fine postural t.
flapping t.
flopping t.
hand t.
head and neck t.
hepatic encephalopathy t.
heredofamilial t.
Hunt t.
hysterical t.
intention t.
intentional t.
kinetic t.
lithium t.
lithium-induced postural t.
medication-induced postural t.
mercurial t.
metabolic t.
metallic t.
methylxanthine-induced postural t.
mine postural t.
neuroleptic-induced parkinsonian t.
neuroleptic-induced postural t.
non-neuroleptic-induced t.
no-no t.
nonparkinsonian t.
nonpharmacologically induced t.
nontoxic lithium t.
t. opiophagorum
orthostatic t.
oscillating t.
parkinsonian t.
passive t.
perioral t.
persistent t.
physiologic t.
pill-rolling t.
positional t.
postural t.
t. potatorum
precipitating t.
preexisting t.
progressive cerebellar t.
psychologic t.
rapid t.
rest t.
resting t.

rhythmic t.
rhythmicity of t.
rubral t.
saturnine t.
senile t.
shaking t.
small-amplitude rapid t.
static t.
stimulant-induced postural t.
stress precipitating t.
striatocerebellar t.
striatocerebral t.
substance withdrawal t.
sustention/intention t.
tardive t.
t. tendinum
terminal t.
to-and-fro t.
toxic lithium t.
transient t.
volitional t.
wing-beating t.
withdrawal t.
writing t.
yes-yes t.
tremorgram
tremulous
  t. cerebral palsy
  t. movement
  t. speech
tremulousness
  alcohol withdrawal t.
trench
  t. lung
  t. warfare
trend
  death t.
  malignant t.
  Mantel-Haenszel Test for Linear T.
  mortality t.
  paranoid t.
  pernicious t.
  phobic t.
  psychiatric t.
  secular t.
  statistical t.
  t. of thought
Trendar
Trendelenburg
  T. position
  T. symptom
trending
  EP t.
  evoked potential t.
trephination, trepanation
trephine, trepan
  t. craniotomy
  D'Errico skull t.
  DeVilbiss skull t.
  Galt skull t.
  Michele vertebral body t.
  Scoville skull t.
trephined
  syndrome of the t.

T

885

trepidans
  abasia t.
trepidant
trepidation
Treponema
  T. denticola
  T. pallidum
  T. pallidum immobilization (TPI)
  T. pallidum immobilization test
Trevor disease
Trexan
TRGI
  teacher's reading global improvement
TRH
  thyrotropin-releasing hormone
TRI
  total response index
triad
  Charcot t.
  cognitive t.
  oral t.
  Sandler t.
triadic
  t. symbiosis
  t. therapy
triage situation
trial
  t. analysis
  clinical t.
  competency to stand t.
  t. court
  t. and error
  t. examiner
  failure of drug t.
  t. home visit
  t. identification
  t. jury
  t. lesson
  lower hook t.
  t. marriage
  medication t.
  placebo medication t.
  randomized clinical t. (RCT)
  t. separation
  therapeutic t.
  upper hook t.
  VA Symptomatic T.
trial-and-error
  t.-a.-e. learning
  Thorndike t.-a.-e.
Trialodine
triamcinolone
  t. acetonide
triamterene
  hydrochlorothiazide and t.
triangle
  t. of fillet
  Glasscock t.
  Gombault t.
  Guillain-Mollaret t.
  hypoglossal t.
  Karpman t.
  Mullan t.
  opticocarotid t.
  paramedian t.

Parkinson t.
Philippe t.
Reil t.
triangular
  t. base transverse bar configuration
  t. lamella
  t. recess
  t. syndrome
  t. therapy
triangulated pedicle screw
Triapin
Triavil
triazolam
triazolobenzodiazepine
triazolopyridine antidepressant
tribade
tribadism
tribal
tribasilar synostosis
tribunal
triceps surae reflex
trichalgia
trichinellosis
trichinophobia
trichinosis
trichlormethiazide
trichloroethanol (TCE)
trichloromonofluoromethane
  dichlorodifluoromethane and t.
trichodynia
trichoepithelioma
trichoesthesia
trichofolliculoma
trichologia
trichology
trichomalacia
trichomania
trichomoniasis
trichopathophobia
trichophagia
trichophagy
trichophobia
trichorrhexis
  t. nodosa
  t. nodosa with mental
  t. nodosa with mental retardation
trichorrhexomania
trichosis sensitiva
Trichosporon beigelii
trichotillomania
trichotillomania-induced alopecia
trichrome
  Gomori t.
  t. stain
triclofos
tricortical iliac crest bone graft
**tricresyl phosphate peripheral
  neuropathy**
tricyclic
  t. antidepressant (TCA)
  t. antidepressant drug (TCAD)
  t. antipsychotic (TCA)
  t. dibenzoxazepine
  t. secondary amine
  t. tertiary amine

tridecaphobia
tridimensional
    t. evaluational scale (TES)
    T. Personality Questionnaire
    t. theory of feeling
Tridione
triethanolamine salicylate
triethiodide
    gallamine t.
triethylene tetramine dihydrochloride
trifacial
    t. nerve
    t. neuralgia
trifluoperazine hydrochloride
trifluorinated
trifluperidol hydrochloride
triflupromazine hydrochloride
trifurcation of middle cerebral artery
Trigant L. Burrow
trigeminal
    t. cavity
    t. cistern
    t. crest
    t. decompression
    t. electrode
    t. evoked potential (TEP)
    t. ganglion
    t. hypesthesia
    t. lemniscus
    t. nerve
    t. nerve neurinoma
    t. neuralgia (TN)
    t. neuroma
    t. neuropathy
    t. nucleus caudalis lesioning
    t. rhizotomy
    t. root
    t. tractotomy
trigeminocerebellar artery
trigeminofacial reflex
trigeminovascular pathway
trigeminus
    nervus t.
Trigesic
trigger
    active t.
    anticipation of t.
    t. area
    chemoreceptors t.
    exposure to t.
    t. finger
    t. point
    t. point neuralgia
    t. reaction
    situational t.
    t. zone
triggering
    t. event
    t. mechanism
    t. stimulus
TriggerWheel Wand
trigona (*pl. of* trigonum)
trigone
    t. of auditory nerve
    collateral t.

    t. of fillet
    t. of habenula
    t. of hypoglossal nerve
    t. of lateral ventricle
    Müller t.
    olfactory t.
    t. of vagus nerve
trigonocephaly
trigonum, pl. **trigona**
    t. acustici
    t. cérébrale
    t. collaterale
    t. habenulae
    t. hypoglossi
    t. lemnisci
    t. nervi hypoglossi
    t. nervi vagi
    t. olfactorium
    t. ventriculi
trigram
trihexoside
    ceramide t.
trihexosyl ceramide
Trihexy
    T.-2
    T.-5
trihexyphenidyl
    t. hydrochloride
triiodobenzoic acid
triiodothyronine (T_3)
Tri-K
Trilafon
trilingual
Trilisate
trilogy
trimeric form
trimethadione
trimethaphan
trimethobenzamide hydrochloride
trimethoprim
trimethoprim-sulfamethoxazole
trimipramine
Trimstat
trinitrate
    glyceryl t.
trinucleotide
    t. repeat
    t. repeat expansion
triolist
triorchid
tri-ortho-cresyl phosphate
Triosil
tripa ida
tripelennamine
triphasic
    t. slow wave activity
    t. wave
triphosphatase
    adenosine t.
triphosphate
    adenosine t. (ATP)
    deoxynucleside t.'s
    guanosine t. (GTP)
    inositol t. (IP_3)

T

triple
  t. alternation
  t. insanity
  t. phase bone scan
triplegia
Triple-H therapy
triple-wire technique
tripole
  guarded t.
  narrow t.
tripped out
TripTone Caplets
trisalicylate
  choline magnesium t.
trisexuality
triskaidekaphobia
trismic
trismoid
trismus
  t. capistratus
  t. dolorificus
  t. nascentium
  t. neonatorum
  t. sardonicus
trisomy
  t. 13–15
  t. 17–18
  autosomal t.
  chromosome 13 t.
  chromosome 18 t.
  chromosome 21 t.
  t. C syndrome
  t. D syndrome
  E t.
  t. syndrome
  t. 8 syndrome
  t. 13 syndrome
  t. 20 syndrome
tristimania
Trites Neuropsychological Test Battery
triton tumor
triventricular hydrocephalus
Trivittatus virus
tRNA
  alanine t.
trocar
  brain t.
  Frazier brain t.
  McCain TMJ t.
  Paulus t.
  pyramidal t.
trochaic stress
trochanter reflex
trochlear
  t. nerve
  t. nerve neoplasm
  t. nerve palsy
  t. nerve paresis
  t. nucleus
trochlearis
  nervus t.
Trofan
Trofan-DS
troilism paraphilia

trois
  folie à t.
  menage à t.
Trolard
  vein of T.
  T. vein
tromethamine
  ketorolac t.
Trömner
  T. percussion hammer
  T. reflex
tromomania
troops
  shock t.
trophesic
trophesy
trophic
  t. change
  t. gangrene
trophicity
trophism
trophodermatoneurosis
trophoneurosis
  facial t.
  lingual t.
  muscular t.
  Romberg t.
trophoneurotic
  t. atrophy
  t. leprosy
trophopathy
trophotropic zone of Hess
tropical
  t. ataxic neuropathy
  t. myeloneuropathy
  t. spastic paraparesis (TSP)
  t. spastic paraparesis/HTLV-I
    associated myelopathy (TSP/HAM)
tropicamide
tropism
troubled relationship
troubling experience
trough
  synaptic t.
Trousseau
  T. point
  T. sign
  T. spot
  T. syndrome
TRPL
  treatment plan
TRRP
  Thackray Reading Readiness Profile
truancy
  school t.
  socialized childhood t.
  unsocialized childhood t.
truant
truculent
Tru-Cut needle biopsy (TCNB)
true
  t. addiction
  t. amnesia
  t. anosmia
  t. anxiety

t. aphasia
t. apnea
t. belief
t. chancre
t. communication stage
t. epilepsy
t. hermaphroditism
t. insight
t. intersex
t. motivation
t. negative
t. nystagmus
t. perception
t. positive
t. self
t. symbolism
t. vertigo
trumped-up
truncal
t. ataxia
t. dysmetria
truncate
truncation artifact
truncus, gen. and pl. **trunci**
t. corporis callosi
trunk
t. of corpus callosum
meningohypophyseal t. (MHT)
sympathetic t.
trust
basic t.
blind t.
interpersonal t.
mistrust versus t.
t. vs. mistrust
trusting relationship
trustworthiness
doubts of t.
unjustified doubts of t.
trustworthy
truth
t. disclosure
support, empathy and t. (SET)
trypanophobia
trypanosome fever
trypanosomiasis
acute t.
African t.
chronic t.
Cruz t.
East African t.
Gambian t.
Rhodesian t.
West African t.
tryptamine derivative
tryptizol hydrochloride
tryptophan hydroxylase allelic genotype
tryptophanuria with dwarfism
tryst
TS
Tourette syndrome
transitional sleep
transsexual
TSA
Test of Syntactic Ability

TSAH, tSAH
traumatic subarachnoid hemorrhage
TSBC
time-sample behavioral checklist
TSCS
Tennessee Self-Concept Scale
TSH
thyroid stimulating hormone
thyrotropin-stimulating hormone
T-shaped
T.-s. Edwards-Barbaro syringeal shunt
T.-s. incision
TSI
Test of Social Inferences
TSP
tropical spastic paraparesis
TSP/HAM
tropical spastic paraparesis/HTLV-I associated myelopathy
TSRH
Texas Scottish Rite Hospital
TSRH buttressed laminar hook
TSRH circular laminar hook
TSRH crosslink stabilization
TSRH double-rod construct
TSRH implant
TSRH instrumentation
TSRH pedicle hook
TSRH pedicle screw-laminar claw construct
TSRH plate
TSRH universal spinal instrumentation system
TSRI
Teacher School Readiness Inventory
TST
total sleep time
Twenty Statements Test
Tsuji laminaplasty
tsutsugamushi
Rochalimaea t.
TTCT
Torrance Tests of Creative thinking
t **test**
TTMAD
Testing-Teaching Module of Auditory Discrimination
TTS
temporary threshold shift
T-tube shunt
TTV
therapeutic trial visit
tube
Adson brain suction t.
air t.
blunt suction t.
Cone suction t.
Dandy suction t.
endoneural t.
endotracheal t.
Ferguson brain suction t.
flow regulated suction t.
Frazier suction t.
Hardy suction t.

T

tube *(continued)*
    malleable multipore suction t.
    medullary t.
    microbore Tygon t.
    nasogastric t.
    neural t.
    Nishizaki-Wakabayashi suction t.
    Rhoton-Merz suction t.
    Sachs brain suction t.
    Sapporo shunt t.
    Silastic t.
    Spetzler Microvac suction t.
    suction t.
    tympanostomy t.
    Yankauer suction t.
    Yasargil suction t.
tuber, pl. **tubera**
    t. anterius
    ashen t.
    t. cinereum
    t. corporis callosi
    t. dorsale
    gray t.
    subependymal t.
    t. valvulae
    t. vermis
tuberal nuclei
tubercle
    acoustic t.
    amygdaloid t.
    anterior t. of thalamus
    ashen t.
    Chassaignac t.
    t. of cuneate nucleus
    gracile t.
    gray t.
    mamillary t. of hypothalamus
    t. of nucleus gracilis
    olfactory t.
    pharyngeal t.
    Rolando t.
    t. of saddle
    wedge-shaped t.
tubercula *(pl. of* tuberculum)
tubercular meningitis
tuberculoma
tuberculomania
tuberculophobia
tuberculosis
    cerebral t.
    Mycobacterium t.
    t. peripheral neuropathy
    spinal t.
tuberculous
    t. abscess
    t. meningitis
    t. spondylitis
tuberculum, pl. **tubercula**
    t. anterius thalami
    t. cinereum
    t. hypoglossi
    t. nuclei cuneati
    t. nuclei gracilis
    t. olfactorium

    t. sellae
    t. sellae meningioma
tuberofundibular
tuberoinfundibular tract
tuberosa
    urticaria t.
tuberothalamic infarction
tuberous sclerosis
Tubex gauze dressing
tubi (*pl. of* tubus)
tubing
    Intramedic PE-50 polyethylene t.
tubocurarine
tubular necrosis
tubulization
tubus, pl. **tubi**
    t. medullaris
tuck position
Tuffier
    T. laminectomy retractor
    T. rib spreader
Tuffier-Raney retractor
tuft
    dendritic t.
tufted cell
Tuinal
Tukey test
tulipmania
tulip pedicle screw
tumarcin crisis
tumefacient
tumescence
    nocturnal penile t. (NPT)
    penile t.
tumor
    acidophilic pituitary t.
    acoustic nerve sheath t.
    adhesio interthalamica t.
    aggressive papillary middle ear t.
      (APMET)
    angioglomoid t.
    anterior cingulate gyrus t.
    aortic body t.
    astrocytic t.
    atypical giant cell t.
    atypical teratoid/rhabdoid t.
      (ATT/RhT)
    basiocciput t.
    basophilic pituitary t.
    t. bed
    benign cranial nerve t.'s
    benign lymphoepithelial parotid t.
    bone t.
    brain t.
    brainstem t.
    t. bulk
    carotid body t.
    cartilaginous t.
    cavernous sinus t.
    cerebellopontine angle t.
    cervical intramedullary t.
    chemoreceptor t.
    childhood primitive
      neuroectodermal t.
    chondromatous t.

chromaffin t.
Collins law of survival after
  brain t.
collision t.
congenital t.
convexity metastatic t.
dermoid t.
diffuse fibrillary astrocytic t.
diffuse intrinsic brainstem t.
dumbbell t.
dysembryoplastic neuroepithelial t.
  (DNT)
eighth nerve t.
enhancing exophytic t.
t. enucleation
epidermoid t.
epidural t.
Erdheim t.
t. extension
t. extirpation
extradural t.
extrameatal intracapsular t.
extramedullary spinal cord t.
germ cell t.
giant cell t.
giant glomus t.
glial t.
glomus jugulare t.
granular cell t.
hourglass t.
inclusion t.
infiltrating t.
infratentorial-Lindau t.
infratentorial neurological t.
interdural t.
intracavernous t.
intracranial t.
intradural t.
intramedullary spinal cord t.
intraorbital granular cell t.
intraventricular t.
intrinsic brainstem t.
invasive t.
Kernohan classification of brain t.
leptomeningeal t.
Lindau t.
lumbar t.
lymphoepithelial parotid t.
lymphomatous t.
malignant germ cell t.
t. marker
McLain-Weinstein classification of
  spinal t.'s
medullary t.
melanotic neuroectodermal t.
meningeal t.
metastatic t.
t. metastatic to spine
mixed germ cell t.
t. necrosis
t. necrosis factor-α
t. necrosis factor (TNF)
t. necrosis factor receptor (TNFR)
Nelson t.
nerve sheath t.

neuroectodermal t.
neuroepithelial t.
neuronal t.
occipital lobe t.
orbital solitary fibrous t.
Pancoast t.
parachiasmal epidermoid t.
parasellar t.
parotid t.
pearl t.
pediatric supratentorial
  hemispheric t.
peripheral nerve sheath t.
petroclival t.
pineal cell t.
pituitary t.
pontine angle t.
potato t. of neck
Pott puffy t.
primary neuroectodermal t. (PNET)
primitive neuroectodermal t.
  (PNET)
Rathke pouch t.
recurrent t.
t. resection
rhabdoid t.
right frontal craniotomy for gross
  total resection of t.
sand t.
sarcomatous t.
sellar t.
small-bowel carcinoid t.
smooth muscle t.
solitary fibrous t.
spinal cord t.
spindle-cell t.
t. stroma
subdural t.
subependymal t.
superior pulmonary sulcus t.
t. suppressor gene
supratentorial primary malignant
  brain t.
supratentorial primitive
  neuroectodermal t.
tectal plate t.
teratoid t.
thalamic t.
thoracic t.
triton t.
turban t.
vascular t.
vasoformative t.
vertebral body t.
visual system t.
t. volume
tumor-associated
  t.-a. rickets
tumor:cerebellum ratio
tumor:healthy tissue ratio
tumorigenesis
  glial t.
tumor-infiltrating lymphocyte (TIL)
tumor-nerve bundle
tumorous involvement

T

Tums
T. E-X Extra Strength Tablet
T. Extra Strength Liquid
tumultuous growth
tuning fork test
tunnel
t. cell
cubital t.
superior-inferior submucous t.
tarsal t.
t. vision
tunnelable ventricular ICP catheter
tunneled ventriculostomy
Tuohy needle
turban tumor
turbid
turbulence
family t.
turbulent flow
turcica
sella t.
Türck
T. bundle
T. column
T. degeneration
T. tract
Turcot syndrome
turgid
turkomania
turmoil
adolescent t.
emotional t.
turn in
turnbuckle jack
Turnbull method
Turner
T. marginal gyrus
T. sulcus
T. syndrome
turning
t. against self (TAS)
saccadic contraversive head t.
turpitude
moral t.
turricephaly
tussive
t. absence
t. syncope
tutamen, pl. tutamina
tutamina cerebri
Tutoplast
T. allograft
T. anterior tibialis tendon
T. auditory ossicle
T. bone
T. costal cartilage
T. Dura
T. fascia lata
T. fascia temporalis
TVD
transmissible virus dementia
TVI
Temperament and Values Inventory
TWCS
Test of Work Competency and Stability

tweak
T1-weighted
T1-w. inversion recovery scan
T1-w. MR image
T1-w. spin echo
T1-w. spin-echo image
T2-weighted
T2-w. MR image
T2-w. spin echo
T2-w. spin-echo image
twelfth cranial nerve
twelve-step program for substance abuse
twenty-minute hour
Twenty Statements Test (TST)
TWF
Test of Word Finding
TWFD
Test of Word Finding in Discourse
twice a day
twilight
t. attack
t. confusional state
t. epilepsy
t. sleep
t. thirst
t. vision
Twilite Oral
twin
biovular t.
t. concordance
conjoined t.
dizygotic t.
fraternal t.
identical t.
t. language
monozygotic t. (MZ)
t. separation
Siamese t.
t. studies
twinge
Twin-K
twirling of object
twist drill
twisted mouth
twitch
Cogan lid t.
facial t.
focal t.
involuntary t.
muscle t.
rhythmical t.
twitching
uremic t.
two
rule of t.
two-column cervical spine injury
two-component microgrip precision control suction unit
two-dimensional (2D)
t.-d. Fourier transform (2DFT)
t.-d. Fourier transform gradient-echo imaging
t.-d. Fourier transform imaging

t.-d. imaging
t.-d. mapping
Two-Dyne
two-person interview team
two-sided message
two-stage procedure
two-word messages stage
Tycolet
tying forceps
Tylenol
T. Allergy Sinus
T. Extended Relief
T. with codeine
Tylox
tympani
chorda t.
tympanic
t. ganglion
t. intumescence
tympanometry
tympanophonia
tympanoplasty
tympanosquamous suture
tympanostomy tube
tympanum
Tyndall effect seen in cerebrospinal fluid
type
t. A behavior
t. A behavior/personality
actively aggressive reaction t.
adenoid t.
affective reaction t.
aggressive predatory t.
amyloidosis-Dutch t.
t. A personality
apoplectic t.
asthenic constitutional t.
athletic constitutional t.
Attention-Deficit/Activity Disorder, Combined T.
Attention-Deficit/Activity Disorder, Predominantly Hyperactive-Impulsive T.
Attention-Deficit/Activity Disorder, Predominantly Inattentive T.
attention-deficit/hyperactivity disorder, combined t.
attitude t.
attitudinal t.
basic personality t.
t. B behavior
t. B behavior/personality
behavior t.
blood t.
blood-injection-injury t.
body t.
t. B personality
Bulimia Nervosa, Nonpurging T.
Bulimia Nervosa, Purging T.
character t.
choleric constitutional t.
complex t.
constitutional t.

Conversion Disorder, Mixed T.
Conversion Disorder, Motor T.
Conversion Disorder, Seizure T.
Conversion Disorder, Sensory T.
dementia of Alzheimer t. (DAT)
Dementia of the Alzheimer's T.
deterioration reaction t.
Don Juan t.
dysplastic constitutional t.
ectomorphic constitutional t.
eidetic t.
endomorphic constitutional t.
erotic t.
Erotomanic T.
explicit t.
exploiting t.
extroverted t.
family t.
functional t.
grandiose t.
hereditary cerebral hemorrhage with amyloidosis, Dutch t. (HCHWA-D)
hypercompensatory t.
Hypochondriasis With Poor Insight T.
t. I alcoholic
idiotropic t.
t. I error
t. II alcoholic
t. II curve pattern
t. II error
t. indicator
introverted t.
intuitive t.
irrational t.
jealous t.
Kretschmer t.
libidinal t.
linear t.
melancholic constitutional t.
mesomorphic constitutional t.
mixed t.
MMPI Code T.
noradrenaline dementia of Alzheimer t.
nosotropic drug dementia of Alzheimer t.
objective t.
obsessional t.
Obsessive-Compulsive Disorder With Poor Insight T.
paranoid reaction t.
Persecutory T.
personality t.
Personality Change Due to a General Medical Condition, Aggressive T.
Personality Change Due to a General Medical Condition, Apathetic T.
Personality Change Due to a General Medical Condition, Disinhibited T.

T

type *(continued)*
Personality Change Due to a General Medical Condition, Labile T.
Personality Change Due to a General Medical Condition, Paranoid T.
phlegmatic constitutional t.
physique t.
primary degenerative dementia of Alzheimer t. (PDDAT)
Primary Hypersomnia, Recurrent T.
pyknic constitutional t.
reaction t.
Reactive Attachment Disorder of Infancy or Early Childhood, Disinhibited T.
Reactive Attachment Disorder of Infancy or Early Childhood, Inhibited T.
receiving t.
sanguine constitutional t.
schizophrenia, catatonic t.
schizophrenia, disorganized t.
schizophrenia, paranoid t.
schizophrenia, residual t.
schizophrenia, undifferentiated t.
senile dementia of Alzheimer t. (SDAT)
social t.
somatic t.
t. specifier
substitutive reaction t.
T. 2 superconductor
thinking t.
t. 1 trauma
t. 2 trauma
undersocialized conduct disorder, aggressive t.
undersocialized conduct disorder, nonaggressive t.

unspecified t.
working t.
typhoid peripheral neuropathy
typhomania
typhosus
status t.
typhus fever
typical
t. absence
t. absence seizure
t. age
t. behavior
t. theme
typing
HLA DR15 (DR2) t.
sex t.
typist's cramp
typity
typology
anxiety t.
typomania
tyramine challenge test
tyramine-induced hypertensive crisis
tyramine-rich food
tyrannical
t. behavior
t. decision making
tyrannism
tyrannophobia
tyranny of silence
tyropanoate
tyropanoic acid
tyrosine
t. hydroxylase
t. hydroxylase-positive
tyrosine-kinase receptor
tyrosinemia aminoaciduria
tyrosinosis
Tzanck smear

UA
   urinalysis
ubiquitous
UCI
   usual childhood illness
UCR
   unconditioned reflex
   unconditioned response
UCS
   unconditioned stimulus
   unicoronal synostosis
UES
   Unpleasant Events Schedule
U74006F
   21-aminosteroid U74006F
UFO
   unidentified flying object
UHMWPE
   ultra high molecular weight polyethylene
   fiber
      UHMWPE cable
Uhthoff
   U. phenomenon
   U. sign
UID/S
   unilateral interfacetal dislocation or
   subluxation
UL
   unauthorized leave
ulcer
      contact u.
      Cushing u.
      decubitus u.
      duodenal u.
      peptic u.
      u. personality
      psychogenic u.
      stress u.
ulceration
      genital u.
      oral u.
ulcerative colitis
ulegyria
Ullmann line
ulnar
      u. nerve
      u. nerve entrapment
      u. nerve lesion
      u. neuropathy
      u. reflex
ulterior transaction
Ulthoff symptom
Ultimate Xphoria
Ultiva
ultradian rhythm
ultradistant
Ultradol
ultrafastidious
ultrafeminine
ultra high molecular weight
   polyethylene fiber (UHMWPE)

ultra-high molecular weight polyethylene
   fiber cable
Ultralente Iletin I
Ultram
ultramarginal zone
ultramicroclip
UltraPower
      U. basic drill system
      U. bur guard
      U. revision drill system
      U. surgical drill system
ultrashort-acting barbiturate
ultrasonic
      u. aspirating device
      u. aspiration
      u. aspirator
      u. dissector
      u. localizer
      u. probe
      u. surgical aspirator
      u. therapy
      u. wave
ultrasonographic
      u. guidance
      u. localization
ultrasonography
      B-mode u.
      Doppler u.
      sequential u.
      transcranial Doppler u.
ultrasonosurgery
ultrasound
      Doppler u.
      intraoperative u.
      intraoperative B-mode u.
      Intrascan u.
      TCD u.
      transcranial B-mode u.
      transfontanel Doppler u.
      u. treatment
ultrasound-guided transfrontal
   transventricular approach
ultraviolet
ultromotivity
ululation
Umbradil
unacceptable
      u. behavior
      u. feeling
      u. impulse
      u. thought
unaggressive
      u. conduct disorder
      u. undersocialized reaction
unaided augmentative communication
unanticipated crisis
unassertive
      u. aggression
      u. expression
unauthorized leave (UL)
unawareness of environment
unbiased information

U

uncal
  u. gyrus
  u. herniation
uncanny emotion
uncertain biological status
uncertainty
  u. factor
  u. level
uncertainty-arousal factor
unci (*pl. of* uncus)
unciform fasciculus
uncinate
  u. attack
  u. aura
  u. bundle of Russell
  u. convulsion
  u. epilepsy
  u. fasciculus of Russell
  u. fit
  u. gyrus
  u. process
  u. seizure
Uncle
  U. Tom
  U. Tomism
uncomplicated
  u. alcohol withdrawal
  u. arteriosclerotic
  u. arteriosclerotic psychosis
  u. bereavement
  u. recovery
  u. sedative, hypnotic, or anxiolytic
    withdrawal
unconditional positive regard
unconditioned
  u. reflex (UCR)
  u. response (UCR)
  u. stimulus (UCS)
unconscious
  u. cerebration
  collective u.
  u. concern
  u. conflict
  u. factor
  familial u.
  u. fantasy
  u. guilt
  u. homosexuality
  impersonal u.
  u. impulse
  u. memory
  u. motivation
  u. need for punishment
  personal u.
  u. process
  u. processing
  u. rage
  u. resistance
  superpersonal u.
unconsciousness
  absolute u.
  conversion u.
unconsummated marriage
uncontrollability
  stressor u.

uncontrollable
  u. action
  u. quality
  u. sleep attack
  u. thought
uncontrolled
  u. laughter
  u. worry
uncoordinated
  u. gait
  u. motor skills
uncoupling
  metabolic flow u.
uncovering technique
uncovertebral joint hypertrophy
uncued
  u. behavior
  u. panic attack
uncus, pl. **unci**
  arachnoid of u.
  u. band of Giacomini
  u. gyri parahippocampalis
  u. of temporal lobe
underachievement disorder
undercontrol
  behavioral u.
  emotional u.
undercutting
  cortical u.
  u. saw
underlying
  u. emotional issue
  u. structure
undermine
underproductive speech
under the skin
undersocialized
  u. conduct behavior
  u. conduct disorder, aggressive
    type
  u. conduct disorder, nonaggressive
    type
  u. disorder
  u. nonaggressive reaction
  u. socialized disturbance
understanding
  shared u.
  word u.
understimulation theory
under-the-counter
under-the-table
undetermined origin (UO)
undiagnosed general medical condition
undifferentiated
  u. attention-deficit disorder
  u. cell adenoma
  chronic u.
  u. schizophrenia
  schizophrenic reaction, acute u.
    (SR/AU)
  schizophrenic reaction, acute, u.
  schizophrenic reaction, chronic, u.
    (SR/CU)
  u. wholeness
undinism

undirected thinking
undisciplined self-conflict
undisturbed nocturnal sleep
undoing defense mechanism
undressing
    paradoxical u.
undue social anxiety
undulant fever
undulate
unemotional thought
unemployable unethical behavior
unencapsulated joint receptor
unequal distribution
unequivocal change in functioning
unethical behavior
unexpected
    u. behavior
    u. panic attack
    u. response
unexplained
    u. absence from work
    u. pain
unfamiliar place
unfocused delirium
unformed
    u. image
    u. visual hallucination
ungiving
    emotionally u.
    u. parent
unguis, pl. ungues
    u. avis
    Haller u.
unhappiness
    u. and misery disorder
    pattern of pervasive u.
    pervasive u.
Uni-Ace
unicoronal synostosis (UCS)
unidentified flying object (UFO)
unidirectional nystagmus
unification in wit
Unified Parkinson Disease Rating Scale
(UPDRS)
Uniform Determination of Death Act
uniformly progressive deterioration
Unilab Surgibone bovine bone graft
unilateral
    u. abductor paralysis
    u. adductor paralysis
    u. anesthesia
    u. brief pulse ECT
    u. chorea
    u. decision
    u. epileptiform activity
    u. focus
    u. focus of activity
    u. hemilaminectomy
    u. hermaphroditism
    u. hydrocephalus
    u. hyperreflexia
    u. hypophysectomy
    u. interfacetal dislocation or
      subluxation (UID/S)
    u. laminotomy

    u. megalencephaly
    u. migraine
    u. migraine headache
    u. nondominant-hemisphere ECT
    u. optic neuritis
    u. organic neglect
    u. pedicle cannulation
    u. seizure
    u. sine wave ECT
    u. spatial neglect
    u. variable screw placement system
    u. visual neglect
uninhibited
    u. behavior
    u. motor planning
    u. neurogenic bladder
unintelligible speech
unintended
    u. effect
    u. sleep
unintentional
    u. daytime sleep episode
    u. death
unintentionally produced symptom
uninterrupted episode
union
    mystic u.
Unipen
unipolar
    u. cell
    u. cutting loop
    u. depression
    u. disorder
    u. double-bind
    u. mania
    u. manic-depressive psychosis
    u. neuron
Uni-Pro
unique
    u. characteristic
    u. trait
unisensory
unisex
Uni-Shunt
UNI-SHUNT hydrocephalus shunt
Unisom
unit
    acute care u. (ACU)
    addictive disease u. (ADU)
    afferent   motor u.
    AME microcurrent TENS u.
    BICAP u.
    Cadwell 5200A somatosensory
      evoked potential u.
    u. clerk
    communication u.
    day treatment u.
    Dial Away Pain 400
      electrotherapy u.
    Eclipse TENS u.
    efferent   motor u.
    family u.
    G5 Fleximatic
      massage/percussion u.

U

unit *(continued)*
>G5 Vibramatic massage/percussion u.
>Hounsfield u. (HU)
>intensive care u. (ICU)
>intensive treatment u. (ITU)
>internal pulse generating u.
>Leksell stereotactic gamma u.
>life change u. (LCU)
>locked hospital u.
>Malis electrocoagulation u.
>Maxima II TENS u.
>maximum security u.
>Mayfield radiolucent base u.
>memory for symbolic u. (MSU)
>motor u.
>Parental Stressor Scale: Neonatal Intensive Care U. (PSS:NICU)
>polyphasic motor u.
>polysensory u.
>psychiatric u.
>psychiatric intensive care u. (PICU)
>Radionics bipolar coagulation u.
>relational u.
>u. restriction
>Sheffield gamma u.
>Signa 1.5 Tesla u.
>201-source cobalt-60 gamma u.
>u. spinal rod
>state hospital children's u. (SHCU)
>stereotactic gamma u.
>teleradiotherapy u.
>training u.
>treatment u.
>two-component microgrip precision control suction u.
>valve u.
>work-for-pay u.
>Wright Care TENS u.
>ZD-Neurosurgical localizing u.

unitary
>u. consciousness
>u. disorder

United
>U. States Pharmacopeia (USP)
>U. States Public Health Service (USPHS)
>U. States-United Kingdom Study

uniting
>u. canal
>u. duct

unitization

unity
>functional u.
>u. and fusion

universal
>u. instrumentation
>u. phobia
>u. symbol

universalis
>alopecia u.

universalization

universals
>formal u.
>substantive u.

University Residence Environment Scale (URES)

unjustified
>u. doubt of loyalty
>u. doubts of trustworthiness

unkempt
>u. appearance
>u. manner

unknown
>u. language
>u. meaning
>u. substance-induced mood disorder

unlawful behavior
unmet dependency need
unmitigated echolalia
unmodified ECT therapy
unmyelinated fiber
unnatural cheerfulness
unobtrusive measure
unpaired electron
unplanned pregnancy
unpleasant
>U. Events Schedule (UES)
>u. hallucination
>u. mood

unpredictable
>u. agitation
>u. mood change

unproductive mania
unprotected
>u. intercourse
>u. sex

unpurposeful behavior
unrealistic worry
unreality
>feelings of u.
>idea of u.

unreasonable
>u. belief
>u. demand
>u. fear
>u. idea

unrefined motor skill
unrelated thought
unrelenting pain
unrelieved agitation
unresolved
>u. bereavement
>u. conflict
>u. grief
>u. loss

unresponsive
>u. patient
>u. state

unrestricted diet
unruptured aneurysm
unsanctioned
>culturally u.
>u. response

unsatisfying relationship
unselective observation

unshakable
u. belief
u. preoccupation
unshunted hydrocephalus
unsocialized
u. childhood truancy
u. disorder
u. disturbance of thought
unspecified
u. aneurysm
bipolar I disorder, most recent episode u.
u. mental disorder, nonpsychotic
u. mental retardation
mental retardation, severity u.
u. mood episode
u. psychological factor
u. schizophrenia
u. substance dependence
u. type
unspecified-type
u.-t. delusion
u.-t. dyssomnia
unstable
u. affect
u. attachment
u. cervical spine injury
emotionally u.
u. personality
u. relationship
u. self-image
unsteady gait
unstructured interview
unsustained clonus
unsystematized delusion
untimely
u. death
u. demise
u. pregnancy
untreated episode
untriggered agitation
unusual
u. behavior
u. detail response (Dd)
u. manner
u. personality
u. rare detail response (dr)
u. sleep posture
Unverricht
U. disease
U. myoclonus epilepsy
Unverricht-Lafora disease
Unverricht-Lundborg
U.-L. disease
U.-L. myoclonus epilepsy
U.-L. syndrome
unvoluntary behavior
unwanted
u. child
u. pregnancy
u. screw torque
unwarranted idea
UO
undetermined origin

u-PA
urokinase-type PA
upbeating nystagmus
upbiting/downbiting pituitary rongeur
up in the clouds
UPDRS
Unified Parkinson Disease Rating Scale
upper
u. abdominal periosteal reflex
u. bound
u. cervical spine anterior construct
u. cervical spine anterior exposure
u. cervical spine fusion
u. cervical spine posterior construct
u. cervical spine procedure
u. hook trial
u. limb areflexia
u. motor neuron
u. motor neuron impairment
u. motor neuron lesion
u. motor neuron paralysis
u. pons
u. radicular syndrome
u. thoracic spine
uprooted psychology
uprooting neurosis
upset
emotionally u.
excessively u.
mental u.
upswap
frontal u.
upward
u. gaze paresis
u. masking
u. mobility
UR
utilization review
Uracel
uranism
uranophobia (*var. of* ouranophobia)
uranoplasty
uranoschisis
Urbach-Wiethe disease
urban
u. crisis
u. psychiatry
urbanite
urchin
ur-defense
urea
u. cycle
u. cycle disorder
Ureaphil Injection
uremia peripheral neuropathy
uremic
u. amaurosis
u. convulsion
u. encephalopathy
u. neuropathy
OKT3 u.
u. polyneuropathy
u. seizure
u. twitching

U

URES
> University Residence Environment Scale

ureter injury
ureterolysis
urethral
> u. anxiety
> u. character
> u. complex
> u. erotism
> u. phase
> u. stage

urethrism, urethrismus
urethritis
urethrospasm
urge
> anomalous sexual u.
> inappropriate u.
> u. incontinence
> intense sexual u.
> intrusive u.
> involuntary premonitory u.
> masochistic sexual u.
> sexual u.

urgency incontinence
uric acid
urinalysis (UA)
urinary
> u. creatinine
> u. incontinence
> u. reflex
> u. sphincter
> u. stuttering
> u. tract

urinate
urine
> dirty u.
> drug-negative u.
> u. drug screen
> white turbid u.

uriposia
Uristix
> Dextrostix U.

uroclepsia
urocrisia, urocrisis
Urografin
urokinase
urokinase-type PA (u-PA)
Uro-KP-Neutral
urolagnia
urologist
Uromiro
Uropac
urophilia
urophobia
urorrhea
Urovision
urticaria
> giant u.
> u. gigans
> u. gigantea
> psychogenic u.
> u. tuberosa

urticate
urtication

US
> Imagent US

usage
> idiomatic u.

use
> adolescent drug u.
> u. of alias
> cannabis u.
> cocaine and cannabis u.
> compulsive substance u.
> crack u.
> u. disorder
> drug u.
> heroin and crack u.
> inhalant u.
> long-term heavy u.
> lysergic acid diethylamide u.
> nonpathological substance u.
> opium u.
> pathologic substance u.
> recreational drug u.

user
> intravenous drug u. (IVDU)

U-shaped scalp flap
Usher syndrome
USP
> United States Pharmacopeia
> extended phenytoin sodium
>   capsules, USP

USPHS
> United States Public Health Service

usual
> u. behavior
> u. childhood illness (UCI)
> u. nondepressed mood

Utah Test of Language Development (UTLD)
uterine curette
utero
> in u.

uteromania
uteroplacental environment
utilitarianism
> act u.
> hedonistic u.
> negative u.
> pluralistic u.
> rule u.

utilitarian principle
utility
> expected u. (EU)

utilization
> evaluation u.
> u. review (UR)
> u. review committee
> u. technique
> Test of Concept U. (TCU)

UTLD
> Utah Test of Language Development

Utopia
utricle
utricular
> u. reflex
> u. spot

utriculosaccular duct
utriculus, pl. **utriculi**
    macula utriculi
utter
utterance
uveitis
    juxtapapillary u.
uveomeningoencephalic syndrome
uveomeningoencephalitis
uvula, pl. **uvuli**

    bifid u.
    u. cerebelli
    u. vermis
uxorial
uxoricide
uxorious
Uzgiris-Hunt Scale

U

V
    V code
    V factor
μV
2-μV
v
    versus
V1 halo ring
VA
    VA Hospital
    vertebral artery
    Veterans Administration
        VA Hospital (VA)
        VA Symptomatic Trial
vacant
    v. spell
    v. stare
vaccination peripheral neuropathy
vaccine
    diphtheria, tetanus toxoids, and
        pertussis v. (DTP)
vaccinophobia
vache
    coitus á la v.
vacillate
VACPAC support
vacuo
    hydrocephalus ex v.
vacuous affect
vacuum
    v. activity
    v. disk
    existential v.
    v. headache
vadum
vagabond neurosis
vagal
    v. attack
    v. nerve implant
    v. part of accessory nerve
vagale
    glomus v.
vagectomy
vagina, gen. and pl. **vaginae**
    v. cellulosa
    v. dentata
vaginal
    v. envy
    v. father
    v. hypesthesia
    v. orgasm
    v. plethysmograph
vaginam
    per v.
vaginate
vaginismus, vaginism
    functional v.
    lifelong-type v.
    psychic v.
vagoaccessory syndrome
vagoglossopharyngeal
    v. neuralgia

vagolysis
vagolytic
vagomimetic
vagotomy
vagotonia
vagotropic
vagovagal
vagrancy
vague
    v. communication
    nouvelle v.
    v. perplexity
    v. speech
vagus
    v. area
    v. nerve
    v. nerve stimulation (VAS, VNS)
    nervus v.
    v. neuropathy
    v. stimulator implant
vail
vain
Vairox high compression vascular
  stockings
valence
    positive v.
Valentin
    V. corpuscle
    V. ganglion
valepotriate
valerate
    ammonium v.
    amyl v.
valerian
validating variable
validation
    v. communication pattern
    consensual v.
    cross v.
    v. therapy
valid consent
validity
    concurrent v.
    construct v.
    content v.
    criterion-related v.
    descriptive v.
    discriminant v.
    ecological v.
    empirical v.
    etiological v.
    external v.
    face v.
    factorial v.
    V. Indicator Profile (VIP)
    internalized v.
    intervening v.
    item v.
    predictive v.
    v. scale
valinemia
Valin hemilaminectomy retractor

Valium
  V. Injection
  V. Oral
vallecula, pl. **valleculae**
  v. cerebelli
  v. sylvii
Valleix point
Valleylab
  V. CUSA CEM system
  V. neurosurgical product
vallis
Valmid
valnoctamide
valor
Valpar Work Sample Battery
valproate
  sodium v.
valproic
  v. acid
  v. acid and derivatives
  v. acid poisoning
valpromide
Valrelease
Valsalva maneuver
value
  acculturation problem with
    expression of political v.
  acculturation problem with
    expression of religious v.
  Adjustment and V.
  aesthetic v.
  Allport-Vernon-Linzey Study
    of V.'s
  being v.
  cocaine v.
  confusion of v.'s
  C-reactive protein v.
  critical v.
  educational v.
  foreign v.
  idealized v.
  internal v.
  v.'s inventory
  V.'s Inventory for Children (VIC)
  v. judgment
  K index v.
  law of initial v.
  Maferr Inventory of Masculine V.'s
    (MIMV)
  moral v.
  nontrivial v.
  p v.
  personal v.
  political v.
  predictive v.
  prognostic v.
  religious v.'s
  sentimental v.
  sharing of v.'s
  social v.
  status v.
  Study of V.'s (SV)
  Survey of Interpersonal V.'s (SIV)
  Survey of Personal V.'s
  Survey of Work V.'s, Revised,
    Form U
  symbolic v.
  traditional v.
  Wilder law of initial v.
valve
  ball-in-cone v.
  Codman-Medos programmable v.
  Codman slit v.
  Cordis-Hakim v.
  cruciform slit v.
  CRx v.
  Delta v.
  Denver v.
  double spring ball v.
  Hakim high-pressure v.
  Hakim precision v.
  Heyer-Pudenz v.
  Heyer-Schulte bur hole v.
  Holter v.
  Holter-Hausner v.
  Holter high-pressure v.
  Holter medium-pressure v.
  Low Profile v.
  Medos v.
  Medos-Hakim v.
  Mishler v.
  Novus hydrocephalic v.
  Novus mini v.
  Orbis-Sigma cerebrospinal fluid
    shunt v.
  v. patency
  Phoenix ancillary v.
  Phoenix cruciform v.
  programmable v.
  prosthetic heart v.
  PS Medical Flow Control v.
  Pudenz v.
  rotating hemostatic v. (RHV)
  safety v.
  slit v.
  Sophy mini programmable
    pressure v.
  v. system (VS)
  Tarin v.
  v. unit
  Vieussens v.
valvula, pl. **valvulae**
  v. semilunaris tarini
valvuloplasty
Vamate
vampirism
  parasitic v.
van
  v. Bogaert-Canavan disease
  v. Bogaert disease
  v. Bogaert encephalitis
  v. Bogaert sclerosing
    leukoencephalitis
  v. der Knaap syndrome
  v. der Kolk law
Vancocin
vancomycin

vandalism
    sexual v.
Vane Evaluation of Language Scale (VELS)
vane-type motor
vanilla mandelic acid
vanquish
vaporize
variability
    behavioral v.
    peak amplitude v.
    trait v.
variable
    antecedent v.
    antecedent-consequence v.
    autochthonous v.
    v. behavior
    biopsychosocial v.
    cognitive v.
    criterion v.
    dependent v.
    experimental v.
    independent v.
    index v.
    v. interval (VI)
    intervening v.
    moderator v.
    organic v.
    organismic v.
    outcome v.
    predictor v.
    quantitative v.
    random v.
    v. ratio (VR)
    v. reinforcement
    v. resistor
    v. screw placement (VSP)
    v. screw placement system
    v. screw placement system instrumentation
    v. screw placement system-instrumented lumbar spine
    v. screw placement system-plated patient
    v. stereotactic image fusion
    v. stiffness microcatheter
    validating v.
variable-interval reinforcement schedule
variance
    analysis of v. (ANOVA)
    between-group v.
    error v.
    multivariate analysis of v. (MANOVA)
Vari-Angle
    V.-A. aneurysm clip
    V.-A. clip applier
    V.-A. clip holder
    V.-A. screw
variant
    anatomical v.
    Becker v.
    epileptic v.
    primitive trigeminal artery v.
    Westphal v.

variate
variation
    cerebral hemodynamic v.
    chance v.
    coefficient of v. (CV)
    conative negative v. (CNV)
    contingent negative v. (CNV)
    cultural v.
    diurnal v.
    negative v.
    physiological functional v.
    reverse diurnal v.
varicella
    v. encephalitis
    v. zoster virus (VZV)
varices (*pl. of* varix)
Varidase
variegate porphyria
Varigrip spine fixation system
VARIMIC 900 microscope
varix, pl. **varices**
    orbital varices
VAS
    vagus nerve stimulation
    visual analog scale
vas, gen. **vasis**, gen. and pl. **vasorum**, pl. **vasa**
    vasa recta
    vasa vasorum
Vasamedics laser Doppler flow probe
VASC
    Verbal-Auditory Screen for Children
    Visual-Auditory Screen for Children
    VASC test
vascular
    v. accident
    v. circle of optic nerve
    v. decompression
    v. dementia
    v. dementia with delirium
    v. dementia with delusions
    v. dementia with depressed mood
    v. depression
    v. endothelial growth factor (VEGF)
    v. erosion
    v. fragility
    v. groove
    v. hamartoma
    v. headache
    v. injury
    v. malformation
    v. neurosyphilis
    v. occlusion
    v. parkinsonism
    v. patch graft
    v. perforation
    v. surgery
    v. territory
    v. tumor
vascularized split calvarial cranioplasty
vasculature
    CNS v.
    systemic v.

V

vasculitic neuropathy
vasculitis, pl. **vasculitides**
    Churg-Strauss v.
    hypersensitivity v.
    leukocytoclastic vasculitides
    mesenteric v.
    necrotizing v.
    pauci-immune necrotizing v.
    radiation v.
    retinal v.
    septic venous v.
    systemic v.
vasculogenic loss of erectile functioning
vasculomotor
vasculomyelinopathy
vasculopathy
    radiation-induced v.
vasculosa
    meninx v.
vasculosum
    punctum v.
vasectomy
Vaseline gauze packing
Vaseretic 10-25
Vasiodone
vasis (*gen. of* vas)
vasoactive
    v. intestinal peptide (VIP)
    v. intestinal polypeptide (VIP)
vasoconstriction
vasoconstrictor
vasodilatation, vasodilation
    mannitol-induced cerebral v.
vasodilator headache
vasodilator-stimulated rCBF single
  photon emission computed
  tomographic measurement
vasoformative tumor
vasogenic
    v. edema
    v. shock
    v. theory
vasomotor
    v. absence
    v. ataxia
    v. epilepsy
    v. headache
    v. imbalance
    v. instability
    v. ischemia
    v. paralysis
    v. rhinitis
    v. spasm
    v. syncope
vasoneuropathy
vasoneurosis
vasopressin
    arginine v.
    desamino-D-arginine v.
    v. receptor agonist
    v. tannate
vasopressor
    v. reflex
    v. syncope

vasoreactivity
    cerebral v.
vasoreflex
vasorum (*gen. and pl. of* vas)
vasosensory
vasospasm
    angiographic v.
    arterial v.
    cerebral v.
    delayed cerebral v.
vasospastic attack
vasostimulant
vasotocin
    arginine v. (AVT)
vasovagal
    v. attack
    v. attack of Gowers
    v. epilepsy
    v. syncope
    v. syndrome
VAT
    Vocational Apperception Test
Vater corpuscle
Vater-Pacini
    V.-P. body
    V.-P. corpuscle
vault
    cranial v.
VBR
    ventricle-to-brain ratio
VC
    visual communication
Vc
    ventrocaudal nucleus
VCDQ
    Verbal Comprehension Deviation
      Quotient
VCR
    vincristine
VD
    venereal disease
VDR
    vitamin D receptor
VDRL
    Venereal Disease Research Laboratory
      VDRL test
VDRS
    Verdun Depression Rating Scale
VDS
    ventral derotating spinal
    ventral derotation spondylodesis
VDT
    visual distortion test
vector
    v. diagram
    v. field
    M v.
    macroscopic magnetization v.
    magnetic field v.
    nuclear magnetization v.
    v. phase
vecuronium bromide
VEE
    Venezuelan equine encephalomyelitis
vegan diet

veganism
vegetarian diet
vegetarianism
vegetate
vegetative
    v. level
    v. life
    v. lifelikelihood
    v. nervous system
    v. neurosis
    v. retreat
    v. state
    v. subscale
    v. symptom
vegetotherapy
    character-analytic v.
VEGF
    vascular endothelial growth factor
vehemence
vehicle
    all-terrain v. (ATV)
    v. for communication
    v. fear
    v. for
vehicular accident
veil
    aqueduct v.
vein
    anterior v. of septum pellucidum
    azygous v.
    basal v. of Rosenthal (BVR)
    brachiocephalic v.
    bridging v.
    Browning v.
    carotid v.
    cerebellar v.
    v. of cerebellum
    cerebral v.
    cervical intersegmental v.
    choroid v.
    v. of corpus striatum
    cortical v.
    deep middle cerebral v.
    diencephalic v.
    diploic v.
    draining v.
    emissary v.
    v. of Galen
    v. of Galen aneurysm
    v. of Galen malformation
    great cerebral v.
    great v. of Galen
    inferior anastomotic v.
    inferior v.'s of cerebellar
      hemisphere
    innominate v.
    intradural draining v.
    jugular v.
    jugulocephalic v.
    Labbé v.
    v. of Labbé
    lingual v.
    linguofacial v.
    maxillary v.
    meningeal v.

    meningorachidian v.
    mesencephalic v.
    myelencephalic v.
    ophthalmic v.
    orbital v.
    v. patch rupture
    posterior callosal v.
    posterior v. of septum pellucidum
    precentral cerebellar v.
    primitive maxillary v.
    radicular v.
    Rosenthal v.
    saphenous v.
    v. of septum pellucidum
    striate v.
    superficial middle cerebral v.
    superficial temporal v.
    superior anastomotic v.
    superior v. of cerebellar
      hemisphere
    superior thyroid v.
    telencephalic v.
    terminal v.
    thalamostriate v.
    thrombosed thick-walled v.
    v. of Trolard
    Trolard v.
vela (*pl. of* velum)
velar assimilation
velars
    backing to v.
Velban
Veley headrest
velleity
vellicate
vellus
    v. olivae inferioris
velnacrine maleate
velocardiofacial syndrome
velocimetry
    laser-Doppler v.
velocity
    average v.
    blood v.
    v. encoding
    flow v. (FV)
    glutamate transport v.
    nerve conduction v. (NCV)
    preserved conduction v.
    v. profile
    saccade v.
    spectral v.
    spin v.
VELS
    Vane Evaluation of Language Scale
velum, pl. **vela**
    anterior medullary v.
    inferior medullary v.
    v. interpositum
    v. medullare inferius
    v. medullare superius
    v. palatinum
    posterior medullary v.
    v. semilunare
    superior medullary v.

V

velum *(continued)*
    v. tarini
    v. terminale
    v. transversum
    v. triangulare
vena, gen. and pl. **venae**
    v. anastomotica inferior
    v. anastomotica superior
    v. basalis
    v. cava injury
    venae cerebelli
    venae cerebelli inferiores
    venae cerebelli superiores
    v. cerebri anterior
    venae cerebri inferiores
    venae cerebri internae
    v. cerebri magna
    v. cerebri media profunda
    v. cerebri media superficialis
    venae cerebri profundae
    venae cerebri superficiales
    venae cerebri superiores
    v. choroidea inferior
    v. choroidea superior
    venae hemispherii cerebelli inferiores
    venae hemispherii cerebelli superiores
    v. petrosa
    venae pontis
    v. precentralis cerebelli
    v. septi pellucidi anterior
    v. septi pellucidi posterior
    venae striatae
    v. terminalis
    venae thalamostriatae inferiores
    v. thalamostriata superior
    v. vermis inferior
    v. vermis superior
venereal
    v. bubo
    v. disease (VD)
    V. Disease Research Laboratory (VDRL)
    V. Disease Research Laboratory test
    v. sore
venereophobia
veneris ardor
Venezuelan
    V. equine encephalitis
    V. equine encephalomyelitis (VEE)
venial sin
venipuncture pain
venlafaxine
    v. HCl
    v. hydrochloride
venography
    digital subtraction v.
    epidural v.
    transosseous v.
    vertebral v.
venorespiratory reflex

venous
    v. aneurysm
    v. angioma
    v. angle
    v. embolism
    v. hypertension
    v. lake
    v. lake configuration
    v. occlusive disease
    v. outflow obstruction
    v. plexus
    v. sinus
    v. stasis
    v. stasis retinopathy
    v. system
    v. thromboembolic disease (VTED)
venous-side embolization
venous-sinus
    thrombocytopenia v.-s.
venter
    abactus v.
ventilate concern
ventilation
    abnormal v.
    assisted v.
    v. of feeling
    high-frequency percussive v. (HFPV)
    mechanical v.
ventilator
    v. alarm
    v. weaning
Ventolin
ventral
    v. amygdalofugal pathway
    v. amygdaloid fugal projection
    v. anterior nucleus of thalamus
    v. column of spinal cord
    v. derotating spinal (VDS)
    v. derotation spondylodesis (VDS)
    v. globus pallidus
    v. horn
    v. intermediate nucleus of thalamus
    v. lateral nucleus of thalamus
    v. medial mesencephalic syndrome
    v. medullary compression
    v. mesencephalon
    v. nucleus of thalamus
    v. nucleus of trapezoid body
    v. pallidum
    v. part of the pons
    v. plate of neural tube
    v. pontine infarction
    v. posterior intermediate nucleus of thalamus
    v. posterior lateral nucleus of thalamus
    v. posterior nucleus of thalamus
    v. posterolateral nucleus (VPL)
    v. posterolateral nucleus of thalamus
    v. posteromedial nucleus of thalamus
    v. putamen
    v. regimental area

v. root
v. spinocerebellar tract
v. spinothalamic tract
v. striatum
v. tegmental area (VTA)
v. tegmental decussation
v. thalamic peduncle
v. tier thalamic nuclei
ventralis
v. intermedius (VIM)
v. lateralis (VL)
v. oralis anterior (Voa)
v. oralis posterior (VOP)
v. posterior lateralis
v. posteromedialis (VPM)
ventricle
Arantius v.
ballooned floor of v.
bulb of lateral v.
cerebral v.
v. of cerebral hemisphere
v. of diencephalon
dilated v.
Duncan v.
v. effacement
fifth v.
fourth v.
lateral v.
left v.
v. of rhombencephalon
right v.
sixth v.
v. size
slit v.
sylvian v.
terminal v.
third v.
Verga v.
Vieussens v.
Wenzel v.
ventricle-to-brain ratio (VBR)
ventricular
v. aqueduct
v. arrhythmia
v. catheter occlusion
v. catheter reservoir
v. decompression
v. drainage
v. dysphonia
v. ependyma
v. fibrillation
v. fluid
v. layer
v. needle
v. Ommaya reservoir
v. peritoneal shunting
v. puncture
v. system
v. tachycardia (VT)
v. wall
ventriculi (*pl. of* ventriculus)
ventriculitis
ventriculoamniotic shunting
ventriculoatrial shunt

ventriculocisternostomy
Torkildsen v.
ventriculofugal artery
ventriculogram
iohexol CT v.
ventriculography
air v.
cerebral v.
stereotactic anteroposterior and
lateral metrizamide v.
water-soluble contrast v.
ventriculojugular (VJ)
ventriculomastoidostomy
ventriculomegaly
progressive posthemorrhagic v.
ventriculoperitoneal (VP)
v. shunt
v. shunting
ventriculopuncture
ventriculoscope
four-channel Aesculap v.
rigid v.
ventriculoscopy
monoportal v.
ventriculostomy
v. catheter
v. needle
straight-in v.
terminal v.
third v.
tunneled v.
ventriculosubarachnoid
ventriculotomy
ventriculus, pl. ventriculi
v. lateralis
fomes ventriculi
v. quartus
v. quintus
v. terminalis
v. tertius
Ventrix
V. fiberoptic ventricular drainage
system
V. fiberoptic ventricular monitoring
system
V. SD fiberoptic subdural ICP
catheter
V. tunnelable ventricular ICP
monitoring and drainage system
V. tunnelable ventricular intracranial
pressure monitoring system
ventrobasal nucleus
ventrocaudal nucleus (Vc)
ventro-intermedius
nucleus v.-i.
ventrolateral (VL)
v. medulla (VLM)
v. nuclear complex
ventrolateralis thalamotomy
ventromedial
v. frontal leukotomy
v. hypothalamic hamartoma
v. hypothalamus
v. nucleus of hypothalamus

ventroposterior medial pallidotomy
ventroposterolateral (VPL)
    v. pallidotomy
venular obstruction
VEP
    visual evoked potential
VER
    visual evoked response
vera
    melancholia v.
    neuralgia facialis v.
    polycythemia v.
veracious
veracity
Veraguth
    fold of V.
verapamil
Veratran
Verax
verb
    auxiliary v.
verbal
    v. abuse
    v. aggression
    v. agraphia
    v. alexia
    v. amnesia
    v. aphasia
    v. apraxia
    v. auditory agnosia
    v. automatism
    v. aversion therapy
    v. behavior
    v. communication
    V. Comprehension Deviation
    Quotient (VCDQ)
    v. comprehension factor
    v. comprehension index
    v. conceptualization ability
    v. expression
    V. Fluency Test
    v. generalization
    v. ifiasochism
    v. intelligence
    V. Intelligence Quotient (VIQ)
    V. IQ score
    V. Language Development Scale
    v. language quotient
    v. leakage
    v. learning
    V. Meaning Test
    v. mediation
    v. and oral language ability
    v. outburst
    v. paraphasia
    v. perceptual speed
    v. perseveration
    v. play
    v. reinforcement
    v. scale (VS)
    V. Scale Score
    v. suggestion
    v. technique
    v. visual agnosia
    v. working memory

Verbal-Auditory
    V.-A. Screen for Children (VASC)
    V.-A. Screen for Children Test
    V.-A. Screen for Children test
verbalis
    asemasia v.
verbalism
verbalization of feeling
Verbalizer-Visualization Questionnaire
    (VVQ)
verbal, numerical, and reasoning (VNR)
verbatim recall
verbiage
verbigeration
    hallucinatory v.
verbochromia
verborum
    delirium v.
verbose
verboten
Verdun
    V. Depression Rating Scale
    (VDRS)
    V. Target Symptom Rating Scale
    (VTSRS)
vergae
    cavum v.
Verga ventricle
verge
    anal v.
vergence
    v. movement
    v. system
Vergon
veridical
    v. dream
    v. memory
verifiable
veritable
verity
vermes (*pl. of* vermis)
vermian
    v. artery
    v. atrophy
    v. medulloblastoma
    v. split
vermicular movement
vermilion border
verminous
vermiphobia
vermis, pl. vermes
Vermont
    V. spinal fixator
    V. spinal fixator articulation
vernacular
vernal encephalitis
Vernet syndrome
Verneuil neuroma
Verocay body
veroomania
VersaPulse holmium laser
versatility
    attachment v.
Versed

versenate
    calcium disodium v.
versicolor
    membrana v.
version
    Career Assessment Inventory, The
       Enhanced V.
    Diagnostic Interview for Children
       and Adolescents-Child V. (DICA-
       C)
    Diagnostic Interview for Children
       and Adolescents-Parent V. (DICA-
       P)
    episode v.
    Family Relations Test,
       Children's V.
    Interest Determination, Exploration
       and Assessment System,
       Enhanced V. (IDEAS)
    Schedule for Affective Disorders
       and Schizophrenia Lifetime V.
    Structured Clinical Interview for
       DSM-III-R-Patient V. (SCID-P)
    Structured Clinical Interview for
       DSM-IV Axis I Disorders:
       Clinician V. (SCID-CV)
    Wechsler Memory Scale,
       Russell V.
    Wechsler Memory Scale, Standard
       and Russell v.'s
    Yale Schedule for Tourette
       Syndrome and Other Behavioral
       Disorders, Hebrew V.
versus (v, vs)
VertAlign spinal support system
vertebra, pl. **vertebrae**
    block v.
    butterfly v.
    cervical v.
    coronal cleft v.
    inferior v.
    limbus v.
    lumbar v.
    lumbosacral v.
    vertebrae spreader
    thoracic v.
    thoracolumbar v.
    transitional v.
vertebral
    v. angiogram
    v. angiography
    v. aplasia
    v. artery (VA)
    v. artery injury
    v. artery occlusion
    v. artery transposition
    v. body anterior cortex
    v. body anterior cortex penetration
    v. body corpectomy
    v. body decompression
    v. body impactor
    v. body tumor
    v. cervical instability
    v. collapse
    v. column

    v. dissection
    v. end-plate enhancement
    v. exposure
    v. fascia
    v. fracture
    v. fusion
    v. ganglion
    v. hemangioma
    v. level
    v. osteosynthesis
    v. osteosynthesis fusion rate
    v. part
    v. plate
    v. plate application
    v. pulp
    v. resection
    v. subluxation
    v. venography
vertebrectomy
    Bohlman anterior cervical v.
    cervical v.
    cervical spondylotic myelopathy v.
    microsurgical thoracoscopic v.
vertebrobasilar
    v. aneurysm
    v. artery
    v. disease
    v. infarction
    v. insufficiency
    v. ischemia
    v. system
vertebrogenic
    v. pain syndrome
    v. symptom complex
vertex sharp wave
vertical
    v. gaze
    v. gaze palsy
    v. gaze paresis
    v. line bisection
    v. midline incision
    v. migration
    v. mobility
    v. nystagmus
    v. pedicle diameter
    v. plane
    v. ring curette
    v. sharp wave
    v. transmission
    v. vertigo
vertiginosa
    epilepsia v.
vertiginosus
    status v.
vertiginous
    v. epilepsy
    v. seizure
vertigo
    benign functional v.
    benign paroxysmal v.
    benign positional paroxysmal v.
    Charcot v.
    chronic v.
    endemic paralytic v.
    epidemic v.

V

vertigo *(continued)*
    epileptic v.
    episodic v.
    essential v.
    galvanic v.
    gastric v.
    height v.
    horizontal v.
    hysterical v.
    labyrinthine v.
    laryngeal v.
    lateral v.
    mechanical v.
    nocturnal v.
    objective v.
    organic v.
    paralyzing v.
    paroxysmal v.
    positional v.
    postural v.
    proprioceptive v.
    psychogenic v.
    rotary v.
    sham-movement v.
    subjective v.
    systematic v.
    true v.
    vertical v.
    voltaic v.
very
    v. high dose phenobarbital (VHDPB)
    v. important person (VIP)
    v. low amplitude
    v. low-density syndrome
Vesalius
    canal of V.
    foramen of V.
vesical reflex
vesica pudica syndrome
vesicle
    cerebral v.
    encephalic v.
    forebrain v.
    hindbrain v.
    midbrain v.
    ocular v.
    optic v.
    pinocytotic v.
    primary brain v.
    synaptic v.
    telencephalic v.
vesicospinal
vesicula, gen. and pl. **vesiculae**
    v. ophthalmica
vesicular stomatitis virus
vesiculation of the Golgi
Vesprin
vessel
    blood v.
    cerebral blood v.
    collateral v.
    crack-like v.
    v. hyperplasia

    nutrient v.
    pial cortical v.
vest
    Bremer AirFlo halo v.
    halo v.
    Minerva v.
    vestibule aqueduct of v.
    vestibuli aqueductus v.
vestibular
    v. area
    v. crest
    v. disorder
    v. end-organ nystagmus
    v. fissure of cochlea
    v. function
    v. ganglion
    v. hair cell
    v. hallucination
    v. hydrops
    v. labyrinth
    v. membrane
    v. migraine
    v. migraine headache
    v. movement
    v. nerve
    v. nerve section
    v. neurectomy
    v. neuronitis
    v. nuclei
    v. nucleus
    v. nystagmus
    v. organ
    v. part of vestibulocochlear nerve
    v. root of vestibulocochlear nerve
    v. schwannoma (VS)
    v. suppressant
    v. system
vestibularis
    nervus v.
vestibule aqueduct of vest
vestibuli aqueductus vest
vestibulocerebellar ataxia
vestibulocerebellum
vestibulocochlear
    v. nerve
    v. neuropathy
    v. organ
vestibulocochlearis
    nervus v.
vestibuloequilibratory control
vestibulogenic epilepsy
vestibuloocular
    v. reflex (VOR)
    v. reflex suppression
vestibulospinal
    v. reflex
    v. tract
veteran
    V.'s Administration (VA)
    V.'s Administration Hospital
VEWA
    Vocational Evaluation and Work Adjustment
vex
vexatious

VFDT
Visual Form Discrimination Test
VGCC
voltage-gated calcium channel
V-groove hollow-ground connection design
VHDPB
very high dose phenobarbital
VI
variable interval
visual imagery
viability
neuronal v.
viable alternative
Viagra
vial
beat v.
blue v.
crack v.
drug v.
VIB
Vocational Interest Blank
vibrant
vibration
forced v.
v. syndrome
vibrator
vibratory
v. massage
v. sensibility
Vibrio parahaemolyticus
vibrotactile
v. response
v. threshold
VIBS
vocabulary, information, block design, similarity
VIC
Values Inventory for Children
visual communication
vicarious
v. function
v. learning
v. living
v. trial and error (VTE)
vice allemand
vice-like pain
Vici agnesis
vicious
v. circle
v. cycle
vicissitude
instinctual v.
vicissitudes of life
Vicodin
V. ES
V. HP
Vicoprofen
Vicq
V. d'Azyr bundle
V. d'Azyr centrum semiovale
V. d'Azyr foramen
Vicryl Rapide suture
victim
v. abuse

v. psychology
v. recidivism
v. role
v. syndrome
victimization
victimology
victorianism
victorious
vidarabine
videocassette recording
video/EEG monitoring
video feedback
video-polysomnographic
videotape assessment
Videx
Vienna Psychoanalytic Society
VIESA
Vocational Interest, Experience, and Skill Assessment
Viet Cong
Vietnam war
Vieussens
annulus of V.
V. ansa
V. centrum
V. ganglion
V. loop
V. valve
V. ventricle
view
field of v.
point of v.
Pollyanna-like v.
stilted v.
swimmer's v.
Waters v.
viewing
tachistoscopy v.
V. Wand
V. Wand image guided system
viewpoint
biologic v.
vigabatrin
vigil
coma v.
fatiguing v.
vigilambulism
vigilance
v. deficit
perceptual v.
visuomotor v.
vigilant
vigilante
vigility of attention
vignette
vigorous
Vigotsky Test
Viking II nerve monitoring device
vile
vilification
vilify
villainous
Villaret-Mackenzie syndrome
Villaret syndrome

V

villa system
villus, pl. **villi**
    arachnoid v.
VIM
    ventralis intermedius
vim
vimentin tumor marker
Vim thalamotomy
vinbarbital sodium
vinblastine sulfate
vinca alkaloid
vincible
vincristine (VCR)
    v. peripheral neuropathy
    v. sulfate
vinculum, pl. **vincula**
    vincula lingulae cerebelli
vindicate
vindictive
Vineland
    V. Adaptive Behavior Scale
    V. percentile scale
    V. Social Maturity Scale (VSMS)
Viñuela cocktail
violation
    boundary v.
    nonsexual boundary v.
    sexual boundary v.
violations of rules
violence
    alcohol-related risk for v.
    alleviating v.
    domestic v. (DV)
    drug-related v.
    family v.
    v. risk
    v. theory
    workplace v.
violent
    v. act
    v. agitation
    v. behavior
    v. death
    v. outburst
    v. personal assault
violinist's cramp
VIP
    Validity Indicator Profile
    vasoactive intestinal peptide
    vasoactive intestinal polypeptide
    very important person
    voluntary interruption of pregnancy
    VIP syndrome
VIQ
    Verbal Intelligence Quotient
    Vocational Interest Questionnaire
Viracept
viraginity
viral
    v. encephalitis
    v. encephalopathy
    v. hypothesis
    v. infection
    v. intracerebral arteritis
    v. leukoencephalitis

    v. meningitis
    v. rhinitis
    v. vector-mediated therapy
    v. vector system
Viramune
Virchow
    V. disease
    V. psammoma
Virchow-Robin
    V.-R. space
    V.-R. space of the brain
virgin
    v. fear
    V. Mary vision
virginal anxiety
virginity
    v. scruple
    v. taboo
virgophrenia
viridans
    Streptococcus v.
virile
virilism
virility
virilization
virtual
    v. probe
    V. Vision heads-up display
virtue
    cardinal v.
    easy v.
virulence
virulent
virus
    BK v. (BKV)
    dengue v.
    DNA v.
    ECHO v.
    v. encephalomyelitis
    enteric cytopathic human orphan v.
    Epstein-Barr v. (EBV)
    hepatitis A v.
    hepatitis B v.
    hepatitis C v.
    hepatitis D v.
    hepatitis E v.
    hepatitis F v.
    hepatitis G v.
    hepatropic v.
    herpes simplex v. (HSV)
    human immunodeficiency v. (HIV)
    human T-cell leukemia v. (HTLV)
    human T-cell lymphoma v.
      (HTLV)
    human T-cell lymphotropic v.
      (HTLV)
    inhibitory v.
    Jamestown Canyon v.
    Japanese encephalitis v.
    JC v. (JCV)
    Junin v.
    Lassa fever v.
    lymphocytic choriomeningitis v.
      (LCMV)
    Machupo v.

Oklahoma tick fever v.
Powassan v.
rabies v.
Rio Bravo v.
RNA v.
rubella v.
Saint Louis encephalitis v. (SLEV)
Seoul v.
slow v.
snowshoe hare v.
Trivittatus v.
varicella zoster v. (VZV)
vesicular stomatitis v.

virus-mediated gene transfer
VIS
vocational interest schedule
VISA
Vocational Interest and Sophistication
Assessment
visage
scanning v.
visceral
v. anesthesia
v. brain
v. disorder
v. epilepsy
v. larva migrans
v. learning
v. motor neuron
v. nervous system
v. neurosis
v. organ
v. pain
v. sense
v. sympathectomy
viscerogenic reflex
visceromotor reflex
viscerosensory reflex
viscerosomatic tone
viscerotonia
viscoelastic action
viscosity
blood v.
v. of libido
v. personality
visibility
visible
vision
altered v.
beatific v.
binocular v.
blurred v.
blurring of v.
central v.
color v.
darkening v.
v. disparity
double v.
entopic v.
facial v.
field of v.
foveal v.
hemifield of v.
hypnagogic v.
impaired v.

inner v.
organ of v.
patterning v.
phantom v.
photopic v.
stereoscopic v.
subjective v.
tunnel v.
twilight v.
Virgin Mary v.
visionary
visit
conjugal v.
home v.
reason for v.
therapeutic trial v. (TTV)
trial home v.
weekend v.
visitant
visitation rights
visiting nurse
vista
V. American Health 0.5 Tesla
MRI scanner
v. response
Vistacon
Vistaject-25
Vistaject-50
Vistaquel
Vistaril
Vistazine
visual
v. accommodation
v. acuity
v. acuity loss
v. agnosia
v. aid
v. alertness
v. alexia
v. allesthesia
v. amnesia
v. analog scale (VAS)
v. aphasia
v. area
v. axis
v. blurring
v. center
v. change
v. choice reaction time test
v. claudication
v. closure
v. communication (VC, VIC)
v. cortex
v. cue
v. discrimination
v. disorientation reaction
v. distortion
v. distortion test (VDT)
v. disturbance
v. epilepsy
v. evoked potential (VEP)
v. evoked response (VER)
v. evoked response test
v. extinction
v. field

V

visual *(continued)*
  v. field construction
  v. field cut
  v. field defect
  v. field deficit
  v. field disturbance
  v. fixation
  V. Form Discrimination Test (VFDT)
  v. hallucination
  v. hallucination denial syndrome
  v. hearing
  v. illusion
  v. image
  v. image inversion
  v. image movement disorder
  v. imagery (VI)
  v. impairment
  v. inattention
  v. letter dysgnosia
  v. literacy
  V. Memory Score (VMS)
  v. memory span (VMS)
  v. memory span task
  v. motor integration (VMI)
  v. motor processing
  V. Motor Test
  v. neglect
  V. Neglect Test
  v. number dysgnosia
  v. obstruction
  v. orbicularis reflex
  v. paraneoplastic syndrome
  v. pathway
  V. Pattern Completion test
  v. pattern recognition
  v. perception
  V. Perception Test
  v. perceptual deficit
  v. perceptual skill
  v. perceptual speed
  v. prodrome
  v. pursuit movement
  v. radiation
  v. receptor cell
  v. reproduction
  V. Retention Test
  V. Search and Attention Test (VSAT)
  v. seizure
  v. sensation
  v. sensory modality
  v. shimmering with aura
  v. shining with aura
  v. sparkling with aura
  v. spatial memory
  v. stimulation
  v. stimulus
  v. subsystem
  v. symptom
  v. system
  v. system tumor
  v. threat test
  v. tracking

  v. training
  v. zone
Visual-Auditory Screen for Children (VASC)
visualization
  endoscopic v.
visually-guided saccade
Visual-Motor
  V.-M. Gestalt Test (VMGT)
  V.-M. Integration Test (VMIT)
  V.-M. Sequencing Test (VMST)
visual-motor
  v.-m. coordination
  v.-m. impairment
  v.-m. task
visual-spatial
  v.-s. acalculia
  v.-s. agnosia
  v.-s. distortion
Visual-Tactile System of Phonetic Symbolization
visuoauditory
visuoconstruction skill
visuognosis
visuomotor
  v. ability
  v. behavior
  v. vigilance
visuoperceptive defect
visuoperceptual
visuopsychic
visuosensory
visuospatial
  v. attention
  v. awareness
  v. construction
  v. constructive cognition
  v. disorder
  v. disorientation
  v. problem solving
  v. processing
  v. scratch pad
  v. skill
  v. stimulus
visuotopic
  vitae arbor v.
VitaCarn Oral
vitae arbor visuotopic
vital
  v. center
  v. energy
  v. knot
  v. node
  v. sign (VS)
  v. statistics
vitality
vitalize
Vitallium
  V. equipment
  V. plate
vitam
  intra v.
vitamin
  v. B1
  v. B6

v. B12
v. B1 deficiency
v. B6 deficiency
v. B12 deficiency
v. B12 deficiency dementia
v. B12 neuropathy
V. D Analog
v. D deficiency
v. D receptor (VDR)
v. E deficiency
v. therapy
water soluble v.
vitrectomy
vitreous
v. disease
v. hemorrhage
primary v.
vitritis
vitro
in v.
v. matrigel model
vitronectin
Vivactil
Vivarin
vivid
v. dream
v. dream image
v. dream recall
v. hallucination
vivo
exposure in v.
in v.
VJ
ventriculojugular
VJ shunt
VL
ventralis lateralis
ventrolateral
VL thalamotomy
VLM
ventrolateral medulla
VM900 Smart Scope
VMETH
volumetric multiple exposure
transmission holography
VMGT
Visual-Motor Gestalt Test
VMI
visual motor integration
VMIT
Visual-Motor Integration Test
VMS
Visual Memory Score
visual memory span
VMST
Visual-Motor Sequencing Test
**V. Mueller McCulloch universal
instrument set**
VNR
verbal, numerical, and reasoning
VNS
vagus nerve stimulation
Voa
ventralis oralis anterior

vocabulary
active v.
auditory v.
V. Comprehension Scale
v. language quotient
passive v.
v. scale
v. test
**vocabulary, information, block design,
similarity (VIBS)**
vocal
v. abuse
v. amusia
v. attack
v. band
v. cord
v. fold approximation
v. pitch abnormality
v. tic
vocal, chronic motor, or tic disorder
vocalization
involuntary v.
motor v.
nonrhythmic v.
rapid v.
recurrent v.
stereotyped v.
sudden v.
vocalize
vocational
v. achievement
v. adjustment
V. Apperception Test (VAT)
v. appraisal
v. choice
v. counseling
v. evaluation
V. Evaluation and Work
Adjustment (VEWA)
v. functioning
v. goal-setting
v. guidance
v. identity
V. Interest Blank (VIB)
V. Interest, Experience, and Skill
Assessment (VIESA)
V. Interest Inventory
V. Interest Inventory and
Exploration Survey
V. Interest Questionnaire (VIQ)
v. interest schedule (VIS)
V. Interest and Sophistication
Assessment (VISA)
V. Interest Survey
V. Learning Styles (LSV2)
v. maladjustment
V. Opinion Index (VOI)
V. Planning Inventory (VPI)
V. Preference Inventory (VPI)
psychological, social, and v. (PSV)
v. rehabilitation (VR)
v. rehabilitation and education
(VR&E)
V. Rehabilitation Services (VRS)

vocational *(continued)*
    v. strain
    v. training
Voc-Tech Quick Screener (VTQS)
Vogt
    V. disease
    V. syndrome
Vogt-Koyanagi-Harada syndrome
Vogt-Spielmeyer
    V.-S. disease
    V.-S. idiocy
VOI
    Vocational Opinion Index
voice
    active v.
    adolescent v.
    altered v.
    breathy v.
    chest v.
    conversational v.
    v. disorder
    esophageal v.
    eunuchoid v.
    falsetto v.
    gravel v.
    hearing v.'s
    high-pitched v.
    negative v.
    pejorative v.
    shaking v.
    soundless v.
    threatening v.
    tone of v.
    transsexual v.
    trembling v.
voiceless
voiceprint
voices
    v. commenting
    v. conversing
    v. inside head
    v. outside head
void
    v. fear
    signal v.
voiding
    inappropriate v.
Voigt line
voila
volatile
    v. disposition
    v. hydrocarbons
    v. personality
    v. solvent
volition
    act and v.
    derailment of v.
    hedonic v.
volitional
    v. drinking
    v. movement
    v. tremor
Volkmann contracture
Volpe criteria

voltage
    transient v.
voltage-activated conductance
voltage-gated
    v.-g. calcium channel (VGCC)
    v.-g. sodium channel
    v.-g. sodium channel blocker
voltage-sensitive protein
voltaic vertigo
Voltaren
    V. Ophthalmic
    V. Oral
Voltaren-XR Oral
volubility
    excessive v.
volume
    blood v.
    caudate v.
    cerebellar v.
    cerebrospinal fluid v.
    v. expansion
    mamillary body v.
    mean corpuscular v. (MCV)
    v. regulation
    v. segmentation
    sensitive v.
    v. transmission
    tumor v.
volumetric
    v. analysis
    v. computed tomography
    v. infusion pump
    v. interstitial brachytherapy
    v. multiple exposure transmission holography (VMETH)
    v. resection
voluntarism
voluntary
    v. admission
    v. behavior
    v. commitment
    v. control
    v. dehydration
    v. euthanasia
    v. hospitalization
    v. hysterical overbreathing
    v. impulse
    v. interruption of pregnancy (VIP)
    v. motion
    v. motor functioning
    v. muscle movement
    v. mutism
    v. napping phenomenon
    v. nystagmus
    v. retention
    v. sensory functioning
volunteer bias
vomer
    posterior v.
vomeronasal
vomiting
    cyclic v.
    v. fear
    nausea and v. (N&V)
    nervous v.

projectile v.
psychogenic v.
psychogenic cyclical v.
v. reflex
self-induced v.
vomiturition
vomitus
von
    v. Domarus principle
    v. Ebner gland
    v. Economo disease
    v. Economo encephalitis
    v. Eulenberg disease
    v. Frey test
    v. Gierke disease
    v. Graefe sign
    v. Graefe strabismus hook
    v. Hippel-Lindau
    v. Hippel-Lindau disease
    v. Hippel-Lindau syndrome
    v. Knorring criterion
    v. Monakow diaschisis concept
    v. Recklinghausen disease
    v. Recklinghausen neurofibromatosis
voodoo death
voodooism
voodooistic
VOP
    ventralis oralis posterior
VOR
    vestibuloocular reflex
voracious appetite
vow
    marriage v.'s
    solemn v.
vowel
    accented v.
    v. assimilation
    back v.
voxel
    cerebral v.
voyeur
voyeurism paraphilia
voyeuristic
    v. activity
    v. behavior
    v. sexual behavior
    v. sexually arousing fantasy
voyeuse
VP
    ventriculoperitoneal
    VP shunt
VPI
    Vocational Planning Inventory
    Vocational Preference Inventory
VPL
    ventral posterolateral nucleus
    ventroposterolateral
    VPL pallidotomy
VPM
    ventralis posteromedialis
VR
    variable ratio
    vocational rehabilitation

VR&E
    vocational rehabilitation and education
VRS
    Vocational Rehabilitation Services
VS
    valve system
    verbal scale
    vestibular schwannoma
    vital sign
        Profile VS
vs
    versus
VSAT
    Visual Search and Attention Test
V-shaped incision
VSMS
    Vineland Social Maturity Scale
VSP
    variable screw placement
        VSP plate instrumentation
VT
    ventricular tachycardia
VTA
    ventral tegmental area
VTE
    vicarious trial and error
VTED
    venous thromboembolic disease
VTQS
    Voc-Tech Quick Screener
VTSRS
    Verdun Target Symptom Rating Scale
vu
    déjà v.
    jamais v.
vulgaris
    Artemisia v.
vulgar language
vulnerability
    emotional v.
    genetic v.
    narcissistic v.
    putative adoptee v.
    v. theory
    v. threshold
vulnerable
    v. child
    v. child syndrome
Vulpe Assessment
Vulpian
    V. atrophy
    V. effect
Vulpian-Bernhardt spinal muscular atrophy
vulvae
    pruritus v.
vulvismus
VVQ
    Verbalizer-Visualization Questionnaire
Vygotsky Concept Formation Test, Modified
VZV
    varicella zoster virus

V

W
    whole response
Waardenburg syndrome
WAB
    Western Aphasia Battery
Wachs Analysis of Cognitive Structures
Wackenheim clivus canal line
Wada test
waddling gait
wafer
    Gliadel w.
    polyanhydride biodegradable
      polymer w.
waggish
wagon
    on the w.
Wahler
    W. Physical Symptoms Inventory
    W. Self-Description Inventory
      (WSDI)
WAIS
    Wechsler Adult Intelligence Scale
WAIS-III
    Wechsler Adult Intelligence Scale-Third
    Edition
WAIS-R Block Design Test
waiter's cramp
waiver
Wakefield Self-Assessment Depression
   Inventory
wakefulness
    w. disorder
    w. epochs
    full w.
    intermittent w.
    midpontine w.
    primary disorder of w.
    w. quiet
    Repeated Test of Sustained W.
      (RTSW)
    w. resting
wakeful state
wake time
waking
    w. EEG
    w. frequency
    w. hypnosis
    w. numbness
Wakoz
Waldenstrom
    macroglobulinemia of W.
    W. macroglobulinemia
Waldeyer
    W. tract
    W. zonal layer
Waldrop Scale
Walker-McConnell Scale of Social
   Competence and School Adjustment
Walker tractotomy
Walker-Warburg syndrome
walking
    w. aid

    bipedal w.
    chromosome w.
    w. stance
    w. swing phase
wall
    w. fistula
    stone w.
    ventricular w.
Wallenberg syndrome
wallerian
    w. degeneration
    w. law
Walther ganglion
wand
    3-dimensional reconstruction w.
    Elekta viewing w.
    ISG viewing w.
    stylus-type sensor w.
    TriggerWheel W.
    Viewing W.
wandering
    aimless w.
    w. attention
    w. cell
    w. impulse
    w. mind
    w. pain
    w. thought
wanderlust
wane
    wax and w.
Wangensteen needle holder
waning discharge
WAQ
    Work Attitudes Questionnaire
war
    w. baby
    w. footing
    gang w.
    w. gas
    limited w.
    w. of nerves
    w. neurosis
    not prisoner of w. (NPOW)
    nuclear w.
    Persian Gulf W.
    w. power
    prisoner of w. (POW)
    Vietnam w.
    world w.
    World W. I (WWI)
    World W. II (WWII)
    w. zone
    W. Zone Exposure Subscale
Warburg syndrome
ward
    W. Atmosphere Scale (WAS)
    W. Behavior Rating Scale (WBRS)
    w. clerk
    disturbed w.
    locked w.

W

ward *(continued)*
    open w.
    psychiatric w.
Wardrop method
Ware instrument
warfare
    biologic w.
    chemical w.
    chemical and biological w. (CBW)
    gang w.
    guerrilla w.
    psychological w. (PW)
    trench w.
warfarin
    w. sodium
    w. syndrome
Waring
    W. blender syndrome
    W. Intimacy Questionnaire (WIQ)
warlock
Warm 'n Form lumbosacral corset
warmth
    paradoxical w.
warm-wire anemometer
warn
    duty to w.
    failure to w.
warning
    Tarasoff w.
warrant
    bench w.
    death w.
    search w.
war-related stress
Warrington Recognition Memory Test
Wartenberg
    W. reflex
    W. symptom
WAS
    Ward Atmosphere Scale
washboard effect
washed out
washer
    plate-spacer w.
Washington
    W. School of Psychiatry
    W. Speech Sound Discrimination
        Test (WSSDT)
    W. University Sentence Completion
        Test (WUSCT)
wash out
WASP
    Weber Advanced Spatial Perception
    white Anglo-Saxon Protestant
wastage
    air w.
wastebasket diagnosis
wasting
    cerebral salt w.
    nitrogen w.
    w. palsy
    w. paralysis
    salt w.

watchfulness
    frozen w.
watchmaker's cramp
watchspring theory
water
    w. balance
    w. balance in schizophrenia
    body w.
    w. deprivation
    w. drinking
    w. intoxication
    w. on the brain
    w. phobia
    w. soluble vitamin
    toilet w.
water-seeking behavior
watershed
    w. area
    w. area paresis
    w. infarct
    w. infarction
    w. region
    w. zone
water-soluble
    w.-s. contrast myelography
    w.-s. contrast ventriculography
Waters view
watertight closure
**Watson-Glaser Critical Thinking
    Appraisal (WGCTA)**
**Watson-Williams intervertebral disk
    rongeur**
wave
    alpha w.
    w. analyzer
    aperiodic w.
    beta w.
    continuous w.
    delta w.
    EEG alpha w.
    electromagnetic w.
    flat top w.
    gamma w.
    generalized periodic sharp w.
    Hering-Traube w.
    Jewett w.
    kappa w.
    M w.
    mu w.
    new w.
    positive sharp w.
    random w.
    rho w.
    sine w.
    square w.
    theta w.
    Traube-Hering-Mayer w.
    triphasic w.
    ultrasonic w.
    vertex sharp w.
    vertical sharp w.
waveform
    w. amplitude
    apiculate w.
    brief pulse w.

dampened w.
early component w.
nondampened w.
out-of-phase w.
pulse w.
signal voltage w.
wavering light with aura
waveshape
waving
hand w.
wax
bone w.
Horsley bone w.
w. and wane
waxen
waxy flexibility
WAY
Who Are You?
WAY technique
WAY test
way
W. of Coping Scale
maladaptive w.
one w.
parting of the w.'s
set in one's w.'s
Wayne laminectomy seat
WBRS
Ward Behavior Rating Scale
WBRT
whole-brain radiation therapy
WBS
Wechsler-Bellevue Scale
WBST
WCS
Wiggins Content Scale
WCST
Wisconsin Card-Sorting Test
weak
w. ego
w. ego control
w. mindedness
W. Opiate Withdrawal Scale
(WOWS)
w. parent
w. stress
weakness
abduction w.
adduction w.
arm w.
color w.
ego w.
eye muscle w.
w. fear
hemifacial w.
infranuclear w.
limb w.
localized w.
neck w.
pharyngeal w.
sternocleidomastoid muscle w.
weaning
ventilator w.
weapon
assault with a deadly w. (ADW)

biologic w.
chemical w.
lethal w.
Weary
W. brain spatula
W. cordotomy knife
W. nerve hook
W. nerve root retractor
weaving
head w.
Weber
W. Advanced Spatial Perception
(WASP)
W. esthesiometer
W. sign
W. syndrome
W. test
Weber-Christian disease
Weber-Fechner law
Weber-Fergusson incision
Weber-Leyden syndrome
webspace incision
Webster needle holder
Wechsler
W. Adult Intelligence Scale
(WAIS)
W. Adult Intelligence Scale-Revised
W. Adult Intelligence Scale-Third
Edition (WAIS-III)
W. digit span
W. Intelligence Scale
W. Intelligence Scale for Children
(WISC)
W. Intelligence Scale for Children-
Revised (WISC-R)
W. Intelligence Scale for Children,
Revised Version and Version III
W. Intelligence Scale for Children-
Third Edition (WISC-III)
W. IQ Scale
W. Memory Scale (WMS)
W. Memory Scale/Memory Quotient
(WMS-MQ)
W. Memory Scale - Revised
(WMS-R)
W. Memory Scale, Russell Version
W. Memory Scale, Standard and
Russell versions
W. Preschool and Primary Scale
of Intelligence (WPPSI)
Wechsler-Bellevue Scale (WBS)
Weck clip
wedding
w. night
shotgun w.
Wedensky facilitation
wedge
Duo-Cline bed w.
wedge-compression fracture
wedge-shaped
w.-s. astrocyte
w.-s. fasciculus
w.-s. tubercle
wedlock
out of w.

W

Wednesday Evening Society
WEE
Western equine encephalitis
Western equine encephalomyelitis
weekend
w. drinker
w. drinking
w. headache
w. hospital
w. neurosis
w. parent
w. pass
w. visit
weepy
Wegener
W. granulomatosis (WG)
W. granulomatosis-associated
neuropathy
we-group
Weigert staining
weight
beta w.
brain w.
w. discrimination
failure to gain w.
w. gain
ideal body w. (IBW)
w. lifter
w. loss
w. loss therapy
w. perception
weight-control program
weighted-harm principle
weighting
item w.
proton density w.
T1 w.
T2 w.
Weight Watchers diet
weighty
Weil-Blakesley intervertebral disk
rongeur
Weinberg rib spreader
Weingrow reflex
Weinstein Enhanced Sensory Test
(WEST)
Weir
W. Mitchell therapy
W. Mitchell treatment
Weiss
W. Comprehensive Articulation Test
W. Intelligibility Test
W. sign
Weitbrecht cord
Weitlaner-Beckman retractor
Weitlaner retractor
Welander
W. disease
W. distal muscular atrophy
W. muscular dystrophy
welding
tissue w.
welfare
w. emotion
w. organization

welfarism
well-articulated speech
well-being
Index of W.-b. (IWB)
w.-b. scale
sense of w.-b.
Wellbutrin SR
Wellcovorin
Weller-Strawser Scales of Adaptive
Behavior for the Learning Disabled
well-formed
w.-f. delusion
w.-f. outcome
Wells stereotaxic apparatus
well-systematized delusional system
Welsh Figure Preference Test
welt
Wender Utah Rating Scale
Wenzel ventricle
Wepman
W. Auditory Discrimination Test
W. Test of Auditory Discrimination
WEPS
Work Environment Preference Schedule
Werdnig-Hoffmann
W.-H. disease
W.-H. spinal muscular atrophy
werewolf
Wermer syndrome
Wernekinck
W. commissure
W. decussation
Wernicke
W. aphasia
W. 22 area
W. 39 area
W. 40 area
W. center
W. cramp
W. dementia
W. disease
W. field
W. fluent encephalopathy
W. hemianopic pupillary
phenomenon
mirror of W.
W. radiation
W. reaction
W. region
W. sign
W. syndrome
W. zone
Wernicke-Korsakoff
W.-K. encephalopathy
W.-K. syndrome
Wernicke-Mann spastic hemiplegia
Werther syndrome
WES
Work Environment Scale
Wesman Personnel Classification Test
WEST
Weinstein Enhanced Sensory Test
West
W. African
W. African sleeping sickness

W. African trypanosomiasis
W. hand and foot nerve tester
W. Nile encephalitis
W. Nile fever
W. syndrome

Westco Neurostat-Mark II
Westergren method
westermani
    Pargonimus w.
Western
W. Aphasia Battery (WAB)
W. blot test
W. equine encephalitis (WEE)
W. equine encephalomyelitis (WEE)
W. Personality Inventory
W. subtype
Westphal
W. disease
W. phenomenon
W. pseudosclerosis
W. pupillary reflex
W. sign
W. variant
Westphal-Erb sign
Westphal-Leyden syndrome
Westphal-Piltz phenomenon
Westphal-Strümpell pseudosclerosis
wet
w. behind the ears
w. beriberi
w. bipolar system
w. brain syndrome
w. dream
Wever-Bray
W.-B. effect
W.-B. phenomenon
WG
    Wegener granulomatosis
WGCTA
    Watson-Glaser Critical Thinking
    Appraisal
WH
    whole head
What I Like to Do: An Inventory of Students' Interests (WILD)
wheal
wheel
    activity w.
wheeze
whimper
whine
whiplash
    acute w.
    w. injury
Whipple
W. disease
W. disease peripheral neuropathy
whirling
whisper
    forced w.
whispered speech
whispering
    w. dystonia
    involuntary w.
whispery

Whitacre spinal needle
Whitaker Index of Schizophrenic thinking (WIST)
Whitcomb-Kerrison laminectomy rongeur
white
w. Anglo-Saxon Protestant (WASP)
w. blood cell
w. commissure
w. ghost
w. horizon
w. iritis
w. knuckling sobriety
w. matter
w. matter disease
w. matter hyperintensity
w. matter hypodensity
w. matter infarction
w. matter lesion (WML)
w. noise
w. noise masking
w. Owsley's
W. and Panjabi criteria
w. substance
w. sugar
w. supremacist
w. turbid urine
whiteout syndrome
Whitesides-Kell cervical technique
WHO
    World Health Organization
    WHO astrocytoma classification
    WHO Handicap Scale
Who
W. Are You? (WAY)
W. Are You? technique
W. Are You? test
whole
w. cranial headache
detail response elaborating the w. (DdW)
w. head (WH)
w. response (W, WR)
whole-body cooling
whole-brain
w.-b. mapping database
w.-b. radiation therapy (WBRT)
whole-cortex MEG/EEG system
wholeness
    undifferentiated w.
whole-spine MRI
whore
whorl
    storiform w.
wick
    Silastic w.
wicket rhythm
wide
w. area network
w. bipole
w. circles of thought
w. range
W. Range Achievement Test (WRAT)
W. Range Achievement Test-Revised (WRAT, WRAT-R)

W

wide *(continued)*
  W. Range Assessment of Memory and Learning (WRAML)
  W. Range Employment Sample Test (WREST)
  W. Range Intelligence and Personality Test (WRIPT)
  W. Range Interest-Opinion Test (WRIOT)
  w. ranging
wide-based gait
wide-necked aneurysm
widespread distribution of activity
widow
widower
widowhood crisis
width
  line w.
  pulse w.
wieldy
wife
  battered w.
wife-beating
wife-to-husband aggression
Wiggins Content Scale (WCS)
Wiggly Block Test
Wigraine
wihtiko
WII
  Work Information Inventory
Wilbrandt knee injury
Wilcoxon rank sum test
WILD
  What I Like to Do: An Inventory of Students' Interests
wild
  w. behavior
  w. psychoanalysis
Wilde cord
Wilder law of initial value
wild-type allele
will
  ambivalence of the w.
  w. to be oneself
  disturbance of the w.
  w. disturbance
  w. factor
  free w.
  general w.
  gesture of good w.
  ill w.
  lack of w.
  w. to live
  living w.
  w. to meaning
  w. to power
  w. to surrender
  w. therapy
williamsii
  Lophophora w.
Williams syndrome
Willis
  W. centrum nervosum
  circle of W.

  W. headache
  W. paracusis
  spontaneous occlusion of the circle of W.
willisii
  accessorius w.
  chordae w.
Willowbrook consent
Wilson
  W. agnesis
  W. disease dementia
  W. frame
  W. hepatolenticular degeneration
  W. hepatolenticular degeneration disease
  W. rib spreader
  W. syndrome
Wilson-Patterson Attitude Inventory (WPAI)
Wiltberger
  W. anterior cervical approach
  W. fusion
  W. spinous process spreader
Wiltse
  W. paraspinal approach
  W. system
  W. system aluminum master rod
  W. system cross-bracing
  W. system double-rod construct
  W. system H construct
  W. system single-rod construct
  W. system spinal rod
Wiltse-Gelpi retractor
wind
  w. contusion
  w. effect
  w. fear
windage
Windigo
  w. culture-specific syndrome
  w. psychosis
windmill illusion
window
  acoustic bone w.
  CT bone w.
  w. glass
  therapeutic w.
wine
  opium w.
wing
  ashen w.
  gray w.
  W. Negative Symptom Scale
  w. plate
  sphenoid w.
  W. symbol
wing-beating tremor
Winkelman disease
winking
  w. spasm
  w. spasmodic syndrome
Winkle
  Rip van W.
Winkler body
wink reflex

Winslow concept
Winston-Lutz method
Winstrol-V
winter depression
Wintrobe method
wipe out
WIPI
Word Intelligibility by Picture
Identification
WIQ
Waring Intimacy Questionnaire
wire
w. contour preparation
Drummond w.
w. extrusion
Kirschner w.
Luque w.
Mullan w.
w. osteosynthesis
w. passage
w. penetration depth
w. removal technique
spinous process w.
w. stabilization
sublaminar w.
w. thrombosis
titanium w.
Wisconsin interspinous w.
Wisconsin spinous process w.
wiring
facet fracture stabilization w.
facet subluxation stabilization w.
posterior interspinous w.
spinous process w.
sublaminar w.
wiry
WISC
Wechsler Intelligence Scale for Children
WISC-III
Wechsler Intelligence Scale for Children-
Third Edition
Wisconsin
W. Card-Sorting Test (WCST)
W. interspinous wire
W. Psychosocial Pain Inventory
W. Scoring Test
W. spinous process wire
WISC-R
Wechsler Intelligence Scale for Children-
Revised
wish
child-penis w.
w. dream
w. fulfillment
fundamental w.
gratification of dependent w.'s
id w.
intense w.
Klein death w.
libido w.
masochistic w.
penis w.
recovery w.
wisher
ill w.

wishful thinking
WIST
Whitaker Index of Schizophrenic
thinking
wit
abstract w.
allusion in w.
characterization w.
displacement w.
ellipsis w.
exaggeration in w.
exhibition w.
harmless w.
indirect w.
naive w.
nonsense in w.
obscene w.
omission in w.
outdoing w.
parody in w.
recognition in w.
tendency w.
thought w.
travesty in w.
unification in w.
word w.
w. work
witchcraft
witch doctor
witchery
withdrawal
w. adjustment
w. adjustment reaction
alcoholic delirium w.
amphetamine w.
anchor signs of w.
anxiolytic w.
apathetic w.
barbiturate w.
benzodiazepine w.
caffeine w.
cocaine w.
w. criteria
w. delirium
w. destructiveness
w. disorder
drug w.
w. dyskinesia
w. dystonia
w. emergent syndrome
ethanol w.
w. from social affair
w. hallucinosis
heroin w.
hypnotic w.
infant narcotic w.
w. insomnia
interpersonal w.
w. method of contraception
morphine w.
w. movement
narcotic w.
neonatal opiate w.
nicotine w.
opioid w.

W

withdrawal *(continued)*
  psychoactive substance w.
  w. reaction of adolescence
  w. reaction of childhood
  w. reflex
  sedative w.
  w. seizure
  w. sign
  social w.
  w. state
  substance intoxication or w.
  substance-specific w.
  sympathomimetic w.
  w. symptom
  w. syndrome alcoholic psychosis
  w. syndrome drug psychosis
  thought w.
  tobacco w.
  w. tremor
  uncomplicated alcohol w.
  uncomplicated sedative, hypnotic, or
   anxiolytic w.
withdrawal-related mood disorder
withdrawn catatonic schizophrenia
withhold
within normal limits (WNL)
withstand
witless
witness
  character w.
  w. credibility
  expert w.
WITT
  Wittenborn Psychiatric Rating Scale
Wittenborn
  W. Psychiatric Rating Scale
   (WITT, WPRS)
  W. Psychiatric Rating Scale Test
wittigo
Wittigo psychosis
Wittmaak-Ekbom syndrome
witzelsucht
  primary affective w.
wizardry
WJAT
  Woodcock-Johnson Achievement Test
WJPTB
  Woodcock-Johnson Psychoeducational
   Test Battery
WMI
  Work Motivation Inventory
WML
  white matter lesion
WMS
  Wechsler Memory Scale
WMS-MQ
  Wechsler Memory Scale/Memory
   Quotient
WMS-R
  Wechsler Memory Scale - Revised
WNAI
  Word and Number Assessment Inventory
WNL
  within normal limits

Wohlfart-Kugelberg-Welander disease
Wolf endoscope
Wolff
  W. headache
  W. vasogenic theory
wolf-man
Wolf-Orton body
Wolfram needle electrode
Wollaston theory
Wolman disease
Woltman sign
woman
  other w.
  phallic w.
  rainy day w.
womanhood
womb
  w. envy
  w. fantasy
women's
  w. liberation movement
  w. role
women who fail syndrome
wonder drug
Wonderlic Personnel Test
wont
Wood Assessment Scale
woodbine
  African w.
Woodcock
  W. Language Proficiency Battery
  W. Reading Mastery Test
Woodcock-Johnson
  W.-J. Achievement Test (WJAT)
  W.-J. Psychoeducational Test
   Battery (WJPTB)
woodcutter's encephalitis
Woodson
  W. dural separator
  W. dural separator-spatula
  W. dura packer
wool hwa-byung
woozy
word
  w. accent
  w. approximation
  w. association
  w. association technique
  W. Association Test
  w. attack
  back-formation w.
  base w.
  w. blindness
  w. cathexis
  w. center
  class w.
  w. coinage
  coin new w.'s
  w. configuration
  w. deafness
  w. debris
  dirty w.'s
  w. discrimination score
  W. Discrimination subtest
  w. dumbness

empty w.
feared w.'s
W. Finding Test
w. fluency
W. Fluency Test
function w.
W. Intelligibility by Picture
  Identification (WIPI)
Jonah w.'s
last w.
microcosm of w.'s
W. and Number Assessment
  Inventory (WNAI)
phonetically balanced w.'s
phonologically irregular w.'s
phonologically regular w.'s
play on w.'s
portmanteau w.
W. Processing Test
W. Processor Assessment Battery
W. Recognition Test
w. rhyming
w. salad
W. Search
w. stimulus
thinking creatively with sounds
  and w.'s (TCSW)
w. understanding
w. wit
word-attack skill
word-building test
word-finding
  w.-f. ability
  w.-f. ability disturbance
  w.-f. difficulty
  w.-f. skill
Word-in-Context Test
word-recognition skill
work
  w. addiction
  W. Attitudes Questionnaire (WAQ)
  Bachelor of Social W. (BSW)
  breath w.
  case w.
  circadian rhythm sleep disorder,
    shift w.
  w. cure
  w. decrement
  w. disability
  dream w.
  w. dysfunction
  W. Environment Preference
    Schedule (WEPS)
  W. Environment Scale (WES)
  w. ethic
  family social w.
  field w.
  w. force
  grief w.
  w. group
  group w.
  W. Information Inventory (WII)
  w. inhibition
  W. Interest Index
  Master of Social W. (MSW)

  w. motivation
  W. Motivation Inventory (WMI)
  mourning w.
  w. paralysis
  w. phobia
  psychiatric social w.
  W. Sample Battery
  W. Skills Series Production (WSS)
  social w.
  W. and Social Adjustment Scale
  testing, orientation, and w.
  w. therapy
  unexplained absence from w.
  W. Values Inventory (WVI)
  wit w.
workable
Workaholics Anonymous
worker
  aftercare w.
  blue-collar w.
  certified social w. (CSW)
  child-care w.
  indigenous w.
  intake w.
  linkage w.
  mental health w.
  psychiatric social w.
  skilled w.
  social w.
work-for-pay unit
workhorse
working
  w. alliance
  w. environment
  w. memory
  w. mother
  w. out
  w. over
  w. relationship
  w. type
work-limit test
workmanship
workplace violence
workshop
  career w.
  employment w.
  sheltered w.
  survival skills w.
  transitional employment w.
workstation
  MKM w.
  SUN w.
work-study program
world
  external w.
  W. Health Organization (WHO)
  on top of the w.
  w. soul
  w. war
  W. War I (WWI)
  W. War II (WWII)
  W. of Work Inventory (WWI)
world-destruction fantasies
wormian bone
worrisome

W

worry
  w. beads
  w. circuit
  constant w.
  w. control
  excessive w.
  hyperresponsible w.
  W. Scale for Children
  uncontrolled w.
  unrealistic w.
worse
  W. Premorbid Adjustment Scale
  w. sleep continuity
worship
  ancestor w.
  devil w.
  hero w.
  Satan w.
  satanic w.
worth
  comparable w.
  inflated w.
worthless
Wortman Social Support Scale
wound
  gunshot w.
  multiple stab w.'s (MSW)
  self-inflicted w. (SIW)
wounded
  w. in action
  w. victim syndrome
Wound-Evac drain
wounding
  narcissistic w.
  symbolic w.
WOWS
  Weak Opiate Withdrawal Scale
WPAI
  Wilson-Patterson Attitude Inventory
WPPSI
  Wechsler Preschool and Primary Scale of
    Intelligence
WPRS
  Wittenborn Psychiatric Rating Scale
WR
  whole response
WRAML
  Wide Range Assessment of Memory and
    Learning
wrap
  cotton w.
  Dura-Kold ice w.
wraparound
wrapping of aneurysm
WRAT
  Wide Range Achievement Test
  Wide Range Achievement Test-Revised
WRAT-R
  Wide Range Achievement Test-Revised
wrench
  Texas Scottish Rite Hospital w.
  T-handle nut w.
  T-handle screw w.
WREST
  Wide Range Employment Sample Test

wretched
Wright Care TENS unit
wringing
  hand w.
  w. of hands
WRIOT
  Wide Range Interest-Opinion Test
WRIPT
  Wide Range Intelligence and Personality
    Test
Wrisberg
  W. ganglia
  nerve of W.
  W. nerve
wrist
  w. clonus
  w. clonus reflex
  w. cutting
  w. drop
  w. restraint
writhe
writing
  w. ability
  w. assignment
  ataxic w.
  automatic w.
  CAP Assessment of W.
  developmental expressive w.
  w. disability
  w. disorder
  w. fear
  w. hand
  mirror w.
  pornographic w.
  spirit w.
  w. tremor
written
  w. expression
  w. language
  W. Language Assessment
  w. language quotient
wrongdoer
wrongdoing
wrong-way deviation
wryneck
wry neck
WSDI
  Wahler Self-Description Inventory
WSS
  Work Skills Series Production
WSSDT
  Washington Speech Sound
    Discrimination Test
Würzburg
  W. implant system
  W. titanium plating system
WUSCT
  Washington University Sentence
    Completion Test
WVI
  Work Values Inventory
WWI
  World War I
  World of Work Inventory

WWII
    World War II
Wyburn-Mason
    W.-M. arteriovenous malformation
    W.-M. syndrome

Wyler cylindrical subdural electrode

W

X

X chromosome
X zone

X25 PCR
Xanax
xanthine oxidase inhibitor
xanthoastrocytoma

pleomorphic x. (PXA)
xanthochromia of cerebrospinal fluid
xanthocyanopsia
xanthogranulomatous cyst
xanthomatosis

cerebrotendinous x. (CTX)
xanthomatous Rathke cleft cyst
xanthosarcoma
X-bar theory
Xe

xenon
¹³³Xe

xenon-133
¹³³Xe intravenous injection
technique
XeCT, Xe-CT

xenon enhanced computed tomography
XeCT scanning
Xe/CT CBF study
Xenical
xenogeneic

x. chromaffin cell
x. graft
xenoglossophilia
xenograft

glioblastoma x.
xenomania
xenon (Xe)

x.-133 (¹³³Xe)
x. computed tomography (Xe-CT)
x. CT
x.-CT
x. CT measurement
x. CT scanning
x. enhanced computed tomography
(XeCT, Xe-CT)
x. method
xenon-enhanced CT
xenophobia
xenorexia
Xerecept
xeroderma pigmentosum
xerodermic idiocy
xerophagia

xerophobia
xerostomia
XeScan

Linde X.
¹³³XeSPECT contrast medium
x **gradient**
X-ing
xiphodynia
xiphoidalgia
XKnife
XL

XL illuminator
Lodine XL
X-linkage
x-linked

X.-l. abnormality
X.-l. anophthalmia
x.-l. cortical migration disorder
X.-l. dominance
X.-l. lymphoproliferative syndrome
X.-l. recessive muscular dystrophy
X.-l. recessive spinobulbar muscular
atrophy
X.-l. spastic paraparesis
Xomed nerve integrity monitor-2
Xomed-Treace nerve integrity monitor-2
X-O test
Xp21 myopathy
Xphoria

Ultimate X.
x-ray

artifact on x.-r.
intraoperative x.-r.
isocentric linear accelerator x.-r.
x.-r. localization
orthogonal x.-r.
XRT

radiotherapy
X-Trel spinal cord stimulation system
X-Trozine
XXXX syndrome
XXXXX syndrome
XXXXY syndrome
XXXY syndrome
XXY syndrome
XXYY syndrome
Xylocaine with epinephrine
Xyrem
xyrospasm
XYY syndrome

X

Y

Y chromosome
Y incision
neuropeptide Y (NPY)

Yale

Y. brace
Y. Global Tic Severity Scale
Y. Revised Developmental Schedule
Y. Schedule for Tourette Syndrome and Other Behavioral Disorders
Y. Schedule for Tourette Syndrome and Other Behavioral Disorders, Hebrew Version

Yale-Brown Obsessive Compulsive Scale (YBOCS)

y-aminobutyric acid

yan

pen y.

yancy

yang

shuk y.
suo y.
yin and y.

Yankauer suction tube

yantra

Yasargil

Y. arachnoid knife
Y. artery forceps
Y. bayonet forceps
Y. bayonet scissors
Y. carotid clamp
Y. clip-applying forceps
Y. craniotomy
Y. dissector
Y. elevator
Y. flat serrated ring forceps
Y. hypophyseal forceps
Y. instrument
Y. knotting forceps
Y. Leyla retractor arm
Y. ligature carrier
Y. ligature guide
Y. microclip
Y. microcurette
Y. micro curette
Y. microdissector
Y. micro dissector
Y. micro forceps
Y. microforceps
Y. microrasp
Y. microscissors
Y. microvascular knife
Y. needle holder
Y. OptiMat floor stand
Y. pituitary rongeur
Y. rasp
Y. retractor
Y. scoop
Y. spring hook
Y. suction tube
Y. tissue lifter

Y. tumor forceps
Y. vessel clip

Yasargil-Aesculap

Y.-A. instrument
Y.-A. spring clip

Yasargil-Leyla brain retractor

yawning

psychogenic y.

yawn-sign approach

YBOCS

Yale-Brown Obsessive Compulsive Scale

YBR

yellow brick road

YBT

Yerkes-Bridges Test

year

y. of birth (YOB)
Disability Adjusted Life Y.'s (DALYs)
quality-adjusted life y. (QALY)

yearbook

Mental Measurements Y. (MMY)

yearning

yeh

yellow

y. brick road (YBR)
y. fever
y. fever encephalitis
y. jacket
y. ligament
y. spot

yen

pin y.
y. sleep

Yerkes-Bridges Test (YBT)

Yerkes-Dodson law

Yersinia enterocolitica

YES

Youth Enjoying Sobriety

yes-no question

yes-yes tremor

y **gradient**

yin and yang

YOB

year of birth

Yocon

yoga

Bhakti y.
Hatha y.
Karma y.
Kundalini y.
tantric y.

yo-he-ho theory

yohimbine

yoke

double y.

yoked control

yong

shook y.

York retreat

You

Who Are Y.? (WAY)

Y

935

young
Y. Adult Behavior Checklist
y. adulthood
Y. Adult self-report
developmentally appropriate self-
stimulatory behaviors in the y.
Y. Mania Rating Scale
young-old
y.-o. patient
youth
y. counselor

y. culture
Y. Enjoying Sobriety (YES)
Y. self-report
youthful
youthquake
yo-yo syndrome
Y-shaped reference arc
yttrium-90

Z

Z code
Z coordinate
zalcitabine
Zange-Kindler syndrome
Zanoli-Vecchi syndrome
Zantac
Zappert syndrome
Zaraflex
Zarontin
Zaroxolyn
Zaxopam
ZD

ZD frame
ZD stereotactic system
ZD-Neurosurgical localizing unit
ZDS

Zung Depression Scale
zealot
zealous
Zeigarnik

Z. effect
Z. effect phenomenon
Zeiss

Z. Image Guided System
Z. MKM microscope
Z. OpMi CS-NC2 surgical microscope
Z. OpMi CS-NC2 surgical microscope system
Z. Super Lux 40 light source
Zeiss-Contraves operating microscope
Zeitgeber

endogenous Z.
exogenous Z.
Zeitgeist
Zeldox
Zellballen
Zellweger cerebrohepatorenal syndrome
zelophobia
zelotypia
Zen

Z. Buddhism
Z. therapy
Zenker

Z. paralysis
Z. solution
Zeppelin micro-motor system
zeppia
Zerit
zero

z. cerebral pseudotumor cerebri
z. drift of the sensor
z. family
z. filling
z. ICP ventricle shunt (ZIPS)
z. population growth (ZPG)
protein z.
zest

loss of z.
Zestoretic
zeta method

Zetran
zeugmatography

Fourier transformation z.
z-gradient

z.-g. coil
z.-g. field
zidovudine and lamivudine
Ziehen-Oppenheim disease
Zielke

Z. bifid hook
Z. instrument
Z. instrumentation
Z. VDS implant
Zieve syndrome
zifrosilone
Zika fever
zimeldine
Zimmer

Z. caudal hook
Z. clip
Z. microsaw
Zimmerman Personality Test
zinc-finger

z.-f. family
z.-f. gene
Zinn

annulus of Z.
Z. corona
Z. vascular circle
ziprasidone hydrochloride
ZIPS

zero ICP ventricle shunt
zoanthropic
zoanthropy

melancholia z.
Zocor
zoetic
zoic
zol
zolazepam
Zollinger-Ellison syndrome
Zollner illusion
zolmitriptan
Zoloft
zolpidem tartrate
Zomax
zombie
zombiism
zomepirac sodium
Zomig
zona, pl. zonae

z. dermatica
z. epithelioserosa
z. incerta
z. medullovasculosa
zonal
Zonalon Topical Cream
zone

anelectrotonic z.
anterior speech z.
body buffer z.
chemoreceptor trigger z.

Z

zone *(continued)*
    color z.
    cortical z.
    dolorogenic z.
    dorsal root entry z. (DREZ)
    entry z.
    ependymal z.
    epileptogenic z.
    erogenous z.
    erotogenic z.
    genital z.
    Head z.
    hyperesthetic z.
    hypnogenic z.
    hysterogenic z.
    intimate z.
    language z.
    latent z.
    limbic z.
    Lissauer marginal z.
    Marchant z.
    motor z.
    Obersteiner-Redlich z.
    peripolar z.
    personal distance z.
    polar z.
    posterior language z.
    primary z.
    reflexogenic z.
    Rolando z.
    social z.
    Spitzka marginal z.
    subplate z.
    subventricular z.
    tender z.
    time z.
    transition z.
    trigger z.
    trophotropic z. of Hess
    ultramarginal z.
    visual z.
    war z.
    watershed z.
    Wernicke z.
    X z.
Zonegran
zonesthesia
zonifugal
zonipetal
zonisamide
zonular layer
zooerastia
zooerasty
zoogenic
zoolagnia
zoolatry
zoomania

zoom microscope
zoomorphism
zoon politikon
zoophagous
zoophile psychosis
zoophilia
zoophilism
    erotic z.
zoophil psychosis
zoophobia
zoopsia
zoosadism
zootic
zopolrestat
Zoroastrianism
ZORprin
zoster
    z. encephalomyelitis
    herpes z.
    measles, rubella and z. (MRZ)
    ophthalmic z.
    z. ophthalmic
zosteriform
zosteroid
Zostrix
Zostrix-HP
Zovirax
ZPG
    zero population growth
Z-plate
    Z-p. anterior thoracolumbar
      instrumentation
    Z-p. fixation system
z score
Zuckerkandl
    Z. convolution
    organ of Z.
zuclopenthixol dihydrochloride
Zulliger Test
Zung
    Z. Anxiety Scale
    Z. Depression Scale (ZDS)
    Z. Self-Rating Depression Scale
Zurich school
zwischenstufe
Zyban
Zydone
zygal fissure
zygapophyseal joint
zygoma
zygomatic fracture
zygomaticoorbital artery
zygon
zygosis
zygosity
zygote
Zyprexa

Appendix 1
Anatomical Illustrations

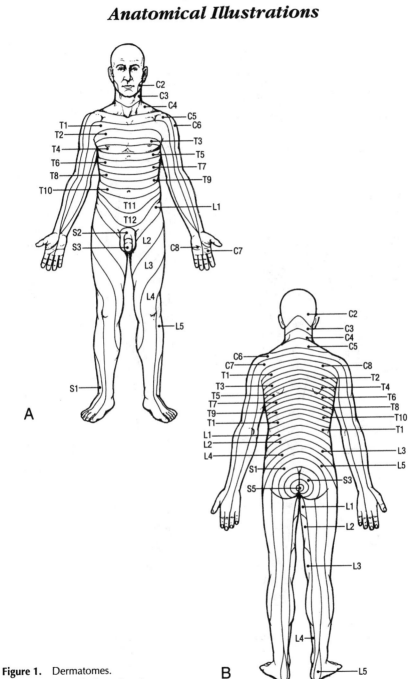

Figure 1. Dermatomes.
A, Anterior view. B, Posterior view.

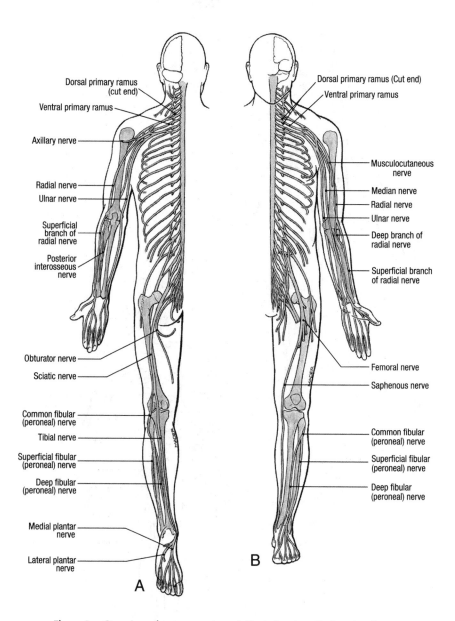

Figure 2. Overview of nervous system. A, Posterior view. B, Anterior view.

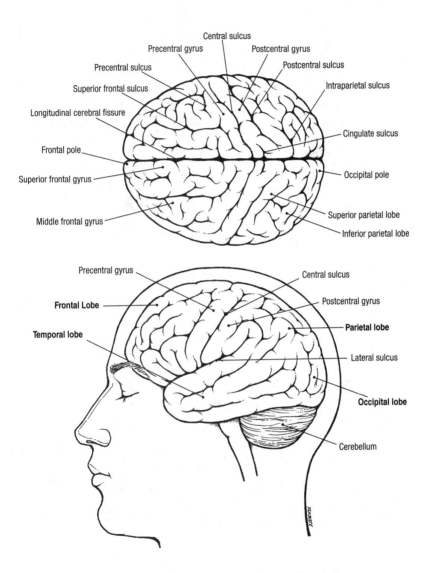

Figure 3. Brain. Top, superior view. Bottom, lateral view.

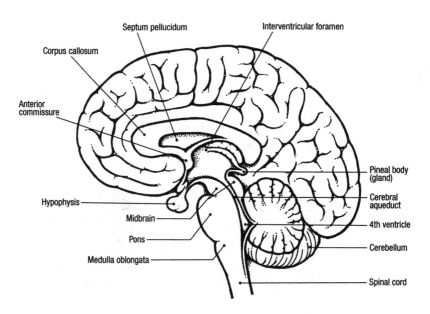

Figure 4. Brain, medial view.

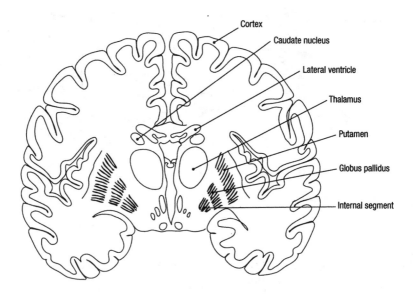

Figure 5. Brain, coronal view.

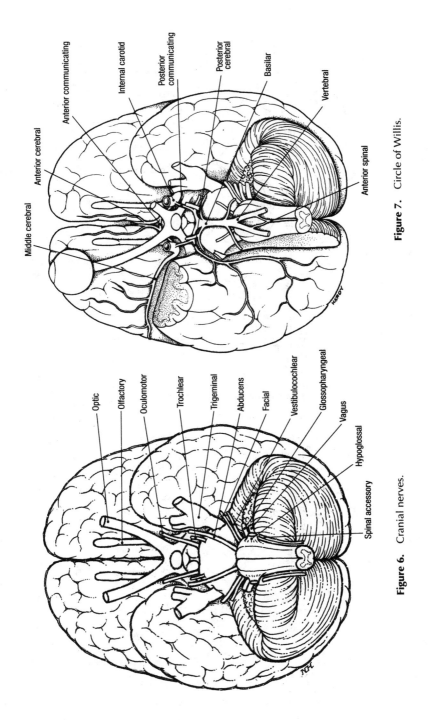

Figure 7. Circle of Willis.

Figure 6. Cranial nerves.

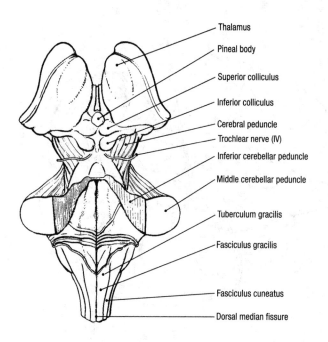

Thalamus
Pineal body
Superior colliculus
Inferior colliculus
Cerebral peduncle
Trochlear nerve (IV)
Inferior cerebellar peduncle
Middle cerebellar peduncle
Tuberculum gracilis
Fasciculus gracilis
Fasciculus cuneatus
Dorsal median fissure

Figure 8. Brainstem, dorsal view.

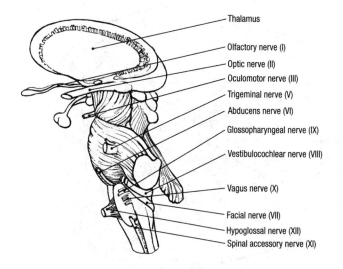

Thalamus
Olfactory nerve (I)
Optic nerve (II)
Oculomotor nerve (III)
Trigeminal nerve (V)
Abducens nerve (VI)
Glossopharyngeal nerve (IX)
Vestibulocochlear nerve (VIII)
Vagus nerve (X)
Facial nerve (VII)
Hypoglossal nerve (XII)
Spinal accessory nerve (XI)

Figure 9. Brainstem, lateral view.

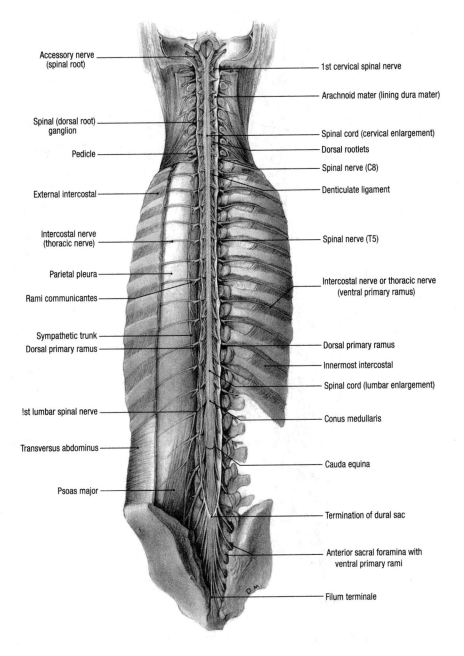

Accessory nerve (spinal root)

1st cervical spinal nerve

Arachnoid mater (lining dura mater)

Spinal (dorsal root) ganglion

Spinal cord (cervical enlargement)

Pedicle

Dorsal rootlets

Spinal nerve (C8)

External intercostal

Denticulate ligament

Intercostal nerve (thoracic nerve)

Spinal nerve (T5)

Parietal pleura

Rami communicantes

Intercostal nerve or thoracic nerve (ventral primary ramus)

Sympathetic trunk

Dorsal primary ramus

Dorsal primary ramus

Innermost intercostal

Spinal cord (lumbar enlargement)

!st lumbar spinal nerve

Conus medullaris

Transversus abdominus

Cauda equina

Psoas major

Termination of dural sac

Anterior sacral foramina with ventral primary rami

Filum terminale

Figure 10. Spinal cord and surrounding structures, posterior view.

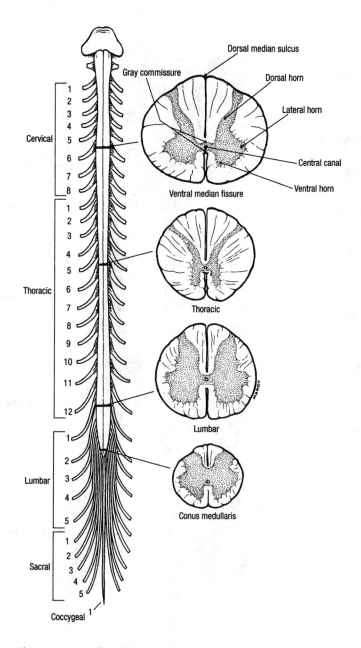

Figure 11. Spinal cord showing cross-sections at various levels.

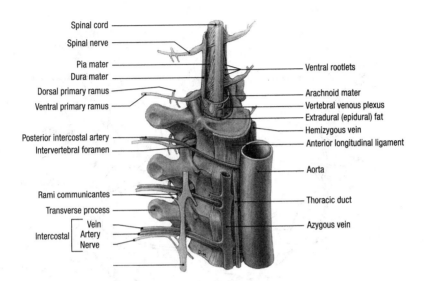

Figure 12. Spinal cord and prevertebral structures.

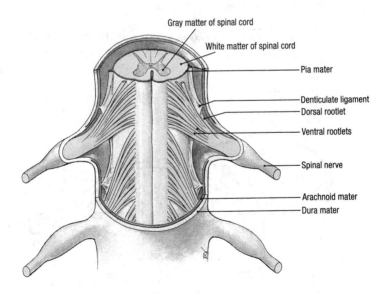

Figure 13. Formation of spinal nerves.

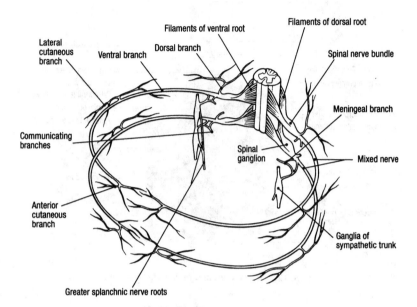

Figure 14. Spinal nerves, with roots and branches.

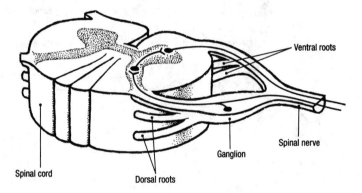

Figure 15. Spinal ganglion.

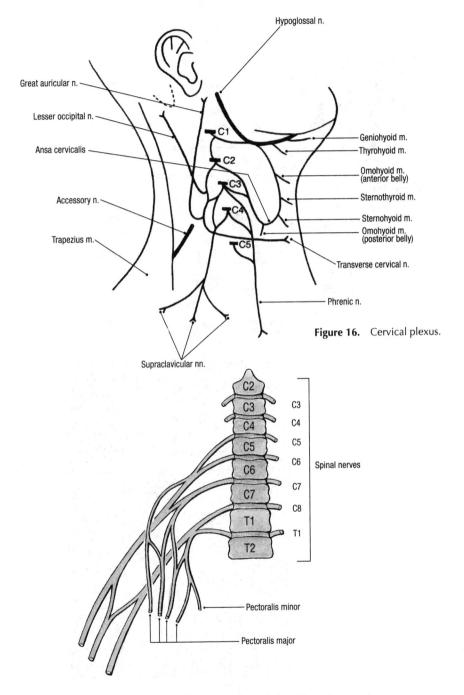

Figure 16. Cervical plexus.

Figure 17. Innervation of pectoral muscles, medial and lateral pectoral nerves.

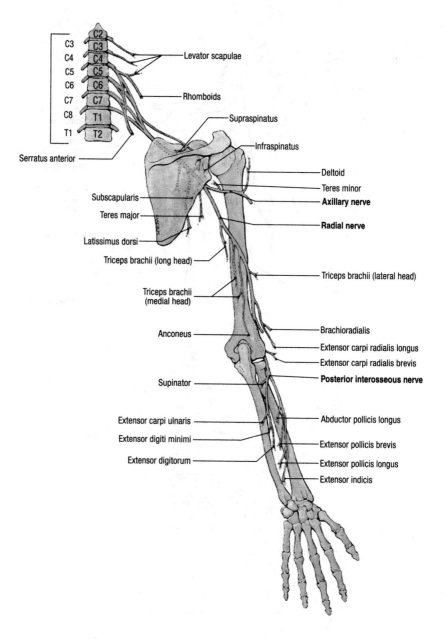

Figure 18. Innervation of upper limb muscles, radial nerve.

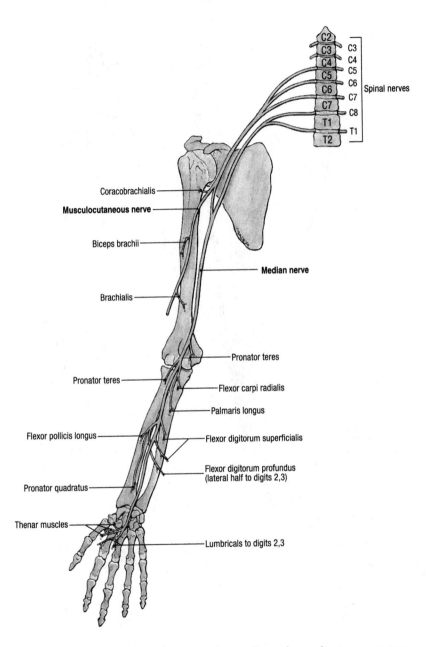

Figure 19. Innervation of upper limb muscles, median and musculocutaneous nerves.

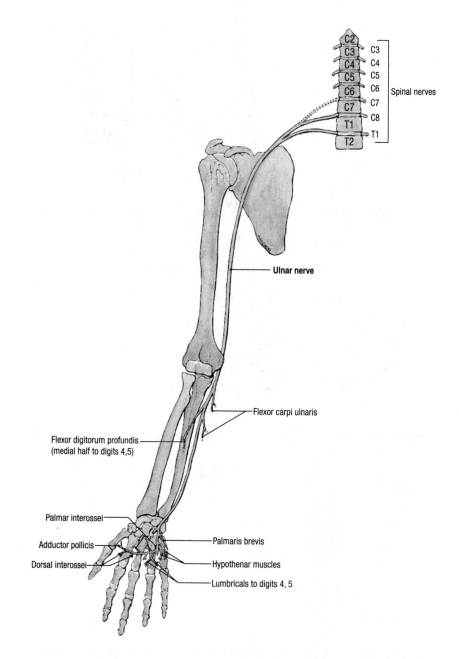

Figure 20. Innervation of upper limb muscles, ulnar nerve.

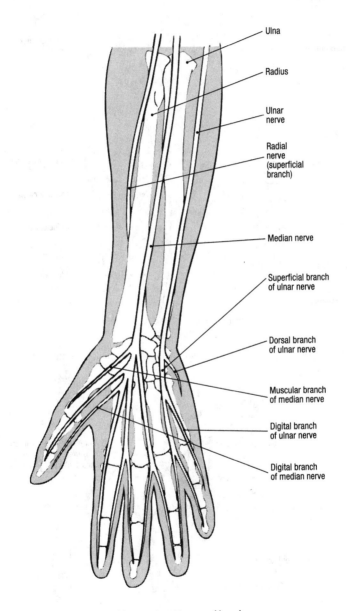

Ulna

Radius

Ulnar
nerve

Radial
nerve
(superficial
branch)

Median nerve

Superficial branch
of ulnar nerve

Dorsal branch
of ulnar nerve

Muscular branch
of median nerve

Digital branch
of ulnar nerve

Digital branch
of median nerve

Figure 21. Nerves of hand.

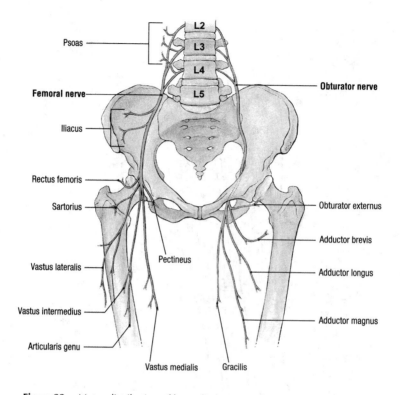

Figure 22. Motor distribution of lower limb nerves, femoral and obturator nerves.

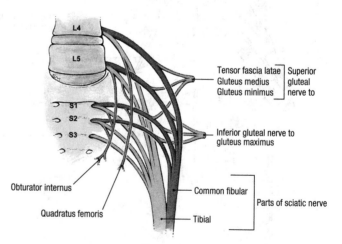

Figure 23. Motor distribution of lower limb nerves, sciatic nerve.

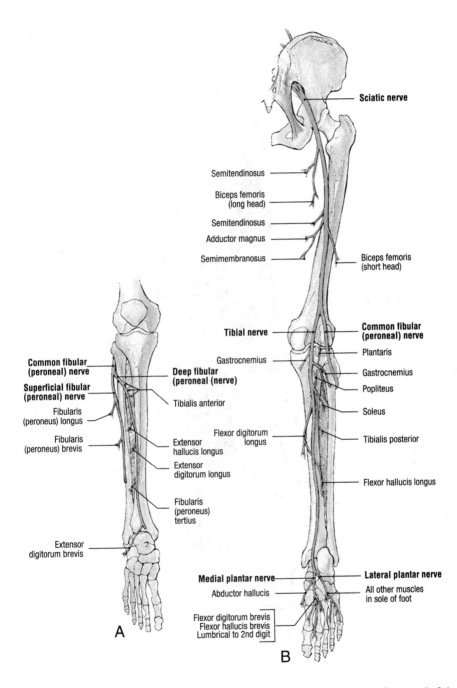

Figure 24. Motor distribution of lower limb nerves. A, common fibular (peroneal) nerve. B, Sciatic nerve.

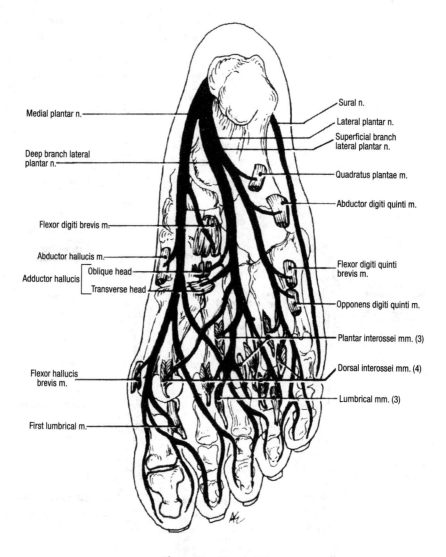

Figure 25. Nerves of foot.

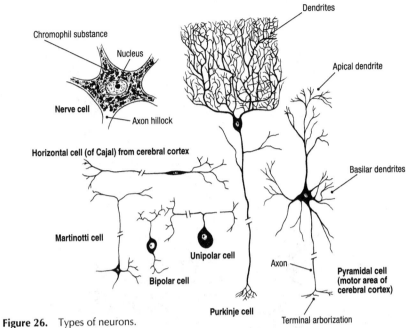

Figure 26. Types of neurons.

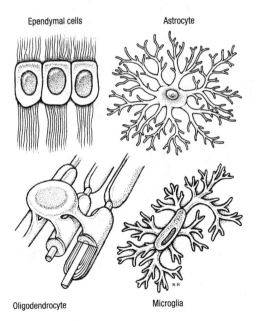

Figure 27. Neuroglia.

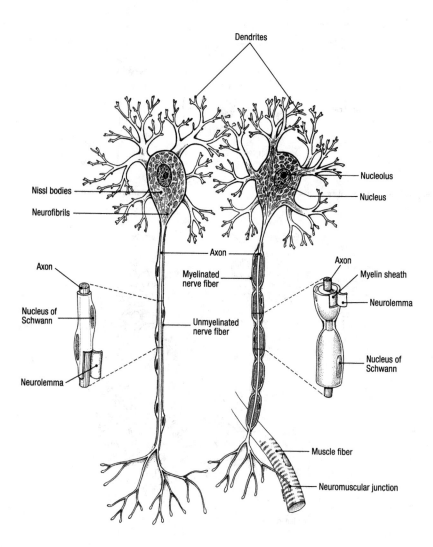

Figure 28. Myelinated and unmyelinated neurons.

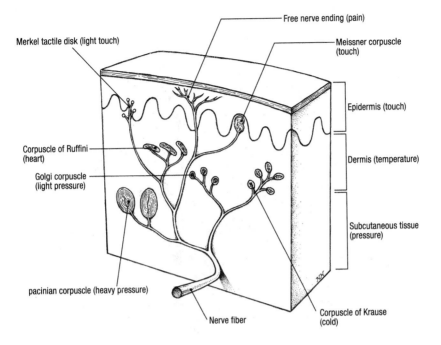

Figure 29. Sensory nerves and bodies.

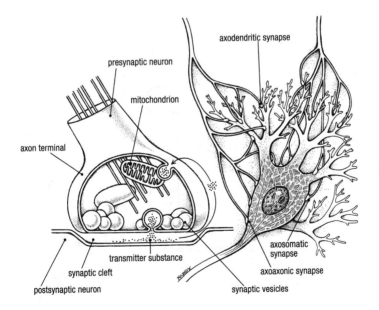

Figure 30. Nerve synapse.

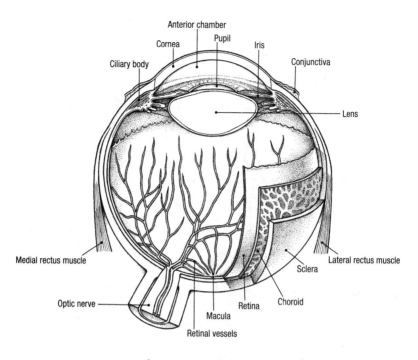

Figure 31. Structures of eye.

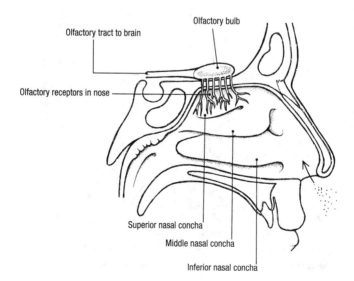

Figure 32. Olfaction.

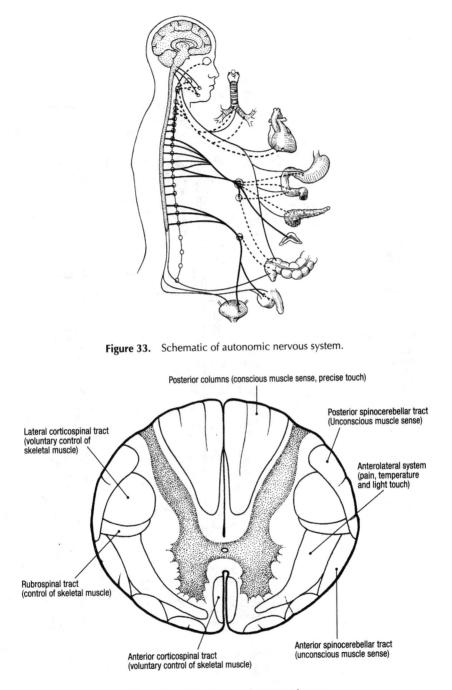

Figure 33. Schematic of autonomic nervous system.

Posterior columns (conscious muscle sense, precise touch)

Posterior spinocerebellar tract
(Unconscious muscle sense)

Lateral corticospinal tract
(voluntary control of
skeletal muscle)

Anterolateral system
(pain, temperature
and light touch)

Rubrospinal tract
(control of skeletal muscle)

Anterior corticospinal tract
(voluntary control of skeletal muscle)

Anterior spinocerebellar tract
(unconscious muscle sense)

Figure 34. Principal conduction pathways.

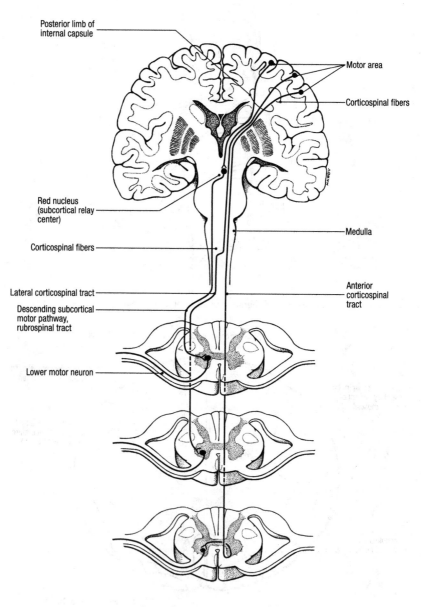

Figure 35. Corticospinal Tract.

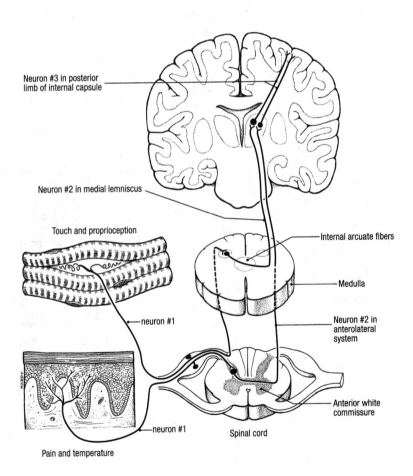

Figure 36. Decussation of nerve fibers.

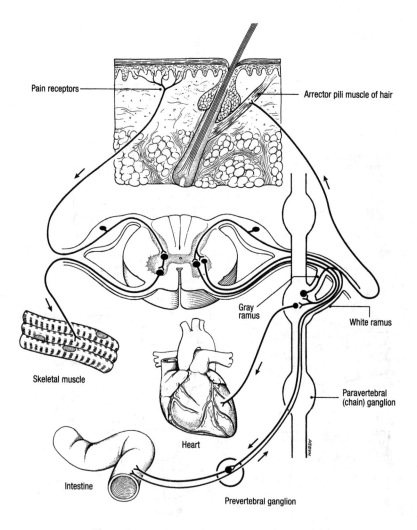

Pain receptors

Arrector pili muscle of hair

Gray ramus

White ramus

Skeletal muscle

Heart

Paravertebral (chain) ganglion

Intestine

Prevertebral ganglion

Figure 37. Somatic and visceral reflex pathways.

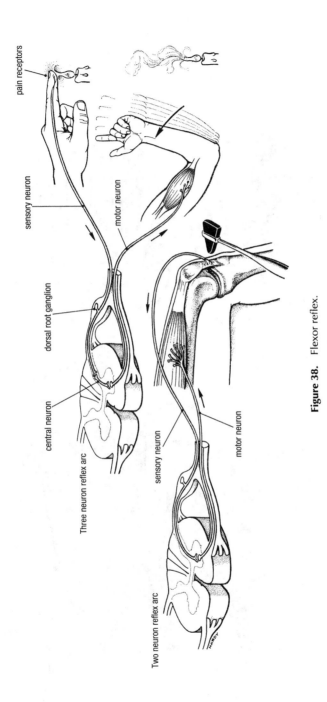

pain receptors

sensory neuron

motor neuron

dorsal root ganglion

central neuron

Three neuron reflex arc

sensory neuron

motor neuron

Two neuron reflex arc

Figure 38.   Flexor reflex.

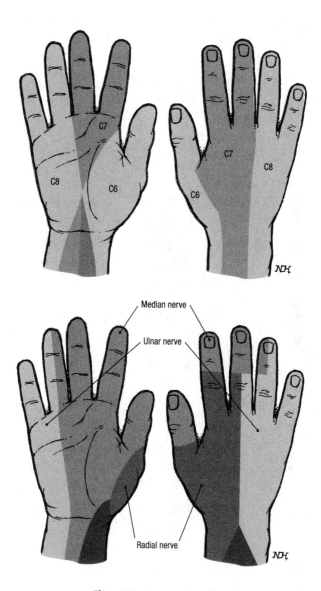

Figure 39. Innervation of hand.

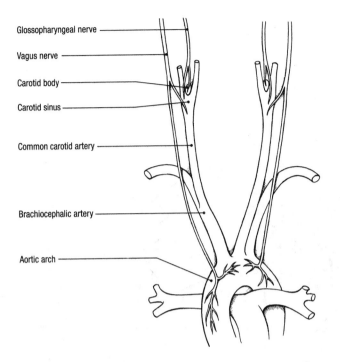

Glossopharyngeal nerve

Vagus nerve

Carotid body

Carotid sinus

Common carotid artery

Brachiocephalic artery

Aortic arch

Figure 40. Baroreceptor.

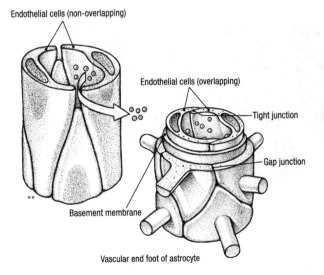

Endothelial cells (non-overlapping)

Endothelial cells (overlapping)

Tight junction

Gap junction

Basement membrane

Vascular end foot of astrocyte

Figure 41. Blood-brain barrier.

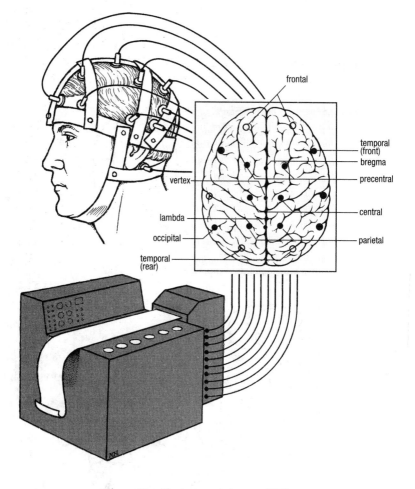

Figure 42. Electroencephalogram (EEG).

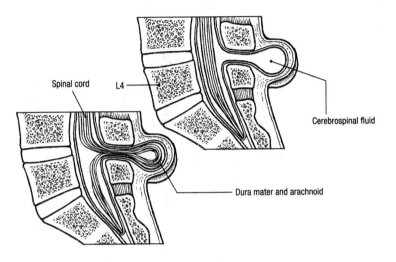

Figure 43. Meningocele.

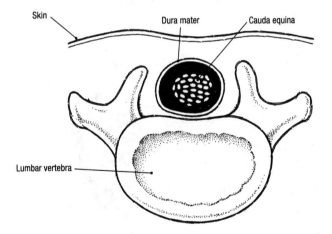

Figure 44. Spina bifida occulta.

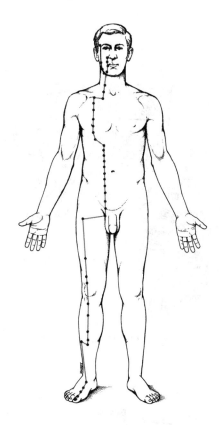

Figure 45. Acupuncture meridians.

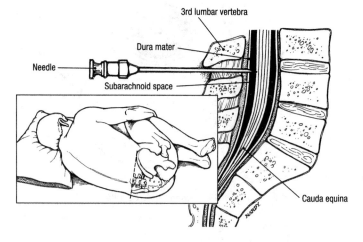

3rd lumbar vertebra

Dura mater

Needle

Subarachnoid space

Cauda equina

Figure 46. Lumbar puncture.

$10 pistol	poisoned heroin
25	LSD
49er	cocaine user
7–14s	methaqualone
A	amphetamines; LSD
a boot	under the influence
Abe	$5 worth of drugs
Abe's cabe	$5 bill
Abolic	veterinary steroid
A-bomb	marijuana and opium
Acapulco gold/red	marijuana
AC-DC	bisexual
ace	marijuana; PCP
acid/acido	LSD
AD	PCP
ad	addict
Adam	MDMA
Afghanistan black	hashish or marijuana
African	marijuana
African black/bush/woodbine	marijuana
age out	age-related diminished drug effect
ager	senior citizen
aimies, ames, amy, amys	amphetamine; amyl nitrite
ah-pen-yen	opium
AIP	heroin from Afghanistan, Iran, Pakistan
air blast	inhalant
air head, airhead	marijuana user
airplane	marijuana
Alice B. Toklas	marijuana brownie
all day and night	life sentence
all lit up	under the influence
all star	user of multiple drugs
all-American drug	cocaine
alley cat	promiscuous woman
alley juice	methyl alcohol
alligator	attractive male
alpha-ET	alpha-ethyltryptamine
ambition	amphetamine
amidone	methadone
ammo	amobarbital
amoeba	PCP
amp	ampule; amphetamine; marijuana dipped in formaldehyde and smokes
amped	under the influence
amped out	fatigue after amphetamine use

amping	accelerated heartbeat
AMT	dimethyltryptamine
Amy-John	lesbian
Anadrol	oral steroid
Anatrofin	injectable steroid
Anavar	oral steroid
angel/angel dust/hair/mist/poke	PCP
angie	cocaine
Angola	marijuana
animal	LSD
animal tranq	PCP
antifreeze	heroin
Apache	fentanyl
apples	fellow addicts
Apple jacks	crack
Are you anywhere?	Do you smoke marijuana?
Are you holding?	Do you have any dope?
Aries	heroin
arm	police
aroma of men	isobutyl nitrite
around the turn	completed withdrawal
artillery	drug paraphernalia
A's	amphetamine
ashes	marijuana
astro turf	marijuana
Asian white	cocaine
at liberty	unemployed
atom bomb	marijuana and heroin
atshitshi	marijuana
attitude	negative affect
aunt(ie)	elderly homosexual male
Aunt Hazel	heroin
Aunt Mary	marijuana
Aunt Nora	cocaine
Auntie, Auntie Emma	opium
aurora borealis	PCP
author	doctor who writes illegal prescriptions
B	matchbox of marijuana
B-bombs	amphetamines
B-40	cigar laced with marijuana and dipped in malt liquor
babe	drug used for detox
baby	small habit; drug beginner; marijuana
baby bhang	marijuana
babysit, babysitter	trip or first use guide
baby T	crack
backbreaker	LSD and strychnine
black dex	amphetamine

back door	pipe residue
back jack	injecting opium
back to back	using heroin after crack or vice versa
backtrack	reinjecting same dose
backup	prepare vein
backwards	tranquilizers; barbiturates; reacquire habit
bad	very good; crack
bad bundle	inferior quality heroin
bad go	bad reaction to drug
bad paper	worthless checks
bad rock	crack
bad seed	peyote; mescaline
badge bandit	police
badger game	extortion
bag, baggage	marijuana or heroin; condom
bag bride	crack-smoking prostitute
bagging	using inhalant
bagman	small habit; drug dealer; money transport
bake	smoke marijuana
baker (the)	electric chair
bale	marijuana
ball	party; genital absorption of drugs; genitalia; testicle; sex; Mexican black tar heroin
balling	vaginally implanted cocaine; sex
balloon	heroin supplier
ballot	heroin
balmy	mental problem, crazy
bam, bambita, bombita	amphetamine; depressant
bammies	inferior marijuana
bamba, bambalacha	marijuana
bambs	depressant
bandit	aggressive/violent homosexual
bang	inject drugs; sex; inhalant
banging	under the influence; sex
bank bandit pills	depressant
bar	marijuana
barb, barbies	barbiturates
barbs	cocaine
bareback rider	unprotected sex
barf tea	peyote
bark at the moon	under the influence
barrels	LSD
Bart Simpson	heroin
base, basing	cocaine; crack
baseball	crack
base crazies	searching on hands and knees for crack
bash	marijuana

baste (to)	battery
basuco	cocaine; coca paste residue sprinkled on marijuana or tobacco
bathtub speed	methcathinone
batt	IV needle
batted out	arrested
battery acid	LSD
batu	smokable methamphetamine
bazooka	cocaine; crack
bazulco	cocaine
BD	belladonna
beagle	detective
beam	cocaine
beam me up Scottie	crack dipped in PCP
beamer, beamers	crack user; crack
beans	Benzedrine; amphetamine; crack; mescaline
bear	a capsule of narcotic
bear in the air	helicopter law enforcement
bear trap	radar trap
beast	heroin; LSD; prostitute; unattractive woman
beat	crack; bogus drug
beat artist	person selling bogus drug
beat the bricks	get out of jail
beat the gong	smoke opium
beat vials	vials containing sham crack to cheat buyers
beautiful bolders	crack
Beavis & Butthead	LSD
bebe	crack
bedazzled	under the influence
bedbugs	fellow addicts
beedies	cigarettes from India
beetle crusher	police
behind the scale	weigh and sell cocaine
beiging	altering appearance of cocaine
belch	inform
belladona	PCP
belly habit	oral ingestion
belongs	drug user
belt	effects of drugs
belted	under the influence
Belushi, Belushi cocktail	heroin and cocaine
belyando spruce	marijuana
bending and bowing	under the influence
benny, bennies	Benzedrine; amphetamine
bent	a drug high; a homosexual
benz	Benzedrine; amphetamine
Bernice, Bernies, Bernie's flake, Bernie's gold dust	cocaine

betsy, Betsy, Betsie	gun
bhang	marijuana
big bag	heroin
big bloke	cocaine
big C	cocaine
big chief	peyote; mescaline
big D	LSD
big 8	1/8 kilogram of crack
big flake	cocaine
big H	heroin
big Harry	heroin
big John	police
big man	drug supplier
big nickel	$5000 bet
Big O	opium
big one	$1000 bet
big rush	cocaine
biker's coffee	methamphetamine and coffee
biker's speed	methamphetamine
Bill Blass	crack
Billie hoke	cocaine
bindle	small packet of drug powder; heroin
bindler	drug dealer
bing	one dose for injection
bingers	crack addicts
bingo	inject drugs
bings	crack
biphetamine	amphetamine
bird cage hype	financially deprived class of addicts
birds	marijuana; young female
bird's eye	extremely small quantity
birdhead	LSD
birdie powder	heroin; cocaine
biscuit	50 rocks of crack
bite	arrest
bite lips	smoke marijuana
biz	drug paraphernalia; portion of drugs
BJs	crack
black and white	patrol car; mixed-race couple or team; amphetamines
black bart	marijuana
blacks, black beauties	amphetamines; depressants
black birds, blackbirds	amphetamine
black bombers	amphetamine
black Cadillacs	amphetamine
black dust	PCP
black ganga	marijuana resin
black gold	high potency marijuana
black gungi	marijuana from India

black gunion	marijuana
black H	black tar heroin
black hash	opium and hashish
black mo, black moat	highly potent marijuana
black Mollies	amphetamine
black mote	marijuana
black pearl	heroin
black pill	opium pill
black rock	crack
black Russian	hashish mixed with opium
black star	LSD
black stuff	heroin
black sundae	heroin cut with cocoa
black sunshine	LSD
black tabs	LSD
black tar	heroin
black whack	PCP
blanca	cocaine
blanco	heroin
blanket	marijuana
blanks	bad narcotics; vasectomized male
blast	party; shoot with a firearm; smoke marijuana or crack; cocaine
blizzard	white cloud in coke pipe
blind munchies	marijuana-induced appetite
bliss out	euphoria
blond, blonde	hashish; marijuana
block	marijuana
block buster	depressant
bloods	street gang
blotter	daily arrest record; LSD; cocaine
blotter acid, blotter cube	LSD
blow	cocaine; inhale; inhale cocaine; smoke marijuana; miss the vein; leave; fellatio
blow a fix, blow a shot, blow the vein	miss the vein
blow blue	inhale cocaine
blowcaine	crack diluted with cocaine
blow Charley	sniff cocaine
blow grass	smoke marijuana
blow one's roof	smoke marijuana
blow smoke	smoke marijuana or hashish; obfuscate
blue	Numorphan; crack; depressant
blue acid	LSD
blue and red	secobarbital
blue angels	amobarbital
blue birds, bluebirds	depressant
blue boy	amphetamine

blue barrels	LSD
blue bullets	depressant
blue caps	mescaline
blue chairs	LSD
blue cheer	LSD
blue devils	amobarbital
blue du Hue	Vietnam marijuana
blued	tattooed
blue dolls	amobarbital
blue flags	LSD
blue heaven	LSD
blue heavens	amobarbital
blue madman	PCP
blue meth	methamphetamine
blue microdot	LSD
blue mist	LSD
blue moons	LSD
blue mollies	amphetamine
blue morph	Numorphan
blue pipe	vein
blues	amobarbital; melancholia; police; oxymorphone
blue sage	marijuana
blue sky	heroin
blue sky blond	Colombian marijuana
blue tips	barbiturates
blue vial	LSD
blue velvet	paregoric and amphetamine; cough preps with codeine
blunt	marijuana inside a cigar; marijuana and cocaine inside a cigar
bo, bo-bo, bobo bush	marijuana
boat	marijuana and PCP
body packer	transporting drugs by ingesting
body stuffer	ingesting drugs to avoid prosecution
body shake	inspect for needle marks
Bogart	salivate on a marijuana cigarette; refuse to share
bohd	marijuana; PCP
bolasterone	injectable steroid
Bolivian, Bolivian marching powder	cocaine
bolt	isobutyl nitrite
bomb	crack; heroin; large marijuana cigarette; high potency heroin
bomber	marijuana cigarette
bombido, bombit, bombito, bombita	injectable amphetamine; heroin; depressant
bombs away	heroin
bomb squad	crack-selling crew
bone breaker	physician

bonecrusher	crack
bones	crack; dice
boneshaker	gambler
bong	drug paraphernalia
bonita	heroin; lactose crystals used to cut or dilute a drug
boo, boo boo bama	marijuana
book	100 LSD doses; one-year prison sentence; entered on police blotter for alleged crime
boom	marijuana
boondagger	an aggressive lesbian
boost	to shoplift; steal; inject drug; crack
boot	inject a drug; repeatedly reinject same dose; to remove from one's residence or end relationship
boot the gong	smoke marijuana
booted	under the influence
boppers	amyl nitrite
boss	excellent quality
BOT	balance of time (remaining time of a prison sentence)
both hands	a ten-year prison sentence
botray	crack
bottles	crack vials; injectable amphetamines
boulya	crack
bouncing powder	cocaine
box man	expert safe cracker
boxcars	sixes on dice
boxed	in jail or prison
boy	heroin
boys uptown (the)	a group of influential criminals
bozo	heroin; epithet
brain bucket	a helmet
brain damage	heroin
brain dead	drug-induced permanent CNS effects
brain ticklers	amphetamine
brand X	inferior-quality marijuana
brea	heroin
breakdowns	$40 crack rock sold for $20
break night	staying up until daybreak
breeder	a heterosexual; female; derogatory
brewery	place where drugs are made
brick	one kilogram of marijuana; crack
brick agent	an FBI agent
brick gum	heroin
bridge up or bring up	prepare vein for injecting
britton	peyote
broccoli	marijuana
brodie, Brodie, Brody	suicide committed by jumping from a high place
broja, bruja	heroin
bromo	2CB

Brompton cocktail	cocaine, alcohol, and morphine
brown	Mexican heroin; marijuana
brown bagger	a physically unattractive person;
brown bombers	LSD
brown crystal	heroin
brown dots	LSD
brown horse	Mexican heroin
brown rhine	heroin
brown sugar	heroin; a black prostitute; heroin
browns, brownies	amphetamine
bubble gum	cocaine; crack
buck	shoot someone in the head; a physically fit male; one dollar; a $100 bet
bud	marijuana
buda	joint filled with crack
bufo	5-hydroxy-N,N-dimethyltryptamine
buffer	crack smoker; woman who trades oral sex for crack
bugged	annoyed; covered with sores and abscesses from needles
bull	federal narcotics agent; police; prison guard
bullet	isobutyl nitrite
bullet bolt	inhalant
bullia capital	crack
bullion, bullyon	crack
bullpen	a holding cell in a jail or prison
bum trip, bummer	unsettling or threatening experience from LSD or PCP trip
bumblebees	amphetamines
bump	crack; fake crack; cocaine; boost a high; $20 hit of ketamine
bundle	twenty-five $5 bags of heroin
burese	cocaine
burn bag	bogus drugs
burn one	smoke marijuana
burned out	collapse of veins; permanent impairment from drug abuse; exhausted
burner	the electric chair
burnie	marijuana
bush	marijuana; female genitalia; cocaine
businessman's acid/high/special	dimethyltryptamine
busy bee	PCP
busters	depressant
butter, butterflower	marijuana
buttons	mescaline
butu	heroin
buzz bomb	nitrous oxide
C, C-dust, C-game	cocaine
CA	cocaine addict
C&H, cold and hot	cocaine and heroin
C&M	cocaine and morphine

C.S.	marijuana
C joint	place where cocaine is sold
C note	$100 bill
caballo	heroin
cabello	cocaine
cabbage	money
caca	inferior or adulterated heroin, cocaine, or marijuana
cache	a hidden supply of drugs
cactus, cactus buttons, cactus head	peyote; mescaline
cadet	a new addict
Cad, Cadillac	one ounce; PCP; cocaine
Cadillac express	methcathinone
caine	cocaine; crack
cake	drugs that are smuggled into a prison or hospital; round disks of crack
calbo	heroin
California cornflakes	cocaine
California sunshine	LSD
California turnarounds	amphetamines
calling card	needle marks
Cambodian red, Cam red	reddish-brown Cambodian marijuana
Cambodian trip weed, Cam trip	potent Cambodian marijuana
came	cocaine
campfire boy	an opium addict
campy	a homosexual
can	a marijuana container; one ounce;
Can you do me good?	Do you have drugs I can buy?
Canadian black	marijuana
Canadian blues	methaqualone
Canadian quail	methaqualone
canamo	marijuana
canappa	marijuana
canary	Nembutal capsule (bright yellow color); an informer
cancelled stick	marijuana
cancer stick	a cigarette
candied	a cocaine addict
candy	cocaine; crack; depressant; amphetamine
candy C	cocaine
candy flipping	combining or sequencing LSD with MDMA
candy flipping on a string	LSD
candy a J	add another drug to a marijuana cigarette
candy canes and gumdrops	LSD
cannabinol	PCP
cannabis tea	marijuana
canned goods	cans containing drugs
cannon	a gun; a pickpocket
cannonball	an injection of mixed drugs

canvas back	a street person
cap	capsule of drugs; packet of heroin; crack; LSD
capital H	heroin
caps	crack; heroin; psilocybin/psilocin
capsula	crack
cap up	transfer bulk form to capsules
captain	an influential drug distributor
carburetor	drug paraphernalia
card	prepared dose of cocaine
carga, cargo	heroin
carmabis	marijuana
carne	heroin
carnie	cocaine
carpet patrol	searching floor for drugs
Carrie, Carrie Nation	cocaine
cartucho	package of marijuana cigarettes
cartoon acid	LSD
cartwheels	amphetamines
cascade	to move to stronger drugs
cashed	a container of marijuana that has been completely used
cashing a script	getting forged or bogus prescription orders dispensed
Casper, Casper the ghost	crack
cast iron horrors	delirium tremens
cat	any male; heroin; methcathinone
catch up	withdrawal process
catcher's mitt	diaphragm
Catholic aspirin	cross-scored amphetamine tablets
catnip	marijuana; adulterant or substitute for marijuana
cattail	a marijuana cigarette
cattle rustler	drug user who steals meat to support habit
cat Valium	ketamine
caught in a snowstorm	under the influence of cocaine
cave	an abscessed or collapsed portion of a vein
cave digging	searching for a suitable site for injecting
caviar	crack
cavite all star	marijuana
CD	glutethimide
Cecil	morphine; cocaine
Cecil Jones	a morphine addict
cement	large quantities of wholesale drugs
cement arm	an addict's heavily scarred arm
cent	one dollar
cha cha	an opium pipe
chalk	methamphetamine; amphetamine; crack
chalked up	under the influence
chalking	chemically altering color of cocaine
chamber pipe	a pipe designed to hold a large amount of marijuana
champ	a captured drug user who will not reveal his drug source

chandoo, chandu	Chinese opium
channel	a drug source; vein favored for injection
channel swimmer	addict who injects drugs
chapapote	heroin
charas, charash, charras	East Indian marijuana
charge	a drug portion; marijuana
charged up	under the influence
Charles, Charlie, Charley	heroin; cocaine; one dollar
Charley Cotton	cotton that is used to strain injectable drug
Charley goon	police
chase	smoke cocaine; smoke marijuana
chase the bag	shop around for best quality street heroin
chase the dragon	smoke crack and heroin
chaser	compulsive crack user
chasing the nurse, chasing the white nurse	morphine
chasing the tiger	smoke heroin
chatarra	heroin
cheap basing	crack
cheaters	marked playing cards
check	personal supply
cheeba, cheeo	marijuana
chef	opium preparer
chemical	crack
chewies	crack
cherry top	LSD
chewing the gum	chewing opium
chiba-chiba	Colombian marijuana
Chicago black, Chicago green	marijuana
Chicago leprosy	tracks from injecting drugs
chicharra	tobacco and marijuana
chick	heroin
chicken	homosexual
chicken hawk	homosexual pedophile
chicken powder	amphetamine
chicken scratch	searching on hands and knees for drug
chicken-shit habit	small drug habit
chicle	heroin
chicory	inferior opium
chief	peyote; mescaline; LSD
chieva	heroin
chill	to ignore; refuse to sell drugs to suspected informer; relax; kill
chill pill	tranquilizer
chillum	drug paraphernalia
China, China cat, China	white heroin
China girl, China town	fentanyl
Chinaman on back	addict's withdrawal

Chinese connection	Chinese drug smugglers
Chinese cure	gradual drug withdrawal
Chinese molasses	raw opium
Chinese needlework	tracks
Chinese red	heroin
Chinese saxophone	an opium pipe
Chinese tobacco	opium
Chino	a Chinese drug dealer
chip	heroin
chipping, chipper	occasional use
chippy, chippie	prostitute; girlfriend
chira	marijuana
chiva	heroin
chlorals	chloral hydrate
chocofan	brown tar heroin
chocolate	opium; amphetamine; marijuana
chocolate chips	LSD
chocolate ecstasy	chocolate milk powder and crack
chocolate powder	mescaline
choe	cocaine
choke	to dilute drugs
Cholly	cocaine
chop	to process heroin or marijuana
chorals	depressant
Christians	cross-scored amphetamine tablets
Christine, Christina	methamphetamine
Christmas rolls or trees	barbiturate capsules; amphetamines; marijuana
chronic	marijuana; marijuana and crack
chuck a Charley, chuck a dummy	to fake withdrawal to obtain drugs
chucks, chuck horrors	voracious craving for food during withdrawal
chunky	marijuana
church key	an opener used to open cans or bottles
churus	marijuana
cibas (CIBAS)	Doriden
cid	LSD
cigarette paper	packet of heroin
cigarrode cristal	PCP
circles	Rohypnol
circus	faking withdrawal drug seeking
citizen	nonuser of drugs
citrol	Nepalese marijuana
CJ, KJ	PCP
clanks	delirium tremens
clarity	MDMA
clay	hashish
clean and manicured	marijuana free of stems and seeds
clear light	superior-quality LSD in gelatin capsule

clicker	crack and PCP; marijuana dipped in formaldehyde and smoked
cliffhanger	PCP
climax	crack; isobutyl nitrite; heroin
climb	marijuana
clip	marijuana butt holder
clips	rows of vials sealed together
clipped	to rob or be robbed
clipped wings	arrested
clocking paper	drug profits
closed	drug source under scrutiny
closet baster	secret crack user
cloud	crack
cloud 9	caffeine and ma huang; ephedra; crack
clouted	arrested
club	a place to smoke marijuana
cluck	crack smoker
Clydesdale	a physically fit or handsome male
coast	Preludin; Ritalin
coast to coast	amphetamine
coasting	under the influence
coca	cocaine
coca paste	a potent form of cocaine
cocaine blues	post-cocaine use depression
cochornis	marijuana
cock pipe	drug paraphernalia
cockleburs	amphetamines
cocktail	tobacco cigarette cocaine, crack, marijuana or hashish; partially smoked marijuana cigarette inserted into regular one
cocoa puff	smoke cocaine and marijuana
coconut	cocaine
coco rocks	crack and chocolate pudding
coco snow	crack cut with benzocaine
cod	large amount of money
cod cock	cough syrup containing codeine
coffee	LSD
coffin dodger	a chain smoker
coffin nail	a cigarette
coke bugs	paresthesias or formication
coke oven	drug house for cocaine
cokeroaches	paresthesias or formication
cokie	cocaine user
cola	cocaine
coli	marijuana
coliflor tostao	marijuana
collar	narrow strip of paper which secures a needle to an eyedropper

collard greens	marijuana
Colombian, Columbian	marijuana
Colombian gold	potent Colombian marijuana
Colombian green	superior-quality Colombian marijuana
Colombian roulette	smuggling cocaine from Colombia by swallowing packets, then excreting upon delivery
Colorado Kool-Aid	Coor's beer
Colorado cocktail	marijuana
Columbo	PCP
Columbus black, Columbus black tea	marijuana
combol	cocaine
comeback	adulterants benzocaine and mannitol in cocaine to convert it to crack
come home	end an LSD trip
communist M&Ms	red Seconal capsules
comp man	a drug dealer
conductor	LSD; LSD trip guide
Congo brown	African marijuana
Congo dirt	superior-quality African marijuana
contact lens	LSD
cook	an opium den attendant; mix heroin with water; preparing heroin for injection; to smoke marijuana or hashish
cook down	liquify heroin to inhale
cook up a pill	to prepare a drug for smoking
cooker	inject a drug; amphetamine manufacturer
cookies	crack
coolie	cigarette laced with cocaine
coolie mud	inferior-quality opium
cookin'	process of manufacturing amphetamine
cooler	jail or prison; cigarette laced with drug
coop	jail or prison
coot	very good; composed; in a mellow state
coozie, coozy, couzie, couzy	female genitalia
coozie stash	drugs concealed in vagina
cop	to get anything; to buy dope
cop a deuceway	to purchase a $2 pack of narcotics
cop a match	to purchase a matchbox of marijuana
cop a pill	to smoke an opium pellet
cop a sneak	to leave a place
cop and blow	to purchase drugs and leave the scene quickly
copilots	amphetamine
copping zone	specific areas to purchase drugs
copper	police
corals	chloral hydrate; depressant
coriander seeds	cash
Corine, Corrine	cocaine
corn	marijuana

cosa	marijuana
cosmic, cozmic	experience on drugs
cosmos, cozmos	PCP
cotics	heroin
coties	codeine
cotton	currency
cotton brothers	cotton used to strain cocaine, heroin, or morphine and actual drugs
cotton catcher, cotton freak, cotton head, cotton top	addict who uses straining cotton to get drugs
cotton fever	illness contracted from cotton used for drug straining
cotton shot	water added to cotton to get more drug
count	purity level
courage pills	barbiturates; heroin
courting Cecil	a morphine addict
cowboy	independent drug dealer
crack	smokable cocaine
crack attack	craving
crack back	crack and marijuana
crack cooler	crack in wine cooler
crack kit	glass pipe and copper mesh
cracker, cracker jacks	crack cocaine user
crackers	LSD; mental problem or crazy
crank	methamphetamine; amphetamine; methcathinone; heroin
crank bugs	paresthesias or formication
cranking up	inject a drug
crap	heroin; inferior-quality heroin
crater	healed abscess from injecting
crazy coke, crazy Eddie	PCP
crazy weed	marijuana
creamed	under the influence
credit card	crack stem
creeper	slow-acting marijuana
creeps	delirium tremens
crib	addict's dwelling; prostitute's place of business; crack
crimmie	cigarette laced with crack
crink	methamphetamine
cripple	marijuana cigarette
crips	street gang
crisp	under the influence
crispo	burned out from drug use
crispy critter	under the influence
cris	methamphetamine
crisscross	amphetamine
crisscrossing	lines of heroin and cocaine each snorted into each nostril
cristal	MDMA
cristina	methamphetamine
cristy	smokable methamphetamine

croak	crack and methamphetamine
croaker	physician
croaker joint	hospital
crock	opium pipe; falsehood
crocked	under the influence
crop	low quality heroin
crosses, crossies, cross tops, crossroads	amphetamine
cross-country hype	drug-seeking
crown crap	heroin
cruise	look for drugs or paid sex partner
crumbs	crack
crunch & munch	crack
crusher	police
crutch	drug paraphernalia
cruz	opium
crying weed	marijuana
cryppie, cryptonie	marijuana
crypto	methamphetamine
crystal	methamphetamine; PCP; amphetamine; cocaine
crystal doe	methamphetamine
crystal joint	PCP
crystal lady	homosexual male amphetamine user
crystal meth	methamphetamine
crystal ship	syringe containing a dissolved crystallized drug
crystal T	PCP
crystal tea	LSD
cube	one ounce; LSD; straight person
cubes	marijuana tablets; crack cocaine
cube juice	morphine
cubehead	sugar cube LSD user
culican	Mexican marijuana
cupcakes	LSD
cura	heroin
curbstones	cigarette butts retrieved from gutters
cushion	vein for injecting a drug
cut deck	heroin or morphine mixed with powedered milk
cycline, cyclones	PCP
D	Dilaudid; LSD; PCP
D&D	drunk and disorderly
D-man	federal drug enforcement officer
DA	drug addict
dagga	marijuana
dagga rooker	marijuana smoker
daisy chaining	simultaneous group sex; sharing injectable drug
dai-yen	opium prepared for smoking
dais	Dalmane
dama blance	cocaine

Dame DuPaw	marijuana
damps	barbiturates
dance fever	fentanyl
dance hall	execution chamber
dank	marijuana
dans	oxycodone or Percodan
darvs	Darvon
date rape drug	Rohypnol
dawamesk	marijuana
DD	deadly dose
dead on arrival	heroin
dead	out of drug money; out of drugs
deadly nightshade	belladonna
deadwood	undercover narcotics agent
deans, deens, deines, denes	codeine
death trips	LSD mixed with another drug
death wish	PCP
death's head	*Amanita muscaria* mushroom
death's herb	belladonna
deazingus	hypodermic syringe or medicine dropper with a needle attached
debs	amphetamines; barbiturates
decadence	MDMA
deca-duabolin	injectable steroid
deck	dose of heroin; packet of drugs
deck up	inject heroin
dees, D's	Dilaudid
deeda	LSD
delatestryl	injectable steroid
Delilah	prostitute
demis, dems, demies	Demerol
demo	crack sample
demolish	crack
dep-testosterone	injectable steroid
desert horse	Camel cigarette
designer drugs	chemically altered drugs
desire	PCP and cocaine
desocin, desocsin, desogtion	methamphetamine
destroyed	heavily under the influence
DET	dimethyltryptamine
Detroit pink	PCP
deuce	$2 worth of drugs; two doses
deuceways	$2 worth of drugs
developing paper	rolling papers
devil	Seconal
devil's apple	jimsonweed
devil's dandruff, devil's drug, devilsmoke	crack

devil's dick	crack pipe
devil's dust	PCP
dew	marijana; hashish
dews	$10 worth of drugs
dex, dexies	Dexedrine; amphetamines
diablito	crack and marijuana in a joint
diambista	marijuana
diamonds	amphetamine
dianabol	veterinary steroid
Diane	meperidine
dib & dab	intermittent drug use
dice	methamphetamines; crack
dick	police officer or detective
diddieums	delirium tremens
dids	Dilaudid
dies	Valium
diesel	heroin
diesel dyke	lesbian
diet pills	amphetamine
digatee	drug-induced rush
digger	pickpocket
digging the bowls	smoking marijuana from a pipe
dihydrolone	injectable steroid
dill	Placidyl
dillie, dillies, dilies, dilly	Dilaudid
dimba	West African marijuana
dime	a ten-year prison sentence; a $1000 bet; crack; $10 worth of crack
dime bag	a $10 drug purchase
dime-dropper	an informer
dime special	crack
dime's worth	amount of heroin to cause death
ding	marijuana
dingbats	delirium tremens
dingers, dinghizen, dingus	drug paraphernalia
dinky dow, dinkie dow	marijuana
dinosaurs	middle-aged heroin users
dip	crack
dipped	narcotics addict
dipper	opium pipe; PCP
dipping out	crack runners taking a portion from vial
dirt	heroin
dirt grass	inferior-quality marijuana
dirty	drug use or possession
dirty arm	needle marks
dirty basing	crack
dirty deed	inject drugs
dirty joints	crack and marijuana

disco biscuits	methaqualone; MDMA
disco drug	vapors from butyl nitrite
disease	drug of choice
dispatcher	killer
ditch	cubital fossa; throw away or hide; marijuana
ditch digger	injectable drug user
ditch weed	inferior-quality marijuana
dithers	delirium tremens
djamba	African marijuana
DLs	hydromorphone
DMT	dimethyltryptamine
DMZ	benactyzine
DOA	PCP; crack
do it Jack	PCP
doctor	MDMA
do up	shoot or inject a drug; smoke marijuana; place a tourniquet
dodo	drug addict
does	methamphetamines
dog	weak opium residue; good friend
dog biscuits	peyote
dog food	heroin
dogie, dojee, dooiee	heroin
dollar	$100 worth of drugs
doll, dolls, dolly, dollie	barbiturates; amphetamines
dolo	methadone
DOM	analog of amphetamine/methamphetamine
domes	LSD; ecstasy
domestic	marijuana grown in the United States
domex	PCP and MDMA
domino	amphetamine and a barbiturate
done	methadone
donjem	hashish
Don Juan, Dona Juana, Dona Juanita	marijuana
doob, doobee, doobie, dubbe, duby	marijuana cigarette
doogie, doojee, dugie	heroin
dool	addict
dooley	heroin
doors	sedative
dope gun	hypodermic needle
dope sick	addict in need of drugs
dopium	opium
doradilla	marijuana
dors and 4's	Doriden and Tylenol No. 4
dossing	sleeping after drug use
dots	LSD
doub	$20 rock of crack

double blue	Amytal
double breasted dealing	dealing cocaine and heroin together
double bubble	cocaine
double cross	amphetamine
double deed	injecting drugs and taking pills
double dome	LSD
double header	two marijuana cigarettes smoked at once
double narky	double dose of drugs
double rock	crack diluted with procaine
double trouble	barbiturates
double up	marketing ploy giving extra product
double ups	a $20 rock that can be broken into two $20 rocks
double yoke	crack
douche	inject a drug
douse the lamp	ejaculation during an opium-induced sexual dream
dove	$25 piece of crack
Dover's powder	opium
down, downie, downs, downers	barbiturate; sedatives; alcohol; tranquilizer
downtown	heroin
DPT	analog of dimethlytryptamine
Dr. Bananas	amyl nitrite
Dr. Feelgood	heroin; physician who prescribes or sells drugs on request
Dr. White	cocaine
draf	marijuana ecstacy with cocaine
draf weed, drag weed	marijuana
dragged	marijuana-induced anxious state
draw up	inject drug
dread weed	marijuana
dream	cocaine
dream beads	opium pellets
dream boat	drug dealer's establishment
dreamer	depressants; morphine
dream gum	opium
dream pipe	opium pipe
dreams	opium
dream stick	opium; marijuana
dreck	heroin
drink	PCP
drink Texas tea	smoke marijuana
dripper	drug paraphernalia
dripping bummer	return from a cocaine high
drive	drug-induced rush
drivers	amphetamines
droopy	effects of sedative drugs
drop, drop a bop	take pills or capsules by mouth
drop a roll	take variety of drugs at one time
drop man	heroin delivery person
dropped	arrested

dropper	drug paraphernalia; to inject a drug
drowsy high	depressant
drug store heroin	Dilaudid
drugstore Johnson	prescription drugs addiction
dry high	marijuana
dub	extra rock of crack as marketing ploy
duct	cocaine
'due	residue from smoking drugs
dugie, duige, duji	heroin
dugout	scarred veins
dummies	propoxyphene
dummy	bogus heroin
dummy dust	bogus PCP
durabolin	injectable steroid
dust	heroin; cocaine; PCP; marijuana mixed with chemicals
dust joint	marijuana and PCP
dust of angels	PCP
dust of Morpheus	morphine
dusted	under the influence
dusted parsley	PCP
duster	heroin and tobacco mixed in a cigarette
dusting	adding PCP, heroin, or other drug to marijuana
Dutch mill	where drugs are sold
Dutchman	drug dealer
dyls	Placidyl
dymethzine	injectable steroid
dynamite	heroin and cocaine; narcotics of high potency
dyno, dyno-pure	heroin
earth	marijuana cigarette
easing powder	morphine
Eastside player	crack
eater, eating	oral drug use
echoes	LSD trip flashbacks
ecstacy	MDMA
Edge City	contemplation of beginning withdrawal
egg	crack
Egyptian driver	drug dealer
eight, eighth	heroin
eight ball	one-eighth ounce of drugs
eightball	crack and heroin
eighth piece	one-eighth ounce
eighty-six	kill; forcibly removed from bar or public place for inappropriate behavior; end relationship
el diablito	marijuana, cocaine, heroin and PCP
el diablo	marijuana, cocaine, and heroin
ekies	Mandrake
elbow	pound of marijuana
Eleanor	narcotic antagonist

electric	hallucinogenic matter
electric butter	marijuana leaves sauteed in butter
electric Kool-Aid; electric wine	LSD
elephant, elephant tranquilizer	PCP
elevator	opium used regularly
eleventh finger	penis
els, L's	Elavil
Elvis	LSD
embalming fluid	PCP
emergency gun	safety pin or sewing machine needle substituted for hypodermic needle
empties	return used capsules to dealer for discount
emsel	morphine
endo	marijuana
ends	money used for drugs
energizer	PCP
enforcer	strongman for dealer
eng shee	alcohol extraction of opium residue
engine	opium smoking outfit
enhanced	under the influence
enoltestovis	injectable steroid
ephedrone	methcathinone
Equipose	veterinary steroid
erth	PCP
esnortiar	snorting
esra	marijuana
essence	MDMA
estuffa	heroin
ET	alpha-ethyltryptamine
Eve	MDMA
everclear	cocaine
experience	LSD trip
explorer's club	group of LSD users
exposures	marijuana cigarettes
eyelid movies	images seen during an LSD trip
eye-opener	first narcotics injection of the day; amphetamines; crack
F-forties, F40s	Seconal
factory	place where drugs are processed
fag, faggot	cigarette or cigarette butt; homosexual male
fair share	drugs shared with others
fairy	opium smoker's lamp; homosexual male
fairy dust	PCP
fairy powder	powdered narcotic
fake	substitute for hypodermic needle
fake a blast	pretend to be under the influence
fake STP	PCP
Fallbrook redhair	marijuana
famine	out of drugs

famous dimes	crack
fang	hypodermic needle
Fantasia	dimethlytryptamine
farm to arm	people who grow, process, and sell drugs
farmer	home marijuana grower
Fastin	amphetamine
fat bags	crack
fat jay	thick marijuana cigarette
fatty	thick marijuana cigarette
feathered	under the influence
feebie	an FBI agent
feeblo	drug addict
feed	drugs; to use drugs
feed and grain man	drug dealer
feed bag	package of drugs
feed my head	take drugs by mouth
feed store	place to buy and use drugs
feeder	hypodermic needle
feeling	marijuana
fen	fentanyl
Felix the Cat	LSD
fender bender	barbiturate
ferry dust	heroin
fi-do-nie	opium
five-oh, 5–0	police
fields	LSD
fiend	drug addict; someone who smokes marijuana alone
fifteen cents, 15¢	$15 worth of drugs
fifty, 50	LSD
fifty-one	crack
figure-8	fake withdrawal, drug seeking
film can	container for marijuana
Finajet/finaject	veterinary steroid
finger	drug-filled condom or finger cot concealed internally
finger wave	digital exam of the rectum for drugs or weapons
fir	marijuana
fire	to inject a drug; crack and methamphetamine
firecracker	marijuana cigarette
fired	marijuana ashes with no remaining active ingredient
firing the antiaircraft gun	tobacco and heroin cigarette
first line	morphine
fish	arrestee
fish scales	crack
fish slip	criminal charge
fishbowl	jail's holding area
fit	drug paraphernalia
five-cent bag	$5 worth of drugs
five-cent paper	$5 worth of heroin

five C note	$500 bill
five dollar bag	$50 worth of drugs
fives	amphetamines
fizzies	methadone
flag	blood appearing in syringe or medicine dropper
flake	cocaine
flakes	PCP
flake acid	LSD
flaky	addict
flame cooking	smoking cocaine base by putting pipe over stove flame
flamethrower	cigarette laced with cocaine and heroin
Flannigan	marijuana
flash	drug rush; hallucination; LSD
flash in the pan	brief rush from heroin cut with quinine
flash out	momentary unconsciousness caused from sniffing
flat blues	LSD
flat chunks	crack cut with benzocaine
flats	LSD
flatten the poker	impotence caused from drug use
flattened	under the influence
flea powder	low purity heroin
flier	drug user who is always high
flip over	stop using temporarily; newly infatuated
floater	congealed blood clogging a hypodermic needle; corpse found in water
floating	under the influence
flogged	under the influence
Florida snow	white powdered drugs; cocaine
flow	hallucinogenic euphoria
flower, flower tops	marijuana
flower power	morning glory seeds
fluff	clean marijuana; run powdered drugs through a nylon stocking; chop up dope to make it bulkier; female
flunk out	move from use to addiction
flunky	drug deliverer; high-risk drug seeking; obtain drugs
flush and mush	flush or swallow drugs to avoid detection
flushing	method of drug sharing
fly	under the influence
fly Mexican Airways	smoke Mexican marijuana
fly swatter	muscle man for a drug dealer
flying saucers	PCP; morning glory seeds
focus	liquid narcotics
fold up	substance-induced unconsciousness; cease drug use or dealing
foo-foo, foo-foo dust	cocaine
foo-foo stuff	heroin; cocaine
foolish powder	heroin
foon	pellet of roasted opium

footballs	amphetamines
foreign mud, foreign smoke	opium
forget pill, forget me drug	Rohypnol
forties, 40s	Seconal
fortnighter	occasional drug user
forty-five minute psychosis	DMT, dimethyltryptamine
forwards	amphetamines
fours	painkillers with codeine in tablets or capsule with a 4
fours and dors	Tylenol No. 4 and Doriden
fourteen	narcotics
fourth degree	withdrawal sickness
four-way hits	cross-scored amphetamine tablets
four-way star	LSD combined with three other substances
forwards	amphetamine
frajo, fraho	marijuana
frame a twister	fake withdrawal; drug seeking
frantic	in need of drugs
freak house	drug house
Freddy, Freddie	stimulant
free trip	flashback
freebase, freebase rocks	smoking cocaine; crack
freeze	refuse to sell drugs to certain individuals; cocaine; renege
French blue	amphetamines
French fries	crack
french fried	under the influence
freon freak	freon gas inhaler
fresh	PCP
fresh and sweet	recently released from prison; new prostitute; new drug user
freshman	new drug user or addict
fried	under the influence; fentanyl
fries	crack
Frisco speedball/special	heroin, cocaine, and LSD
frisky, frisky, friskie powder	cocaine
frios	marijuana and PCP
frog	drug seeking
frontloading	syringe used to measure distribute doses
frosty	under the influence
frozen	under the influence
fruit salad	combination of pills
fry	executed in the electric chair; crack
fry daddy	crack and marijuana; cigarette laced with crack
Fu, Fu Manchu	marijuana
fuck the hop	sexual fantasies while under the influence
fuel	PCP; marijuana mixed with insecticides
fuete	hypodermic needle
full moon	peyote top
fuma D'Angola	marijuana

fun joint	drug house
funny paper	marijuana concealed in a newspaper
fur	law enforcement agents
furra	heroin
G	$1000 or 1 gram of drugs; term for an unfamiliar male
G.B.	depressant
GHB	gamma hydroxybutyrate
G-rock	one gram rock cocaine
G-shot	small dose used to hold off withdrawal symptoms
gaffle	fake cocaine
gaffus	improvised hypodermic needle
gag	heroin
gage, gauge, gage butt	marijuana cigarette
gagers, gaggers	methcathinone
gaggler	amphetamine
Gainesville green	marijuana
galhead	drug addict
gallery	location to buy drugs and drug paraphernalia
gallon distemper	delirium tremens
galloping horse	heroin
Gallup	heroin
gammon	one microgram of LSD
gamot	heroin; morphine
gange, ganga, ganja	marijuana
gangster	marijuana; user or manufacturer of amphetamines
gangster pills	barbiturates
gank	fake crack
gap	drug craving symptoms
gapper	in drug withdrawal
garbage	bad drugs; food
garbage freak, garbage head	addict who uses anything available
garbage rock	crack
Garden of Eden	female genitalia
garden variety	middle class
gargoyle	drug user or addict
gas	sniff gaseous substances; nitrous oxide
gash	marijuana; female genitalia
gasket	hypodermic needle seal
gasper, gasper stick	marijuana
gassing	inhaling through a drug-saturated cloth
gate	vein used to inject drugs
gato	heroin
gay	homosexual
gazer	federal law enforcement agent
gear	drug paraphernalia; drugs in general
gee	narcotics
gee fat	smoked opium residue
gee gee	opium pipe

gee head	paregoric user
gee rag	drug paraphernalia
gee stick	opium pipe
gee yen	opium residue
geed up	opium high
geek	crack and marijuana
geek joint	cigarettes or cigars filled with tobacco and crack
geekers	crack user
geez, geeze	inhale cocaine
geezed up	under the influence
geezer	inject a drug
geezin a bit of dee gee	injecting a drug
gelatin	LSD
gems	narcotics
George, George smack	heroin
Georgia home boy	GHB
Geronimo	heroin and barbiturates
Gestapo	police; IRS agents; those in charge
get a gage up	smoke marijuana
get a gift	obtain drugs
get lifted	under the influence
get one's nose cold	snort cocaine
get one's wings	become addicted
get the wind	smoke marijuana
getting roached	using Rohypnol
get through	obtain drugs
get up	first drug dose of the day
Ghana	marijunana
ghost	opium addict; LSD
ghost busting	smoking cocaine; searching for white particles in the belief that they are crack
GI gin	terpin hydrate
gick monster	crack smoker
gift-of-the-sun	cocaine
gig	drug high; job
giggle smoke, giggle weed	marijuana
gimmicks	drug paraphernalia
gimmie	crack and marijuana
gin	cocaine
girl, girly	cocaine; heroin; crack
girlfriend	cocaine
giro house	non-bank financial institutions for drug money laundering
gismo	drug paraphernalia
give birth	opium-induced constipation
give the go-by	refuse to sell drugs
give wings	introduce to heroin by injection
gizzy	marijuana

glacines, glassine	heroin
glad rag	drug-saturated cloth
glad stuff	cocaine
gladiator school	maximum security
Gladeing, glading	using inhalants
glass	hypodermic; amphetamine; heroin
glass gun	hypodermic syringe
glo	crack
globetrotter	drug-seeking behavior; homeless wanderer
glom	steal drugs
glooch	deranged sensorium from drug use
glory hole	hole in the wall for gay male sex
glory seeds	morning glory seeds
glove	condom
glow	mild intoxication
glued	arrested
gluey	glue sniffer
go, go pills	amphetamines
go fast, go fasters	amphetamines, methcathinone, crank; methamphetamine
go on a sleighride	inhale cocaine
go into the sewer	inject drugs into a vein
go loco	smoke marijuana
go on the boot	method of injecting drugs
go on the wagon	refrain from alcohol
go talk to Al and Herbie	drink alcohol and smoke marijuana
go to the cathedral	smoke hashish
go up	under the influence
goblet of jam	marijuana
God's drug	morphine
God's flesh	psilocin/psilocybin
God's medicine	opium; morphine
gold	marijuana; crack; heroin
gold bud	marijuana
gold dust	cocaine
gold star	marijuana
golden	marijuana
golden dragon	LSD
golden girl	heroin
golden leaf	very high quality marijuana
golden crescent	heroin-producing area in Middle East
golden grain	Lebanese hashish
golden spike	hypodermic syringe
golden triangle	opium-producing area of Far East
goldfinger	synthetic heroin
golf ball	crack
golf balls	depressant
golpe	heroin
goma	opium; black tar heroin

gong	opium; marijuana
gong beater	opium smoker
gonga smudge; gonj	marijuana cigarette
gongola, gondola	opium; opium pipe
goob	methcathinone
good	PCP; heroin
good and plenty	heroin
good H	heroin
goodhorse	heroin
good lick	good drugs
good go	proper amount of drugs for the money paid
good time man	drug dealer
goodfellas	fentanyl
goody-goody	marijuana
goof artist	prefers unusual drugs
goof butt	marijuana cigarette
goofballs	cocaine and heroin; barbiturates
goofers	barbiturates
Goofys	LSD
goofing	under the influence; aimless behavior
goofy dust	cocaine
goon, goon dust	PCP
gopher	person paid to pick up drugs
goric	opium
gorilla	powerfully addicted
gorilla biscuits, gorilla tab	PCP
gorilla pills	barbiturates
got it going on	fast sale of drugs
gouch off	drug-induced loss of consciousness
gouger	marijuana smoker
gow cellar	opium den
gow, ghow	opium
gozniks	addictive drugs
GQ	good quality
grads	amphetamines
graduate	stop using completely; move to more addictive/powerful drugs
gram	hashish
granulated orange	methamphetamine
granny	drug paraphernalia
grape parfait	LSD
grapes of wrath	wine hangover
grass, grass brownies	marijuana
grasshopper	marijuana
grass mask	drug paraphernalia
grass pipe	pipe used for smoking marijuana
grata	marijuana
gravel	crack

gravy	to inject drug; heroin and coagulated blood in a hypodermic syringe
gray dust	stale PCP
grease	currency
grease pit	dealer's place of business
greasy bag	bag in which heroin is kept
great bear	fentanyl
great Scott	opium pipe
great tobacco	opium
greefa, greefo	marijuana
greefer	marijuana smoker
green	inferior marijuana; PCP; ketamine
green acorn acid	LSD
green and blacks	Librium
green and clears	Dexamyl
green angelfish	LSD
green ashes	usable opium residue
green beauty	Dexamyl
green bud	home-grown marijuana
green caps	green LSD capsules
green dragons	depressant; LSD
green dots, green double domes	LSD
green frog	depressant
green goddess	marijuana
green gold	cocaine
green goods	paper currency
green hornets	Dexamyl
green hype	new addict
green leaves	PCP
green meanies	amphetamines
green moroccan	marijuana grown in Morocco
green mud	usable opium residue
green rot	inferior-quality opium
green single domes	LSD
green stuff	money
green swirls	LSD combined with another drug
green tea	PCP
green wedge	LSD
greenies	Dexedrine and amobarbital
greens	Dexamyl
greeter	marijuana
grey shields	LSD
griefo, grief, grifa, griff, griffa, griffo	marijuana
greta	marijuana
grievous bodily harm	GHB
grit	crack
groceries	crack

grocery boy	hungry addict
ground control	LSD trip guide
gulf	Persian Gulf heroin
gum, guma	opium
gumball	heroin; light bar on top of a police car
gumdrop	Seconal
gun	syringe or needle; to inject
gunga, gungeon, gungun, gunja	marijuana
gunk	morphine
gunny	African or Jamaican marijuana
gunpowder	raw opium
guns	drug paraphernalia
guru	LSD trip guide
gutter	cubital fossa
gutter hype, gutter junky	destitute addict
guttersnipe	child who lives on the streets
guy	marijuana
gweebo	epithet
gyve, gyve stick	marijuana
H	heroin
H&C	heroin and cocaine
H&R	hit and run; quick drug purchase and exit)
H caps	powdered heroin in gelatin capsules
hair of the dog	drink taken as a hangover cure
hairy	heroin
half bundle	twelve $5 bags of heroin
half kee	fraction of a kilogram
half load	fifteen $3 bags of heroin
half moons	hashish; peyote
half piece	one-half ounce of powdered drugs
half spoon	one-half spoon of cocaine
halvah	illicit drugs
halves	one-half ounce of heroin
hand-to-hand	drug delivery
happy cigarette	marijuana
happy dust	powdered drugs; cocaine
happy grass	marijuana
happy medicine	morphine
happy pills	barbiturates
happy powder	powdered drugs
happy sticks	marijuana cigarettes dusted with powdered drugs
happy-time weed	marijuana
hard candy	heroin
hard hat	epithet
hard nail	hypodermic needle
hard stuff	morphine, cocaine, heroin, or other opiates
hard time	sentence without parole
hardware	-butyls/isobutyl nitrate

harness bulls	uniformed police
harpoon	hypodermic needle
Harry	heroin; morphine
Harvey Wallbanger	STP and LSD
hash cannon	drug paraphernalia
have a Chinaman on back	withdrawal symptoms; heroin or opium habit
have a monkey on back	withdrawal symptoms
have a snake in boots	delirium tremens
have an orangutan on back	withdrawal symptoms
Hawaiian, Hawaiian grass	marijuana
Hawaiian pods	potent hallucinogen
Hawaiian sunshine	LSD
hawk	LSD
hay	inferior-quality marijuana
hay burner	marijuana smoker
hay butt	marijuana cigarette
hay head, hay puffer	marijuana smoker
haze	LSD
head drugs	drugs that affect the mind
head kit	drug paraphernalia
head rush	dizziness from drugs
head shop	shop for drug-related items and paraphernalia
heaped	under the influence
hearts	heart-shaped amphetamine sulfate; amphetamine tablets; dextroamphetamine sulfate
heaven	cocaine
heaven and hell	PCP
heaven dust	powdered drugs
heavenly blue	LSD; morning glory seeds
heavies	addictive drugs
heavy artillery	drug paraphernalia
heavy joint	marijuana and PCP
heavy metal	music style
heebie jeebies	delirium tremens
Helen	heroin
hell dust	powdered heroin or morphine
helpers	amphetamines
hemp	marijuana
hemp humper, hemp roller	marijuana smoker
her	cocaine
herb	marijuana
Herbal Ecstacy	caffeine and ma huang;ephedra
Hercules	superior-quality PCP
herms	PCP
hero	heroin
hi-fi	morphine and cocaine
high baller	amyl nitrite
high hat	prepared opium pellet

high kick	drug rush
high tea	marijuana smoking party
hikori, hikuli	peyote; mescaline
him	heroin
hip layer	opium smoker
hiroppon	methamphetamine (methamphetamine hydrochloride)
hit spike	substitute hypodermic needle
hit the flute	smoke opium
hit the hay	smoke marijuana
hit the mainline	inject drugs into a vein
hit the pipe	smoke opium
hitch	prison sentence
hitch up the reindeer	prepare to inject or inhale cocaine
hocus	liquor laced with drugs; morphine
Hoffmann's bicycle	LSD
hog	PCP
hog	one who requires large doses of drugs to sustain a habit; PCP; Harley-Davidson
holding	in possession of narcotics
hole in one	bullet wound in orifice
holy week	menstrual period
home	vein targeted for injection
homegrown	marijuana
honey oil	hashish extract
honeymoon	the stage of drug use before addiction occurs
hong yen	heroin in red pill form
hook, hookah	drug paraphernalia
hop head	a drug addict
horn	to inhale, snort, or sniff a drug
horror drug	belladonna
horrors	delirium tremens
hors d'oeuvres	Seconal
horse	heroin; condom
horse and buggy	hypodermic needle and medicine dropper used for injecting drugs
horse hearts	Dexedrine
horsed	under the influence
horseradish	heroin
hot and cold	heroin and cocaine
hot heroin	bag containing heroin
hotshot	fatal dose; an injection of poison instead of drugs
hot stick	marijuana cigarette
housewife's delight	tranquilizers
How does your garden grow	Are you growing marijuana?
huatari	peyote; mescaline
huffing	inhaling a solvent or glue
humming	under the influence
hungry croaker	a physician who accepts a bribe for prescription drugs

hunk	small amount of hashish
hygelo	addict
hyke	cough syrup that contains codeine
hype stick	hypodermic syringe and needle
ice	kill someone; diamonds; methamphetamine sulfate
ice cream	drugs in crystallized form
ice cream man	drug dealer
ice pack	marijuana packed in dry ice to make it more potent
ice tong doc	physician who refuses to give drugs to an addict
ice tray	drug paraphernalia
ice water doc	physician who refuses to give drugs to an addict
icicles	crystallized cocaine
idiot pills	barbiturates
Illinois green	marijuana
I'm looking.	Do you have drugs you can sell to me?
I'm way down.	I need drugs.
in betweens	barbiturates and amphetamines
in flight, in orbit	under the influence
in transit	to be on an LSD trip
Inca message	cocaine
Indian hay, Indian hemp	marijuana
instant Zen	LSD
iron cure	withdrawal from drugs while imprisoned
J	marijuana
J. Edgar Hoover	police officers; federal agents
J pipe	a pipe used to smoke marijuana
jab	to inject drugs
jab artist	injectable drug user
jab joint	where to buy and use drugs
jab stick, jabber	a hypodermic needle
Jack Ketch	a killer
jack off shot	injecting a drug in a manner that prolongs the rush
jack up	to inject a drug; barbiturate
jackal	an undercover narcotics officer
jacked up	under the influence
jacking off the spike	to release pressure on the syringe before all the liquid has gone into the vein, allowing blood to re-enter the hypodermic syringe
jag	drug party; a prolonged period of drug or alcohol use
jam	cocaine
Jamaican red	Jamaican marijuana
jammed up	overdose; broke
Jane	marijuana
jar wars	drug testing controversy
jazz	heroin
Jefferson airplane	drug paraphernalia
jell	heroin
jelly babies	amphetamines

jelly beans	amphetamines (amphetamine sulfate)
jelly roll	sex; penis
jerks	delirium tremens
Jersey green	marijuana thought to grow in New Jersey
jet	amphetamines; methamphetamines; dextroamphetamines
jet fuel	PCP
Jim Jones	marijuana cigarette and PCP
jim-jams, jimmies	delirium tremens
Jimmy	a subcutaneous injection of drugs; amphetamines
Jimmy Valentine	a thief or robber
jimson	a weed containing hallucinogenic substances
jingo	marijuana
jive	marijuana; dishonest; not trustworthy
job pop	to inject drugs
Job's antidote	a hypodermic needle
jock	-butyls/isobutyl nitrate
jockey	an addictive drug
Joe Blakes	delirium tremens
Johnny be good	police
Johnny Law	police
Johnson	marijuana
join the stream	to inject drugs
joint	a marijuana cigarette; prison; syringe and needle
jolly beans	amphetamines
jolly pop	a dose of heroin
jolt	to inject drugs
Jones	a heroin habit
joy dust	Vietnamese heroin
joy juice	chloral hydrate
joy pop	intermittent use of heroin by a nonaddict
joy powder	powdered drugs
joy prick	an injection of drugs
Juanita	marijuana
jug	jugular vein; jail or prison
jug man	injecting into jugular vein
juggler	an addict who sells drugs
jugs	injectable amphetamines
juice	alcohol; respect; power; illegally obtained money; gasoline
juiced	under the influence
juicehead	alcoholic
juju	marijuana
jumpy Stevie	drug-induced jumpiness
junk	narcotics; heroin
junk picker	a street person
junk squad	narcotics agents
junk tank	jail cell in which addicts are held
junkie	drugs or heroin addict

junkie pro	a prostitute who sells drugs or who is addicted
juvie	juvenile hall
juvies	law enforcement agents and social workers who deal with juveniles
K blast	PCP
Kansas grass	inferior-quality marijuana
katzenjammer	delirium tremens
kaya	marijuana
kee, key	one kilogram
keef	marijuana
keeler	chloral hydrate drops
keister plant	drugs that are concealed in the rectum or vagina
Ken dolls	barbiturates
Kentucky blue	marijuana thought to be grown in Kentucky
Kentucky fried	under the influence
key, kee	one kilogram
khat	milder than amphetamines
Kibbles and Bits	Ritalin and Talwin
kick the clouds	under the influence
kick the engine around	to smoke opium
kicked by a horse	heroin addict
kicked out in the snow	under the influence
kif	marijuana
killer weed	potent marijuana; PCP
kilo	one kilogram
kilo brick	marijuana packed into a brick shape that weighs approximately one kilogram
kilter	a marijuana cigarette
King Kong	$200 or more a day drug habit
King Kong pills	barbiturates
king of the road	a homeless person who wanders from place to place
kingdom weed	superior-quality marijuana
Kipper Lane	urban opium district
kiss Mary, kiss the fish	to smoke marijuana
kit	drug paraphernalia
kite	one ounce of drugs
KJ	PCP
knockout drops	chloral hydrate and alcohol
kokomo	cocaine addict or user
Kona gold	Hawaiian marijuana
kools	PCP
KW	PCP
L	LSD
L's	Elavil
LA	long-acting amphetamines
LA glass	smokable amphetamine
LA ice	smokable methamphetamine
LA turnabouts	amphetamines

lace	cocaine and marijuana; add a drug or alcohol to ordinary drink or food
lady, lady caine, lady snow	cocaine
lady in white	powdered drugs
Lady White	powdered drugs
ladyfinger	marijuana cigarette
ladykiller	a gigolo
lag	a prisoner
lakbay diva	marijuana
Lamborghini	crack pipe from plastic rum bottle and rubber sparkplug cover
lamp habit	addiction to opium
La Roche	Rohypnol
Las mujercitas	psilocybin
Lason sa daga	LSD
late night	cocaine
Latin lettuce	marijuana
laugh and scratch	to inject drugs
laughing gas	nitrous oxide
laughing grass, laughing weed	marijuana
launching pad	a place to use drugs
lay back	depressant
lay out	drug paraphernalia; to kill
lay up	to stay off the streets after a large drug supply has been obtained
LBJ, LBL	JB-336-N-methyl-3-piperidyl benzilate HCl; a hallucinogen; LSD; PCP; heroin
leaf	marijuana; cocaine
leaky bolla, leaky leak	PCP
leapers	amphetamines
leaping	under the influence of drugs
Lebanese red	marijuana
legal speed	over the counter asthma drug; trade name MiniThin
lemon 714	PCP
lemon bowl	an opium pipe that has a lemon rind covering the bowl
lemon drop	methamphetamine with dull yellow tint
lemonade	heroin; inferior-quality drugs
lemons	methaqualone
lens	LSD
lenos	PCP
lenno	marijuana
leper grass	potent Colombian marijuana
Let me hold something	an inquiry from one seeking to buy drugs
lethal weapon	PCP
let sunshine do	LSD
lettuce	money
libs	Librium

lick up a tab	to swallow a tablet or capsule
licorice	opium
lid	approximately one ounce of marijuana
lid poppers	amphetamines
lie in state with the girls	to smoke marijuana
lift pills	amphetamines
light artillery	drug paraphernalia
light green	inferior-quality marijuana
light somebody	to introduce someone to marijuana
light stuff	marijuana; nonaddictive drugs
lightning	amphetamine
lightweight	minimally addicted
lilly	amobarbital
Lima	marijuana
limbo	Colombian marijuana
lime acid	LSD
line	a vein in the arm; cocaine
line shot	an injection of drugs
liner	injectable drug user
lint	morphine in fibrous or cotton form
lip	test airtightness of drug apparatus
Lipton tea	inferior-quality drugs
liquid bam	injectable amphetamines
liquid ecstacy	GBH
lit, lit up	under the influence
little bomb	amphetamine; heroin; depressant
little boy blue	a male police officer
little D	Dilaudid
little ones	PCP
little smoke	marijuana; psilocybin/psilocin
live in grass huts	to smoke marijuana
live ones	PCP
llesca	marijuana
load	an injection of drugs; a drug supply; a large drug purchase; 25 bags of heroin
loaded for bear	ready for a fight
loads	glutethimide mixed with codeine
loaf	marijuana
lobo	marijuana
loco	marijuana
locker room	isobutyl nitrite
locoweed, loco weed	marijuana
locust point	a place from which to buy drugs
log	an opium pipe; PCP
logor	LSD
loose joint	a single marijuana cigarette
lords, lorphs	hydromorphone
lotes	butabarbital

loused	covered by sores and abscesses from repeated use of unsterile needles
love affair	cocaine
love boat	marijuana dipped in formaldehude; PCP; blunts mixed with marijuana and heroin
love blow	marijuana
love drug	aphrodisiac; methaqualone; MDMA
love pearls, love pills	alpha-ethyltryptamine
love trip	MDMA
love weed	marijuana
lovely	PCP
lovelies	PCP and marijuana
lover	marijuana smoker
low rider	drug addict who is on the skids
LT	living together
lubage	marijuana
Lucy in the sky with diamonds	LSD
lude out	methaqualone and alcohol
ludes	methaqualone
luggage	LSD
lunch-hour trip	DMT taken on one's lunch break
lunch money drug	Rohypnol
lung duster	cigarette
M	morphine; marijuana
M.O.	marijuana
M.S.	morphine
M.U.	marijuana
M&M, M&Ms	depressant; barbiturate
M&C	morphine and codeine
machinery	drug paraphernalia; marijuana
Machu Picchu	Peruvian marijuana
macon, maconha	marijuana
mad dog, madman	PCP
mafu	marijuana
Maggie, maggot	a cigarette butt
magic	PCP; psilocin/psilocybin
magic dust	PCP
magic flake	high-quality cocaine
magic mushrooms	psilocybin/psilocin
magic pumpkin	mescaline
magic smoke	marijuana
mainline	inject drugs into a vein
make a croaker for a reader	obtain a prescription drug from a physician
make a spread	set up drug paraphernalia
make up	need to find more drugs
mama coca	cocaine
mama's mellow	sedative drug effect
man about town	gigolo

Manhattan silver	marijuana
manteca	heroin
manicure	prepare marijuana
MAO	amphetamines
marathons	amphetamines
marbles	Placidyl
marching dust/powder	cocaine
margie wanna	marijuana
mari	marijuana
mariholic	marijuana addict
marimba	marijuana
Mary, Mary and Johnny, Mary Ann, Mary Jane, Mary Jonas, Mary Warner, Mary Weaver	marijuana
marshmallow reds	depressant
Maserati	crack pipe made from plastic rum bottle and rubber sparkplug cover
mash Allah	opium
matchbox	1/4 ounce of marijuana or 6 marijuana cigarettes
matsakow	heroin
Maui wauie	marijuana from Hawaii
Maui-wowie	marijuana; methamphetaminem
max	gamma hydroxy butyrate dissolved in water and mixed with amphetamines
Maxibolin	oral steroid
Mayo	cocaine; heroin
McCoy	pure drugs or alcohol
MDM, MDMA	methylenedioxy-methamphetamine
mean green	PCP
medical hype	addicted to appropriately prescribed drugs
medusa	inhalant
Meg, Megg, Meggie	marijuana
mellow yellow	LSD
mellow yellows	tranquilizers
melt wax	smoke opium
melter	morphine
mepro	meprobamate
Merck, Merk	cocaine
mesc, mese	mescaline
mescal beans, mescal buttons	peyote; mescaline
messorole	marijuana
meth	methamphetamine
meth monster	violent reaction to or from methamphetamine
meth speed ball	methamphetamine and heroin
Methatriol	injectable steroid
methedrine	amphetamin
methlies Quik	methamphetamine

methyltesosterone	oral steroid
metros	police officer
Mexican brown	heroin
Mexican crack	methamphetamine which appears to be crack
Mexican green	marijuana
Mexican jumping beans	Mexican barbiturates
Mexican horse	heroin
Mexican locoweed	marijuana
Mexican mud	Mexican heroin
Mexican mushrooms	psilocybin
Mexican reds	secobarbital
Mexican Valium	Rohypnol
mezc	mescaline
Michael	chloral hydrate
Michoacán, Mishwacan	Mexican marijuana
Mickey, Mickeys	chloral hydrate
Mickey Finn	chloral hydrate and alcohol
Mickey Mouse	LSD
Mickey Mouse ears	lights and siren on top of a police car
microdot	LSD
midget	underage drug runner
midnight oil	opium
mig	marijuana cigarette
Mighty Joe Young	large heroin habit; depressant
mighty mezz	marijauana
mighty Quinn	LSD
mike, mic	one microgram
milk a rush	method of injecting drug
mind bender	hallucinogen
mind detergent	LSD
mind fuck	secretly give drug and watch
mind spacer	hallucinogen
ming	marijuana cigarette made from leftover butts
minibennies, mini beans	amphetamines
miniwhite	amphetamine in tablet form
minstrels	amphetamine and barbiturate
mint leaves, mint weed	PCP
mired in the mud	opium addict
miser	drug paraphernalia
miss	inject a drug; missing vein
Miss Carrie	carrying drugs
Miss Emma	morphine
Miss Emma Jones	morphine addiction
Miss Freeze	doesn't share marijuana
missile basing	crack liquid and PCP
missionary	turns on new addicts
Mississippi marbles	dice
mist	PCP; crack smoke

Mister Blue	morphine; hydromorphone
mixed jive	crack
mo, modams, mohasky	marijuana
mojo	cocaine; heroin
Molotov cocktail	homemade bomb
monkey	drug dependency; cigarette made from cocaine paste and tobacco
monkey bait	free sample of addictive drug
monkey drill	hypodermic needle
monkey dust	PCP
monkey jumps	addicts' disordered gait
monkey meat	drug addict
monkey medicine	morphine
monkey pump	hypodermic needle
monkey talk	addict's distorted speech
monkey tranquilizer	PCP
monkey wagon	drug addiction
monos	cigarette made cocaine paste and tobacco
monolithic	heavily under the influence
Monroe in a Cadillac	morphine and cocaine
monster	CNS effects of drugs
monster weed	potent marijuana
monte	South American marijuana
mooca, moocha	marijuana
mooch joint	where drugs are sold
moocher	drug addict
moody blues	pentazocine mixed with tripelennamine
moon	peyote; mescaline
moonbeams	PCP
moon gas	inhalant
moonrock	crack and heroin
mooster, moota, mutah, moota, mutah, mooters, mootie, mootos	marijuana
morals	Demerol
mor a grifa	marijuana
more	PCP
morning	wake-up first blast of crack from the pipe
morning glory	first injection of the day
morning shot	amphetamine
morph, morf, morpho, morphie	morphine
morpho moron	morphine addict
morotgara	heroin
mortal combat	high potency heroin
moscop	morphine and scopolamine
mosquitos	cocaine
mosquito bit	cocaine addiction
mota, moto	marijuana

mother	drug dealer; marijuana
mother dear	methadone
mother nature	marijuana
Mother's Day	first of month, welfare check arrives
mother's little helper	depressant
mountain dew	illicit liquor
mouth habit, mouth worker	oral drug addiction
movie star drug	cocaine
mow the grass	smoke marijuana
MPPP, MPTP	synthetic meperidine
Mr. Twenty-Six	26-gauge hypodermic needle
Mr. Warner	marijuana smoker
Mr. Whiskers	federal narcotics agent
Mrs. Warren	prostitute
Mrs. White	drug dealer
mu	marijuana
mud	heroin; unprocessed opium
mud wiggler	opium addict
mug	assault during robbery
muggie, muggles	marijuana
mugglehead	marijuana smoker
mujer	cocaine
mule	marijuana; illegal drug carrier
mule skinner	recruits mules
munchies	drug-induced appetite
muscle pop	use IM route when veins are ruined
mushrooms	wounded or killed bystanders; psilocin/psilocybin
murder one	heroin and cocaine
murder 8	fentanyl
murotugora	heroin
musk	psilocybin/psilocin
muta ,mootah, mutha	marijuana
muzzle	heroin
nail, nail in the coffin	tobacco or marijuana cigarette; to arrest
Nam black	Vietnamese marijuana
nance	homosexual
nanoo	heroin
nanny goat sweat	illicit liquor
narc, nark, narco	undercover narcotics agent; informer
narco card	methadone registration card
narcotic bull	federal narcotics agent
Nazi vitamins	crystal meth
nebbies, nemmies	Nembutal; depressant
necessities	drug supplies
needle candy	drugs taken by injection
needle flash	short high
nemish	Nembutal
Nepalese hash	hashish

new acid	PCP
new addition	crack
new Jack Swing	heroin and morphine
new magic	PCP
nexus	2C-B
nice and easy	heroin
nicked	arrested
nickel	five-year sentence; $5 supply of drugs
nickel bag, nickel deck	$5 supply of drugs; heroin
nickel note	$5 bill
nickelonian	crack addict
niebal	PCP
nieve	cocaine
night on the rainbow	night spent under the influence
nightingale	informer
nightshade	belladonna
nigra	marijuana
nimbly, nimble nimby, nimbies	Nembutal
nineteen	amphetamine
nitrous	nitrous oxide
nix	stranger among group
Nixon	bad street drugs
noble princess of the waters	hallucinogenic mushrooms
nod	effects of heroin
nodded out	under the influence
noise	heroin
nontoucher	crack user who doesn't want affection during or after smoking
noodlelars	methyprylon
nose	heroin or cocaine;snorted or sniffed drug
nose candy, nose powder, nose stuff	cocaine
nose drops	liquified heroin
Ns	Darvocet-N
nubs	peyote
nugget	amphetamine
nuggets	crack
number	marijuana cigarette
number 1	liquid hashish
number 3	cocaine; heroin
number 4, number 8	heroin
number 13	morphine
nurse	powdered drugs
O	opium; ounce
oboy	marijuana
octane	PCP laced with gasoline
ogoy	heroin
oil	hashish oil; heroin; PCP

oil burner	expensive drug habit
oiled	under the influence; to be injected with drugs
oiler	drug addict
oink	police
OJ	marijuana cigarette dipped in opium
old lady White, old Madge	powdered drugs
Old Smoky	electric chair
old Steve	heroin
olive	cotton strainer
on a mission	searching for crack
on the bricks	walking the streets
on the nod	under the influence, esp. heroin
one and one	inhale cocaine
one hitter	Single-dose pipe
one-hit grass	DMT smoked with tobacco, marijuana, or parsley
one-on-one	Talwin and pyribenzamine; drug house
one-toke weed	potent marijuana
one box tissue	one ounce of crack
one fifty one	crack; crazy
one plus one sales	selling cocaine and heroin together
one way	LSD
oolies	marijuana cigarettes laced with crack
O.P., Ope	opium
operator	drug dealer
O.P.P.	PCP
optical illusions	LSD
orange barrels	LSD
orange bowl	opium pipe fitted with an orange rind
Orange County	methaqualone
orange crystal	PCP
orange cube, orange haze, orange micro, orange mushrooms, orange sunshine, orange wedges	LSD
orange cupcakes	LSD, usually added to other drugs
oranges	amphetamines
oregano	hashish
ounce man	drug dealer
outer limits	crack and LSD
outfit	drug paraphernalia
outside of myself	effect of hallucinogen
overcharged	semiconscious from overdose
overs and unders	amphetamines and barbiturates
owl	night-shift narcotics agent
Owsley, Owslet's acid	LSD
oyster stew	cocaine
Oz	amyl nitrite; inhalant
Oz man	drug dealer

ozone	under the influence; PCP
ozzy, ozzie	LSD
P	peyote; mescaline; pure heroin; PCP
P-dope	20% to 30% pure heroin
P funk	heroin; crack and PCP
P-head	phenobarbital user
P stuff	PCP
pacifier	homemade hypodermic needle
pack	heroin; marijuna
pack a bowl	marijuana
pack of rocks/rockets	marijuana cigarettes
pack one's coozie	conceal parcel of drugs in vagina
pack one's keister	conceal parcel of drugs in vagina or rectum
pack one's nose	snort cocaine
packed up	under the influence
packs	glutethimide with codeine
pad	residence; drug house
pad money	admission fee to drug house
padded	drugs concealed on body
paid torch	hired arsonist
paisley caps	LSD capsules or pills
pakalolo	marijuana
Pakistani black	marijuana
pan up	prepare injectable drug
Panama cut/gold/red	marijuana
panatella	large marijuana cigarette
pancakes and syrup	gluthethimide and codeine cough syrup
pangonadalot	heroin
pane	LSD
panic	shortage of drugs
panic man	addict who cannot obtain drugs
panic trip	adverse LSD reaction
panther piss	liquor
paper	dosage of heroin; prescription; drug-saturated paper; money; counterfeit bills
paper acid	LSD
paper bag	container for drugs
paper boy	heroin peddler
paper blunts	marijuana in paper casing
paper fiend	amphetamine-soaked paper user
paper hanger	bad check or counterfeit money passer
Parabolin	veterinary steroid
parackie	paraldehyde
parachute	PCP and crack smoked together; heroin; Rohypnol
paradise, paradise white	cocaine
parakeet	paraldehyde
paraphernalia	items involved in drug use
Park Lane No. 2	marijuana sold and used during the Vietnam War

parlay	crack
parsley	marijuana; PCP
pass	successful drug exchange
paste	physical violence; crack
pasto	marijuana
pat	marijuana
patico	crack
pattern	drug-induced hallucination
pay street	expensive drug habit
paz	PCP
PCP	phencyclidine
PCPA, PCE, PCPy	PCP
peace	LSD; PCP
peace pills/tablets	LSD
peace weed	PCP
peaches	amphetamines
peanut	depressant
peanut butter	PCP mixed with peanut butter; methamphetamine
pearls	amyl nitrite
pearly gates	morning glory seeds; LSD
pears	amyl nitrite
pebbles	crack
peep	PCP
pee wee	thin marijuana cigarette; crack; $5 worth of crack
peg	heroin
pekoe	high-quality opium
pellets	LSD
pen shot	injection of drugs
pen yan	opium
penitentiary highball	strained shellac and milk
penitentiary shot	injection of drugs via a pin and medicine dropper
peppermint swirl	LSD combined with another drug
Pepsi Cola habit	occasional use; small habit
per	prescription
Percs, perkers, perkies, perks	Percodan; oxycodone
percia, percio	cocaine
perfect high	heroi
period hitter	occasional drug user
perlas	heroin street dealer
perp	fake crack made of candle wax and baking soda
Persian brown	Middle Eastern heroin
Peruvian, Peruvian flake/ lady/rock	cocaine
peth	depressant
Peter	chloral hydrate
Peter Jay	police
Peter Pan	PCP
Peter, Paul, and Mary	ménage à trois

peyote	*Lophophora williamsii;* mescaline
PG	paregoric; pregnant
phennies, phenies, phenos	phenobarbital
piano-ing	using fingers to find lost crack
picking the poppies	opium addict
pickup	injection
piece	gun; one ounce of a cocaine or crack; female sex partner
piedra	crack
pie-eyed	under the influence
pig killer	police killer; PCP
piggie	opium pellets
piles	crack
pill cooker	opium addict
pill peddler	physician
pillows	knockout drops; opium; methaqualone; a bag containing pills
pimp, pimp dust	cocaine
pimp your pipe	lending or renting crack pipe
pin	drug paraphernalia; marijuana
pinch hitter	hired drug injector
pineapple	grenade or small bomb
ping a pill	portion of a pill for a small dose
pin gon	opium
pin gun	drug paraphernalia
pingus	Rohypnol
pinhead	injectable drug user
pin-in-wing, ping in wing	inject drug into arm
pink	Seconal; morphine
pink blotters	LSD
pink elephants	delirium tremens
pink hearts	amphetamine
pink lady, pink ladies	depressant
pink panther, pink robots	LSD
pinks and greens	amphetamines
pink spiders	delirium tremens
pink swirl, pink wedge, pink witches	LSD
pin yen	opium
pinned eyes	pinpoint pupils
pins and needles	morphine
pipe	large vein; drug paraphernalia; mix drugs with other substances
pipe dream	opium-induced altered consciousness
piped	under the influence
pipero	crack user
pit	cubital fossa; PCP
pixies	amphetamine
playing the harmonica	inhaling heroin through matchbox cover

PMA	analog of amphetamine/methamphetamine
PO	paregoric
pocket rocket	marijuana
pod	marijuana
pogo	cocaine
point	a needle
point shot	injection with broken sewing needle
poison	heroin; fentanyl
poke	marijuana
polo	mixture of heroin and motion sickness drug
pollutants	amphetamines
polvo	heroin; PCP
polvo blanco	cocaine
polvo de angel, polvo do estrellas	PCP
pony	crack
poor man's pot	inhalant
popcorn machine	lights bar on a police car
poppers	amyl nitrite; isobutyl nitrite
poppy	heroin
poppy alley	opium den location
poppy grove	opium den
poppy puffer	opium addict
popstick	opium pipe
pork	police
potato	LSD
potato chips	crack cut with benzocaine
potlikker	marijuana
potten bush	marijuana
powder	heroin; amphetamine; cocaine HCL
power puller	rubber piece attached to crack stem
powder monkey	powdered drug dealer
powder room	room where drugs are bought or sold
powdered diamonds	cocaine
powdered joy	powdered narcotics
power hitter	drug paraphernalia
pox	opium
preacher	informer
predator	heroin
prescription	marijuana cigarette
press	cocaine; crack
pretendica, pretendo	marijuana
prime time	crack
primo	crack; marijuana mixed with crack
Primobolan	injectable and oral steroid
primos	tobacco laced with cocaine and heroin
prod	hypodermic needle
product	LSD combined with another drug; crack

Proviron	oral steroid
prunes	testicles
pseudocaine	phenylproanolamine
psychedelic drug	hallucinogen
puff the dragon	smoke marijuana
puffer	crack smoker
puffy	PCP
pulborn	heroin
pullers	crack users who pull at parts of their bodies excessively
pumping	selling crack
pumpkin seed	mescaline
puna butter	Hawaiian marijuana
punchboard	promiscuous female
puppy	gun
pure	heroin
pure love	LSD
purple	ketamine
purple barrels, purple haze, purple flats, purple microdot, purple ozoline	LSD
purple hearts	LSD; amphetamine; depressant; phenobarbital
purple passion	stimulant and depressant
purple rain	PCP
push shorts	to cheat or sell short amounts
pusher	drug seller; metal hanger or umbrella rod used to scrape residue in crack stems
put it on paper	saturate a paper with drugs
put on a circus	fake withdrawal or drug-seeking behavior
Qs, quas	methaqualone (Quaalude)
qat	methcathinone
quacks	methaqualone
quad	depressant
quarter, quarter bag, quarter piece	$25 drug supply or quarter-ounce
quarter kee, key	fraction of a kilogram
quarter moon	hashish
quarter trip	LSD
quartermaster	quarter bag dealer
quartz	smokable methamphetamine
Queen Ann's lace	marijuana
quicksilver	isobutyl nitrite
quill	matchbook cover used for sniffing; methamphetamine; heroin; cocaine
R-2, R2	Rohypnol (flunitrazepam)
racehorse Charley	cocaine; heroin
rag and bones man, rag picker, ragman	street person
Raggedy Ann	LSD

ragweed	inferior marijuana; heroin
railroad tracks	needle marks
railroad weed	marijuana
railroader	intravenous drug user
rainbow	LSD
rainbow roll, rainbows	barbiturates
raincoat	condom
rainy day woman	marijuana
ram	male
Rambo	heroin
rane	cocaine; heroin
rangood	wild marijuana
raspberry	abscessed injection; female who trades sex for crack or money to buy crack
rasta weed	marijuana
ration	drug dose or stash
raw	crack
raw fusion, rawhide	heroin
rave party	enhancement of hallucinogens through music and behavior
RDs	secobarbital
ready rock	cocaine; crack; heroin
reader	prescription
reader with tail	forged prescription
Reagans	amobarbital
recompress	change shape of flake cocaine to resemble rock
recycle	LSD
red, reds	secobarbital
red and blues	Tuinal; depressants
red angelfish	LSD
red birds, redbird, red bullets	barbiturates
red bud	marijuana
red caps	crack
red cross	marijuana
red chicken	heroin
red devils	barbiturates
red dimple	LSD combined with another drug
red dirt	marijuana
red dolls	barbiturates
red dot	LSD tablet
red dragon	LSD
red eagle	heroin
red flag	anger inducing
red hots, red jackets	barbiturates
red lips	LSD
red lilies	barbiturates
red phosphorous	smokable speed
red pipe	artery
redneck cocaine	methamphetamie

reefer	marijuana
register	confirm entry into a vein by pulling up blood
regular P	crack
reindeer dust	heroin
rest in peace	crack
Reynolds	Rohypnol
rhapsody	amphetamine, methamphetamine
rhythm	amphetamines
Rhine	heroin
rib, Rib Roche	Rohypnol
Rice Krispies	amyl nitrite
rich man's aspirin	cocaine
ride the poppy train	smoke opium
riding a white horse	powdered heroin use
riding a witch's broom	powdered heroin use
riding the thorn	injecting drugs
riding the wave	under the influence
rifle range	where drugs are purchased and injected
rig	drug paraphernalia
right croaker	physician who provides drugs or sells prescriptions to addicts
righteous	superior-quality drugs
righteous bush	marijuana
ringer	good hit of crack
rip	marijuana
ripper	killer; amphetamine
rits	Ritalin
roach	butt of a marijuana cigarette; police
roach-2	Rohypnol
roach clip, roach pin	holder for marijuana butt
roacha	marijuana
roach bender	marijuana smoker
roached out	under influence of Rohypnol
roaches, roachies	Rohypnol
road dope	amphetamines
roapies, ropies	Rohypnol
roasting	smoking marijuana
Robbie, Robby	cough preparations with codeine
robin eggs	blue capsules of LSD
robutal	Rohypnol
roca	crack; MDMA
rochas dos	Rohypnol
Roche	Rohypnol
rock, rocks, rox	crystallized heroin or cocaine; crack
rock attack	crack
rocket caps	caps on crack vials
rocket fuel	PCP
rockets	marijuana

rockette	female crack user
rocks of hell	crack
rock star	female who trades sex for crack or money to buy crack
Rocky III	crack
rod	gun
rogues gallery	criminals' photos
roid rage	aggressive behavior from steroid abuse
roll	rob unconscious or sleeping person
roll of reds	barbiturate capsules
roll the boy	smoke opium
roller	inject a drug
rollers	veins that move while injecting; police
rolling	MDMA
rolling buzz	moderate length drug high
rolling stone	homeless wanderer
roofies, roofenol	Rohypnol
rooms	psilocin/psilocybin
rooster	crack
root	marijuana
rope	marijuana; Rohypnol
ropies, rophies, rophys, roples	Rohypnol
rosa, roses	amphetamines
Rose Marie	marijuana
roto rooter	penis
rough stuff	marijuana
row of coke	cocaine dose
Row-shay	Rohypnol
Roxanne	cocaine
royal blue	LSD
roz	crack
RPMs	amphetamines; dextroamphetamines
rubia	marijuana
Ruderalis	cannabis species
ruffies	Rohypnol
run	drug continuously injected over time
runner	drug sellers
running	MDMA
rush snappers	isobutyl nitrite
Russian sickles	LSD
S&M	sadomasochism
sacrament	LSD
sack	heroin
sacred mushrooms	psilocin/psilocybin
sadie-maisie	sadomasochism
safety pin mechanic	safety pin and medicine dropper to inject drugs
sagebrush whacker	marijuana smoker
Salmon River Quiver	marijuana
salt	heroin

salt and pepper	marijuana; police car; mixed-race couple or team
Sam or Sam and Dave	federal narcotics agent; police
sancocho	to steal
San Francisco bomb	cocaine, heroin, and LSD
San Quentin quail	minor or underage female
sandbag	physical violence; check a bet and raise it
sandos, sandoz	LSD
Santa Marta, Santa Marta gold	marijuana
sasfras	marijuana
Satan's secret	inhalant
satch	drug-saturated paper or clothing used to smuggle drugs into hospitals or prisons
satch cotton	fabric to filter narcotic solution before injection
sativa	marijuana
saxophone	an opium pipe
scab	heroin
scaffle, scuffle	PCP
scag, skag, scat, scate	heroin
scagged, skagged	heroin addict
scarf a joint	detection avoidance byswallowing
scattered	under the influence
schlock	drugs; junk
schmack	drugs
schmeck, shmeck	cocaine
schmeek	heroin
schnozzler	cocaine user
schoolboy	paregoric; codeine; cough preps; cocaine
schoolcraft	crack
scissors	marijuana
Scooby snacks	MDMA
scoop	GHB; folded matchbook cover for snorting
score	acquire drugs or sex; blood show in eyedropper
scorpion	cocaine
scott	heroin
Scottie, Scotty	cocaine; crack, the high from crack
scramble	worthless or near-worthless heroin; crack
scrape and snort	share crack
scruples	crack
screaming meemies	delirium tremens
scribe	prescription forger
script doc	physician who writes ethically questionable prescriptions
script writer	sympathetic physician; prescription forger
scroll	rolling papers
scrubwoman's kick	inhaled naphtha
sealed stuff	canned or bottled opium
sec, seco-8,seccy, seggy	secobarbital; depressant
second-story man	thief or burglar
second to none	heroin

seeds	morning glory or marijuana seeds
send it home	inject a drug
sen	marijuana
seni	peyote; mescaline
serenity	STP
serial speedballing	sequencing cocaine, cough syrup and heroin over a 1–2 day period
sernyl	PCP
serpent	hypodermic syringe
Serpico 21	cocaine
server	crack dealer
ses, sess, sezz	marijuana
set	places where drugs are sold; amphetamine and barbiturate
sevenup	cocaine; crack
sewer	median cephalic vein or other vein for injecting
sex	barbiturates
shabu	ice; crack; methamphetamine
shaker/baker/water	shaker bottle, baking soda, water for freebasing cocaine
sharp shooter	always hits the vein
sharps	hypodermic needles
she	cocaine
Sherlock Holmes	police
sheet rocking	crack and LSD
sheets	PCP
Shermans	PCP; crack
shit	drugs; heroin
shoot	heroin
shoot below the belt	inject into a vein in the lower part of the body
shoot gravy	cooked blood and a dissolved drug
shoot skin	inject into the skin
short piece	small amount or weak drug
shot down	under the influence; insulted
shotgun	pipe used to in blowing marijuana smoke from one mouth to another
shovel	drug paraphernalia
shovel snow	snort cocaine
shrooms	psilocin/psilocybin
sick dizzies	peyote
siddi	marijuana
Sidney	LSD
sightball	crack
silk and satin	amphetamines and barbiturates
silly putty	psilocin/psilocybin
silo	psilocin/psilocybin
sinse, sinsemilla	marijuana
sip	puff of marijuana cigarette
sitter	LSD trip guide

sitting well	under the influence
sixty-two	2–1/2 ounces poor quality crack
Skag Jones	heroin addict
skag, scag	heroin
skagged out	under the influence
Skagtown	a neighborhood inhabited by addicts
skee	opium
skeegers/skeezers	crack-smoking prostitute
sketch	methamphetamine
sketching	coming down from speed-induced high
skid	heroin
skied	under the influence
skin	rolling papers; nudity
skin pop, skin shot	subcutaneous injection
skin pumping	subcutaneous or intramuscuiar injection
skinhead	Neo-Nazi gang member
skinner	subcutaneous injection
skuffle	PCP
skunk, skunk number 1	marijuana; heroin
sky river	LSD mixed with another drug
skyrockets	amphetamines
slab	crack
slack	a bag that does not weigh out
slag	heroin; drug addict
slam	inject a drug
slammin, slamming	amphetamine
slammed	caught or arrested
slanging	selling drugs
sleepers	heroin; barbiturates
sleepwalker	heroin addict
sleet	crack
sleigh ride	cocaine party
slick superspeed	methcathinone
slime	heroin
slow boat	marijuana cigarette
slum	narcotics use
slum dump	opium den
slumber party	drug party
slut	epithet
smack	heroin
smash	marijuana and hashish
smears	LSD
smell it up	snorting
smell the reindeer dust	snorting
smizz	heroin
smoke	heroin and crack; crack; marijuana
smoke Canada	marijuana
smoke a joint	marijuana cigarette

smoked	under the influence; killed
smoke-out	under the influence
smoking	PCP
smoking gun	heroin and cocaine
smudge	small amount of heroin
smurf	cigar dipped in embalming fluid
snakes	delirium tremens
snap	amphetamine
snapped up	under the influence
snappers	isobutyl nitrite
snatcher	police
snerf	snorting cocaine
sniff	inhale cocaine; inhalant; methcathinone
sniffer bags	$5 bag of heroin to inhale
snipe	marijuana butt
snop	marijuana
snork	smoke marijuana
snorts	PCP
snot	residue from smoked amphetamine
snot balls	rubber cement rolled into balls, burned and inhaled
snow	cocaine; heroin; amphetamine
snowball	cocaine and heroin
snowbank	place to buy or use powdered drugs
snow bird, snowbird	cocaine; user
snowcones	cocaine
snow drifter	cocaine dealer
snow eagle	primary figure in a drug ring
snowfall	snorting
snowflake	cocaine
snow flower	female snorter
snowmobiling	snorting
snow pallets	amphetamine
snow seals	cocaine and amphetamine
snow scoop	spoon to hold powdered drugs
snow smoke	crack
snowstorm	large amount of powdered drugs
snow white	cocaine
snozzle	snorting
soapers, sopors, sopers	methaqualone
society high	cocaine
softballs	barbiturates
soles	hashish
soma	PCP
songbird	informer
soot the chimney	snorting
sophisticated lady	cocaine
soul searching	looking for a vein
spaceball	PCP used with crack

space base	crack dipped in PCP; hollowed out cigar with PCP and crack
space cadet	crack dipped in PCP; under the influence
space dust	crack dipped in PCP
space ship	glass crack pipe
space ships	LSD
spangles	Librium
spark an owl	smoke a gigantic joint
Sparkle Plenty, sparklers	amphetamine
Sparky	electric chair
spear	needle
Special K	ketamine
special la coke	ketamine
speckled eggs	amphetamines
speed	methamphetamine; amphetamine; crack
speedball	cocaine-heroin combination; amphetamine, methylphenidate mixed with heroin
speedballs-nose style	snorting cocaine
speed boat	marijuana, PCP, and crack
speed demon	amphetamines; methamphetamines
speed for lovers	MDMA
speedster	amphetamine user
spider blue	heroin
spike	needle for injecting drugs; injecting
spit ball	mouthful of free-base vapors puffed into someone else's mouth
spivias	amphetamines
splash	liquid amphetamine or methamphetamine
splay	marijuana
spliff	marijuana rolled in newspaper
splim	marijuana
split	half and half marijuana and cocaine
splits	tranquilizers
splivins	amphetamines
sploff	marijuana cigarette
spook	long-time addict
spoon	drug paraphernalia; two grams of heroin
spores	PCP; mushrooms
sport of the gods, sporting	cocaine use
spray	inhalant
spread the good news	sharing drug supply
sprouting	injecting drugs from one syringe into another
sprung	person just starting to use
spur	one gram
square mackerel	marijuana
square-time Bob	crack
square John	non-user
squealer	informer

squirrel	smoking cocaine, marijuanae and PCP; LSD; mentally ill
stack	marijuana
stacking	taking steroids without prescription
stackola	stacking money
stall	finger cot or condom package used for powdered drugs
star	methcathinone; cocaine; methamphetamine
stardust	heroin with cocaine; PCP
star-spangled powder, star stuff	cocaine
start cooking	begin injecting drugs
stat	methcathinone
steamboat	drug paraphernalia
steamroller	toilet paper roll used to smoke marijuana
steel and concrete cure	abstinence from drugs while in prison
steerer	drug dealer's scout
Stella	rolling papers
stem	opium pipe; crack pipe
stencil	thin marijuana cigarette
step on	dilute drugs
stepping high	under the influence
Steve's mission	place to buy or use drugs
Stevie	drug-induced hallucination
stick	marijuana; PCP
stinger	hypodermic needle
stink weed	marijuana
stoms	barbiturates
stone wall horrors	delirium tremens
stones	crack
stony bush, stoney weed	marijuana
stoppers	barbiturates
STP	PCP
stove top	crystal methamphetamine
straddle the spike	inject drugs
strawberry	peyote; mescaline; trade sex for drugs
strawberries	depressant
strawberry fields, strawberry hill	LSD
strawberry shortcake	methamphetamine
street ounce	diluted heroin sold on the street
stretch	dilute a drug
strike	dose of drugs
studio fuel	cocaine
stum	marijuana
stumblers	barbiturates
stung by a viper	marijuana addiction
stung by the hop	opium addiction
stung by the white nurse	morphine addiction
stung by white mosquitos	cocaine addiction
submarine	large marijuana cigarette

sugar	cocaine; crack; LSD; heroin
sugar block	crack
sugar cube, sugar lump	LSD
sugar daddies	amphetamines
sugar down	dilute powdered drugs
sugar weed	marijuana
summer sky	morning glory seeds
sunflower seeds	amphetamines
sunshine	LSD
super	PCP
super acid, super C	ketamine
supercharged	under the influence
Super Grass	PCP
supergrass	marijuana
super ice	smokable methamphetamine
Super-Jaded	blitzed from drugs; unable to think clearly
super joint, super kools	PCP
Superman	LSD
super weed, superweed	PCP, marijuana or PCP and LSD
surfer	PCP
sweat	butyl/isobutyl nitrate
sweet dreams	heroin
sweet Jesus	morphine
sweet Lucy, sweet lunch, sweet Mary	marijuana
sweet Morpheus	morphine
sweet stuff	heroin; cocaine
sweeties	amphetamines;Preludin
sweets	amphetamines
swell up	crack
swing	sell drugs
swinger	user of variety of drugs in all forms
swishers	cigars emptied of tobacco and filled with marijuana
Swiss purple	LSD
switch hitter	bisexual
syndicate acid	LSD; PCP
synthetic heroin	analog of fentanyl/meperidine
synthetic cocaine, synthetic THT	PCP
syrup	Mexican heroin
syrup head	ingesting cough syrup with codeine and depressant
T	cocaine; marijuana
TT1, TT2, TT3	PCP
T-buzz	PCP
T man	narcotics or treasury agent; marijuana smoker
tab, tabs	LSD; tablet or pill
TAC	PCP
tag	drug-induced euphoria

tail lights	LSD
taima	marijuana
take a Brody	fake drug withdrawal or attempt suicide
take-a-too	drug paraphernalia
take a dive	suicide
take a Duffy	fake drug withdrawal
take a sweep	snort cocaine
take it in line	injecting drugs into the median cephalic vein
take the gas	suicide
taking a cruise	PCP
takkouri	marijuana
talcum powder	bogus powdered drug
talco	cocaine
tall	under the influence
tals	Talwin
tamale	large marijuana cigarette
tang	drug addiction
Tango & Cash	fentanyl
tanks	PCP
tap the bag	short weight of drugs; cheat buyer
tar	opium; heroin
tar dust	cocaine
tarred and feathered	opium addict
tattoos	track marks
taxing	price paid to enter a crackhouse; charging more per vial depending on race of customer or if not a regular customer
TCP	synthetic PCP
tea	marijuana; PCP
team meeting	marijuana party
teardrops	dosage units of crack packaged in cut-off corners of plastic bags
tecata	heroin
tecatos	Hispanic heroin addicts
Teddies and Betties	Talwin and Pyribenzamine
teenager	cocaine
teeth	cocaine; crack; bullets
tens, 10s	amphetamine
ten pack	1,000 units of LSD
tension	crack
tester	judge of the strength of diluted heroin
Texas leaguer	marijuana smoker
Tex-mex, Texas pot, Texas tea	marijuana
Thai sticks	bundles of marijuana soaked in hashish oil; marijuana buds bound on short sections of bamboo
the animal	LSD
the beast	heroin

the bad seed	peyote; mescaline
the C	methcathinone; amphetamine
the devil	crack
the witch	heroin
Therobolin	injectable steroid
thing	heroin; cocaine; main drug of the moment
thirst monsters	heavy crack smokers
thirteen	marijuana
thorn	hypodermic needle
thoroughbred	prostitute; prisoner; dealer of pure narcotics
$3 bill	homosexual
threes	Tylenol No. 3
thrill pills	barbiturates
thriller	marijuana cigarette
thrust	isobutyl nitrite
thrusters	amphetamines
thumb	marijuana
thunder	heroin
thunder cookie, thunder weed	marijuana
Tic or Tic Tac	PCP
ticket	LSD
ticket agent	drug dealer
tie	inject drug
tighten up	give drugs
tigre, tigre de blanco, tigre de norte	heroin
tish, titch	PCP
tissue	crack
TMA	analog of amphetamine/methamphetamine
T.N.T.	heroin; fentanyl
toilet water	inhalant
tom cat	sewing machine needle used to open vein
Tom Mix	injection of drugs
toncho	octane booster which is inhaled
tongs	heroin
tongue	injecting into vein beneath the tongue
tooies, tuies, tootsie	Tuinal
tooles	depressant
toot	cocaine; snort, sniff, inhale
tooter	tube used for snorting cocaine
tooties	depressant
tootsie roll	heroin
top gun	crack
topi	peyote; mescaline
topo	crack
tops	marijuana; peyote
tops and bottoms	Talwin and pyribenzamine

tornado	crack cocaine
torpedo	hired killer; drink with chloral hydrate; crack and marijuana mixed
tossed	body search
toss up	female who trades sex for crack or money to buy crack
totally spent	MDMA hangover
toucher	crack user who wants affection before, during, or after smoking
tout	person who introduces buyers to sellers
tough	injecting into vein beneath the tongue
tour guide	LSD trip guide
toy, toys	prepared opium; drug paraphernalia
toxy	opium
TR-6s	amphetamines
Track One	houses of prostitution
Track Two	homosexual houses of prostitution
tracked up	needle marks and abscess scars
tracking	re-experiencing drug-induced hallucination; repetitive verbalization while under the influence
tragic magic	crack dipped in PCP
trade	sex partner
trail	needle marks
trails	LSD induced perception that moving objects leave multiple images or trails behind them; cocaine
train	gang rape; serial sex
trained nurse	hospital or prison drug smuggler
trank	PCP
tranks, tranx, tranq	tranquilizers
tranquility	hallucinogen; mescaline; amphetamines
trash picker	street person
trays	bunches of vials
travel agent	LSD seller or trip guide
tree jumper	rapist
tree of knowledge	marijuana
trees	pills and capsules
triangles	delirium tremens
trick track	injectables-addicted prostitute
tricycles and bicycles	Talwin and pyribenzamine
trim	physical violence
trip	LSD; alpha-ethyltryptamine; effect of hallucinogen
trip grass	marijuana and amphetamines
triple line	marijuana with heroin
tripper	hallucinogen user
trips	amitriptyline; LSD
trojan horse	hospital- or prison-employee or visitor drug smuggler
troop	crack
Trophobolene	injectable steroid
truck drivers	amphetamines

trupence bag	marijuana
truth serum	amobarbital or thiopental sodium
Ts and blues	Talwin and pyribenzamine
tuies	Tuinal
turbo	potent form of ecstasy; crack and marijuna
turd	drugs concealed in rectum
turkey	cocaine; amphetamine
Turkish green	marijuana
turkey trots	needle marks
turnabout, turnabouts	amphetamine
turn a cartwheel	drug seeking behavior
turnip greens	marijuana
turps	terpin hydrate with codeine
Tustin	marijuana
tuti-frutti	flavored cocaine
TV	transvestite
tweak mission	a mission to find crack
tweaker	crack user looking for rocks on the floor after a police raid
tweaks	crack cocaine
tweaking	drug-induced paranoia; peaking on speed
tweek	methamphetamine-like substance
tweeker	methcathinone
twenty, twenty rock	$20 rock of crack
twenty-five	LSD
twig	marijuana cigarette
twirl	to sell drugs
twist, twistum	marijuana cigarette
twisted	extreme intoxication
twists	small plastic bags of heroin secured with a twist tie
Two for nine	two $5 vials or bags of crack for $9
2-for-1 sale	a marketing scheme designed to promote and increase crack sales
typpie	tattooed young professional
U boat	drugs concealed in rectum
uglies	delirium tremens
ultimate	crack
Ultimate Xphoria	caffeine and ma huang; ephedra
umbilical cord	methadone
uncle	federal agents
Uncle Milty	depressant
under the white cross	under the influence of cocaine
unkie	morphine
Unotque	marijuana
up and down	inject drugs and take pills
up against the stem	addicted to smoking marijuana
uptown	cocaine
Utopiates	hallucinogens
U.S.P.	amphetamine

Uzi	crack; crack pipe
V	Valium
valley	cubital fossa
Valo	nasal inhalant
vals	Valium
vanilla	heterosexual
Vega	a cigar wrapping refilled with marijuana
Vidrio	heroin
vegetarian	marijuana smoker
vipe, viper, viper's weed	marijuana
vitamins	amphetamines
vivor	street person
vodka acid	LSD
void	under the influence
vons	Darvon
vroomed	under the influence
wac	PCP on marijuana
wack	PCP
wacky backy, whackatabacky, wacky weed	marijuana
wake and bake	marijuana
wafers	ecstasy; cookies and LSD
wakeups	amphetamines
wakowi	mescaline
Waldorf Astoria	solitary confinement
wall hangers	methaqualone
warped	under the influence
water	methamphetamine; PCP; a mixture of marijuana and other substances within a cigar
wave	crack
weasel	informer
wedding bells	morning glory seeds; LSD
wedge	LSD
wedge series	STP and LSD
weed tea	marijuana
weight	weekly habit
weightless	high on crack
west coast	Preludin; Ritalin
West Coast turnarounds	amphetamines
wet	PCP and marijuana;methamphetamines
wet dog shakes	delirium tremens
whack	dilute a narcotic; to kill; crack
wheat	marijuana
wheels	amphetamine
wen-shee	opium
whiff	cocaine
whiffle dust	amphetamine
whippets	nitrous oxide

whips and jangles	symptoms of withdrawal
whiskers	federal agent
white	amphetamine; heroin
whites, whities	amphetamines
white angel	healthcare drug smuggler
white ball	crack
white boy	heroin
white cloud	crack smoke
white crosses	amphetamines
white domes	LSD
white dust	LSD or PCP
white ghost	crack
white girl	cocaine; heroin
white goddess	morphine
white-haired lady	marijuana
white horse	cocaine;heroin
white junk	heroin
white lady	heroin;cocaine
white lightning	raw liquor;LSD
white merchandise	powdered drugs
white mosquito	cocaine
white nurse	heroin
White Owsley's	LSD
white powder	cocaine; PCP
white silk	morphine crystals
white stuff	heroin
white sugar	crack
white tornado	crack
whitey	heroin
white out	isobutyl nitrite
whiz bang	cocaine and heroin
whizz	amphetamines
wicked	a potent brand of heroin
whoops and jangles	drug withdrawal
wide	under the influence
widows	amphetamines
wig out	drug-induced psychosis
wig picker	psychiatrist
wild cat	methcathinone and cocaine
wild Geronimo	barbiturates and alcohol
window glass, window pane	LSD
wings	heroin; cocaine
Winstrol	oral steroid
Winstrol V	veterinary steroid
wisdom weed	marijuana
witch	heroin; cocaine
witch Hazel	heroin
witches' brew	LSD mixed with Datura

wobble weed	marijuana; PCP and crack
wokowi	peyote; mescaline
wolf	PCP
wollie	rocks of crack rolled into marijuana
Wolminic nasal spray	methamphetamine
Wonder star	methcathinone
woodpecker of Mars	*Amanita muscaria* mushroom
woolaha	hollowed out cigar refilled with marijuana
woolas	cigarette laced with cocaine; marijuana cigarette sprinkled with crack
woolies	marijuana and crack or PCP; delirium tremens
wooly blunts	marijuana and crack or PCP
working	selling crack
working half	crack rock weighing half gram or more
working man's cocaine	methamphetamine
works	drug paraphernalia
world traveler	homeless wanderer
worm	PCP
wrangled	stop using drugs
wrecking crew	crack
X	ecstasy (MDMA); marijuana; aphetamine
X-ing	MDMA
XTC	MDMA
Xmas	drug-induced euphoria
XTC	ecstasy (MDMA)
yahoo, yeaho yeah-O, yeo	crack
Yale	crack
yam yam	opium
yancy	opium
yayoo	crack
yanked	arrested
yeh	marijuana
yellow, yellows	LSD; depressants; barbiturates
yellow bam	methamphetamine
yellow birds, yellow bullets	pentobarbital
yellow dimples	LSD
yellow dolls	pentobarbital
yellow fever	PCP
yellow jack speed	amphetamines
yellow jackets	pentobarbital; depressants
yellow powder	methamphetamine
yellow submarines	marijuana
yellow sunshine	LSD
yen pop	marijuana
yen shee	opium ash
yen shee suey	opium wine
yen sleep	restless drowsy state after LSD use
Yerba	marijuana

Yerba mala	marijuana and PCP
yerhia	marijuana
yesca, yesco	marijuana
yeyo	cocaine
yimyom	crack
ying	marijuana
ying yang	LSD
yuppie flu	ongoing effects from cocaine-snorting habit
Z	1 ounce of heroin
Zacatecas purple	Mexican marijuana
zambi	marijuana
Zay	mixture of marijuana and other substances within a cigar
Zen	LSD
Zero	opium
zings	amphetamines
Zig Zag Man	LSD; marijuana; rolling papers
zings	amphetamines
zip	cocaine
zip gun	homemade gun
zips	one ounce any drug
zol	marijuana cigarette
zombie	heavy user; PCP
zombie buzz, zombie dust, zombie weed	PCP
zooie	holds butt of marijuana cigarette
zoom	ecstasy; cocaine; PCP; marijuana laced with PCP
zoomers	sellers of fake crack who flee
Zoquete	heroin (Spanish)
Zulu	bogus crack

NOTES

NOTES

NOTES

NOTES

NOTES

NOTES

NOTES

NOTES

NOTES

NOTES

NOTES

NOTES

NOTES

NOTES

NOTES

NOTES

NOTES

NOTES

NOTES

NOTES

NOTES

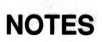

NOTES

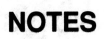

NOTES

NOTES

NOTES

NOTES

NOTES

NOTES